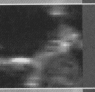

Echocardiography
in Pediatric and Adult Congenital Heart Disease

EDITORS

Benjamin W. Eidem, MD, FACC, FASE

Associate Professor of Pediatrics
Director, Pediatric and Fetal Echocardiography Laboratory
Divisions of Pediatric Cardiology and Cardiovascular Diseases
College of Medicine, Mayo Clinic
Rochester, Minnesota

Frank Cetta, MD, FACC, FASE

Professor of Pediatrics and Medicine
Divisions of Pediatric Cardiology and Cardiovascular Diseases
College of Medicine, Mayo Clinic
Rochester, Minnesota

Patrick W. O'Leary, MD, FACC, FASE

Associate Professor of Pediatrics
Divisions of Pediatric Cardiology and Cardiovascular Diseases
College of Medicine, Mayo Clinic
Rochester, Minnesota

 Wolters Kluwer | Lippincott Williams & Wilkins
Health

Philadelphia • Baltimore • New York • London
Buenos Aires • Hong Kong • Sydney • Tokyo

Acquisitions Editor: Frances R. DeStefano
Product Manager: Leanne McMillan
Production Manager: Bridgett Dougherty
Senior Manufacturing Manager: Benjamin Rivera
Marketing Manager: Kimberly Schonberger
Design Coordinator: Stephen Druding
Production Service: KnowledgeWorks Global Limited

Printed in China

Library of Congress Cataloging-in-Publication Data

Echocardiography in pediatric and adult congenital heart disease / editors, Benjamin W. Eidem, Frank Cetta, Patrick W. O'Leary.
     p. ; cm.
   Includes bibliographical references.
   ISBN-13: 978-0-7817-8136-7
   ISBN-10: 0-7817-8136-1
   1. Congenital heart disease—Ultrasonic imaging. 2. Congenital heart disease in children–Ultrasonic imaging. 3. Echocardiography. I. Eidem, Benjamin W. II. Cetta, Frank. III. O'Leary, Patrick W.
   [DNLM: 1. Heart Defects, Congenital–ultrasonography. 2. Echocardiography—methods. WG 220 E185 2010]
   RC687.E26 2010
   616.1'207543—dc22

                                                                2009029035

Care has been taken to confirm the accuracy of the information presented and to describe generally accepted practices. However, the authors, editors, and publisher are not responsible for errors or omissions or for any consequences from application of the information in this book and make no warranty, expressed or implied, with respect to the currency, completeness, or accuracy of the contents of the publication. Application of the information in a particular situation remains the professional responsibility of the practitioner.

    The authors, editors, and publisher have exerted every effort to ensure that drug selection and dosage set forth in this text are in accordance with current recommendations and practice at the time of publication. However, in view of ongoing research, changes in government regulations, and the constant flow of information relating to drug therapy and drug reactions, the reader is urged to check the package insert for each drug for any change in indications and dosage and for added warnings and precautions. This is particularly important when the recommended agent is a new or infrequently employed drug.

    Some drugs and medical devices presented in the publication have Food and Drug Administration (FDA) clearance for limited use in restricted research settings. It is the responsibility of the health care provider to ascertain the FDA status of each drug or device planned for use in their clinical practice.

To purchase additional copies of this book, call our customer service department at (800) 638-3030 or fax orders to (301) 223-2320. International customers should call (301) 223-2300.

Visit Lippincott Williams & Wilkins on the Internet: at LWW.com. Lippincott Williams & Wilkins customer service representatives are available from 8:30 am to 6 pm, EST.

                    10 9 8 7 6 5 4 3 2

CCS0410

Preface

Evolution of Echocardiography in Congenital Heart Disease

The editors are indebted to the historic and ground-breaking work that Drs. James B. Seward and A. Jamil Tajik performed in the 1970s and 1980s as pioneers of the use of echocardiography in congenital heart disease. The editors were educated by these two great echocardiographers and much, if not all, of what follows in this text is a result of the genius and perspiration of Drs. Seward and Tajik.

In 1987, Drs. Seward and Tajik in conjunction with Dr. William D. Edwards (Mayo Clinic Department of Pathology) and Dr. Donald J. Hagler (Mayo Clinic Division of Pediatric Cardiology) published one of the earliest textbooks dedicated to the field of congenital echocardiography, entitled *Two-Dimensional Echocardiographic Atlas of Congenital Heart Disease*. In the introduction of that textbook, the following quote appeared:

> The tomographic approach to congenital anomalies is the imaging modalities of the 1980s and is applicable to echocardiography, computerized tomography and magnetic resonance imaging. It is the building block from which the expected three dimensional imaging techniques of the 1990s will be developed. The widespread application of these imaging modalities has rekindled interest in cardiac anatomy and pathology, particularly in the evaluation of patients with congenital heart disease. Each clinical cardiologist now has the tools at hand to make preliminary, if not detailed, morphologic diagnoses. No longer is it necessary to refer a patient to the cardiac catheterization laboratory or surgical amphitheater with less than a near complete evaluation of the underlying congenital anomaly. This capability has led to and will continue to contribute to the rationale and expeditious management of patients with congenital heart disease.

These statements from the 1980s have become fact in this century. Advances in resolution of two-dimensional imaging with techniques such as harmonic imaging, advances in Doppler technology including spectral, color, and tissue Doppler techniques and the advent of three-dimensional echocardiography have all added to the clinical echocardiographer's ability to properly assess anatomy and physiology and impact clinical care for patients with congenital heart disease. Currently, the vast majority of children who are born with heart disease and require surgery within the first 6 months of life generally go to surgery with only echocardiographic assessment of their cardiac anatomy and physiology. It is rare in the current clinical era for cardiac catheterization to be performed for diagnostic purposes in young infants. In fact, congenital cardiac catheterization has become more interventional and has evolved as an alternative to surgical procedures rather than a field of pure diagnosis. Echocardiographic and, to a large extent, magnetic resonance imaging advances in the past three decades have streamlined the evaluation of these patients and made noninvasive assessment the cornerstone of diagnosis.

Similar to the *Atlas* that Drs. Seward, Tajik, Edwards, and Hagler constructed in the 1980s, this textbook will provide a comprehensive review of congenital anomalies that shall serve as a reference for echocardiographers at all levels of interest and expertise.

The editors and all those who practice congenital echocardiography are indebted to the immense contributions by Drs. Seward and Tajik.

Special mention should also be made to the current contributions of Drs. Edwards and Hagler. Dr. Edwards is a renowned cardiac pathologist who for many years has served as an invaluable resource to the Mayo Clinic Echocardiography Laboratory. Dozens of photographs of pathologic specimens from his collection have been used in this textbook. Dr. Hagler has been instrumental in the development of noninvasive imaging in fetuses, children, and adults with congenital heart disease and has been a pioneer in the use of echocardiography as a complementary imaging modality in the congenital cardiac catheterization laboratory. His contribution to this textbook is demonstrated by the number of authors who he has mentored during his career. Both Dr. Hagler's and Dr. Edward's work at Mayo have significantly impacted the assessment and management of thousands of patients with congenital heart disease.

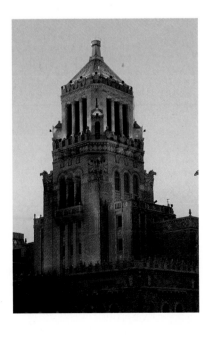

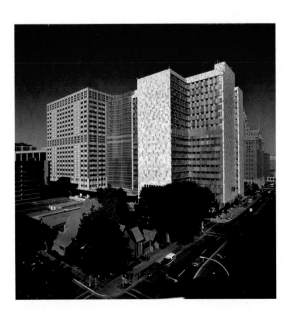

Contributors

Naser M. Ammash, MD
Associate Professor of Medicine
Department of Cardiovascular Diseases
College of Medicine, Mayo Clinic
Rochester, Minnesota

Nancy Ayres, MD
Assistant Professor
Department of Pediatrics (Cardiology)
Baylor College of Medicine
Director of Non-Invasive Imaging and
    Perinatal Cardiology
Texas Children's Hospital
Houston, Texas

Peter J. Bartz, MD
Assistant Professor of Pediatrics and
    Medicine
Departments of Pediatric Cardiology and
    Cardiovascular Medicine
Medical College of Wisconsin
Children's Hospital of Wisconsin
Milwaukee, Wisconsin

Stuart Berger, MD
Professor
Department of Pediatrics
Medical College of Wisconsin
Medical Director
Herma Heart Center
Children's Hospital of Wisconsin
Milwaukee, Wisconsin

William L. Border, MD
Pediatric Cardiology
Cincinnati Children's Hospital Medical
    Center
Cincinnati, Ohio

Allison K. Cabalka, MD
Associate Professor of Pediatrics
Mayo Clinic College of Medicine
Consultant
Division of Pediatric Cardiology
Mayo Clinic
Rochester, Minnesota

Frank Cetta, MD, FACC, FASE
Professor of Pediatrics and Medicine
Divisions of Pediatric Cardiology and
    Cardiovascular Diseases
College of Medicine, Mayo Clinic
Rochester, Minnesota

Heidi M. Connolly, MD
Cardiologist
Division of Cardiovascular Diseases
Mayo Clinic
St. Mary's Hospital and Rochester Methodist
    Hospital
Rochester, Minnesota

David J. Driscoll, MD
Professor of Pediatrics
Departments of Cardiovascular Diseases
    and Pediatrics
College of Medicine, Mayo Clinic
Mayo Clinic Transplant Center
Rochester, Minnesota

Michael G. Earing, MD
Associate Professor of Internal Medicine and
    Pediatrics
Divisions of Adult Cardiovascular Medicine
    and Pediatric Cardiology
Medical College of Wisconsin
Director of the Adult Congenital Heart
    Disease Program
Children's Hospital of Wisconsin
Froedtert Memorial Lutheran Hospital
Milwaukee, Wisconsin

William D. Edwards, MD
Professor of Pathology
Laboratory Medicine and Pathology
College of Medicine, Mayo Clinic
Consultant, Anatomic Pathology
Laboratory Medicine and Pathology
Mayo Clinic
Rochester, Minnesota

Benjamin W. Eidem, MD, FACC, FASE
Associate Professor of Pediatrics
Director, Pediatric and Fetal
    Echocardiography Laboratory
Divisions of Pediatric Cardiology and
    Cardiovascular Diseases
College of Medicine, Mayo Clinic
Rochester, Minnesota

Gregory Ensing, MD
Professor of Pediatrics
Department of Pediatrics
University of Michigan
Pediatric Cardiologist
Department of Pediatrics
C.S. Mott Children's Hospital
Ann Arbor, Michigan

Malek M. El Yaman, MD
Pediatric Cardiology Fellow
Department of Pediatrics
Mayo Clinic
Rochester, Minnesota

Bernadette Fenstermaker, RDCS
Technical Director
Echocardiography Laboratory,
    The Heart Center
Nationwide Children's Hospital
Columbus, Ohio

Mark A. Fogel, MD, FACC, FAAP
Associate Professor of Pediatrics, Cardiology
    and Radiology
Director of Cardiac MR
The University of Pennsylvania School of
    Medicine
The Children's Hospital of Philadelphia
Philadelphia, Pennsylvania

Michele A. Frommelt, MD
Assistant Professor
Department of Pediatric Cardiology
Medical College of Wisconsin
Director
Fetal Echocardiography
Children's Hospital of Wisconsin
Milwaukee, Wisconsin

Peter C. Frommelt, MD
Professor
Department of Pediatric Cariology
Medical College of Wisconsin
Director
Pediatric Echocardiography
Children's Hospital of Wisconsin
Milwaukee, Wisconsin

Javier Ganame, MD, PhD
Assistant Professor
Cardiology Department
Catholic University of Leuven
Staff Cardiologist
Cardiology/Radiology Departments
University Hospital Leuven
Leuven, Belgium

Sarah Gelehrter, MD
Assistant Professor, Clinical
Department of Pediatrics
University of Michigan
Pediatric Cardiologist
Department of Pediatrics
C.S. Mott Children's Hospital
Ann Arbor, Michigan

Edmund Gillis, BS, RDCS

Martha Grogan, MD
Assistant Professor of Medicine
Division of Cardiovascular Diseases
Mayo Foundation
Rochester, Minnesota

Donald J. Hagler, MD
Consultant, Professor of Pediatrics
Departments of Pediatric Cardiology
Mayo Clinic
Rochester, Minnesota

Frederick D. Jones, RDCS
Pediatric Cardiac Sonographer
Echocardiography Laboratory
Kentucky Children's Heart Center
Kentucky Children's Hospital
Lexington, Kentucky

Thomas R. Kimball, MD
Professor of Pediatrics
University of Cincinnati College of Medicine
Director, Echocardiography
Cincinnati Children's Hospital Medical Center
Cincinnati, Ohio

John P. Kovalchin, MD
Associate Professor
Department of Pediatrics
The Ohio State University
Director of Echocardiography
The Heart Center at Nationwide Children's
    Hospital
Columbus, Ohio

Mark Lewin, MD
Professor of Pediatrics and Chief of
Cardiology
University of Washington School of Medicine
Co-Director, Heart Center
Department of Pediatrics
Seattle Children's Hospital
Seattle, Washington

Robert Lichtenberg, MD, FACC
Director, Adult Congenital Heart Clinic
Department of Medicine
Heart Care Centers of Illinois
Mokena, Illinois

Leo Lopez, MD
Associate Professor
Department of Clinical Pediatrics
Albert Einstein College of Medicine
Director, Pediatric Cardiac Noninvasive
Imaging
Pediatric Cardiology Division
Children's Hospital at Montefiore
Bronx, New York

William T. Mahle, MD
Staff Pediatric Cardiologist
Children's Healthcare of Atlanta, Emory
University School of Medicine
Atlanta, Georgia

Colin J. McMahon, MD
Consultant Paediatric Cardiologist
Department of Paediatric Cardiology,
Our Lady's Hospital for Sick Children
Dublin, Ireland

Shaji Menon, MD
Assistant Professor of Pediatrics
Adjunct Professor of Radiology
Department of Pediatric Cardiology
University of Utah
Salt Lake City, Utah

Luc Mertens, MD, PhD
Associate Professor
Department of Paediatrics
University of Toronto
Section Head, Echocardiography
Department of Cardiology
The Hospital for Sick Children
Toronto, Ontario, Canada

Erik C. Michelfelder, MD
Associate Professor
Department of Pediatrics
University of Cincinnati College of Medicine
Director, Fetal Heart Program
The Heart Institute
Cincinnati Children's Hospital Medical Center
Cincinnati, Ohio

Fletcher A. Miller, MD
Department of Cardiovascular Diseases
Mayo Clinic
Rochester, Minnesota

L. LuAnn Minich, MD
Professor of Pediatrics
Pediatric Administration
University of Utah
Director of Clinical Research/Cardiologist
Department of Pediatric Cardiology
Primary Children's Medical Center
Salt Lake City, Utah

Shobha Natarajan, MD
Attending Cardiologist
Assistant Professor of Pediatrics
The Children's Hospital of Philadelphia
Philadelphia, Pennsylvania

Patrick W. O'Leary, MD, FACC, FASE
Associate Professor of Pediatrics
Divisions of Pediatric Cardiology and
Cardiovascular Diseases
College of Medicine, Mayo Clinic
Rochester, Minnesota

Jae K. Oh, MD
Professor of Medicine
Co-Director, Echocardiography Laboratory
Department of Cardiovascular Diseases
Mayo Clinic
Rochester, Minnesota

Angira Patel, MD, MPH
Pediatric Cardiology Fellow
Department of Pediatrics
Northwestern University, Feinberg School of
Medicine
Department of Pediatric Cardiology
Children's Memorial Hospital
Chicago, Illinois

Sabrina D. Phillips, MD
Assistant Professor of Medicine
Department of Cardiovascular Disease
Mayo Clinic
Rochester, Minnesota

Ricardo H. Pignatelli, MD
Assistant Professor of Pediatrics
Department of Pediatrics
Baylor College of Medicine
Texas Children's Hospital
Houston, Texas

Jack Rychik, MD
Professor of Pediatrics
The Children's Hospital of Philadelphia
University of Pennsylvania School of
Medicine
Director, Fetal Heart Program
The Cardiac Center at The Children's
Hospital of Philadelphia
Philadelphia, Pennsylvania

Ritu Sachdeva, MBBS, FACC
Associate Professor
Department of Pediatrics, Division of
Pediatric Cardiology
University of Arkansas for Medical
Sciences
Medical Director, Heart Station
Arkansas Children's Hospital
Little Rock, Arkansas

Ivan Salgo, MD
Chief, Cardiovascular Investigations
Fellow
Ultrasound Research and Development
Philips Healthcare
Andover, Massachusetts

Amy H. Schultz, MD
Assistant Professor
Department of Cardiology
University of Washington
Attending Physician
Department of Cardiology
Seattle Children's Hospital
Seattle, Washington

James B. Seward, MD
Consultant, Division of Cardiovascular
Diseases
Mayo Clinic
John M. Nasseff, Sr., Professor in Cardiology
in Honor of Dr. Burton Onofrio
Professor of Medicine and of Pediatrics
Mayo Clinic College of Medicine
Rochester, Minnesota

Girish S. Shirali, MBBS
Professor
Departments of Pediatrics and Obstetrics &
Gynecology
Medical University of South Carolina
Director, Pediatric Echocardiography
Medical University of South Carolina
Children's Hospital
Charleston, South Carolina

**Jeffrey F. Smallhorn, MBBS, FRACP,
FRCP(C)**
Professor
Department of Pediatrics
University of Alberta
Head, Section of Echocardiography
Pediatric Cardiology
Stollery Children's Hospital
Edmonton, Alberta, Canada

Ronald Springer, BS, RDCS

Anita L. Szwast, MD
Assistant Professor of Pediatric Cardiology
Department of Pediatrics, Division of
Cardiology
University of Pennsylvania School of
Medicine
Attending Cardiologist
Department of Pediatrics, Division of
Cardiology
Children's Hospital of Philadelphia
Philadelphia, Pennsylvania

Lloyd Y. Tani, MD
Professor of Pediatrics
Department of Pediatrics
University of Utah School of Medicine
Division Chief, Pediatric Cardiology
Primary Children's Medical Center
Salt Lake City, Utah

Himesh V. Vyas, MD
Assistant Professor
Department of Pediatric Cardiology
University of Arkansas for Medical Sciences
Assistant Professor
Department of Pediatric Cardiology
Arkansas Children's Hospital
Little Rock, Arkansas

Luciana T. Young, MD
Associate Professor
Department of Pediatrics
Northwestern University, Feinberg School of
Medicine
Department of Pediatric Cardiology
Children's Memorial Hospital
Chicago, Illinois

Robert Young, BA, RDCS
Academic Instructor
Echo Program
Mayo School of Health Sciences
Cardiac Sonographer
Mayo Echo Lab
Mayo Clinic
Rochester, Minnesota

Acknowledgments

To my wife, Debbie, my daughter, Katie, and my family for their love, support, and sacrifices throughout my medical career.—BWE

I am extremely thankful to my children, Cate, Michael, and Matt, for the sacrifices they have made for my career.—FC

To my mentors, patients, and, most of all, my family. Thank you for the examples you have provided, the patience you have shown, and the love you have given.—PWO

The editors would like to sincerely thank Mark Zangs, Jeff Stelley, and Vern Weber for their significant efforts in the preparation of many of the figures and videos throughout this textbook.

Contents

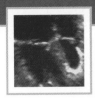

Chapter 1
Principles of Cardiovascular Ultrasound

Robert Young • Patrick W. O'Leary

Echocardiography has revolutionized the diagnostic approach to patients with congenital heart disease. A comprehensive cardiovascular ultrasound imaging and hemodynamic evaluation is the initial diagnostic test used in the assessment of any congenital cardiac malformation. Since echocardiography became a part of clinical practice in the 1970s, the technology used for cardiac imaging has been in a nearly constant state of change. New techniques have been introduced at an increasingly rapid pace, especially since the 1990s. In this chapter, we will review the basic physical properties of ultrasound and the primary modalities used in clinical imaging. These discussions will provide an important foundation that will allow us to understand the more advanced methods of imaging and functional assessment, which will be covered in more detail later.

WHAT IS ULTRASOUND?

Diagnostic ultrasound generates images of internal organs by reflecting sound energy off the anatomic structures being studied. An ultrasound imaging system is designed to project sound waves into a patient and detect the reflected energy, then converting that energy into an image on a video screen. The types of sound waves used are given the name "ultrasound" because the frequencies involved are greater than the frequencies of sound that can be detected by the human ear. The average human ear can respond to frequencies between 20 and 20,000 Hz. Therefore, it stands to reason that ultrasound waves have frequencies greater than 20,000 Hz. In clinical practice, most imaging applications actually require frequencies in excess of 1 MHz. Current cardiac imaging systems have the ability to produce ultrasound beams varying between 2 and 12 MHz. A typical diagnostic ultrasound system consists of a central processing unit (CPU), the video image display screen, a hard drive for storage of the digital images, and a selection of transducers. The transducers both transmit and receive ultrasound energy.

Some Definitions

Sound wave: Series of cyclical compressions and rarefactions of the medium through which the wave travels (Fig. 1.1).
Cycle: One alternation from peak compression through rarefaction and back to peak compression in a sound wave.
Wavelength (λ): Distance from one peak (or trough) of the wave to the next (one complete cycle of sound).
Velocity (v): Speed with which sound travels through a medium. The ultrasound propagation velocity in human tissue is 1540 m/s.
Period (p): Time duration required to complete one cycle of sound.

Amplitude (A): Magnitude of the sound wave, representing the maximum change from baseline to the peak of compression or a rarefaction in a cycle.
Frequency (f): Number of sound cycles occurring in 1 second.
Power: Rate at which energy is transferred from the sound wave to the medium. This is related to the square of the wave amplitude.
Fundamental or carrier frequency (f_0): Frequency of the transmitted sound wave.
Harmonic frequency (f_x): Sound waves that are exact multiples of the carrier frequency. The first harmonic frequency is twice the frequency of the carrier wave.
Bandwidth: Range of frequencies that a piezoelectric crystal can produce and/or respond to.

IMAGE GENERATION

Diagnostic ultrasound imaging relies on the ability of high-frequency sound waves to propagate (travel) through the body *and* be partially reflected back toward the sound source by target tissues within the patient (Fig. 1.2). The imaging system generates the imaging beam by electrically exciting a number of piezoelectric crystals contained within a transducer. The imaging beam is then focused and projected into the patient. As the ultrasound beam travels through the patient, some of the energy will be scattered into the surrounding tissue (attenuation), and some will be reflected back toward the source by the structures in the beam's path. These reflected waves will provide the information used to create images of the internal organs. This is the same imaging strategy used in sonar technology to detect objects below the water's surface. The intensity (amplitude) of the reflected energy wave is proportional to the density of the reflecting tissue (see later). The reflected ultrasound energy induces vibrations in the transducer crystals and an electric current is created. This current is sensed by the CPU and converted into a video image.

The ultrasound image generation is based primarily on the amount of energy contained in the reflected wave and the time between transmission of the ultrasound pulse and detection of the reflected waves by the transducer crystals. The interval between transmission and detection of the reflected waves is referred to as **"time of flight."** The depth at which the ultrasound image is displayed is determined by this time interval. Reflections from structures in the far field take longer to return to the transducer than do reflections from objects close to the sound source. This time interval is sensed by the CPU and directly converted into distance from the sound source based on the speed of ultrasound propagation within tissue.

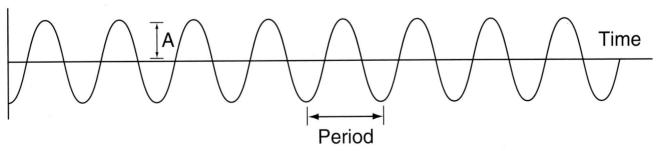

FIGURE 1.1. Graphic depiction of a sound wave. The portions of the wave above the dashed baseline represent compression of the medium by the energy in the wave. Conversely, the portions of the wave shown below the baseline represent rarefaction. The portion of the wave that lies between one peak in the next, or one valley and the next, is referred to as the *period*. Wavelength is the distance covered by one period. Amplitude (A) refers to the maximum change from baseline caused by the wave (by either compression or rarefaction).

1

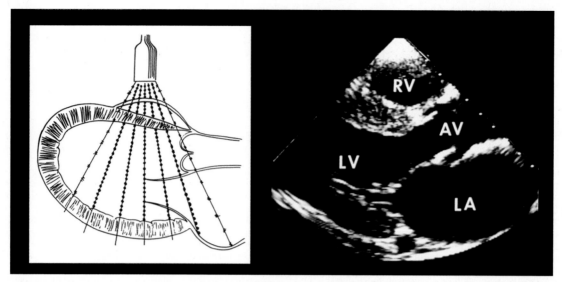

FIGURE 1.2. Ultrasound transducer transmitting a plane of ultrasound through a heart in a parasternal, sagittal, or long-axis plane (left). The myocardial and valvar structures reflect the ultrasound energy back to the transducer. The crystals within the transducer detect the returning energy, and the processors within the ultrasound system quantitate the intensity of the reflected waves and the time required for the ultrasound energy to travel from the transducer to the reflector and back. The intensity of the returning signal determines the brightness of the display (**right**), and the time defines the depth at which the signal is displayed. The central processing unit filters and then converts this information into a video display (**right**), which corresponds to the anatomy encountered by the plane of sound as it traversed the chest. AV, aortic valve; LA, left atrium; LV, left ventricle; RV, right ventricle.

The energy contained within the reflected waves is related to the **amplitude** of those waves. The amplitude of the reflected waves can be measured based on the amount of electric current produced by the receiving crystals. The brightness of the image created by the ultrasound system is determined by the amplitude of the reflected waves. Bodily fluids, such as blood, effusions, and ascites, will transmit nearly all of the energy contained within the imaging beam. Because there is little reflected energy, these areas are displayed as black (or nearly black) on the imaging screen. Air is not dense enough to allow transmission of sound frequencies in the ultrasound range. Therefore, all of the imaging energy present in the beam will be reflected at an air–tissue interface, such as at the edge of a pneumothorax or of the normal lung. This nearly 100% reflection is translated into a very bright (usually white) representation on the imaging screen. Other very dense tissues, like bone, will also reflect virtually all of the energy and be displayed as very bright echo returns. Structures beyond these very bright "echos" cannot be displayed, because no ultrasound energy reaches them. These areas are often referred to as acoustic shadows. Fat, muscle, and other tissues will transmit some of the imaging beam and reflect a fraction of the sound wave. The amount reflected is related to the density of the tissue, and the amount of returning energy sensed by the crystals in the transducer will determine how brightly an image will be displayed on the video screen.

During a clinical examination, echocardiographers are usually less conscious of amplitude than they are of the frequency of the transmitted sound beam. The frequency of the ultrasound waves has a tremendous impact on the ability to produce images of anatomic structures. The greater the frequency, the greater is the resolution of the resulting image. However, high-frequency sound beams lose more of their energy to surrounding tissues (attenuation) and, therefore, do not penetrate human tissue as well as low-frequency beams. Thus, the echocardiographers must always balance penetration (lower frequencies) and resolution (higher frequencies). For example, the heart of an adult patient will have structures that are positioned farther from the transducer than they are in the heart of a child. Therefore, lower imaging frequencies are usually required to produce adequate images in older patients.

The advent of *harmonic imaging* has significantly enhanced the ability to examine these older patients with surface echocardiography. Human tissue is not homogeneous in character. As a result, when an imaging beam is reflected by the target, the reflected sound energy exists not only in an unaltered state but also in multiples of the carrier frequencies (harmonic waves). Modern ultrasound transducers now have sufficiently broad bandwidths to vibrate not only at the carrier or fundamental frequency but also at the first harmonic frequency of the transmitted wave. The first harmonic frequency has twice the number of alternating cycles of compression/rarefaction relative to the transmitted frequency. For example, the first harmonic frequency of a 4-mHz ultrasound beam will be 8 mHz. This allows the ultrasound system to transmit at a relatively low frequency but to detect (to image with) reflected waves of a much higher frequency than the original wave. Thus, harmonic imaging combines the advantages of low-frequency transducers (penetration) with the improved resolution associated with higher-frequency imaging.

 ## COMMON IMAGING FORMATS AND IMAGING ARTIFACTS

The earliest echocardiograms displayed either the amplitude or the brightness of the reflected waves on an oscilloscope. These were referred to as either A-mode (amplitude) or B-mode (brightness) echocardiograms. When video screens were linked to echocardiographic systems, it became possible to display the information in "real-time." These "echocardiograms in motion" were referred to as motion mode studies, or M-mode. **M-mode** scans display the brightness of the ultrasound reflections, as well as the distance from the transducer and the time at which the reflection occurs. This allows the examiner to visualize cardiac activity as it occurs. M-mode scanning interrogates targets along a single line within the patient. Advances in transducer construction, image processing, and video display allowed multiple M-lines to be fused into a sector of scanning, including usually 80 to 90 degrees of arc. Two-dimensional sector scanning produced a "flat" tomographic display of the areas being interrogated. **Two-dimensional** imaging remains the primary imaging modality in modern anatomic echocardiography (Fig. 1.2). However, additional advances in transducer and image processing capabilities now allow real-time volumetric three-dimensional interrogation of the cardiovascular system (Fig. 1.3). As this technology continues to progress, it is likely to, once again, revolutionize the way in which echocardiographic data are acquired.

Ultrasound, like any imaging technique, will occasionally produce an erroneous image. These are referred to as *artifacts*. The echocardiographer must be aware of these imaging anomalies to avoid misinterpretation of the images. Image formation depends on the reflection of ultrasound energy. As a result, the most common artifact

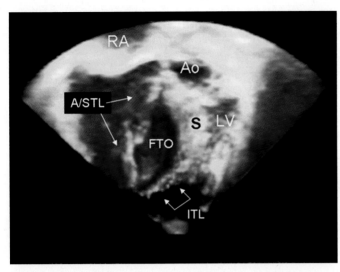

FIGURE 1.3. Improved transducer and processing capabilities allow ultrasound systems to scan in "volumes" of interest rather than just in planes. This image was obtained during real-time three-dimensional imaging. The patient had significant Ebstein malformation. The transducer was positioned at the right ventricular apex, and the resulting volume of sound was cropped to display the ventricular cavity at the level of the functional tricuspid orifice (FTO). The abnormalities of the tricuspid valve leaflets are clearly seen. The large anterior leaflet and remnant of the septal leaflets (A/STL) are highlighted (*long arrows*), and the smaller inferior tricuspid leaflet can be seen parallel to the diaphragm (ITL) (*short connected arrows*). Ao, aorta; LV, left ventricle; RA, right atrium; S, ventricular septum.

encountered is due to the fact that structures that lie parallel to the beam of sound produce no return. The structures do not appear on the video image. This is referred to as **parallel dropout**. Imaging areas from multiple angles of interrogation is a way to avoid this problem. Very dense, and therefore bright, structures produce echocardiographic shadows that lie beyond the intense return and parallel to the plane of sound. This **shadowing** reduces or eliminates the information obtainable in these areas. Imaging from multiple windows and angles of interrogation is the most effective strategy when faced with such shadows. In extreme cases, such as shadowing caused by a prosthetic valve, the transducer may need to be placed posterior to the heart to avoid the shadow. These are situations in which transesophageal echocardiography can be extremely useful. Echo-dense structures can also distort the image lateral to the bright reflector. This occurs due to scattering of the ultrasound energy in nonparallel directions to the original beam. This distortion has been referred to as **side-lobing**. This effect can artificially broaden the appearance of a bright structure, such as a calcified valve or thickened pericardium. Enhanced focusing and filtering capabilities have sig-

nificantly reduced this issue in modern equipment. Other unusual echo returns can be encountered. These returns often have an arc-like appearance on the video screen. Alterations in frequency, depth of image, or video frame rate will frequently eliminate these returns from the image, confirming their artifactual nature.

THE DOPPLER EFFECT AND CARDIOVASCULAR HEMODYNAMICS

Structures of interest to the echocardiographer are generally not stationary. It is well known that objects in motion reflect sound energy differently than do objects at rest. When an energy wave reflects off or is produced by a moving target, the frequency of the resulting wave is altered based on the direction and speed of the target. This phenomenon was first described by Austrian scientist Christian Doppler in 1843 while he was studying distant stars. Doppler found that the change (or shift) in the frequency of the wave produced or reflected by an object in motion is directly proportional to both its speed and the direction of the motion relative to the observer. This shift has become known as the *Doppler effect* in honor of its discoverer. A classic example of the Doppler effect is the change in the perceived pitch of a train horn as it approaches and then passes by a stationary observer. The train's horn produces a sound of a single, constant pitch, defined by the frequency of the sound waves. However, when the train is in motion, the frequency/pitch that will be "heard" by the observer will be greater or less than the transmitted frequency, depending on the direction of motion. If the train is traveling toward the observer, the perceived frequency is greater than the transmitted frequency (more cycles per second). Conversely, the pitch is lower than the transmitted frequency if the train is moving away from the observer.

These shifts in frequency occur because targets in motion toward an observer will physically encounter and reflect the wave more often than will a stationary target. This increase in "encounter rate" compresses the reflected wave and thereby increases the number of cycles per second in the "reflection," increasing the frequency (Fig. 1.4). If the target is moving away from the observer, the energy wave will encounter the target, and be reflected, less often (Fig. 1.5). The frequency of the reflected wave will therefore be reduced. In the case of cardiac ultrasound, the transducer is the stationary observer and the moving reflector is either the red blood cells within the vascular system or myocardial tissue in motion. The changes in frequency that occur due to target motion are referred to as the *Doppler shift*, or Δf.

$$\Delta f = f_t - f_r$$

The shift from the original frequency (Δf) can be determined by measuring the frequency of the reflected wave (f_r) and determining the difference between *that* value and the transmitted frequency (f_t). This difference is routinely calculated by ultrasound systems.

FIGURE 1.4. Doppler shift: Impact of a reflector moving toward the transducer. The motion of the targets (red blood cells) toward the ultrasound source compresses the reflected waves, reducing its period ($-\Delta P$) and wavelength. The frequency of the reflected wave (f_r) is thereby increased relative to the transmitted wave (f_t) of ultrasound.

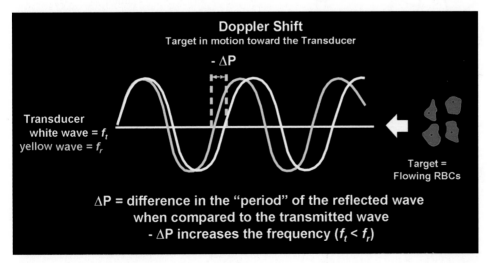

FIGURE 1.5. Doppler shift: Impact of a reflector moving away from the transducer. The motion of the targets (red blood cells) away from the ultrasound source decreases their interaction with the transmitted wave. As a result, the reflected wave has an increase in its period (+ΔP) and wavelength. The frequency of the reflected wave (f_r) is thereby reduced relative to the transmitted wave (f_t) of ultrasound.

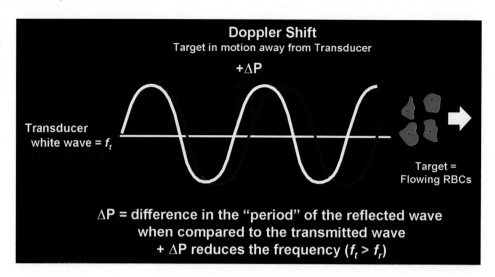

THE DOPPLER EQUATION

Additional studies of these frequency shifts have shown that the speed (velocity) of the moving target can be determined mathematically. This mathematical relationship is known as the *Doppler equation*. The components of the Doppler equation are the frequency shift (Δf), the speed of the wave within the medium (c), the original transmitted frequency (f_t), and the cosine of the angle between the original wave and the direction of the moving reflector. This angle is referred to as the *angle of interrogation*, or is designated by the Greek letter theta, θ. If Δf is known, then the Doppler equation can be easily solved for velocity as shown in the following equation:

$$\Delta f = 2f_t \times [(V \times \cos\theta)/c]$$

$$\text{Velocity} = (\Delta f \times c)/[(2f_t) \times \cos\theta]$$

The influence of the *angle of reflection* (also referred to as the angle of interrogation) can be minimized by aligning the transducer's beam nearly parallel to the flow being investigated (angle = 0 degrees, cos θ = 1; Fig. 1.6). In clinical practice, one strives to maintain the angle of interrogation at less than 20 degrees, because the cosine values of all angles less than 20 degrees are essentially equal to 1 (Fig. 1.6). If the Doppler beam can be aligned with the flow in this way, the angle of reflection will not influence the calculation of velocity by the Doppler equation and it can be ignored. Because the speed of sound in tissue is constant, the only remaining variable in the Doppler equation is the frequency shift, which is measured by the ultrasound system. This relationship allows a nearly direct calculation of the velocity of any moving reflector in the path of the sound wave.

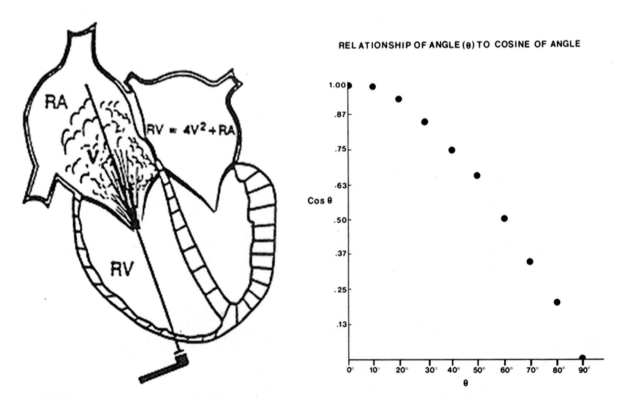

FIGURE 1.6. Influence of the angle of interrogation (θ) on calculated Doppler velocity. The Doppler equation relates to velocity to the frequency shift of the reflected wave but also includes the cosine of the angle that the ultrasound beam makes with the flow direction. The angle term (cosine θ) in the Doppler equation can be neglected when the angle is less than 20 degrees. This is because the cosine values of angles less than 20 degrees are approximately 1 (**right**). Therefore, when using Doppler echocardiography, the examiner should use two-dimensional and color flow guidance to achieve directions that are parallel to the blood flow being evaluated or at least minimize the angle of interrogation. RA, right atrium; RV, right ventricle; V, velocity.

RELATIONSHIP BETWEEN VELOCITY AND PRESSURE DIFFERENCES

Bernoulli was an Italian physicist who had an interest in fluid dynamics. He found that flow velocities were directly related to the pressure difference ($P_1 - P_2$, or ΔP) across a flow restrictor (analogous to a stenosis; Fig. 1.7). It was Bernoulli's work that allowed the Doppler effect to be used in assessing cardiovascular hemodynamics. Bernoulli's equation states that the pressure difference between two points on opposite sides of a restrictor within a flow stream is related to the difference between the squares of the flow velocities at those two points. His mathematical description of this relationship included terms related to convective acceleration, flow acceleration, and viscous friction (Fig. 1.7). For clinical purposes, we can simplify this relationship by making a few assumptions. First, one assumes that the influence of friction between the flowing column of blood and the vessel/chamber wall is negligible. This is a reasonable assumption because we are usually interrogating flows in the center of relatively large vessels or chambers. Similarly, the flow acceleration term can usually be ignored because the flow in the area of interest is not accelerating significantly. These two assumptions simplify the Bernoulli relationship to the following equation:

$$\Delta P = \tfrac{1}{2}\,\rho\,(V_2^2 - V_1^2)$$

V_2 represents the flow velocity beyond the flow restrictor (valve or other stenosis), V_1 represents the flow velocity just proximal to the restrictor, and ρ represents the mass density of the fluid—in this case, blood, which is constant. In the human, with a relatively normal hemoglobin concentration, $\tfrac{1}{2}\rho$ is equal to 4. Therefore, the Bernoulli equation as it relates to Doppler echocardiography is usually expressed as $\Delta P = 4(V_2^2 - V_1^2)$. If the proximal velocity (V_1) is relatively low (<1 m/s), then it, too, can be ignored without altering the results of the calculation significantly. In clinical practice, this "very" simplified Bernoulli equation, $\Delta P = 4(V_2^2)$, is actually the equation that is most commonly used. Neglecting the proximal velocity is almost always appropriate when evaluating a velocity profile produced by regurgitation. However, in valvar or vascular stenosis, the accuracy of ΔP is improved by including V_1 in the relationship. Whenever such assumptions are made, one must make a conscious

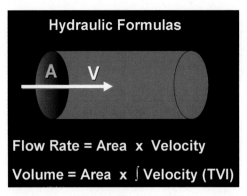

FIGURE 1.8. Hydraulic formulas. These equations show the relationships of flow rate and velocity to the cross-sectional area of a column of moving fluid, the velocity of the fluid, and the integral (time-weighted average) of that velocity. A, cross-sectional area; TVI, time-velocity integral; V, velocity; ∫ velocity, integral of velocity.

effort to beware of clinical situations in which the assumptions are being violated. The most common clinical situation that violates these assumptions is encountered with prosthetic aortic–to–pulmonary artery shunts. These prosthetic tubes are small. Therefore, their walls do exert friction on the column of moving blood and the acceleration within the area of interest can also be important in "vessels" of such a small size. Cyanotic patients with significant polycythemia also create a problem for the Bernoulli equation because their blood viscosity is greater than normal, altering the value of ρ.

The principles of fluid dynamics allow Doppler echocardiography to do more than evaluation pressure differences. It is also possible to calculate the volume of blood that flows past a specific point in the cardiovascular system using a combination of imaging and range-gated Doppler techniques. The hydraulic formula states that the rate of flow within a tube is equal to the product of the tube's cross-sectional area (CSA) and the flow velocity of the fluid (Fig. 1.8). Flow volume can be calculated as the product of the CSA and the "stroke distance" traveled by the flowing fluid. Stroke distance is the integral of the fluid flow velocity over time. Flow volume is equal to CSA multiplied by the time-velocity intergral (TVI) of the fluid's velocity (Fig. 1.8). This concept is easily applied to the determination of flow volume within blood vessels or across cardiac valves (Figs. 1.9 and 1.10). Most vessels and valves are relatively circular, and CSA is used in the geometric equation for the area of a circle [CSA = $\pi \times$ (radius)^2]. The examiner measures the diameter (D, in cm) from a two-dimensional scan. The radius (R) is one-half the diameter and $\pi = 3.14$. Some prefer to simplify the relationship by combining the constant numerical terms into one value and simply using the measured

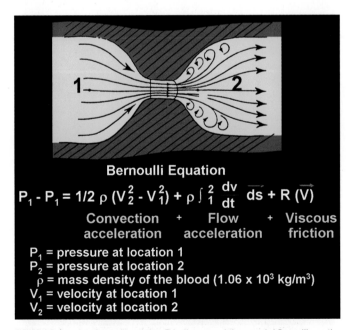

FIGURE 1.7. Complete Bernoulli equation. This diagram and the expanded Bernoulli equation describe how the flow velocities of a fluid moving through a restriction are related to the pressure difference across that restriction. For most situations in clinical echocardiography, the flow of acceleration and viscous friction terms can be ignored (see text). In most human subjects, the term "½ρ" is approximately equal to 4. The resulting "expanded" Bernoulli equation predicts that the pressure "drop" ($P_1 - P_2$) across the restriction can be estimated by the difference between the squares of the flow velocities proximal and distal to the restriction or $P_1 - P_2 = 4(V_2^2 - V_1^2)$.

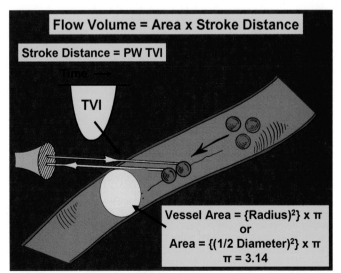

FIGURE 1.9. Use of Doppler echocardiography in calculating flow volume in a blood vessel. TVI is obtained by tracing the Doppler signal from a PW Doppler sample volume positioned within the "area" of interest. PW, pulsed wave; TVI, time-velocity integral.

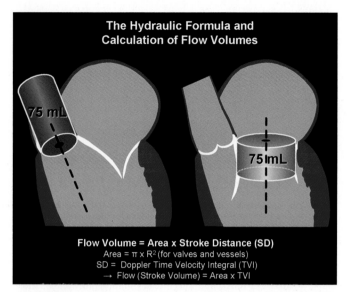

The Hydraulic Formula and Calculation of Flow Volumes

75 mL

75 mL

Flow Volume = Area × Stroke Distance (SD)
Area = π × R² (for valves and vessels)
SD = Doppler Time Velocity Integral (TVI)
→ Flow (Stroke Volume) = Area × TVI

FIGURE 1.10. Use of the hydraulic formula to calculate the stroke volume crossing the aortic (left) and mitral (right) valves. Cross-sectional area is determined by measuring the two-dimensional diameter of the valve at the annular hinge points. Radius (R) is determined by dividing the diameter by 2. Cross-sectional area is calculated using the formula for the area of a circle (πR²). The pulsed-wave Doppler sample volume is placed between the annular hinge points of the valve being examined. In this way, one can be certain that the Doppler flow time-velocity integral (TVI) corresponds directly to the "area" of interest. R, radius; SD, stroke distance.

diameter in the equation rather than the radius. This results in the following relationship: $CSA = 0.785 \times D^2$. The other component of the hydraulic relationship, stroke distance, is determined by tracing the pulsed-wave (PW) Doppler signal to "integrate" the velocity profile (determine the average flow velocity during the period being examined, usually one cardiac cycle). The product of this TVI and the CSA is equal to the volume of blood flow. This technique can be used to determine chamber stroke volumes, cardiac outputs, and regurgitant or shunt volumes. Specific applications of these relationships will be covered in more detail in later chapters of this text.

 ## DOPPLER ECHOCARDIOGRAPHIC MODALITIES

The most common Doppler modalities used during an echocardiographic examination are color flow, PW, and continuous-wave (CW) Doppler. These techniques are focused on the description of blood flow. Other Doppler techniques, such as tissue Doppler imaging, color kinesis, and Doppler-derived myocardial deformation imaging (strain), are used to describe myocardial activity. The remainder of this chapter will focus on the mechanics of the Doppler techniques used to describe blood flow. The topics of myocardial Doppler examinations will be addressed in later chapters.

Use of the Doppler equation allows determination of blood flow velocities within the heart and central blood vessels. Spectral Doppler techniques (CW and PW) are used to describe relatively discrete flowing streams of blood. By convention, blood flows that are directed toward the transducer have their velocities displayed as positive (upward) deflections above a zero-velocity baseline (red signal, Fig. 1.11). Conversely, flows that are directed away from the transducer's position are displayed as negative (downward) deflections below the baseline (blue signal, Figure 1.11). The oldest Doppler echocardiographic technique is CW Doppler. This type of Doppler interrogation is performed using two independent ultrasound crystals within the transducer. One crystal continuously transmits a beam of ultrasound (Fig. 1.12), usually at a relatively low frequency (2 MHz). The other crystal acts as a continuous receiver for the reflected ultrasound waves. Because the sound beam is continuously produced and detected, this type of Doppler will detect velocity profiles from all moving targets in the beam's path. Because the sound beam is generated continuously, the pulse repetition frequency is essentially infinite (see later discussion of Nyquist limit). The continuous nature of beam generation and sensing allows detection of large frequency shifts and therefore very high velocity flows.

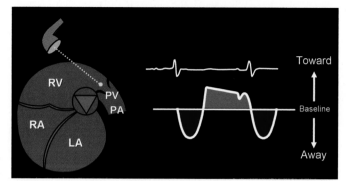

FIGURE 1.11. Continuous-wave (CW) Doppler interrogation of the right ventricular outflow tract (RVOT) (left) and representation of the resulting Doppler tracing. The tracing is shown with a simultaneous, single-lead electrocardiogram to allow accurate timing of Doppler events to the phases of the cardiac cycle. The baseline of the Doppler tracing represents a velocity of zero, or no flow. Blood flow directed toward the transducer is displayed above the baseline, as a positive velocity profile (*red shaded area*). In this case, the positive signal represents pulmonary valve (PV) regurgitation. Blood flow directed away from the transducer is displayed below the baseline; as a negative velocity profile (*blue shaded area*). In this case, the negative flow signal represents right ventricular (RV) ejection across the pulmonary valve (PV). LA, left atrium; PA, pulmonary artery; RA, right atrium.

CW Doppler is therefore the primary modality used to define the rapid blood flows encountered in valvular regurgitation or stenoses of any etiology. The continuous nature of CW Doppler also means that there is no spatial information contained in the signals. In other words, this method cannot be used to localize the flow being interrogated. As a result, postprocessing and signal filtering are usually optimized to display the maximum velocity profile encountered. As a general rule, CW Doppler is best recorded with both high gain and filter settings.

Unlike CW Doppler, PW Doppler only transmits the interrogating sound beam intermittently. Once the pulse of ultrasound is generated, the crystal then "listens" for the reflected wave. This characteristic allows the examiner to specifically interrogate flows within an area of interest, often referred to as the *sample volume* (Fig. 1.12). For this reason, PW Doppler is referred to as "range

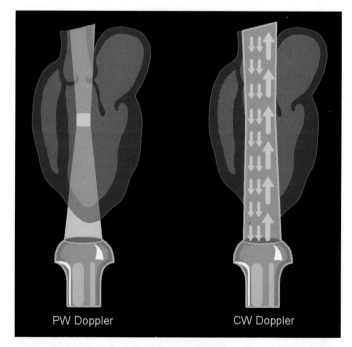

PW Doppler

CW Doppler

FIGURE 1.12. Physical difference between pulsed-wave (PW) Doppler (left) and continuous-wave (CW) Doppler (right). CW Doppler uses a constant interrogating beam of ultrasound (*large arrows*) and continuously senses the reflected ultrasound energy (*small arrows*). In contrast, PW Doppler intermittently transmits the interrogating beam in pulses and detects the reflected energy between those pulses. This allows the ultrasound system to focus on the reflections occurring within a single area of interest, at a specified distance from the transducer. This characteristic, unique to PW Doppler, is referred to as range gating and allows definition of Doppler flow profiles at specific points within the cardiovascular system.

gated." This means that PW Doppler will detect frequency shifts/velocity profiles that occur only within a defined region of interest, allowing one to localize the origin of the flow pattern. The advantage that range gating provides is offset by the limited ability of PW Doppler to assess high-velocity flows without distorting the flow envelope. This limitation stems from the intermittent or "pulsed" nature of the Doppler beam. The highest velocities that can be displayed by PW Doppler are determined by the pulse repetition frequency (PRF) of the interrogating sound beam. If the frequency shift is greater than 50% of the PRF, the resulting signal will "alias." These aliased signals are displayed as if the reflector was moving in a direction opposite to its actual motion, or on the incorrect side of the tracing's baseline (Fig. 1.13). The maximum velocity that can be displayed without aliasing is referred to as the **Nyquist limit** (NL = 0.5 × PRF). The continuous nature of the ultrasound beam used for CW Doppler results in an essentially infinite PRF, and therefore there is no theoretical limit to the maximum velocity that could be recorded by CW Doppler techniques.

Color flow Doppler is based on PW Doppler technology. Color Doppler creates a "map" of velocity data, coded in shades of red and blue. This map is then displayed over an image of the cardiovascular structures within a defined region of interest (Fig. 1.14). Color Doppler data can be displayed with images obtained using any imaging format—M-mode, two-dimensional, or even three-dimensional volumetric scans. The choice of background imaging is made based on the imaging task being performed. Color mapping allows the echocardiographer to "see" both normal and abnormal blood flow patterns and directly relate them to the structures involved (Fig. 1.15). In essence, color flow Doppler is the echocardiographic equivalent to angiography, but with added value. Color Doppler maps have both direction and velocity data encoded in the signals. By convention, flows that are directed toward the interrogating transducer will be shown in shades of red. Flows that are directed away from the transducer are seen in blue (Fig. 1.16). Students often use a simple mnemonic (BART) to assist in remembering the directionality of color coding. BART stands for "blue away—red toward."

Because color Doppler is based on PW technology, it shares the ability of PW Doppler to localize flow velocities in space, but it also has an upper velocity limit beyond which the flow pattern becomes aliased. When a flow velocity exceeds the Nyquist limit during color flow imaging, the color map will take on characteristics of flows that are opposite the actual direction of the flow stream. This phenomenon is also referred to as "aliasing." Disordered or turbulent blood flows are displayed by the inclusion of variance in the color map. This variance is displayed by adding shades of green to the color coding for the direction of flow and is often perceived as "speckling" in the flow stream (Figs. 1.16 and 1.17).

Color flow Doppler is particularly useful for detecting the sources of abnormal blood flows (Fig. 1.17). Most normal cardiovascular flow patterns are relatively laminar, low velocity, and undisturbed. Flows generated by septal defects, valvar regurgitation, and stenoses of

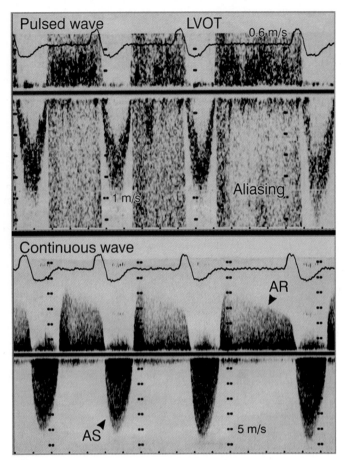

FIGURE 1.13. Aliasing. These pulsed-wave (**top**, PW) and continuous-wave (**bottom**, CW) Doppler recordings were taken from an examination of a patient with both aortic stenosis (AS) and regurgitation (AR). Both tracings were obtained with the transducer at the cardiac apex. The PW sample volume was placed in the left ventricular outflow tract (LVOT), just proximal to the aortic annulus. The PW tracing shows both the relatively laminar, systolic LVOT flow profile, as well as the turbulent, diastolic, high-velocity flow associated with AR. Since the AR velocity (4 to 5 m/s) is greater than the Nyquist limit (NL), much of the PW signal is displayed below the baseline. This occurs even though the AR flow is actually directed toward the transducer at the apex. This phenomenon where a velocity profile "wraps around" to the inappropriate side of the zero-velocity baseline is referred to as *aliasing*. The CW tracing displays both the high-velocity systolic (AS) and diastolic (AR) signals correctly and unambiguously. The AS flow signal, traveling away from the apex, is all displayed below the baseline. Conversely, the AR flow signal is seen entirely above the zero-velocity baseline, as expected for a flow stream moving away from the transducer. The continuous transmission/detection of the ultrasound beam creates an essentially infinite NL, allowing accurate display of very high velocity profiles but eliminating the ability limit flow detection to a single region of interest.

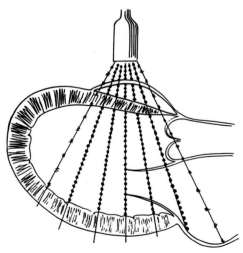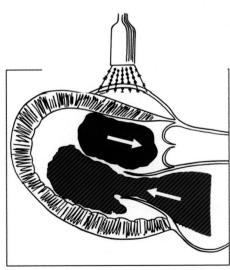

FIGURE 1.14. Production of a two-dimensional ultrasound image (left) and a color flow Doppler map obtained in the same parasternal long-axis projection (right). The color flow Doppler encodes flows that are directed, even partially, toward the transducer in shades of red. Conversely, flows away from the transducer are coded in blue.

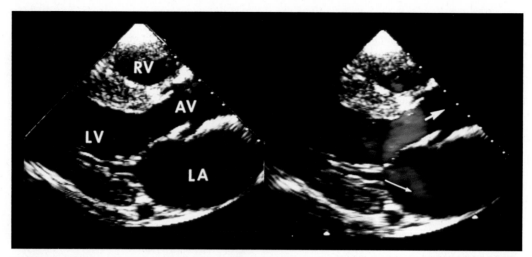

FIGURE 1.15. Two systolic, parasternal long-axis echocardiographic images displaying the color flow principles described in Figure 1.14. The regurgitant flow crossing the mitral valve is moving at an angle to the plane of sound (*thin arrow*) that is directed away from the transducer. Therefore, the mitral regurgitation flow is coded in blue. The flow generated by systolic ejection of the left ventricle (LV) is moving toward (*thick arrow*) the position of the transducer and is coded in red. AV, aortic valve; LA, left atrium; RV, right ventricle.

FIGURE 1.16. Color palette used during color flow Doppler mapping. The color coding includes information regarding not only direction but also velocity and turbulence. Velocity is indicated by decreasing intensity of color shade. Turbulence is displayed by adding shades of green to the dominant red or blue directionally determined color.

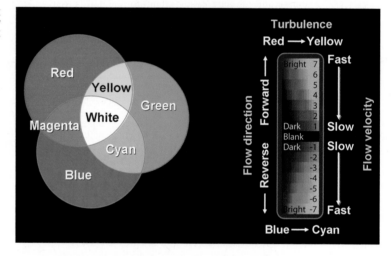

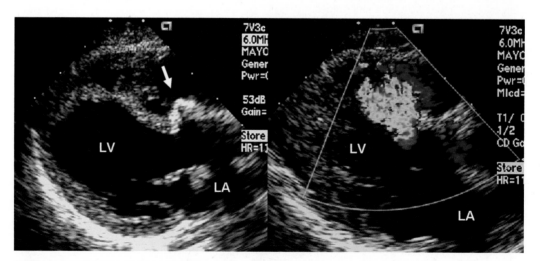

FIGURE 1.17. Parasternal long-axis images acquired from a patient after patch closure of a ventricular septal defect (VSD). The VSD patch is shown (**left**, *arrow*). There is no obvious gap detected on two-dimensional imaging. The addition of color flow Doppler interrogation (**right**) allowed rapid recognition of an abnormal flow arising from the junction of the patch and the muscular ventricular septum. This flow has high velocity (note the speckled pattern and variance coding) and a narrow origin from the left ventricular cavity. These features suggest that the defect is actually small, despite the broad color flow disturbance seen within the right ventricular cavity. LA, left atrium; LV, left ventricle.

any kind generally will display greater velocity and variance. These features make these flow streams stand out from the more laminar background, allowing them to be quickly and easily recognized. When interpreting color flow Doppler signals, the echocardiographer must remember that, unlike spectral Doppler techniques, color flow does not demonstrate peak or maximal velocities. Rather, the color flow Doppler velocity is a representation of the mean flow velocity in the area being interrogated. While this makes prediction of pressure differences difficult, it is actually an advantage when determining flow volumes. The fact that color Doppler velocities represent the mean flow velocity is one of the major reasons that proximal isovelocity surface area (PISA) analysis of regurgitant and stenotic flows is possible.

Although many of the concepts outlined in this chapter are old ones, they provide an essential foundation for anyone investigating the cardiovascular system with ultrasound technology. The chapters that follow will build on these foundations, but when one encounters confusing or inconsistent information during an echocardiographic examination, it is often useful to reflect on these basic principles of ultrasound imaging to determine what portion of the acquired data may be based on an inaccurate assumption or influenced by a technical limitation of ultrasound imaging.

Acknowledgment

The authors gratefully recognize the generous contributions of Dr. Jae Oh to this chapter. He has generously contributed many of the figures used in this chapter from his teaching library. His zeal for echocardiographic education and investigation is an example to us all.

SUGGESTED READING

Currie PJ, Hagler DJ, Seward JB, et al. Instantaneous pressure gradient: a simultaneous Doppler and dual catheter correlative study. *J Am Coll Cardiol.* 1986;7:800–806.

Currie PJ, Seward JB, Chan KL, et al. Continuous wave Doppler determination of right ventricular pressure: a simultaneous Doppler-catheterization study in 127 patients. *J Am Coll Cardiol.* 1985;6:750–756.

Edler I, Hertz CH. The use of ultrasonic reflectoscope for the continuous recording of the movements of heart walls. 1954. *Clin Physiol Funct Imaging.* 2004;24:118–136.

Hatle L, Angelsen B. *Doppler ultrasound in cardiology.* 2nd ed. Philadelphia, Pa: Lea & Febiger; 1985.

Hatle L, Brubakk A, Tromsdal A, et al. Noninvasive assessment of pressure drop in mitral stenosis by Doppler ultrasound. *Br Heart J.* 1978;40:131–140.

Houch RC, Cooke J, Gill EA. Three-dimensional echo: transition from theory to real-time, a technology now ready for prime time. *Curr Probl Diagn Radiol.* 2005;34:85–105.

Kremkau FW, ed. *Diagnostic ultrasound: principles and instruments.* 6th ed. Philadelphia, Pa: WB Saunders; 2002.

Omoto R, Kasai C. Physics and instrumentation of Doppler color flow mapping. *Echocardiography.* 1987;4:467–483.

Tajik AJ, Seward JB, Hagler DJ, et al. Two-dimensional real-time ultrasonic imaging of the heart and great vessels: technique, image orientation, structure identification, and validation. *Mayo Clin Proc.* 1978;53:271–303.

Zamorano J, Cordeiro P, Sugeng L, et al. Real-time three-dimensional echocardiography for rheumatic mitral valve stenosis evaluation: an accurate and novel approach. *J Am Coll Cardiol.* 2004;43:2091–2096.

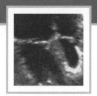

Chapter 2
Practical Issues Related to the Examination, Anatomic Image Orientation, and Segmental Cardiovascular Analysis

Ed Gillis • Ronald Springer • Patrick W. O'Leary

An echocardiographic examination can and should be much more than a simple definition of cardiac anatomy. A thorough evaluation not only defines cardiovascular anatomy but also describes myocardial performance, valvar function, and overall hemodynamics. Therefore, our approach to the echocardiographic examination must allow complete and efficient definition of all of these factors, while also taking into account patient comfort, age, and clinical situation. In this chapter, we will review some of the practical issues surrounding the performance of congenital and pediatric echocardiography. These issues involve everything from patient cooperation to complex hemodynamic analyses and digital image archiving. In this chapter, we hope to provide the reader with a solid foundation on which to build their understanding of echocardiography and its use. We will review a general approach to the examination, image acquisition, archiving, and report generation. A standardized method of image orientation and an outline of the segmental analysis of cardiovascular anatomy will also be presented.

 ## GENERAL EXAMINATION GUIDELINES

The examination process should begin even before the examiner meets the patient. The first step is to understand the events that led to a referral for the study. This can be accomplished by reviewing the patient's history and/or interviewing the patient and/or family before acquiring any images. Particular attention should be paid to prior cardiovascular events, symptoms, and/or treatments (if any). Review of the written operative notes is crucial for the patient with a history of surgical intervention. Precise knowledge of the details of the preceding "repairs" allows the echocardiographer to perform a more thorough and efficient study. It is also prudent to confirm the details of what is learned from written records by discussing the history with the patient and/or accompanying family members before beginning the examination. When no information is available, inspection of the patient's color, respiratory status, and chest can be helpful. A cyanotic or distressed infant is more likely to have complex malformations than is the school-age child presenting for evaluation of a murmur. If sternotomy or lateral thoracotomy scars are present, they confirm previous surgical interventions, even though they do not define the specific procedure. In the remainder of this chapter, we will focus primarily on the approach to a comprehensive echocardiographic study. However, there are times when a more goal-directed approach is prudent or even required. These limited examinations are appropriate when the primary anomaly has been well defined and/or the patient is presenting for a "re-check" of a residual abnormality, such as a pericardial effusion.

The advent of digital imaging, archiving, and reporting systems has simplified the process necessary to obtain historical information and compare current findings with the patient's prior status. There are many commercially available systems that provide all of these features. During an echocardiographic examination, it is important to have access to not only the electronic medical record but also any previous imaging studies. Ideally, the electronic reporting and archiving tool used will not only display current and past images but also allow for creation of the clinical echocardiographic report within the same program. These reports should be reviewed before beginning an examination. The quantitative measurements obtained should be compared to historical baselines before the conclusion of the study. The ability to quickly perform side-by-side comparison of current images with previous examinations has been a major advance associated with digital echocardiography, allowing for easier and more accurate assessment of changes in cardiac findings over time.

The second phase of the examination also occurs before scanning begins. This is when the examiner assesses the patient's clinical status. This information should be documented in the patient's clinical report and should include definition of the patient's heart rate and rhythm, blood pressure, and state of consciousness during the examination. This information is required because hemodynamic data obtained from a sedated patient need to be interpreted differently from those obtained from the agitated or awake "but calm" patient. When the state of consciousness is anything other than awake and calm, this should be documented within the formal report. Additional pieces of information that should be included in the report relate to the patient's body size. Height, weight, body mass index, and body surface area should all be documented on the report and linked to the measurements obtained. These biometric values become especially important when determining whether specific chamber sizes or wall thicknesses are normal or abnormal relative to the general population.

When measuring blood pressure, it is important to use cuffs of appropriate size. The width of the inflatable bladder should cover most of the upper arm between the elbow and shoulder. Smaller cuffs will result in artificially elevated readings. It is advisable to use the right arm for these determinations, because the right arm will be upstream from a coarctation in the majority of patients. Occasionally, the patient's state changes between the initial measurement and the time that important Doppler measurements are made. In these cases, a repeat blood pressure measurement should be obtained. For example, if the patient is initially agitated or anxious but becomes more relaxed during the examination, repeating the blood pressure measurement will give a more accurate picture of the patient's hemodynamic state at the time of the Doppler measurements.

Finally, the scan can begin. The ultrasound system and examination room in a pediatric/congenital cardiac ultrasound laboratory must have features that would not normally be found in a laboratory solely devoted to the care of adults with acquired cardiac disorders. The echocardiographic system must have a wide range of transducers to allow for the variation in body habitus and image quality associated with congenital heart disease. In a single day, the system may be used to study neonates, fetuses, and adults with histories of multiple complex surgical repairs (and the challenging acoustic windows that accompany that history). Three or four phased-array transducers, with frequencies ranging from 3 to 12 mHz, represent a minimal complement for a congenital echocardiographic system. A 2-mHz, nonimaging continuous-wave Doppler transducer is often needed to clearly define weak Doppler signals. Linear and curvilinear probes, in addition to phased-array transducers, are helpful for vascular and fetal studies, respectively.

The waiting and examination rooms should be nonthreatening, comfortable, and spacious (Fig. 2.1). Several family members often accompany patients with congenital heart defects to their appointments. It is best to include the family in the examination, avoiding issues of separation anxiety in both the children and their parents. The examination room should be kept at a comfortable temperature, remembering that the patient will be partially undressed for the study. Providing entertainment/distractions, both in the waiting room and during the examination, is extremely helpful in achieving a complete examination of complex cardiac malformations. Television monitors or digital video players can be strategically positioned so that the patient can be watching a movie of his or her choice while the echocardiographic data are being obtained. We have found that patient cooperation and comfort are enhanced by having the person who is to perform the initial examination meet the patient/family in the waiting area, assist them with choosing music or a video to play during the test, and then escort them to the examination room.

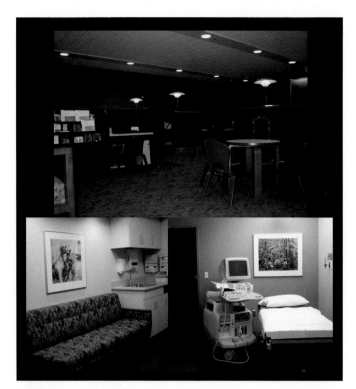

FIGURE 2.1. A congenital echocardiographic laboratory can accommodate the needs of a wide variety of patients. Top: A waiting area with space for families and activities for all ages. Bottom: One way of arranging an echocardiographic examination room to meet both the medical needs of the patient and the needs of the patient's family members. Examination rooms in the congenital suite must be somewhat larger than those found in a standard adult laboratory. Comfortable seating for accompanying family members, a child-friendly environment, and videos for distraction during the examination make an otherwise intimidating process less threatening. The ultimate purpose, of course, is to improve the information obtained during the echocardiographic examination.

In the very young patient (about 2 months to 2 years of age) or for more invasive procedures (such as transesophageal echocardiography), even these measures may not be enough to relieve the patient's anxiety. In these situations, it is appropriate to consider the use of conscious sedation or even monitored anesthesia care. Complete guidelines for use of conscious sedation have been provided by the American Academy of Pediatrics. The method of sedation should be chosen such that both patient safety and the quality of the examination are maximized. Common sense suggests and the Academy guidelines require that, regardless of the agent(s) used, a practitioner who is not involved in the procedure be present and responsible for monitoring the patient's well-being and vital signs while sedated. Pulse oximetry, in addition to heart rate, rhythm, and blood pressure, are mandatory components of monitoring when using sedative agents. Additional information regarding equipment and training necessary for conscious sedation can be found in the American Academy of Pediatrics guideline document (see Suggested Reading).

Transesophageal echocardiography in pediatric patients will often require deep sedation or general anesthesia. Some teenage patients may be mature enough to allow a transesophageal examination using standard conscious sedation. The choice of sedation protocol must be tailored to the patient, the reason for the examination, and the availability of appropriate personnel and anesthesia equipment. A complete discussion of the training required for and the practical aspects of performing transesophageal echocardiography can be found later in this book and in *The Echo Manual*.[2]

Echocardiographic examinations have become indispensible in several hospital settings. Intraoperative echocardiography is now an integral part of surgical care. Intensive care unit patients often benefit from hemodynamic evaluations provided by a detailed echocardiogram. However, these environments are not the quiet controlled spaces that we are accustomed to in the echocardiographic laboratory. Once the examiner is at the bedside or in the operating room,

he or she must be certain to not interfere with the other cares being provided. Hand and probe hygiene must be meticulous, and use of sterile, ultrasound transparent, barriers should be considered in the postsurgical suite, when scans near surgical wounds are required. One advantage of the bedside examination is that the continuous hemodynamic monitoring available often makes hemodynamic conclusions even more accurate. Certainly, measured central venous or arterial pressures are superior to an assumed atrial pressure or a cuff-determined blood pressure. In most cases, the challenges associated with inpatient, bedside examinations are easily overcome with patience and communication with the bedside staff.

 ## IMAGE ACQUISITION

Image acquisition should be gated and synchronized with the electrocardiogram. When cardiac rhythms are irregular or when performing fetal examinations, digital clips of specified times can be used. The length of the digital clip should be determined by the patient's heart rate and the information being recorded. For standard images, we prefer a clip that includes three cardiac cycles. Although a three-cycle clip requires more storage space than a single beat, the longer clip usually results in more satisfactory playback and less "stitch artifact" as the recording loops from the final to the initial frame. When acquiring sweeps (to display spatial relationships of one structure to another), a longer acquisition is more effective (6 to 10 beats, or 5 seconds). These longer clips are especially helpful when searching for intricately subtle defects or demonstrating the relationships of the supracardiac great vessels.

In general, the examination of children and patients with congenital heart disease follows a relatively set pattern. All patients must have a determination of blood pressure at least once during the examination. In uncooperative patients, this may occur after the images are acquired to avoid further aggravating the child. A continuous, single-lead electrocardiogram is recorded and displayed simultaneously with the ultrasound image. The electrocardiogram is a mandatory part of the complete examination; without it, accurate timing of the cardiac events visualized is not possible.

At each transducer position, the examination should initially focus on a clear demonstration of the two-dimensional anatomy. Images should be recorded in the classic planes (see image orientation section later in this chapter). However, the examination is not complete unless the scans include all of the areas visible from each transducer position, even those that do not conform to standard imaging planes. For example, when scanning in a sagittal plane, one must sweep the beam as far to the right and left as the acoustic window will allow. Once the examiner is familiar with the structures seen from that transducer position, more focused anatomic scans of abnormal areas, color and spectral Doppler recordings, and three-dimensional acquisitions can be performed. At the conclusion of the echocardiographer's examination, the images should be reviewed, ideally by both the echocardiographer and the reviewing physician, to ensure completeness. If immediate physician review is not possible, the images should still be reviewed by the examiner to ensure that the recording accurately displays all of the information that was acquired. When this initial review reveals missing or poorly displayed information, additional images can be obtained while the patient is still in the laboratory.

The order in which images are recorded should be standardized, but the precise sequence is determined by local preferences and patient behavior. When dealing with a cooperative patient, we prefer to begin with the subcostal position. In neonates and young infants, this window will often provide visualization of nearly the entire cardiovascular system. More anterior and superior structures can be difficult to assess from the subcostal window in older patients. In these cases, images from the subcostal position will focus primarily on the inferior and superior venae cavae, the atrial septum, and the ventricular chambers themselves. An effort to visualize the pulmonary venous connections should also be made from this position. This will be more successful in younger patients, but a surprising number of mature patients can be extensively evaluated from this transducer position.

Once all of the information available from the subcostal window has been obtained, our attention usually shifts to the anterior chest wall. Initial scans are oriented in the sagittal (long-axis) plane. The initial focus is on the left ventricular inflow and outflow tracts, noting the size and position of each chamber and the valves and their relationships to one another. The plane of sound is then oriented toward the right ventricular inflow tract, demonstrating the inferior vena cava–right atrial junction, right atrium and its appendage, and the tricuspid valve. The right ventricular inflow view often allows an advantageous alignment with tricuspid regurgitant flow.

Parasternal sagittal scanning is followed by horizontal sweeps (short-axis scans) in the same area. Doppler evaluation of the right ventricular outflow tract and pulmonary arteries is often optimal from these positions. Images obtained from this window have been used to define many of our normal quantitative values related to atrial and annular dimensions, as well as left ventricular cavity diameters and wall thickness. Coronary arterial anomalies are best detected using horizontal plane scans near the base of the heart. Definition of the ventricular septum and exclusion of ventricular septal defects (VSDs) require focused color flow Doppler examinations in this area. These can be recorded as sweeps, or as a sequence of adjacent clips, flowing from the cardiac base to its apex or vice versa. The relationships of the great arteries (particularly the pulmonary vessels and the aorta) are best displayed in high parasternal short-axis image sweeps.

The right parasternal border should also be interrogated in a similar fashion. If the patient lies on his or her right side, images from this window are often improved. The superior and inferior venae cavae, right atrium, atrial septum, and pulmonary veins can be visualized in many patients from this transducer position. Image quality at the right parasternal border is more variable between patients than the other standard transducer positions. However, when the right heart is enlarged, this area often provides images of surprisingly high quality.

Our attention then shifts to the cardiac apex. Coronal images (four-chamber views) are usually obtained first. Size, position, and relationships of the atria, atrioventricular (AV) valves, and ventricles are documented. Volumetric assessments, whether derived from two-dimensional or three-dimensional scans, of ventricles are performed. Many spectral Doppler recordings are made from the apical window because beam alignment is optimal for the right and left ventricular inflow tracts, the pulmonary veins, and the left ventricular outflow tract. Sagittal plane images (apical long-axis and two-chamber views) are the next to receive attention. These scans provide anatomic and Doppler data related to the left ventricular inflow and outflow tracts.

Finally, the transducer is positioned at or near the suprasternal notch. This position is often saved until the end of the examination, because most children are somewhat threatened by the slight pressure on their necks required to image here. Taking a moment to prepare the child, by describing what is about to happen, is time well spent in most cases. Images from the suprasternal notch usually begin with a sagittal orientation. However, combinations of sagittal and coronal plane scans are required to clearly define the right–left relationships of the great vessels. The aortic arch, its arterial branching pattern, and sidedness should be determined. Superior systemic veins, pulmonary arteries, left atrium, and pulmonary venous structures can also be seen, even in most adults, from these positions. Doppler interrogation of the descending aorta is often optimal from this position. However, two-dimensional determinations of descending aortic diameters should not be performed from the suprasternal notch. From the notch, the plane of sound is parallel with the aortic walls. We prefer high left parasternal images (the ductal/coarctation view; Fig. 2.2) for determination of upper descending aortic size.

Although these standard acoustic windows are used in all patients, there are many other possible transducer positions that provide views of the cardiovascular system.

Oblique or hybrid transducer positions can often be found if one searches for them. These windows can be particularly helpful in postoperative patients, whose acoustic characteristics are often altered by their surgical procedures.

The examination sequence just described applies to comprehensive transthoracic echocardiography. A transesophageal examination should also follow an organized pattern. In the operating room with an anesthetized patient, it is often helpful to begin the examination from the transgastric transducer position. Coronal plane images allow definition of right- and left-sided structures and provide spatial orientation for the rest of the examination. The transducer can then be slowly withdrawn to the distal, mid-, and proximal esophageal positions to complete the examination. Two- and three-dimensional scans, color Doppler interrogation, and spectral Doppler flow maps should be obtained at all levels. When a patient is not anesthetized but is sedated and responsive, the examination must be modified. After esophageal intubation, it is often advisable to begin the examination at the distal esophagus. While imaging in this position, the cardiologist can also assess the level and adequacy of sedation before advancing the probe into the stomach.

The echocardiographic examination of the fetus has many unique characteristics. One is that an organized sequence of imaging is often impossible. Due to fetal motion, the examiner should obtain the most advantageous images available at the time. All of the same information should be obtained during fetal examinations. However, the order in which the tasks are accomplished cannot be standardized.

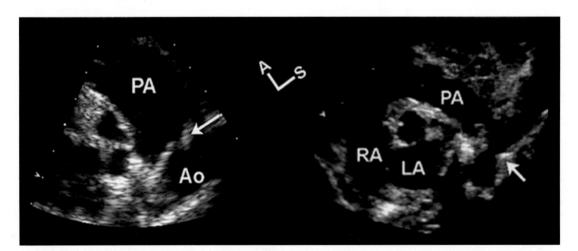

FIGURE 2.2. The ductal/coarctation view. These two echocardiographic images were obtained from an oblique high left parasternal transducer position. The plane of sound was moved toward the patient's left shoulder and was rotated clockwise from the parasternal long-axis view to visualize these structures. **Left:** The distal main pulmonary artery (PA), ductus (*arrow*), and upper descending aorta (Ao). **Right:** Same area but in a patient with coarctation of the aorta (*arrow*). This view is not only an excellent position for interrogation of ductal flows but also the best plane for evaluating the size of the upper descending aorta. The luminal narrowing associated with coarctation is clearly defined because the plane of sound is perpendicular to the vessels walls in this position (**right**). This view should also be used to define the size of the upper descending aorta in patients with connective tissue disorders, such as Marfan syndrome. A, anterior; LA, left atrium; RA, right atrium; S, superior.

THE ECHOCARDIOGRAPHIC REPORT

The echocardiographic report requires careful construction. The reports must convey all of the pertinent information to the referring physician in an efficient, yet understandable manner. It is usually preferable to organize a report into sections. These sections would include (a) patient demographics, biometrics, and vital signs, (b) a section summarizing the most important positive and pertinent negative diagnoses/findings, (c) a section describing all of the normal or noncontributory findings documented by the examination, (d) a section detailing the quantitative measurements made during the imaging and Doppler components of the examination, and (e) a section that directly compares current with historical quantitative data pertinent to the patient's primary diagnosis. We refer to this last section as the "serial summary." Not all measurements are included in this area. For example, a serial summary related to aortic valvar stenosis would include a table summarizing historical values for and trends in aortic annulus diameter, left ventricular size, wall thickness, Doppler velocities and gradients, cardiac index, and valve areas.

As mentioned earlier, the report should be directly linked to the digital echocardiographic images, so that the surgeon and/or referring physician can simultaneously review both the report and the images that generated it.

 ## IMAGE ORIENTATION AND NOMENCLATURE IN CONGENITAL HEART DISEASE

A standardized method of assessment is necessary if one is to obtain a complete understanding of even the most straightforward congenital cardiac malformations. In the setting of very complicated cardiovascular anomalies, it becomes essential. The first step in this evaluation is to consistently present echocardiographic images of the anomaly in a straightforward and reproducible way. The American Society of Echocardiography's Pediatric Council has defined a method for "preferred" image orientation in studies involving congenital heart disease.[1]

We will base the remainder of this chapter on these tomographic imaging conventions. These guidelines result in echocardiographic images that are displayed in an anatomic format. Sagittal plane images are displayed with superior structures to the viewer's right and anterior structures at the top of the video screen (Fig. 2.3). Thus, we view these images as if we are looking through the heart from the left side toward the right of a supine patient (Fig. 2.4). Horizontal plane images are displayed with anterior structures at the top of the video screen and left-sided structures to the viewer's right (Fig. 2.5). These views simulate examining the heart of the supine patient from below, looking toward the head (Fig. 2.4). Coronal plane images, such as the apical

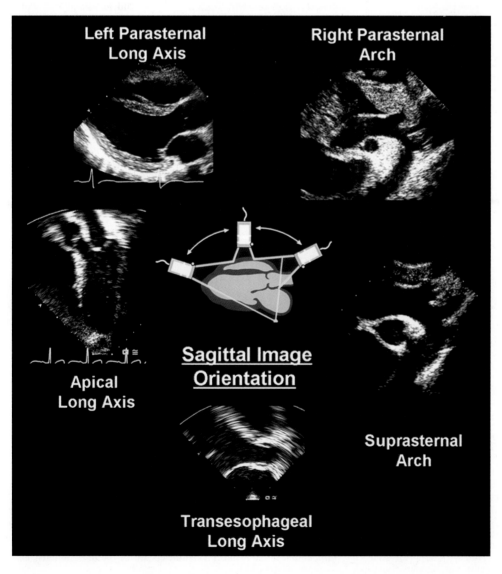

FIGURE 2.3. Standard image orientations used when scanning in sagittal planes. The left ventricular long-axis images (**top left** and **bottom**) are shown as if the patient were supine. Images obtained from the cardiac apex (**middle left**), suprasternal notch (**middle right**), or high parasternal (**top right**) positions are oriented as if the patient was standing. These choices are made based on the fact that the two-dimensional image cannot be rotated. Therefore, the orientation that most closely approximates one of the standardized views described in Figure 2.4 is used. The paired images (right parasternal/suprasternal and left parasternal/transesophageal) demonstrate the fact that practitioners strive to display anatomy in a consistent manner, even when the image is obtained from a different acoustic window. This consistency helps avoid confusion when dealing with complex spatial relationships and anomalies of cardiac position and simplifies the use of echocardiographic data by nonechocardiographic medical providers.

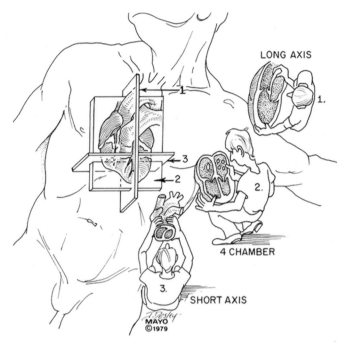

FIGURE 2.4. Convention used to orient echocardiographic images. This is the same convention applied in all forms of tomographic imaging. The examiner in the diagram is observing the patient/echocardiographic images as if the patient were either lying in a supine position (positions 1 and 3) or standing in front of the examiner (position 2). Position 1 corresponds to images taken in sagittal planes. The examiner is looking at the patient/image from the patient's left side. Because the patient is supine, anterior structures will be "up," and superior structures will be to the observer's right. Position 2 corresponds to coronal images. Here, the images displayed as if the patient were standing upright, facing the examiner. Therefore, superior structures will now be "up," and left-sided structures will be seen to the observer's right. Position 3 represents horizontal plane scanning. Again, the images displayed as if the patient were supine, but now the examiner is looking at the heart from below, as if standing at the foot of the bed. This results in an image orientation with anterior structures at the top of the video screen, while left-sided structures are again shown to the examiner's right.

four-chamber view (Fig. 2.6), and the suprasternal view of the pulmonary venous confluence ("crab-view," Fig. 2.7) are displayed with superior structures at the top of the video screen and left-sided structures to the viewer's right. These views simulate looking through the front of the heart toward the patient's back (Fig. 2.4). The common theme among all of these orientations is that the anatomy is displayed in a classic anatomic format, as if the patient was in front of and facing the examiner in either an upright or a supine position.

The figures and text that follow will familiarize the reader with this approach. We believe that it is best to use this system of image orientation regardless of the method used to create the image. In other words, the same anatomic features should be displayed in the same orientation whether the images are a part of a transthoracic, transesophageal, or intracardiac ultrasound examination (Figs. 2.3, 2.5, and 2.6). Occasionally, complete consistency is not possible. This is due to the fact that most two-dimensional image displays can only be "flipped" top to bottom and/or left to right. The best examples of situations requiring more than one orientation are the sagittal views. Parasternal sagittal images follow the convention and display superior structures to the examiner's right and anterior anatomy at the top of the video screen. Subcostal, right parasternal, and suprasternal sagittal images cannot be shown as if the patient was supine. Therefore, we opt to display the image as if the patient was standing, similar to the coronal image convention, with superior structures at the top and anterior to the viewer's left. For many images, like the four-chamber (Fig. 2.6) and the aortic arch (Fig. 2.8), this creates no inconsistency, because these images are not available in the parasternal window. However, the subcostal, suprasternal notch, right parasternal, and esophageal transducer positions all provide images of the venae cavae, atria, and atrial septum the "bicaval" views (Fig. 2.9). These are parasagittal images and, according to the convention, they should be displayed with superior structures to the examiner's right and anterior anatomy at the top

of the video screen. Esophageal bicaval views conform to this convention (bottom, Fig. 2.9). However, the angle of the interrogating plane of sound from the right parasternal, subcostal, and suprasternal positions is such that the image becomes tilted (top, Fig. 2.9). The subcostal images are often displayed with superior structures "closest" to the top of the screen (top left, Fig. 2.9). Mid-right parasternal images are shown with the anterior surface toward the top of the screen. The display of high-right parasternal (top right, Fig. 2.9) and suprasternal images requires a hybrid approach, with the apex of the sector representing a transition point from anterior to superior orientations.

There are two primary advantages to using the image orientations just described.

First, use of the apex down orientations maintains a relatively consistent approach to the display of anatomy imaged in the sagittal, horizontal, and coronal planes, regardless of where the transducer is positioned (Figs. 2.3, 2.5, and 2.6). Therefore, it becomes easier to determine and to understand the appropriate image orientations for nonstandard views. For example, coronal images taken from the cardiac apex in patients with dextrocardia (still a coronal apical four-chamber view) should be displayed with the apex down and left-sided structures to the right. Such consistency of presentation is vital to understanding the complex anatomy found in some patients with congenital heart disease.

Second, nonechocardiographers (surgeons, nonimaging cardiologists) have difficulty understanding anatomy when it is displayed in a nonanatomic format. The widely used "apex up" format simulates the anatomy of a patient who is standing on his or her head and facing away from the examiner. Therefore, apex down imaging not only displays echocardiographic data in a more anatomic format, but also allows echocardiographers to communicate more effectively with their colleagues.

A last word about image orientation: The consistent approach described for the orientation of transthoracic images should also be applied to images obtained using other echo technology (transesophageal or intravascular). A simple way to achieve this while performing transesophageal echocardiography is to display all images (except the four-chamber view) with the "point" of the sector at the bottom of the video screen. This requires inverting the electronic image. Images that are recorded in this way will automatically display posterior structures (those close to the esophagus) at the bottom of the screen and place anterior structures at the top. The only exception to this rule is the esophageal four-chamber view. Here, one would want to leave the apex at the bottom of the image to maintain a consistent anatomic orientation. This would require the examiner to invert the image, placing the sector's apex (and the atria) at the top of the screen.

NOMENCLATURE OF CONGENITAL HEART DISEASE

One of the areas of recent controversy in congenital cardiology concerns the language used to describe the anatomy of the heart and great vessels. Some cardiac morphologists and physicians, led by Professor Robert Anderson, have adopted language that uses English terms instead of the more classic Latin nomenclature. Unfortunately, this can create a great deal of confusion for those attempting to understand congenital heart disease. What follows is an attempt to define the terms used to describe congenital heart disease using the standard, Latin terms and the more recently proposed, but already widely adopted, Anglicized language.

Situs or Sidedness

This concept applies to structures/organ systems that are not bilaterally symmetric. It describes the position of the organs in the system and usually has three possible arrangements: normal or solitus, inverted or inversus (mirror image of normal), and ambiguous (something else).

Visceral situs or sidedness

- *Solitus,* or *normal:* Liver and cecum to the right, stomach and spleen to the left.
- *Inversus,* or *inverted:* Liver and cecum to the left, stomach and spleen to the right.

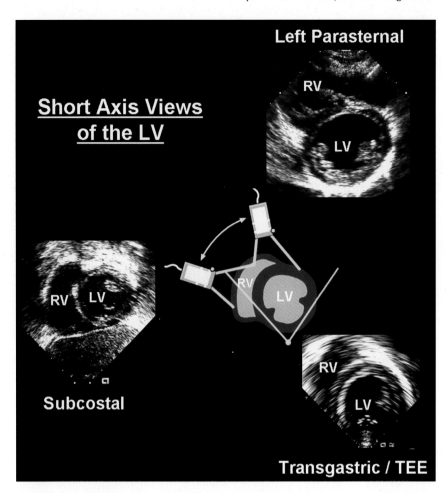

Short Axis Views of the LV

Left Parasternal

RV

LV

RV LV

Subcostal

RV

LV

Transgastric / TEE

FIGURE 2.5. **Short-axis images of the right and left ventricles and the central diagram illustrate a consistent approach to image orientation in the horizontal plane.** The three echocardiographic images shown here were obtained in very different ways. The transducer was placed on the anterior chest wall near the left border of the sternum to obtain the first image (**top right**). In contrast, the transducer was placed on the upper abdomen, below the xyphoid, to obtain the subcostal image (**bottom left**). The transesophageal echocardiographic probe was advanced into the stomach and the plane of sound was angled back across the diaphragm to produce the transgastric image (**bottom right**). Despite the variety of maneuvers and transducer positions, the images produced can easily be seen to demonstrate the same anatomic structures. LV, left ventricle; RV, right ventricle; TEE, transesophageal echocardiogram.

- *Ambiguous:* Any other patterns—frequently the liver is bilateral and there is intestinal malrotation; gastric position is variable (the spleen, when present, is always posterior to the stomach).

Atrial situs or sidedness: Also referred to as cardiac situs or sidedness. It is determined by the position of the morphologic right and left atria.

- *Solitus,* or *normal:* Morphologic left atrium is posterior and to the left of right atrium.
- *Inversus,* or *inverted:* Morphologic left atrium is posterior and to the right of right atrium.
- *Ambiguous:* Confident assignment of morphologic left and right atria cannot be made, usually in common atrium.

Cardiac position (top, Fig. 2.10): This represents the gross position of "most" of the heart relative to the midline.

- *Levoposition:* Most of the cardiac mass is to the left of midline.
- *Dextroposition:* Most of the cardiac mass is the right of midline.
- *Mesoposition:* The heart is evenly distributed around the midline.

Cardiac orientation (Fig. 2.10, lower panel): This represents the orientation of the base to apex axis of the heart, not its position within the mediastinum (although the two usually go together).

- *Levocardia:* Base-to-apex axis is "pointed" from upper right to lower left.
- *Dextrocardia:* Base-to-apex axis is "pointed" from the upper left to the lower right.
- *Mesocardia:* Base-to-apex axis is "pointed" nearly directly from superior to inferior and usually is in the midline.

The distinction between orientation and position is usually not important because they tend to go together. In other words, levopositioned hearts usually also have a leftward base-to-apex axis (levocardia). However, when other pathology (diaphragmatic hernia or unilateral lung hypoplasia) causes a shift in cardiac position; the difference

between position and orientation can become significant. For example, most infants with left-sided diaphragmatic hernias have levocardia with dextroposition because the hernia has "pushed" a normal heart into the right chest.

Assessment of cardiac location is most efficiently performed using coronal plane imaging (four-chamber view) from the subcostal window. Figure 2.11 provides an example of the maneuver used to determine cardiac position and axis in a normal patient. The scan begins with a midline horizontal plane image of the upper abdomen (left, Fig. 2.11). The plane of sound is maintained in the midline and angled superiorly (across the diaphragm) to a coronal view of the heart, usually in a four-chamber orientation (middle, Fig. 2.11). Once the axis and position of the heart have been determined, the image is re-formated into a standard anatomic orientation (right, Fig. 2.11). Figure 2.12 illustrates the same sweep from a patient with osteogenic sarcoma, in whom the tumor has shifted the heart into the right hemithorax. Despite the abnormal position, it is clear that the base-to-apex axis is still slightly oriented to the left, resulting in a case of dextroposition with levocardia.

TERMS USED TO DESCRIBE CARDIOVASCULAR SEGMENTS AND CONNECTIONS

Segment: Section of the cardiovascular system (i.e., great veins or the ventricles).
Connections: Junction between two cardiovascular segments.
Overriding: Function of a valve annulus and a VSD. The term describes an annulus that crosses the plane of a VSD and is therefore "over" more than one ventricle. Any of the cardiac valves can potentially be described as overriding.

FIGURE 2.6. "Four-chamber" images and the central diagram illustrate a consistent approach to image orientation in the coronal plane. The three echocardiographic images shown here were obtained in very different ways. The transducer was placed at the cardiac apex, near the left anterior axillary line, to obtain the first image (**bottom right**). In contrast, the transducer was placed on the upper abdomen, below the xyphoid, to obtain the subcostal image (**bottom left**). The transesophageal echocardiographic probe was placed in the distal esophagus and the plane of sound entered the heart from behind to produce the last image (**top left**). Despite the variety of maneuvers and transducer positions, the images produced can easily be seen to demonstrate the same anatomic structures. TEE, transesophageal echocardiogram.

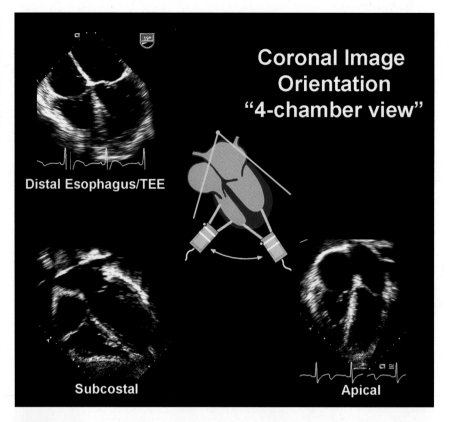

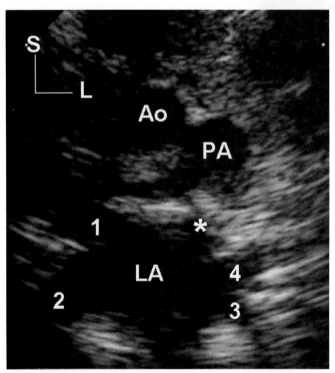

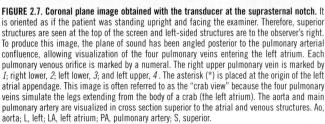

FIGURE 2.7. Coronal plane image obtained with the transducer at the suprasternal notch. It is oriented as if the patient was standing upright and facing the examiner. Therefore, superior structures are seen at the top of the screen and left-sided structures are to the observer's right. To produce this image, the plane of sound has been angled posterior to the pulmonary arterial confluence, allowing visualization of the four pulmonary veins entering the left atrium. Each pulmonary venous orifice is marked by a numeral. The right upper pulmonary vein is marked by *1*; right lower, *2*; left lower, *3*; and left upper, *4*. The asterisk (*) is placed at the origin of the left atrial appendage. This image is often referred to as the "crab view" because the four pulmonary veins simulate the legs extending from the body of a crab (the left atrium). The aorta and main pulmonary artery are visualized in cross section superior to the atrial and venous structures. Ao, aorta; L, left; LA, left atrium; PA, pulmonary artery; S, superior.

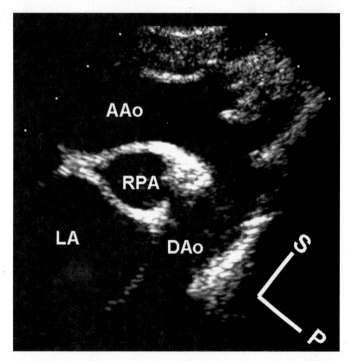

FIGURE 2.8. Sagittal plane image obtained with the transducer at the suprasternal notch. The plane of sound cannot be directed in a completely superior-interior direction from this position. However, because the plane of interrogation is closer to the body's superior-inferior axis than it is to an anterior-posterior plane, the image is oriented as if the patient was standing "nearly" upright with the examiner to the patient's left. Although the image is slightly tilted, superior structures are seen toward the top of the screen and anterior structures are toward the observer's right. In reality, the apex of the sector represents the transition point between superior structures (**top right**) and anterior structures (**top left**). To produce this image, the plane of sound has been angled to the left, allowing visualization of the aortic arch and its brachiocephalic arterial branches. AAo, ascending aorta; DAo, descending aorta; LA, left atrium; P, posterior; RPA, right pulmonary artery; S, superior.

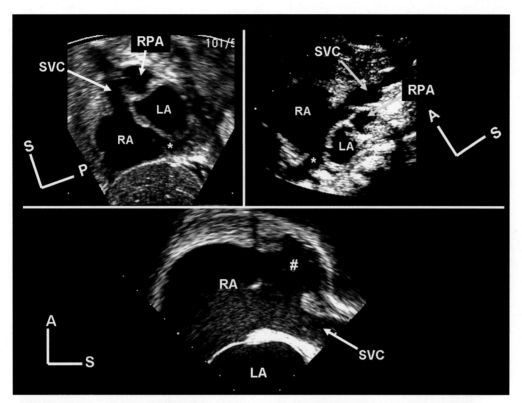

FIGURE 2.9. "Bicaval" views. These three images demonstrate similar anatomy. All are sagittal plane images focused on the atrial septum and the junctions of the superior and inferior venae cavae with the right atrium. **Top left:** The image was obtained from the subcostal transducer position. The plane of sound enters the body along a path a slight angle to the true inferior-superior axis. **Top right:** Similarly, the plane of sound that created this high right parasternal image traveled through the thorax at an angle to both the true superior-inferior and the anterior-posterior planes. The subcostal image achieves a nearly vertical orientation and therefore is displayed as if the patient were upright. The more oblique nature of the right parasternal image requires use of a hybrid of the two acceptable orientations for sagittal images. The apex of the sector represents the transition point between superior structures **(top right)** and anterior structures **(top left)**. The asterisk (*) in the two top panels is positioned at the junction of the inferior vena cava and right atrium. The esophageal bicaval view **(bottom)** represents the ideal orientation for a sagittal image. The interrogating plane of sound crosses the chest in a nearly direct posterior-anterior route. It has been angled slightly to the right to produce this image. Anterior structures are at the top of the viewing screen and superior structures are seen to the observer's right. Note: The thicker superior limbus of the atrial septum (seen clearly in the **top left** and **bottom**) will always be associated with the morphologically right atrium. The thinner, more inferior-posterior, component of the atrial septum (valve of the fossa ovalis) is a reliable marker for the position of the morphologically left atrium. **Bottom:** Position of the right atrial appendage (#). A, anterior; LA, left atrium; P, posterior; RA, right atrium; RPA, right pulmonary artery; S, superior; SVC, superior vena cava.

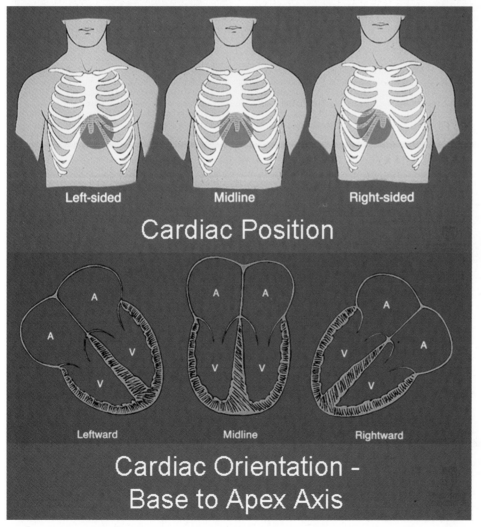

FIGURE 2.10. Difference between the concepts of cardiac position and cardiac orientation. Cardiac position is determined only by the overall location of the heart relative to the anatomic midline **(top)**. It has no relationship to the internal organization of the cardiac structures. If the majority of the heart is to the left, then the heart is in levo-position. Conversely, if most of the heart is to the right of midline, then we refer to the patient as having dextro-position. When the heart is located centrally in the chest, the patient is said to have meso- or midline position. Determination of cardiac orientation requires knowledge of the internal arrangement of the heart. Orientation refers to the right-left direction of the so-called base-to-apex axis. The apex of heart is the ventricular apex, and the base is at the great arterial origin(s). The normal base-to-apex axis is directed inferiorly and to the left **(bottom right)**. This orientation is referred to as levocardia. When the heart is vertically oriented and in the midline, the apex is directly inferior to the base. This situation is illustrated by the central diagram in the bottom panel and is referred to as mesocardia. The diagram on the bottom right illustrates the concept of dextrocardia. In this situation, the cardiac apex is inferior and to the right relative to the base. Clinically, most patients will have concordant cardiac positions and orientations. In other words, hearts with levoposition will also display a leftward base-to-apex axis (levocardia). However, extracardiac processes can shift the cardiac position resulting in discrepancies between position and orientation.

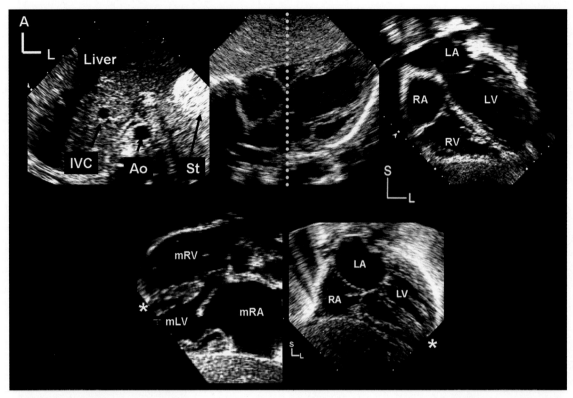

FIGURE 2.11. Normal cardiac orientation and axis. This series of images were obtained from the same patient and demonstrate the determination of cardiac position and axis. **Left:** This image is a subcostal horizontal plane view of the upper abdomen. The apex of the sector is positioned in the midline. The liver and inferior vena cava (IVC) are seen on the patient's right. The aorta (Ao) and stomach (St) are to the patient's left. **Middle:** This image was obtained by angling the interrogating plane of sound superiorly into the chest. The apex of the sector was maintained in the midline (*dashed yellow line*). Most of the cardiac structures are to the left of the patient's midline, including the cardiac (ventricular) apex. This confirms the presence of both levoposition and levocardia. The apex-up image **(middle)** is used only to confirm cardiac position and axis. Once this determination is complete, we can reorient the image into the more anatomic format **(right)**. The two echocardiographic images **(bottom)** illustrate the different appearances of levocardia **(right)** and dextrocardia **(left)** when associated with congenital heart disease. Both images were obtained from the subcostal transducer position and demonstrate four-chamber coronal views. **Left:** This image was taken during examination of the patient with atrioventricular discordance, ventricular septal defect, and pulmonary stenosis. The majority of the heart is to the right of the midline. Chamber enlargement has rotated this heart into a nearly horizontal orientation. The apex (*) is clearly to the right of the base, consistent with dextrocardia. **Right:** This image was taken from an examination of a patient with tricuspid valve atresia. In this case, both cardiac orientation and position are normal (leftward). The cardiac apex (*) is to the left and inferior to the cardiac base, consistent with levocardia. A, anterior; L, left; LA, left atrium; LV, left ventricle; mLV, morphologically left ventricle; mRA, morphologically right atrium; mRV, morphologically right ventricle; RA, right atrium; RV, right ventricle; S, superior.

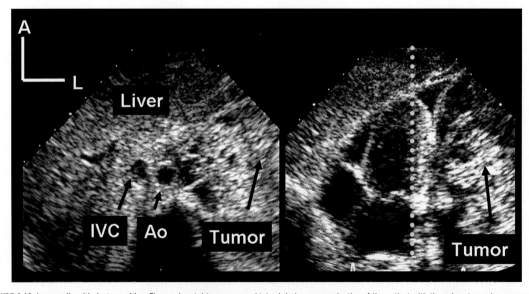

FIGURE 2.12. Levocardia with dextroposition. These subcostal images were obtained during an examination of the patient with thoracic osteogenic sarcoma. The tumor is visualized above the diaphragm in both images. **Left:** Normal spatial arrangement of the organs in the upper abdomen. The stomach is not as apparent as usual due to the presence of the tumor near the left diaphragm. The abdominal aorta (Ao) has been shifted slightly to the right but is still generally recognizable as a left-sided structure. As the plane of sound is swept superiorly to reveal the heart **(right)**, it is obvious that the majority of the cardiac chambers lie to the right of the midline (yellow dashed line). This represents a situation in which there is dextroposition due to an extracardiac mass occupying most of the left hemithorax. The cardiac base-to-apex axis remains slightly leftward, despite the positional shift that has occurred. A, anterior; IVC, in inferior vena cava; L, left.

Straddling: Function of the chordae tendineae of an AV valve and a VSD. The term describes chordae that cross a VSD and have their myocardial attachments within the opposite ventricle. This can create difficulties for the surgeon trying to close a VSD. An AV valve can both straddle and override, but a semilunar valve cannot straddle because it does not have chordae.

Concordant: This refers to a normal connection between segments. For example, when the right atrium connects to the right ventricle, the connection is described as concordant.

Discordant: This refers to the opposite of the normal connection. For example, when the left ventricle connects to the pulmonary artery, the connection is discordant.

Univentricular: A special form of AV connection in which all atria are committed to only one functional ventricle.

Transposition: The prefix *trans-* means "across," in this case "across the septum." Therefore, transposition refers to the semilunar valves only and occurs when the great arteries (and therefore the semilunar valves) are on the opposite side of the ventricular septum relative to normal (aorta on the morphologically right ventricular side of the septum and pulmonary artery on the morphologically left ventricular side).

Malposition: This term also refers to the semilunar valves and great arteries. It is applied to any position/connection of the great arteries to the ventricles that is not normal and not transposition. For example, the great arteries are always malpositioned in double-outlet right ventricle, and the term "transposition" should never be applied to a double-outlet right ventricle because the great arteries are on the same side of the septum (not "across" it).

Some Synonyms

Superior vena cava = superior caval vein
Inferior vena cava = inferior caval vein
Foramen ovale = fossa ovalis = oval fossa
Endocardial cushion defect = AV canal defect = AV septal defect
Truncus arteriosus = persistent truncal artery
Ductus arteriosus = ductal artery

SEQUENTIAL SEGMENTAL ANALYSIS OF CARDIOVASCULAR ANATOMY AND CONGENITAL CARDIAC MALFORMATIONS

One of the more intimidating aspects of congenital heart disease is the large number and broad spectrum of anomalies that can be found in a single patient. As a result, congenital cardiologists have developed a standardized approach to the description of cardiovascular anatomy and pathology. This process has been called the "sequential segmental approach" to congenital heart disease. Simply described, this approach divides the patient's cardiovascular system into a sequence of individual segments and the connections between those segments (Fig. 2.13). One then describes the position, anatomy, and function of all the structures within each segment, as well as the connections between the segments. Using this approach, one can be confident that a complete assessment has been obtained even in the most unusual cases. In the setting of very complicated anomalies, this type of rigorous and organized approach becomes essential. This is not to say that every echocardiographic examination follows the sequence of the segmental approach. Image acquisition still follows the pattern described earlier in this chapter. Segmental analysis is not a physical action but rather a thought process that provides the congenital echocardiographer with a checklist or framework for categorizing any cardiovascular malformation.

DETERMINATION OF CARDIAC LOCATION AND SITUS (SIDEDNESS)

Before specifically describing the structures that are found within the cardiovascular segments, the general positions of the major thoracic and abdominal organ systems must be defined. In congenital cardiology, one must specifically describe the position and orientation of the

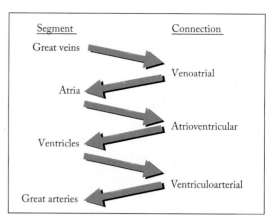

FIGURE 2.13. Sequential segmental analysis of cardiovascular anatomy.

heart within the chest and the positions of the two major organ groups that affect the location of cardiovascular structures. These organ groups are (a) the abdominal viscera and (b) the atria. Each of these organ groups has an asymmetric arrangement of their structures and therefore can be described as having situs (or sidedness). In other words, the right half of the organ group is not the same as the left. The nomenclature describing these asymmetric organ groups, cardiac position, and orientation was described in the preceding section.

Abdominal Situs

The echocardiographic assessment of abdominal (or visceral) situs focuses on the positions of the liver, stomach, spleen and abdominal great vessels, aorta, and inferior vena cava. Horizontal plane images of the upper abdomen are most useful for most of this assessment, although the spleen is more easily seen from the flank (lateral and posterior to the stomach). Examples of three common abdominal patterns are shown in Figure 2.14. When the liver and inferior vena cava are to the right and the stomach, spleen, and abdominal aorta are to the left, the patient has abdominal situs solitus. Abdominal situs inversus is just the opposite, with the stomach, spleen, and aorta to the right and liver and inferior vena cava to the left. There are several recognized forms of abdominal situs ambiguous. The most common ambiguous pattern is seen in the asplenia syndrome. There is a large midline liver. The inferior vena cava and aorta are located on the same side of the spine (can be right or left). Stomach position is variable and the spleen is absent. In this setting, some of the hepatic veins may connect directly to the atrium instead of entering the inferior vena cava. These independently connecting veins are important to identify because they need to be incorporated into the systemic venous pathway of a modified Fontan procedure.

Atrial Situs

Atrial situs, sometimes referred to as cardiac situs, refers to the arrangement of the atria. In atrial situs solitus, the morphologically right atrium is located anterior and to the right of the morphologically left atrium. Atrial situs inversus results in the morphologically right atrium being to the left of (but still slightly anterior to) the morphologically left atrium. True atrial situs ambiguous is rare. When present, it is usually associated with a large common atrium in which there are no clear differences between the right and left portions of the atrium. This is most often seen in patients with asplenia, and the two halves of the common atrium both tend to resemble a morphologically right atrium.

To distinguish a morphologically right from a morphologically left atrium, a variety of anatomic landmarks can be used. The most reliable is the anatomy of the atrial septum (Fig. 2.15). The thicker limbus of the foramen ovale is always located on the same side of the septum as the morphologically right atrium. Conversely, the thin valve of the foramen ovale is always on the same side as the morphologically left atrium. This information can be most clearly visualized in subcostal, right parasternal, or esophageal images of the atrial septum (Fig. 2.16).

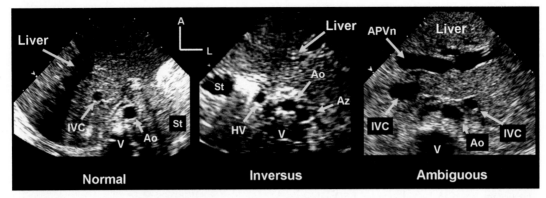

FIGURE 2.14. Different spatial arrangements of the upper abdominal viscera. Left: Normal anatomy. The central image was taken during examination of the patient with the polysplenia syndrome and shows an arrangement of the abdominal organs that is the mirror image of normal. The liver, abdominal aorta (Ao), and azygous vein (Az) are all found to the patient's left. The stomach (St) and the hepatic venous confluence (HV) are on the patient's right. This arrangement is consistent with abdominal situs inversus, or mirror image sidedness. The azygous vein is quite prominent in this case, because there was interruption of the inferior vena cava. **Right:** This image was obtained during the examination of a newborn with asplenia syndrome, subdiaphragmatic total anomalous pulmonary venous connection, and bilateral inferior venae cavae. The spatial arrangement of the abdominal organs in this case is "ambiguous." The liver is found in both upper quadrants; the stomach was found to be right-sided. When scans of the upper abdomen reveal unusual spatial relationships of the liver, stomach, and abdominal great vessels **(middle and right)**, the examiner is alerted to the fact that the patient's cardiovascular anatomy is also likely to be complex. A, anterior; APVn, anomalous pulmonary vein; IVC, inferior vena cava; L, left; V, vertebral body.

Unfortunately, in patients with large atrial septal defects, this landmark is absent. In others with suboptimal image quality, one may not be able to resolve the septum well enough to make this distinction. In these situations, we rely on the connection of the coronary sinus, suprahepatic portion of the inferior vena cava, the size and shape of the atrial appendages, and/or the pattern of the atrial wall (muscular or not) to determine which atrium is which. The coronary sinus, when present, will always connect to the morphologically right atrium. The suprahepatic portion of the inferior vena cava (upstream from the entrance of the hepatic veins) will also almost invariably connect to the morphologically right atrium. The only times that these findings become difficult to interpret are when the inferior vena cava connects to one side of an atrium and an independently connecting hepatic vein connects to the other or the inferior vena cava connects to an unroofed coronary sinus. The connection of the superior vena cava is not a reliable indication of atrial morphology.

The atrial appendages have also been used to identify atrial situs. The appendage of a morphologically right atrium tends to be broad, somewhat pyramidal in shape. In contrast, the morphologically left atrial appendage is usually smaller and more "finger-like" (Fig. 2.15). When using these criteria, one must remember that atrial dilation and/or hypoplasia can distort the size and shape of either appendage. The last and least reliable feature involves the atrial walls. The morphologically right atrium has coarse, muscular

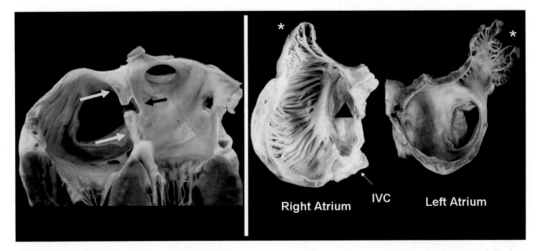

FIGURE 2.15. Anatomic specimens display features that distinguish the morphologically right from the morphologically left atrium. Left: The four-chamber view shows the normal arrangement of the atrial septum. Note that the thicker, muscular limbus (*yellow arrows*) is positioned to the right. The presence of this limbus is the most reliable echocardiographic marker associated with the morphologically right atrium. Just to the left of the thick limbus is the thin fossa ovalis membrane (*black arrow*). This thin segment of the atrial septum was the "flap valve" of the fetal foramen ovale and is always associated with the morphologically left atrium. When the atrial septum is absent, other anatomic features must be relied on to distinguish the morphologically right atrium from the morphologically left atrium. The specimens to the right of the white line are the free walls and appendages of a normal, morphologically right atrium (specimen in the center of the figure) and a normal, morphologically left (specimen on the far right) atrium. The right atrium is far more muscular than the left. There are a series of pectinate muscles radiating outward from a thick muscular ridge, called the christa terminalis (*black arrowhead*). These muscular ridges are absent from the morphologically left atrium because it is derived primarily from the common pulmonary vein. Note the smooth walls present in the body of the left atrium. These features are often difficult to assess echocardiographically, especially when the chambers are enlarged. If the atrial septum does not provide adequate information to assign atrial morphology, the next most reliable echocardiographic marker for the position of the morphologically right atrium is the entrance of the coronary sinus and/or the suprahepatic inferior vena cava (IVC). This segment of the IVC will always relate to either to the right atrium or the coronary sinus. Historically, cardiologists had focused on the shape of the atrial appendages (*s) to distinguish atrial morphology. The morphologically right atrium generally has a broad-based, pyramidal appendage. In contrast, the left atrial appendage is narrower and often has multiple small side lobes (as in this figure). The left atrial appendage has also been described as "finger-like," because of its narrow base. Unfortunately, the shape of the appendages can change, especially with chamber dilation. As a result, appendage shape is less reliable than the other features listed here.

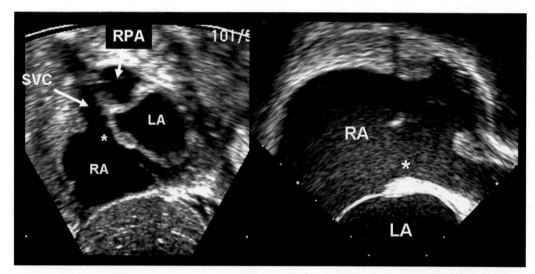

FIGURE 2.16. Normal anatomy of the atrial septum in a patient with normal cardiac situs (sidedness). Left: Subcostal, bicaval view. The superior, thicker limbus of the atrial septum is seen on the right (*). Even without knowledge of other anatomic features, this confidently classifies the right-sided atrial chamber as a morphologically right atrium in this case. **Right:** Also a bicaval view but obtained from the distal esophageal transducer position during transesophageal echocardiography. The asterisk (*) again marks the position of the thick superior limbus. The thinner "flap valve" of the atrial septum is found posterior to the limbus. This relationship identifies the anterior chamber as the morphologically right atrium and the posterior chamber as the left atrium. LA, left atrium; RA, right atrium; RPA, right pulmonary artery; SVC, superior vena cava.

appearing walls due to its pectinate muscles and the crista terminalis. The morphologically left atrium, because it is derived primarily from the common pulmonary vein, has a smoother appearance to its walls. Although these differences are quite clear to the pathologist, echocardiographically, they are rather subjective and understandably less reliable than the other features used to determine atrial situs.

 ## SEGMENTS AND CONNECTIONS

Once the cardiac location, orientation, and situs have been determined, the echocardiographer then examines each of the cardiovascular segments and the connections between them. Because the determination of location and situs was made using the subcostal transducer position, the remainder of the examination usually begins in that position and progresses from there to the parasternal, apical, and suprasternal views in a sequential fashion. Obviously, multiple segments and connections can, and should, be interrogated from each window. Furthermore, information obtained from one plane of imaging may prompt a return to a previous window to clarify or reexamine a finding. Therefore, while our thought processes follow the segmental approach toward a final diagnosis, the scans providing the information may not. Nevertheless, for the purposes of this discussion, we will assume that both our thoughts and our scans will follow a segmental path toward the final diagnosis.

The examination of each segment must describe the anatomy, function, and physiology (i.e., shunts, stenoses, etc.) present within it. In addition, and sometimes most important, the connections between segments must be described. Connections can be concordant (normal) or discordant (opposite of normal). In some situations, other designations are needed for connections that are not normal but are also not the opposite of normal (i.e., double-outlet right ventricle or univentricular AV connection).

The Venous Segment

Both systemic and pulmonary venous anomalies play important roles in the presentation and treatment of congenital heart disease. The systemic veins that we are most concerned with are the inferior and superior venae cavae, the coronary sinus, and the hepatic veins. The inferior vena cava and hepatic veins are imaged from the subcostal position. Horizontal plane scans that progress gradually from the infrahepatic region of the upper abdomen toward the diaphragm provide the best delineation of these structures. Normally, veins draining both the right and left lobes of the liver

can be easily identified and followed to their connections to the inferior vena cava. The inferior vena cava will then be seen to enter the morphologically right atrium, just posterior to the Eustachian valve. In cases where one or more hepatic veins connect to the morphologically right atrium independently, the anomalous vein will travel in a more superiorly directed course than normal and will enter the morphologically right atrium through a separate orifice. These independently connecting veins will usually, but not always, enter the morphologically right atrium near the orifice of the true inferior vena cava. Patients with interruption of inferior vena cava (frequently associated with the polysplenia syndrome) will have a large azygous vein, seen along the spine in the abdomen. This vessel can be either right or left sided and will enter the superior vena cava within the thorax, allowing inferior venous return to reach the heart. In this situation, there will still be a vein (or veins) entering the floor of the morphologically right atrium. This vessel is the "suprahepatic inferior vena cava" that was mentioned in the discussion of atrial situs. This vessel can be distinguished from a normal inferior vena cava by its generally smaller size and by the fact that it does not extend inferior to the liver. It should be noted that in defining the anatomy of these veins, one has simultaneously described their venoatrial connections.

Venous drainage from the upper body usually is directed to a single, right-sided superior vena cava and from there to the right atrium. A right-sided superior vena cava can be visualized in several planes from the subcostal window (Fig. 2.16), high parasternal views, or the suprasternal notch. It is not generally seen from the apex. One of the most common variations in systemic venous anatomy is the persistence of a left-sided superior vena cava, resulting in the presence of bilateral great veins from the upper body. When present, a left superior vena cava will usually connect to the coronary sinus at the posterior/lateral border of the left atrium (Fig. 2.17). Therefore, a clue to the presence of a left superior vena cava is dilation of the coronary sinus (due to the increased flow passing through it). Direct visualization of the left superior vena cava can be obtained in a long-axis plane—where it is seen coursing superiorly from the coronary sinus into the upper left mediastinum. In parasternal short-axis images, the left superior vena cava appears as a circular vessel just anterior to the left pulmonary artery, near the pulmonary artery bifurcation (Fig. 2.17). When abnormalities of situs exist, superior vena caval connections are frequently abnormal. Bilateral superior venae cavae may be present and both may connect directly to the superior aspect of the atria due to absence of the coronary sinus. In other patients, there may be only one superior vena cava present. Unfortunately, it is difficult to predict which superior vena cava will persist in these patients.

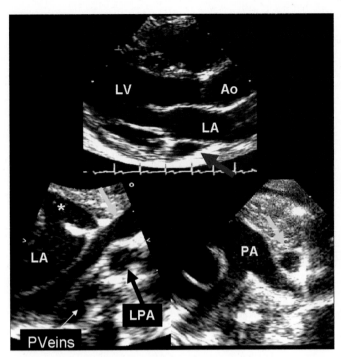

FIGURE 2.17. Common echocardiographic presentation of a left-sided superior vena cava. **Top:** Parasternal long-axis image. *Blue arrow* points to an enlarged coronary sinus. This is often the first indication of a persistent left superior vena cava (LSVC). **Bottom:** High parasternal images that directly visualize the LSVC. **Bottom left:** Sagittal plane view parallel to the long axis of the LSVC (*yellow arrow*). **Bottom right:** Horizontal plane view of the LSVC (*yellow arrow*) at the level of the pulmonary arterial confluence (PA). Both images reveal that the LSVC is positioned anterior to the left pulmonary artery (LPA). The sagittal plane image **(bottom left)** also shows that this vessel passes posterior to the left atrial appendage (*) and anterior to the left pulmonary veins before merging with the coronary sinus.

Similar to the systemic veins, the pulmonary veins can be seen in a number of views. The most useful images tend to be from the subcostal, apical, and suprasternal coronal planes (Fig. 2.7). Color flow Doppler is often helpful in defining the position of the

pulmonary veins and distinguishing them from the atrial appendage. Most patients have four pulmonary veins, two from each lung. However, variations from this pattern can still be normal. The left veins frequently join before entering the atrium, resulting in only three venous entries at the atrial level. Alternatively, the most common variant of right pulmonary veins is for there to be three separate veins connecting to the atrium.

There are two general categories of anomalous pulmonary venous connection: total and partial. Total anomalous connection of the pulmonary veins is further subdivided into supracardiac, cardiac, and infradiaphragmatic types. The anatomy and echocardiographic features of both partial and total anomalous connections have been extensively described elsewhere.

The Atrial Segment

We have already discussed the features that distinguish a morphologically right atrium from a morphologically left atrium. In addition to the size and position of each atrium, the status of the atrial septum requires definition when describing the atrial segment. The assessment of atrial septal defects is discussed in Chapter 6.

The Atrioventricular Connection

There are a large number of terms used to describe the spectrum of AV connections that exist in patients with congenital cardiac malformations. This creates at least some degree of unnecessary confusion. If one uses a simple description of the connection, most of the confusion can be avoided (Figs. 2.18 and 2.19). The first point should be to define whether there is a biventricular or univentricular connection. In biventricular hearts, the connection will usually be composed of two AV valves. These valves will then connect the atria to the ventricles in either a concordant (or normal) or discordant (opposite of normal) manner (Fig. 2.18). A concordant AV connection exists when the morphologically right atrium connects to the morphologically right ventricle through a tricuspid valve and the morphologically left atrium connects to the morphologically left ventricle through a mitral valve. AV discordance implies that the morphologically right atrium connects to the morphologically left ventricle. When it does, the valve associated with this connection will always be a morphologically mitral valve. The morphologically left atrium will then connect to the morphologically right ventricle through a morphologically tricuspid valve.

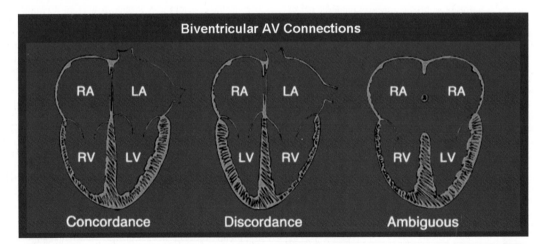

FIGURE 2.18. Three potential atrioventricular connections seen with biventricular circulations. The connection is normal and described as concordant **(left)** when the morphologically right atrium connects to the morphologically right ventricle, and vice versa. The two other connections in this illustration are abnormal. **Middle:** Discordant atrioventricular connections, with the morphologically right atrium associated with the morphologically left ventricle. Conversely, the morphologically left atrium is connected to the morphologically right ventricle in this case. The septal insertions of the two atrioventricular files provide an excellent echocardiographic marker of this connection. This will be illustrated further in the subsequent figures. **Far right:** Ambiguous connection that is difficult to assign. There is a common nature atrioventricular valve with no attachments to the septum, the atrial septum is absent, and the atria appear anatomically similar. In these situations, one must rely on the connection of the coronary sinus and suprahepatic inferior vena cava to determine the position of the morphologically right atrium. Occasionally even this criterion is difficult to apply (bilateral hepatic veins or inferior cavae). In these complex hearts, it is better to simply describe the anatomy of the heart and function of the valves and chambers and refer to the connection as ambiguous. AV, atrioventricular; LA, left atrium; LV, left ventricle; RA, right atrium; RV, right ventricle.

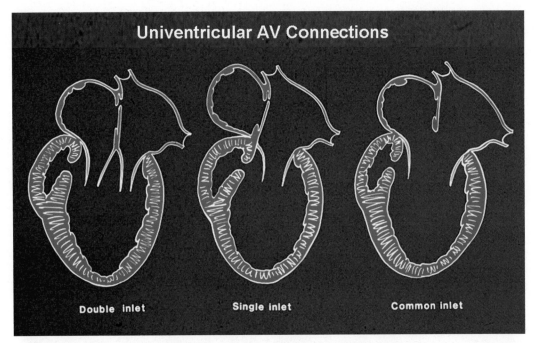

FIGURE 2.19. Three of the potential atrioventricular (AV) connections associated with univentricular circulations. These connections are described based on the number and type of atrioventricular valve(s) that are related to the dominant ventricle. **Left:** Two separate atria, each with its own atrioventricular valve, that connect to a single ventricular cavity. This connection is described as a double inlet, univentricular AV connection. **Middle:** Situation in which there is atresia of one atrioventricular valve. This connection exists in both tricuspid and mitral atresia. When the anatomy does not fall simply into one of these two categories, the connection is described as a single inlet, univentricular AV connection.

The type of connection present in a biventricular heart is most easily defined using a four-chamber view. The internal cardiac crux (the area at which the septal leaflets of both AV valves insert) is asymmetric. At the annulus, the septal leaflet of the morphologic tricuspid valve will always insert at a point that is slightly apical to the insertion of the septal component of the mitral valve (Figs. 2-18 and 2.20). Because the AV valves are invariably associated with their appropriate ventricle (mitral with the left ventricle and tricuspid with right ventricle), the internal crux can be used not only as a marker for AV connection but also for defining ventricular morphology. Occasionally, the AV connection in a biventricular heart will involve a common valve, as in the complete form of AV septal defect. In these cases, one can think of the connection as ambiguous because the internal crux cannot be used. Alternatively, one can rely on the positioning of the atria relative to the ventricular inflow to define the connection. An atrium with an "outflow" orifice positioned more than 50% over one ventricular inflow tract is, by convention, said to be committed or connected to that ventricle (Fig. 2.21). The appropriateness of the connection is then determined by the morphology of the two chambers in question (see sections on atrial and ventricular segments).

Univentricular connections are more variable. However, they can still be described in a straightforward way. When there is only a single functional ventricle, there can be either a double inlet, single inlet, or common inlet connection. The dominant ventricular morphology is usually described in conjunction with the classification of the AV connection. For example, the most common forms of univentricular AV connections are found in patients with hypoplastic left heart syndrome and tricuspid atresia (Figs. 2.22 and 2.23). These connections can be thought of as "single inlet univentricular connections with atresia of one atrioventricular valve." Although this seems to be a cumbersome designation for tricuspid atresia, the true utility of this approach becomes apparent in more complex patients. A diagnosis such as "common inlet univentricular connection to a dominant right ventricle" clearly describes the anatomy present, even to those unfamiliar with these malformations or unaware that many patients with this type of connection have a heterotaxy syndrome.

Functional assessment of the AV connection consists primarily of defining the status of the valves in terms of hypoplasia, obstruction, and/or stenosis. Again, more complete descriptions of these evaluations are found in the appropriate chapters later in the text.

The Ventricular Segment

Obviously, it is important to initially define whether the patient has biventricular or functionally univentricular anatomy. In patients with biventricular hearts, the most reliable feature distinguishing a morphologically right ventricle from a morphologically left ventricle is the asymmetric arrangement of the internal cardiac crux (the septal insertions of the two AV valves). If this landmark is unavailable or difficult to visualize, one then relies on the inherent differences in the myocardial structure of the ventricles (Figs. 2.22 and 2.23). A morphologically right ventricle will have coarse apical trabeculations and a moderator band (Fig. 2.22). The morphologically left ventricular apex will have a relatively smooth endocardial surface (Fig. 2.23). There are multiple, small papillary muscles associated with the AV valve support apparatus in a morphologically right ventricle, and some of the chordae will insert directly onto the ventricular septum. In a morphologically left ventricle, the papillary muscles will be large and discrete (Fig. 2.23). In addition, there will usually be only two papillary muscles (univentricular hearts of left ventricular type may have four papillary muscles). The AV valve support apparatus in a morphologically left ventricle does not insert onto the ventricular septum, unless there is a common valve. In terms of relative position, the right ventricular outflow tract will always be the most anterior ventricular structure in the heart, even in patients with congenitally corrected transposition of the great arteries. Many authors have used shape to distinguish between the ventricles. A normal morphologically right ventricle is somewhat crescent shaped and the normal morphologically left ventricle is round in the short-axis plane and somewhat bullet shaped three-dimensionally. However, these shapes can be altered dramatically by pressure or volume overload (not to mention positional anomalies). Therefore, ventricular shape is probably the least reliable feature available to determine ventricular morphology.

In the functionally univentricular heart, many of these criteria are not available. In this setting, the most reliable way to

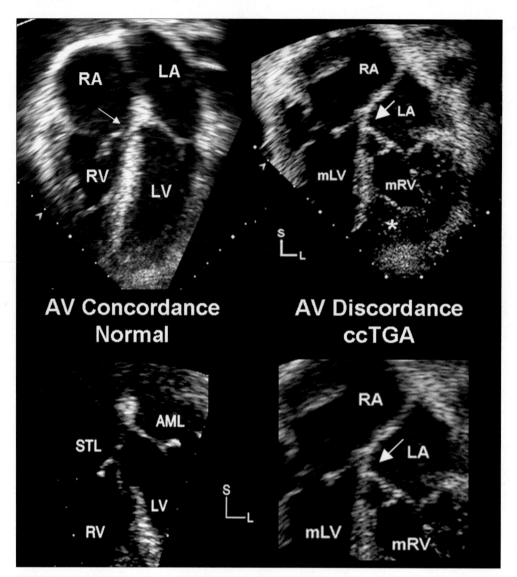

FIGURE 2.20. Echocardiographic anatomy associated with normal and discordant atrioventricular connections and focus on the septal insertions of the two atrioventricular valves (***white arrows***). **Left:** Images from patients with normal hearts. The right atrium relates to the right ventricle, and the left atrium, to the left ventricle. **Bottom left:** Magnified image is centered on the insertions of the septal tricuspid leaflet (STL) and the anterior mitral leaflet (AML) at the internal cardiac crux. The STL will always attach to the ventricular septum at a point that is slightly apical to the insertion of the AML. This offset between the septal insertions can be used to reliably identify the morphology of the atrioventricular valves. Because these valves developed from the ventricular myocardium, this relationship can also be used to identify the morphology of the ventricle that is associated with the atrioventricular valve. **Right:** Example displays the relationships seen in a patient with congenitally corrected transposition of the great arteries. The atrioventricular connections are discordant. The right atrium is associated with a right-sided but morphologically left ventricle. The valve connecting these two chambers is a morphologically mitral valve as evidenced by the basal position of its septal insertion. Conversely, the left atrium is related to a left-sided, morphologically right ventricle. The atrioventricular valve on the left is morphologically a tricuspid valve. Its septal insertion is apically positioned relative to the valve on the opposite side of the septum (*white arrow*). Although this finding alone identifies that the chamber and valve morphologically have a right ventricle and tricuspid valve, this conclusion is confirmed by the presence of a moderator band at the apex of the left-sided morphologically right ventricle (*). AV, atrioventricular; L, left; LA, left atrium; LV, left ventricle; mLV, morphologically left ventricle; mRV, morphologically right ventricle; RA, right atrium; RV, right ventricle; S, superior.

determine ventricular morphology is to determine the type of "rudimentary ventricle" present. Patients with single ventricles of the right ventricular type will have a hypoplastic left ventricular remnant that is positioned posterior to the main ventricular chamber. These left ventricular remnants usually do not connect to great arteries and are generally very small (Fig. 2.22). The findings characteristic of a morphologically right ventricle (coarse apical trabeculation and chordal insertions onto the septum) will still be present. However, they will often be difficult to detect with certainty because of coexisting chamber enlargement and myocardial hypertrophy. In a univentricular heart of left ventricular type, the rudimentary right ventricle will be

found anteriorly and, unlike the rudimentary left ventricle, will frequently connect to a great artery.

The examination of the ventricular segment must also include assessment of the ventricular septum and ventricular function. These topics are well covered later in the text.

The Ventricular–Great Arterial Connection

Similar to the assignment of the AV connection, there are several types of ventricular–great arterial connections. Concordant connections imply that the morphologically left ventricle gives rise to the

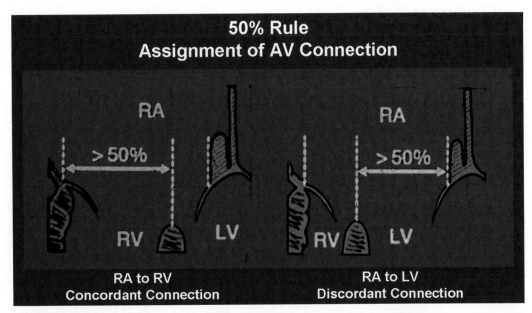

FIGURE 2.21. The 50% rule. Assignment of the atrioventricular and ventriculoarterial connection in the presence of the ventricular septal defect (VSD) and annular override. The valvar annulus may not be perfectly aligned with the ventricular chamber in patients with a septal defect. When a valve annulus overlies more than one ventricle, it is said to override the VSD. In these cases, we assign the connection of the valve and its proximal atrium or distal artery to the ventricle over which more than half (50%) of the annulus is found. The diagram illustrates this concept for two atrioventricular valves that override inlet VSDs. **Left:** Example shows a right atrium with a valve that is more than 50% committed to the right ventricular inlet. Therefore, despite the override, the atrioventricular connection is concordant. **Right:** In contrast, the valve associated with the right atrium has an annulus that is primarily committed to the left ventricular inlet. As a result of this severe override, the atrioventricular connection is now discordant (the right atrium is committed to the left ventricle). AV, atrioventricular, LV, left ventricle, RA, right atrium, RV, right ventricle.

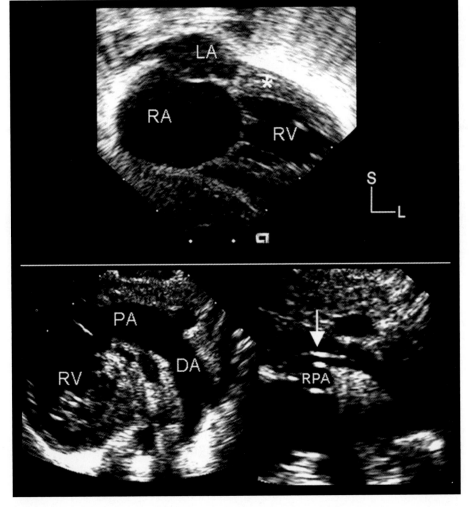

FIGURE 2.22. Determining ventricular morphology in hearts with univentricular circulations (morphologically right ventricles). These echocardiographic images were taken from an infant with hypoplastic left heart syndrome. **Top:** Subcostal "four-chamber" view of this heart. The right ventricle (RV) is supporting the systemic circulation and has become enlarged and hypertrophied. As a result, the anatomic features normally associated with right ventricular morphology are not as easily appreciated. The severe abnormality of the mitral valve makes determination of the septal offset difficult. In these situations, we rely on the fact that a morphologically tricuspid valve and right ventricle will display atrioventricular chordal attachments to the ventricular septum, the presence of a moderator band in the right ventricular apex (not seen here), and the relationship of the dominant ventricle to the hypoplastic ventricular remnant. In this case, there were septal chordal attachments of the only sizable atrioventricular valve, and the hypoplastic ventricular remnant (*) was posterior to the dominant ventricle. This spatial relationship alone identifies the dominant ventricle as a morphologically right ventricle. **Bottom:** Classic arterial anatomy associated with hypoplastic left heart syndrome. **Left:** Main pulmonary artery (PA) continuing through the "ductal arch" (DA) to supply flow to the aortic circulation. **Right:** Diminutive descending aorta (*white arrow*) just anterior to the right pulmonary artery (RPA). L, left; LA, left atrium; RA, right atrium; RV, right ventricle; S, superior.

FIGURE 2.23. Determining ventricular morphology in hearts with univentricular circulations (morphologically left ventricles). The echocardiographic images in this figure were taken during examinations of patients with tricuspid valve atresia (top) and a univentricular heart with left ventricular morphology and double inlet atrioventricular connection, the so-called double-inlet LV. Because the anatomy of the internal cardiac crux lacks the asymmetry of the biventricular heart, one must rely on other anatomic markers to determine ventricular morphology. The ventricular chamber can be seen in multiple planes. In both of these cases, the ventricles have a relatively smooth endocardial lining and large discrete papillary muscle groups (top right) that do not attach to the ventricular septum. However, the most reliable indicator that the dominant ventricle is a structurally left ventricle is the anterior position of the hypoplastic right ventricular remnant (* in the bottom right image). Top left: Area of the expected, but absent, right atrioventricular connection (white arrow). A, anterior; L, left; LA, left atrium; LV, left ventricle; RA, right atrium; S, superior.

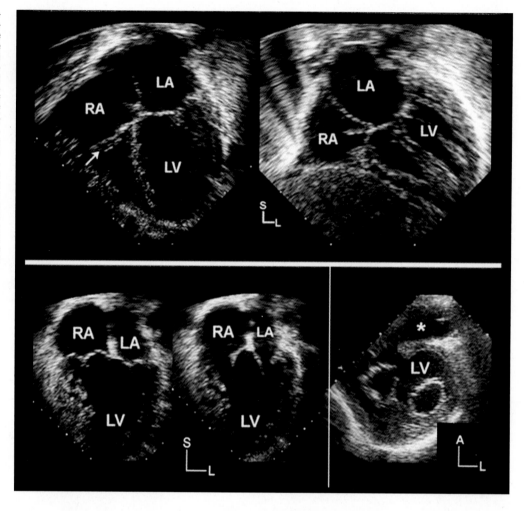

aorta and the morphologically right ventricle connects to the pulmonary artery. Discordant connections are characterized by the pulmonary artery arising from the morphologically left ventricle and the aorta originating from the morphologically right ventricle. It should be noted that there are no anatomic features of the semilunar valves themselves that can be used to make these assignments. The aortic and pulmonary valves are anatomically identical. Therefore, the "morphology" of the valve is determined by the downstream artery. So, a semilunar valve that is connected to the pulmonary arteries becomes the pulmonary valve, and the valve in continuity with the aorta, the aortic valve.

When VSDs are present, the assignment of both the AV and ventriculoarterial connections can be more difficult. In this setting, the simplest rule to follow has been called the "50% rule." This "rule" can be applied to both connections and states that if a valve annulus overlies a ventricular cavity by 50% or more, then it is assigned to the ventricular cavity that is associated with the majority of the annulus. Figure 2.21 shows this relationship for two AV valves. This assignment is best made using the apical four-chamber view in most cases. The same process can be applied to the semilunar valves. However, the parasternal long-axis projection provides the optimal visualization of these relationships (Fig. 2.24). Ventriculoarterial connections can be more difficult to assign from the subcostal window (Fig. 2.25). Careful definition of the plane of the ventricular septum is required to use the 50% rule accurately from this transducer position. An additional useful anatomic clue for assigning the left ventricle to an arterial connection is the presence of fibrous continuity between a semilunar valve and the morphologically mitral valve. The semilunar valve that originates from the left ventricle will usually (but not always) be in direct continuity with the anterior hinge of the morphologically mitral valve.

Some complex forms of congenital heart disease will have absence of one great arterial connection (i.e., pulmonary atresia or truncus

arteriosus). Others will result in both great arteries originating from the incorrect ventricle or even the same ventricle, most commonly a morphologically right ventricle (Fig. 2.25). In these cases, the spatial relationship of the aorta must be described relative to the pulmonary artery and valve, as well as any VSDs that may be present. For example, in AV concordance with VA discordance (complete transposition of the great arteries), the aorta is usually found anterior and to the right of the pulmonary valve. This can be referred to simply as "AV concordance with VA discordance and an anterior and rightward aorta."

The relationship of the great arteries to the VSD is most important in cases of double-outlet right ventricle, because this relationship will in large part determine the type of surgical repair. Subaortic and "double committed" VSDs can be repaired using a relatively simple patch technique. Patients with double-outlet right ventricle and a subpulmonary VSD require more complex surgical maneuvers, involving either a Rastelli approach (intraventricular baffle, right ventricle-to-pulmonary artery conduit, and ligation of the native main pulmonary artery) or an arterial switch operation to achieve a biventricular repair. VSDs that are "remote" from both great arteries present perhaps the greatest surgical challenge and may be more appropriately treated with a Fontan protocol as if they were a univentricular heart.

As with all of the preceding components of the segmental approach, the status, anatomy, and function of each connection (i.e., semilunar valve) must be specifically examined and described.

The Great Arterial Segment

Descriptions of this segment are relatively self-explanatory. Individual vessels that must be examined include the aorta, pulmonary arteries (main, right, and left), coronary arteries (usually limited to the

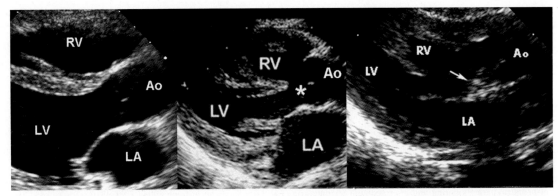

FIGURE 2.24. Echocardiographic images demonstrate normal (concordant) left ventricular to aortic connection (left and middle). **Left:** There is no ventricular septal defect, and thus the connection is unambiguous. **Middle:** Taken from the examination of an infant with tetralogy of Fallot. The aortic annulus is centrally positioned above an outlet for ventricular septal defect (*). There is roughly 50% of the aortic annulus committed to each ventricle, a common situation in patients with tetralogy. The muscular ventricular septum is almost perfectly aligned with the central coaptation point of the aortic valve leaflets. In this situation, we assign the aortic connection to the left ventricle because there is no conal muscle separating the posterior hinge point of the aortic valve from the anterior hinge of the mitral valve (fibrous continuity). **Right:** The long-axis image was taken during an examination of the patient with double-outlet right ventricle (DORV). Here, there is no evidence of a semilunar valve near the anterior hinge point of the mitral valve. Instead, the aorta (Ao) is positioned anterior to the ventricular septal defect and is completely separated from the left ventricle and mitral valve by infundibular/conal muscle (*arrow*). As a result, the aortic valve connection is assigned to the right ventricle. The pulmonary valve also arose from the right ventricle and was positioned even farther from this subaortic ventricular septal defect. LA, left atrium; LV, left ventricle; RV, right ventricle.

left main, and the proximal parts of the left anterior descending, circumflex, and right coronary arteries), and ductus arteriosus. Complete assessment describes the presence/absence, size, origin, position, and any dilations or stenoses of these arteries.

Because the echocardiographic evaluation of a patient with congenital heart disease can be a challenging and complex task, it is best approached in a systematic manner. The guidelines for performing an examination, orienting the images, and the sequential segmental approach provide a framework that can support the understanding of any cardiovascular malformation. It should be reemphasized that the order of images obtained during an examination will not correspond exactly to the segments described. For example, because

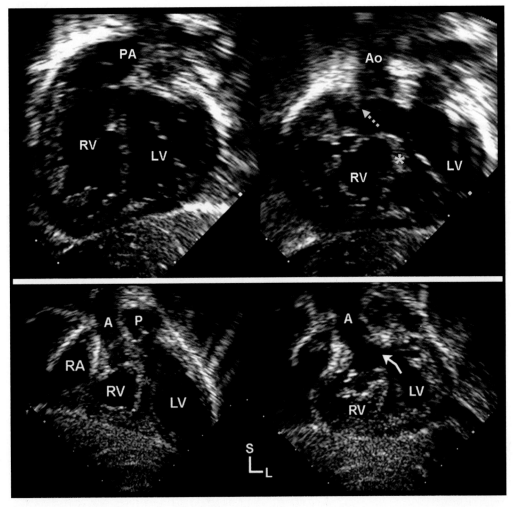

FIGURE 2.25. Relationship of the aorta and pulmonary artery to the ventricular septal defect in double-outlet right ventricle (DORV). These echocardiographic images are of two different patients with DORV. **Top left:** Subcostal image demonstrates that the pulmonary artery is distant from the interventricular communication. It is supported by a fully developed, circumferential sleeve of infundibular muscle. **Top right:** Nearly direct relationship of the aorta to the outlet for ventricular septal defect (*yellow arrow*). The muscular portion of the upper ventricular septum is marked (*yellow asterisk*). Continuity between the left ventricle and the aorta can be achieved by insertion of a patch from the superior aspect of this muscular ventricular septum to the anterior aspect of the subaortic conus (*yellow arrow*). **Bottom:** Subaortic ventricular septal defect with double outlet from the right ventricle but with a greater length separating the left ventricle from the aortic annulus (**bottom right**). **Bottom left:** Completely intact anterior ventricular septum (*red asterisk*), with both great arteries completely committed to the right ventricular outflow tract, and the side-by-side orientation of the great arteries (aorta to the right). Although this patient can also have patch redirection of left ventricular outflow to the aorta, the likelihood of postoperative subaortic stenosis is greater. A or Ao, aorta; L, left; LV, left ventricle; P or PA, pulmonary artery; RA, right atrium; RV, right ventricle; S, superior.

children frequently dislike suprasternal imaging, the superior veins are usually imaged last—even though they should be included in the "beginning" (the venous segment) of any sequential segmental description.

Acknowledgment

We gratefully acknowledge the generosity of Dr. William D. Edwards in contributing anatomic images and diagrams to better illustrate this chapter. Thank you very much.

SUGGESTED READING

American Academy of Pediatrics, American Academy of Pediatric Dentistry, Cote CJ, Wilson S. Work Group on Sedation. Guidelines for monitoring and management of pediatric patients during and after sedation for diagnostic and therapeutic procedures: an update. *Pediatrics.* 2006;118(6):2587–2602.

Anderson RH, Becker AE, Freedom RM, et al. Sequential segmental analysis of congenital heart disease. *Pediatr Cardiol.* 1984;5(4):281–287.

Edwards WD. Cardiac anatomy and examination of cardiac specimens. In: Allen HD, Driscoll DJ, Feltes TF, Shaddy RE, eds. *Moss and Adams' Heart disease in infants, children and adolescents.* Philadelphia, PA: Lippincott Williams & Wilkins; 2008:2–33.

Edwards WD. Classification and terminology of cardiovascular anomalies. In: Allen HD, Driscoll DJ, Feltes TF, Shaddy RE, eds. *Moss and Adams' Heart disease in infants, children and adolescents.* Philadelphia, PA: Lippincott Williams & Wilkins; 2008:34–57.

Hance-Miller W, Fyfe DA, Stevenson JG, et al. Indications and guidelines for performance of transesophageal echocardiography in the patient with pediatric acquired or congenital heart disease. A report from the Task Force of the Pediatric Council of the American Society of Echocardiography. *J Am Soc Echocardiogr.* 2005;18:91–98.

Jacobs JP, Anderson RH, Weinberg PM, et al. The nomenclature, definition and classification of cardiac structures in the setting of heterotaxy. *Cardiol Young.* 2007;17(suppl 2):1–28.

Lai WW, Geva T, Shirali GS, et al. Task Force of the Pediatric Council of the American Society of Echocardiography. Guidelines and standards for performance of a pediatric echocardiogram: a report from the Task Force of the Pediatric Council of the American Society of Echocardiography. *J Am Soc Echocardiogr* 2006;19(12):1413–1430.

O'Leary PW. The segmental approach to congenital heart disease. *Pediatr Ultrasound Today.* 2005;5(10):107–132.

Rychik J, Ayres N. Cunco B, et al. American Society of Echocardiography guidelines and standards for performance of the fetal echocardiogram. *J Am Soc Echocardiogr.* 2004;17:803–810.

REFERENCES

1. Lai WW, Geva T, Shirali GS, et al. Task Force of the Pediatric Council of the American Society of Echocardiography. Guidelines and standards for performance of a pediatric echocardiogram: a report from the Task Force of the Pediatric Council of the American Society of Echocardiography. *J Am Soc Echocardiogr.* 2006;19(12):1413–1430.

2. Oh JK, Seward JB, Tajik AJ. *The echo manual.* 3rd ed. Philadelphia, Pa: Lippincott Williams & Wilkins; 2006.

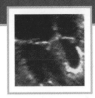

Chapter 3
Quantitative Methods in Echocardiography—Basic Techniques

Benjamin W. Eidem • Patrick W. O'Leary

The noninvasive echocardiographic evaluation of ventricular performance is an essential tool in the clinician's assessment and management of children and adults with congenital heart disease. As noninvasive methods have continued to evolve, the importance of global and regional ventricular function has become better appreciated. Alterations in both ventricular geometry and loading conditions are the hallmarks of congenital heart disease and can often make the quantitative assessment of ventricular function challenging. This chapter will discuss traditional echocardiographic techniques in the evaluation of ventricular function in patients with congenital heart disease. Newer modalities for functional assessment, including three-dimensional echocardiography, strain and strain rate imaging, and cardiac magnetic resonance imaging, will be covered in greater detail in subsequent chapters in this text.

ECHOCARDIOGRAPHIC ASSESSMENT OF GLOBAL SYSTOLIC VENTRICULAR FUNCTION

Left Ventricular Shortening Fraction

One-dimensional wall motion analysis, or M-mode echocardiography, has traditionally been one of the most commonly used methods to measure the extent of LV shortening. Shortening fraction represents the change in LV short-axis diameter that occurs during systole:

$$SF\% = [LVEDD - LVESD]/LVEDD \times 100$$

where LVEDD represents LV end-diastolic dimension and LVESD represents LV end-systolic dimension (Fig. 3.1). Normal values for shortening fraction range between 28% and 44%. The short-axis view at the mid-papillary level is the echocardiographic view most frequently used to make these measurements. Similar to shortening fraction, fractional area change can also be measured in this orientation by determining the change in LV area that occurs during the cardiac cycle:

$$[(LV\ end\text{-}diastolic\ area) - (LV\ end\text{-}systolic\ area)]/(LV\ end\text{-}diastolic\ area)$$

Normal values have been reported to be greater than 36% for fractional area change in adults. LV fractional shortening and fractional area change have been reported to be independent of changes in heart rate and age but are significantly affected by changes in ventricular preload and afterload.

Left Ventricular Ejection Fraction

LV ejection fraction (LVEF) is the most commonly measured parameter of ventricular function. Global estimation LVEF is often determined in a qualitative fashion; however, using transthoracic or transesophageal echocardiography, two-dimensional echocardiography allows quantitative measurement of LVEF by assessing changes in ventricular volume during the cardiac cycle. The geometric model most commonly used to measure LVEF is the modified Simpson's biplane method (Fig. 3.2). By using orthogonal apical four-chamber and two-chamber views of the left ventricle, this geometric model calculates LV end-diastolic (LVEDV) and LV end-systolic volume (LVESV) by summing equal sequential slices of LV area from each of these scan planes. LVEF can then be calculated as:

$$LVEF\ (\%) = [LVEDV - LVESV]/LVEDV \times 100$$

Normal values for LVEF range between 56% and 78%. Similar to shortening fraction, LVEF has been shown to be dependent on changes in ventricular loading conditions.

Accurate calculation of LV volume can occasionally be challenging due to foreshortening of the LV cavity. To circumvent this limitation, the area-length method to derive LVEF can also be used (Fig. 3.3). One of the more commonly used methods, termed the "bullet" method, uses the short-axis area of the left ventricle and the long-axis major LV length (from the apical four-chamber view):

$$LV\ volume = 5/6\ [LV\ area] \times [LV\ length]$$

Determination of ventricular volume and EF by this method has been shown to correlate well with invasively measured parameters of ventricular function.

New echocardiographic technology and advancements in image processing have allowed improved acquisition of ventricular volume. Recent studies have validated the ability of three-dimensional echocardiography to obtain accurate and reproducible estimates of LV and right ventricular (RV) volumes and EF. While this imaging modality has historically been limited by the time-consuming reconstruction of acquired images, the introduction of real-time three-dimensional imaging will significantly enhance the quantitative assessment of ventricular volume and function.

Automated border detection (ABD) is another recent advancement in imaging technology that uses acoustic quantification to differentiate the myocardium from the blood pool and thereby allows enhanced visualization of the endocardial border. End-diastolic and end-systolic LV area can be continuously displayed with this modality, enabling determination of ventricular volume, fractional

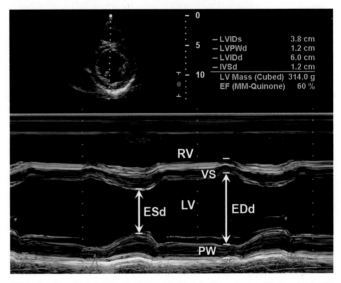

FIGURE 3.1. Parasternal short-axis image at level of papillary muscles of left ventricle with M-mode measurement of left ventricular shortening.
M-mode–derived shortening fraction (FS%) of left ventricle:

$$FS\% = [LVEDD - LVESD]/LVEDD$$
$$= [60\ mm - 38\ mm]/60\ mm$$
$$= 37\%$$

Left ventricular ejection fraction (EF%) can be obtained as follows:

$$EF\% = [(LVEDD)^2 - (LVESD)^2]/[LVEDD]^2 \times 100\%$$
$$= [(60)^2 - (38)^2]/[60]^2 \times 100\%$$
$$= 60\%$$

(FROM OH JK, SEWARD JB, TAJIK AJ. *The echo manual.* 3rd ed. [Figure 7-1, p. 110]. Philadelphia, Pa: Lippincott Williams & Wilkins; 2006. Used with permission.)

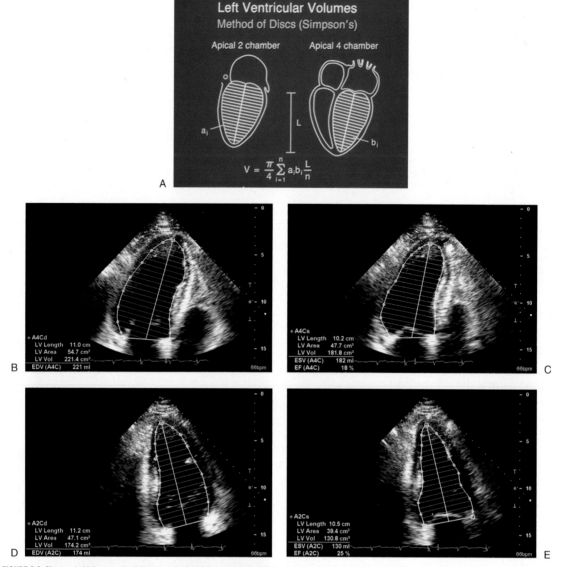

FIGURE 3.2. Simpson's biplane methodology to calculate left ventricular (LV) ejection fraction. A: Apical four-chamber and two-chamber views are used to calculate LV volume. LV ejection fraction is assessed from apical four-chamber (**B** and **C**) and two-chamber (**D** and **E**) views. (**A,** Adapted from Shiller NB, et al. American Society of Echocardiography Committee on Standards, Subcommittee on Quantitation of Two-dimensional Echocardiograms. Recommendations for quantitation of the left ventricle by two-dimensional echocardiography. *J Am Soc Echocardiogr.* 1989;2:358–367. **B–E,** From Oh JK, Seward JB, Tajik AJ. *The echo manual.* 3rd ed. [Figure 7-10, p. 115]. Philadelphia, Pa: Lippincott Williams & Wilkins; 2006. Used with permission.)

area change, and even pressure-volume or pressure-area loops. Excellent correlation of ABD with other noninvasive and invasive measurements of ventricular function has been reported in some adult studies, but data are lacking in patients with congenital heart disease with altered ventricular geometry.

Left Ventricular Mass

LV mass can be calculated using several echocardiographic methodologies. The unifying principle behind these various measurements is to subtract the volume of the LV cavity from the volume encompassed by the LV epicardium—leaving a "shell" of myocardial muscle volume that can be converted to LV mass by factoring in the specific gravity of myocardium. Devereux and colleagues (1986) have described an M-mode formula to derive LV mass using the short-axis LV dimension as follows:

$$1.04[(LVID + PWT + IVST)^3 - LVID^3] \times 0.8 + 0.6g$$

where 1.04 is the specific gravity of myocardium, LVID is the LV internal dimension, PWT is the posterior wall thickness, IVST is the interventricular septal wall thickness, and 0.8 is a correction factor. Two-dimensional echocardiographic and, more recently, three-dimensional echocardiographic methodologies have been shown to be superior to M-mode–derived measures of LV mass. The two most common two-dimensional approaches include the area-length and the truncated ellipsoid methods. Both of these methodologies use a short-axis view of the left ventricle at the papillary muscle level and an apical four-chamber or two-chamber view to measure the LV long-axis length. LV mass is calculated using LV dimensions and wall thicknesses (measured in centimeters) at end diastole (Fig. 3.4). Normal values for both pediatric and adult cohorts have been published using the area-length or truncated ellipsoid methods.

 VELOCITY OF CIRCUMFERENTIAL FIBER SHORTENING AND THE STRESS-VELOCITY INDEX

The rate of LV fiber shortening can be noninvasively assessed by M-mode echocardiography. This measurement, termed the mean

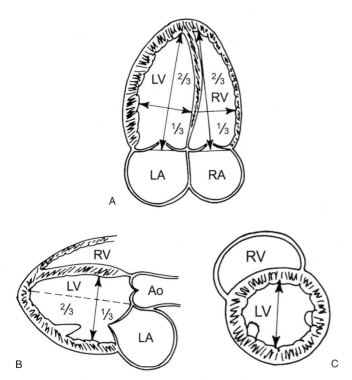

FIGURE 3.3. Left ventricular (LV) dimensions. A: Measurement of the major long-axis and minor short-axis dimension of the left ventricle from the apical four-chamber view. **B:** Similar measurements of the LV long-axis and short-axis dimensions can be obtained from the parasternal long-axis view. **C:** LV short axis measured in the parasternal short-axis view. (Adapted from Shiller NB, et al. American Society of Echocardiography Committee on Standards, Subcommittee on Quantitation of Two-dimensional Echocardiograms. Recommendations for quantitation of the left ventricle by two-dimensional echocardiography. *J Am Soc Echocardiogr.* 1989;2:358–367.)

velocity of circumferential fiber shortening (Vcf), is normalized for LVEDD and can be obtained from the following equation:

$$Vcf = [LVEDD - LVESD]/[LVEDD \times LVET]$$

where LVET represents LV ejection time. Reported normal values for mean Vcf are 1.5 ± 0.04 circumferences (circ)/sec for neonates and 1.3 ± 0.03 circ/sec for children between 2 and 10 years of age. This index assesses not only the degree of fractional shortening but also the

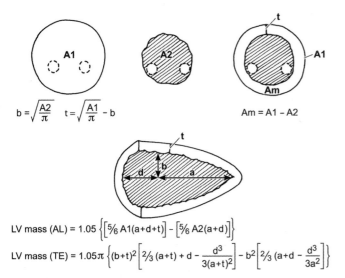

LV mass (AL) = $1.05 \left\{ \left[\frac{5}{6} A1(a+d+t) \right] - \left[\frac{5}{6} A2(a+d) \right] \right\}$

LV mass (TE) = $1.05\pi \left\{ (b+t)^2 \left[\frac{2}{3}(a+t) + d - \frac{d^3}{3(a+t)^2} \right] - b^2 \left[\frac{2}{3}(a+d - \frac{d^3}{3a^2}) \right] \right\}$

FIGURE 3.4. Calculation of left ventricular (LV) mass. Calculation of LV mass by the area-length method and truncated ellipsoid method (see text). (Adapted from Shiller NB, et al. American Society of Echocardiography Committee on Standards, Subcommittee on Quantitation of Two-dimensional Echocardiograms. Recommendations for quantitation of the left ventricle by two-dimensional echocardiography. *J Am Soc Echocardiogr.* 1989;2:358–367.)

rate at which this shortening occurs. To normalize Vcf for variation in heart rate, LVET is divided by the square root of the RR interval to derive a rate-corrected mean velocity of circumferential fiber shortening (Vcf_c). Normal Vcf_c has been reported to be 1.28 ± 0.22 and 1.08 ± 0.14 circ/sec in neonates and children, respectively. Because Vcf_c values are corrected for heart rate, a significant decrease in Vcf_c between neonates and children has been attributed to increased systemic afterload with advancing age. Vcf is sensitive to changes in contractility and afterload but relatively insensitive to changes in preload. Similar to fractional shortening, this parameter relies on the elliptical shape of the left ventricle and is invalid with altered LV geometry.

Because the majority of ejection phase indices, including shortening fraction, EF, and Vcf_c, are dependent on the underlying loading state of the left ventricle, measures of wall tension, namely circumferential and meridional end-systolic wall stress, have been proposed to assess myocardial performance in a relatively load-independent fashion. Colan and colleagues (1984) have previously described a stress-velocity index that is an inverse linear relationship between Vcf_c and end-systolic wall stress (Fig. 3.5). This stress-velocity index is independent of preload, is normalized for heart rate, and incorporates afterload resulting in a noninvasive measure of LV contractility that is independent of ventricular loading conditions. This index can therefore differentiate states of increased ventricular afterload from decreased myocardial contractility. While the stress-velocity index is appealing, the clinical application of this index has been limited by its cumbersome acquisition and its time-consuming off-line. This index is also limited in patients with altered ventricular geometry and wall thickness, features that are hallmarks of congenital heart disease.

Doppler Paramenters of Left Ventricular Systolic Function

Echocardiographic evaluation of systolic dysfunction has primarily relied on one-dimensional measures of LV shortening or two-dimensional measures of LV volume change that are often difficult to assess in patients with distorted ventricular geometry. Doppler measures of global ventricular function have been reported to be a potentially more reproducible and sensitive measure of ventricular function.

Left Ventricular dP/dt

Doppler echocardiography can be used in the quantitative evaluation of LV systolic function. If mitral regurgitation (MR) is present, the peak and mean rate of change in LV systolic pressure (dP/dt) can be derived from the ascending portion of the continuous-wave MR Doppler signal. This rate of change of ventricular pressure is determined during the isovolumic phase of the cardiac cycle before opening of the aortic valve. Using the simplified Bernoulli equation, two velocity points along the MR Doppler envelope are selected from which a corresponding LV pressure change can be derived (Fig. 3.6). This change in LV pressure can then be divided by the change in time between the two Doppler velocities to derive the LV dP/dt. Normal values for mean dP/dt have been reported to be greater than 1200 mm Hg/sec for the left ventricle. While more time consuming to perform, peak dP/dt correlates more accurately with invasive cardiac catherization measurements. To ascertain peak LV dP/dt noninvasively, the MR signal is digitized to obtain the first derivative of the pressure gradient curve from which peak positive and peak negative LV dP/dt as well as the time constant of relaxation (Tau) can be calculated. While reflective of myocardial contractility, LV dP/dt is significantly affected by changes in preload and afterload.

Myocardial Performance Index (Tei Index)

The myocardial performance index (MPI) is a Doppler-derived quantitative measure of global ventricular function that incorporates both systolic and diastolic time intervals. The MPI is defined as the sum of isovolumic contraction time (ICT) and isovolumic relaxation time (IRT) divided by ejection time (ET): MPI = (ICT + IRT)/ET (Fig. 3.7). The components of this index are measured from routine pulsed-wave Doppler signals at the atrioventricular (AV) valve and ventricular outflow tract of either the left or right ventricle. To derive the sum of ICT and IRT, the Doppler-derived ejection time for either ventricle is subtracted from the Doppler interval between cessation

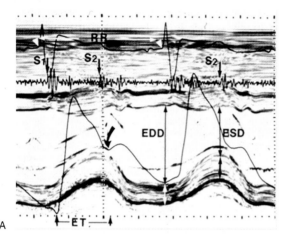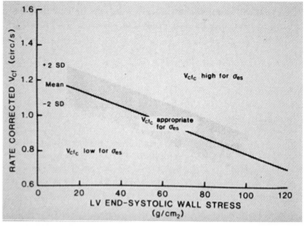

FIGURE 3.5. Stress-velocity index for assessment of left ventricular (LV) systolic function. A: Parameters used to calculate the stress-velocity index. Note the simultaneous phonocardiogram (identifying the first (S1) and second (S2) heart sounds), ECG, carotid pulse tracing (*arrow*), and M-mode echocardiogram. Parameters measured include LV end-diastolic (EDD) and end-systolic (ESD) dimensions and LV ejection time (ET). **B:** Graphic representation of the relationship between the mean rate-corrected velocity of circumferential LV fiber shortening (Vcf$_c$) and the LV end-systolic wall stress (œ es). To normalize Vcf for variation in heart rate, it is divided by the square root of the RR interval to derive a rate-corrected mean velocity of circumferential LV fiber shortening (Vcf$_c$). Values above the upper limit of the mean relationship imply an increased inotropic state, whereas values below the mean imply depressed contractility. (From Colan SD, Borow KM, Neumann A. Left ventricular end-systolic wall stress-velocity of fiber shortening relation: A load independent index of myocardial contractility. *J Am Coll Cardiol.* 1984;4:715–724. Used with permission.)

and onset of the respective AV valve inflow signal (from the end of the Doppler A wave to the beginning of the Doppler E wave of the next cardiac cycle). Increasing values of the MPI correlate with increasing degrees of global ventricular dysfunction.

Both adult and pediatric studies have established normal values for the MPI. In adults, normal LV and RV MPI values are 0.39 ± 0.05 and 0.28 ± 0.04, respectively. In children, similar values for the LV and RV are reported to be 0.35 ± 0.03 and 0.32 ± 0.03, respectively. The MPI has been shown to be a sensitive predictor of outcome in adult and pediatric patients with acquired and congenital heart disease. Because the MPI incorporates measures of both systolic and diastolic performance, this index may be a more sensitive early measure of ventricular dysfunction in the absence of other overt changes in isolated systolic or diastolic echocardiographic indices. In addition, because the MPI is a Doppler-derived index, it has been reported to be easily applied to the assessment of both LV and RV function as well as complex ventricular geometries found in patients with congenital heart disease. The MPI, however, does have significant limitations. It is significantly affected by changes in loading conditions and has a paradoxical change with high filling pressure or severe semilunar valve regurgitation ("pseudo-normalization"). In addition, the combined nature of this index fails to readily discriminate between abnormalities of systolic or diastolic performance.

ECHOCARDIOGRAPHIC ASSESSMENT OF REGIONAL SYSTOLIC VENTRICULAR FUNCTION

Two-dimensional Imaging

Both transthoracic and transesophageal echocardiography are ideally suited to evaluate regional wall motion abnormalities. These wall motion abnormalities are characterized by reduced systolic thickening and decreased inward endocardial excursion. Echocardiographic assessment of regional systolic function is best facilitated in the LV short-axis view at the level of the papillary muscles. In the American Society of Echocardiography's 17-segment model, the left ventricle is divided into six myocardial segments at this level: anterior, anteroseptal, anterolateral, inferolateral, inferior, and inferoseptal (Fig. 3.8). Qualitative visual assessment of wall thickening is graded as normal, hypokinetic

(reduced systolic thickening), akinetic (absent systolic thickening), or dyskinetic (paradoxical thinning). Additional views are needed to evaluate all myocardial segments.

Tissue Doppler Imaging and Strain Rate Imaging

Quantitative assessment of regional systolic LV function, as detailed earlier, has centered on the evaluation of segmental endocardial excursion and LV wall thickening. These semiquantitative methods often fail to discriminate between active and passive myocardial motion. Newer echocardiographic modalities, including tissue Doppler imaging and strain rate imaging, offer a potentially more quantitative and accurate approach to the assessment of regional myocardial contraction and relaxation.

Tissue Doppler echocardiography is a more recent addition to the armamentarium of the echocardiographer. By incorporating a high pass filter, tissue Doppler allows the display and quantitation of the low-velocity high-amplitude Doppler shifts present within the myocardium as opposed to the higher-velocity lower-amplitude Doppler signals more commonly measured within the blood pool (Fig. 3.9). Tissue Doppler is less load dependent than corresponding Doppler velocities from the blood pool and has systolic and diastolic components. These velocities are heterogenous depending on ventricular wall and position.

Measurement of myocardial wall velocities by TDI has been shown to be a promising modality for assessment of longitudinal systolic performance. Recent studies have demonstrated significant changes in mitral annular systolic TDI velocities in adult patients with LV dysfunction and elevated LV filling pressures.

Tissue Doppler velocities, however, cannot differentiate between active contraction and passive motion, which is a major limitation when assessing regional myocardial function. Regional strain rate corresponds to the rate of regional myocardial deformation and can be calculated from the spatial gradient in myocardial velocity between two neighboring points within the myocardium. Regional strain represents the amount of deformation (expressed as a percentage) or the fractional change in length caused by an applied force and is calculated by integrating the strain rate curve over time during the cardiac cycle. Strain measures the total amount of deformation in either the radial or longitudinal direction, while strain rate calculates the velocity of shortening (Fig. 3.10). These two measurements reflect different aspects of myocardial function and therefore provide complementary information. In contrast to tissue Doppler velocities, these newer indices of myocardial deformation are not influenced by global heart motion or tethering of adjacent

MEASUREMENT OF dp/dt

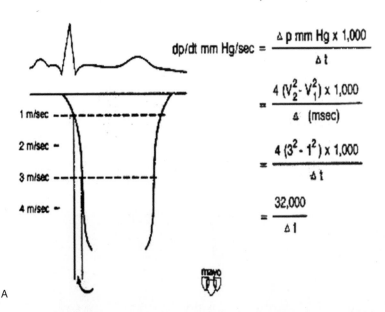

$$dp/dt \; mm \; Hg/sec = \frac{\Delta p \; mm \; Hg \times 1{,}000}{\Delta t}$$

$$= \frac{4 (V_2^2 - V_1^2) \times 1{,}000}{\Delta \; (msec)}$$

$$= \frac{4 (3^2 - 1^2) \times 1{,}000}{\Delta t}$$

$$= \frac{32{,}000}{\Delta t}$$

A

FIGURE 3.6. Measurement of dP/dt (A) and calculation of left ventricular (LV) dP/dt from the mitral regurgitation jet (B). This still frame demonstrates the Doppler velocity curve of the mitral regurgitation jet obtained during transesophageal echocardiography in a child with dilated cardiomyopathy and severe LV dysfunction. Using the modified Bernoulli equation, the LV dP/dt is the change in LV pressure measured from 1.0 m/sec to 3.0 m/sec divided by the change in time between these two LV pressure points:

LV dP/dt = (36 mm Hg − 4 mm Hg)/63 msec = 508 mm Hg/sec (normal >1200 mm Hg/sec)

(**A,** Used with permission from Mayo Clinic.)

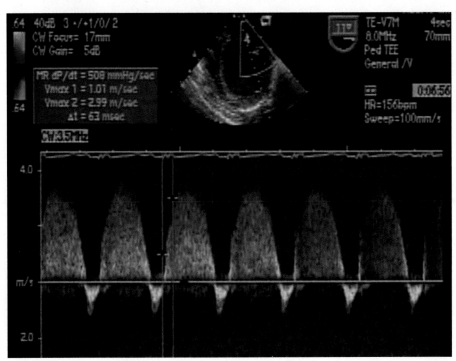

B

segments and therefore are better indices of true regional myocardial function.

ECHOCARDIOGRAPHIC ASSESSMENT OF DIASTOLIC VENTRICULAR FUNCTION

Doppler echocardiography has historically been an essential noninvasive tool in the quantitative assessment of LV diastolic function. Abnormalities of ventricular compliance and relaxation can be demonstrated by characteristic changes in mitral inflow and pulmonary venous Doppler patterns. The addition of newer methodologies, including tissue Doppler echocardiography and flow propagation velocities, enhances

the ability of echocardiography to define and quantitate these adverse changes in diastolic performance. Because diastolic dysfunction often precedes systolic dysfunction, careful assessment of diastolic function is mandatory in the noninvasive characterization and serial evaluation of patients with congenital heart disease.

Noninvasive evaluation of diastolic function in normal infants and children is influenced by a variety of factors, including age, heart rate, and the respiratory cycle. Reference values detailing both mitral and pulmonary venous Doppler velocities in a large cohort of normal children have been established (Table 3-1). Similar to many echocardiographic parameters, these Doppler velocities are also significantly affected by loading conditions, making determination of diastolic dysfunction by using these parameters alone very challenging in patients with congenital heart disease.

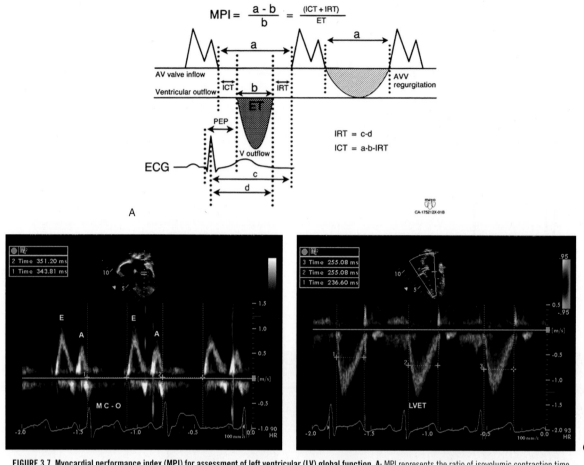

FIGURE 3.7. Myocardial performance index (MPI) for assessment of left ventricular (LV) global function. A: MPI represents the ratio of isovolumic contraction time (ICT) and isovolumic relaxation time (IRT) to ventricular ejection time (ET): MPI = (ICT + IRT)/ET. **B:** Pulsed-wave Doppler interrogation in the apical four-chamber view at the level of the mitral valve leaflets. The duration of ICT + IRT is measured from the cessation of mitral valve inflow to the onset of AV valve inflow of the next cardiac cycle (interval a). **C:** Pulsed-wave Doppler interrogation within the LV outflow tract in the apical five-chamber view. Ventricular ejection time is measured from the onset to cessation of LV ejection (interval b).

$$MPI = (a - b)/b = (ICT + IRT)/ET$$
$$= (347 - 249)/249$$
$$= 0.39$$

(**A,** From Eidem BW, et al. Non-geometric quantitative assessment of right and left ventricular function:myocardial performance index in normal children and patients with Ebstein anomaly. *J Am Soc Echocardiogr.* 1998;11:849–856. Used with permission.)

Evaluation of Diastolic Ventricular Function—Technical Considerations

A complete Doppler assessment of a ventricle's diastolic performance *must* include analysis of the flow signals across the AV valve and within the proximal central venous system (either pulmonary veins for the left ventricle or systemic veins for the right ventricle). Inaccurate assessment will result from attempts to draw conclusions from only one or the other of these flow signals. It is also critically important to obtain these flow signals appropriately or all subsequent conclusions drawn from them will be erroneous. The ultrasound instrument should be set at the lowest frequency and with the smallest sample volume (for pulsed Doppler) possible. This will maximize axial and lateral flow velocity resolution. Low-velocity filtering is used to eliminate tissue motion artifacts. These filters need to be set lower (200 to 600 Hertz) for pulsed-wave interrogation than for continuous-wave Doppler studies (800 to 1200 Hertz). For all signals, the Doppler beam must be aligned as close to parallel as possible with the interrogated flow. Color flow Doppler mapping is extremely useful in achieving optimal alignment.

For AV valve evaluation, the pulsed-wave sample volume is positioned between the tips of the open valve leaflets (Fig. 3.11). This will place the sample volume "below" the anatomic AV valve annulus, at a point within the proximal ventricular inflow tract. In many patients, the apical four-chamber view may *not* the best position to record AV valve signals. In fact, for the mitral valve, the best alignment is often achieved from the apical long-axis ("two-chamber") view. This is because normal mitral flow is directed somewhat laterally and posteriorly to the cardiac apex. This flow direction becomes even more pronounced in the dilated heart. Tricuspid inflow signals are often best recorded from a parasternal transducer position. Medial rotation and inferior angulation from the long-axis image will produce a "tricuspid inflow" view that can be used to sample this valve.

Recordings of central venous flow signals must be made within the vein, not at the junction of the vein and the receiving atrium or vena cava. In adults, it is generally recommended that the sample volume be at least 1 cm "upstream" from the venous orifice. In children, shorter distances must be accepted due to their smaller size, but the sample volume must be placed within the body of the vein to accurately record the flows, especially reversal flows.

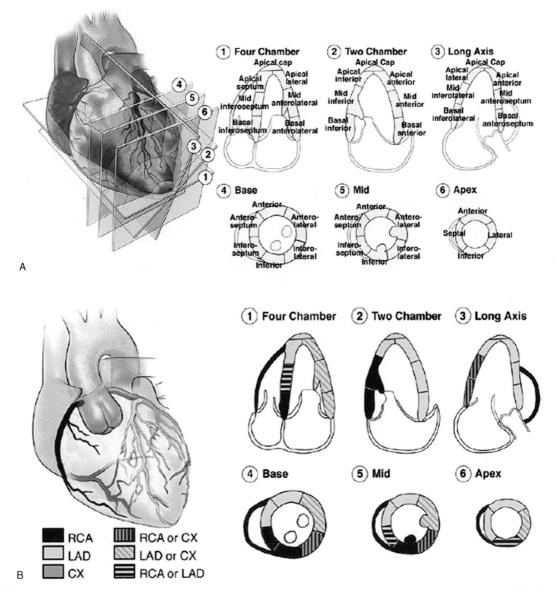

FIGURE 3.8. Seventeen-segment model for analysis of left ventricular wall motion proposed by the American Society of Echocardiography. A: Apical (four-, three-, and two-chamber) and parasternal short-axis views demonstrate the 16 myocardial segments + apical cap. **B:** Typical coronary artery distribution pattern to these myocardial segments. *Note:* Coronary arterial suppy is variable and may differ from the distribution pattern demonstrated. (From Lang RM, Bierig M, Devereux RB, et al. Recommendations for chamber quantification: a report from the American Society of Echocardiography's Guidelines and Standards Committee and the Chamber Quantification Writing Group, developed in conjunction with the European Association of Echocardiography, a branch of the European Society of Cardiology. *J Am Soc Echocardiogr.* 2005;18:1440–1463. Used with permission.)

The mitral valve inflow signal (Fig. 3.11) is divided into early (E wave) and atrial (A wave) components at the point where the mid-diastolic flow velocity curve changes from a negative to a positive slope (the E-at-A velocity). If no change in slope occurs or if the E-at-A velocity occurs at a velocity greater than one-half of the peak E velocity, then the signal should be considered fused. Deceleration time and total A wave duration should not be measured from fused signals. Mitral A wave duration includes the interval from the E-at-A velocity to cessation of forward flow.

Similarly, division of the pulmonary vein forward flow signal (Fig. 3.11) is made at the point where the flow-velocity curve changes slope. Systolic flows occur before and diastolic flows occur after the slope change. Pulmonary vein atrial reversal (PVAR) duration is measured from the onset to cessation of reversed flow occurring after the P wave on the simultaneously recorded, single-lead surface electrocardiogram (ECG). These measurements can be made in the same manner for flow signals recorded at the tricuspid valve and in the systemic (usually hepatic) veins.

The intrathoracic pressure changes associated with normal respiration markedly alter the filling of the right ventricle. Therefore, it is generally recommended that evaluation of right heart flow patterns be made at end-expiration. Alternatively, multiple sequential cycles can be averaged to account for the respiratory variation. Respiration has less affect on LV filling, but it is still wise to average the values from at least three consecutive signals.

Mitral Inflow Doppler

Mitral inflow obtained by pulsed-wave Doppler echocardiography represents the diastolic pressure gradient between the left atrium and left ventricle (Fig. 3.11). The early diastolic filling wave, or E wave, is the dominant diastolic wave in children and young adults and represents the peak left atrium–to–LV pressure gradient at the onset of diastole. The deceleration time of the mitral E wave reflects the time period needed for equalization of left atrial (LA) and LV pressure. The late diastolic filling wave, or A wave,

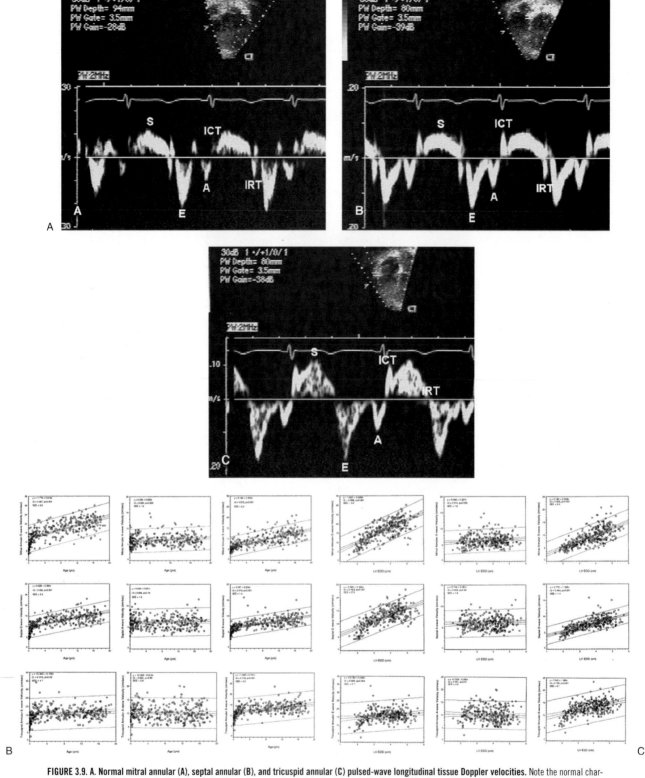

FIGURE 3.9. A. Normal mitral annular (A), septal annular (B), and tricuspid annular (C) pulsed-wave longitudinal tissue Doppler velocities. Note the normal characteristic pattern of a larger early diastolic velocity (E wave) compared with late diastolic velocity (A wave). The S wave is the systolic wave. **B:** Impact of increasing age on tissue Doppler velocities. **C:** Impact of increasing left ventricular end-diastolic dimension on tissue Doppler velocities. (From Eidem BW, et al. Clinical impact of altered left ventricular loading conditions on Doppler tissue imaging velocities: a study in congenital heart disease. *J Am Soc Echocardiogr.* 2005;18:830–838.)

represents the peak pressure gradient between the left atrium and the left ventricle in late diastole at the onset of atrial contraction. Normal mitral inflow Doppler is characterized by a dominant E wave, a smaller A wave, and a ratio of E and A waves (E:A ratio) between 1.0 and 3.0. Normal duration of mitral deceleration time and

isovolumic relaxation time vary with age and have been reported in both pediatric and adult populations. Mitral inflow Doppler velocities are affected not only by changes in LV diastolic function but also by a variety of additional hemodynamic factors, including age, altered loading conditions, heart rate, and changes in atrial and

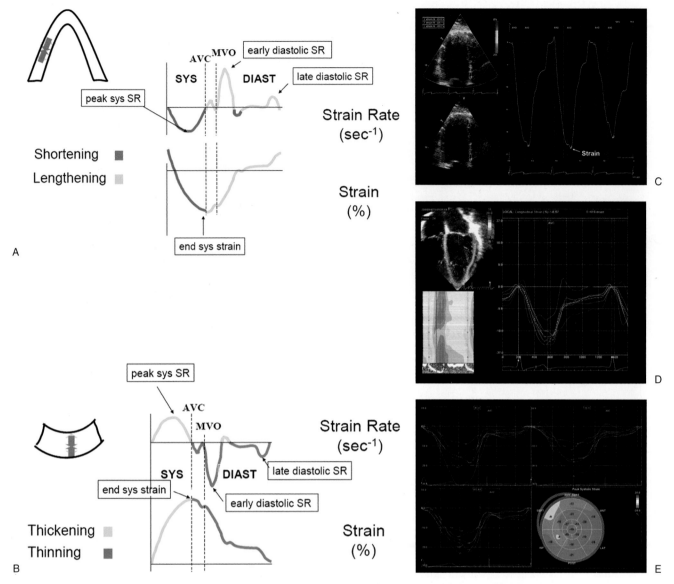

FIGURE 3.10. Schematic representation of longitudinal (A) and radial (B) strain and strain rate imaging. In the longitudinal direction, strain represents myocardial shortening (systole) and lengthening (diastole), whereas strain rate represents the rate at which shortening or lengthening occurs. Similarly, radial strain represents myocardial thickening (systole) and thinning (diastole), whereas strain rate represents the rate at which thickening or thinning occurs. AVC, aortic valve closure; MVO, mitral valve opening; sys, systolic; diast, diastolic. **C:** Normal Doppler-based strain acquired in an apical four-chamber orientation at the basal septum. **D:** Two-dimensional strain obtained in an apical four-chamber view in a normal child. Note the multiple colored curves that represent the various strain patterns in each myocardial segment. **E:** Two-dimensional strain in a patient with hypertrophic cardiomyopathy. Strain is determined from the apical four-, three-, and two-chamber views. Bull's eye diagram (*bottom right*) demonstrates strain in each myocardial segment. Note the decreased strain in the anterior septal, inferior, and septal wall segments. (**A** and **B**, Used with permission from Luc Mertens, MD.)

ventricular compliance. Interpretation of characteristic patterns of mitral inflow must be carefully evaluated, with particular attention paid to the potential impact of each of these hemodynamic factors on mitral inflow Doppler velocities.

Pulmonary Venous Doppler

Pulmonary venous Doppler, combined with mitral inflow Doppler, provides a more comprehensive assessment of LA and LV filling pressures. Pulmonary venous inflow consists of three distinct Doppler waves: a systolic wave (S wave), a diastolic wave (D wave), and a reversal wave with atrial contraction (Ar wave) (Fig. 3.11). In normal adolescents and adults, the characteristic pattern of pulmonary venous inflow consists of a dominant S wave, a smaller D wave, and a small Ar wave of low velocity and brief duration. In neonates and younger children, a dominant D wave is often present with a similar brief low-velocity, or even absent, Ar wave.

With worsening LV diastolic dysfunction, LA pressure increases leading to diminished systolic forward flow into the left atrium from the pulmonary veins with relatively increased diastolic forward flow resulting in a diastolic dominance of pulmonary venous inflow (Fig. 3.12). More important, both the velocity and duration of the pulmonary venous atrial reversal wave are increased. Pediatric and adult studies have demonstrated that an Ar-wave duration greater than 30 msec longer than the corresponding mitral A-wave duration or a ratio of pulmonary venous Ar wave to mitral A wave duration greater than 1.2 is predictive of elevated LV filling pressure (Fig. 3.13).

Patterns of Diastolic Dysfunction

Before attempting to analyze Doppler data regarding diastolic ventricular function, one must assess the general cardiac status of the patient. In the absence of abnormal anatomic/functional findings or clinical symptoms, Doppler data that exist slightly outside the 95% confidence limits may simply represent normal variation. However,

Table 3-1	NORMAL DIASTOLIC DOPPLER DATA IN CHILDREN		
	Age (y)		
	3–8 (n = 75)	9–12 (n = 72)	13–17 (n = 76)
Mitral valve			
E velocity (cm/s)	92 (14)	86 (15)	88 (14)
A velocity (cm/s)	42 (11)	41 (9)	39 (8)
A duration (ms)	136 (22)	142 (21)	141 (22)
E to A velocity ratio	2.4 (0.7)	2.2 (0.6)	2.3 (0.6)
Deceleration time (ms)	145 (18)	157 (19)	172 (22)
LV IVRT (ms)	62 (10)	67 (10)	74 (13)
Pulmonary vein			
Systolic velocity (cm/s)	46 (9)	45 (9)	41 (10)
Diastolic velocity (cm/s)	59 (8)	54 (9)	59 (11)
Atrial reversal velocity (cm/s)	21 (4)	21 (5)	21 (7)
Atrial reversal duration (ms)	130 (20)	125 (20)	140 (28)
Difference data			
PVAR duration − MV A duration (ms)	−8 (26)	−17 (24)	−6 (33)

Values in parentheses represent 1 SD.
From A, atrial filling wave; E, early filling wave; IVRT, isovolumic relaxation time; LV, left ventricle; MV, mitral valve; PVAR, pulmonary vein atrial reversal.
Modified from O'Leary PW et al. Diastolic ventricular function in children: a Doppler echocardiographic study establishing normal values and predictors of increased ventricular end-diastolic pressure. *Mayo Clin Proc* 1998;73:616–28 and reproduced with permission.

in the presence of symptoms or clear cardiac abnormalities, these deviations are much more likely to represent clinically significant diastolic dysfunction.

In discussions of diastolic function, two distinctive abnormal patterns of ventricular filling are usually recognized: abnormal relaxation and restrictive filling. However, the Doppler manifestations of diastolic dysfunction are probably better thought of as a continuum of gradually changing filling patterns, beginning with normal and ending with irreversible restrictive filling (Fig. 3.12). It is possible for a patient to move toward either a more or less severe level over time. Successful therapy may lead the patient to display a lesser degree of dysfunction. Alternatively, disease progression may move the filling patterns toward the more severe end of the spectrum.

Using this concept of diastolic disease, one can identify four "grades" of diastolic dysfunction. Normal filling can be thought of as grade "0" dysfunction. Figure 3.12 displays representative normal mitral valve and pulmonary vein flow tracings. Exact values will depend on both age and heart rate at the time of the recording. These

diagrams demonstrate the Doppler flow patterns observed at the AV valve and in the central veins for the various grades of diastolic dysfunction. Grade 0 is the normal flow pattern and is shown on the far left. As ventricular diastolic function deteriorates, flow patterns shown farther to the right of the figure become apparent. These filling patterns represent a continuum of ventricular compliance and function. A single patient can display a variety of patterns depending on loading conditions, their stage of disease, and the success of therapeutic maneuvers. Only grade 4 dysfunction (irreversible restrictive filling) implies a permanent change in ventricular function.

Abnormal relaxation is considered to be grade 1 diastolic dysfunction. This is the initial abnormality seen in most forms of heart disease, and ventricular compliance is usually still normal. Abnormal relaxation is especially common in disorders producing myocardial hypertrophy. The AV valve early filling velocity is reduced and the atrial component of ventricular filling becomes dominant (E/A ratio <1.0). Diastolic ventricular relaxation is slowed, resulting in prolongation of the isovolumic relaxation time and the mitral deceleration time. Venous diastolic velocity decreases in parallel with the E wave. A slight increase in the systolic velocity can be observed. Venous atrial reversals are variable but usually remain within normal limits at this stage (Fig. 3.12).

As the patient transitions from the early/mild stage of abnormal relaxation to more advanced diastolic dysfunction, the AV valve E-wave velocity will increase. This increase in early velocity is due primarily to increasing atrial pressure, caused by deterioration of diastolic function (reduced ventricular compliance). This increase in pressure "restores" the trans-AV valve flow gradient in early diastole and creates an AV valve inflow pattern with a normal E/A ratio, leading to the term "pseudo-normalization." In our schema for grading diastolic disease, this is referred to as grade 2 diastolic dysfunction and can be distinguished from truly normal filling in one of two ways. A patient has grade 2 dysfunction when he demonstrates a "normal" AV valve filling pattern and has an atrial reversal in the central vein that is abnormally large and long (velocity greater than 95% confidence limit and reversal duration usually 20 msec longer than the AV valve A wave; Fig. 3.14). This is usually associated with moderate diastolic impairment, mildly to moderately elevated atrial mean pressure, and rising ventricular end-diastolic pressure. In patients where venous flow signals are poor or confusing, one can acutely reduce ventricular preload and then reassess the filling patterns. This is most conveniently done by having the patient perform a Valsalva maneuver. In the setting of grade 2 dysfunction, E-wave velocity will decrease, the A wave will increase, and deceleration time will lengthen during Valsalva, unmasking the underlying relaxation abnormality by decreasing atrial filling (preload). A truly normal patient will display symmetrical reductions in E- and A-wave velocity and deceleration time will not change significantly after a Valsalva maneuver.

The filling pattern associated with the most advanced stage of diastolic disease is restrictive filling. Flow signals in this group display a high-velocity, but abbreviated, AV valve E wave, shortened deceleration time, and little additional ventricular filling with

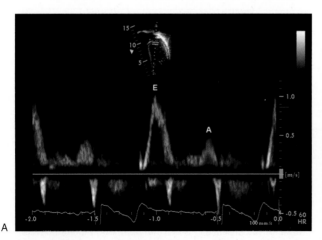
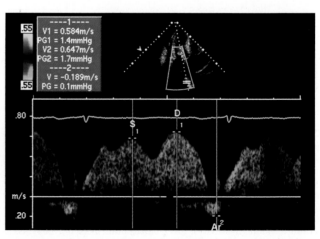

FIGURE 3.11. Normal mitral inflow (A) and pulmonary venous inflow Doppler (B). E, early diastolic wave; A, atrial filling wave; S, systolic venous wave; D, diastolic venous wave; Ar, atrial reversal wave.

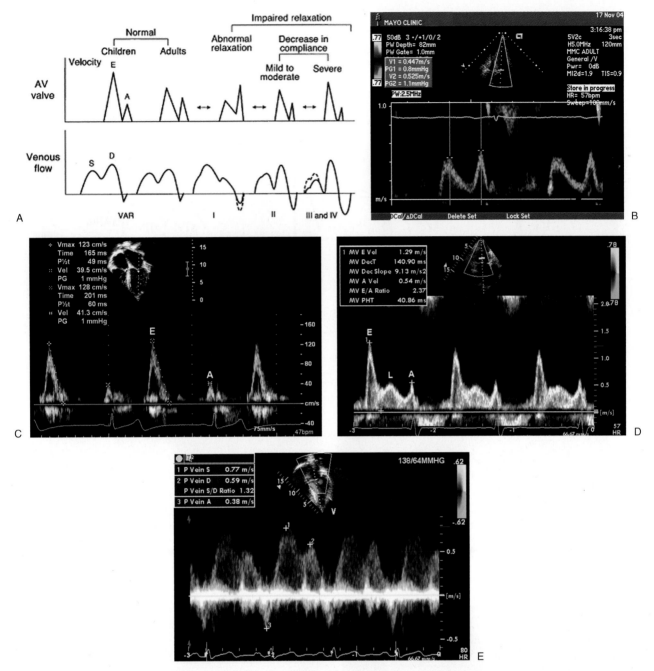

FIGURE 3.12. Inflow in children and adults. A: Spectrum of mitral and pulmonary venous inflow patterns in diastolic dysfunction in children (see text). **B:** Pulsed-wave mitral inflow Doppler in an adult demonstrating abnormal relaxation pattern with E:A ratio of less than 1. **C:** Pulsed-wave mitral inflow Doppler demonstrating restrictive filling pattern with increased E-wave velocity, decreased A-wave velocity, and E:A ratio greater than 3. **D:** Mitral inflow Doppler in adolescent with hypertrophic cardiomyopathy. Note the prominent mid-diastolic filling wave ("L wave") consistent with severely impaired left ventricular relaxation. **E:** Pulsed-wave pulmonary venous inflow Doppler. Note prominent atrial reversal velocity and prolonged duration. AV, atrioventricular; E, early filling wave; A, atrial filling wave; S, systolic filling wave; D, diastolic filling wave; VAR, atrial reversal wave. (A, From Olivier M, O'Leary PW, Pankranz S, et al. Serial Doppler assessment of diastolic function before and after the Fontan operation. *J Am Soc Echocardiogr.* 2003;16:1136–1143. Used with permission.)

atrial contraction (Fig. 3.13). Central venous flows are decreased in systole due to increased mean atrial pressure. Early diastolic flow velocities are increased due to elevated venous pressure "rushing" flow to cross the AV valve as it opens, but duration of diastolic flow is reduced, reflecting the abbreviated AV valve E wave and markedly reduced ventricular compliance. Atrial reversal is now quite prominent, assuming sinus rhythm and normal atrial contractility. Venous atrial reversal duration is now much longer than the AV valve A wave (greater than 30 msec).

Both grade 3 and 4 diastolic dysfunction are characterized by restrictive filling patterns. The difference between these stages of diastolic dysfunction has to do with reversibility, bringing us back to

the concept of a continuum. The patient who presents with restrictive filling and improves with treatment (later displays a filling pattern consistent with either grade 1 or 2 dysfunction) initially had grade 3 dysfunction. The patient who retains a restrictive filling pattern, despite all treatments has the most severe form of diastolic dysfunction and is classified as grade 4 dysfunction (irreversible restrictive filling).

Clinical Utility of Diastology

Many common cardiac disorders can result in impaired diastolic ventricular function. In children and adults, diastolic dysfunction

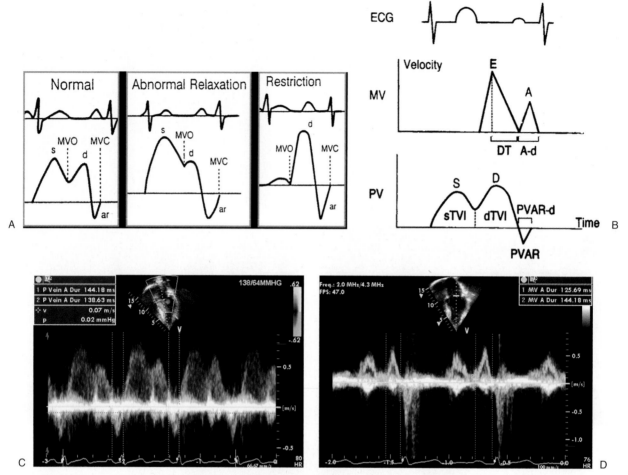

FIGURE 3.13. Pulmonary venous Doppler in the assessment of left ventricular (LV) diastolic function. A: Changes in pulmonary venous Doppler with diastolic dysfunction. Note the significant increase in atrial reversal velocity and duration with increasing degrees of diastolic dysfunction. Significant changes in systolic and diastolic filling also occur (see text). MVO, mitral valve opening; MVC, mitral valve closure. **B:** Diagram depicts mitral valve and pulmonary vein Doppler flow tracings. Diastolic dysfunction with increased LV filling pressure leads to increased duration and velocity of pulmonary venous atrial reversal wave. A, atrial filling wave; A-d, duration of atrial filling wave; D, pulmonary vein diastolic flow wave; DT, mitral deceleration time; dTVI, time-velocity integral of pulmonary vein diastolic flow wave; E, early filling wave; ECG, electrocardiogram; PVAR, pulmonary vein atrial reversal wave; PVAR-d, duration of pulmonary vein atrial reversal flow; S, pulmonary vein systolic flow wave; sTVI, time-velocity integral of pulmonary vein systolic flow wave. **C:** Measurement of pulmonary venous atrial reversal duration. **D:** Measurement of duration of mitral atrial filling wave. (From O'Leary PW, Durongpisitkul K, Cordes TM, et al. Diastolic ventricular function in children: a Doppler echocardiographic study establishing normal values and predictors of increased ventricular end-diastolic pressure. *Mayo Clin Proc.* 1998;73:616–628. Used with permission.)

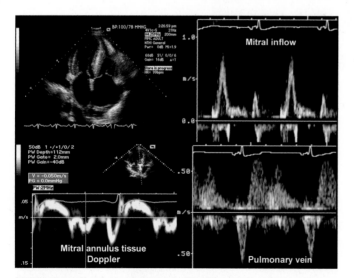

FIGURE 3.14. Pseudonormal (grade 2) diastolic filling abnormality. Top left: Two-dimensional image in adult with hypertrophic cardiomyopathy. **Top right:** Mitral inflow Doppler suggestive of normal early (E) and atrial (A) filling velocities with normal E:A ratio. **Bottom right:** Pulmonary venous Doppler with prominent atrial reversal velocity and duration. **Bottom left:** Tissue Doppler at the medial septal annulus with significantly decreased early annular and septal velocities.

can even precede the onset of systolic dysfunction. As a result, serial examinations demonstrating increasing diastolic dysfunction provide a valuable marker of disease progression. For example, in patients with aortic regurgitation, diastolic filling patterns will remain normal or at a grade 1 level (abnormal relaxation) until ventricular compliance decreases. This decrease in compliance will be manifested by a change to a pseudo-normalized filling pattern (grade 2 dysfunction). This change in Doppler pattern indicates that the ventricle has exceeded the limits of its Starling curve and can be used by the clinician as a guide to timing for surgical intervention.

Qualitative versus Quantitative Diastology

The concepts described thus far have focused on outlining Doppler patterns that are associated with normal or abnormal ventricular diastolic performance. The grading continuum provides a "semi-quantitative" approach to classifying the severity of the abnormal filling pattern observed. Researchers have also tried to develop formulae to quantitate diastolic cardiac pressures. However, clinicians are not yet able to truly perform quantitative assessments of diastolic function in most children.

There are two exceptions. First, it is possible to indirectly "measure" LA mean pressure in the patient with a restrictive atrial septal defect. This is done by recording the maximal LA–to–right atrial (RA) flow signal with continuous-wave Doppler. The signal is then traced

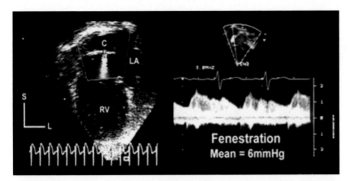

FIGURE 3.15. Fenestrated Fontan connection with continuous "right atrial (RA)"–to–neo-left atrial (LA) shunt. The Doppler flow pattern, assessed for mean gradient, is helpful to quantitate the pressure difference between the two "atrial" chambers. In this patient, the RA-to-LA mean pressure difference was 6 mm Hg. This is consistent with a low (normal) transpulmonary gradient. The patient's central venous pressure was 14 mm Hg, which would predict a mean LA pressure of 8 mm Hg. LA, left atrium; RV, right ventricle; C, Fontan connection.

to determine the mean "gradient" between the atria. It is best to trace multiple, consecutive cycles, to account for respiratory variation. The gradient across the atrial septum can then be added to the assumed (or measured) RA pressure to give the mean LA pressure. The most common clinical scenarios in which this can be applied are the neonate with hypoplastic left heart syndrome (HLHS) and a restrictive PFO and, less commonly, the patient with mitral stenosis and a small atrial septal defect. This concept can also be applied to the patient with a "fenestrated" Fontan circulation (Fig. 3.15). In this case, the gradient indicates by how much the mean "RA" pressure exceeds the neo-LA pressure. If the patient's central venous pressure is known, the LA pressure can be determined by subtracting the mean "fenestration" gradient from the central venous pressure value. This can be helpful in the cardiac intensive care unit, allowing noninvasive assessment of both transpulmonary gradient and LV preload.

Second, a gross estimation of LV end-diastolic pressure can be made by examining the relative durations of the mitral A wave and the pulmonary vein atrial reversal (Fig. 3.13). It has been demonstrated that a pulmonary vein atrial reversal duration that exceeds the A-wave duration by more than 29 msec provides a relatively reliable marker for elevated end-diastolic pressure (18 mm Hg or greater). It must be noted that the sensitivity and specificity for this value were 90% and 86%, respectively. This reemphasizes the need to interpret Doppler data in conjunction with the overall assessment of cardiac status. Clearly some *normal* children can have "abnormal" Doppler flow patterns. The presence of these flow patterns in a patient with cardiac disease will have much greater predictive value than when they are seen in an otherwise normal child.

Limitations and Pitfalls of Doppler Evaluation of Diastolic Ventricular Function

Although Doppler echocardiography can provide tremendous insights into diastolic ventricular function, there are limits to our current understanding. Almost all of the preceding discussion assumes that the patient is in a regular sinus rhythm at the time of the evaluation. Irregular rhythms are difficult to analyze and require that the cardiac cycle length be "matched" when comparing venous and AV valve flow variables. Junctional or ventricular rhythms make assessments invalid that depend on atrial contraction.

The most significant pitfall inherent to this type of diastolic evaluation is the fact that AV valve and venous flow patterns are significantly influenced by variations in ventricular preload. Conditions of reduced volume loading (prolonged fasting, diuretic use) can potentially make significant diastolic dysfunction appear less severe (analogous to the Valsalva maneuver when used to detect "pseudo-normal" filling). Markedly increased volume loads (regurgitation, left-to-right shunts) can produce flow patterns suggestive of severe diastolic dysfunction even when the ventricular compliance is nearly normal. The echocardiographer must take into

account the loading conditions present at the time of the evaluation before making a final assessment of the ventricle. As a result, we can only state the diastolic function is normal or abnormal if loading conditions are normal. Conservely, if loading is abnormal (especially if there are increased volume loads present), then we are really able to evaluate diastolic filling pressures, not the underlying myocardial function, with these techniques.

Some congenital heart defects can make diastolic evaluation difficult. AV valve stenosis makes this method of assessment nearly meaningless. It is impossible to separate the disturbed AV valve and venous flows caused by the stenosis from those caused by the ventricle. One must then rely on other techniques (isovolumic relaxation time, tissue Doppler, or automated border detection) to assess diastolic function. Significant AV valve regurgitation can alter systolic flow in the central veins. In these cases, one must rely on AV valve flow patterns and venous atrial reversals more heavily. Tissue Doppler imaging can also be very helpful in these patients. Large atrial septal defects result in equilibration of atrial pressures and make it impossible to separate RV from LV diastolic activity. The flow patterns will reflect the function of the more compliant ("healthier") ventricle in the presence of a large atrial septal defect. This is not a problem in the functionally univentricular heart because both atria are committed to the same ventricle. Also, in keeping with the concept of diastolic disorders presenting as a continuum, not all patients with diastolic abnormalities display flow patterns that are easily placed into one of the four broad categories of dysfunction. In these cases, one may not be able to specifically "grade" the degree of disease, but it is usually possible to identify the patient as abnormal.

Last, some patients may not have optimal signals available for analysis. In these cases, it is best to state that the examination was not adequate to comment on diastolic function. Attempts to use signals obtained from poor sample volume positions or of inadequate clarity will usually result in incorrect conclusions about the status of the ventricle.

NEWER ECHOCARDIOGRAPHIC TECHNIQUES TO EVALUATE DIASTOLIC VENTRICULAR FUNCTION

Tissue Doppler Imaging

Tissue Doppler imaging is particularly well suited to the quantitative evaluation of LV diastolic function. Both early (Ea) and late (Aa) annular diastolic velocities can be readily obtained with the use of tissue Doppler echocardiography (Fig. 3.9). Similar to systolic tissue Doppler velocities, differences in diastolic velocities exist between (a) the subendocardium and subepicardium, (b) from cardiac base to apex, and (c) between various myocardial wall segments. Previous studies have reported an excellent correlation between the early annular diastolic mitral velocity and simultaneous invasive measures of diastolic function at cardiac catheterization. Early annular diastolic velocities also appear to be less sensitive to changes in ventricular preload compared with the corresponding early transmitral Doppler inflow velocity. These diastolic tissue Doppler velocities, however, are affected by significant alterations in preload. The impact of afterload on tissue Doppler velocities is less controversial, with many studies documenting significant changes in systolic and diastolic annular velocities with changes in ventricular afterload. Therefore, the clinical use of tissue Doppler velocities in patients with valvar stenosis or other etiology of altered ventricular afterload needs to be interpreted carefully in light of this limitation.

Tissue Doppler velocities have been shown to be clinically helpful in the discrimination between normal and pseudo-normal transmitral Doppler filling patterns. In addition to changes incurred by loading conditions, alterations in LA pressure and LVEDP also affect the early transmitral diastolic velocity. However, the corresponding tissue Doppler velocity is characteristically decreased in patients with pseudo-normal filling, allowing differentiation of this abnormal filling pattern from one of normal transmitral Doppler inflow. Clinical reports have suggested a ratio of the early transmitral inflow Doppler signal to the lateral mitral annular early diastolic velocity (mitral E/Ea) as a noninvasive measure of LV filling pressure. Nagueh and colleagues (1997) demonstrated a significant correlation of mitral

E/Ea with invasively measured mean pulmonary capillary wedge pressure, whereas subsequent studies have further validated this ratio and reported its applicability in a variety of hemodynamic settings. Additional novel indices of LV diastolic function using tissue Doppler echocardiography have recently been reported that may further expand the role of this modality in the clinical evaluation of LV filling pressures.

Tissue Doppler has also been shown to be of considerable clinical value in the differentiation of constrictive from restrictive LV filling. Evaluation of patients with constrictive pericarditis and restrictive cardiomyopathy with two-dimensional echocardiography and even invasive cardiac catheterization may fail to confidently differentiate these two disease states. Because the myocardium in patients with constrictive pericarditis is most commonly normal, the corresponding tissue Doppler velocities are also normal. However, patients with restrictive cardiomyopathy have been shown to have significantly decreased early diastolic as well as systolic tissue Doppler velocities, allowing separation of these two distinct clinical entities.

Tissue Doppler Studies in Normal Children

To date, a number of transthoracic echocardiographic studies have been performed in children to establish normal reference values of tissue Doppler velocities in this cohort (Table 3-2). Similar to previously published reports for adults, pediatric tissue Doppler velocities vary with age, heart rate, wall location, and myocardial layer. In addition, pulsed-wave tissue Doppler velocities are also highly correlated with parameters of cardiac growth, most notably LVEDD and LV mass, with the most significant changes in these velocities occurring during the first year of life (Fig. 3.9). In a recently published large series of infants and children, tissue Doppler velocities did not correlate significantly with other more commonly used measures of systolic and diastolic ventricular performance including LV shortening fraction, LV and RV myocardial performance indices, and transmitral inflow Doppler. This lack of correlation in part is likely due to pulsed-wave tissue Doppler assessing longitudinal ventricular function while other more traditional two-dimensional and Doppler methods assess radial and global measures of ventricular performance.

Similar to previously published adult normative data, normal values for the E/Ea ratio in children have also been reported. These values are also affected by age, heart rate, ventricular wall location, LV dimension, and LV mass. Values for E/Ea are highest in neonates and decrease with advancing age primarily due to an increased Ea velocity over this time period. Simultaneous echo:cath measurements correlating the E/Ea ratio in children with invasive measures of LV filling pressure are lacking to date. In a small cohort of children, invasive cardiac catheterization measures of LV function were compared with simultaneously obtained color M-mode and Doppler parameters of LV performance. The ratio of early diastolic mitral annular tissue Doppler velocity to flow propagation velocity (Ea/Vp) correlated closely with invasive LV end diastolic pressure while the septal Ea velocity correlated with the time constant of relaxation (tau).

Table 3-2 | **PULSED WAVE DOPPLER TISSUE VELOCITIES AND TIME INTERVALS IN HEALTHY CHILDREN BY AGE GROUP**

Age group	N	E'-wave velocity	A'-wave velocity	S'-wave velocity	ICT	IRT	E/E ratio
Mitral annular							
<1 y	63	9.7 ± 3.3 (8.8 – 10.5)	5.7 ± 1.8 (5.3 – 6.2)	5.7 ± 1.6 (5.3 – 6.1)	77.4 ±18.4 (72.7 – 82.0)	57.0 ± 14.8 (53.1 – 60.8)	8.8 ± 2.7 (8.1 – 9.5)
1–5y	68	15.1 ± 3.4† (14.3 – 15.4)	6.5 ± 1.9 (6.1 – 7.0)	7.7 ± 2.1† (7.2 – 8.2)	76.9 ± 15.9 (72.8 – 80.9)	62.1 ±13.2 (58.9 – 65.4)	6.5 ± 2.0† (6.0 – 7.0)
6–9y	55	17.2 ± 3.7† (16.2 – 18.3)	6.7 ± 1.9 (6.2 – 7.3)	9.5 ± 2.1† (8.9 – 10.1)	77.9 ± 18.9 (72.4 – 83.4)	62.9 ± 11.9 (59.5 – 66.3)	5.8 ± 1.9 (5.3 – 6.4)
10–13y	58	19.6 ± 3.4† (18.7 – 20.5)	6.4 ± 1.8 (5.9 – 6.9)	10.8 ± 2.9* (10.0 – 11.5)	79.6 ± 16.2 (72.4 – 80.9)	62.6 ± 12.4 (59.4 – 65.9)	4.9 ± 1.3 (4.6 – 5.2)
14–18y	81	20.6 ± 3.8 (19.7 – 21.4)	6.7 ± 1.6 (6.3 – 7.1)	12.3 ± 2.9† (11.6 – 12.9)	78.9 ± 15.4 (75.4 – 82.3)	69.5 ± 15.5* (66.1 – 73.0)	4.7 ± 1.3 (4.4 – 5.0)
Total	325	16.5 ± 5.3 (16.0 – 17.1)	6.4 ± 1.9 (6.2 – 6.6)	9.3 ± 3.4 (8.9 – 9.7)	77.5 ± 16.7 (75.7 – 79.5)	63.2 ± 14.4 (61.7 – 64.9)	6.1 ± 2.4 (5.9 – 6.4)
Septal							
<1y	63	8.1 ± 2.5 (7.5 – 8.7)	6.1 ± 1.5 (5.7 – 6.4)	5.4 ± 1.2 (5.1 – 5.7)	77.5 ± 17.5 (73.0 – 82.0)	53.0 ± 11.7 (50.0 – 56.0)	10.3 ± 2.7 (9.7 – 11.0)
1–5y	68	11.8 ± 2.0† (11.3 – 12.3)	6.0 ± 1.3 (5.7 – 6.4)	7.1 ± 1.5† (6.8 – 7.5)	80.1 ± 15.5 (76.3 – 83.9)	59.8 ± 12.0 (56.9 – 62.7)	8.1 ± 1.8† (7.7 – 8.5)
6–9y	55	13.4 ± 1.9† (12.8 – 13.9)	5.9 ± 1.3 (5.5 – 6.3)	8.0 ± 1.3 (7.6 – 8.4)	82.8 ± 15.3 (78.4 – 87.2)	65.6 ± 10.7 (62.5 – 68.7)	7.2 ± 1.6 (6.8 – 7.7)
10–13y	58	14.5 ± 2.6 (13.8 – 15.2)	6.1 ± 2.3 (5.6 – 6.7)	8.2 ± 1.3 (7.9 – 8.5)	87.9 ± 16.4* (83.6 – 92.2)	72.5 ± 12.3 (69.3 – 75.8)	6.6 ± 1.4 (6.3 – 7.0)
14–18y	81	14.9 ± 2.4 (14.3 – 15.4)	6.2 ± 1.5 (5.9 – 6.6)	9.0 ± 1.5 (8.7 – 9.3)	88.4 ± 15.6 (84.9 – 91.9)	77.5 ± 14.5 (74.3 – 80.8)	6.4 ± 1.5 (6.1 – 6.8)
Total	325	12.6 ± 3.4 (12.2 – 13.0)	6.1 ± 1.6 (5.9 – 6.3)	7.6 ± 1.9 (7.4 – 7.8)	83.5 ± 16.5 (81.7 – 85.4)	66.1 ± 15.3 (64.4 – 67.9)	7.7 ± 2.3 (7.5 – 8.0)
Tricuspid annular							
<1y	63	13.8 ± 8.2 (11.7 – 15.9)	9.8 ± 2.4 (9.1 – 10.5)	10.2 ± 5.5 (8.8 – 11.7)	68.7 ± 18.2 (63.9 – 73.5)	52.0 ± 12.9 (48.5 – 55.4)	4.4 ± 2.3 (3.8 – 5.0)
1–5y	68	17.1 ± 4.0† (16.1 – 18.1)	10.9 ± 2.7 (10.2 – 11.6)	13.2 ± 2.0† (12.7 – 13.7)	77.7 ± 15.0 (73.9 – 81.5)	59.0 ± 13.9 (55.4 – 62.5)	3.8 ± 1.1 (3.5 – 4.1)
6–9y	55	16.5 ± 3.0 (15.7 – 17.4)	9.8 ± 2.7 (9.0 – 10.6)	13.4 ± 2.0 (12.8 – 14.0)	91.8 ± 21.5† (85.5 – 98.0)	58.5 ± 17.5 (53.4 – 63.6)	3.6 ±0.8 (3.4 – 3.9)
10–13y	58	16.5 ± 3.1 (15.7 – 17.4)	10.3 ±3.4 (9.3 – 11.2)	13.9 ± 2.4 (13.2 – 14.5)	98.1 ± 21.7 (92.2 – 103.9)	61.7 ± 19.9 (56.4 – 67.1)	3.5 ± 1.4 (3.2 – 3.9)
14–18y	81	16.7 ± 2.8 (16.0 – 17.3)	10.1 ± 2.6 (9.5 – 10.7)	14.2 ± 2.3 (13.7 – 14.7)	101.9 ± 20.4 (97.2 – 106.6)	63.9 ± 18.9 (58.5 – 67.3)	3.7 ± 1.0 (3.5 – 3.9)
Total	325	16.1 ± 4.7 (15.6 – 16.7)	10.2 ± 2.8 (9.9 – 10.5)	13.0 ± 3.4 (12.6 – 13.4)	88.2 ± 23.1 (85.6 – 90.8)	59.0 ± 17.2 (57.0 – 60.9)	3.8 ± 1.4 (3.6 – 4.0)

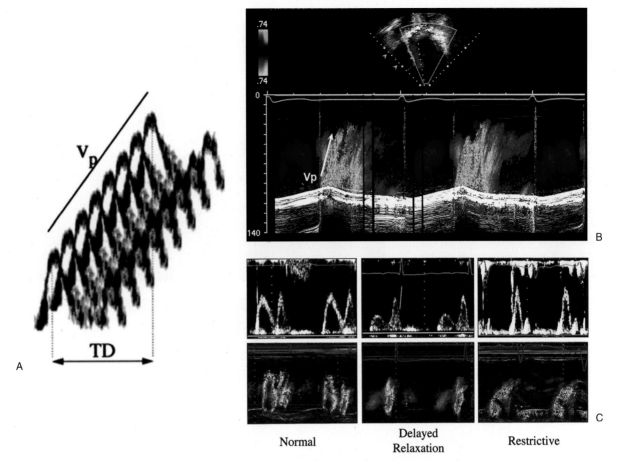

FIGURE 3.16. Measurement of flow propagation velocity (Vp) from color M-mode Doppler in the assessment of left ventricular (LV) diastolic function. **A:** Diagram demonstrating sequential pulsed Doppler mitral inflow signals as they are propagated from the base to the apex. **B:** Vp is determined by the slope of the first clearly demarcated aliasing velocity (white line) during early LV filling. **C:** Paired examples of mitral inflow pulsed Doppler and color Doppler flow propagation. Note that as diastolic dysfunction worsens, the slope of Vp decreases. E, early filling wave; A, atrial filling wave; TD, time delay in ventricular filling. (**A** and **C**, From Garcia MJ, Thomas JD, Klein AL. New Doppler echocardiographic applications for the study of diastolic function. *J Am Coll Cardiol.* 1998;32:865–875. Used with permission.)

Color M-mode Flow Propagation Velocity

Flow propagation of early diastolic filling from the mitral annulus to the cardiac apex can be quantitated by color M-mode echocardiography (Fig. 3.16). As opposed to mitral inflow Doppler, this propagation velocity has been shown to be significantly less affected by changes in heart rate, LA pressure, and loading conditions and therefore may more accurately reflect changes in myocardial relaxation. Numerous studies have demonstrated a significant decrease in flow propagation velocity in patients with diastolic dysfunction of varying etiology. In addition, Ea/Vp has also been shown to be a significant predictor of congestive heart failure and outcome in patients after myocardial infarction. This ratio of flow propagation and Doppler tissue imaging velocity may also be helpful in distinguishing a normal mitral inflow pattern from one of pseudo-normalized mitral inflow. In a small cohort of children undergoing simultaneous cardiac catheterization and transthoracic echocardiography, Border and colleagues (2003) showed a significant correlation between invasively measured LVEDP and the ratio of peak early transmitral Doppler flow velocity to flow propagation velocity (E/Vp). Similar studies have been published for adult data.

Left Atrial Volume

LA volume (LAV) has been identified as a marker of chronically increased LV filling pressure and has been increasingly appreciated as a clinical predictor of adverse cardiovascular outcomes in adults with cardiac disease. Studies evaluating LAV in normal infants and children and in young patients with hypertrophic cardiomyopathy have recently been published.

Several methods to measure LAV have been reported, including the biplane area-length method, the prolate ellipse method, the biplane Simpson method, and three-dimensional echocardiographically derived LAV. The biplane area-length method is demonstrated in Figure 3.17. Maximal LA area is planimetered at end ventricular systole just before opening of the mitral valve in the orthogonal apical four-chamber and two-chamber views. Care is taken to exclude the confluence of the pulmonary veins and the LA appendage. The length of the left atrium is measured in each of these orthogonal planes using a perpendicular line from the midpoint of the plane of the mitral annulus to the superior aspect of the LA free wall. LAV is calculated as follows:

$$LAV = 0.85[(\text{LA four-chamber area}) \times (\text{LA two-chamber area})]/ \text{shorter measured LA length}$$

LAV is most commonly indexed to body surface area. The normal range for LAV in adults is 22 ± 6 ml/m^2. Similar indexed values for LAV in normal children over 3 months of age have also been recently reported.

 ECHOCARDIOGRAPHIC ASSESSMENT OF RIGHT VENTRICULAR FUNCTION

Echocardiographic assessment of RV function has been limited due to the geometric shape of the right ventricle. Doppler echocardiography has historically been useful in the noninvasive prediction of RV systolic and pulmonary artery pressures. However, quantification of RV systolic function by M-mode or two-dimensional echocardiography has relied on the visual assessment

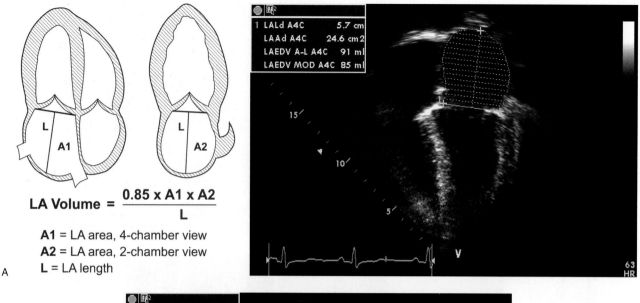

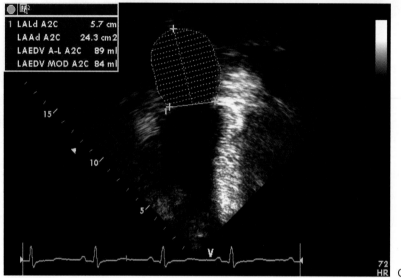

FIGURE 3.17. Left atrial volume (LAV). A: Calculation of LAV using the biplane area-length method. Left atrial length is measured in two orthogonal planes (apical four-chamber and two-chamber views) with the shorter length used to calculate LAV. LA area is traced in both views with care taken to exclude the LA appendage and entrance of the pulmonary veins. Example of LAV measured in the apical four-chamber (**B**) and two-chamber views (**C**). (From Oh JK, Seward JB, Tajik AJ. The echo manual. 3rd ed. [Figure 7-6, p. 112]. Philadelphia, Pa: Lippincott Williams & Wilkins; 2006. Used with permission.)

of relative RV wall motion or semiquantitative measurements of fractional area change in RV dimension or volume. Newer echocardiographic modalities that have shown promise in quantifying RV function include additional Doppler measures of RV performance (myocardial performance index, RV dP/dt, and Doppler tissue imaging) and acoustic quantification and three-dimensional echocardiography.

Right Ventricular Myocardial Performance Index

As described previously, the MPI is a Doppler-derived measure of global ventricular function that can be applied to any ventricular geometry (Fig. 3.7). Studies have validated the ability of the MPI to quantitatively assess RV function in adults and patients with congenital heart disease. In addition, the MPI has demonstrated prognostic power in discriminating outcome in patients with either RV or LV failure. Care, however, must be exercised in using this index in patients with congenital heart disease with altered RV preload or afterload. The RV MPI has been shown to be relatively independent of changes in chronic loading conditions, but the impact of acute changes in physiologic loading are significant and need further definition.

Right Ventricular dP/dt

Similar to the left ventricle, the rate of pressure change over time can also be used as a measure of RV systolic function in patients with tricuspid regurgitation. RV dP/dt has been shown to have correlation with invasive measures of RV performance. RV dP/dt has also been shown to be helpful in the serial assessment of RV function in children with HLHS. Similar to LV limitations with this parameter, RV dP/dt is affected by changes in loading conditions.

Right Ventricular Tissue Doppler Imaging

A relatively new addition to the quantitative evaluation of RV function is tissue Doppler imaging. Tricuspid annular motion has been shown to correlate with RV function in previous studies. TDI has been shown to be a reproducible noninvasive method of assessing systolic and diastolic annular motion and RV function (Fig. 3.10). While affected by both afterload and preload, studies in adults and children with TDI have demonstrated these velocities to be less influenced by altered preload than corresponding mitral or tricuspid inflow Doppler.

Acoustic Quantification and Right Ventricular Function

Acoustic quantification uses ABD techniques to measure the absolute change and rate of change in RV volume. This modality has been shown to correlate with other invasive methods of RV functional assessment in adults with abnormalities of global RV function. Automated border methods have also shown good correlation with magnetic resonance imaging in assessing changes in RV volume and systolic function. Feasibility of acoustic quantification in the noninvasive transthoracic evaluation of RV function in normal children has also been reported. Ongoing investigation is needed to establish the potential of this technique for the identification and serial evaluation of RV dysfunction in children.

Three-dimensional Echocardiography and Right Ventricular Function

Recent advances in three-dimensional echocardiography have enabled the noninvasive evaluation of RV volume and function. Because three-dimensional echocardiography can be used to evaluate RV geometry in multiple spatial planes, accurate assessment of changes in RV volume during the cardiac cycle is now possible. Application of this new modality to the evaluation of RV volume and systolic function in adults and children appears promising, and is discussed in detail later in this text.

Evaluation of Right Ventricular Diastolic Function

When RV compliance is significantly reduced (a "stiff" ventricle) and pulmonary pressures are low, it is possible for even atrial contraction to "open" the pulmonary valve and cause forward flow into the pulmonary artery. This can be seen on either continuous- or pulsed-wave Doppler signals obtained from the main pulmonary artery (Fig. 3.18). This phenomenon is most often observed in patients with chronic RV outflow obstruction. In the early postoperative period, this pattern can reflect reduced cardiac output in patients on mechanical positive pressure ventilation. The positive intrathoracic pressures generated by the ventilator impair the RA's ability to contribute to forward flow. Paradoxically, in the late follow-up of patients after tetralogy of Fallot repair, this pattern (pulmonary arterial forward flow due to atrial contraction) has been associated with improved exercise performance. This is likely due to the fact that a poorly compliant right ventricle will "accept" less regurgitant flow, and thereby has more effective "forward" output, than a normally compliant ventricle. In either situation, the presence of this atrial forward flow in the pulmonary artery is a reliable sign of reduced RV compliance and represents significantly abnormal diastolic function (usually grade 2 or greater).

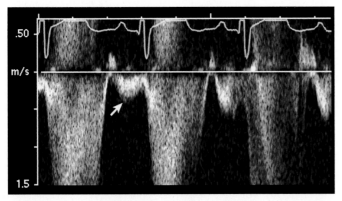

FIGURE 3.18. Restrictive right ventricular (RV) filling in postoperative tetralogy of Fallot. Parasternal short-axis scan with pulsed-wave Doppler interrogation in the main pulmonary artery. Note the antegrade forward flow (*arrow*) into the pulmonary artery with atrial contraction. This Doppler pattern is consistent with decreased RV compliance.

ECHOCARDIOGRAPHIC ASSESSMENT OF SINGLE VENTRICLE FUNCTION IN PATIENTS WITH COMPLEX CONGENITAL HEART DISEASE

Quantitative measurement of ventricular function in patients with functional single ventricles can be challenging. In most cases, a visual estimate of systolic function from two-dimensional images is used. Quantitative echocardiographic assessment is limited by complex ventricular geometry, often with associated abnormalities of wall motion.

Similar to novel techniques used to assess RV function, Doppler echocardiography holds promise in the potential evaluation of global single ventricle function. However, only limited studies to date have addressed either dP/dt or the MPI in patients with functional single ventricles. Data are lacking on the ability of these new Doppler indices to predict outcome in patients with complex single ventricle anatomy. Finally, three-dimensional echocardiography and cardiac magnetic resonance imaging hold promise in the nongeometric assessment of ventricular volume and function but have yet to be comprehensively evaluated in patients with congenital heart disease.

SUGGESTED READING

Anconina J, Danchin N, Selton-Suty C, et al. Noninvasive estimation of right ventricular dP/dt in patients with tricuspid valve regurgitation. *Am J Cardiol*. 1993;71:1495–1497.

Appleton CP, Galloway JM, Gonzalez MS, et al. Estimation of left ventricular filling pressures using two-dimensional and Doppler echocardiography in adult patients with cardiac disease. *J Am Coll Cardiol*. 1993;22:1972–1982.

Appleton CP, Hatle LK, Popp RL. Relation of transmitral flow velocity patterns to left ventricular diastolic function: new insights from a combined hemodynamic and Doppler echocardiographic study. *J Am Coll Cardiol*. 1988;12:426–440.

Baran AO, Rogal GJ, Nanda NC. Ejection fraction determination without planimetry by two-dimensional echocardiography: a new method. *J Am Cardiol*. 1983;1:1471–1478.

Basnight MA, Gonzalez MS, Kershenovich SC, et al. Pulmonary venous flow velocity: relation to hemodynamics, mitral flow velocity and left atrial volume, and ejection fraction. *J Am Soc Echocardiogr*. 1991;4:547–548.

Border WL, Michelfelder EC, Glascock BJ, et al. Color M-mode and Doppler tissue evaluation of diastolic function in children: simultaneous correlation with invasive indices. *J Am Soc Echocardiogr*. 2003;16:988–994.

Borow KM, Neumann A, Marcus RH, et al. Effects of simultaneous alterations in preload and afterload on measurements of left ventricular contractility in patients with dilated cardiomyopathy: comparisons of ejection phase, isovolumetric and end systolic force velocity indexes. *J Am Coll Cardiol*. 1992;20:787–795.

Brower RW, van Dorp WG, Vogel JA, et al. An improved method for quantitative analysis of M-mode echocardiograms. *Eur J Cardiol*. 1975;3:171–179.

Brun P, Tribouilloy C, Duval AM, et al. Left ventricular flow propagation during early filling is related to wall relaxation: a color M-mode Doppler analysis. *J Am Coll Cardiol*. 1992;20:420–432.

Chen C, Rodriguez L, Guerrero JL, et al. Noninvasive estimation of the instantaneous first derivative of left ventricular pressure using continuous-wave Doppler echocardiography. *Circulation*. 1991;83:2101–2110.

Chen C, Rodriquez L, Lethor RA, et al. Continuous wave Doppler echocardiography for noninvasive assessment of left ventricular dP/dt and relaxation time constant from mitral regurgitation spectra in patients. *J Am Coll Cardiol*. 1994;23:970–976.

Cheung YF, Penny DJ, Redington AN. Serial assessment of left ventricular diastolic function after Fontan procedure. *Heart*. 2000;83:420–424.

Chung N, Nishimura RA, Holmes DR Jr, et al. Measurement of left ventricular dP/dt by simultaneous Doppler echocardiography and cardiac catheterization. *J Am Soc Echocardiogr*. 1992;5:147–152.

Colan SD, Borow KM, Neumann A. Left ventricular end systolic wall stress velocity of fiber shortening relation. A load independent index of myocardial contractility. *J Am Coll Cardiol*. 1984;4:715–724.

Denault AY, Gorcsan J III, Mandarino WA, et al. Left ventricular performance assessed by automated border detection and arterial pressure. *Am J Physiol*. 1997;272:H138–H147.

Devereaux RB, Alonso DR, Lutas EM, et al. Echocardiographic assessment of left ventricular hypertrophy: Comparison to necropsy findings. *Am J Cardiol*. 1986;57:450–458.

D'hooge J, Heimdal A, Jamal F, et al. Regional strain and strain rate measurements by cardiac ultrasound: principles, implementation and limitations. *Eur J Echocardiogr*. 2000;1:154–170.

Donovan CL, Armstrong WF, Bach DS. Quantitative Doppler tissue imaging of the left ventricular myocardium: validation in normal subjects. *Am Heart J.* 1995;130:100–104.

Eidem BW, McMahon CJ, Ayres NA, et al. Impact of chronic left ventricular preload and afterload on Doppler tissue imaging velocities: a study in congenital heart disease. *J Am Soc Echocardiogr.* 2005;18:830–838.

Eidem BW, McMahon CJ, Cohen RR, et al. Impact of cardiac growth on Doppler tissue imaging velocities: a study in healthy children. *J Am Soc Echocardiogr.* 2004;17:212–221.

Eidem BW, O'Leary PW, Tei C, et al. Usefulness of the myocardial performance index for assessing right ventricular function in congenital heart disease. *Am J Cardiol.* 2000;86:654–658.

Eidem BW, Tei C, O'Leary PW, et al. Nongeometric quantitative assessment of right and left ventricular function: myocardial performance index in normal children and patients with Ebstein anomaly. *J Am Soc Echocardiogr.* 1998;11:849–856.

Fisher EA, DuBrow IW, Hastreiter AR. Comparison of ejection phase indices of left ventricular performance in infants and children. *Circulation.* 1975;52:916–925.

Fleming AD, Xia X, McDicken WN, et al. Myocardial velocity gradients detected by Doppler imaging. *Br J Radiol.* 1994;67:679–688.

Franklin RC, Wyse RK, Graham TP, et al. Normal values for noninvasive estimation of left ventricular contractile state and afterload in children. *Am J Cardiol.* 1990;65:505–510.

Frommelt PC, Ballweg JA, Whitstone BN, et al. Usefulness of Doppler tissue imaging analysis of tricuspid annular motion for determination of right ventricular function in normal infants and children. *Am J Cardiol.* 2002;89:610–613.

Frommelt PC, Snider AR, Meliones JN, et al. Doppler assessment of pulmonary artery flow patterns and ventricular function after the Fontan operation. *Am J Cardiol.* 1991;68:1211–1215.

Fujimoto S, Mizuno R, Nakagawa Y, et al. Estimation of the right ventricular volume and ejection fraction by transthoracic three-dimensional echocardiography. A validation study using magnetic resonance imaging. *Int J Card Imaging.* 1998;14:385–390.

Garcia MJ, Ares MA, Asher C, et al. Color M-mode flow velocity propagation: an index of early left ventricular filling that combined with pulse Doppler peak E velocity may predict capillary wedge pressure. *J Am Coll Cardiol.* 1997;29:448–454.

Garcia MJ, Rodriguez L, Ares M, et al. Myocardial wall velocity assessment by pulsed Doppler tissue imaging: characteristic findings in normal subjects. *Am Heart J.* 1996;132:648–656.

Garcia MJ, Smedira NG, Greenberg NL, et al. Color M-mode Doppler flow propagation is a preload insensitive index of left ventricular relaxation: animal and human validation. *J Am Coll Cardiol.* 2000;35:201–208.

Geva T, Powell AJ, Crawford EC, et al. Evaluation of regional differences in right ventricular systolic function by acoustic quantification echocardiography and cine magnetic resonance imaging. *Circulation.* 1998;98:339–345.

Gorcsan J III, Romand JA, Mandarino WA, et al. Assessment of left ventricular performance by on-line pressure area relations using echocardiographic automated border detection. *J Am Coll Cardiol.* 1994;23:242–252.

Graham TP Jr, Franklin RCG, Wyse RKH, et al. Left ventricular wall stress and contractile function in childhood: normal values and comparison of Fontan repair versus palliation only in patients with tricuspid atresia. *Circulation.* 1986;74 (Suppl I):I-61–I-69.

Greenberg NL, Firstenberg MS, Castro PL, et al. Doppler-derived myocardial systolic strain rate is a strong index of left ventricular contractility. *Circulation.* 2002;105:99–105.

Gulati VK, Katz WE, Follansbee WP, et al. Mitral annular descent velocity by tissue Doppler echocardiography as an index of global left ventricular function. *Am J Cardiol.* 1996;77:979–984.

Gutgesell HP, Paquet M, Duff DF, et al. Evaluation of left ventricular size and function by echocardiography. Results in normal children. *Circulation.* 1977;56:457–462.

Ha JW, Ommen SR, Tajik AJ, et al. Differentiation of constrictive pericarditis from restrictive cardiomyopathy using mitral annular velocity by tissue Doppler echocardiography. *Am J Cardiol.* 2004;94:316–319.

Haendchen RV, Wyatt HL, Maurer G, et al. Quantitation of regional cardiac function by two-dimensional echocardiography. I. Patterns of contraction in the normal left ventricle. *Circulation.* 1983;67:1234–1245.

Hagler DJ, Seward JB, Tajik AJ, et al. Functional assessment of the Fontan operation: combined two-dimensional and Doppler echocardiographic studies. *J Am Coll Cardiol.* 1984;4:745–764.

Harada K, Suzuki T, Tamura M, et al. Role of age on transmitral flow velocity patterns in assessing left ventricular diastolic function in normal infants and children. *Am J Cardiol.* 1995;76:530–532.

Harada K, Suzuki T, Tamura M, et al. Effect of aging from infancy to childhood on flow velocity patterns of pulmonary vein by Doppler echocardiography. *Am J Cardiol.* 1996;77:221–224.

Harada K, Suzuki T, Tamura M, et al. Role of age on transmitral flow velocity patterns in assessing left ventricular diastolic function in normal infants and children. *Am J Cardiol.* 1995;76:530–532.

Harada K, Takahashi Y, Shiota T, et al. Changes in transmitral and pulmonary venous flow patterns in the first day of life. *J Clin Ultrasound.* 1995;23:399–405.

Heimdal A, Stoylen A, Torp H, et al. Real-time strain rate imaging of the left ventricle by ultrasound. *J Am Soc Echocardiogr.* 1998;11:1013–1019.

Helbing WA, Bosch HG, Maliepaard C, et al. On-line automated border detection for echocardiographic quantification of right ventricular size and function in children. *Pediatr Cardiol.* 1997;18:261–269.

Helle-Valle T, Crosby J, Edvardsen T, et al. New noninvasive method for assessment of left ventricular rotation: speckle tracking echocardiography. *Circulation.* 2005;112(20):3149–3156.

Henry WL, Gardin JM, Ware JH. Echocardiographic measurements in normal subjects from infancy to old age. *Circulation.* 1980;62:1054–1061.

Henry WL, Ware J, Gardin JM, et al. Echocardiographic measurements in normal subjects. Growth-related changes that occur between infancy and early adulthood. *Circulation.* 1978;57:278–285.

Igarashi H, Shiraishi H, Endoh H, et al. Left ventricular contractile state in preterm infants: relation between wall stress and velocity of circumferential fiber shortening. *Am Heart J.* 1994;127:1336–1340.

Isaaz K, Munoz del Romeral L, Lee E, et al. Quantitation of the motion of the cardiac base in normal subjects by Doppler echocardiography. *J Am Soc Echocardiogr.* 1993;6:166–476.

Isaaz K, Thompson A, Ethevenot G, et al. Doppler echocardiographic measurement of low velocity motion of the left ventricular posterior wall. *Am J Cardiol.* 1989;64:66–75.

Jiang l, Siu C, Handschmacher S, et al. Three-dimensional echocardiography: in vitro validation for right ventricular volume and function. *Circulation.* 1994;89:2342–2350.

Johnson GL, Moffett CB, Noonan JA. Doppler echocardiographic studies of diastolic ventricular filling patterns in premature infants. *Am Heart J.* 1988;116(6 Pt 1):1568–1574.

Kanzaki H, Nakatani S, Kawada T, et al. Right ventricular dP/dt (max), not dP/dt (max), noninvasively derived from tricuspid regurgitation velocity is a useful index of right ventricular contractility. *J Am Soc Echocardiogr.* 2002;15:136–142.

Kapusta L, Thijssen JM, Cuypers MH, et al. Assessment of myocardial velocities in healthy children using tissue Doppler imaging. *Ultrasound Med Biol.* 2000;26:229–237.

Kaul S, Tei C, Hopkins JM, et al. Assessment of right ventricular function using two-dimensional echocardiography. *Am Heart J.* 1984;107:526–531.

Klein AL, Tajik AJ. Doppler assessment of pulmonary venous flow in healthy subjects in patients with heart disease. *J Am Soc Echocardiogr.* 1991;4:379–392.

Kreulen TH, Bove AA, McDonough MT, et al. The evaluation of left ventricular function in man. A comparison of methods. *Circulation.* 1975;51:677–688.

Lang RM, Bierig M, Devereux RB, et al. Recommendations for chamber quantification: a report from the American Society of Echocardiography's Guidelines and Standards Committee and the Chamber Quantification Writing Group, developed in conjunction with the European Association of Echocardiography, a branch of the European Society of Cardiology. *J Am Soc Echocardiogr.* 2005;18:1440–1463.

Langeland S, D'hooge J, Wouters PF, et al. Experimental validation of a new ultrasound method for the simultaneous assessment of radial and longitudinal myocardial deformation independent of insonation angle. *Circulation.* 2005;112:2157–2162.

Mahle WT, Coon PD, Wernovsky G, et al. Quantitative echocardiographic assessment of the performance of functionally single right ventricle after the Fontan operation. *Cardiol Young.* 2001;11:399–406.

Martins TC, Rigby ML, Redington AN. Left ventricular performance in children: transthoracic versus transesophageal measurement of M mode derived indices. *Br Heart J.* 1992;68:485–487.

Mercier JC, DiSessa TG, Jarmakani JM, et al. Two-dimensional echocardiographic assessment of left ventricular volumes and ejection fraction in children. *Circulation.* 1982;65(5):962–969.

McDicken WM, Sutherland GR, Moran CM, et al. Colour Doppler velocity imaging of the myocardium. *Ultrasound Med Biol.* 1992;18:651–654.

McMahon CJ, Nagueh SF, Eapen RS, et al. Echocardiographic predictors of adverse clinical events in children with dilated cardiomyopathy: a prospective clinical study. *Heart.* 2004;90:908–915.

McMahon CJ, Nagueh SF, Pignatelli RH, et al. Characterization of left ventricular diastolic function by tissue Doppler imaging and clinical status in children with hypertrophic cardiomyopathy. *Circulation.* 2004;109:1756–1762.

Michelfelder EC, Vermillion RP, Ludomirsky A, et al. Comparison of simultaneous Doppler- and catheter-derived right ventricular dP/dt in hypoplastic left heart syndrome. *Am J Cardiol.* 1996;77:212–214.

Mulvagh S, Quinones M, Kleiman N, et al. Estimation of left ventricular end-diastolic pressure from Doppler transmitral flow velocity in cardiac patients independent of systolic performance. *J Am Coll Cardiol.* 1992;20(1):112–119.

Nagueh SF, Middleton KJ, Kopelen HA, et al. Doppler tissue imaging. A noninvasive technique for evaluation of left ventricular relaxation and estimation of filling pressures. *J Am Coll Cardiol.* 1997;30:1527–1533.

Nishimura RA, Abel MB, Hatle LK, et al. Assessment of diastolic function of the heart: background and current applications of Doppler echocardiography. Part II. Clinical studies. *Mayo Clin Proc.* 1989;64:181–204.

Nishimura RA, Abel MD, Hatle LK, et al. Relation of pulmonary vein to mitral flow velocities by transesophageal Doppler echocardiography: effect of different loading conditions. *Circulation.* 1990;81:1488–1497.

Nishimura RA, Abel MD, Housman, PR, et al. Mitral flow velocity curves as a function of different loading conditions: evaluation by intraoperative transesophageal Doppler echocardiography. *J Am Soc Echocardiogr*. 1989;2:79–87.

Oh JK, Appleton CP, Hatle LK, et al. The noninvasive assessment of left ventricular diastolic function with two-dimensional and Doppler echocardiography. *J Am Soc Echocardiogr*. 1997;10(3):246–270.

O'Leary PW, Durongpisitkul K, Cordes TM, et al. Diastolic ventricular function in children: a Doppler echocardiographic study establishing normal values and predictors of increased ventricular end-diastolic pressure. *Mayo Clin Proc*. 1998;73:616–628.

Olivier M, O'Leary PW, Pankranz S, et al. Serial Doppler assessment of diastolic function before and after the Fontan operation. *J Am Soc Echocardiogr*. 2003;16:1136–1143.

Pai RG, Bansal RC, Shah PM. Doppler-derived rate of left ventricular pressure rise. *Circulation*. 1990;82:514–520.

Pai RG, Yoganathan AP. Toomes C, et al. Mitral E wave propagation as an index of left ventricular diastolic function. I: its hydrodynamic basis. *J Heart Valve Dis*. 1998;7:438–444.

Penny DJ, Rigby ML, Redington AN. Abnormal patterns of interventricular flow and diastolic filling after the Fontan operation: evidence for incoordinate ventricular wall motion. *Br Heart J*. 1991;66:375–378.

Perez JE, Waggoner AD, Barzilai B, et al. On-line assessment of ventricular function by automatic boundary detection and ultrasonic backscatter imaging. *J Am Coll Cardiol*. 1992;19:313–320.

Quinones MA, Gaasch WH, Alexander JK. Influence of acute changes in preload, afterload, contractile state and heart rate on ejection and isovolumic indices of myocardial contractility in man. *Circulation*. 1976;53:293–302.

Quinones MA, Gaasch WH, Cole JS, et al. Echocardiographic determination of left ventricular stress-velocity relations. *Circulation*. 1975;51:689–700.

Quinones MA, Pickering E, Alexander JK. Percentage of shortening of the echocardiographic left ventricular dimension. Its use in determining ejection fraction and stroke volume. *Chest*. 1978;74:59–65.

Quinones MA, Waggoner AD, Reduto LA, et al. A new, simplified and accurate method of determining ejection fraction with two-dimensional echocardiography. *Circulation*. 1981;64:744–753.

Rankin LS, Moos S, Grossman W. Alterations in preload and ejection phase indices of left ventricular performance. *Circulation*. 1975;51(5):910–915.

Reeder GS, Currie PJ, Hagler DJ, et al. Use of Doppler techniques (continuous-wave, pulsed-wave, and color flow imaging) in the noninvasive hemodynamic assessment of congenital heart disease. *Mayo Clin Proc*. 1986;61:725–744.

Riggs TW, Rodriguez R, Snider AR, et al. Doppler echocardiographic evaluation of right and left ventricular diastolic function in normal neonates. *J Am Coll Cardiol*. 1989;13(3):700–705.

Riggs TW, Snider AR. Respiratory influence on right and left ventricular diastolic function in normal children. *Am J Cardiol*. 1989;63:858–861.

Rowland DG, Gutgesell HP. Noninvasive assessment of myocardial contractility, preload, and afterload in healthy newborn infants. *Am J Cardiol*. 1995;75:818–821.

Royse CF, Royse AG. Afterload corrected fractional area change (FACac): a simple, relatively load-independent measurement of left ventricular contractility in humans. *Ann Thorac Cardiovasc Surg*. 2000;6:345–350.

Rychik J, Tian ZY (1996) Quantitative assessment of myocardial tissue velocities in normal children with tissue Doppler imaging. *Am J Cardiol*. 1996;77:1254–1257.

Silverman NH, Ports TA, Snider AR, et al. Determination of left ventricular volume in children: echocardiographic and angiographic comparisons. *Circulation*. 1980;62(3):548–557.

Sluysmans T, Sanders SP, van der Velde M, et al. Natural history and patterns of recovery of contractile function in single left ventricle after Fontan operation. *Circulation*. 1992;86:1753–1761.

Sonnenblick EH, Parmley WW, Urschel CW, et al. Ventricular function: evaluation of myocardial contractility in health and disease. *Prog Cardiovasc Dis*. 1970;27:449–466.

Stoddard MF, Pearson AC, Kern MJ, et al. Influence of alteration in preload on the pattern of left ventricular diastolic filling assessed by Doppler echocardiography in humans. *Circulation*. 1989;79:1226–1236.

Sutherland GR, Stewart MJ, Groundstroem WE, et al. Color Doppler myocardial imaging: a new technique for the assessment of myocardial function. *J Am Soc Echocardiogr*. 1994;7:441–458.

Takatsuji H, Mikami T, Urasawa K, et al. A new approach for evaluation of left ventricular diastolic function: spatial and temporal analysis of left ventricular filling flow propagation by color M-mode Doppler echocardiography. *J Am Coll Cardiol*. 1996;27:365–371.

Tei C, Dujardin KS, Hodge DO, et al. Doppler echocardiographic index for assessment of global right ventricular function. *J Am Soc Echocardiogr*. 1996;9:838–847.

Tei C, Ling LH, Hodge DO, et al. New index of combined systolic and diastolic cardiac performance index: correlation with simultaneous measurements of cardiac catheterization measurements. *J Am Soc Echocardiogr*. 1995;26:357–366.

Tei C. New noninvasive index for combined systolic and diastolic ventricular function. *J Cardiol*. 1995;26:135–136.

Tynan M, Reid DS, Hunger S, et al. Ejection phase indices of left ventricular performance in infants, children, and adults. *Br Heart J*. 1975;37:196–202.

Vasan RS, Benjamin EJ, Levy D. Prevalence, clinical features and prognosis of diastolic heart failure: an epidemiologic perspective. *J Am Coll Cardiol*. 1995;21(7):1565–1574.

Weidemann F, Eyskens B, Jamal F, et al. Quantification of regional left and right ventricular radial and longitudinal function in healthy children using ultrasound-based strain and strain imaging. *J Am Soc Echocardiogr*. 2002;15:20–28.

Weidemann F, Jamal F, Sutherland GR, et al. Myocardial function defined by strain rate and strain during alterations in inotropic states and heart rate. *Am J Physiol Heart Circ Physiol*. 2002;283:H792–H799.

Williams RV, Ritter S, Tani LY, et al. Quantitative assessment of ventricular function in children with single ventricles using the Doppler myocardial performance index. *Am J Cardiol*. 2000;86:1106–1110.

Zoghbi WA, Habib JB, Quinones MA. Doppler assessment of right ventricular filling in a normal population: comparison with left ventricular filling dynamics. *Circulation*. 1990;82:1316–1324.

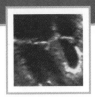

Chapter 4
Quantitative Methods in Echocardiography—Advanced Techniques in the Assessment of Ventricular Function

Javier Ganame • Luc Mertens

THREE-DIMENSIONAL ECHOCARDIOGRAPHY

Reliable echocardiographic evaluation of left ventricular (LV) and right ventricular (RV) function and volumes is important in the management of patients with congenital and acquired heart disease. This has generally relied on two-dimensional (2D) imaging. Two-dimensional echocardiography uses several geometric assumptions to calculate ventricular volumes and ejection fraction. These assumptions may not be representative of patients with congenital heart defects. Furthermore, these assumptions, such as a uniform, elliptical ventricular cavity, do not apply to the right ventricle, which has a different shape. In addition, inadequate acoustic windows may further limit the ability of 2D echocardiography to image the entire heart. Three-dimensional (3D) echocardiography overcomes most of these limitations.

From Reconstruction Techniques to Real-Time Three-dimensional Imaging

The development of 3D echocardiographic imaging was a logical but difficult step to solve the difficulties inherent in cross-sectional 2D imaging. Initial attempts to record and display images of the heart in three dimensions were reported in the 1970s. At that time, off-line 3D reconstruction from serial electrocardiogram (ECG)-gated acquisitions of multiple 2D planes was performed either by free-hand scanning or a mechanically driven transducer that sequentially recorded images at predefined intervals. With freehand scanning, a series of images were obtained by manually tilting the transducer along a fixed plane, and a spatial locator attached to the transducer translated the 3D spatial location into a Cartesian coordinate system. The main disadvantage of this approach was the relative bulk of the spatial locator device, which made transducer manipulation difficult. An alternative to freehand scanning was the use of a mechanized transducer to obtain serial images at set intervals in a parallel fashion or by pivoting around a fixed axis in a rotational, fanlike manner. Because the intervals and angles between the 2D images were defined, a 3D coordinate system could be derived from the 2D images in which the volume was more uniformly sampled than with the freehand scanning approach. This approach, although accurate, required long acquisition and postprocessing times. The quality of 3D reconstruction from 2D images depended on a number of factors, including the intrinsic quality of the 2D data set, the number (density) of the 2D images used, the ability to limit motion artifacts, and adequate ECG and respiratory gating. In addition, this 3D reconstruction relied on the assumption that all planes would be acquired at the same phase of the respiratory cycle to ensure identical shape and position of the heart within the chest. Also, the need to shorten the acquisition time to minimize motion artifacts made image quality often suboptimal. Later, the use of multiplane probes emerged as a readily available method to obtain rotational images at defined interval angles around a fixed axis.

In the 1990s, a different approach has been pursued to eliminate the need for tedious multiplane acquisition. This approach is based on real-time volumetric 3D imaging. This advance in 3D imaging saves computer interpolation of cross-sectional images and thus could avoid spatial motion artifacts. Real-time 3D echocardiography uses transducers containing arrays of piezoelectric elements capable of acquiring pyramidal data sets. Processing the information obtained by these transducers required computational power that was beyond what was available at that time. More recently, further improvements in multiplane probe design to obtain rotational

images together with increased computational power have led to more widespread commercialization of real-time 3D systems. It is now possible to depict cardiac motion at sufficient frame rate during a single breath hold without the need for off-line reconstruction, thus eliminating motion artifacts known to adversely affect the reconstruction methodologies.

Technical Aspects

Real-time 3D echocardiography uses matrix array transducers with elements arranged in a grid fashion, typically containing more than 3000 imaging elements transmitting at 2.5 or 3.5 MHz for adult applications. More recently, the clinical availability of a higher frequency probe (7 MHz) made it possible to obtain real-time 3D images with improved spatial resolution even in small infants. These probes can acquire data sets at 360-degree focusing and have electronic steering for volumetric acquisition at satisfactory spatial resolution (voxel size, $0.5 \times 0.5 \times 0.6$ mm) with acceptable temporal resolution (20 to 25 frames/s). Real-time 3D systems generally have three acquisition modes: real-time, narrow angle; zoom, magnified; and wide angle. The real-time mode displays a pyramid of approximately 50×30 degrees. The zoom mode displays a magnified pyramid of 30×30 degrees. The wide angle shows a pyramidal data set of approximately 90×90 degrees (Fig. 4.1). This allows inclusion of a larger cardiac volume but still requires ECG gating because the full-volume data set is compiled by merging four narrower wedge-shaped subvolumes obtained over four consecutive heartbeats (Fig. 4.2). To minimize reconstruction artifacts, data should be acquired during breath holding if possible. Wide-angle data sets provide larger pyramidal scans at the cost of lower spatial resolution compared with narrow-angle acquisition. More recent developments resulted in a smaller transducer footprint, improved side lobe suppression, and harmonic capabilities that may be used for contrast imaging.

Recognizing and avoiding potential artifacts are critical for an accurate interpretation of 3D data. Artifacts are mainly related to respiratory motion in patients unable to hold their breath, like young children. Inability to maintain a breath hold may result in stitching artifacts when the four subvolumes are merged. ECG gating can be challenging in patients with arrhythmias including normal sinus arrhythmia. Importantly, in real-time 3D echocardiography, image quality is closely related to the intrinsic 2D images used to produce the 3D data set. The use of optimal gain settings is essential for accurate diagnosis. Low gain settings can artificially eliminate certain structures that will not be viewable during postprocessing. Therefore, it is recommended to use some overcompensation of gain during acquisition. This maneuver will allow maximum flexibility during postprocessing.

Imaging Protocols

A complete 3D echocardiogram should include assessment of ventricular morphology, volumes, and function, as well as valvular morphology and hemodynamic status. In general, 3D echocardiography is performed as a complement to a 2D study. For example, focused 3D imaging for LV volume quantification typically can be performed with an apical four-chamber wide-angle acquisition complementing standard 2D imaging (Fig. 4.3). An advantage of 3D echocardiography compared with 2D echocardiography is that quantitative analysis does not rely on the ability of the operator to acquire images positioned properly in certain standard views relative to cardiac anatomy. Unlike 2D echocardiography, in which standard views are described based on the plane through which

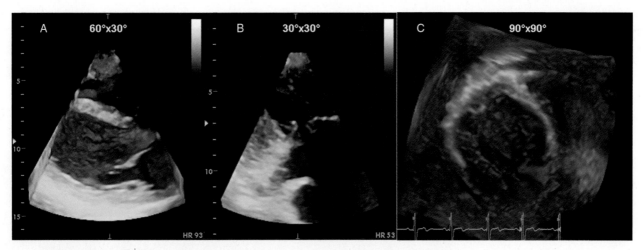

FIGURE 4.1. Three different three-dimensional data acquisition modes. A: Real-time narrow-angle imaging mode. **B:** Zoom mode, which allows visualization of small structures such as a coaptation abnormality of the tricuspid valve. **C:** Wide-angle full-volume data set; this data set is acquired over four to seven heartbeats.

they pass, 3D echocardiography is inherently volumetric. As such, full-volume data sets of the beating heart, which can be rotated and sliced in any plane, allow the reader both an external view of the heart and multiple internal views with the use of cropping.

Essential components of a full 3D echocardiogram for assessment of ventricular function include wide-angle acquisition of a parasternal long-axis view, an apical 4-chamber view, and a subcostal view including color interrogation of all valves. Visualization, description, and analysis of images are generally performed in three orthogonal planes: (a) the sagittal plane, which corresponds to a vertical long-axis view of the heart; (b) the coronal plane, which corresponds to a four-chamber view; and (c) the transverse plane, which corresponds to a short-axis view. Each plane can be viewed from two sides representing opposite perspectives. For example, the transverse plane can be viewed from the apex or the base of the heart.

The choice of narrow- or wide-angle acquisition depends on the structure to be visualized. For smaller structures, such as the valves, a narrow-angle acquisition is more appropriate. For imaging the ventricles, it is best to use a wide-angle acquisition in the apical window so that the entire volume of the ventricles can be covered.

Acquisition is followed by off-line analysis with dedicated 3D software. This requires cropping and tilting of the data set. Because a data set comprises the entire ventricular volume, multiple slices can be obtained from base to apex to evaluate wall motion. An advantage of 3D over 2D imaging is the possibility to manipulate the plane to align the true long and short axis of the left ventricle, avoiding foreshortening and oblique imaging planes.

Clinical Applications

Chamber Quantification – One of the main reasons for performing echocardiograms in clinical practice is the assessment of regional and global LV function. To date, this has generally been performed with visual interpretation (eye-balling) of dynamic 2D images of the beating heart. This is highly subjective and requires adequate training and experience to estimate ventricular function and wall motion accurately. The limitations of this subjective interpretation have long been recognized; consequently, the use of quantitative techniques has been recommended. Multiple methods for measuring LV size and function have been developed for both M-mode and 2D echocardiography. The relative inaccuracy of these one-dimensional

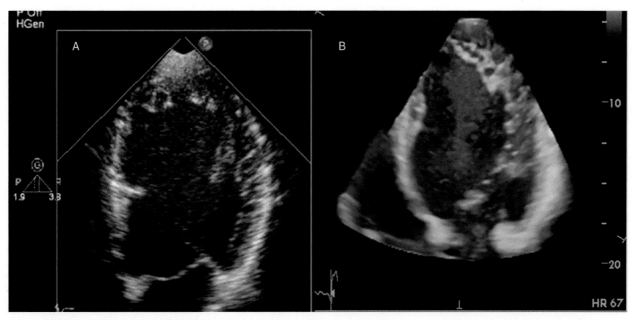

FIGURE 4.2. A two-dimensional (2D) (A) and a full-volume three-dimensional (3D) (B) data sets cropped to view cardiac structures of interest in a patient with left ventricular noncompaction. Compared with the 2D image, the 3D image shows depth information at the cost of lower spatial resolution.

FIGURE 4.3. A full-volume data set (bottom right) cropped into coronal, sagittal, and transverse planes. Such data sets are used to delineate endocardial and epicardial borders and calculate ventricular volumes, mass, and ejection fraction.

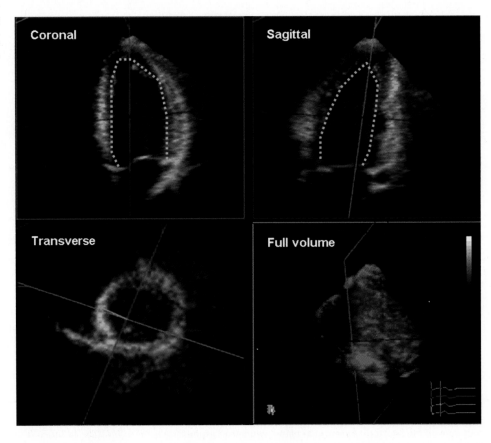

(1D) and 2D approaches has been attributed to the need for geometric modeling of the ventricle assuming the left ventricle is an ellipsoid. The lack of information on one dimension, the *"missing dimension,"* has been considered the main source of the wide intermeasurement variability of the echocardiographic estimates of LV size and function. This is particularly true in children with congenital heart disease whose ventricles have distorted morphology and do not follow geometric models that are generally used. A particular advantage of 3D echocardiography over 2D imaging is that it provides full-volume data sets, so there is no need for geometric modeling of the left ventricle. Several studies comparing 3D echocardiography with magnetic resonance imaging (MRI) as a gold standard have shown the quantification of LV volumes and function with 3D echocardiography is feasible, accurate, and highly reproducible in both children with morphologically normal ventricles, as well as in patients with abnormal geometry (Fig. 4.4).

Visualization of the endocardial surface can be challenging, especially in the apical-lateral myocardial segments. This is commonly compensated for by tilting the transducer. This maneuver generally improves endocardial visualization at the expense of generating foreshortened views of the left ventricle, resulting in an additional source of error when calculating LV volumes. In this regard, an added advantage of 3D echocardiography is the lack of dependence on geometric modeling and image plane positioning, which should result in more accurate chamber quantification.

In the past, 3D echocardiographic quantification of LV volumes and function required tedious manual delineation of subendocardial border in multiple planes. Today, this has been replaced by a nearly fully automated frame-by-frame detection of the endocardial surface that only requires indicating the septal, lateral, anterior, and inferior annuli. Then commercially available customized software can calculate LV volume in each frame, endocardial wall motion, and ejection fraction with the use of almost no geometrical assumptions (Fig. 4.5 & 4.6).

Another clinically important parameter that is frequently assessed by echocardiography is LV mass. Two-dimensional echocardiography derives LV mass from measurements taken at a single point within the myocardial wall. This leads to inaccuracies, especially when there is inhomogeneous wall thickness as occurs in hypertrophic cardiomyopathy. It is well known that 1D and 2D echocardiography overestimate LV mass compared with autopsy and MRI studies. Three-dimensional echocardiography seems to overcome this limitation because it allows calculation of wall thickness in all myocardial segments. Three-dimensional echocardiographic measurement of LV mass requires the delineation of endocardial as well as epicardial borders, with the latter being challenging because it is often difficult to identify the epicardial border.

The assessment of regional wall motion is common practice in adult cardiology because a large number of patients have coronary artery disease, which first affects regional function and only in a later stage affects global ventricular function. The relevance of assessing regional function in pediatric heart disease has gained more interest recently because it may well be that in pediatric heart disease regional dysfunction also precedes global ventricular dysfunction. Volumetric imaging with 3D echocardiography makes it possible to obtain the complete dynamic information on all myocardial segments from a single data set. From these data sets one can quantify wall motion and thickening in all myocardial segments. Additionally, 3D echocardiography during stress echocardiography has been found to be feasible and useful for the detection of stress-induced wall motion abnormalities. A reduction in acquisition time makes 3D echocardiography particularly suited to stress echocardiography in which there is a narrow temporal window to acquire images at peak stress. The benefit of this methodology in pediatric heart disease awaits further studies.

The presence of dyssynchronous electrical and mechanical activation of the myocardium causes a deleterious effect on ventricular performance. Cardiac resynchronization therapy has emerged as a solution to electrical and mechanical dyssynchrony. A clinically useful byproduct of the 3D quantification of regional LV wall motion is the ability to quantify the temporal aspects of regional systolic wall thickening. The standard deviation of regional ejection times (interval between the R wave and peak systolic endocardial motion) has been used as an index of myocardial synchrony (Fig. 4.7 & 4.8).

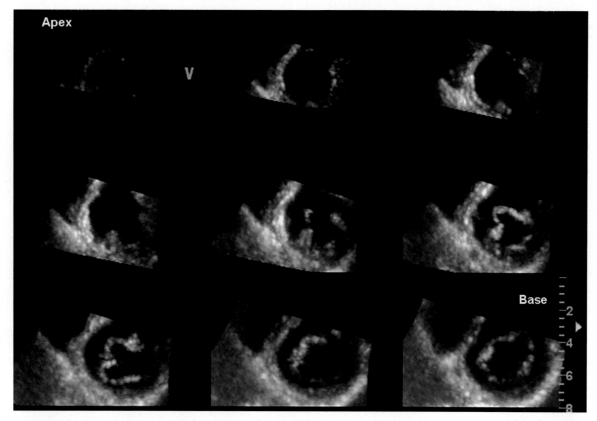

FIGURE 4.4. Multislice short-axis display of a full-volume data set. Cropping and rotation in any desired plane allow the operator to render the true short-axis views covering the entire left ventricle from base to apex. This display is useful to evaluate wall motion abnormalities because it allows direct comparison among different myocardial segments.

This index can also be used to select candidates and to guide resynchronization therapy.

An accurate evaluation of RV size and function is of great importance in patients with congenital heart disease. Conventional methods for LV volume estimation assume a prolate ellipsoid shape of the ventricle; these geometric assumptions do not hold for the right ventricle because the right ventricle has a complex, asymmetrical, crescent shape. This has made the estimation of RV volumes based on geometric modeling from 2D images extremely challenging. Using MRI, one can visualize the entire RV and measure RV volumes and function. Cardiac MRI, however, requires sedation in young children, cannot be done at the bedside, and is not widely available. Real-time 3D echocardiography has emerged as an alternative to MRI for the assessment of RV shape and function. In theory, visualization of the entire RV chamber from either the subcostal or a slightly more medial apical view should be possible with 3D echocardiography, thereby overcoming the inherent limitations of tomographic methods (Fig. 4.9). Visualization of the entire right ventricle from a single data set, however, is often not possible. Notwithstanding this limitation, initial studies show 3D echocardiography compares well with MRI for the calculation of RV volumes and ejection fraction in patients with congenital heart disease. The added clinical value of 3D echocardiography for the assessment of RV function remains to be determined.

Additional potential applications of real-time 3D echocardiography in pediatric heart disease that are beyond the scope of this chapter include (a) accurate measurement of left atrial volume, which is considered to reflect chronic diastolic function and left atrial pressure; (b) quantification of ventricular volumes in the fetal heart; (c) visualization of valve morphology, calculation of valve area, and quantification of regurgitant volumes; (d) guidance of transcatheter interventions such as atrial septal defect device closure, electrophysiologic studies, and intraoperative monitoring; and (e) description of complex congenital heart lesions. The ability to record and analyze all cardiac structures and display complex spatial relationships are

potential advantages of 3D imaging over 2D echocardiography. In addition, the shorter examination time may reduce the need for sedation in some children.

Future Directions

Future advances in transducer and computer technology should focus on allowing wider angle acquisition to be completed in a single cardiac cycle with a smaller footprint transducer; this would reduce artifacts. Also, increased temporal resolution and higher spatial resolution would bring additional diagnostic benefit. Fully automated tracking of the myocardium in real-time may provide approaches to quantifying myocardial mechanics in 3D and obtain information on regional deformation and wall stress. Finally, combining 3D echocardiography with MRI or computed tomography (CT) images may yield fusion imaging data sets with unsurpassed anatomic, functional, and physiologic information.

 ## TISSUE DOPPLER IMAGING FOR THE EVALUATION OF MYOCARDIAL FUNCTION

Most of the echocardiographic techniques used to assess ventricular function evaluate dimensional changes caused by ventricular contraction or study the effect of cardiac events on blood pool Doppler. All this indirectly reflects what is happening within the cardiac wall during the cardiac cycle. A different approach is to try to look directly into the myocardium using echocardiography and to measure regional function by quantifying myocardial properties like velocity and deformation. Initially, Doppler techniques were applied to measure myocardial velocities, and subsequently, these myocardial

FIGURE 4.5. Calculation of left ventricular end-diastolic and end-systolic volumes, stroke volume, and ejection fraction in a 4-year-old with aortic stenosis and heart failure. Note that ventricular volumes are increased and ejection fraction is reduced. Also, significant heterogeneity in regional volumes indicating differences in regional myocardial function is seen (**bottom left**).

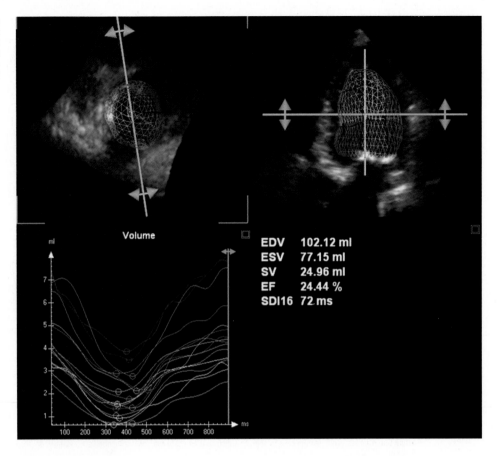

EDV	102.12 ml
ESV	77.15 ml
SV	24.96 ml
EF	24.44 %
SDI16	72 ms

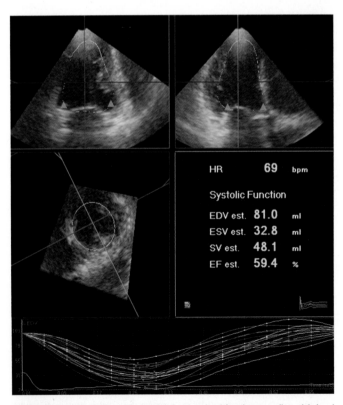

HR	69	bpm

Systolic Function

EDV est.	81.0	ml
ESV est.	32.8	ml
SV est.	48.1	ml
EF est.	59.4	%

FIGURE 4.6. Analysis of left ventricular global and regional function, as well as global and regional volume curves with three-dimensional echocardiography. The endocardial border is semiautomatically traced after manual indication of the mitral annuli and apex in two orthogonal views (*triangles*) at end diastole and end systole.

velocities were used to measure myocardial velocity gradients, which reflect the velocity of deformation or strain rate. From the velocities of deformation, regional deformation or strain can be calculated. Modern techniques like 2D speckle tracking no longer depend on Doppler techniques but directly study deformation.

Tissue Velocities in Pediatric and Congenital Heart Disease

The use of Doppler to evaluate the velocity of blood within vessels as well as cardiac motion has been reported as early as the 1950s and 1960s. With the advent of pulsed-wave Doppler in the late 1960s, the introduction of Doppler methodologies for measurement of myocardial velocity and novel applications to the quantitative assessment of ventricular function soon followed. Tissue Doppler imaging, also known as *Doppler myocardial imaging* or *myocardial velocity imaging*, is a technique that allows measurement of regional myocardial motion and deformation. The technique is based on the physical difference between motion in the blood pool and motion in the myocardial tissue. Blood is poorly reflective (low amplitude) but is rapidly moving (range, 50 to 150 cm/s for normal flow), while tissue is highly reflective (high amplitude) but moves more slowly (range, 3 to 25 cm/s). The introduction of adapted thresholds and clutter filters made it possible to measure myocardial velocities within a segment (Fig. 4.10). The initial description did not raise an immediate clinical interest, but when experimental data confirmed that, in normal myocardium, changes in segmental systolic velocities were linked to changes in regional contractility, there was a renewed interest in the technique. Several clinical studies subsequently investigated the value of regional myocardial velocities in various diseases such as ischemic heart disease, aortic insufficiency, and hypertrophic cardiomyopathy. Especially for ischemic heart disease, it was demonstrated that tissue velocities changed very quickly (within 5 seconds) and consistently after the induction of ischemia in a pig model. Also, for pediatric and congenital heart disease, this technique was

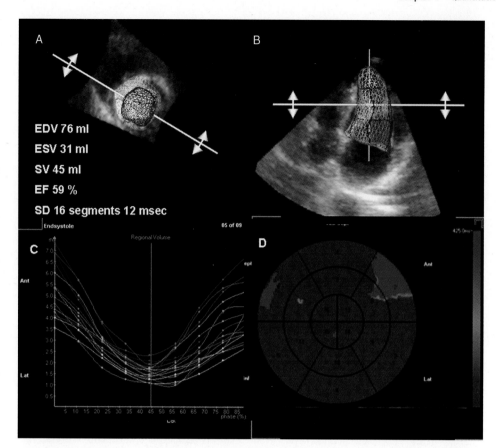

FIGURE 4.7. Assessment of left ventricular synchrony in a normal subject. A & B: Ventricular volumes, ejection fraction, and synchronicity index calculated as standard deviation in time from R wave to minimal regional volume in 16 myocardial segments. Note small variation among myocardial segments. **C:** Regional myocardial volume curves throughout the cardiac cycle. **D:** Bull's eye representation of the same data. Note homogeneous activation pattern with slightly more delayed activation of the basal septal and basal laeral myocardial segments.

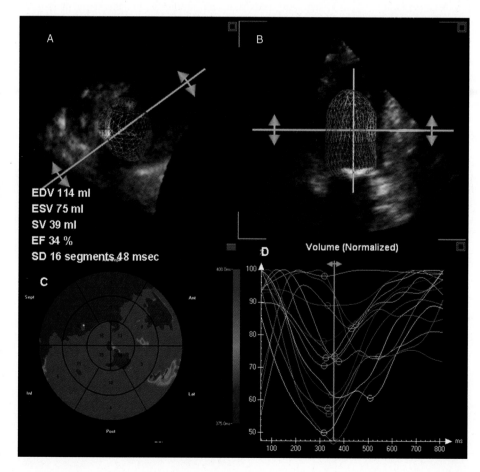

FIGURE 4.8. Assessment of left ventricular synchrony in a child with dilated cardiomyopathy. Note enlarged left ventricular volumes with reduced ejection fraction and large standard deviation of time from R wave to minimal regional volume; this indicated dyssynchrony **(A & B)**. **C:** Bull's eye representation demonstrating earlier activation of the interventricular septum and inferior wall with delayed activation of the basal anterior and lateral myocardial segments. **D:** Curves with marked dispersion of time to minimal regional volume.

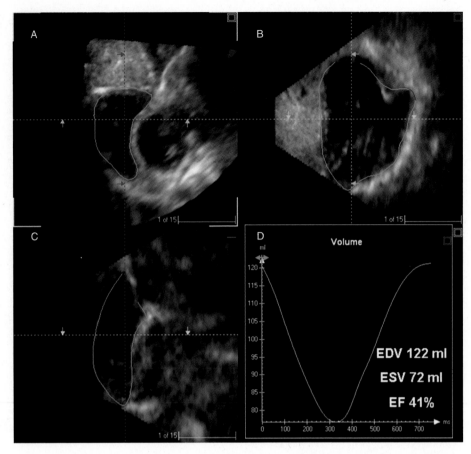

considered to be of potential benefit as it directly looks into the myocardial wall and does not require analysis of chamber geometry, which can be highly variable.

Technical Aspects

Initially myocardial velocities were measured using pulsed-wave Doppler technology. With *pulsed-wave tissue Doppler imaging*, a pulsed Doppler sample volume of 4 to 8 mm is placed within the myocardium while trying to align the myocardial wall as parallel as possible to the ultrasound beam. Alignment is important as all Doppler-based techniques are angle dependent. The velocity waveform obtained by pulsed Doppler represents the peak instantaneous velocity in the region of interest throughout the cardiac cycle. Pulsed Doppler has a very high temporal resolution (250 to 300 frames/s) but a low spatial resolution. The spatial resolution is limited because the sample volume does not track the moving underlying myocar-

dial segment. Thus, not only motion within the segment is measured but also global cardiac motion within the chest. A normal pulsed-wave tissue Doppler imaging trace as obtained in the basal septum is shown in Figure 4.11. Different peaks in the tracing can be observed. During the isovolumetric contraction period, there is a short-lived peak corresponding to the myocardial shape change that occurs during this period. When the myocardial fibers contract against closed valves, there is a change from a more spherical to an ellipsoid shape. During ejection, a longer systolic peak can be

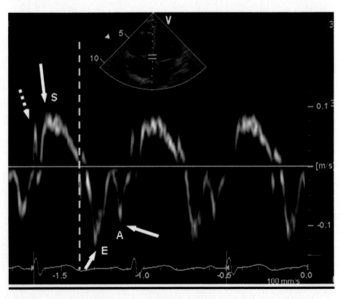

FIGURE 4.11. Pulsed Doppler tracing obtained in the basal septum. Different peaks can be recorded: an isovolumetric contraction peak during the isovolumetric contraction period (*dotted arrow*), followed by a systolic peak during ejection (S), an early diastolic peak (E), and a late diastolic peak occurring during atrial contraction (A).

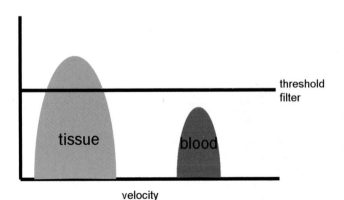

FIGURE 4.10. Principles of tissue Doppler. The tissue signals have a high amplitude but lower frequency, whereas the blood pool signals have a lower amplitude but higher velocity.

measured that corresponds to the base-to-apex motion of the myocardium during systole. During the isovolumetric relaxation period, another short-lived velocity peak can be recorded. In diastole, two peaks can be recorded: an early diastolic peak corresponding to early filling and a late diastolic peak occurring during atrial contraction. These velocities represent the opposite motion of the atrioventricular valve plane from the apex toward the base in diastole when the left ventricle fills. As with all Doppler techniques, by convention, motion toward the transducer is represented as a positive wave and motion away from the transducer as a negative wave.

Color Doppler myocardial imaging (CDMI) is the second technique that can be used to measure tissue velocities. It was introduced in the early 1990s and is based on the same principles as color Doppler blood pool imaging. Using autocorrelation techniques, regional mean velocities, instead of peak tissue velocities, are measured. The difference in measurement technique explains why CDMI-derived myocardial velocities are, on average, 15% to 20% lower than pulsed wave–derived myocardial velocities. Different displays are possible, with the most obvious one being color-coded 2D images. The same color-coding compared to blood pool Doppler imaging is used so that myocardial velocities toward the transducer are displayed in red, while velocities away from the transducer are displayed in blue. From the color-coded images, any velocity curve can be displayed by indicating a region of interest at any point within the myocardial wall in the 2D image. Using anatomical M-mode, a color-coded M-mode velocity map can also be displayed (Fig. 4.12). With current imaging machines and technology, relatively high frame rates can be obtained. Especially when narrowing the sector and optimizing the settings, frame rates of greater than 250 frames/s can be obtained. This is important when one wants to resolve very short-lived myocardial events (e.g., isovolumetric events). The technique also has good spatial resolution. As with any Doppler technique, alignment is an important issue as the technique is angle dependent. The sector has to be aligned as optimally as possible with the wall of interest. An advantage of CDMI is that velocities are recorded simultaneously in different myocardial segments during the same cardiac cycle. This allows the comparison of regional wall motion and timing of cardiac events between different myocardial segments during the same cardiac cycle. This also allows one to calculate differences in velocity within the same segment, a principle that was used as the basis for calculating myocardial velocity gradients. This principle was further applied in Doppler velocity–based deformation imaging (strain and strain rate imaging).

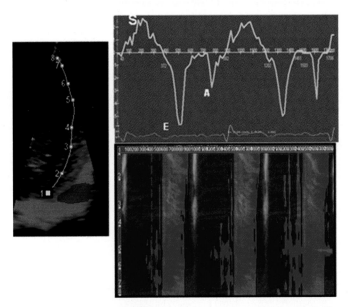

FIGURE 4.12. Color Doppler myocardial imaging. This technique is based on color Doppler imaging. Tissue velocity curves can be extracted from the color data, and on these traces the same velocity peaks can be identified as on the pulsed-wave traces. The advantage of color Doppler myocardial imaging is that velocities in different segments can be recorded during the same cardiac cycle. This allows comparison of velocities in different segments as represented on the color M-mode through the lateral wall of the left ventricle.

Current Clinical Applications of Tissue Velocities

Multiple experimental and clinical studies have been performed to characterize the myocardial velocity profile in normal subjects. Systolic myocardial velocities have been used to evaluate systolic function, while diastolic velocities have been used for assessment of diastolic function. Currently, tissue Doppler velocities are clinically applied mainly in the assessment of diastolic function; however, there may still be some added value in evaluating systolic velocities as well. Velocities are vectors, and these vectors are expressed relative to a certain coordinate system. The most commonly used is the cardiac coordinate system, where motion is described relative to the longitudinal, radial, and circumferential directions (Fig. 4.13). This differs from an intrinsic coordinate system, which is based on actual fiber orientation. Myofibers are predominantly longitudinally oriented like a left-handed helix in the epicardium, their orientation changing gradually to circumferential in the mid-wall and to a right-handed longitudinally oriented helix in the endocardium. This fiber orientation influences the velocities measured in a certain direction.

In the longitudinal direction, systolic and diastolic myocardial velocities are higher at the base of the heart and decrease toward the apex, which remains almost stationary. When analyzing radial myocardial function, myocardial velocities are higher at the endocardium than at the epicardium. For these reasons, a gradient in myocardial velocities exists between the base and the apex (in the longitudinal direction), and between the endocardium and epicardium.

Use of Tissue Doppler Velocities in Children

First, it was necessary to establish normal values for tissue velocities in children. A number of studies have been published in children to establish normal reference values of tissue Doppler velocities. In these studies, it was demonstrated that tissue velocities vary with age, heart rate, myocardial segment, and myocardial layer. A very large study published by Eidem et al. included 325 children from different ages. They showed that pulsed-wave tissue Doppler velocities correlate with parameters of cardiac growth, especially LV end-diastolic dimension and LV mass. This indicates that tissue velocities are not entirely geometry independent and that ventricular geometry might influence indices of wall mechanics. This has important implications when applying this methodology to children with congenital heart disease where there is a large variability in ventricular geometry. Another important issue for congenital heart disease is the load-dependency of tissue velocities. In initial adult studies, tissue velocities were reported to be relatively load independent. Later studies could demonstrate the load-dependency of tissue velocities. In this context, a distinction has to be made between acute load changes and the chronically adapted ventricles where preload and afterload can normalize due to the hypertrophic response. Acute preload changes clearly affect tissue velocities, while this is less clear for the

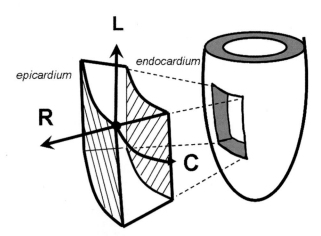

FIGURE 4.13. The cardiac coordinate system. This is the cardiac coordinate system used as a reference system for tissue Doppler vector velocities. Velocities are expressed in the longitudinal (L), radial (R), and circumferential (C) directions.

effect of chronic loading conditions. Studies in children with congenital heart disease with chronic increases in LV preload have documented minimal changes in tissue Doppler velocities compared with normal pediatric control subjects. In a large study by Eidem et al., the effect of different congenital abnormalities on tissue Doppler velocities was studied. In patients with dilated cardiomyopathy, systolic tissue velocities were shown to be reduced in the different myocardial segments. This is consistent with reduced ventricular function. In children with ventricular septal defects, basal velocities were only mildly reduced, especially in the basal septum, while normal in the lateral wall. This is consistent with a preserved ventricular function in these patients. In patients with aortic valve stenosis, systolic basal velocities were reduced in the septum and lateral wall. This suggests that longitudinal systolic function is decreased in this group. This was also demonstrated by Kiraly and colleagues. They published data on 24 children with aortic valve stenosis and demonstrated decreased systolic and diastolic tissue velocities in the lateral and posterior LV walls with longitudinal velocities more significantly reduced compared with radial velocities. All data seem to indicate that load changes differentially affect systolic and diastolic tissue velocities; therefore, they should be used with care under these conditions.

Data on RV systolic velocities in patients with congenital heart disease have also been published. Eyskens et al. showed that RV systolic velocities were elevated in patients with atrial septal defects before closure of the defect. These values normalized within 24 hours after closure of the defect. Pauliks et al. had similar findings in their study, including 39 children with atrial septal defects before and after interventional device closure. At baseline, children with atrial septal defects had increased tricuspid and mitral annular velocities compared with control subjects, whereas isovolumic RV acceleration (which is explained later) was similar between the two groups. Following atrial septal defect closure, a transient immediate decrease in tissue Doppler velocities in all myocardial segments was demonstrated, whereas no change was evident in isovolumic acceleration (IVA). Tissue Doppler velocities normalized at 24 hours postprocedure while IVA remained unchanged, demonstrating the likely load dependence of tissue Doppler velocities and the relative load independence of IVA in children undergoing atrial septal defect device closure. Quantitative assessment of RV performance after repair of tetralogy of Fallot has also been the subject of considerable investigation. Tissue Doppler velocities are decreased in tetralogy of Fallot patients post repair with some regional wall motion abnormalities detectable in the right ventricle (Fig. 4.14). At the apex, the direction of myocardial velocities is opposite compared with the base. This correlates with the duration of the QRS complex, which indicates this is a parameter for the degree of dyssynchrony within the right ventricle (Fig. 4.15).

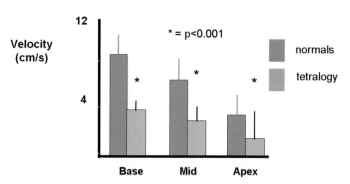

FIGURE 4.14. Systolic tissue Doppler velocities in the right ventricular lateral wall in patients after tetralogy of Fallot correction. Systolic velocities were measured using color Doppler myocardial imaging in the basal, mid, and apical segments of the right ventricular free wall. Systolic velocities are significantly lower in the different segments in the tetralogy of Fallot patients compared with the normal control subjects.

Myocardial Acceleration During IVA – This is a recently described index of contractility. IVA is calculated as the average rate of myocardial acceleration during the isovolumic contraction period (Fig. 4.16) expressed in cm/s^2. Because isovolumic contraction is a short-living event (30 to 40 ms), calculation of IVA requires obtaining images at high temporal resolution (greater than 200 frames/s). In experimental studies, IVA has been validated as a sensitive noninvasive index of RV and LV contractility that is unaffected by preload and afterload within the physiologic range. Subsequently, the value of IVA has been evaluated in clinical conditions. In patients with repaired tetralogy of Fallot, IVA was reduced, indicating a reduced contractile function related to the degree of pulmonary regurgitation. It has also been shown to be a useful noninvasive marker of allograft rejection in pediatric heart transplant patients. The value of IVA as a regional measure of contractility was questioned by Lyseggen et al. In their experimental animal study, they showed that IVA is preload dependent when LV end-diastolic pressure is elevated. Moreover, there was no consistent relationship between regional IVA measurements and regional myocardial contractility in ischemic heart segments. IVA, when calculated from longitudinal velocities near the LV base, should only be used as an index for global systolic function. An important aspect in the use of IVA is its heart rate dependency. This partly explains the relatively large variability in baseline measurements. However, due to its relationship with heart rate, this methodology can be used to study the force-frequency relationship. This was applied by Cheung et al. in the perioperative period in patients after congenital heart surgery. These authors could demonstrate that the

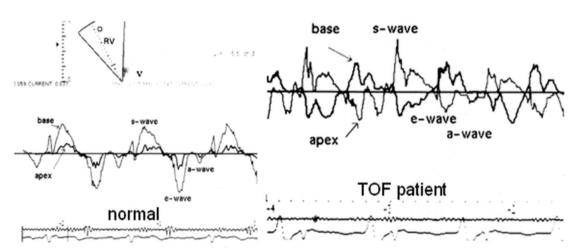

FIGURE 4.15. Regional wall motion abnormalities in tetralogy of Fallot patients as detected by tissue Doppler. Myocardial velocity tracings at base and apex of right ventricular (RV) free wall in a patient with normal regional wall motion (**left**). There is a systolic velocity (s wave) and an early (e wave) and late (a wave) velocity in opposite direction during diastole. Velocities at the apex are lower than at the base. **Right:** Tracings from a tetralogy of Fallot patient are represented with diastolic and systolic wall-motion abnormalities at the RV apex, with both apical s and e waves directed in opposite direction of normal. (From Vogel M, Sponring J, Cullen S, et al. Regional wall motion and abnormalities of electrical depolarization and repolarization in patients after surgical repair of tetralogy of Fallot. *Circulation* 2001; 103:1669–1673.)

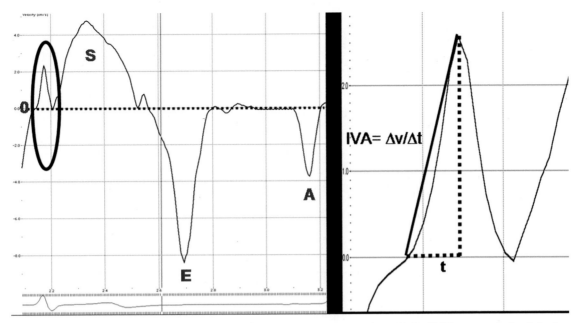

FIGURE 4.16. Measurement of isovolumic acceleration. On the tissue velocity tracing, the isovolumic velocity peak is identified. The mean acceleration starting from the baseline to its maximal velocity is calculated. This measurement requires a high temporal resolution and high frame rate as the isovolumic period is a short-lived event, especially at high heart rates.

force-frequency relationship, as measured by IVA, is preserved in patients after atrial septal closure but severely blunted in patients after the arterial switch operation. The same principle could be used during stress echocardiography. Certainly, further data are required to confirm the applicability of this technique in children with congenital heart disease.

Apart from the dependency on age, heart rate, geometry, and load, tissue Doppler velocities have additional inherent limitations. Like other Doppler modalities used in echocardiography, tissue velocities are angle dependent and currently unidimensional, relying on a 1D assessment of myocardial velocity (typically in either the longitudinal or radial direction). An intrinsic problem of tissue velocities is that when measuring velocities the movement of the heart within the thorax (*cardiac translation)* is also measured. Therefore, measurement is influenced by regional myocardial events as well as global cardiac motion within the chest. Also, the motion and velocity of a myocardial segment are influenced not only by its own intrinsic contractility but also by adjacent myocardial segments (defined as *tethering*). The identification of regional myocardial dysfunction by tissue Doppler echocardiography is therefore significantly limited when regional disease exists (e.g., a localized myocardial infarction) because these diseased segments may continue to move relatively normally due to the influence of healthy adjacent myocardium.

DEFORMATION IMAGING IN PEDIATRIC AND CONGENITAL HEART DISEASE

Strain Rate/Strain Imaging: The Principles

Myocardial velocities are influenced not only by wall thickening and thinning but also by displacement due to global heart translation/rotation and tethering to adjacent segments. Therefore, myocardial velocities cannot differentiate between active contraction and passive motion, which is a major limitation when assessing regional myocardial function. To overcome this limitation, Uematsu and Myatake evaluated gradients in myocardial velocities within a myocardial wall. The authors demonstrated, that in the LV posterior wall, the endocardium moved faster than the epicardium in the radial direction. This myocardial velocity gradient was shown to be reduced in patients with dilated cardiomyopathy and ischemic

heart disease. As this concept was further explored, it led to the development of ultrasound-based strain rate and strain imaging (deformation imaging). Regional strain rate corresponds to the rate of regional myocardial deformation and can be calculated from the spatial gradient in velocities between two neighboring points in the myocardium (Fig. 4.17). The underlying principle is that instantaneous differences in tissue velocity between two adjacent segments reflect either expansion or compression of the tissue in between. Regional strain rate is the rate of deformation (/s) and can be measured from the velocity difference between two segments of myocardium divided by the distance between them (*area of computation*). For paediatrics, we use computational distances of 4 to 5 mm in the radial direction and 8 to 9 mm for the longitudinal direction. Regional strain represents the amount of deformation (percent) or the fractional change in length caused by an applied force and is calculated by integrating the strain rate curve over time during the cardiac cycle. Strain measures the amount of deformation and strain rate measures the velocity of shortening, two measurements that reflect different aspects of myocardial function and provide complementary information.

This echo-based technique measures natural strain, which is the instantaneous deformation of a myocardial segment over an infinitesimal small time interval, in contrast to MRI tagging where Lagrangian strain (change in length compared with the original length) is measured. Deformation can be compression (i.e., shortening) in the longitudinal direction (systole) and thinning in the radial direction (diastole), or expansion (i.e., lengthening) in the longitudinal direction (diastole) and thickening in the radial direction (systole). Shortening is either active contraction or passive recoil after stretching. Similarly, elongation can be relaxation after contraction or passive stretching. Conventionally, compression is characterized by negative strain rate and strain and expansion by positive strain rate and strain (Fig. 4.18). In contrast to myocardial velocities, these novel indices of deformation, namely strain rate and strain, are not influenced by global heart motion and motion in adjacent segments and therefore are better indices of true regional myocardial function.

Strain and strain rate curves can be obtained from different myocardial segments. In our echocardiography laboratory, we measure peak systolic strain rate and end-systolic strain in the radial direction in the inferolateral wall (parasternal short and long axis) and in the longitudinal direction in the basal, mid, and apical segments of the LV lateral wall, the interventricular septum, and the RV free wall (apical four-chamber view).

FIGURE 4.17. Strain and strain rate definitions. Strain rate represents the rate of myocardial deformation, which peaks early during ejection. Strain is the total amount of regional myocardial deformation and peaks at the end of systole.

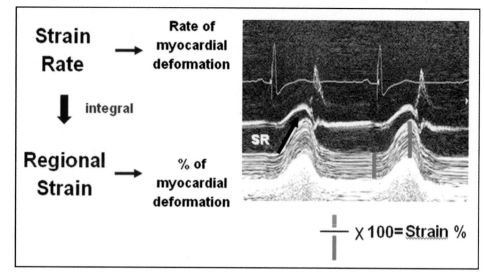

When analyzing regional function, it is always important to compare the local measurements to global timing events, because when inhomogeneities in contraction pattern are present within the heart (bundle branch block, ischemia, asynchronous contraction pattern), a significant amount of thickening or shortening can occur after aortic valve closure (postsystolic deformation). Therefore, timing of mechanical events (aortic valve closure and mitral valve closure) is important to recognize the presence of postsystolic events. An example is given in Figure 4.19. In a patient with hypertrophic cardiomyopathy, there is severely reduced strain and a significant amount of postsystolic shortening in the basal part of the septum. In the mid-apical part, which is less hypertrophied, deformation is higher and there is much less postsystolic shortening. Postsystolic events occur when there are regional differences in myocardial function between different segments. This is the case in patients with ischemic heart disease or any disorder where regional differences in function can be found.

Experimental Validation

Urheim et al. validated Doppler myocardial strain imaging as a new method to quantify regional myocardial function. They compared microcrystal measurements with ultrasound measurements in various conditions, including volume loading and coronary occlusion, and demonstrated that the Doppler-derived strain values approximated those measured by sonomicrometry. Volume loading increased systolic strain and strain rate, which implied that both parameters are load dependent. During coronary artery occlusion, systolic myocardial velocities decreased in the nonischemic segments, whereas regional strain and strain rate values remained unchanged. This suggests that Doppler-derived strain and strain rate are more direct measures of true regional myocardial function than tissue velocities, which are also influenced by contractile function of adjacent segments due to tethering. In an experimental study in normal porcine myocardium, Weidemann et al. studied radial systolic strain rate and strain during alterations in inotropic states and heart rates. Strain was load dependent, decreased with increasing heart rate, and was correlated best with stroke volume. Strain rate is relatively independent of heart rate and better reflects contractility. An experimental canine study performed by Greenberg et al. demonstrated a strong correlation between systolic strain rate and maximal elastance, which is used as the gold standard for global contractility. Correlation between systolic velocities and elastance was weaker. These findings suggest that echo-Doppler derived strain rate can be used as a noninvasive index of contractility.

FIGURE 4.18. Radial and longitudinal strain and strain rate. Left: Radial myocardial deformation estimation from the inferolateral wall. From a short-axis view containing myocardial velocity data, the radial strain rate is calculated. Wall thickening in systole is displayed as positive values, whereas wall thinning in diastole is displayed as negative values. Temporal integration of the strain rate curve results in the local strain profile. Note strain rate peaks early in systole, whereas strain peaks late in systole. S, systole; *dotted lines* indicate aortic valve closure. **Right:** Longitudinal myocardial deformation estimation in the interventricular septum from apical four-chamber view. Shortening in systole is displayed as negative values, whereas lengthening in diastole is displayed as positive values.

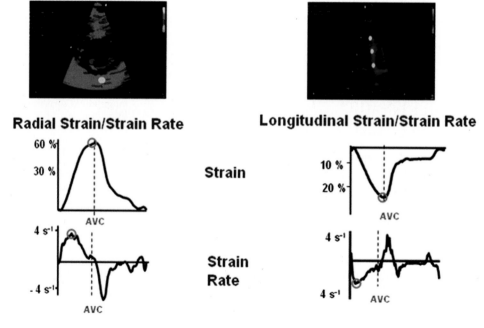

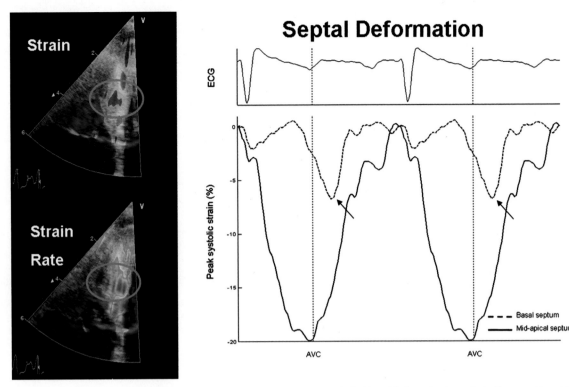

FIGURE 4.19. Postsystolic shortening in hypertrophic cardiomyopathy. Deformation pattern in the interventricular septum in a patient with asymmetric septal hypertrophic cardiomyopathy. Severely reduced systolic strain (also with abnormal systolic lengthening) and presence of postsystolic shortening occur after aortic valve closure in the basal septum (*arrows*). The mid-apical septal myocardial segment shows relatively preserved systolic deformation and no postsystolic shortening. AVC, aortic valve closure. (From Ganame J, Mertens L, Eidem BW, et al. Regional myocardial deformation in children with hypertrophic cardiomyopathy: Morphological and clinical correlations. *Eur Heart J* 2007;28:2886–2894.)

Clinical Applications in Children

Normal Data – The first report on normal strain rate and strain data in children was published by Weidemann et al. They obtained normal strain and strain rate measurements in 33 healthy children (aged 4 to 16 years). They also demonstrated an intraobserver and interobserver variability of 10% to 13% for the different measurements. A recent report by Boettler et al. looked at the values in different age groups and could demonstrate that strain and strain rate values are influenced by heart rate.

Regional RV Deformation in Congenital Heart Disease – One of the most important challenges in congenital heart disease is the assessment of RV function. In current clinical practice, there is no good, easily accessible technique that allows quantification of RV function. The complex geometry of the right ventricle makes the evaluation of RV function extremely difficult. In daily practice, echocardiographers often rely on eyeballing to assess RV systolic function. Nevertheless, the assessment of RV function is often very important, such as in postoperative tetralogy of Fallot patients, patients after Senning or Mustard operations for transposition of the great arteries, and in patients with congenitally corrected transposition of the great arteries. Quantitative assessment of RV function using strain and strain rate imaging has been performed in a number of congenital malformations.

In patients with tetralogy of Fallot, Weidemann et al. demonstrated that in the basal, mid, and apical segments of the RV free wall and interventricular septum, peak systolic strain and strain rate values were reduced (Fig. 4.20). The degree of reduction in peak systolic strain rate in the basal part of the RV free wall correlated significantly with QRS duration on the ECG. This is considered to be a parameter for RV dilatation. It was also demonstrated that in postoperative Fallot patients, there is a reduction in deformation parameters in the LV as well. Interestingly, a recent paper by Geva et al. demonstrated that LV function, as assessed by cardiac MRI, was an important predictor for clinical status in this patient population. Abd El Rahman et al. showed evidence of LV asynchrony in patients after tetralogy of Fallot repair by measuring the time interval between the onset of the QRS complex and peak strain in different segments. They showed a relationship between the degree of asynchrony and different parameters for global and regional myocardial function. The same group demonstrated an increased paradoxical septal motion in these patients that correlated with global LV function. Based on these recent findings, it is suggested that in right heart disease the effect of RV abnormalities on LV function through ventricular interaction are important and that strain and strain imaging could be helpful for this assessment. To further study the effect of pulmonary regurgitation on RV function, our group studied 48 patients after tetralogy of Fallot repair

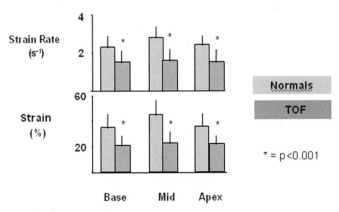

FIGURE 4.20. Strain and strain rate measurements in postoperative patients with tetralogy of Fallot. Peak systolic strain rate and end-systolic strain values are reduced in the different right ventricular lateral wall segments (basal, mid, and apical segments).

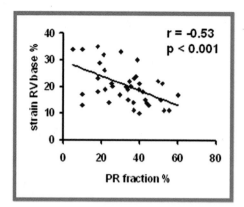
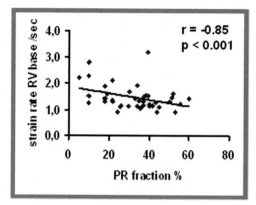

with both MRI and tissue Doppler. We could demonstrate that there was an inverse relationship between peak systolic strain and strain rate at the RV base and the degree of pulmonary regurgitation. This also correlated with impaired clinical status as assessed by exercise testing. This suggests that pulmonary regurgitation has a negative effect on RV deformation (Fig. 4.21).

Another important potential application of this technology is the use of strain and strain rate imaging in patients with a systemic right ventricle such as post Senning or Mustard repair. A study published by Eyskens et al. showed that regional peak systolic strain and strain rate values were reduced in the basal, mid, and apical segments of the RV free wall. The peak systolic strain values measured in the RV basal septum correlated well with ejection fraction measurements obtained using cardiac MRI. This suggests that, in this particular patient population, deformation imaging could be used for serial follow-up, eliminating the need for repetitive evaluation of RV function using MRI. Similar to these data, reduced longitudinal RV deformation has been demonstrated in patients with congenitally corrected transposition of the great arteries.

Regional LV Deformation in Pediatric Heart Disease

– In ischemic heart disease in adults, there is obvious importance in studying regional LV myocardial function. This is less obvious in children with acquired or congenital heart disease, where it is thought that only global ventricular function is affected. Nevertheless, there is growing evidence that assessment of regional myocardial function using deformation imaging may give additional valuable information in this cohort. In routine clinical practice, often only fractional shortening or ejection fraction, based on M-mode echocardiography, is assessed. This essentially looks at only radial ventricular function in the basal part of the left ventricle and assesses only geometrical changes of the LV cavity and not what is happening within the LV wall. There have been a number of publications evaluating LV function in children using deformation imaging that demonstrate its clinical value.

Di Salvo et al. evaluated patients after surgical repair of anomalous left coronary artery from the pulmonary artery (ALCAPA). They studied 13 patients (age at study [SD], 10 ± 8 years; age range, 1.6 to 22 years) at a period of 7.5 ± 5 years after successful surgical repair (coronary reimplantation). All patients had normal LV function when assessed by conventional echocardiographic techniques. In addition, radial function, as measured with deformation imaging, was interpreted to be completely normal. However, longitudinal LV function was significantly decreased using mitral ring motion as well as strain and strain rate imaging. These data suggest that radial function normalizes after coronary reimplantation but that longitudinal LV function is decreased, possibly related to endomyocardial fibrosis resulting from initial neonatal ischemia. The endomyocardial fibers are longitudinally oriented so that subendocardial dysfunction might be reflected, particularly in longitudinal ventricular shortening (Fig. 4.22). This is missed when only radial function is studied.

Deformation imaging has also been used for studying LV regional function in other conditions. Some recent publications focused on regional systolic function in patients with hypertrophic

cardiomyopathy. Weidemann et al. showed that in Friedreich ataxia patients with hypertrophic cardiomyopathy, reduced radial and longitudinal deformation is present in different LV myocardial segments. They could also demonstrate that the reduction in systolic deformation is more pronounced in the more hypertrophic segments. Similar findings were reported in patients with asymmetrical hypertrophic cardiomyopathy. This suggests that in this patient population, regional inhomogeneity in function is present. The prognostic significance of this needs further study. Buyse et al. used deformation imaging to study the effect of treatment with a strong antioxidant on regional myocardial deformation in Friedreich ataxia patients. They could demonstrate an early improvement in regional strain and strain rate before changes in LV wall mass could be detected. This illustrates that this technology could potentially be used to monitor the effect of medical treatment on LV function. A similar application of the technique was used by Weidemann et al. in Fabry patients who were treated with enzyme replacement therapy.

In addition, in dilated cardiomyopathy, the clinical value of regional functional studies has been reported. A number of studies have evaluated the use of deformation imaging in young asymptomatic patients with genetically proved Duchenne muscular dystrophy. Because these boys are born with this genetic mutation in the dystrophin gene, it is surprising that cardiac function has been generally interpreted as being normal at a young age. This cohort has been reported to develop overt myocardial dysfunction only during adolescence. It has been shown that in very young patients with normal conventional echocardiographic measures of function, early diastolic strain rate as measured by myocardial velocity gradients was reduced in the LV inferolateral wall. Moreover, this reduced strain rate at young age was shown to predict an adverse outcome with the development of cardiomyopathy later in life. The abnormal

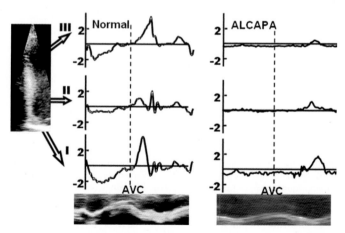

FIGURE 4.22. Reduced longitudinal deformation in postoperative anomalous left coronary artery from the pulmonary artery (ALCAPA) patients. Left ventricular longitudinal myocardial deformation at three levels in a normal control subject and a patient after coronary reimplantation for ALCAPA. The latter shows reduced longitudinal shortening.

deformation pattern was recently confirmed by MRI tagging, as well as in an animal model, where it was shown to correlate with microscopic damage in the myocardium. The detection of early dysfunction might be important in other pediatric conditions affecting LV function like anthracycline toxicity. The acute effect of anthracycline administration on LV deformation was recently explored by Ganame et al., who could demonstrate that reduced LV deformation was noted in all patients receiving anthracyclines within a few hours after administration of the first dose. In some patients, LV deformation further deteriorated after subsequent doses, while in others, LV dysfunction stabilized or even improved. The prognostic value of these findings warrants further investigation.

NEW DEVELOPMENTS IN DEFORMATION IMAGING: FROM DOPPLER-BASED TECHNIQUES TO SPECKLE TRACKING

Doppler-based deformation analysis uses myocardial velocity estimates, making the technique angle dependent as only velocities parallel to the ultrasound scan line can be estimated accurately. Thus, clinical interpretation is difficult and requires a high level of operator expertise. Especially in dilated ventricles and complex congenital heart disease, it can be extremely difficult to obtain good alignment of the ventricular walls in the direction of cardiac motion. This angle-dependency limits the applicability of the technique in children. Moreover, this approach provides only one component of the true 3D deformation of a myocardial segment. Cardiac deformation occurs in three dimensions at the same time. In addition, Doppler-based methodologies require considerable off-line processing, which is time consuming and highly operator dependent, influencing the reproducibility of the technique. In the early era of deformation analysis, it was necessary to manually track a myocardial segment throughout the cardiac cycle to obtain reliable deformation estimates. To try to resolve these issues, new echocardiographic techniques were developed to analyze cardiac deformation that are not Doppler based but are based on gray-scale imaging. Because of scattering, reflection, and interference of the ultrasound beam in myocardial tissue, speckle formations in gray-scale echocardiographic images represent tissue markers that can be tracked from frame to frame throughout the cardiac cycle (Fig. 4.23). Two experimental studies have validated a 2D technique based on speckle tracking that is independent of the insonation angle, allowing the acquisition of both radial and longitudinal deformation in single data sets. This technique also avoids the need for manual tracking, which currently slows the analysis of 1D data sets. It is hoped that the introduction of this new technology will increase the clinical acceptance of deformation imaging, especially in pediatric and congenital heart disease. Further validation studies in children need to be performed as the temporal resolution of the technique is lower compared with the Doppler-based technology. This may be an issue in smaller children with higher heart rates. Another issue is the temporal resolution in smaller hearts.

The advantage of speckle tracking technology is that it allows studying radial and longitudinal deformation in the same cardiac cycle. Also circumferential deformation and torsion can be calculated based on speckle tracking. Thus, ventricular rotational mechanics can be evaluated using echocardiography as validated by Notomi et al. and Helle-Valle et al. It was demonstrated that rotational mechanics in infants are different from these in adults with a progressive increase in torsion occurring with growth and maturation of the heart. It is thought that twisting, and especially untwisting dynamics, are important determinants in diastolic function. It is hoped that this will lead to new methods for assessing diastolic function in children.

An important limitation of deformation imaging that needs to be taken into account when applying it clinically is that deformation is intrinsically load dependent. Changes in both preload and afterload affect these measurements. Increased afterload results in decreased deformation while increased preload has the opposite effect on deformation parameters. Myocardial deformation results from an interaction between intrinsic myocardial force development, elastic myocardial properties, and loading. Loading of a myocardial segment is the result of segment interaction influencing prestretch and wall stress. The clinical relevance of the load-dependency certainly needs further clinical study. As most techniques in cardiology are load dependent, this does not preclude the clinical use of these deformation parameters especially for the quantitative longitudinal follow-up of certain patient populations.

MAGNETIC RESONANCE IMAGING FOR THE ASSESSMENT OF VENTRICULAR FUNCTION

Echocardiography is the principal noninvasive imaging tool in children with congenital and acquired heart disease because it is capable of providing comprehensive anatomic and hemodynamic information in many patients. However, its diagnostic utility is limited primarily by acoustic windows and its high dependency on operator experience. Cardiovascular MRI overcomes many of these limitations. For this reason, cardiovascular MRI has become a more often used imaging modality to assess anatomy, physiology, and function in children with heart disease. MRI often overlaps ventricular functional assessment normally obtained by echocardiography but also provides the clinician with very unique features such as calculating flow within a vessel and depicting the anatomy of all cardiovascular structures within the chest. With current cardiovascular MRI techniques, investigators and clinicians can obtain unique insights into fluid dynamics and ventricular function including regional myocardial deformation in three dimensions as well as increased accuracy of widely accepted measures of ventricular function such as cardiac output and ventricular volumes. Because of the rapid developments in technology, many MRI techniques are still experimental; however, many others are clinically useful. Because many of these techniques

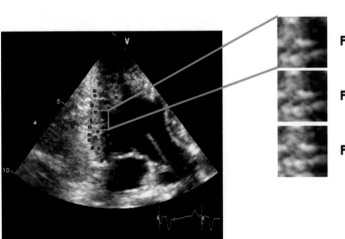

FIGURE 4.23. Principles of speckle tracking. In speckle tracking, speckle formations in gray-scale echocardiographic images are used as tissue markers that can be tracked from frame to frame throughout the cardiac cycle. Relative changes in position of these speckles are used to quantify regional deformation in a more automated fashion.

Frame N

Frame N+1

Frame N+2

are or will be used in clinical practice, physicians should be aware of the full spectrum of MRI capabilities. This section will review the role, advantages, and limitations of cardiac MRI in the assessment of ventricular function in children with heart disease.

Cardiac Magnetic Resonance Techniques Used for the Assessment of Ventricular Function: Cine Magnetic Resonance Imaging, Phase-encoded Velocity Mapping, and Myocardial Tagging

Three cardiac MRI techniques are most commonly used to assess cardiac function in patients with heart disease.

1. **Cine MRI:** This gradient-echo, steady-state free precession (SSFP), ECG-gated cine sequence yields images with high spatial and temporal resolution, excellent blood-to-myocardium contrast, and short acquisition time without the use of contrast agents (Fig. 4.24). Fast acquisition enables multiple phases of the cardiac cycle to be acquired. These can then be reconstructed into a cine MR image representing one full cardiac cycle using retrospective gating techniques at a temporal resolution of 20 to 25 ms. Multiple, contiguous cross-sectional, multiphase (cine loop) 2D slices are obtained across the region of interest to yield a spatially defined 3D data set at multiple levels and phases.

   Cine MRI also allows evaluation of cardiovascular anatomy and function. Cine MRI is unique in that it creates images over several heartbeats, thus averaging ventricular performance in the process. This is in contrast to images obtained with echocardiography, in which each image represents ventricular performance at that instant in time. Readers must then view many heartbeats and average the ventricular performance in their minds. Delineation of the endocardial and epicardial borders makes it possible to calculate ejection fraction, ventricular mass, stroke volume, cardiac output, wall thickness, and wall thickening with cardiac MR. The SSFP sequence is, however, relatively insensitive to flow disturbances and highly sensitive to inhomogeneities in the field of view and metallic artifacts. Alternatively, the older spoiled-gradient technique (with lower contrast) can be used when delineation of abnormal flow jets is desirable or when implanted metallic devices produce significant imaging artifacts.

   Recently, a 3D SSFP technique has been developed. Fast imaging of the entire cardiac volume at slightly reduced spatiotemporal

resolution but almost isotropic voxel size allows multiplanar reformatting. This is particularly useful in the assessment of complex congenital heart disease as it allows off-line reconstruction of often difficult anatomy in any desired plane.

2. **Velocity-Encoded Phase-Contrast MRI:** Quantification of blood flow and velocity can provide relevant information for the management of patients with congenital heart disease. Velocity-encoded phase-contrast MRI uses phase information to encode velocity. In the images parallel to blood flow (in-plane), one can measure peak flow velocity. In the images perpendicular to flow (through-plane), the product of the velocity in each pixel by the area of the blood vessel will yield flow at that given period of time (Fig. 4.25). The addition of flow information across all phases of the cardiac cycle will yield flow during one heartbeat. Direct quantification of stroke volume, flow, pulmonary-to-systemic ratio (Q_p/Q_s), valvular regurgitation fraction, severity of valvular stenosis, and differential lung perfusion can be performed with velocity-encoded phase-contrast MRI (Fig. 4.25).

   In addition, one can assess mitral and tricuspid inflow and pulmonary venous patterns with velocity-encoded phase-contrast MRI, making it possible to evaluate diastolic function. Because the MRI plane can be oriented in any direction, cardiac MRI avoids the difficulty sometimes encountered with Doppler techniques of being parallel to a flow jet. This method has been validated against Doppler echocardiography. Further improvements in temporal resolution as well as introduction of real-time MRI imaging may increase the relevance of MRI in assessing diastolic function in patients with heart disease. Current indications of MRI to assess flow include quantification of pulmonary regurgitation after repair of tetralogy of Fallot, measurement of transaortic valve gradient when there are difficulties with echocardiography, and quantification of (re)coarctation severity.

3. **Myocardial Tagging:** MRI is unique among imaging modalities in its ability to magnetically tag tissue. This is accomplished by applying thin saturation pulses immediately after the R wave. These saturation pulses destroy all the spins in a given plane resulting in a line of signal void in the image. Similarly, two sets of orthogonal tags can be placed to produce a grid across the image. This is followed by a standard but lower spatial resolution cine MRI sequence dividing the myocardial wall into cubes of magnetization. These lines or grids are distorted by myocardial motion, rotation, and deformation throughout the cardiac cycle (Fig. 4.26). Images can be obtained as frequently as every 15 to 20 ms in a given scan yielding high temporal resolution. The tradeoff for this high temporal resolution is that the stripes tend to degrade and blur so the assessment of myocardial wall mechanics in late diastole becomes less accurate.

   To perform calculations with tagged images, the initial step is to track the grid intersections through the phases of interest. This can be done manually or, as more recently described, semiautomatically. Tracking the translation, rotation, and deformation of these cubes in 2D or 3D allows calculation of wall motion, regional radii of curvature, regional wall thickening, and shortening as indicators of myocardial contractility. Of course, the myocardial regions should be divided into (arbitrary) anatomic regions (septal, anterior, lateral, and inferior walls) to perform the analysis. Full 3D analysis of circumferential, radial, longitudinal, and shearing myocardial forces is possible by collectively modeling numerous smaller elements (Fig 4.27). This has led to a better understanding of myocardial mechanics. Through-plane motion, which echocardiography is not able to take into account, can be compensated for by myocardial tagging.

   Despite all the above-mentioned advantages, myocardial tagging has remained a research tool as a result of the lack of automated postprocessing software. A recently described technique for the analysis of myocardial tagging data, harmonic phase imaging (HARP), appears promising because it does not require manual tracing of the tags and so shortens the analysis time.

   In the clinical scenario, myocardial tagging has provided useful information in patients with ischemic heart disease. It has been shown that strain analysis can discriminate viable from necrotic myocardium. In patients with congenital heart disease, Fogel et al. have used myocardial tagging to characterize the pattern of wall motion and deformation in patients with functionally single ventricles. Myocardial tagging has demonstrated a shift in the systemic right ventricle pattern of contraction from

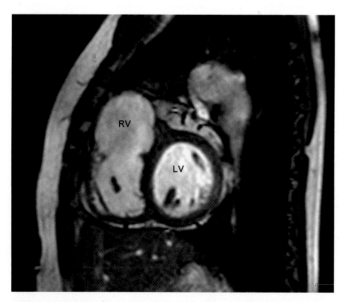

FIGURE 4.24. Balance steady-state free precession (b-SSFP) cine magnetic resonance imaging in short-axis view in a patient after repair of tetralogy of Fallot. The right ventricle is dilated, and the right ventricular outflow tract is thinned and dyskinetic.

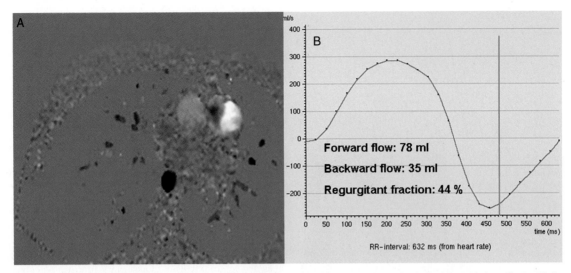

FIGURE 4.25. Phase encoded velocity mapping used to quantify flow and velocities of flow. Forward systolic flow in the right ventricular outflow tract in the cranial direction is displayed as white pixels. Flow-velocity curve is obtained by measuring the flow profile over time.

predominantly longitudinal shortening of the subpulmonary RV to predominantly circumferential shortening with loss of torsion in the systemic RV.

Cardiac Magnetic Resonance to Assess Ventricular Function

Quantitative assessment of ventricular dimensions and function is an important part of MRI evaluation of children with heart disease because the evaluation of cardiac function provides valuable diagnostic and prognostic information. Cardiac MRI has the advantage of being a volumetric technique allowing 3D reconstructions. Cardiac MRI provides highly accurate and reproducible measurements of ventricular mass, volume, and function that have made it the reference standard against which other techniques are measured (Fig. 4.28). This makes cardiac MRI ideal to follow-up patients with heart disease and to monitor the response to therapies because minor changes in volume/function can be detected

with high accuracy. Normal MRI values of ventricular volume and mass in adolescents and adults normalized to body surface area have been extensively reported. Unfortunately, data on adjusting MRI-derived parameters to body size in the pediatric population come from very small studies (Table 4.1).

Cardiac MRI is noninvasive and uses no ionizing radiation. It produces 3D data sets with high signal-to-noise ratio, high spatial resolution, and reasonable temporal resolution. This allows for accurate volume measurements of any cardiac chamber regardless of its morphology and without geometric assumptions. Independence from geometric assumptions is particularly important in patients with congenital heart disease because the ventricles often have complex shapes that do not follow geometric assumptions used in formulas to calculate volumes from 2D data sets.

Quantitative evaluation of biventricular function can be achieved by obtaining a series of contiguous cine slices that cover the ventricles in the short-axis plane. By tracing the endocardial border, the slice volume is calculated as the product of its cross-sectional area and thickness. Then ventricular volume is determined based

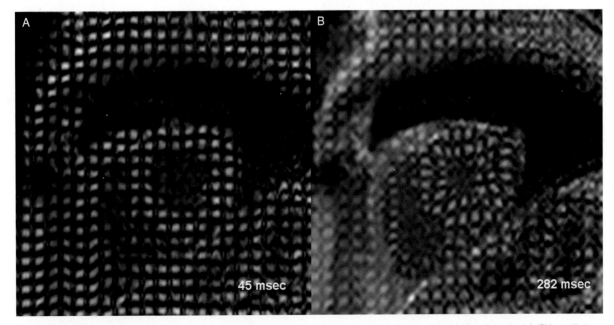

FIGURE 4.26. Myocardial tagging creates a grid on the myocardium. Example of short-axis myocardial tagging at end diastole (A) and at end systole (B) in a patient with congenital aortic stenosis. At end systole, the original grid is distorted by myocardial deformation. Myocardial deformation is larger in the subendocardial than in the subepicardial layers. Note that the grids on the chest wall remain unchanged.

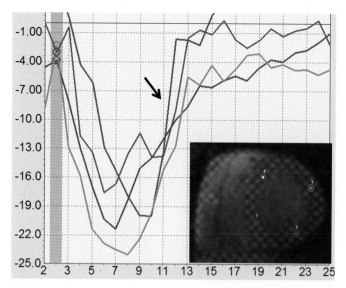

FIGURE 4.27. Analysis of circumferential myocardial deformation in a healthy 14-year-old boy. A short-axis view image is used to perform analysis in four myocardial walls: septal (*1*), inferior (*2*), lateral (*3*), and anterior (*4*). Note that there is a homogeneous amount and timing of systolic myocardial deformation with rapid early diastolic recoil (*arrow*) in all myocardial segments.

on Simpson's rule by simply adding the volumes of all slices. The process can be repeated for each frame in the cardiac cycle to obtain a continuous time-volume loop or may more simply be performed on only an end-diastolic and end-systolic frame to calculate end-diastolic and end-systolic volumes. Subtracting the end-systolic volume from the end-diastolic volume yields the stroke volume. The stroke volume divided by the end-diastolic volume gives the ejection fraction. Because the patient's heart rate at the time of image acquisition is known, one can calculate LV and RV output. Ventricular mass is calculated by tracing the epicardial borders, subtracting the endocardial volumes, and multiplying the resultant muscle volume by the specific gravity of the myocardium (1.05 g/cm^3).

Gradient-echo cine MRI is the technique of choice to assess RV volumes and function. RV volumes and function as well as pulmonary flow can be measured by MRI with a high rate of technical success in comparison with echocardiography. The location of the RV immediately behind the sternum often leads to limited image quality when using echocardiograpy. Also, the complex RV shape makes it extremely difficult to obtain reproducible RV volume calculations. Therefore, visual inspection or measurements of single-plane indices are commonly used to assess RV function by echocardiography. However, these approaches are limited by their lack of standardization and failure to describe the entire RV. At present, MRI using Simpson's rule is considered the gold standard for the evaluation of RV function, providing noninvasive accurate RV volume assessment without geometric assumptions.

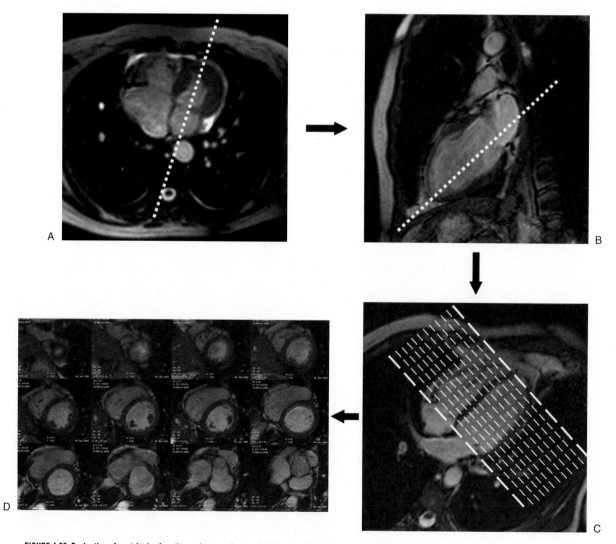

FIGURE 4.28. Evaluation of ventricular function, volume, and mass. A: Using a localizing image in the axial plane, a two-chamber (also known as vertical long-axis) plane is prescribed. **B:** From the two-chamber image, the four-chamber (or horizontal long-axis) plane is defined. **C:** From the four-chamber image, a 12-slice short-axis stack covering the ventricle entirely is prescribed. **D:** Resulting short-axis stack showing end-diastolic phase.

Table 4.1	VENTRICULAR PARAMETERS NORMALIZED TO BODY SURFACE AREA IN THE PEDIATRIC POPULATION
Parameter	**Mean, standard deviation, and 95% confidence interval**
LVEDV/BSA (ml/m^2)	67 ± 9 (49-85)
RVEDV/BSA (ml/m^2)	70 ± 11 (49-91)
SV/BSA (ml/m^2)	44 ± 7 (31-57)
CI (L/min/m^2)	3.2 ± 0.5 (2.2-4.3)
LV mass/BSA (g/m^2)	81 ± 13 (56-106)

LVEDV, left ventricular end-diastolic volume; BSA, body surface area; RVEDV, right ventricular end-diastolic volume; SV, stroke volume; CI, cardiac index.

Assessment of the contribution of different areas of the ventricular wall to global ventricular performance is important in many cardiac diseases. With cardiac MRI one can visualize and evaluate all myocardial segments in different planes. Clinically used parameters to express regional myocardial function are wall thickness, systolic wall thickening, and circumferential and longitudinal wall shortening. Wall thickening can be quantified by delineating the endocardial and epicardial borders at end diastole and end systole. Visual analysis of wall motion using semiquantitative scoring for regional wall motion is often used clinically. Different grades are used: normokinesis (normal wall motion), hypokinesis (decreased wall motion), akinesis (absent wall motion), dyskinesis (wall motion in the opposite direction of expected), and hyperkinesis (increased wall motion). With cardiac MRI, one can also quantify wall motion by measuring the amount of centripetal motion throughout systole.

Myocardial function at rest can be normal; however, during periods of increased oxygen demand, myocardial ischemia resulting in regional myocardial dysfunction, expressed as wall motion abnormalities, may ensue. This can be assessed with gradient-echo cine MRI. Dobutamine stress cine MRI has been reported to be a useful test in adults with coronary artery disease, particularly in patients with poor acoustic windows. More recently, the use of an MRI-compatible supine cycle ergometer has been reported in patients with congenital heart disease to allow assessment of ventricular function and valve regurgitation response to exercise. Stress MRI also allows evaluation of contractile reserve. Contractile reserve is the magnitude of augmentation of ventricular performance with stress. The study of contractile reserve with stress MRI demonstrates functional abnormalities that remain occult at rest and thereby helps to detect early ventricular dysfunction. This may be particularly useful in the evaluation of RV function after correction of tetralogy of Fallot or after the atrial switch procedure. Stress MRI may also detect the functional consequences of coronary anomalies.

Clinical Applications

Cardiac MRI examinations combine a comprehensive description of anatomy together with the quantitative evaluation ventricular function in patients with heart disease. The evaluation of ventricular volumes and function in patients after repair of tetralogy of Fallot is the most common referral for cardiac MRI examinations in pediatric patients. An accurate assessment of ventricular volumes and function is particularly helpful in these patients because timely detection and monitoring of changes in RV volume have prognostic implications. It has been shown that there is a lower likelihood of postoperative reduction in RV end-diastolic volume if pulmonary valve replacement is performed when preoperative RV end-diastolic volume is larger than 160 ml/m^2. Also, cardiac MRI can provide detailed delineation of RV outflow tract anatomy, which is important for planning surgical or interventional valve replacement. In addition, velocity-encoded phase-contrast MRI can be used to quantify pulmonary regurgitation in these patients.

Quantifying systemic RV volumes and systolic function in patients after atrial switch operation or patients with congenitally corrected TGA can be challenging because these ventricles are dilated and hypertrophied with multiple prominent trabeculations. MRI is the only technique that allows acquisition of full-volume data sets encompassing the entire right ventricle. In addition, cardiac MRI can be used to demonstrate the 3D anatomy of the atrial switch baffle and assess flow.

Patients with arrhythmogenic RV cardiomyopathy develop RV dysfunction and are at increased risk of sudden death. Although often challenging and subjective, cardiac MRI can detect subtle wall motion abnormalities, which occur in the early phase of the disease. Also, fatty fibrous tissue infiltration of the RV free wall can also be demonstrated with a T1 fast-spin echo sequence.

Because of its robustness, cardiac MRI is especially well suited for follow-up of patients with valvular heart disease in which an accurate evaluation of ventricular volumes and ejection fraction is crucial for surgical timing.

In patients with simple congenital heart lesions such as atrial septal defects, ventricular septal defects as well as patent ductus arteriosus, cardiac MRI can be used to quantify Q_p/Q_s and to calculate ventricular volume as an indicator of the hemodynamic burden imposed by the defect.

Other situations in which cardiac MRI examinations are performed in the assessment of ventricular function include patients with univentricular hearts with limited acoustic windows. Cardiac MRI allows evaluation of ventricular volumes and function, detection of Fontan baffle fenestration, presence of thrombi, and measurement of pulmonary blood flow. It can also be optimal to detect pulmonary venous obstruction, evaluate atrioventricular valve function, and rule out outflow tract obstruction.

Acquisition Protocols

Detailed preexamination MRI planning is crucial given the wide array of imaging sequences available and the complex nature of the clinical, anatomic, and functional issues in patients with congenital heart disease. As with echocardiography, cardiac MRI examination of patients with congenital heart disease is an interactive diagnostic procedure that requires online review and interpretation of the data by the supervising physician. The imaging specialist need not be deterred by the anatomic variability found in these patients. Discussions with a pediatric cardiologist can clarify the clinical questions to be answered, enabling a comprehensive anatomic and diagnostic examination.

To aid in reproducibility and accelerate clinical scanning, MRI assessment of ventricular function is performed in a highly standardized manner producing two long-axis cine images and a stack of 10 to 12 short-axis cines (Fig. 4.28). A cine image can be acquired in one breath hold of about 8 to 10 seconds. Therefore, a typical set of ventricular images can be acquired in less than 5 minutes. Initially, a series of transverse pilot views are obtained. From these, the mitral valve and LV apex can be identified. The vertical long-axis (VLA) cine image can then be obtained. The VLA is then used to plan the horizontal long-axis (HLA) image, which shows all four chambers and the mitral and tricuspid valves. The HLA and VLA views are then used to plan the short axis. The first short-axis plane should be placed using the end-diastolic image at the base of the heart covering the most basal portion of the left and right ventricles just forward of the atrioventricular ring. It is vital that the basal slice is acquired in a consistent and standardized manner to optimize reproducibility. Further short-axis images are acquired sequentially every 6 to 8 mm in children and every 8 to 10 mm in adults along the long axis to the cardiac apex. All cines should be acquired during breath holding. The expiratory phase of respiration has shown to provide more reproducible diaphragmatic position, but acquiring the images in inspiration is better tolerated.

RV "short-axis" volume data are available as a byproduct of the LV volume short-axis acquisition. However, this is not true RV short-axis data. For true RV short-axis data, the stack of short-axis slices should be specifically planned so that they are parallel to the tricuspid valve. As a result, extra care is needed when defining and analyzing the most basal slice of the above conventional RV "short-axis" data. The RV volume measurements can alternatively be made from data sets acquired in the axial orientation. We acquire these data from the coronal localizing images, which demonstrate the gross cardiac anatomy, by planning an orthogonal stack of slices to cover the heart from a level just below the diaphragm to the pulmonary bifurcation (Fig. 4.29).

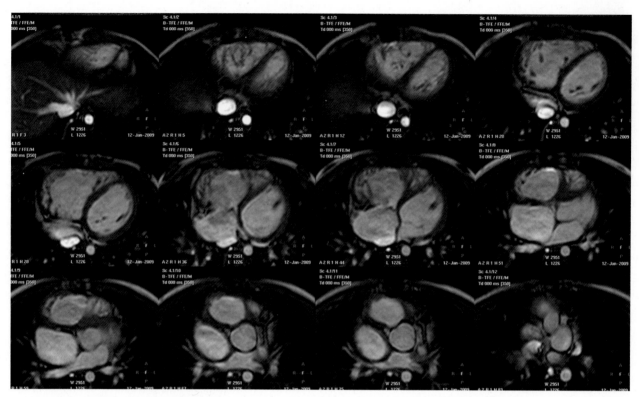

FIGURE 4.29. Right ventricular axial scan in a patient after arterial switch operation for transposition of the great arteries. Plane scans extend from the diaphragm (**top left**) to above the pulmonary artery (**bottom right**).

Additionally, velocity-encoded cine MRI can be acquired in the transverse plane crossing the proximal ascending aorta or proximal pulmonary artery. This makes it possible to quantify the hemodynamic severity of shunts and calculate stroke volume in a way independent of the volumetric calculation, and thus can be used as an internal control of the accuracy of the measurements. Care should be taken to set the limit of the velocity encoding range above the expected values to avoid aliasing. The velocities within the myocardium have recently been measured in 3D using velocity-encoded cine MRI by setting low velocity encoding ranges (15 to 30 cm/s). This method, however, lacks sufficient temporal resolution and has blood-related artifacts. These problems may be resolved by future improvements in image acquisition techniques.

Data Analysis

Cardiac MRI image analysis is usually performed off-line using commercially available analysis software. This remains a time-consuming process requiring manual delimitation of multiple images. For LV and RV volume analyses, end diastole and end systole are visually defined as the phase with the largest area (generally the first) and the phase with the smallest LV and RV areas, respectively. The endocardial contour has to be drawn in each slice at end diastole and end systole. Also, the epicardial boundary has to be delimited (generally in end diastole) to calculate LV mass. Ideally, the papillary muscles should be outlined separately and excluded from the ventricular volume but included in the myocardial mass. This, however, is not always possible. At the base of the heart, slices are considered to be within the left ventricle if the blood volume is surrounded by 50% or more ventricular myocardium. If the basal slice contains both ventricular and atrial tissue, the ventricular contours are drawn to the junction with the atrium and joined by a straight line through the blood pool. The workstation computes the LV and RV end-diastolic volume, end-systolic volume, stroke volume, ejection fraction, and LV mass using a modified Simpson's rule equation.

The manual delineation of LV endocardial and epicardial borders takes 10 to 15 minutes per data set. Development of algorithms for automatic border detection has facilitated the application of these techniques, but further refinements are required to improve their efficiency.

Through-plane motion represents a major challenge to achieve accurate volume measurements during the cardiac cycle. Through-plane motion results from a 15% to 18% longitudinal shortening in normal hearts while the base of the heart moves toward the apex. As a consequence of this long-axis shortening, a short-axis slice positioned through the base of the left ventricle at end diastole will be located in the atrium at end systole. Without correction for through-plane motion, end-systolic volumes are overestimated and ejection fraction is underestimated. Although correction for through-plane motion can be achieved with slice tracking techniques, this promising feature is not clinically available. So, correction techniques need to be applied during postprocessing.

Problems and Potential Solutions

Despite many advantages, the use of cardiac MRI for the evaluation of cardiac function in pediatric patients with heart disease is still limited by several factors. MRI cannot be performed in patients with pacemakers or defibrillators or with recent (within 6 weeks) implantation of vascular coils. Sternal wires, vascular coils, prosthetic heart valves, and intracardiac devices will induce imaging artifacts, mainly when using gradient-echo sequences.

Cardiac MRI evaluation under general anesthesia or deep sedation is needed in patients younger than 7 to 8 years or in subjects with claustrophobia. Other patients may be unable to hold their breath for long periods (longer than 10 seconds). Performing cardiac MRI with free breathing can be performed in patients who are unable to hold their breath using two approaches. The first is to use a diaphragmatic navigator so that an image is only acquired when the diaphragm, and therefore the heart, is in a preset location. More recently, "real-time" imaging has been used. In this case, images are acquired in one cardiac cycle, rather than across several. Real-time images are of lower resolution but still able to render reproducible information.

Irregular heart rhythms such as atrial fibrillation or frequent ectopy pose a challenge to the MRI acquisition because images are acquired over several heartbeats. This requires acquiring the images at comparable RR intervals. Blurred images result from acquiring images when the RR intervals are irregular. The use of real-time imaging can overcome these problems.

Future Applications

Future applications of MRI in the setting of pediatric heart disease include optimization of current sequences to make acquisition faster while maintaining spatial resolution. More interactive planning with more "on-line" information and shorter postprocessing time would be desirable as well.

In addition, the use of new sequences may provide additional valuable information. Postcontrast myocardial enhancement has been extensively validated and proved to be helpful in defining viable myocardium in patients with ischemic heart disease and demonstrating the presence of myocardial scar in various conditions such as dilated and hypertrophic cardiomyopathies. The value of this technique to detect areas of myocardial fibrosis in patients with congenital heart disease warrants further evaluation. Also, evaluation of contractile reserve and myocardial perfusion with stressors may help to identify early cardiac dysfunction and areas of abnormal perfusion, respectively. Finally, high field-strength magnets (3 T) with multiple channels and faster gradients will allow better imaging of small children and smaller structures like the coronary arteries.

Interventional MRI is a new exciting field. The combination of 3D information with high spatial resolution and real-time imaging makes MRI particularly appealing as a guide to intravascular procedures such as (re)coarctation or pulmonary valve stenting. MRI-guided cardiac catheterization allows simultaneous acquisition of MRI flow data and invasive pressure measurements and thus accurate measurements of pulmonary vascular resistance.

 ## CONCLUSIONS

Significant recent technological developments allow the clinician to use a wide array of different methods and techniques to assess systolic ventricular function in children. No technique, however, allows the easy quantification of intrinsic myocardial contractility. Most techniques used in daily clinical practice are load dependent and/or geometry dependent. An individualized approach considering the clinical question to be answered and the benefits and drawbacks of each technique appears appropriate.

SUGGESTED READINGS

Abd El Rahman MY, Hui W, Dsebissowa F, et al. Quantitative analysis of paradoxical interventricular septal motion following corrective surgery of tetralogy of Fallot. *Pediatr Cardiol.* 2005;26:379–384.

Abd El Rahman MY, Hui W, Yigitbasi M, et al. Detection of left ventricular asynchrony in patients with right bundle branch block after repair of tetralogy of Fallot using tissue-Doppler imaging-derived strain. *J Am Coll Cardiol.* 2005;45:915–921.

Ahmad M, Xie T, McCulloch M, et al. Real-time three-dimensional dobutamine stress echocardiography in assessment stress echocardiography in assessment of ischemia: Comparison with two-dimensional dobutamine stress echocardiography. *J Am Coll Cardiol.* 2001;37:1303–1309.

Altmann K, Shen Z, Boxt LM, et al. Comparison of three-dimensional echocardiographic assessment of volume, mass, and function in children with functionally single left ventricles with two-dimensional echocardiography and magnetic resonance imaging. *Am J Cardiol.* 1997;80:1060–1065.

Amundsen BH, Helle-Valle T, Edvardsen T, et al. Noninvasive myocardial strain measurement by speckle tracking echocardiography: Validation against sonomicrometry and tagged magnetic resonance imaging. *J Am Coll Cardiol.* 2006;47:789–793.

Arai K, Hozumi T, Matsumura Y, et al. Accuracy of measurement of left ventricular volume and ejection fraction by new real-time three-dimensional echocardiography in patients with wall motion abnormalities secondary to myocardial infarction. *Am J Cardiol.* 2004;94:552–558.

Ashford MW Jr, Liu W, Lin SJ, et al. Occult cardiac contractile dysfunction in dystrophin-deficient children revealed by cardiac magnetic resonance strain imaging. *Circulation.* 2005;112:2462–2467.

Baker GH, Hlavacek AM, Chessa KS, et al. Left ventricular dysfunction is associated with intraventricular dyssynchrony by 3-dimensional echocardiography in children. *J Am Soc Echocardiogr.* 2008;21:230–233.

Balestrini L, Fleishman C, Lanzoni L, et al. Real-time 3-dimensional echocardiography evaluation of congenital heart disease. *J Am Soc Echocardiogr.* 2000;13:171–176.

Barkhausen J, Ruehm SG, Goyen M, et al. MR evaluation of ventricular function: True fast imaging with steady-state precession versus fast low-angle shot cine MR imaging: Feasibility study. *Radiology.* 2001;219:264–269.

Be'eri E, Maier SE, Landzberg MJ, et al. In vivo evaluation of Fontan pathway flow dynamics by multidimensional phase-velocity magnetic resonance imaging. *Circulation.* 1998;98:2873–2882.

Beerbaum P, Körperich H, Barth P, et al. Noninvasive quantification of left-to-right shunt in pediatric patients: Phase-contrast cine magnetic resonance imaging compared with invasive oximetry. *Circulation.* 200;103:2476–2482.

Boettler P, Hartmann M, Watzl K, et al. Heart rate effects on strain and strain rate in healthy children. *J Am Soc Echocardiogr.* 2005;18:1121–1130.

Bogaert J, Dymarkowski S, Taylor AM, eds. *Clinical Cardiac MRI.* Heidelberg: Springer; 2005.

Borlaug BA, Melenovsky V, Redfield MM, et al. Impact of arterial load and loading sequence on left ventricular tissue velocities in humans. *J Am Coll Cardiol.* 2007;50:1570–1577.

Bos JM, Hagler DJ, Silvilairat S, et al. Right ventricular function in asymptomatic individuals with a systemic right ventricle. *J Am Soc Echocardiogr.* 2006;19:1033–1037.

Buyse G, Mertens L, Di Salvo G, et al. Idebenone treatment in Friedreich's ataxia: neurological, cardiac, and biochemical monitoring. *Neurology.* 2003;60:1679–1681.

Caiani EG, Corsi C, Sugeng L, et al. Improved quantification of left ventricular mass based on endocardial and epicardial surface detection with real-time three dimensional echocardiography. *Heart.* 2006;92:213–219.

Chetboul V, Escriou C, Tessier D, et al. Tissue Doppler imaging detects early asymptomatic myocardial abnormalities in a dog model of Duchenne's cardiomyopathy. *Eur Heart J.* 2004;25:1934–1939.

Cheung MM, Smallhorn JF, Vogel M, et al. Disruption of the ventricular myocardial force-frequency relationship after cardiac surgery in children: Noninvasive assessment by means of tissue Doppler imaging. *J Thorac Cardiovasc Surg.* 2006;131:625–631.

Corsi C, Lang RM, Veronesi F, et al. Volumetric quantification of global and regional left ventricular function from real-time three-dimensional echocardiographic images. *Circulation.* 2005;112:1161–1170.

Dekker DL, Piziali RL, Dong E Jr. A system for ultrasonically imaging the human heart in three dimensions. *Comput Biomed Res.* 1974;7:544–553.

Derumeaux G, Ovize M, Loufoua J, et al. Doppler tissue imaging quantitates regional wall motion during myocardial ischemia and reperfusion. *Circulation.* 1998;97:1970–1977.

Di Salvo G, Eyskens B, Claus P, et al. Late post-repair ventricular function in patients with origin of the left main coronary artery from the pulmonary trunk. *Am J Cardiol.* 2004;93:506–508.

Didier D, Ratib O, Beghetti M, et al. Morphologic and functional evaluation of congenital heart disease by magnetic resonance imaging. *J Magn Reson Imaging.* 1999;10:639–655.

Eidem BW, McMahon CJ, Ayres NA, et al. Impact of chronic left ventricular preload and afterload on Doppler tissue imaging velocities: A study in congenital heart disease. *J Am Soc Echocardiogr.* 2005;18:830–838.

Eidem BW, McMahon CJ, Cohen RR, et al. Impact of cardiac growth on Doppler tissue imaging velocities: A study in healthy children. *J Am Soc Echocardiogr* 2004;17:212–221.

Eyskens B, Ganame J, Claus P, et al. Ultrasonic strain rate and strain imaging of the right ventricle in children before and after percutaneous closure of an atrial septal defect. *J Am Soc Echocardiogr.* 2006;19:994–1000.

Eyskens B, Weidemann F, Kowalski M, et al. Regional right and left ventricular function after the Senning operation: An ultrasonic study of strain rate and strain. *Cardiol Young.* 2004;14:255–264.

Flachskampf FA, Chandra S, Gaddipatti A, et al. Analysis of shape and motion of the mitral annulus in subjects with and without cardiomyopathy by echocardiographic 3-dimensional reconstruction. *J Am Soc Echocardiogr.* 2000;13:277–287.

Fogel MA, Weinberg PM, Chin AJ, et al. Late ventricular geometry and performance changes of functional single ventricle throughout staged Fontan reconstruction assessed by magnetic resonance imaging. *J Am Coll Cardiol* 1996;28:212–221.

Fogel MA, Weinberg PM, Gupta KB, et al. Mechanics of the single left ventricle: A study in ventricular-ventricular interaction II. *Circulation.* 1998;98:330–338.

Fogel MA. Assessment of cardiac function by magnetic resonance imaging. *Pediatr Cardiol.* 2000;21:59–69.

Frigiola A, Redington AN, Cullen S, et al. Pulmonary regurgitation is an important determinant of right ventricular contractile dysfunction in patients with surgically repaired tetralogy of Fallot. *Circulation.* 2004;110:II-153–II-157.

Ganame J, Claus P, Eyskens B, et al. Acute cardiac functional changes after subsequent anthracycline infusions in children. *Am J Cardiol.* 2007;99:974–977.

Ganame J, Mertens L, Eidem BW, et al. Regional myocardial deformation in children with hypertrophic cardiomyopathy: Morphological and clinical correlations. *Eur Heart J.* 2007;28:2886–2894.

Garot J, Bluemke DA, Osman NF, et al. Fast determination of regional myocardial strain fields from tagged cardiac images using harmonic phase MRI. *Circulation.* 2000;101:981–988.

Geva T, Sandweiss BM, Gauvreau K, et al. Factors associated with impaired clinical status in long-term survivors of tetralogy of Fallot repair evaluated by magnetic resonance imaging. *J Am Coll Cardiol.* 2004;43:1068–1074.

Giatrakos N, Kinali M, Stephens D, et al. Cardiac tissue velocities and strain rate in the early detection of myocardial dysfunction of asymptomatic boys with Duchenne's muscular dystrophy: Relationship to clinical outcome. *Heart.* 2006;92:840–842.

Gorcsan J 3rd, Strum DP, Mandarino WA, et al. Quantitative assessment of alterations in regional left ventricular contractility with color-coded tissue Doppler echocardiography. Comparison with sonomicrometry and pressure-volume relations. *Circulation.* 1997;95:2423–2433.

Greenberg NL, Firstenberg MS, Castro PL, et al. Doppler-derived myocardial systolic strain rate is a strong index of left ventricular contractility. *Circulation.* 2002;105:99–105.

Greil G, Geva T, Maier SE, Powell AJ. Effect of acquisition parameters on the accuracy of velocity encoded cine magnetic resonance imaging blood flow measurements. *J Magn Reson Imaging.* 2002;15:47–54.

Grothues F, Smith GC, Moon JC, et al. Comparison of interstudy reproducibility of cardiovascular magnetic resonance with two-dimensional echocardiography in normal subjects and in patients with heart failure or left ventricular hypertrophy. *Am J Cardiol.* 2002;90:29–34.

Haber I, Metaxas DN, Axel L. Three-dimensional motion reconstruction and analysis of the right ventricle using tagged MRI. *Med Image Anal.* 2000;4:335–355.

Heimdal A, Stoylen A, Torp H, et al. Real-time strain rate imaging of the left ventricle by ultrasound. *J Am Soc Echocardiogr.* 1998;11:1013–1019.

Helbing WA, Rebergen SA, Maliepaard C, et al. Quantification of right ventricular function with magnetic resonance imaging in children with normal hearts and with congenital heart disease. *Am Heart J.* 1995;130:828–837.

Helle-Valle T, Crosby J, Edvardsen T, et al. New noninvasive method for assessment of left ventricular rotation: Speckle tracking echocardiography. *Circulation.* 2005;112:3149–3156.

Hiarada K, Orino T, Yasuoka K, et al. Tissue Doppler imaging of left and right ventricles in normal children. *Tohoku J Exp Med.* 2000;191:21–29.

Hozumi T, Yoshikawa J, Yoshida K, et al. Three-dimensional echocardiographic measurement of left ventricular volumes and ejection fraction using a multiplane transesophageal probe in patients. *Am J Cardiol.* 1996;78:1077–1080.

Hung J, Lang R, Flachskampf F, et al. 3D echocardiography: A review of the current status and future directions. *J Am Soc Echocardiogr.* 2007;20:213–233.

Isaaz K, Thompson A, Ethevenot G, et al. Doppler echocardiographic measurement of low velocity motion of the left ventricular posterior wall. *Am J Cardiol.* 1989;64:66–75.

Jacobs LD, Salgo IS, Goonewardena S, et al. Rapid online quantification of left ventricular volume from real-time three-dimensional echocardiographic data. *Eur Heart J.* 2006;27:460–468.

Jenkins C, Bricknell K, Hanekom L, et al. Reproducibility and accuracy of echocardiographic measurements of left ventricular parameters using real-time three-dimensional echocardiography. *J Am Coll Cardiol.* 2004;44:878–886.

Kapetanakis S, Kearney MT, Siva A, et al. Real-time three-dimensional echocardiography: A novel technique to quantify global left ventricular mechanical dyssynchrony. *Circulation.* 2005;112:992–1000.

Kapusta L, Thijssen JM, Groot-Loonen J, et al. Tissue Doppler imaging in detection of myocardial dysfunction in survivors of childhood cancer treated with anthracyclines. *Ultrasound Med Biol.* 2000;26:1099–1108.

Keenan NG, Pennell DJ. CMR of ventricular function. *Echocardiography.* 2007;24:185-193.

Kim RJ, Wu E, Rafael A, et al. The use of contrast-enhanced magnetic resonance imaging to identify reversible myocardial dysfunction. *N Engl J Med.* 2000;343:1445–1453.

Kiraly P, Kapusta L, Thijssen JM, et al. Left ventricular myocardial function in congenital valvar aortic stenosis assessed by ultrasound tissue-velocity and strain-rate techniques. *Ultrasound Med Biol.* 2003;29:615–620.

Kuhl HP, Bucker A, Franke A, et al. Transesophageal 3-dimensional echocardiography: in vivo determination of left ventricular mass in comparison with magnetic resonance imaging. *J Am Soc Echocardiogr.* 2000;13:205–215.

Kukulski T, Voigt JU, Wilkenshoff UM, et al. A comparison of regional myocardial velocity information derived by pulsed and color Doppler techniques: An in vitro and in vivo study. *Echocardiography.* 2000;17:639–651.

Lamb HJ, Singleton RR, van der Geest RJ, et al. MR imaging of regional cardiac function: Low-pass filtering of wall thickness curves. *Magn Reson Med.* 1995;34:498–502.

Lang RM, Mor-Avi V, Sugeng L, et al. Three-dimensional echocardiography: The benefits of the additional dimension. *J Am Coll Cardiol.* 2006;48:2053–2069.

Langeland S, D'Hooge J, Wouters PF, et al. Experimental validation of a new ultrasound method for the simultaneous assessment of radial and longitudinal myocardial deformation independent of insonation angle. *Circulation.* 2005;112:2157–2162.

Lorenz CH. The range of normal values of cardiovascular structures in infants, children, and adolescents measured by magnetic resonance imaging. *Pediatr Cardiol.* 2000;21:37–46.

Lyseggen E, Rabben SI, Skulstad H, et al. Myocardial acceleration during isovolumic contraction: relationship to contractility. *Circulation.* 2005;111:1362–1369.

Matsumura Y, Hozumi T, Arai K, et al. Non-invasive assessment of myocardial ischaemia using new real-time three-dimensional dobutamine stress echocardiography: Comparison with conventional two-dimensional methods. *Eur Heart J.* 2005;26:1625–1632.

McDicken WN, Sutherland GR, Moran CM, et al. Colour Doppler velocity imaging of the myocardium. *Ultrasound Med Biol.* 1992;18:651–654.

Mor-Avi V, Sugeng L, Weinert L, et al. Fast measurement of left ventricular mass with real-time three-dimensional echocardiography: Comparison with magnetic resonance imaging. *Circulation.* 2004;110:1814–1818.

Nagel E, Lehmkuhl HB, Bocksch W, et al. Non-invasive diagnosis of ischemia induced wall motion abnormalities with the use of high-dose dobutamine stress MRI: Comparison with dobutamine stress echocardiography. *Circulation.* 1999;99:763–770.

Niemann PS, Pinho L, Balbach T, et al. Anatomically oriented right ventricular volume measurements with dynamic three-dimensional echocardiography validated by 3-Tesla magnetic resonance imaging. *J Am Coll Cardiol.* 2007;50:1668–1676.

Notomi Y, Lysyansky P, Setser RM, et al. Measurement of ventricular torsion by two-dimensional ultrasound speckle tracking imaging. *J Am Coll Cardiol.* 2005;45:2034–2041.

Notomi Y, Srinath G, Shiota T, et al. Maturational and adaptive modulation of left ventricular torsional biomechanics: Doppler tissue imaging observation from infancy to adulthood. *Circulation.* 2006;113:2534–2541.

Oosterhof T, van Straten A, Vliegen HW, et al. Preoperative thresholds for pulmonary valve replacement in patients with corrected tetralogy of Fallot using cardiovascular magnetic resonance. *Circulation.* 2007;116:545–551.

Papavassiliou DP, Parks WJ, Hopkins KL, et al. Three-dimensional echocardiographic measurement of right ventricular volume in children with congenital heart disease validated by magnetic resonance imaging. *J Am Soc Echocardiogr.* 1998;11:770–777.

Pauliks LB, Chan KC, Chang D, et al. Regional myocardial velocities and isovolumic contraction acceleration before and after device closure of atrial septal defects: A color tissue Doppler study. *Am Heart J.* 2005;150:294–301.

Pauliks LB, Pietra BA, DeGroff CG, et al. Non-invasive detection of acute allograft rejection in children by tissue Doppler imaging: Myocardial velocities and myocardial acceleration during isovolumic contraction. *J Heart Lung Transplant.* 2005;24:S239–S248.

Pauliks LB, Vogel M, Madler CF, et al. Regional response of myocardial acceleration during isovolumic contraction during dobutamine stress echocardiography: A color tissue Doppler study and comparison with angiocardiographic findings. *Echocardiography.* 2005;22:797–808.

Pettersen E, Helle-Valle T, Edvardsen T, et al. Contraction pattern of the systemic right ventricle shift from longitudinal to circumferential shortening and absent global ventricular torsion. *J Am Coll Cardiol.* 2007;49:2450–2456.

Plein S, Bloomer TN, Ridgway JP, et al. Steady-state free precession magnetic resonance imaging of the heart: Comparison with segmented k-space gradient echo imaging. *J Magn Reson Imaging.* 2001;14:230–236.

Poutanen T, Jokinen E, Sairanen H, et al. Left atrial and left ventricular function in healthy children and young adults assessed by three-dimensional echocardiography. *Heart.* 2003;89:544–549.

Powell AJ, Geva T. Blood flow measurement by magnetic resonance imaging in congenital heart disease. *Pediatr Cardiol.* 2000;21:47–58.

Razavi RS, Hill DL, Muthurangu V, et al. Three-dimensional magnetic resonance imaging of congenital cardiac anomalies. *Cardiol Young.* 2003;13:461–465.

Roberson DA, Cui W, Chen Z, et al. Annular and septal Doppler tissue imaging in children: Normal z-score tables and effects of age, heart rate, and body surface area. *J Am Soc Echocardiogr.* 2007;20:2076–2084.

Roest AA, Helbing WA, Kunz P, et al. Exercise MR imaging in the assessment of pulmonary regurgitation and biventricular function in patients after tetralogy of Fallot repair. *Radiology.* 2002;223:204–211.

Rychik J, Tian ZY. Quantitative assessment of myocardial tissue velocities in normal children with Doppler tissue imaging. *Am J Cardiol.* 1996;77:1254–1257.

Sapin PM, Schroeder KM, Gopal AS, et al. Three-dimensional echocardiography: Limitations of apical biplane imaging for measurement of left ventricular volume. *J Am Soc Echocardiogr.* 1995;8:576–584.

Sengupta PP, Korinek J, Belohlavek M, et al. Left ventricular structure and function: Basic science for cardiac imaging. *J Am Coll Cardiol.* 2006;48:1988–2001.

Sengupta PP, Krishnamoorthy VK, Korinek J, et al. Left ventricular form and function revisited: applied translational science to cardiovascular ultrasound imaging. *J Am Soc Echocardiogr.* 2007;20:539–551.

Sheikh K, Smith SW, von Ramm O, et al. Real-time, three-dimensional echocardiography: Feasibility and initial use. *Echocardiography.* 1991;8:119–125.

Sohn DW, Chai IH, Lee DJ, et al. Assessment of mitral annulus velocity by Doppler tissue imaging in the evaluation of left ventricular diastolic function. *J Am Coll Cardiol.* 1997;30:474–480.

Sugeng L, Weinert L, Thiele K, et al. Real-time three-dimensional echocardiography using a novel matrix array transducer. *Echocardiography*. 2003;20:623–635.

Sutherland GR, Di Salvo G, Claus P, et al Strain and strain rate imaging: A new clinical approach to quantifying regional myocardial function. *J Am Soc Echocardiogr*. 2004;17:788–802.

Tsai-Goodman B, Geva T, Odegard KC, et al. Clinical role, accuracy, and technical aspects of cardiovascular magnetic resonance imaging in infants. *Am J Cardiol*. 2004;94:69–74.

Uematsu M, Miyatake K, Tanaka N, et al. Myocardial velocity gradient as a new indicator of regional left ventricular contraction: Detection by a two-dimensional tissue Doppler imaging technique. *J Am Coll Cardiol*. 1995;26:217–223.

Urheim S, Edvardsen T, Torp H, et al. Myocardial strain by Doppler echocardiography. Validation of a new method to quantify regional myocardial function. *Circulation*. 2000;102:1158–1164.

van den Bosch AE, Robbers-Visser D, Krenning BJ, et al. Real-time transthoracic three-dimensional echocardiographic assessment of left ventricular volume and ejection fraction in congenital heart disease. *J Am Soc Echocardiogr*. 2006;19:1–6.

Vicario ML, Caso P, Martiniello AR, et al. Effects of volume loading on strain rate and tissue Doppler velocity imaging in patients with idiopathic dilated cardiomyopathy. *J Cardiovasc Med (Hgerstown, Md)*. 006;7:852–858.

Vinereanu D, Florescu N, Sculthorpe N, et al. Differentiation between pathologic and physiologic left ventricular hypertrophy by tissue Doppler assessment of long-axis function in patients with hypertrophic cardiomyopathy or systemic hypertension and in athletes. *Am J Cardiol*. 2001;88:53–58.

Vinereanu D, Ionescu AA, Fraser AG. Assessment of left ventricular long axis contraction can detect early myocardial dysfunction in asymptomatic patients with severe aortic regurgitation. *Heart*. 2001;85:30–36.

Vogel M, Cheung MM, Li J, et al. Noninvasive assessment of left ventricular force-frequency relationships using tissue Doppler-derived isovolumic acceleration: Validation in an animal model. *Circulation*. 2003;107:1647–1652.

Vogel M, Schmidt MR, Kristiansen SB, et al. Validation of myocardial acceleration during isovolumic contraction as a novel noninvasive index of right ventricular contractility: Comparison with ventricular pressure-volume relations in an animal model. *Circulation*. 2002;105:1693–1699.

Vogel M, Sponring J, Cullen S, et al. Regional wall motion and abnormalities of electrical depolarization and repolarization in patients after surgical repair of tetralogy of Fallot. *Circulation*. 2001;103:1669–1673.

Weidemann F, Breunig F, Beer M, et al. Improvement of cardiac function during enzyme replacement therapy in patients with Fabry disease: A prospective strain rate imaging study. *Circulation*. 2003;108:1299–1301.

Weidemann F, Eyskens B, Mertens L, et al. Quantification of regional right and left ventricular function by ultrasonic strain rate and strain indexes after surgical repair of tetralogy of Fallot. *Am J Cardiol*. 2002;90:133–138.

Weidemann F, Eyskens B, Mertens L, et al. Quantification of regional right and left ventricular function by ultrasonic strain rate and strain indexes in Friedreich's ataxia. *Am J Cardiol*. 2003;91:622–626.

Weidemann F, Eyskens B, Sutherland GR. New ultrasound methods to quantify regional myocardial function in children with heart disease. *Pediatr Cardiol*. 2002;23:292–306.

Weidemann F, Jamal F, Sutherland GR, et al. Myocardial function defined by strain rate and strain during alterations in inotropic states and heart rate. *Am J Physiol Heart Circ Physiol*. 2002;283:H792–H799.

Yang H, Sun JP, Lever HM, et al. Use of strain imaging in detecting segmental dysfunction in patients with hypertrophic cardiomyopathy. *J Am Soc Echocardiogr*. 2003;16:233–239.

Zeidan Z, Erbel R, Barkhausen J, et al. Analysis of global systolic and diastolic left ventricular performance using volume-time curves by real-time three-dimensional echocardiography. *J Am Soc Echocardiogr*. 2003;16: 29–37.

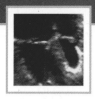

Chapter 5
Anomalies of the Pulmonary and Systemic Venous Connections

Frank Cetta • Naser Ammash

 ANOMALOUS PULMONARY VENOUS CONNECTIONS

Introduction and Embryogenesis

Abnormalities associated with connections of the pulmonary veins are rare and make up a small percentage of cases of congenital heart disease (CHD). These abnormalities have traditionally been divided into two major subgroups. *Total anomalous pulmonary venous connections* (TAPVCs) occur when *all* of the pulmonary veins from both lungs do not connect normally to the left atrium (LA) but instead connect to other veins or the right atrium (RA). With very rare exception, it is obligatory for patients with TAPVC to have an atrial septal defect (ASD) or patent foramen ovale (PFO) to sustain life. *Partial anomalous pulmonary venous connections* (PAPVCs) constitute the abnormal connection of one or several pulmonary veins. However, in PAPVCs, at least one pulmonary vein connects normally to the LA. PAPVCs can have a large variety of connections to systemic veins or the RA. Many, but not all, patients with PAPVC have an ASD.

There are important clinical differences between the two subgroups. Patients with a TAPVC will usually present early in life with cyanosis and severe pulmonary hypertension secondary to pulmonary venous obstruction, whereas patients with a PAPVC will usually be asymptomatic in childhood. These patients may be discovered incidentally in adulthood or present with signs and symptoms similar to an ASD with left-to-right shunting. Meticulous echocardiographic assessment from multiple imaging planes is essential to confidently establish that the pulmonary venous connections are normal. If one cannot identify all of the pulmonary veins, then an exhaustive search for the pulmonary venous connections must ensue. If transthoracic echocardiography (TTE) is not completely diagnostic, then other imaging modalities, such as transesophageal echocardiography (TEE), computed tomography (CT), magnetic resonance imaging (MRI), or, rarely, cardiac catheterization, need to be used.

Normally, there are two right-sided and two left-sided pulmonary veins. Although the normal right lung has three lobes, the right middle and upper veins usually join before entering the LA. The most common variation in normal pulmonary venous anatomy is to have a single pulmonary vein from either lung (the left is more common). Healey reported in 1952 that this may occur in as many as 24% of anatomic specimens. To understand the variety of pulmonary venous anomalies, one must understand the embryologic origin of the pulmonary veins. During early embryogenesis, part of the splanchnic plexus forms the pulmonary vascular bed. The pulmonary vascular bed is connected to the umbilicovitelline and cardinal venous systems. The pulmonary vascular bed is not connected to the heart during early development. Eventually, an evagination from the LA joins the interparenchymal pulmonary veins to form the "common pulmonary vein." The common pulmonary vein, also termed a *pulmonary venous confluence,* becomes incorporated completely into the LA during the first month of gestation. Once this connection to the heart is established, the original pulmonary venous attachments to the splanchnic plexus involute. All abnormalities of pulmonary venous connections can be understood based on the original development of the pulmonary veins from the splanchnic plexus (Fig. 5.1). Geva and van Praagh recently provided an excellent review of pulmonary venous anomalies (2001, pp. 736–772). This chapter is recommended reading for those interested in further description of the embryogenesis of pulmonary venous anomalies.

A distinction should also be made between the exact anatomic "connection" of a pulmonary vein to the LA or other vessel/chamber and the "drainage" of a pulmonary vein. Although a pulmonary vein may "connect" normally to the LA, if malposition of the atrial septum (Fig. 5.2) or an ASD is present, pulmonary venous flow may actually "drain" across the interatrial defect into the RA. The echocardiographer should therefore use this terminology carefully when communicating with the surgeon.

Transthoracic Imaging of Pulmonary Venous Connections

Accurate delineation of the pulmonary venous connections to the LA requires clear two-dimensional imaging from multiple imaging

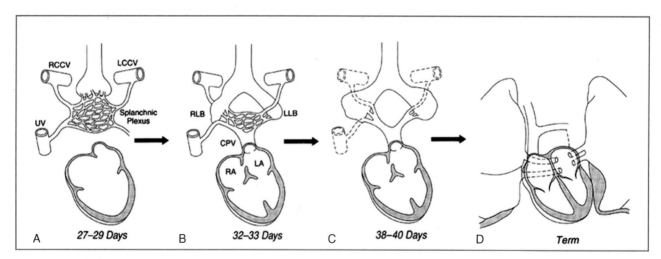

FIGURE 5.1. Embryologic development of the pulmonary veins from the splanchnic plexus during the first month of embryogenesis. A: Lung buds connected to the splanchnic plexus. No connection to heart exists at this point. LCCV, left common cardinal vein; RCCV, right common cardinal vein; UV, umbilicovitelline vein. **B:** Later in development, the common pulmonary vein (CPV) has evaginated from the left atrium (LA) and connected to the pulmonary venous plexus. The pulmonary veins are connected to the splanchnic plexus and the heart at this point in development. LLB, left lung bud; RLB, right lung bud. **C:** The connections to the splanchnic plexus involute. **D:** By term, the common pulmonary vein has become completely incorporated into the LA and the individual veins connect to the LA. (From Geva T, Van Praagh S. Anomalies of the pulmonary veins. In: Allen HD, Gutgesell HP, Clark EB, Driscoll DJ, eds. *Moss and Adams' Heart disease in infants, children and adolescents.* 6th ed. Philadelphia, Pa: Lippincott Williams & Wilkins; 2001:736–772. Originally adapted from work by R. C. Anderson, with permission.)

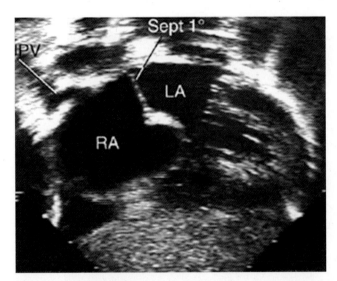

FIGURE 5.2. Subcostal frontal plane view (four-chamber) demonstrating normal "connection" of the right upper pulmonary vein (PV) to the left atrium (LA). However, due to malposition of the primum atrial septum (Sept 1°), the "drainage" from this vein is directed to the right atrial (RA) side of the septum.

windows. Color and spectral Doppler imaging is required to demonstrate flow from each vein into the LA. Suspicion of APVC should be raised if right-sided volume is demonstrated, especially if no interatrial communication is observed. In newborns, suspect TAPVC if the left atrial size is reduced.

Subcostal Frontal (Four-Chamber) and Sagittal Views – The subcostal frontal and sagittal views offer excellent imaging of the connections of the pulmonary veins, especially in children or thin adults. These views also are critical to the assessment of the atrial septum. Frequently, a sinus venosus ASD can be adequately assessed from the subcostal sagittal plane, obviating the need for alternative imaging. The subcostal sagittal view with rightward angulation offers a unique view of the right upper pulmonary vein as it travels between the superior vena cava (SVC) (anterior) and the right pulmonary artery (posterior) (Fig. 5.3A). When one rotates the transducer 90 degrees back to the frontal view, the SVC will no longer be visualized, but assessment of the right lower pulmonary vein (Fig. 5.3B) can occur. The os of the coronary sinus can also be evaluated from the subcostal frontal plane image; dilation of the coronary sinus may suggest APVC.

Parasternal Long- and Short-Axis (PSLA and PSSA) Views – PSLA images with leftward angulation will demonstrate the connection of one or both left pulmonary veins to the LA. Color flow interrogation at the posterior aspect of the cardiac border can demonstrate these flows (Fig. 5.3C). PSSA images demonstrate the anterior and posterior aspects of the atrial septum. The connection of the right lower pulmonary vein to the LA can be demonstrated with rightward angulation when one focuses on the posterior edge of the atrial septum. PSSA at the level of the main pulmonary artery demonstrates the connection of the left pulmonary veins to the LA. A dilated coronary sinus may also be detected in the PSSA scans as well as the os of the coronary sinus between the tricuspid inlet and the inferior vena cava (IVC)–RA junction. The high right parasternal window offers a unique view of the relationship of the SVC and the right pulmonary veins. Figure 5.3D demonstrates three right-sided pulmonary veins connecting to the LA in a normal fashion.

Apical Four-Chamber View – The apical four-chamber image clearly demonstrates the connection of the right lower and left lower pulmonary veins (Fig. 5.3E). A common misconception is that the right upper pulmonary vein is demonstrated in this scanning plane. However, the apical four-chamber image is not oriented in an anterior-to-posterior plane. Instead, the scan is entirely posterior from a superior-to-apical perspective, providing excellent imaging

of the posteriorly positioned atrioventricular valves, the entrance of the IVC into the RA, and the respective lower pulmonary veins.

Suprasternal Notch Short-Axis or "Crab View" – The "crab" view (Fig. 5.4A–C) permits the identification of all pulmonary veins connecting to the LA and should be part of all routine TTE assessments. This image usually provides excellent imaging of the normal pulmonary veins in small children. Adult echocardiography laboratories do not typically obtain this view. Recently, the Mayo Clinic congenital echocardiography laboratory demonstrated in 200 consecutive adult patients that the suprasternal notch short-axis view was obtained in 74% of patients. However, two-dimensional images adequately demonstrated the connection of all pulmonary veins in only 46% of these patients. In this assessment, parameters of body habitus (body mass index, body surface area, height, and weight) did not correlate with ability to adequately evaluate the pulmonary venous connections (P. Katanyuwong, Mayo Clinic, unpublished data). An imaging pitfall is that the LA appendage can also be visualized in this window and should not be mistaken for the left upper pulmonary vein (Fig. 5.4D).

Total Anomalous Pulmonary Venous Connection

TAPVC is usually classified according to the position of the anomalous connection relative to the heart, and TAPVCs are divided into four major subtypes (Fig. 5.5).

- Supracardiac
- Cardiac
- Infracardiac
- Mixed

In the *supracardiac* type of TAPVC, the pulmonary veins come together to form a confluence that does not enter the left side of the heart but instead enters a "vertical vein" (usually on the left side of the chest), which drains to the innominate vein (Fig. 5.6A). This is the most common type of TAPVC. The anomalous vertical vein is an embryologic remnant of the splanchnic and cardinal systems. Children come to medical attention due to an abnormal chest radiograph and enlargement of the right side of the heart. The chest radiograph is classically described as having a "snowman" appearance (Fig. 5.6B). These children generally have difficulty gaining weight and are tachypneic. In the more common anatomic form of supracardiac TAPVC, the left vertical vein originates from the pulmonary venous confluence and travels anterior to the left pulmonary artery (LPA), left mainstem bronchus, and aortic arch before it joins the innominate vein just proximal to where the left internal jugular and left subclavian veins join (Fig. 5.7). However, when the left vertical vein passes *between* the LPA and the left mainstem bronchus, it may become obstructed. This is referred to as a "vascular vise" (Fig. 5.8). The vertical vein is not referred to as a "left superior vena cava." The term "left superior vena cava" should be used when a left-sided chest vessel connects the innominate vein to the coronary sinus or LA (Fig. 5.9). In *cardiac* TAPVCs, all pulmonary veins connect to a vein that directly enters the right side of the heart (usually the coronary sinus). These connections are usually unobstructed (Fig. 5.10). In *infracardiac* TAPVCs, all of the pulmonary veins connect to a vertical vein that descends below the diaphragm (Fig. 5.11). This connection below the diaphragm occurs due to failed involution of the connection to the unbilicovitelline system. This form of TAPVC is associated with severe pulmonary hypertension and obstruction of the vertical vein as it crosses the diaphragm or enters the relatively smaller-caliber veins in or near the liver. Most commonly, the infracardiac vertical vein enters the portal vein system and that is the site of obstruction. Connection to the ductus venosus, hepatic veins, or IVC has also been observed. Infracardiac TAPVC usually requires emergent surgery in the first hours after birth. Rarely, angiography (Fig. 5.12A) is needed to better delineate the course of the pulmonary veins before surgical repair. Infracardiac TAPVC should be suspected in newborns who present with respiratory distress and diffuse bilateral pulmonary venous congestion on chest radiography (Fig. 5.12B).

The diagnosis of infracardiac TAPVC may be particularly challenging in the newborn with lung disease and may be misinterpreted as persistent pulmonary hypertension. Echocardiographic

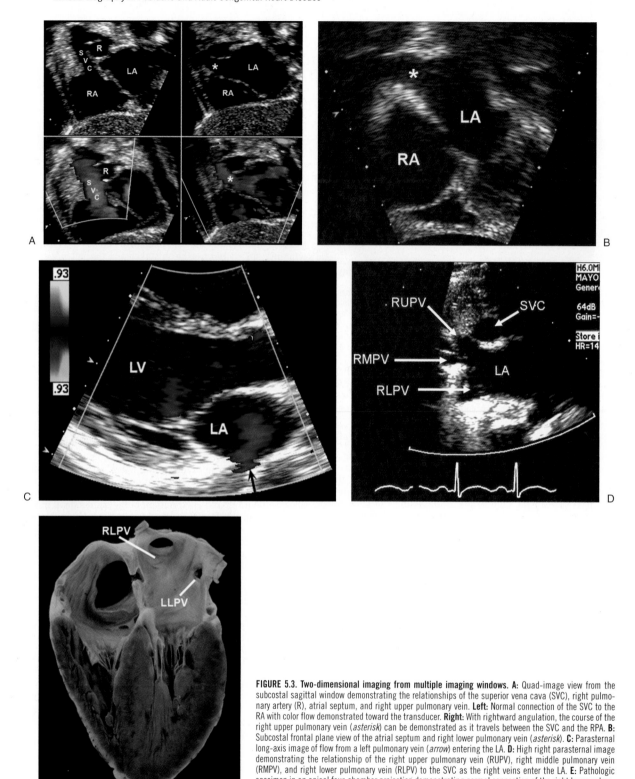

FIGURE 5.3. Two-dimensional imaging from multiple imaging windows. A: Quad-image view from the subcostal sagittal window demonstrating the relationships of the superior vena cava (SVC), right pulmonary artery (R), atrial septum, and right upper pulmonary vein. **Left:** Normal connection of the SVC to the RA with color flow demonstrated toward the transducer. **Right:** With rightward angulation, the course of the right upper pulmonary vein (*asterisk*) can be demonstrated as it travels between the SVC and the RPA. **B:** Subcostal frontal plane view of the atrial septum and right lower pulmonary vein (*asterisk*). **C:** Parasternal long-axis image of flow from a left pulmonary vein (*arrow*) entering the LA. **D:** High right parasternal image demonstrating the relationship of the right upper pulmonary vein (RUPV), right middle pulmonary vein (RMPV), and right lower pulmonary vein (RLPV) to the SVC as the right veins enter the LA. **E:** Pathologic specimen in an apical four-chamber projection demonstrating normal connection of the right lower pulmonary vein (RLPV) and left lower pulmonary vein (LLPV) to the left atrium.

imaging can be especially difficult if the patient is intubated and requires aggressive ventilator management. Clear two-dimensional images of the pulmonary veins may be limited. In these patients, both color and spectral Doppler techniques need to used extensively to ensure that flow from the pulmonary veins is demonstrated into the LA.

In some situations, these neonates deteriorate rapidly. Resuscitation may include extracorporeal membrane oxygenation (ECMO). If the diagnosis of TAPVC is not established before initiation of ECMO, it may be difficult to wean the child from the circuit. In these circumstances, an alternative imaging method, such as angiography, has been used

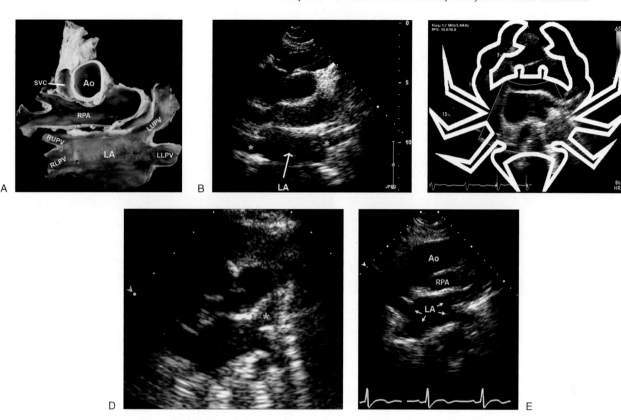

FIGURE 5.4. "Crab" views. A: Pathologic specimen similar to the suprasternal notch short-axis view demonstrating normal pulmonary venous connections. Coined the "crab view," all four pulmonary veins can usually be identified from this scanning plane. This view is usually diagnostic in small children. This imaging window may not be as accessible in adults. Ao, aorta; LA, left atrium; LLPV, left lower pulmonary vein; LUPV, left upper pulmonary vein; RLPV, right lower pulmonary vein; RPA, right pulmonary artery; RUPV, right upper pulmonary vein; SVC, superior vena cava. B: Corresponding two-dimensional echocardiograph demonstrating the LA and the relative positions of the four pulmonary vein entrances (*asterisks*). C: Diagram of the "crab" superimposed on a suprasternal short-axis image demonstrating an abnormal "crab view." The RLPV is not demonstrated entering the LA in this patient with scimitar syndrome. D: Suprasternal short-axis view demonstrating an imaging pitfall. In this image, the *asterisk* depicts the LA appendage and *not* the LUPV. E: A "true" crab view in which the pulmonary veins (*arrows*) are clearly identified connecting to the LA. The course of the proximal RPA just posterior to the ascending Ao is also demonstrated.

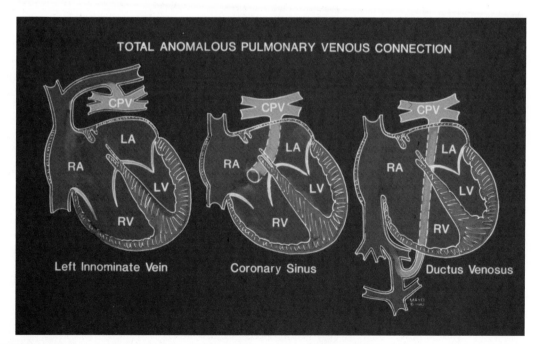

FIGURE 5.5. Three forms of total anomalous pulmonary venous connection (TAPVC): *supracardiac* type (left), *cardiac* type to the coronary sinus (middle), *infracardiac* type (right). CPV, pulmonary venous confluence.

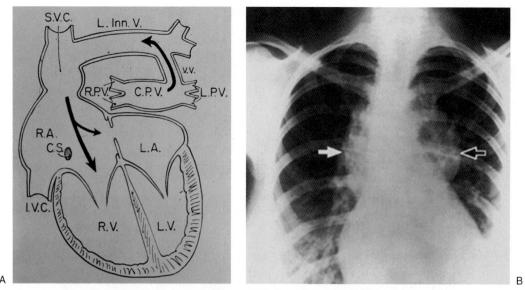

FIGURE 5.6. Supracardiac total anomalous pulmonary venous connection (TAPVC). A: Diagram depicting supracardiac TAPVC. The respective right (RPV) and left (LPV) pulmonary veins connect to a confluence (CPV) that is superior to the dome of the left atrium (LA). The pulmonary venous confluence connects to a dilated vertical vein (VV). In turn, the vertical vein connects to the left innominate vein (L. Inn. V.) and ultimately the superior vena cava (SVC). Both the SVC and innominate vein will appear dilated. CS, coronary sinus; IVC, inferior vena cava. **B:** Chest radiograph in a child with supracardiac TAPVC demonstrating the "snowman" sign. The left-sided mediastinal shadow (*black arrow*) is the dilated VV. The right-sided mediastinal shadow (*white arrow*) is the dilated SVC.

FIGURE 5.7. More common anatomic form of supracardiac total anomalous pulmonary venous connections (TAPVC). Top: Apical four-chamber view demonstrating right atrial (RA) and right ventricular (RV) dilation in a child with supracardiac TAPVC. **Bottom left:** Two-dimensional suprasternal notch image of a left-sided vertical vein (VV) connecting to the innominate vein (Inn V). Ao, aorta. **Bottom right:** Color Doppler image in the same plane demonstrating cephalad (red) flow in the vertical vein as it joins the innominate vein. SVC, superior vena cava.

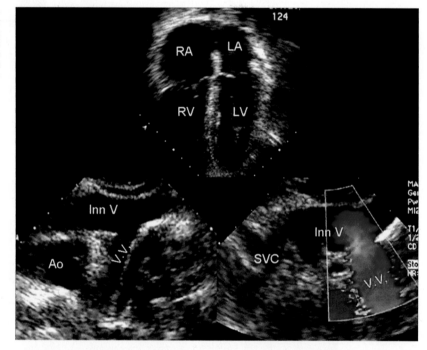

FIGURE 5.8. "Vascular vise." Left: Subcostal coronal image demonstrating the pulmonary venous confluence (*asterisk*) with the appearance of a "hat" on top of the superior aspect of the left atrium (LA). **Right:** Suprasternal short-axis view with color Doppler demonstrating a left vertical vein with aliased flow (*arrow*) at the point of a "vascular vise." The vertical vein is partially obstructed as it passes between the left mainstem bronchus and the left pulmonary artery.

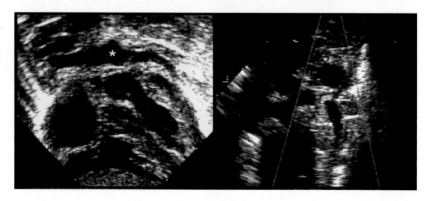

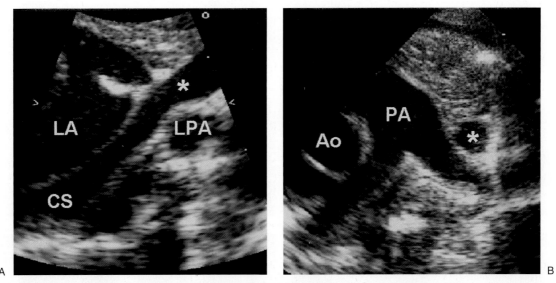

FIGURE 5.9. Left superior vena cava (LSVC) (*asterisk*) connecting to the right atrium (RA) via the coronary sinus (CS). Left: High parasternal short-axis view with clockwise rotation to visualize the course of an LSVC connecting to the CS. **Right:** Parasternal short-axis scan at the level of the pulmonary artery (PA) bifurcation demonstrating an LSVC (*asterisk*) coursing anterior to the left pulmonary artery (LPA). Ao, aorta.

to discover obstructed infracardiac TAPVC. Relief of the pulmonary venous obstruction is mandatory before weaning from ECMO.

The fourth type of TAPVC is generically referred to as "mixed." This form represents a combination of at least two of the other types. In the mixed form of TAPVC, there is no true pulmonary venous confluence. Imaging errors can easily be made in patients with this anatomy. Patients with heterotaxy syndromes may be predisposed to mixed APVCs. Also, patients with heterotaxy syndromes with

situs ambiguous of the atria may have "ipsilateral" APVCs, in which the right and left veins connect to the respective sides of the common atrium.

Partial Anomalous Pulmonary Venous Connections

PAPVC, first described by Winslow in 1739, is an uncommon congenital anomaly found in 0.4% to 0.7% of autopsies. Both

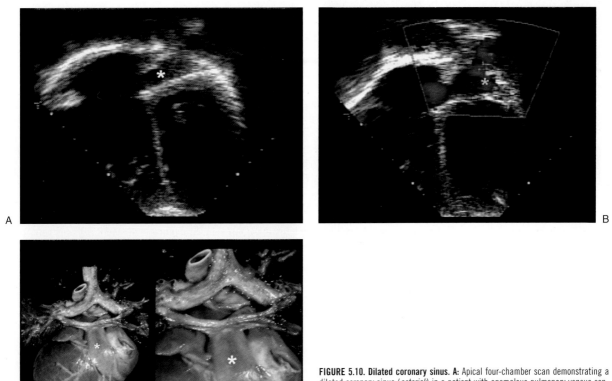

FIGURE 5.10. Dilated coronary sinus. **A:** Apical four-chamber scan demonstrating a dilated coronary sinus (*asterisk*) in a patient with anomalous pulmonary venous connection to the coronary sinus. **B:** Color Doppler image in the same projection as A, demonstrating antegrade flow in the coronary sinus. **C:** Pathologic specimen from a posterior view demonstrating a pulmonary venous confluence connecting to a dilated coronary sinus (*asterisk*) in a *cardiac* form of total anomalous pulmonary venous connections (TAPVC).

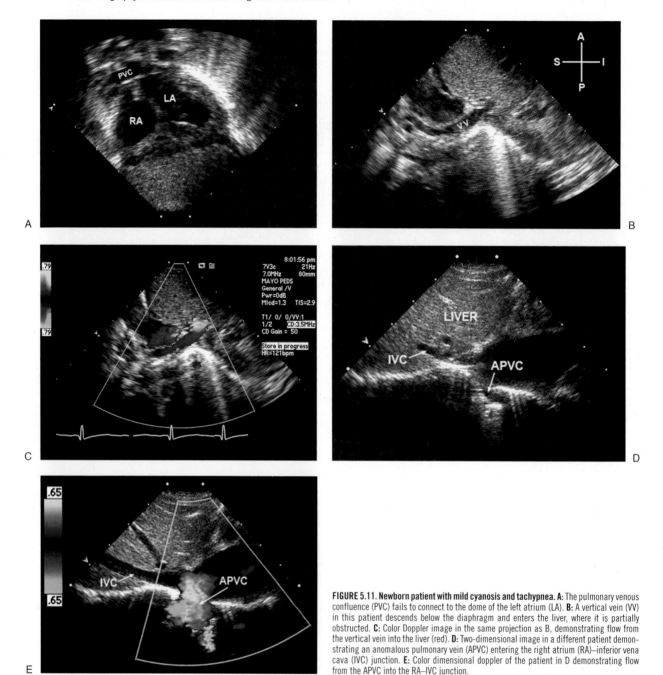

FIGURE 5.11. Newborn patient with mild cyanosis and tachypnea. A: The pulmonary venous confluence (PVC) fails to connect to the dome of the left atrium (LA). **B:** A vertical vein (VV) in this patient descends below the diaphragm and enters the liver, where it is partially obstructed. **C:** Color Doppler image in the same projection as B, demonstrating flow from the vertical vein into the liver (red). **D:** Two-dimensional image in a different patient demonstrating an anomalous pulmonary vein (APVC) entering the right atrium (RA)–inferior vena cava (IVC) junction. **E:** Color dimensional doppler of the patient in D demonstrating flow from the APVC into the RA–IVC junction.

TTE and TEE are commonly used in the detection of PAPVC. Echocardiography also plays an important role in the evaluation of associated hemodynamic changes such as volume overload of the right heart chambers, tricuspid regurgitation, and pulmonary hypertension. Children with PAPVC may be asymptomatic and escape detection until adulthood. When symptomatic, patients with PAPVC present with dyspnea, fatigue, atrial arrhythmia, pulmonary hypertension, unexplained cardiomegaly on chest radiograph, or unexplained right ventricular volume overload on TTE. PAPVC can be an isolated defect with an intact atrial septum or associated with a PFO or secundum ASD. PAPVC has been described in up to 85% of patients with a sinus venosus ASD.

PAPVC can involve the right- or left-sided pulmonary veins and rarely can arise from both lungs in the same patient. The most common variety of PAPVC is a right-sided pulmonary vein connecting to the SVC or RA. Anomalous connection of left-sided pulmonary veins to a vertical vein that connects to the innominate vein and SVC is less common. In addition, there are many reports of PAPVC to the

left subclavian vein, brachiocephalic vein, azygous vein, portal vein, and coronary sinus. Essentially, PAPVC may occur to any thoracic systemic vein.

Right Pulmonary Veins to the RA or SVC – Two-dimensional TTE combined with color flow Doppler are excellent diagnostic tools for visualization of PAPVC, particularly in children and young adults. Using TTE, the most common form of PAPVC (right upper pulmonary vein [RUPV] to the SVA), can be seen from the suprasternal short-axis view. This scanning plane allows visualization of the innominate vein, SVC, aorta, and right pulmonary artery. In the presence of PAPVC of the right upper and/or middle pulmonary vein to the SVC, an abnormal color flow Doppler can be seen entering the wall of the SVC with the flow directed toward the suprasternal notch (Fig. 5.13). Spectral Doppler assessment of that signal will confirm the presence of a systolic and diastolic flow pattern typical of pulmonary venous flow.

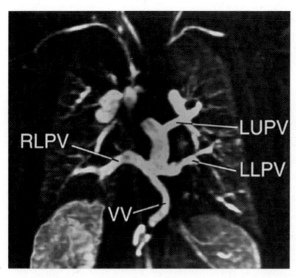
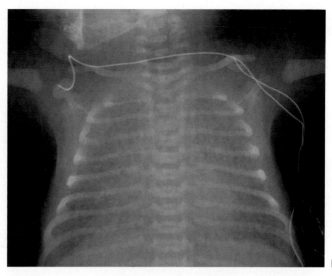

FIGURE 5.12. Infracardiac total anomalous pulmonary venous connection (TAPVC). A: Typical angiogram of an infant with infracardiac TAPVC demonstrating the descending vertical vein (VV), right lower pulmonary vein (RLPV), left lower pulmonary vein (LLPV), and left upper pulmonary vein (LUPV). **B:** Typical chest radiograph in a newborn with obstructed infracardiac TAPVC demonstrating diffuse pulmonary venous congestion.

Most patients with a so-called "sinus venosus ASD" will also have partial anomalous connection of the right pulmonary veins (usually upper and middle) to the RA and/or SVC. In children and thin adults, this can be adequately evaluated from the subcostal window (Fig. 5.14). The use of the term "ASD" is actually a misnomer in these patients. Many pathologists believe that the true defect is between the SVC and the right pulmonary veins as they cross each other. Surgeons frequently use the "ASD" to baffle the right pulmonary venous flow to the LA.

Isolated anomalous connection of the right upper pulmonary vein to the SVC may occur in the absence of an ASD. The anomalous connection of the RUPV to the SVC may occur cephalad of the level azygous vein. When associated with a sinus venosus

ASD, the connection of the RUPV is more typically below the level of the azygous vein connection to the SVC, at the SVC–RA junction, or directly to the RA. A "high" connection of an anomalous RUPV to the SVC may be missed with TTE and with TEE. During TEE, the probe should be withdrawn far enough in the esophagus to allow imaging cephalad of the azygous vein–SVC junction.

Scimitar Syndrome – Scimitar syndrome is a rare association of (a) anomalous right pulmonary vein(s) to the IVC, (b) right lung hypoplasia, and (c) aberrant arterial supply to the affected lobe of the right lung. It occurs in 1 to 3 of 100,000 births, and the clinical presentation is quite variable. The lesion was first described by Cooper in 1836 and is termed "scimitar" because of the later described unique chest radiograph finding of the anomalous right pulmonary vein descending toward the IVC–it resembles a Turkish sword. Seventy-five percent of the time, scimitar syndrome occurs without addition congenital heart defects. Associated lesions that occur in the other 25% of patients include ASD, ventricular septal defect (VSD), patent ductus arteriosus (PDA), tetralogy of Fallot, and coarctation. Neonatal presentation is dramatic because these children may have severe pulmonary hypertension and cyanosis. Surgical results for neonates with scimitar syndrome have historically been poor. More commonly, these patients present in adulthood with dyspnea, right-sided volume overload, or new-onset atrial arrhythmia. Subcostal images are uniquely suited for imaging scimitar syndrome. The anomalous right vein(s) can be demonstrated entering the IVC just below the IVC–RA junction. In scimitar syndrome, the heart may be shifted to the right due to the associated hypoplasia of a portion of the right lung (Fig. 5.15).

Left Pulmonary Veins to the Innominate Vein – When the PAPVC involves the left lung, one or more left-sided pulmonary veins connect into the innominate vein through a left vertical vein (a remnant of the left anterior cardinal system) (Fig. 5.16). This is best seen with surface echocardiography imaging from the suprasternal window. During the examination, attention should be paid to the area on the left side of the aortic arch. Color flow and spectral Doppler will confirm that pulmonary venous flow is directed from the chest, cephalad into the innominate vein and subsequently the SVC.

Right atrial and right ventricular enlargement are typically seen when the left-to-right shunt created by the PAPVC is significant. Right ventricular enlargement will be associated with abnormal septal motion. The main pulmonary artery and its branches also enlarge depending on the volume of the shunt and the presence of

FIGURE 5.13. Transthoracic short-axis view from the suprasternal notch demonstrating anomalous connection of a right pulmonary vein to the superior vena cava (SVC) *(arrow).* Inn, innominate vein, Ao, aorta; LA, left atrium; RPA, right pulmonary artery.

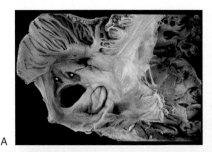
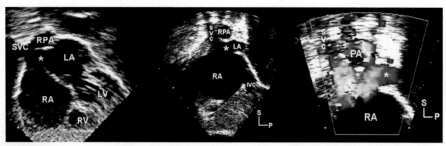

A

B

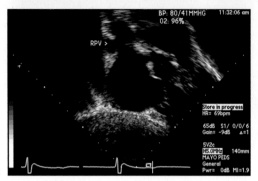

C

FIGURE 5.14. Sinus venosus atrial septal defect (ASD). A: Pathologic specimen of anomalous connection of two right pulmonary veins (*asterisks*) to the right atrium (RA). **B: Left:** Subcostal frontal image with superior angulation demonstrating a sinus venosus ASD (*asterisk*). **Center:** Subcostal sagittal orientation demonstrates the sinus venosus ASD (*asterisk*) just inferior to the right pulmonary artery (RPA). Note the location of the superior vena cava (SVC). **Right:** Color Doppler demonstrates the large left-to-right shunt through the sinus venosus ASD. **C:** Frontal subcostal image with slight rotation in a 10-year-old demonstrating anomalous connection of the right pulmonary vein (RPV) to the SVC just cephalad of the RA–SVC junction.

pulmonary hypertension. In addition, in the case of PAPVC of the left pulmonary vein(s), the innominate vein and SVC are enlarged. Enlargement of the SVC and innominate vein may be the first echocardiographic clue to the presence of PAPVC. On the other hand, in the rare case of PAPVC of the left-sided pulmonary vein(s) into the coronary sinus, the coronary sinus is noted to be enlarged on standard parasternal long-axis images and apical views with posterior angulation.

TEE Evaluation of Normal Pulmonary Venous Connections –
Alternative imaging is indicated if surface echocardiography does not completely delineate the connections of all pulmonary veins to the LA and signs of right-sided volume overload are present. CT, MRI, or TEE imaging fulfills this role, and the choice of modality will be dictated by patient age, size, and comorbidities and the need for the study to be performed at the patient's bedside. Due to the posterior location of the probe, TEE is well suited to allow direct visualization of the PV connections as they enter the LA. In 1997, Ammash and colleagues described techniques that can be used to visualize the normal PV connections. A consistent and systematic examination of normal pulmonary venous connections begins with the tip of the TEE probe posterior to the LA. The right pulmonary veins are seen in the longitudinal plane by flexing a biplane TEE probe tip medially or rotating a multiplane array to approximately 70 to 80 degrees (a foreshortened short-axis view of the left ventricular outflow tract is obtained). One then rotates the probe to the patient's right off the medial wall of the LA. A Y-appearing image of the normal right upper and lower pulmonary veins entering the LA is thus obtained (Fig. 5.17). The left pulmonary veins are imaged by (a) flexing a biplane TEE tip laterally or rotating a multiplane array to approximately 110 to 120 degrees (a foreshortened long-axis view of the left ventricular outflow tract is obtained) and (b) rotating the probe to the patient's left off the free wall of the LA. A Y-shaped appearing image of the normal left upper and lower pulmonary veins entering the LA is thus obtained. The normal pulmonary venous connections can be also confidently visualized in short-axis views at the base of the heart using the transverse plane of a biplane probe or 0 or 45 degrees of a multiplane probe. The left upper pulmonary vein is seen adjacent to the left atrial appendage by rotating the probe to the patient's left. The left lower pulmonary vein is imaged by advancing the probe into the esophagus or with more retroflexion of the shaft. On the other hand, the right pulmonary veins are imaged by rotating the

probe medially to the patient's right and withdrawing to the level of the right pulmonary artery projected in long axis. Medial to the SVC is the short-axis view of the right upper pulmonary vein (Fig. 5.18). By slowly advancing the probe into the esophagus, the right upper pulmonary vein is seen as it enters the medial aspect of the LA. By advancing the probe farther with mild rotation to the patient's right, the right lower pulmonary vein is seen entering the LA. This technique accurately identifies the normal pulmonary vein connections into the LA but also demonstrates the normal size and shape of the SVC. If normal pulmonary vein connections are not visualized with these maneuvers or if the SVC appears dilated, then PAPVC must be suspected.

TEE Evaluation of Partial Anomalous Pulmonary Venous Connections – Anomalous connection of the right pulmonary vein(s) to the SVC can be visualized by using a short-axis view of the SVC at the level of the right pulmonary artery. The right upper pulmonary vein enters the free wall of the SVC, resulting in a teardrop appearance to the normally round-appearing SVC (Fig. 5.19 and 5.20). Connections to the RA–SVC junction and the free wall of the RA are best visualized by slowly advancing the probe into the esophagus while in the same short-axis plane. Color Doppler will help identify the anomalous pulmonary vein flow. When the anomalous connection of the right-sided pulmonary vein is visualized emptying into the SVC, then attention should be paid toward the presence of an ASD and specifically a sinus venosus defect. The longitudinal scanning plane of a biplane TEE probe or the 90-degree angle on a multiplane probe can be used to carefully visualize the atrial septum. If the left-sided pulmonary vein cannot be easily visualized entering the LA, then PAPVC should be suspected. Instead of entering the LA, the left pulmonary veins typically enter a vertical vein lateral to the LA (Fig. 5.21). Rightward rotation of the probe will result in a long-axis view of the SVC that is typically dilated with this defect. Finally, anomalous connection of left pulmonary veins to the coronary sinus should be suspected when the coronary sinus is dilated for no other obvious reason. This can be visualized in the longitudinal plane, starting with the dilated coronary sinus and rotating the probe to the patient's left, demonstrating one or more left-sided pulmonary veins connecting to the coronary sinus.

TEE can confidently visualize the normal pulmonary vein connections and detect the most common forms of PAPVC. Stumper

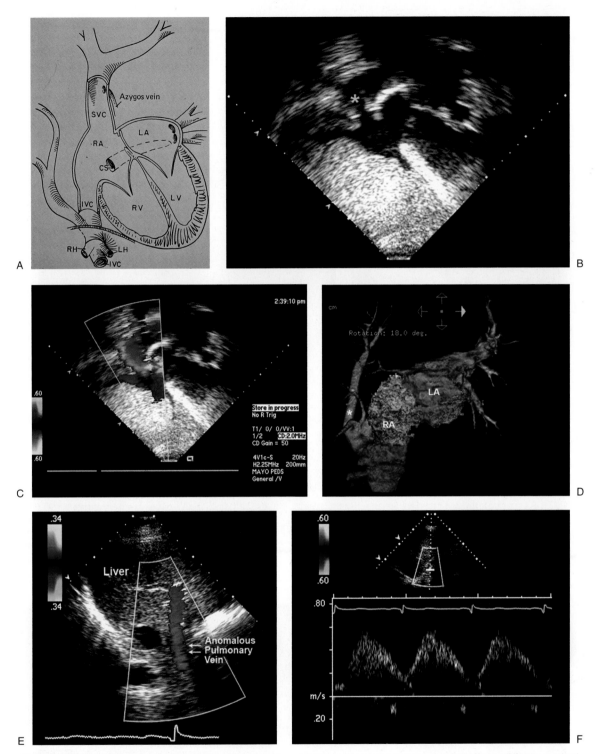

FIGURE 5.15. Scimitar syndrome. A: Diagram of scimitar syndrome. Anomalous connection of right pulmonary vein(s) to the inferior vena cava (IVC), also associated with right lower lobe hypoplasia and aberrant arterial supply to the right lower lobe. **B:** Subcostal frontal image demonstrating a large pulmonary vein from the right lung (*asterisk*) entering the IVC just below the right atrium (RA)–IVC junction. **C:** Color Doppler image from the same projection as **B** demonstrating flow (red) from the right lung toward the IVC. **D:** Computed tomography in same patient with scimitar syndrome demonstrating a large anomalous right pulmonary vein (*asterisk*) that enters the IVC just below the RA–IVC junction. **E:** In another patient with scimitar syndrome, an anomalous right pulmonary vein has flow toward the liver (red) as it enters the intrahepatic portion of the IVC. **F:** Spectral Doppler flow in the same patient depicted in **E**, confirming that a pulmonary venous flow pattern is demonstrated below the diaphragm.

et al. (1991) demonstrated all pulmonary venous connections in 91% of patients studied. But, Sutherland (1989) reported that defining normal pulmonary veins by TEE varied. The detection rate was 100% for the left upper pulmonary vein, 62% for the left lower pulmonary

vein, 90% for the right upper pulmonary vein, and 23% for the right lower pulmonary vein. Conversely, in a Mayo Clinic study, (1997) 45 patients (age range, 2 to 75 years; mean age, 41 years) with PAPVC underwent TEE. A total of 66 PAPVCs were detected in 43 patients.

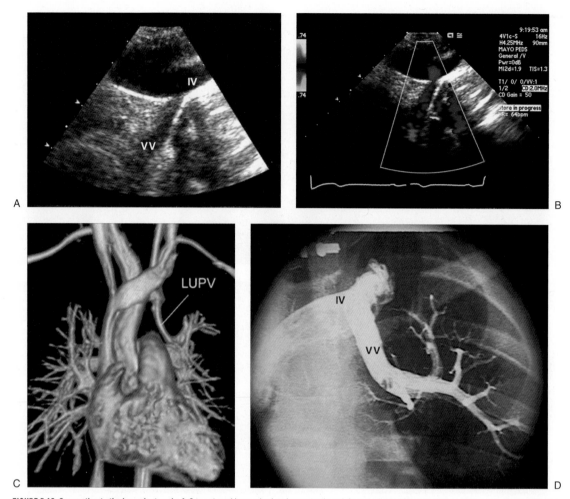

FIGURE 5.16. Connection to the innominate vein. A: Suprasternal long-axis view demonstrating a left vertical vein (VV) connecting to the innominate vein (IV). This VV connected to the left upper pulmonary vein (LUPV). **B:** Color Doppler image from the same window as in **A** demonstrating cephalad flow (red) of the VV connecting to the IV. **C:** Magnetic resonance angiogram demonstrating connection of the LUPV to a VV, which then connects to the IV. **D:** Angiogram demonstrating anomalous connection of the LUPV to a VV, which then connects to the IV.

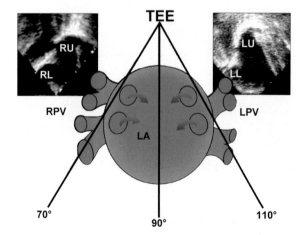

FIGURE 5.17. Transesophageal echocardiographic (TEE) views. Top left: Normal right pulmonary venous connections are most consistently imaged from the transesophageal approach by orienting the array to approximately 70 degrees or medial flexion of the scope tip and then rotating the probe rightward (medially). The right upper (RU) and right lower (RL) pulmonary veins form a typical Y configuration as they enter the left atrium. **Top right:** Normal left pulmonary venous connections are most consistently imaged from the TEE approach by orienting the array to approximately 110 degrees or lateral flexion of the scope tip and then rotating the shaft leftward (laterally). The left upper (LU) and left lower (LL) pulmonary veins form a typical Y configuration as they enter the left atrium. Ammash NM, Seward JB, Warnes CA, et al. Partial anomalous pulmonary venous connection: diagnosis by transesophaged echocardiography. *J Am Coll Cardiol* 1997; 29:1351–1358. (With permission from Elsevier.)

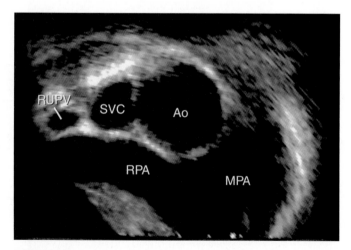

FIGURE 5.18. With the transesophageal array in the horizontal orientation (0 degrees) and withdrawn to the level of the right pulmonary artery (RPA), the RPA is visualized in its long axis. Anterior to the RPA are three ovoid-appearing vessels, and farthest to the patient's right is the right upper pulmonary vein (RUPV) lying immediately adjacent to the superior vena cava (SVC). The ascending aorta (Ao) is leftward from the SVC and medial to the main pulmonary artery (MPA). (From Ammash NM, Seward JB, Warnes CA, et al. Partial anomalous pulmonary venous connection: diagnosis by transesophaged echocardiography. *J Am Coll Cardiol* 1997; 29:1351–1358. (With permission from Elsevier.)

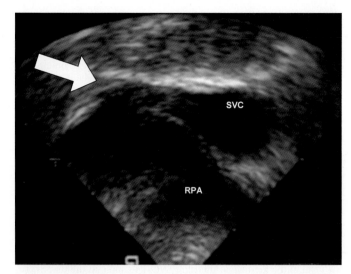

FIGURE 5.19. Transesophageal echocardiographic image in short axis at the cardiac base demonstrating anomalous connection of the right upper pulmonary vein (RUPV) to the superior vena cava (SVC). The conjoined structures form a "tear-drop" appearance (arrow). RPA, right pulmonary artery.

In the remaining 2 patients, TEE was suggestive but not diagnostic of PAPVC. Right-sided anomalous pulmonary veins were identified in 35 patients (81%), left-sided in 7 patients (16%), and bilateral in 1 patient (2%). There was a single anomalous pulmonary vein in 23 patients (53%) and multiple anomalous veins in the other 47%. The anomalous connection site was the SVC in 59% of patients, RA–SVC junction in 9%, RA in 12%, IVC in 1 patient, and the coronary sinus in 2 (3%) patients. Sinus venosus ASD was the most common associated anomaly in 22 (49%) patients, followed by secundum ASD or PFO in 10 (23%) patients. PAPVC was confirmed at the time of surgery in all patients including the two patients whose TEE was only suggestive of PAPVC. Therefore, this retrospective study demonstrated that, using proper techniques, identification of APVCs, especially in patients with unexplained right ventricular volume overload, can be made with confidence with the use of TEE. In addition, with the current instrumentation and techniques described earlier, the identification of normal pulmonary venous connections with TEE should be virtually 100%. APVC should always be considered as a potential cause for unexplained right ventricular volume overload.

Postoperative Echocardiography in APVCs – Surgical repair of PAPVCs is indicated in the presence of symptoms of dyspnea, fatigue, or exercise intolerance. In addition, the presence of

right-sided volume overload or atrial arrhythmias and, less commonly, development of pulmonary hypertension or heart failure are indications for intervention. Anomalous right-sided PAPVCs are commonly repaired with the Warden procedure, whereby the anomalous veins are channeled into the LA, using the floor of the SVC and a pericardial patch. This pathway is constructed through an existing or surgically created ASD, thereby allowing the right-sided pulmonary veins to drain into the LA (Fig. 5.22). If the surgically constructed baffle is large and obstructs the SVC, then the SVC could also be enlarged using a pericardial patch. Alternatively, the SVC could be transected above the baffle and surgically connected to the right atrial appendage. Long-term complications of surgical repair of anomalous right-sided pulmonary veins include SVC obstruction, baffle leak or stenosis, and atrial arrhythmias (especially if present preoperatively and in older patients). Left-sided PAPVCa may be repaired through a left thoracotomy. The vertical vein draining the anomalous left-sided vein(s) is transected and connected to the left atrial appendage. The proximal end of the vertical vein is then closed with suture. The success of surgical repair is usually confirmed with intraoperative TEE. Periodic echocardiographic surveillance, typically using TTE with color Doppler, is needed to ensure the adequacy of repair and the absence of potential long-term complications. Meticulous postoperative scans in these patients need to include evaluation of SVC flow by color and spectral Doppler, two-dimensional demonstration of the pulmonary vein pathway entering the LA, and finally interrogation of the atrial septum.

 ## ANOMALIES OF THE SYSTEMIC VEINS

Introduction

Isolated anomalies of the systemic venous connections are rare. The most common isolated lesion is a persistent left SVC that enters the RA via the coronary sinus. This isolated anomaly creates no physiologic derangement and may be considered a variant from normal. The incidence of a persistent left SVC in the general population is less than 0.5%. It becomes important only if placement of a central venous catheter or pacemaker lead becomes necessary. In patients with CHD, the occurrence of a left SVC is higher and may be observed in 10% to 20% of patients with tetralogy of Fallot and atrioventricular septal defects. Embryologically, this occurs due to failure of regression of the left anterior and common cardinal veins.

The vast majority of patients with complex CHD and heterotaxy syndromes have systemic venous anomalies. Bilateral SVCs are

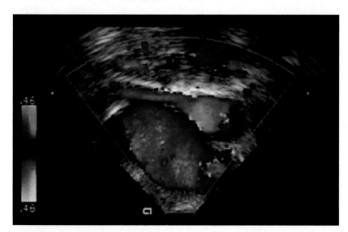

FIGURE 5.20. Color Doppler of the same image in Figure 5.19 demonstrating flow (red) from the right upper pulmonary vein (RUPV) to the superior vena cava (SVC).

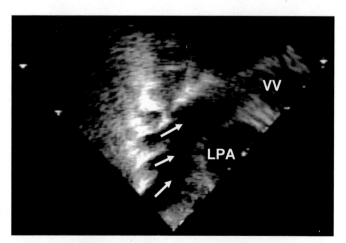

FIGURE 5.21. Left pulmonary veins (arrows) connecting to a left-sided vertical vein (VV) illustrated in this short-axis transesophageal echocardiographic view. In this adult patient, the vertical vein passes anterior to the left pulmonary artery (LPA) and is unobstructed. The patient may have presented earlier in life if the course of the vertical vein was posterior to the LPA, thereby entrapping the vessel in a "vascular vise."

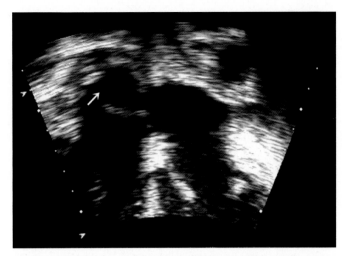

FIGURE 5.22. Zoomed four-chamber image of a surgically created baffle (*arrow*) after a Warden operation. This enables the anomalous right pulmonary veins to drain to the left atrium (LA).

common in patients with heterotaxy syndromes (asplenia, greater than 70%; polysplenia, 50%). Rarely, a left SVC may directly enter the LA; in these cases, the coronary sinus may be partially or completely unroofed. Abnormalities of the coronary sinus are common in patients with heterotaxy syndromes. Very rarely, the right SVC connects to the LA, resulting in cyanosis. If the left SVC is large, then usually there is a diminutive or absent "bridging" or innominate vein connecting the right and left SVCs (Fig. 5.23). Conversely, if the innominate vein is of normal caliber, then a left SVC, if present, is likely small. Knowledge of the connections of the systemic veins to the heart is important in patients with complex heart disease when

considering vascular access for cardiac catheterization and cannulation in the operating room. Patients with single ventricle physiology requiring a cavopulmonary connection may be at increased risk of thrombosis if bilateral SVCs are present, particularly if the SVCs are discrepant in size. Similar to the discussion of pulmonary venous anomalies, the reader is referred to the excellent review by Geva and van Praagh (2008) of the embryology and anatomy of the systemic venous anomalies, entitled "Abnormal Systemic Venous Connections."

An interrupted IVC is another example of a systemic venous anomaly usually encountered in patients with complex CHD including heterotaxy syndromes. It occurs in less than 0.5% of the general population, but more than 75% of patients with polysplenia have an interrupted IVC. An interrupted IVC results from failure of the right subcardinal and vitelline veins to merge, causing the right supracardinal vein to dilate. When the IVC is interrupted, no intrahepatic portion exists. The hepatic veins usually connect independently to the right-sided atrium. Abnormalities of hepatic venous connections to the heart may occur in up to 25% of patients with heterotaxy syndromes. When an interrupted IVC occurs, the abdominal systemic venous return travels cephalad via the azygous vein. The azygous vein connects the IVC drainage above the level of the kidneys to the right SVC. Its course at the diaphragm is posterior to the peritoneal reflection and posterior to the aorta. In the thorax, the azygous vein passes through the diaphragm behind the heart and then arches over the right bronchus and right pulmonary artery to join the posterior aspect of the SVC. In cases of bilateral SVCs, bilateral azygous veins may also be present. The left-sided azygous vein is sometimes referred to by the misnomer "hemiazygous vein." The presence of an interrupted IVC and azygous "continuation" is important in patients with single-ventricle physiology that requires a Fontan operation. In these patients, creation of the cavopulmonary connection nearly completes the Fontan pathway with the exclusion of only the hepatic venous flow, which still connects to the atrium. The hepatic venous flow can be routed via a tube to the pulmonary artery to complete the Fontan circuit, thereby excluding the systemic venous blood from the heart.

The os of the coronary sinus, when present, is a useful anatomic landmark to identify the morphologic RA. The coronary sinus is involved with many of the systemic and pulmonary venous abnormalities discussed in this chapter. Sometimes referred to as the "forgotten systemic vein," the coronary sinus serves to drain the coronary veins to the RA. Its course is typically in the posterior left atrioventricular groove. An unroofed coronary sinus has been discussed elsewhere in this textbook and serves as a rare form of an atrial level shunt. An unroofed coronary sinus usually has an associated left SVC. An exceedingly rare anomaly is atresia of the os of the coronary sinus. In this lesion, coronary venous blood may drain to the LA if the coronary sinus is unroofed or via a left SVC to the innominate vein. The coronary sinus may be dilated in several situations–lesions in which RA pressure is elevated (tricuspid stenosis/atresia), eccentric tricuspid regurgitation that is directed into the os of the coronary sinus, anomalies of systemic (persistent left SVC) or pulmonary (cardiac form of TAPVC) venous connections, and lesions in which coronary blood flow is increased. The importance of the anatomic location of the os and course of the coronary sinus has increased in the modern era as cardiac resynchronization therapy with biventricular pacing becomes more widely used in patients with CHD.

Echocardiographic Assessment of Systemic Venous Anomalies

Left SVC to Coronary Sinus – The parasternal long-axis view readily demonstrates a dilated coronary sinus that may be the first clue to the presence of a persistent left SVC connecting to the RA (Fig. 5.24A). The parasternal short-axis view at the level of the pulmonary artery bifurcation demonstrates the anterior course of the left SVC over the LPA (Fig. 5.24B). Further clockwise rotation will demonstrate the "long axis" of the left SVC as it courses into the coronary sinus (Fig. 5.24B). Subcostal scans demonstrate the os of the coronary sinus and can be used to evaluate the roof of the coronary sinus. TEE imaging, especially in the operating room, is useful to alert the surgeon to the presence of a left SVC and the status of the coronary sinus (Fig. 5.25). Color Doppler assessment from the

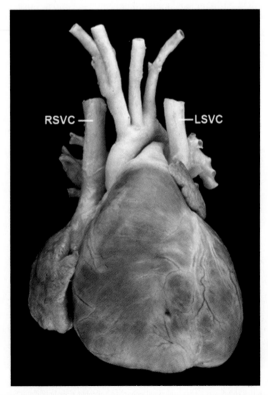

FIGURE 5.23. Pathologic specimen demonstrating right (RSVC) and left (LSVC) superior venae cavae with no obvious bridging vein.

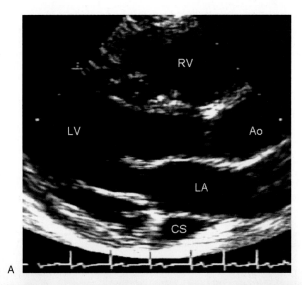

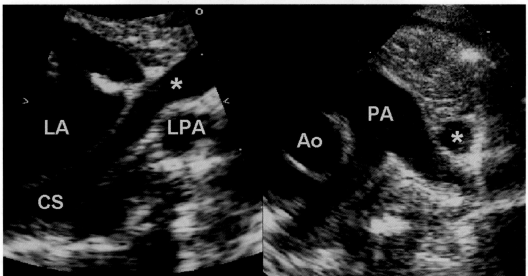

FIGURE 5.24. Parasternal long-axis and short-axis views. A: Parasternal long-axis projection demonstrating a dilated coronary sinus (CS). **B:** Parasternal short-axis images in the same patient. **Right:** Note the anterior location of the left superior vena cava (SVC) (*asterisk*) as it is viewed in short axis anterior to the left pulmonary artery (PA). **Left:** With clockwise rotation, one can develop the length of the left SVC (*asterisk*) as it connects to the CS.

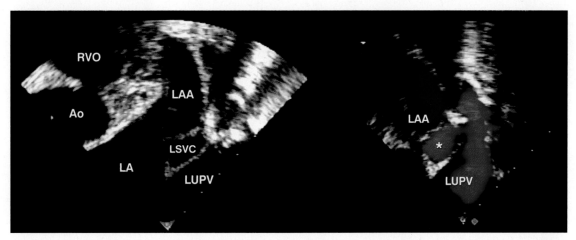

FIGURE 5.25. Transesophageal echocardiographic images of a left superior vena cava (SVC) entering the coronary sinus. Left: The left SVC enters the coronary sinus and is apparent posterior to the left atrial appendage (LAA) and anterior to the left upper pulmonary vein (LUPV). Ao, aorta; RVO, right ventricular outflow tract. **Right:** Color Doppler demonstrating flow (red) in the left SVC traveling posteriorly into the coronary sinus. Also noted is the posteriorly directed flow in the LUPV connecting normally to the LA.

suprasternal notch window with leftward angulation may demonstrate a blue flow indicative of flow away from the innominate vein into the left SVC as it courses toward the coronary sinus. This is in contradistinction to a levoatriocardinal vein, referred to earlier in this chapter as a "left vertical vein." A levoatriocardinal vein may course posterior to the LPA and may become obstructed as it passes between the bronchus and pulmonary artery. When imaging from the suprasternal notch, color Doppler flow in a levoatriocardinal vein or left vertical vein will be red since anomalous pulmonary venous flow is connecting to the innominate vein.

Interrupted IVC with Azygous Continuation

– The lack of an intrahepatic IVC when scanning in the subcostal plane is the first clue to probable interruption of the IVC and presence of a large azygous vein that connects the suprarenal systemic venous return to the SVC. Sagittal images of the abdomen will fail to demonstrate an IVC within the hepatic mass, and a large venous structure may be visualized posterior to the peritoneal reflection. This is the azygous vein, and typically it lies near the midline and posterior to the aorta. The echocardiographer should be suspicious of an azygous vein if color Doppler demonstrates a venous flow in a cephalad direction posterior to the pulsatile abdominal aorta. Once identified, the azygous can be followed along its entire course above the diaphragm as it arches from a posterior to anterior direction over the right pulmonary artery. This can best be viewed in the subcostal sagittal plane when one visualizes the "bicaval" view (Fig. 5.26).

Retroaortic Innominate Vein

– This is a rare anomaly of the innominate vein where it courses posterior to the ascending aorta. It can be identified from the suprasternal long-axis view during

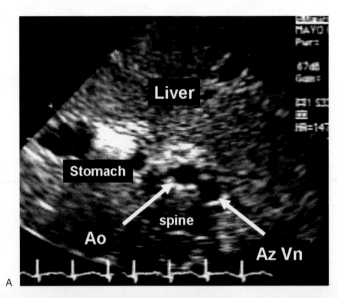

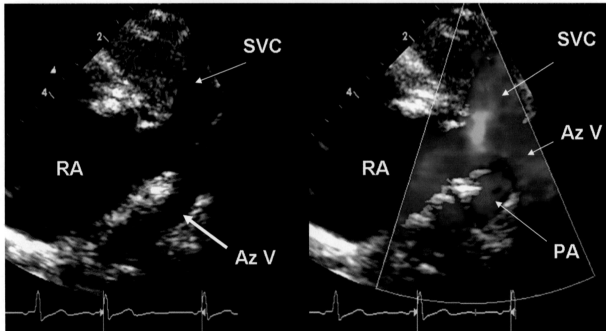

FIGURE 5.26. Subcostal sagittal plane views. A: Cross-sectional image of the abdomen in patient with polysplenia and situs inversus demonstrating an azygous vein (Az vn) positioned posterior to the aorta (Ao) and the peritoneal reflection. No intrahepatic inferior vena cava (IVC) is present. **B:** High right parasternal images in this patient with pulmonary atresia demonstrating that the azygous vein (Az V) arches from posterior to anterior around a diminutive right pulmonary artery (PA) to enter the posterior aspect of the superior vena cava (SVC) just above the right atrium (RA)–SVC junction.

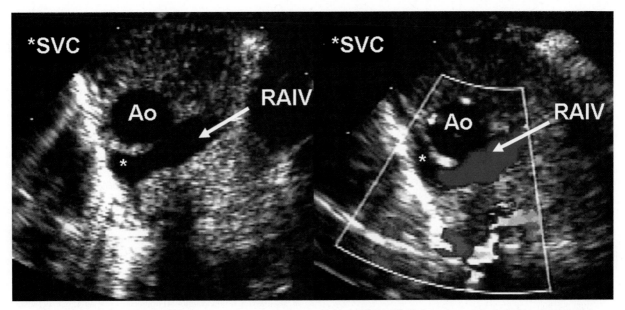

FIGURE 5.27. In these suprasternal short-axis images, a large retroaortic innominate vein (RAIV) is identified coursing posterior to the ascending aorta (Ao) joining the superior vena cava (SVC) (*asterisk*).

assessment of the ascending aorta. Normally, only one vessel (the right pulmonary artery) is visualized posterior to the ascending aorta. If a second vessel is present beneath the ascending aorta, one should be alerted to the presence of a retroaortic innominate vein (Fig. 5.27). In this situation, the innominate vein–SVC connection lies just cephalad of the RA–SVC junction. Retroaortic innominate veins may occur in up to 1% of patients with CHD, most commonly in conotruncal lesions. The location of the innominate vein–SVC junction may be of surgical importance, especially in operations involving creation of cavopulmonary connections.

Imaging the Coronary Sinus – The coronary sinus in the normal heart can be readily assessed in the subcostal frontal (four-chamber) view. Although diminutive in the normal heart, the coronary sinus can be identified in the parasternal long-axis projection in the

left atrioventricular groove just anterior to the echogenic pericardial strip. It should not be confused with the descending thoracic aorta, which lies posterior to the pericardial strip (Fig. 5.28). In the parasternal long-axis projection, gradually scanning toward the tricuspid inflow view will typically provide a smooth assessment of the roof of the coronary sinus and the entrance to the RA (Fig. 5.29). The coronary sinus can also be identified in the apical four-chamber projection by scanning posteriorly. Once the leaflets of the mitral valve are not visualized, the posterior left atrioventricular groove becomes apparent and the course of the coronary sinus can be visualized. TEE can also adequately visualize the coronary sinus when the probe is retroflexed in the four-chamber projection, providing a view of the left posterior atrioventricular groove. Saline contrast injection in a left arm vein can assist in identifying the connection of a left SVC to the coronary sinus.

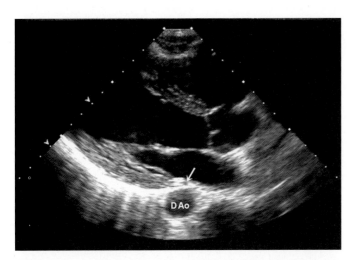

FIGURE 5.28. Parasternal long-axis image demonstrating a normal descending thoracic aorta (*asterisk*) located posterior to the pericardial strip. This should not be confused with the coronary sinus or circumflex coronary artery (*arrow*) that travels in the left atrioventricular groove.

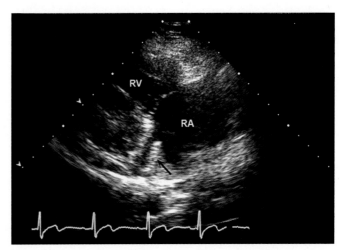

FIGURE 5.29. Parasternal tricuspid inflow view demonstrating an intact roof of the coronary sinus (*arrow*). This view is particularly helpful if an unroofed coronary sinus or left superior vena cava (SVC) connecting to a coronary sinus is suspected.

SUGGESTED READING

Ammash NM, Connolly HM, Julsrud PR, et al. Transesophageal echocardiography: unusual case of anomalous pulmonary venous connection to the azygous vein. *J Am Soc Echocardiogr.* 1997;10:738–744.

Ammash NM, Seward JB, Warnes CA, et al. Partial anomalous pulmonary venous connection: diagnosis by transesophageal echocardiography. *J Am Coll Cardiol.* 1997;29:1351–1358.

Attenhofer-Jost CH, Connolly HM, Danielson GK, et al. Sinus venosus atrial septal defect: Long-term postoperative outcome for 115 patients. *Circulation.* 2005;112:1953–1958.

Brody H. Drainage of the pulmonary veins into the right side of the heart. *Arch Pathol Lab Med.* 1942;33:221–240.

Ferrara N, Zarra AM, Vigorito C, et al. Combined contrast echocardiographic and hemodynamic evaluation of atrial septal defect associated with persistent left superior vena cava and partial anomalous pulmonary venous connection. *J Clin Ultrasound.* 1987;15:64–67.

Fish FA, Davies J, Graham TP, Jr. Unique variant of partial anomalous pulmonary venous connection with intact atrial septum. *Pediatr Cardiol.* 1991;12:177–180.

Geva T, Van Praagh S. Abnormal systemic venous connections. In: Allen HD, Gutgesell HP, Clark EB, Driscoll DJ, eds. Moss and Adams' Heart disease in infants, children and adolescents. 6th ed. Philadelphia, Pa: Lippincott Williams & Wilkins; 2001:792–817.

Geva T, Van Praagh S. Anomalies of the pulmonary veins. In: Allen HD, Gutgesell HP, Clark EB, Driscoll DJ, eds. Moss and Adams' Heart disease in infants, children and adolescents. 6th ed. Philadelphia, Pa: Lippincott Williams & Wilkins; 2001:736–772.

Gupta SR, Reddy KN, Abraham KA, et al. Partial anomalous pulmonary venous connection (PAPVC): left upper lobe pulmonary vein draining into coronary sinus. *Indian Heart J.* 1986;38:489–490.

Gustafson RA, Warden HE, Murray GF, et al. Partial anomalous pulmonary venous connection to the right side of the heart. *J Thorac Cardiovasc Surg.* 1989;98:861–868.

Healey JE, Jr. An anatomic survey of anomalous pulmonary veins: their clinical significance. *J Thorac Surg.* 1952;23:433–434.

Hughes CW, Rumore PC. Anomalous pulmonary veins. *Arch Pathol Lab Med.* 1944;37:364–366.

Kirklin JW. Surgical treatment of anomalous pulmonary venous connection (partial anomalous pulmonary venous drainage). *Proc Staff Meet Mayo Clin.* 1953;28:476–479.

Mehta RH, Jain SP, Nanda NC, et al. Isolated partial anomalous pulmonary venous connection: echocardiographic diagnosis and a new color Doppler method to assess shunt volume. *Am Heart J.* 1991;122:870–873.

Nugent EW, Plauth WH, Jr., Edwards JE, et al. The pathology, clinical recognition, and medical and surgical treatment of congenital heart disease. In: Hurst JW, Schlant RC, Rackley CE, et al, editors. The heart. 7th ed. New York: McGraw-Hill; 1990:655–794.

Pinheiro L, Nanda NC, Jain H, et al. Transesophageal echocardiographic imaging of the pulmonary veins. *Echocardiography.* 1991;8:741–748.

Satomi G, Takao A, Momma K, et al. Detection of the drainage site in anomalous pulmonary venous connection by two-dimensional Doppler color flow-mapping echocardiography. *Heart Vessels.* 1986;2:41–44.

Schatz SL, Ryvicker MJ, Deutsch AM, et al. Partial anomalous pulmonary venous drainage of the right lower lobe shown by CT scans. *Radiology.* 1986;159:21–22.

Senocak F, Ozme S, Bilgic A, et al. Partial anomalous pulmonary venous return. Evaluation of 51 cases. *Jpn Heart J.* 1994;35:43–50.

Stumper O, Vargas-Barron J, Rijlaarsdam M, et al. Assessment of anomalous systemic and pulmonary venous connections by transoesophageal echocardiography in infants and children. *Br Heart J.* 1991;66:411–418.

Sutherland GR. The role of transesophageal echocardiography in adolescents and adults with congenital heart disease. In: Erbel R, Khandheria BK, Brennecke R, et al, eds. Transesophageal echocardiography. New York: Springer-Verlag; 1989:47.

Vargas-Barron J, Rijlaarsdam M, Romero-Cardenas A, et al. Transesophageal echocardiography in adults with congenital cardiopathies. *Am Heart J.* 1993;126:426–432.

Vesely TM, Julsrud PR, Brown JJ, et al. MR imaging of partial anomalous pulmonary venous connections. *J Comput Assist Tomogr.* 1991;15:752–756.

Warden HE, Gustafson RA, Tarnay TJ, et al. An alternative method for repair of partial anomalous pulmonary venous connection to the superior vena cava. *Ann Thorac Surg.* 1984;38:601–605.

Winslow J. *Mem Acad R Sci.* 1739:113.

Wong ML, McCrindle BW, Mota C, et al. Echocardiographic evaluation of partial anomalous pulmonary venous drainage. *J Am Coll Cardiol.* 1995;26:503–507.

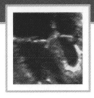

Chapter 6
Abnormalities of Atria and Atrial Septation

Allison K. Cabalka

Atrial septal defects (ASDs) account for approximately 7% to 10% of all congenital heart disease; secundum defects, comprising 60% to 75% of all, are the most common. Two-dimensional, Doppler, and color Doppler echocardiography play a key role in confirmation of the clinical diagnosis of an ASD, providing definitive evaluation of abnormalities of atrial septation. An ASD may exist in isolation or in association with other congenital cardiac abnormalities. It is important to recognize abnormalities of atrial septation; such defects may affect clinical management as whether as catheter-based or surgical treatment is preferred. Cor triatriatum, a very rare type of septation abnormality, will also be reviewed. Primum ASD, which is within the spectrum of atrioventricular septal defects, will be considered in a separate chapter.

ATRIAL SEPTAL ANATOMY AND EMBRYOLOGY

A defect in the atrial septum results in a direct communication between the left atrium (LA) and right atrium (RA). To characterize the location of ASDs, an understanding of septal anatomy is critical. An ASD is typically classified by its location in relationship to the fossa ovalis (Fig. 6.1). During embryologic development, the primitive atrium undergoes a complex septation process, with the septum primum extending inferiorly from the middle of the atrium toward the region of the endocardial cushions, initially leaving an opening called the ostium primum. The inferior portion of the septum primum subsequently fuses with the developing endocardial cushions to close the inferiorly located ostium primum (Fig. 6.1A–B). Tissue reabsorption (or programmed cell death) in the middle of this septum primum leads to a second, central, opening, or ostium secundum. Concurrently, development of the septum secundum occurs, and once joined with the endocardial cushions, the inferior portions of the two atria are separated. The remaining defect in the septum secundum is the foramen ovale, which allows flow from the fetal RA to LA during gestation. Once birth occurs, fusion of these two septa should occur, functionally closing the foramen ovale; however, probe patency is present in approximately 25% to 30% of the population. Secundum ASDs, occurring in the central or secundum portion of the atrial septum, therefore, actually result from a true deficiency in the septum primum (Fig. 6.1D).

Both venae cavae (superior and inferior) and the coronary sinus (CS) enter the more posterior smooth-walled portion of the RA. Defects within this superior/posterior portion of the atrial septum are termed sinus venosus defects (Fig. 6.1D) and result from an abnormality of right pulmonary vein incorporation into the developing atrium. These defects typically occur in conjunction with an abnormality of pulmonary venous return from the right lung. Geva and Van Praagh propose that sinus venosus ASD is not a true ASD but an unroofing of the right pulmonary vein into the superior vena cava (SVC) with the interatrial communication being the left atrial orifice of the unroofed pulmonary veins.

A CS defect, or unroofed CS syndrome, results from an abnormality in the development of the left atrioventricular fold. In this spectrum of abnormalities, complete or partial unroofing of the CS, with direct communication to the LA, is present and is uniformly associated with a left SVC (Fig. 6.1D).

Cor triatriatum sinister, another very rare form of abnormal atrial septation, occurs within the LA. Cor triatriatum may result from abnormal incorporation of the common pulmonary vein into the LA, causing obstruction between the pulmonary vein confluence and the LA; however, not all variants of this rare lesion are embryologically consistent with this theory.

ATRIAL SEPTAL DEFECT

Clinical Presentation

Clinical presentation of the patient with an ASD varies with patient age, size of the defect, and the presence of associated lesions. In the infant with an isolated ASD, presentation with symptomatic pulmonary overcirculation is unusual as right ventricular (RV) compliance is low and atrial shunting may be minimal early in life. An ASD may be found as part of complete evaluation of the infant with other cardiac anomalies. As right ventricular (RV) compliance improves, during infancy and early childhood, left-to-right shunting at the atrial level typically increases. The child or adolescent with a hemodynamically significant ASD usually presents with a cardiac murmur or, less commonly, with symptoms of exercise intolerance or fatigue. The physical examination characteristically reveals a hyperdynamic RV impulse in a patient with a large shunt. A systolic ejection murmur is heard over the left sternal border in association with a widely fixed split second heart sound. A diastolic flow rumble over the tricuspid valve inflow area is present with a significant shunt at the atrial level due to the large volume of blood returning through the tricuspid valve. The chest radiograph may show cardiomegaly with increased pulmonary vascular markings and prominence of the main pulmonary artery segment and central pulmonary arteries.

Atrial level shunting tends to increase with age. The older patient may present with more significant symptoms of exercise intolerance or fatigue and very rarely with overt right heart failure. Atrial arrhythmias are uncommon before adulthood but may persist following late repair unless a surgical arrhythmia procedure is performed concurrently. Pulmonary hypertension or pulmonary vascular obstructive disease is uncommon in the setting of an isolated ASD but must be evaluated carefully before treatment recommendations can be made.

Physiology

Communication between the LA and the RA allows oxygenated pulmonary venous blood to enter the RA via the defect in the atrial septum. Left atrial pressure is typically higher than right atrial pressure through most of the cardiac cycle, so the predominant shunt is left to right. A very transient right-to-left shunt is commonly observed due to variability in atrial compliance. A patent foramen ovale (PFO), particularly redundant septal flaps, may allow right-to-left shunting and a potential for paradoxical embolism to the systemic circulation. Most commonly in the setting of an ASD, left-to-right shunting at the atrial level produces right-sided volume overload, causing progressive right atrial and RV enlargement and pulmonary overcirculation. In the patient with pulmonary vascular disease or RV outflow obstruction, right-to-left shunting at the atrial level may be significant as RV compliance worsens over time.

A patient with a CS ASD and connection of the left SVC to the roof of the LA may have variable degrees of cyanosis due to mixing of systemic venous return with the oxygenated pulmonary venous return. The amount of desaturation is proportional to the amount of systemic venous blood carried by the left SVC.

Complications

A small ASD will typically undergo spontaneous closure (complete or nearly complete) and should not require treatment or produce long-term complications. A moderate (6 to 12 mm) or large (greater

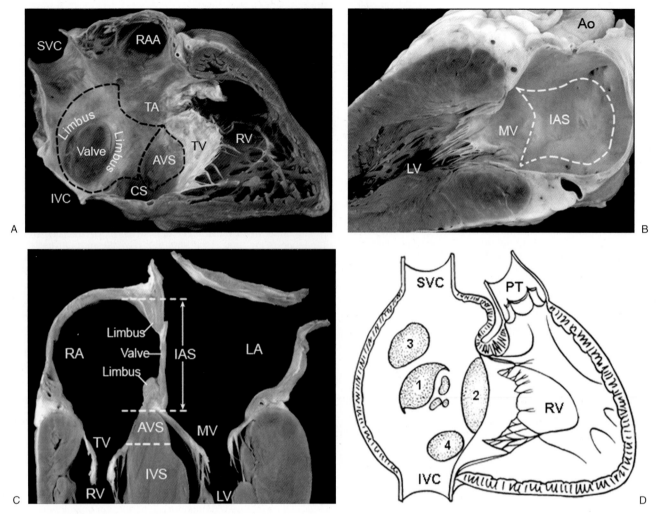

FIGURE 6.1. Atrial septal anatomy. A: Right-sided, two-chamber view of right atrium (RA) and right ventricle (RV). The interatrial septum (IAS) is outlined *(dotted line)*; the superior limbus and inferior limbus surround the valve of the fossa ovalis. The atrioventricular septum (AVS) is shown just above the tricuspid valve. **B:** Left-sided, two-chamber view of left atrium with IAS depicted within the dotted line. **C:** Four-chamber view of the crux of the heart, demonstrating IAS (between the RA and LA) with superior limbus, inferior limbus, and valve of the fossa ovalis. The AVS lies between the RA and the left ventricle (LV). **D:** Diagrammatic representation of the different types of atrial septal defects (ASDs), numbered in decreasing frequency according to rates of occurrence: secundum ASD *(1)*, primum ASD *(2)*, sinus venosus ASD *(3)*, coronary sinus ASD *(4)*. CS, coronary sinus; IVC, inferior vena cava; IVS, interventricular septum; MV, mitral valve; PT, pulmonary trunk; RAA, right atrial appendage; SVC, superior vena cava; TV, tricuspid valve. (Reprinted by permission of Mayo Foundation.)

than 12 mm) ASD may not cause significant symptoms or complications early in life, but as left ventricular compliance decreases over time the volume of intracardiac shunt will steadily increase. It is unlikely that a defect larger than 8 mm will undergo spontaneous closure; in fact, the anatomic size of a moderate or large ASD may increase over time. Also, chronic RV volume overload may produce tricuspid annular dilation, resulting in progressive tricuspid valve regurgitation. Longstanding right atrial dilation contributes to an increased risk of atrial arrhythmias. Although atrial flutter and atrial fibrillation are uncommon in childhood, the prevalence increases with age in a patient with untreated or undiagnosed ASD. Arrhythmias may persist after repair, particularly with repair at an older age or in the setting of elevated pulmonary artery pressure or resistance. Natural history studies suggest that repair of a hemodynamically significant ASD before age 25 years should allow a normal life expectancy.

Pulmonary hypertension and pulmonary vascular obstructive disease in association with ASD is uncommon, occurring in a small percentage of patients. Additional complications of right-to-left shunting may include paradoxical emboli and risk of stroke. Less commonly seen in the setting of unroofed CS is cerebral embolization and risk of brain abscess.

 EVALUATION OF ATRIAL SEPTAL DEFECT: OVERVIEW

Right-sided chamber enlargement is the hallmark of an atrial level shunt. When seen on echocardiographic imaging, this should prompt a comprehensive evaluation of the atrial septum pulmonary venous return.

Because the atrial septum is a complex three-dimensional structure, it must be imaged from multiple planes. Portions of the atrial septum may be quite thin and difficult to visualize; therefore, definitive imaging of the atrial septum with transthoracic echocardiography can be challenging, particularly in the older adolescent or adult. Orthogonal views are needed in order to resolve tissue rims. Diagnostic images are typically obtained with the imaging transducer perpendicular to the structures of interest, so as to not produce artificial dropout or the appearance of a defect where there is not an ASD. The echocardiographer needs to provide an assessment of defect location, size, and distance from surrounding cardiac structures. In addition, a complete assessment of potential associated cardiac abnormalities is indicated. Complete spectral Doppler and color Doppler assessment is important in evaluation of the primary defect as well as to provide hemodynamic evaluation, including quantification of RV systolic and pulmonary artery pressure. Noninvasive shunt quantification is not typically performed.

The goals of imaging should be to provide definitive information for the clinician, to assess the hemodynamic significance of the defect(s), and to aid in planning for catheter-based intervention or surgical treatment. If image quality from the transthoracic approach is suboptimal and the echocardiographer suspects an atrial level shunt or abnormality of pulmonary venous return, then transesophageal echocardiography is warranted. In some cases, cardiac magnetic resonance imaging (MRI) may be needed to definitively evaluate abnormalities of pulmonary venous return, particularly if the abnormal connection is high in the superior vena cava.

Subcostal Imaging

Subcostal imaging is ideal for evaluation of the atrial septum when image quality is adequate. From this orientation, the transducer beam is relatively perpendicular to the atrial septum in both the four-chamber (coronal) and short-axis (sagittal) views, so that tissue structures can be resolved to be sure that artifactual dropout is not present. Key echo findings include the presence of true, dropout in the atrial septum, and right-sided structural enlargement (RA, right ventricle, and pulmonary artery). The edges of the defect may produce additional reflections known as a "T-artifact," allowing identification of defect rims.

Subcostal Four-Chamber (Coronal) Views – Four-chamber or coronal plane imaging provides images of the atrial septum along an anterior-to-posterior axis and are useful to identify the location and size of an ASD. Imaging is carried out with transducer sweeps from anterior to posterior, providing evaluation of the ASD in the long axis of the defect. The location of the defect in the septum and its relationship to the right-sided SVC and right upper pulmonary vein should be ascertained. Scanning anteriorly and superiorly provides evaluation of the atrial septum immediately behind the aorta. The posterior-inferior portion of the atrial septum can be evaluated by angling the transducer more posteriorly in the four-chamber plane, but artifactual dropout may occur. Short-axis imaging is preferred for evaluation of posterior and inferior rims. In the normal heart, the atrial septum should be seen inferiorly/posteriorly extending to the level of the atrioventricular valves (Fig. 6.2A).

The addition of color Doppler typically reveals a continuous left-to-right shunt (Fig. 6.2C), although a transient, brief amount of right-to-left shunting may occur with variations in respiratory cycle.

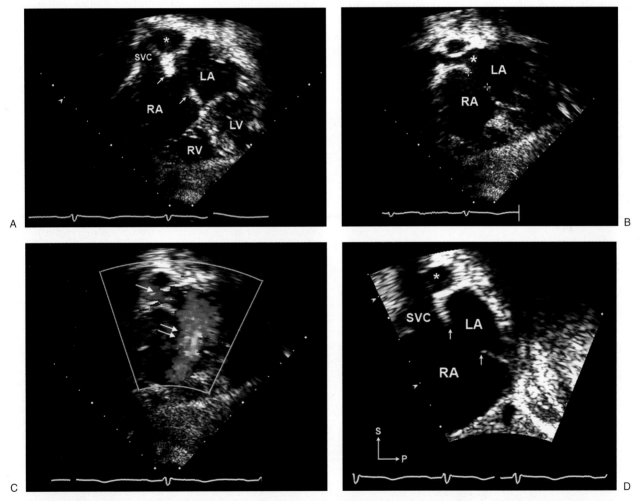

FIGURE 6.2. Subcostal imaging of a moderate-sized secundum atrial septal defect (ASD). A: Subcostal coronal plane focused on biatrial view, showing dropout in mid-septum between the left atrium (LA) and right atrium (RA) consistent with moderate-sized secundum ASD. The rims of the defect in this plane appear well developed (*single arrow,* superior edge; *double arrow,* inferiorly). **B:** Slight anterior angulation of the transducer from the coronal view (shown in **A**) will bring into view the right upper pulmonary vein (large asterisk) entering the LA. **C:** Addition of color Doppler shows left-to-right shunt through the ASD (*double arrow*) and the right pulmonary vein flow to the LA (*single arrow*). **D:** Rotating the transducer approximately 90 degrees from coronal view provides a short-axis (sagittal) view, demonstrating the secundum ASD with adequate superior (near superior vena cava [SVC]) and inferior/posterior rims (*single arrows*) for consideration of device closure. (Imaging note: Farther rightward movement of the transducer to achieve a bicaval view will show the entrance of the inferior vena cava into the RA anteriorly to the inferior rim.) The right pulmonary artery (*asterisk*) can be seen just posterior to the SVC. LV, left ventricle; RV, right ventricle.

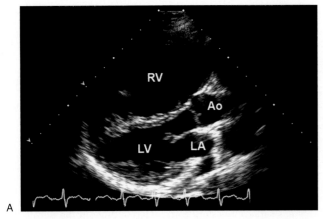
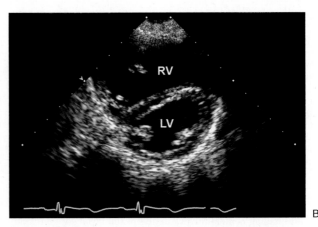

FIGURE 6.3. A: Parasternal long-axis view with severe right ventricular (RV) enlargement due to a large secundum. B: Parasternal short-axis demonstrating RV enlargement and diastolic flattening of the interventricular septum, consistent with RV volume overload. Ao, aorta; LA, left atrium; LV left ventricle.

Pulsed-wave Doppler at the level of the ASD will demonstrate low-velocity, phasic, left-to-right flow; very transient right-to-left flow may be detected. Lack of phasic flow or increased velocity with continuous flow suggests a significant gradient between the LA and RA caused by a restrictive defect (depending on the direction of flow).

Subcostal Short-Axis (Sagittal) Views – Subcostal short-axis (SAX) imaging is obtained in an orthogonal imaging plane to the four-chamber (coronal) view, providing imaging in a superior-inferior axis (Fig. 6.2D). Sweeping the transducer from right to left allows evaluation of the relationship of the right-sided SVC, pulmonary veins (particularly right), and the septal rims of an ASD. One must be careful to note the position of the Eustachian valve, which is located anteriorly at the entrance of the inferior vena cava to the RA; this is most easily accomplished from the subcostal sagittal imaging plane. Short-axis imaging allows imaging of the anterior-superior and posterior-inferior atrial septa. In addition, excellent images of the right ventricle (RV), RV outflow tract (RVOT), and pulmonary valve can be obtained from the subcostal short axis. Doppler interrogation can be performed to evaluate RVOT velocities to determine if a significant outflow tract gradient exists.

Parasternal Views

Parasternal Long-Axis View – Characteristic signs of RV enlargement, volume overload, and paradoxical septal motion are seen in the parasternal long-axis plane when there is a significant atrial

level shunt (Fig. 6.3A). Mitral valve prolapse, seen in association with ASD, is best demonstrated in the long-axis plane. Angling the transducer inferiorly toward the tricuspid inflow view may demonstrate color flow across the atrial septum, although this view is often insufficient for visualization of an ASD. Color Doppler should also be used to evaluate tricuspid valve regurgitation, and, if present, pulsed-wave Doppler can be used to obtain an estimation of RV systolic pressure (RVSP).

Angling the transducer superiorly toward the left shoulder will demonstrate the RVOT, the pulmonary valve leaflets, and main pulmonary artery. Dilation of the main pulmonary artery is seen with significant atrial level shunting. The pulmonary valve leaflets should be examined for morphology and function. In the RVOT, pulsed-wave Doppler velocities as high as to 2.5 m/s may be seen with large atrial level shunts; velocities greater than 2.5 m/s suggest an additional component of valvular pulmonary stenosis. Doming or restricted motion of the pulmonary valve will be seen with valve stenosis and should be evaluated carefully with two-dimensional imaging for correlation with Doppler findings.

Parasternal Short-Axis View – Parasternal short-axis imaging is also very useful for evaluating RV volume overload and flattening or paradoxical motion of the interventricular septum (Fig. 6.3B). Diastolic flattening of the septum is common with volume overload; systolic flattening is seen with pressure overload. Doppler evaluation of tricuspid regurgitation, including assessment of RVSP, is important for comprehensive hemodynamic assessment and to rule out possible

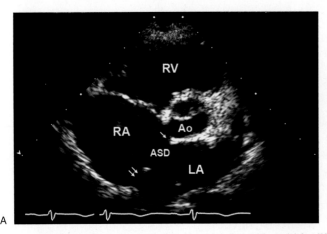
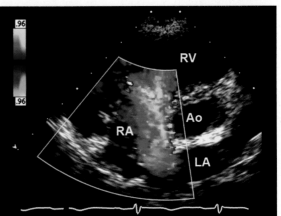

FIGURE 6.4. Parasternal short-axis view of large secundum atrial septal defect (ASD). A: Right atrial (RA) and right ventricular (RV) enlargement are consistent with atrial level shunting. RA is significantly more enlarged than the left atrium (LA). The diminutive anterior, retroaortic rim *(single arrow)* of the ASD is well visualized in this image. The posterior rim is well demonstrated in this view *(double arrow)* as it is not parallel to the imaging plane. Ao, aorta. B: The addition of color Doppler shows a large shunt from LA to RA consistent with the secundum ASD.

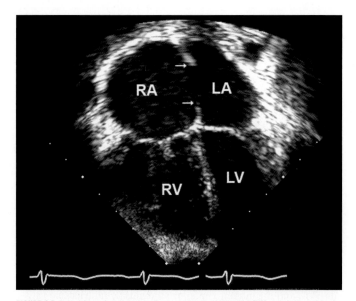

FIGURE 6.5. Apical four-chamber view shows moderate right atrial (RA) and right ventricular (RV) enlargement. There is a large secundum atrial septal defect (ASD) with well-developed superior rim and inferior rims *(single arrows)*. (Imaging note: One must be careful to define the rims of tissue carefully as they are typically more perpendicular to the plane of imaging from the apex and artificial dropout should be avoided.)

coexistent pulmonary hypertension. RA enlargement is also appreciated from this view. As the atrial septum is somewhat perpendicular to the plane of imaging, care must be taken to image the septal rims accurately. Color Doppler will show left to right shunting from LA to RA in a typical secundum ASD (Fig. 6.4A, 6.4B). The RVOT, pulmonary valve, and main pulmonary artery are well seen from the SAX view. Anatomic evaluation of the infundibulum and pulmonary valve is also recommended to correlate with Doppler findings.

Apical Four-Chamber View

RA and RV enlargement can be easily seen from the apical four-chamber orientation (Fig. 6.5). One should use color Doppler to evaluate the degree of tricuspid regurgitation and use pulsed-wave Doppler to provide an accurate estimation of RVSP (Fig. 6.6). Associated mitral valve abnormalities can also be evaluated, taking care to rule out mitral valve stenosis that may accentuate an atrial level shunt due to elevation of left atrial pressure. Because the four-chamber imaging plane is parallel to the atrial septum, the suggestion of dropout in the thinner mid-portion of the atrial septum must be confirmed from additional views. The apical four-chamber view can be used for evaluation of the inferior-most portion of the atrial septum at the level of the crux of the heart.

Angling the transducer anteriorly from the four-chamber view brings the left ventricular outflow tract into view; further anterior angulation (or para-apical) provides another excellent view of the pulmonary valve and RVOT. Doppler determination of any important RVOT obstruction is important with respect to planning therapeutic catheterization or surgery.

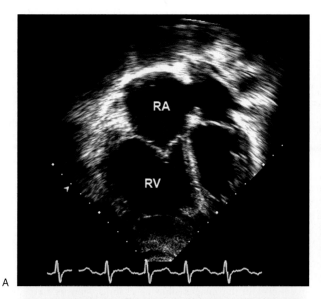

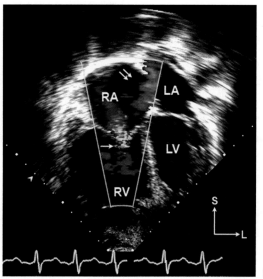

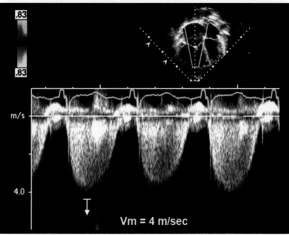

FIGURE 6.6. Apical four-chamber images in patient with pulmonary hypertension and moderate secundum atrial septal defect (ASD). A: Severe right atrial (RA) and right ventricular (RV) enlargement with right ventricular hypertrophy is seen. **B:** Left-to-right shunt is seen through the ASD *(double arrows)* with associated tricuspid valve regurgitation *(single arrow)*. **C:** Quantitative hemodynamic assessment with tricuspid regurgitation velocity of 4 m/s predicting elevated RV systolic pressure (64 mm Hg plus RA pressure). LA, left atrium; LV, left ventricle.

Suprasternal Notch Views

The right and left branch pulmonary arteries are seen well from suprasternal notch imaging. In a short-axis or coronal plane, the LA can be visualized inferior to the right pulmonary artery. Sweeping the transducer from left to right should demonstrate all four pulmonary veins connecting to the LA (the "crab" view). Rotating the transducer 90 degrees to the long-axis plane is helpful to rule out an anomalous left upper pulmonary vein to a vertical vein. From this imaging plane, color Doppler flow coursing superiorly toward the transducer, entering the innominate vein, should alert the echocardiographer to the possibility of an anomalous left pulmonary vein.

Additional Imaging

High right parasternal imaging can provide an additional window to evaluate the SVC–RA junction and superior portion of the atrial septum. In some patients, this imaging plane may provide a "bicaval" view and further assessment of the superior and inferior septal rims of a secundum defect optimally visualizes a high sinus venosus ASD.

In the patient with right-sided cardiac enlargement on transthoracic imaging but no identifiable ASD or abnormality of pulmonary venous return, a transesophageal echocardiogram (TEE) is indicated. TEE imaging of the atrial septum is usually of sufficient quality to demonstrate most defects; however, one must be attentive to the very inferior/posterior portion of the atrial septum as proximity to the imaging probe may obscure visualization. Cardiac MRI may also be of benefit if the atrial septum is adequately visualized from TEE but the pulmonary venous connections cannot be resolved.

CLASSIC TWO-DIMENSIONAL ECHO ANATOMY AND IMAGING

Patent Foramen Ovale

A PFO is located immediately beneath the superior limbus and is typically a small defect. In the majority of neonates undergoing echocardiography, a small amount of left-to-right shunting is present through the PFO with color Doppler echocardiography. Spontaneous closure occurs in the majority of patients, although probe patency persists in approximately 25%. In the older patient with clinical evidence of paradoxical embolism, a small defect or larger redundant septal flap, with a tunnel, may be seen. In such patients, TEE will usually be needed to document septal anatomy in detail, with injection of agitated saline through an intravenous line to confirm a right-to-left shunt if not seen on baseline color Doppler interrogation.

Secundum Atrial Septal Defect

A secundum ASD produces characteristic dropout in the centralmost portion of the atrial septum. Most defects are relatively elliptical in shape. Assessment from multiple views is needed to fully evaluate the maximum ASD dimensions, septal rims, and relationship of the ASD to surrounding cardiac structures. With the widespread availability of transcatheter device closure of secundum ASD, the echocardiographer plays a critical role in assessment and patient selection for catheter-based therapy. One must also exclude the presence of fenestrations or aneurysmal septal tissue in association with a secundum ASD, although these often remain amenable to device closure. It is very important to rule out any defects that would require surgical attention (i.e., anomalies of pulmonary veins).

A typical secundum ASD is seen in the subcostal four-chamber imaging (Fig. 6.7) and in short-axis imaging as a central area of septal dropout within the atrial septum with surrounding rims of tissue present. From the subcostal four-chamber imaging plane, a rim of tissue should separate the SVC entrance to the RA and the right upper pulmonary venous entrance to the LA from the ASD. More inferiorly with leftward and posterior angulation toward the crux of the heart, there is typically a larger rim of tissue separating the atrial defect from the atrioventricular valves and CS. Angling anteriorly, the defect can be seen posterior to the aorta; however,

the retroaortic rim of tissue will be seen more definitively in the parasternal short-axis view. Subcostal short-axis imaging shows the superior/anterior rim of the defect just beneath the SVC–RA junction. The normally connected right upper pulmonary vein is seen entering the LA posterior to this rim. One of the rims that may be most difficult to visualize adequately in patients with secundum ASD is the posterior/inferior rim. Subcostal short-axis imaging is often diagnostic when image quality is adequate (Fig. 6.7C). It is important to remember that the eustachian valve tissue, which may be prominent and often confused with an ASD septal rim, enters the RA *anterior* to the inferior vena cava (Fig. 6.8A).

Parasternal long-axis views do not typically show the ASD adequately, even when angling inferiorly toward the tricuspid inflow view. However, parasternal short-axis views are very useful for visualization of the anterior (retroaortic) and posterior septal rims. These views may also be helpful in patients with difficult subcostal windows before the consideration of TEE. An absent "retroaortic" rim may not prevent successful device closure if other adequate rims are present; however, an adequate posterior septal rim should be present. Complete absence of the posterior/superior rim will preclude successful device closure of a secundum ASD (Fig. 6.8).

Imaging of a secundum ASD from the apical four-chamber view shows the superior rim between the right upper pulmonary vein and SVC, and the inferior rim above the mitral and tricuspid valves (Fig. 6.5). Total atrial septal length, as well as superior and inferior rims, should be measured from this view when considering device closure of a secundum ASD.

Sinus Venosus Defect with Partial Anomalous Pulmonary Venous Connection

A sinus venosus ASD is located in the superior/posterior region of the atrial septum and will be seen directly adjacent to the SVC without an intervening superior rim. Sinus venosus ASD is typically associated with anomalous drainage of the right upper and/or middle lobe pulmonary veins to the SVC–RA junction. The lower right pulmonary vein is rarely involved. Although the connection of the anomalous pulmonary vein(s) may be "high" in the SVC, their connection is not typically present above the entry of the azygous vein to the SVC. Subcostal imaging in the four-chamber plane can be used to visualize this defect, with angling of the transducer superiorly and anteriorly to bring in the atrial septum between the SVC and RA (Fig. 6.9A). One or two of the right pulmonary veins can be seen entering the SVC or superior portion of the RA from this imaging plane and must be identified (Fig. 6.9C). The entrance of the SVC may appear enlarged as a result and may even appear to "override" the defect into the LA, but the SVC remains normally connected to the RA.

In the subcostal short-axis plane, there is dropout of tissue immediately below the entrance of the SVC to the RA, and again there is absence of the superior rim (Fig. 6.9B). The entrance of an anomalous right pulmonary vein to the SVC–RA junction may also be seen from this sagittal imaging plane during sweeps from right to left. If the pulmonary veins are not easily identified in conjunction with the images showing a sinus venosus ASD, then TEE or MRI/magnetic resonance angiography (MRA) may be necessary to completely define the pulmonary venous anatomy in preparation for surgery (as in the case of high connection near the level of the azygous vein).

TEE imaging in sinus venosus ASD shows dropout in the superior portion of the atrial septum immediately beneath the SVC entrance (Fig. 6.10). Withdrawing the probe to a more superior position in the mediastinum, the anomalous right pulmonary vein can be identified from a short-axis view by visualization of a key hole (or "teardrop") sign where the pulmonary vein enters the cava; normally, the SVC would appear as a complete circle in this view (Fig. 6.11A). Color Doppler confirms the venous flow into the SVC from the anomalous pulmonary vein (Fig. 6.11B).

Coronary Sinus Atrial Septal Defect (Unroofed Coronary Sinus)

When there is a CS ASD, an enlarged CS ostium is seen and might be confused with a simple left-sided SVC to the CS. However, the

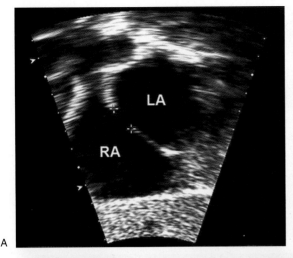

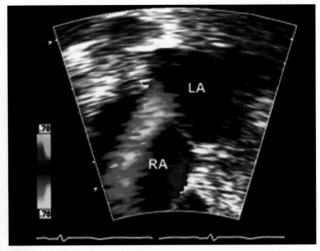

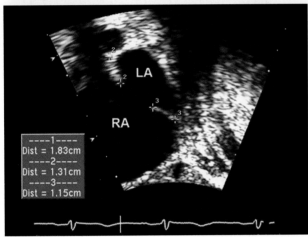

FIGURE 6.7. Subcostal imaging of a moderate-sized secundum atrial septal defect (ASD) amenable to catheter-based device closure. A: Adequate rims are seen in the subcostal coronal view (defect indicated by *asterisks*). **B:** Color Doppler with left-to-right shunt through the ASD. **C:** Corresponding subcostal sagittal view with measurements of superior rim (1.3 cm) and inferior-posterior rim (1.2 cm). The ASD in this plane measured 1.8 cm. LA, left atrium; RA, right atrium.

right-sided cardiac structures will be enlarged because of the atrial level shunt. Parasternal long-axis views can be used to confirm an unroofed CS as there is an absent rim of tissue between the floor of the LA and the CS (Fig. 6.12A–B). Color Doppler examination shows flow going away from the transducer, as the shunt is from the LA to the CS through the defect in the roof of the CS (Fig. 6.12C). A CS ASD is almost always associated with connection of the left SVC to the roof of the LA. It is important to identify the drainage of the left SVC for purposes of surgical intervention. As an adjunct to imaging, an agitated saline injection through an intravenous line in the left arm will demonstrate bubbles appearing initially in the LA and subsequently the RA. If the left SVC is missed or is allowed to remain anomalously connected to the LA following surgical repair of the CS ASD, the patient will have persistent cyanosis due to systemic venous return to the LA.

Associated Defects

Anomalous Pulmonary Venous Connection – One of the critical issues in evaluation of a patient with an ASD is a potential anomalous pulmonary venous connection. A sinus venosus ASD is usually associated with anomalous connection of the right upper/middle pulmonary veins to the SVC or right atrial junction. However, pulmonary vein anomalies can also be seen with secundum ASD and, if present, would be a contraindication to device closure of the ASD in the cardiac catheterization laboratory. Pulmonary veins may be difficult to visualize definitively with transthoracic echocardiography (TTE), especially in the older teenager or adult patient. Further imaging with TEE or cardiac MRI should be used for definitive

documentation of all pulmonary vein connections when they cannot be defined by conventional TTE.

Pulmonary Valve Stenosis – Valvular pulmonary stenosis is identified by typical doming or thickening of the pulmonary valve leaflets, usually with restricted motion. Doppler velocities of up to 2.5 m/s can be seen with a significant left-to-right shunt at the atrial level, but velocities greater than this are more consistent with associated pulmonary valve stenosis. The pulmonary valve annulus and leaflets should be carefully evaluated with two-dimensional imaging. Accentuated poststenotic dilation of the main pulmonary artery may be seen in ASD with pulmonary valve stenosis. Catheter-based treatment is possible for both defects and can be planned accordingly.

Tricuspid Regurgitation – Annular dilation from longstanding atrial level shunting may result in progressive tricuspid regurgitation. Valve coaptation may be adversely affected. Assessment of the degree of tricuspid regurgitation is important in planning for treatment, as the patient with significant tricuspid regurgitation may require surgery rather than catheter-based intervention, if concomitant tricuspid valve repair is indicated.

Pulmonary Hypertension – Assessment of RV systolic pressure is an important part of the evaluation of all patients with an ASD (Fig. 6.6). The tricuspid regurgitant velocity must be carefully evaluated from multiple imaging planes. In the absence of RV outflow obstruction, this Doppler velocity will reflect pulmonary artery systolic pressure. With significant pulmonary hypertension, there will be RV hypertrophy and eventually decreased RV systolic function.

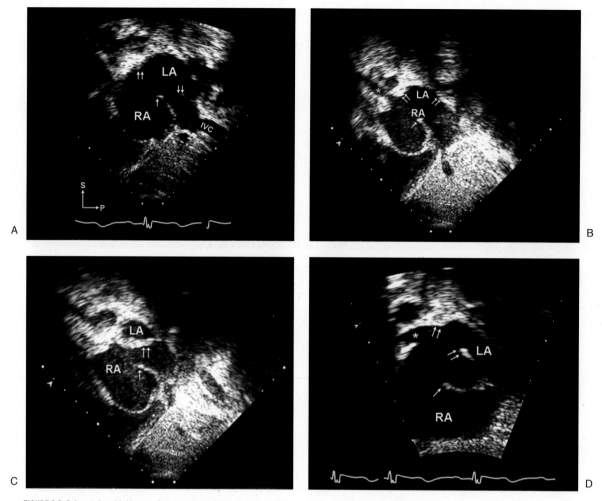

FIGURE 6.8. Subcostal sagittal images from a patient with a very large atrial septal defect (ASD) and associated anomalous connection of right pulmonary veins to the right atrium. **A:** There is no superior rim (*double arrows* pointing superiorly). A very prominent eustachian valve (*single arrow*) is seen entering the right atrium (RA) anterior to the inferior vena cava (IVC). The posterior-inferior rim is seen near the IVC entrance (inferiorly directed double arrows). **B:** Further angulation of the transducer rightward in this sagittal plane demonstrates the right superior vena cava (*asterisk*) entering the right atrium normally. However, there are absent superior and inferior/posterior rims in this part of the defect, seen only with careful sweeps of the transducer rightward (bordered by *double arrows*). The prominent eustachian valve is seen anteriorly to hepatic vein return to the RA (*single arrow*). **C:** Leftward angulation of the transducer in the short sagittal does show the rim of the defect to be present (*double arrow*). A large eustachian valve is seen again (*single arrow*). **D:** Rotating the transducer 90 degrees to a coronal plane shows the prominent eustachian valve (*single arrow*) and the extent of the defect (*double arrows*). In this imaging plane, the superior rim appears to be absent and a right pulmonary vein (*asterisk*) is seen entering the right atrial aspect of the superior portion of the defect. (Imaging note: An ASD with absent rims and potential anomalous pulmonary venous return will require multiple imaging planes for confirmation of this cardiac anatomy. This type of defect is not suitable for device closure.) LA, left atrium.

Interventional and Postinterventional Imaging

Secundum ASD – If catheter-based device closure is undertaken for secundum ASD, echocardiography is a crucial adjunct for guidance. Various modalities may be applicable (transthoracic, transesophageal, or intracardiac), depending on patient size and other factors. In some settings, such as with the smaller child, TTE may be all that is needed for guidance, provided that images are of diagnostic quality. Subcostal imaging is optimal for visualization of septal rims and device position with additional imaging planes such as allowing visualization of the ASD device in relationship to the atrioventricular valves. In general, however, for device closure, TEE or intracardiac echocardiography are more commonly used. With TEE, care must be taken to adequately visualize all septal rims, as it may be difficult to see the most posterior portion of the defect with the probe in proximity to the posterior rim and LA. Regardless of the imaging modality chosen, a careful examination will again be necessary to evaluate septal rims and static defect size from multiple imaging planes (Figs. 6.13 and 6.14). In a setting where balloon sizing is performed, echocardiography is crucial for evaluation of the stretched diameter of the ASD at the point where shunt from left to right ceases ("stop-flow" technique). Continuous visualization during careful balloon inflation is used so as to not overstretch the defect; this allows selection of the smallest size device for ASD closure. During device delivery and deployment, careful imaging is warranted to be sure that the left and right atrial discs of the device are in their proper locations, do not prolapse (i.e., LA disc into RA), and do not interfere with surrounding cardiac structures (Fig. 6.15). In addition, once the left side of the closure device is deployed within the LA, shadowing of the RA may occur, so careful imaging is needed. Transgastric imaging may avoid some of the interference from the ASD device and is often helpful after device placement. TEE will usually require general anesthesia due to the potential for airway compromise, in addition to consideration of patient comfort.

In our laboratory, we generally prefer the use of intracardiac echocardiography for catheter-based device closure of secundum ASD or PFO. The smallest probe with four-way steerability (AcuNav; Acuson, Mountain View, CA) can be introduced through an 8 French sheath in the femoral vein. Image quality is excellent, typically allowing a 8.5- to 10-mHz frequency. With the intracardiac echocardiographic catheter positioned in the RA, evaluation of defect rims and pulmonary veins is easily accomplished. The use of intracardiac echocardiography is covered more extensively in elsewhere in this text.

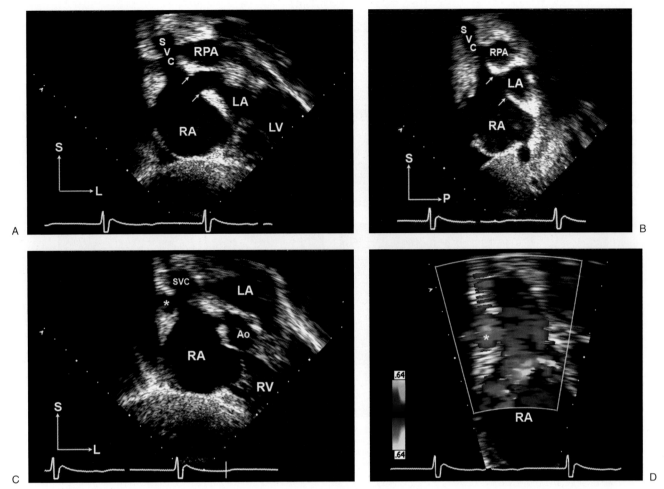

FIGURE 6.9. Subcostal imaging of sinus venosus atrial septal defect (ASD) (*arrows*). **A:** Coronal view showing superiorly located venosus defect adjacent to the superior vena cava (SVC) entry into the enlarged right atrium (RA). **B:** Sagittal view showing left atrium (LA) posteriorly and the superiorly located sinus venosus ASD in proximity to the SVC. Right pulmonary artery (RPA) is seen posterior to the SVC. **C:** In coronal view, transducer is angled slightly anterior to view obtained in **A**; the entry of the anomalous right upper and middle lobe pulmonary veins to the SVC can be seen (*asterisk*). **D:** Addition of color Doppler showing flow from anomalous right pulmonary veins (*asterisk*) entering the SVC. Ao, aorta; L, leftward; LV, left ventricle; P, posterior; RV, right ventricle; S, superior.

If surgery is required for closure of a secundum ASD, TEE typically will be used intraoperatively to evaluate immediate results (Fig. 6.16).

Following intervention, echocardiography is used to evaluate the postintervention anatomy and function. Right-sided cardiac enlargement often improves immediately and continues to improve over time. There should be no evidence of residual shunt at atrial level by color Doppler. It is important to assess for a pericardial effusion in those patients undergoing closure of ASD, particularly in those who have had surgical intervention early in the course of recovery or in those having relatively large devices in place, as there is a very small risk of long-term device erosion. Longer-term monitoring of the closure device and relationship to surrounding cardiac structures is needed during serial follow-up examinations. In rare situations, there may be a residual shunt around the device (Fig. 6.17). Longer-term noninvasive monitoring will demonstrate the device position and rule out any interference with surrounding cardiac structures, valves, or venous drainage (Figs. 6.18 and 6.19).

Sinus Venosus Defect with Partial Anomalous Pulmonary Venous Return – The goal of surgical correction is to restore the original connection of the right pulmonary veins to the LA, functionally closing the interatrial communication. In addition, unobstructed drainage of the right SVC to the RA must be maintained, either within the original vessel or by reattaching the SVC to the right atrial appendage, sometimes using an interposition graft (Warden procedure). Intraoperative TEE is used for preoperative and postoperative

assessment of the patient undergoing complete repair. Postbypass TEE is useful for evaluation of the pulmonary venous pathway and to ensure patency and absence of residual shunt through the pulmonary vein baffle to the RA (Fig. 6.20A–B). In addition, the flow from the SVC to the RA should be laminar with no gradient (Fig. 6.20C–D).

Longer-postoperative follow-up requires ongoing TTE surveillance for vena cava obstruction and pulmonary vein obstruction. In the adult patient with challenging TTE images, additional TEE or MRI may be required to evaluate the anatomy and physiology definitively.

Coronary Sinus ASD (Unroofed Coronary Sinus) – Surgical repair of CS ASD incorporates patch closure of the roof of the CS, excluding it from the LA, and baffling of the left SVC to the CS. If the left SVC is very small and there is an adequate bridging innominate vein, this left SVC may be surgically ligated. Alternatively, a very large left SVC may be directly connected to the left pulmonary artery (left bidirectional cavopulmonary anastomosis) if there appears to be risk of obstruction with a long baffle to the CS. Using TEE in the operating room, the echocardiographer should no longer see flow from the LA to the CS. Agitated saline injection from an intravenous line in the left arm may aid in imaging of the surgical repair to ensure the absence of residual shunt. Follow-up of the patient with repaired CS ASD should reveal no detectable gradient within the CS if the left SVC is baffled to the RA through this pathway. Imaging of a left bidirectional cavopulmonary anastomosis can be accomplished from a suprasternal or high left parasternal window.

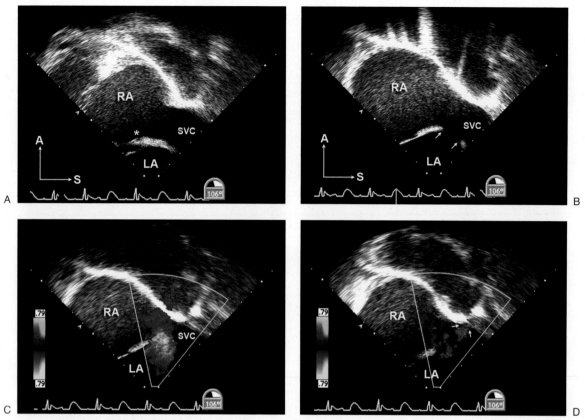

FIGURE 6.10. Transesophageal echocardiographic (TEE) images of sinus venosus atrial septal defect (ASD) associated with anomalous connection of right upper pulmonary vein to superior vena cava (SVC). A: Longitudinal plane imaging in region of inferior edge of superior limbus (*asterisk*) shows intact atrial septum. Note the SVC dilation. **B:** Rotation of the transducer farther rightward shows dropout in the superior portion of the atrial septum (*arrows*) consistent with sinus venosus ASD. **C:** Color Doppler showing left-to-right shunt (*blue*) through the large sinus venosus ASD from left atrium (LA) to right atrium (RA). **D:** Color flow into the SVC from anomalous right pulmonary vein (*red flow with arrows*); this view is not diagnostic and further imaging to confirm the anomalous pulmonary vein connection will be needed. A, anterior; S, superior.

 COR TRIATRIATUM

Background

Cor triatriatum, an unusual form of abnormal atrial septation, occurs within the LA. Cor triatriatum may result from abnormal incorporation of the common pulmonary vein into the LA, causing obstruction between the pulmonary vein confluence and the LA;

however, not all variants of this rare lesion are consistent with this embryologically.

Clinical Presentation

Cor triatriatum may produce signs and symptoms of pulmonary venous obstruction. Timing of presentation depends on the size of the communication between the proximal venous chamber and the distal LA, as well as the location and size of associated communicat-

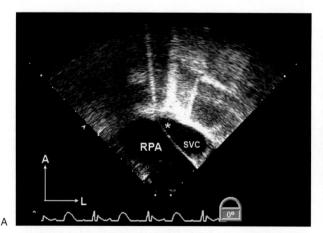
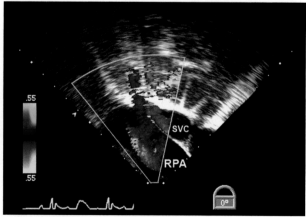

FIGURE 6.11. Transesophageal echocardiographic (TEE) images of anomalous connection of right upper pulmonary vein to superior vena cava (SVC) in patient with sinus venosus ASD as seen in Figure 6.10. A: Short-axis imaging from at level of right pulmonary artery (RPA) showing the teardrop "sign" (*asterisk*) where the anomalous right pulmonary vein enters the SVC, causing elongation of the normal circular-appearing vessel at this level. **B:** Color flow Doppler imaging shows red flow from right pulmonary vein into the SVC; flow in the RPA is away from the transducer (*blue*). A, anterior; L, leftward.

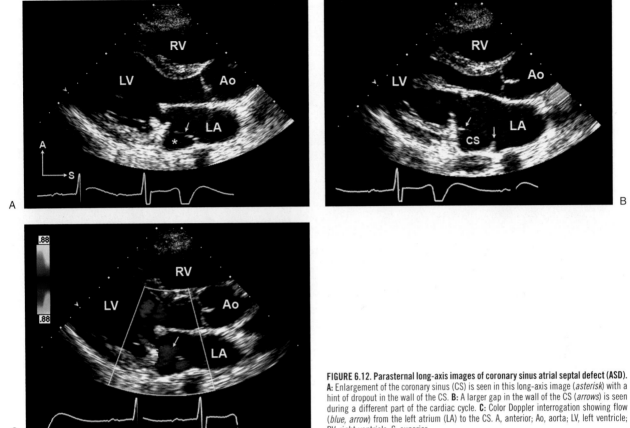

FIGURE 6.12. Parasternal long-axis images of coronary sinus atrial septal defect (ASD). **A:** Enlargement of the coronary sinus (CS) is seen in this long-axis image (*asterisk*) with a hint of dropout in the wall of the CS. **B:** A larger gap in the wall of the CS (*arrows*) is seen during a different part of the cardiac cycle. **C:** Color Doppler interrogation showing flow (*blue, arrow*) from the left atrium (LA) to the CS. A, anterior; Ao, aorta; LV, left ventricle; RV, right ventricle; S, superior.

ing ASDs to the RA. The volume of left-to-right shunting from the proximal LA chamber to the RA is proportional to *both* the size of the ASD between this chamber and the RA, and to the size of the opening within the cor triatriatum to the distal LA.

In the absence of a proximal ASD, a severely obstructed cor triatriatum membrane produces early signs of severe pulmonary venous obstruction. The clinical presentation is similar to the infant with *obstructed* total anomalous pulmonary venous connection. Cardiovascular collapse, due to RV failure, may result from unrecognized critical obstruction. On physical examination, there are signs of severe pulmonary hypertension and poor perfusion.

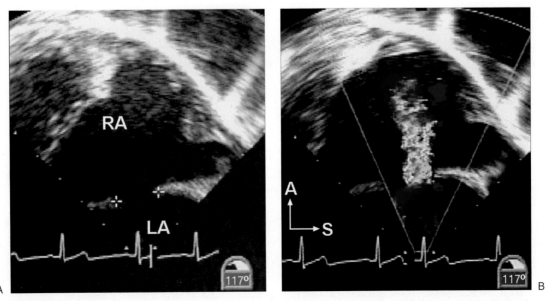

FIGURE 6.13. Transesophageal echocardiographic imaging in patient with moderate secundum atrial septal defect (ASD). A: Longitudinal plane imaging demonstrates central ASD (*asterisks*) with superior (S) and inferior rims. **B:** Color Doppler demonstrating left-to-right shunt (*blue flow*) from left atrium (LA) to right atrium (RA). A, anterior.

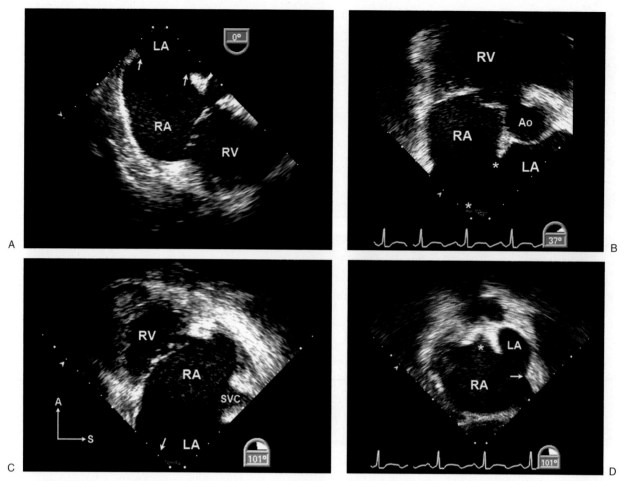

FIGURE 6.14. Transesophageal echocardiographic (TEE) imaging in an adult patient with a large secundum atrial septal defect (ASD). Assessment of septal rims is performed in multiple imaging planes and confirms that the defect is not suitable for device closure due to absence of the inferior and posterior rims. **A:** Apical four-chamber view with probe rotated toward right-sided structures. There is a large secundum ASD (*arrows*) with a small superior rim and adequate inferior rim seen in this imaging plane. Right atrial (RA) and right ventricular (RV) enlargement are seen. **B:** Rotation to 37 degrees in short-axis plane reveals the ASD (*asterisks*) with visible retroaortic rim but no visible posterior rim. **C:** Further rotation of the imaging plane to a longitudinal view shows absence of posterior/inferior rim. Care must be taken to fully evaluate this rim from TEE as the imaging transducer is in very close proximity to the rim. **D:** Deep transgastric imaging in a longitudinal plane confirms the absence of the posterior/inferior rim of this large ASD (*arrow*), making it unsuitable for consideration of device closure. The entry of the SVC to the RA is just seen anteriorly to the superior rim (*asterisk*). A, anterior; Ao, aorta; LA, left atrium; S, superior.

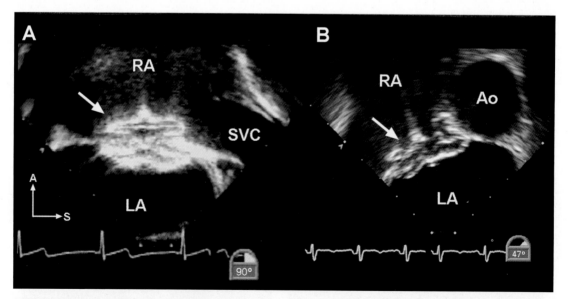

FIGURE 6.15. Transesophageal echocardiographic imaging in patient after implantation of AMPLATZER Septal Occluder (AGA Medical, Inc., Plymouth, Minn). **A:** Longitudinal plane TEE image showing normal device position following delivery; right atrial (RA) disc (*arrow*) in good position without interference in superior vena caval (SVC) drainage. Septal rims appear appropriate between the left and right discs of the device. **B:** Modified short-axis image showing device with anterior rims in proximity behind the aortic root, right atrial disc (*arrow*) in good position. Ao, aorta; LA, left atrium.

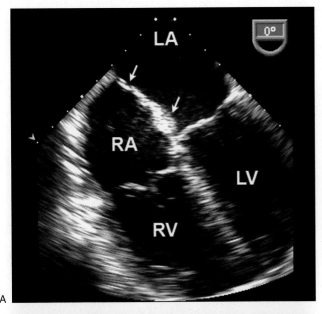

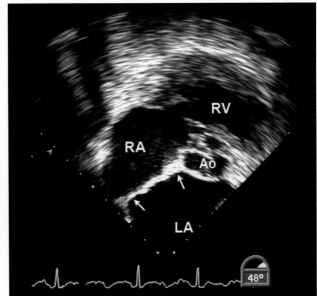

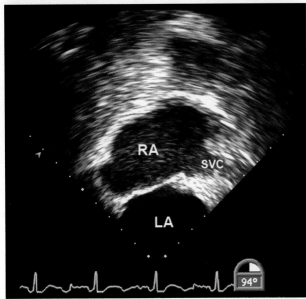

FIGURE 6.16. Transesophageal echocardiographic (TEE) images from the patient in Figure 6.14, following pericardial patch repair of large secundum atrial septal defect (ASD). **A:** Apical four-chamber TEE views showing intact pericardial patch repair of ASD (*arrows*). **B:** Short-axis view of patch between left atrium (LA) and right atrium (RA). **C:** Intact patch seen in longitudinal plane imaging. A, anterior; Ao, aorta; LV, left ventricle; RV, right ventricle; S, superior; SVC, superior vena cava.

Less severe obstruction may produce signs of tachypnea, feeding difficulties, poor weight gain, and a predisposition to respiratory illnesses. In the patient with a large communication between the proximal chamber and the RA, the clinical presentation resembles a patient with *unobstructed* total anomalous pulmonary venous connection (with an additional defect providing "right-to-left" communication between the RA and distal LA). Untreated, severely obstructed cor triatriatum will lead to progressive pulmonary vascular disease due to pulmonary venous and arterial hypertension, RV failure, and possible death.

Classic Two-dimensional Echo Anatomy and Imaging

A membrane is seen within the LA as a linear echo, located above the mitral valve in orthogonal views. As the membrane is somewhat curvilinear, it should be visualized from multiple imaging planes. It is important to note that the left atrial appendage is located between the obstructive membrane and the mitral valve, in contrast to a supravalvular mitral ring, where the left atrial appendage is above

the obstructive tissue. In classic cor triatriatum, the proximal chamber communicates only with the LA and not with the RA. There may be a PFO or an ASD between the lower LA chamber and the RA. Another variant of cor triatriatum exists in which all of the pulmonary veins return to the proximal chamber, which does not communicate with the distal LA directly. In this setting, an ASD provides egress to the RA, and a separate more inferior PFO/septal defect allows flow from the RA back to the LA.

Right-sided cardiac structural enlargement is characteristic of cor triatriatum. The RV is typically hypertrophied. RV function may be severely reduced if cardiac decompensation is present with severe membrane obstruction and little atrial communication for decompression of the proximal LA chamber. Quantification of pulmonary artery pressure can be obtained from tricuspid regurgitant velocity measurement using the modified Bernoulli equation.

Subcostal Views

Subcostal Coronal Views – In the subcostal "coronal" view, an abnormal line of tissue is visualized within the LA. The pulmonary veins connect proximal to this line of tissue, and may be distended.

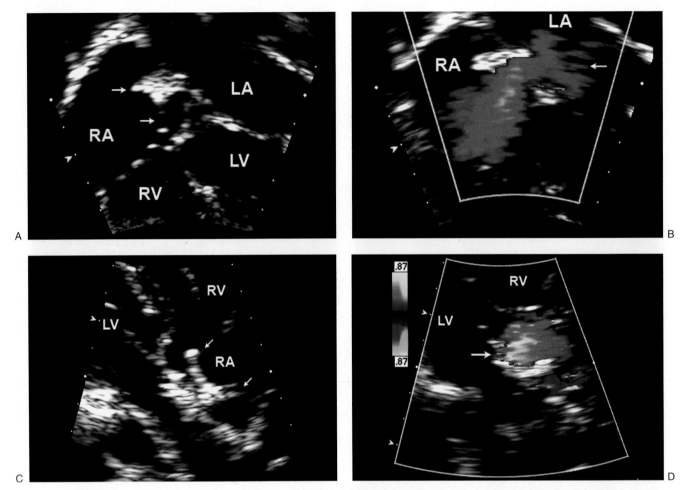

FIGURE 6.17. Images from patient who previously underwent implantation of a CardioSEAL device (NMT, Medical, Inc., Boston, Mass) for closure of a moderate-sized secundum atrial septal defect (ASD), Subcostal coronal view. **A:** The right atrial arms are more everted than normal in this patient. Left atrial arms are well opposed to the septum. **B:** Color flow Doppler interrogation shows moderate shunt (*arrow*) from left atrium (LA) to right atrium (RA) through the inferior portion of the device. **C:** Parasternal long-axis, tricuspid inflow view showing everted right atrial arms of the device (*arrows*). **D:** Color flow Doppler demonstrating left-to-right shunt (*single arrow*) through the inferior part of the defect, which remains patent secondary to the position of the device. LV, left ventricle; RV, right ventricle.

When the membrane is patent, and communicates with the distal LA, color Doppler interrogation will reveal turbulent continuous flow across the obstructed membrane within the LA. Imaging of the atrial septum should be carefully performed to evaluate the presence and location of any interatrial communication, including a Doppler determination of shunt direction and potential gradients. In the absence of a communication between the proximal chamber and the LA, there may be a large ASD between the proximal chamber and the RA with a large left-to-right shunt; a PFO communication between the RA and the distal LA is necessary for maintaining cardiac output and consequently shunts from right to left.

Subcostal Sagittal View – Short-axis imaging demonstrates an abnormal horizontal line of tissue separating the LA into two functional chambers. The atrial septum should be evaluated from both subcostal views, to determine from orthogonal planes the presence or absence of communication between the RA and either the proximal or distal chambers. The RVOT can be easily visualized in the short-axis view, typically showing a dilated main pulmonary artery. If pulmonary regurgitation is present, the end-diastolic velocity can be used to predict pulmonary artery diastolic pressure.

Parasternal Views

The enlarged right ventricle can be seen in both the parasternal long-axis and short-axis views. Septal motion is abnormal, depending on

the degree of pressure overload, again directly related to the degree of obstruction and to the presence of a decompressing atrial communication between the proximal pulmonary venous chamber and the RA. In the long-axis view, there is a linear membrane visualized in the mid-portion of the LA, again seen above the appendage and below the pulmonary veins (Fig. 6.21). Color Doppler may be used to demonstrate the communication with the distal chamber.

Apical View

Imaging of the left atrial membrane from the apical view will show a linear echo appearing above the base of the left atrial appendage and the mitral valve. From this view, the membrane may have a funnel-like appearance and be somewhat mobile. Color Doppler is used to evaluate the communication between the proximal and distal portions of the LA and to visualize fenestrations (Fig. 6.22A–B). This view usually provides the best alignment of the Doppler beam parallel with the opening in the left atrial membrane to the distal LA chamber and allows an estimate of the venous gradient (Fig. 6.22C). If there is a large ASD communicating with the proximal LA chamber, the majority of flow will enter the RA, rather than the distal LA, and may reduce the measured gradient. If there is no communication between this proximal chamber and the LA, an ASD will be seen decompressing from left to right into the RA. In addition, an inferiorly located PFO will be seen with right-to-left shunting. The mitral valve should appear normal, in contrast to supramitral ring, where leaflet mobility is affected.

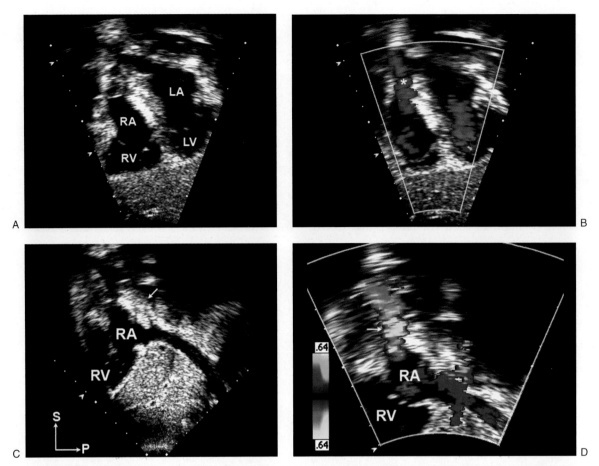

FIGURE 6.18. Subcostal imaging in patient following closure of a large secundum atrial septal defect (ASD) with the AMPLATZER Septal Occluder (AGA Medical, Inc., Plymouth, Minn). A: Coronal view showing the device in good position in the atrial septum. **B:** Slightly anterior angulation of the probe, with color Doppler, shows normal, nonaliased superior vena caval (*asterisk*) flow into the right atrium (RA). **C:** Rotating the transducer 90 degrees to a short-axis view shows the right atrial disc in relationship to the right atrial structures. The left atrium is foreshortened in this view (*arrow*). The RA and right ventricle (RV) are normal in size. The inferior vena cava (IVC) entry is widely patent. **D:** Additional color Doppler flow imaging shows normal, laminar flow into the RA from the SVC (*arrow*) and the IVC (*blue flow*). The right atrial disc does not impinge on right atrial inflow despite the large size of the device. LV, left ventricle; S, superior.

Suprasternal Notch Views

Confirmation of pulmonary venous return to the proximal left atrial chamber should be performed from the suprasternal notch view. A high parasternal short-axis view may be used to evaluate for the presence of a patent ductus arteriosus.

Postoperative Assessment of Cor Triatriatum

Surgical repair of this lesion involves resection of the obstructing membrane within the LA, with pericardial patch repair of any associated ASDs. Postoperative evaluation should include a full assessment of left atrial anatomy and visualization of unobstructed

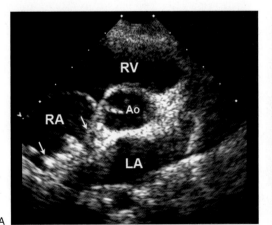
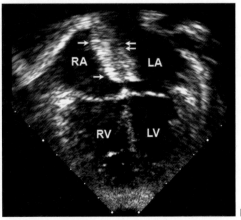

FIGURE 6.19. Transthoracic images from same patient as in Figure 6.18. Parasternal short-axis image showing normal right atrial (RA) and right ventricular (RV) size. **A:** The AMPLATZER Septal Occluder (AGA Medical, Inc., Plymouth, Minn) device sits in a normal position in the atrial septum (arrows), without impingement upon the anterior aortic root (Ao). **B:** Apical four-chamber view shows no device interference with atrioventricular valves. Left atrial (double arrow) and right atrial discs (arrows) are in good position. LA, left atrium; LV, left ventricle.

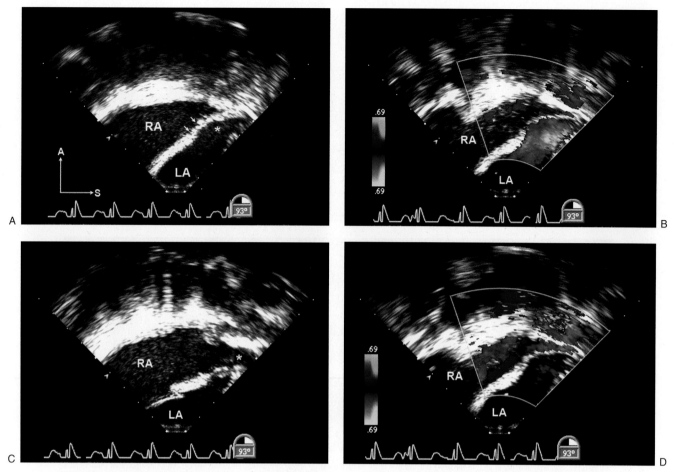

FIGURE 6.20. Intraoperative transesophageal echocardiogram (TEE) following repair of sinus venosus atrial septal defect (ASD) associated with partial anomalous pulmonary venous return to the superior vena cava (SVC) (preoperative images shown in Figs. 6.10 and 6.11). The repair incorporated a graft between the SVC and the right atrium (RA) (Warden technique). **A:** Longitudinal plane imaging shows the patch (*small arrows*) that directs right pulmonary veins (*asterisk*) to the left atrium (LA) through the ASD. **B:** Color Doppler shows laminar flow from unobstructed pulmonary vein baffle to the LA. This baffle serves two purposes: the ASD is functionally closed and the right pulmonary veins are directed to the LA. **C:** Further rightward and slightly superior imaging in the longitudinal plane brings the superior vena caval (*asterisk*) connection to the RA into view. **D:** Color Doppler from this imaging plane is foreshortened, although there is no obvious turbulence that would suggest a venous gradient. Imaging from additional planes would be needed to confirm baffle patency. Again, the pulmonary venous pathway appears widely patent. A, anterior; S, superior.

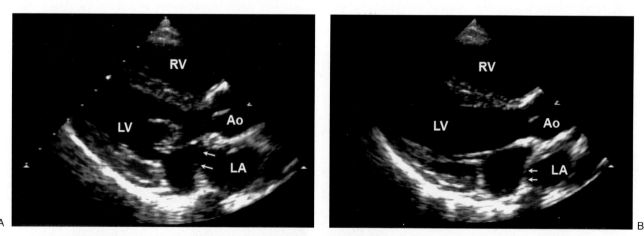

FIGURE 6.21. Parasternal long-axis images in a patient with cor triatriatum. A: Diastolic frame showing membrane within the left atrium (LA). The opening in the membrane is seen anteriorly (*double arrows*). **B:** Systolic frame with mitral valve closed; there is distance between the membrane (*double arrow*) and the mitral valve, which suggests cor triatriatum rather than supramitral ring. Ao, aorta; LV, left ventricle; RV, right ventricle.

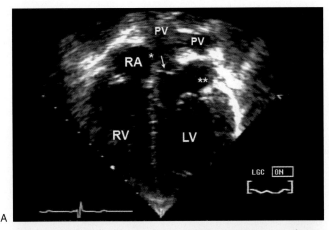

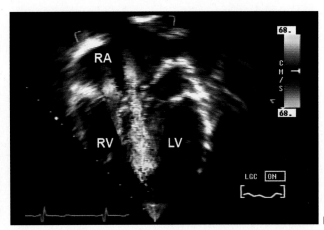

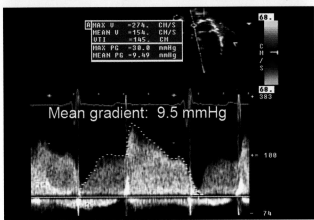

FIGURE 6.22. Apical four-chamber images in cor triatriatum. A: Characteristic linear shadow is seen within the left atrium (LA), separating the pulmonary vein (PV) entrance from the base of the left atrial appendage (*double asterisk*). There is a suggestion of septal dropout (*single asterisk*) between the proximal left atrial chamber and the right atrium (RA). Orthogonal plane imaging is suggested for confirmation. Shadowing within the RA prevents visualization of the tricuspid valve; the right ventricle (RV) is enlarged. **B:** The addition of color Doppler shows flow convergence medially, with turbulence extending into the distal LA chamber and through the mitral valve into the left ventricle (LV). **C:** Pulsed-Doppler tracing demonstrating a mean gradient of approximately 10 mm Hg between the proximal chamber and the distal chamber, consistent with significant obstruction. The gradient will depend on the size of the proximal communication with the RA, which provides decompression.

pulmonary venous return. There should be no Doppler gradient at the level of membrane resection and no evidence of atrial level shunt. RV hemodynamics should improve immediately, although pulmonary hypertension and RVH may take some time to resolve, depending on the age of the infant and preoperative course. It is unlikely that there will be long-term cardiac sequelae/residua following successful neonatal repair of cor triatriatum.

SUGGESTED READING

Alphonso N, Norgaard M, Newcomb A, et al. Cor triatriatum: Presentation, diagnosis and long-term surgical results. *Thorac Surg.* 2005;80:1666–1671.

Ammash N, Seward J, Warnes C, et al. Danielson G. Partial anomalous pulmonary venous connection: Diagnosis by transesophageal echocardiography. *J Am Coll Cardiol.* 1997;29:1351–1358.

Azhari N, Shihata M, Al-Fatani A. Spontaneous closure of atrial septal defects within the oval fossa. *Cardiol Young.* 2004;14:148–155.

Cabanes L, Mas J, Cohen A, et al. Atrial septal aneurysm and patent foramen ovale as risk factors for cryptogenic stroke in patients less than 55¡years of age. A study using transesophageal echocardiography. *Stroke.* 1993;24:1865–1873.

Cetta F, Seward J, O'Leary P. Echocardiography in congenital heart disease: An overview. In: Oh J, Seward J, Tajik A, eds. *The Echo Manual,* 3rd Ed. Philadelphia, Pa: Lippincott Williams & Wilkens, 2006:334–339.

Craig R, Selzer A. Natural history and prognosis of atrial septal defect. *Circulation.* 1968;37:805–815.

Earing M, Cabalka A, Seward J, et al. Intracardiac echocardiographic guidance during transcatheter device closure of atrial septal defect and patent foramen ovale. *Mayo Clinic Proc.* 2004;79:24–34.

Ettedgui J, Siewers R, Anderson R, et al. Diagnostic echocardiographic features of the sinus venosus defect. *Br Heart J.* 1990;64:329–331.

Gatzoulis M, Freeman M, Siu S, et al. Atrial arrhythmia after surgical closure of atrial septal defects in adults. *N Engl J Med.* 1999;340:839–846.

Geva T, Van Praagh R. Abnormal systemic venous connections. In: Allen H, Driscoll D, Shaddy R, Feltes T, eds. *Moss and Adams' Heart Disease in Infants, Children, and Adolescents.* Philadelphia, Pa: Lippincott, Williams & Wilkins, 2007:792–817.

Geva T, Van Praagh R. Anomalies of the pulmonary veins. In: Allen H, Driscoll D, Shaddy R, Feltes T, eds. *Moss and Adams' Heart Disease in Infants, Children, and Adolescents.* Philadelphia, Pa: Lippincott, Williams & Wilkins, 2007:791–792.

Hagen P, Scholz D, Edwards W. Incidence and size of patent foramen ovale during the first 10 decades of life: An autopsy study of 965 normal hearts. *Mayo Clin Proc.* 1984;59:17–20.

Hanslik A, Pospisil U, Salzer-Muhar U, et al. Predictors of spontaneous closure of isolated secundum atrial septal defect in children: A longitudinal study. *Pediatrics.* 2006;118:1560–1565.

Kearney D, Titus J. Cardiovascular anatomy. In: Garson A, ed. *The Science and Practice of Pediatric Cardiology.* Baltimore, Md: Williams & Wilkins, 1998:127–153.

Kirklin J, Barratt-Boyes B. Unroofed coronary sinus syndrome. In: Kirklin J, Barratt-Boyes B, eds. *Cardiac Surgery.* New York: Churchill-Livingstone, 1993:683–692.

Mathewson J, Bichell D, Rothman A, et al. Absent posteroinferior and anterosuperior atrial septal defect rims: Factors affecting nonsurgical closure of large secundum defects using the Amplatzer occluder. *J Am Soc Echocardiogr.* 2004;17:62–69.

Mazic U, Gavora P, Masura J. Role of transesophageal echocardiography in transcatheter closure of secundum atrial septal defects by the Amplatzer septal occluder. *Am Heart J.* 2001;142:482–488.

McMahon C, Feltes F, Fraley J, et al. Natural history of growth of secundum atrial septal defects and implications for transcatheter closure. *Heart.* 2002;87:256–259.

Murphy J, Gersh B, McGoon M, et al. Long-term outcome after surgical repair of isolated atrial septal defect. Follow-up at 27 to 32 years. *N Engl J Med.* 1990;13:1645–1660.

Patel A, Cao Q, Koenig P, et al. Intracardiac echocardiography to guide closure of atrial septal defects in children less than 15 kilograms. *Catheter Cardiovasc Interv.* 2006;68:287–291.

Porter C, Edwards W. Atrial septal defect. In: Allen H, Driscoll D, Shaddy R, Feltes T, eds. *Moss and Adams: Heart Disease in Infants, Children, and Adolescents.* Philadelphia, Pa: Lippincott Williams & Wilkins, 2007.

Quaegebeur J, Kirklin JP, Bargeron L. Surgical experience with unroofed coronary sinus. *Ann Thorac Surg.* 1979;27:418–425.

Raghib G, Ruttenberg H, Anderson R, et al. Termination of left superior vena cava in left atrium, atrial septal defect, and absence of coronary sinus: A developmental complex. *Circulation.* 1965;31:906–918.

Shahriari A, Rodefeld M, Turrentine MB. Caval division technique for sinus venosus atrial septal defect with partial anomalous pulmonary venous connection. *Ann Thorac Surg.* 2006;81:224–229.

Snider A, Serwer G, Ritter S. *Echocardiography in Pediatric Heart Disease.* 2nd Ed. St. Louis, Mo: Mosby, 1997.

Steele P, Fuster V, Cohen M, et al. Isolated atrial septal defect with pulmonary vascular obstructive disease: Long-term follow-up and prediction of outcome after surgical correction. *Circulation.* 1987;76:1037–1042.

Van Praagh S, Carrera M, Sanders S. Sinus venous defects: Unroofing of the right pulmonary veins, anatomic and echocardiographic findings and surgical treatment. *Am Heart J.* 1994;128:365–379.

Vick G III. *Defects of the Atrial Septum Including Atrioventricular Septal Defects.* Baltimore, Md: Williams & Wilkins, 1998.

Wahl A, Windecker S, Meier B. Evaluation and treatment of abnormalities of the interatrial septum. *Cathet Cardiovasc Interv.* 2004;63:94–103.

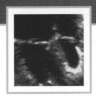

Chapter 7
Atrioventricular Septal Defects

Malek El Yaman • William D. Edwards • Frank Cetta

Atrioventricular septal defects (AVSDs) comprise a spectrum of lesions characterized by deficient atrioventricular (AV) septation and a variety of AV valve anomalies. AVSDs occur due to failure of fusion of the embryonic endocardial cushions. AVSDs represent 5% of congenital heart disease. Other terms have been used to describe this group of defects, including "AV canal," "persistent common AV canal," "atrioventricular defect," and "endocardial cushion defect." For the purposes of this chapter, the term "AVSD" will be used. The severity of AVSD is determined by many factors, including the size of atrial and ventricular level shunts, the extent of AV valve abnormalities, the presence of associated cardiac anomalies, and discrepancy in ventricular sizes. Long-term survival after surgical repair has been excellent and cumulative 20-year survival of 95% has been reported. However, long-term postoperative echocardiographic surveillance is required. Reoperation awaits 15% to 25% of patients due to progressive left AV valve regurgitation or development of left ventricular outflow tract (LVOT) obstruction.

TERMINOLOGY AND CLASSIFICATION

Many classification schemes have been used to describe AVSDs, resulting in confused terminology (Figs. 7.1 and 7.2). There is general agreement that AVSDs can be subdivided into two forms: *complete* and *partial*. *Complete AVSD* is characterized by a primum ASD that is contiguous with an inlet VSD, and the presence of a common AV valve. The common AV valve is composed of five leaflets: anterior and posterior bridging leaflets, anterior leaflet (present on the right side), and right and left lateral leaflets.

The typical *partial AVSD* is distinguished from complete forms of the malformation by the absence of an inlet VSD. The anatomic hallmarks of partial AVSD are the primum ASD and a cleft in the anterior

mitral valve leaflet. This type of AVSD has distinct mitral and tricuspid valves, each with a complete and separate annulus.

Two other subtypes, the *intermediate* and *transitional* forms, have been described. *Intermediate AVSD* is considered a variant of complete AVSD and is characterized by a single AV valve annulus that is divided by a tongue of tissue into right and left orifices. Because of the single annulus, it is preferred to use the terms "right and left components of the AV valve" in complete and intermediate AVSDs rather than "tricuspid" and "mitral" valves.

A *transitional AVSD* has two separate AV valve annuli and is considered a variant of partial AVSD. In addition to a primum ASD and a cleft mitral valve, there is a small inlet VSD that is often restricted or obliterated by dense attachments of the AV valves to the crest of the ventricular septum.

Complete and intermediate AVSDs have the physiology and clinical features of an ASD and a VSD. In contrast, partial and transitional AVSDs have the clinical picture of a large ASD (Table 7.1).

CHARACTERISTIC ANATOMIC FEATURES OF ATRIOVENTRICULAR SEPTAL DEFECTS

A number of characteristics are shared by all forms of AVSDs. These features aid in making the echocardiographic diagnosis of AVSD and have important clinical implications (Table 7.2).

Level of Atrioventricular Valve Insertion

In normal hearts, the tricuspid valve inserts onto the ventricular septum more apically than the mitral valve. With this "offset" in the level

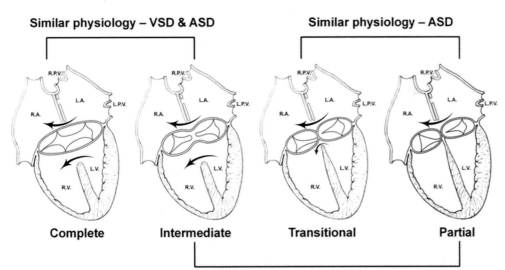

FIGURE 7.1. Summary of atrioventricular septal defects (AVSDs). Anatomic and physiologic similarities between the different forms of AVSD are illustrated. *Complete* AVSD has one annulus with a large atrial septal defect (ASD) and a large ventricular septal defect (VSD). *Intermediate* defects (one annulus, two orifices) are a subtype of complete AVSD. Complete AVSD has physiology of a VSD and an ASD. *Partial* AVSD has physiology of an ASD. *Transitional* defects are a subtype of partial AVSD in which a small inlet VSD is also present. Partial defects and the intermediate form of complete AVSD share a similar anatomic feature: a tongue of tissue divides the common AV valve into distinct right and left orifices. AV, atrioventricular; LA, left atrium; LPV, left pulmonary vein; LV, left ventricle; RA, right atrium; RPV, right pulmonary vein; RV, right ventricle.

FIGURE 7.2. Embryologic development of the atrioventricular canal region and the spectrum of atrioventricular septal defects (AVSDs). The diagrams in the middle of the figure illustrate the normal embryonic development of the AV valves leading to formation of the normal mitral and tricuspid valves (upper left). Abnormal development of the embryonic AV canal can lead to partial (upper middle), transitional (upper right) and complete (lower row of diagrams) forms of AVSD. Complete AVSD can be further subclassified into types A–C and intermediate AVSD; as described in the text and illustrated in the lower row of diagrams. A, anterior leaflet; AB, anterior bridging leaflet; DDCC, dextrodorsal conus cushion; IEC, inferior endocardial cushion; LEC, lateral endocardial cushion; P, posterior leaflet; PB, posterior bridging leaflet; S, septal leaflet; SEC, superior endocardial cushion, L, lateral leaflet.

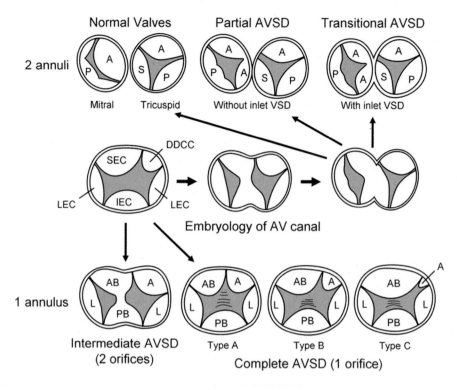

of insertion, a portion of septum, called the AV septum (Fig. 7.3A), separates the right atrium (RA) and the left ventricle. In AVSDs, both right and left AV valve components insert at the same level, and this is echocardiographically best appreciated from an apical four-chamber view. Apical four-chamber imaging demonstrates the crux of the heart, which has been referred to as the most reliable and consistent intracardiac landmark. A unifying feature of all forms of AVSDs is the complete absence of the AV septum (Fig.7.3B).

Unwedging of the Aortic Valve

In normal hearts, the aortic valve is "wedged" between the mitral and tricuspid valves (Fig. 7.4). In AVSDs, the aortic valve is "sprung" and displaced anteriorly. This contributes to elongation of the LVOT. This is best appreciated from the parasternal long-axis and subcostal outflow views.

Elongation of the Left Ventricular Outflow Tract

In normal hearts, the distance from the left ventricular (LV) apex to the aortic annulus is equal to the distance from the LV apex to the mitral annulus (Fig. 7.5). The inlet and outlet portions of the left ventricle are approximately equal in length. In contrast, the deficiency of the AV septum and apical displacement of the left AV valve insertion in AVSDs lends a scooped-out appearance to the ventricular septum and results in a shorter inlet portion. In addition, the anterior displacement of the unwedged aortic valve leads to an elongated and narrowed LVOT. The narrow, long LVOT has been classically described as having a "goose neck" appearance. This can be identified on angiographic and echocardiographic long-axis views of the left ventricle. This anatomic feature is clinically important as it provides a setup for the development of LVOT obstruction, especially when present with other findings such as aberrant left AV valve chordal insertions or displacement of a papillary muscle anteriorly into the LVOT.

Cleft of the Left Atrioventricular Valve

In partial AVSDs, the anterior mitral leaflet inserts onto the crest of the ventricular septum (Fig. 7.6). A cleft is invariably present in the anterior mitral leaflet and it is directed toward the midportion of the ventricular septum. In complete AVSDs, the common AV valve

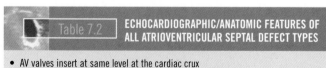

Table 7.1	DISTINGUISHING FEATURES OF THE VARIOUS TYPES OF ATRIOVENTRICULAR SEPTAL DEFECTS (AVSDs)
Type of AVSD	**Features**
Partial	Primum ASD Cleft anterior mitral leaflet
Transitional	Primum ASD Cleft anterior mitral leaflet Inlet VSD (small), mostly obliterated by chordal attachments to the septum
Intermediate	Primum ASD Inlet VSD (large) Common AV valve annulus, separated by a tongue of tissue into two orifices
Complete	Primum ASD Inlet VSD (large) Common AV valve with five leaflets

ASD, atrial septal defect; AV, atrioventricular; VSD, ventricular septal defect.

Table 7.2	ECHOCARDIOGRAPHIC/ANATOMIC FEATURES OF ALL ATRIOVENTRICULAR SEPTAL DEFECT TYPES

- AV valves insert at same level at the cardiac crux
- Absence of the AV septum
- Unwedging and anterior displacement of the aortic valve
- Elongated LVOT
- Counterclockwise rotation of LV papillary muscles
- Cleft of left AV valve component, directed towards the ventricular septum

AV, atrioventricular; LV, left ventricle; LVOT, left ventricular outflow tract.

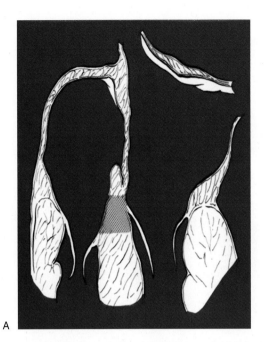

A

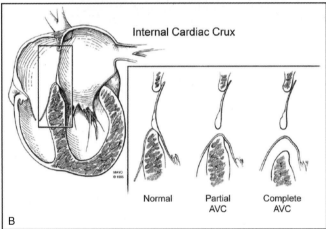

Internal Cardiac Crux

Normal   Partial AVC   Complete AVC

B

FIGURE 7.3. Atrioventricular septum (AVS). A: Diagram of the AVS (*shaded area*) in the normal heart (four-chamber view). The AVS lies between the right atrium and the left ventricle. The interatrial septum is above and the interventricular septum is below the AVS. The septal tricuspid leaflet normally inserts at a lower (more apical) level than the anterior mitral leaflet. **B:** Line drawing demonstrating the deficiency of the AVS in all forms of AVSD. (With permission of Mayo Foundation.)

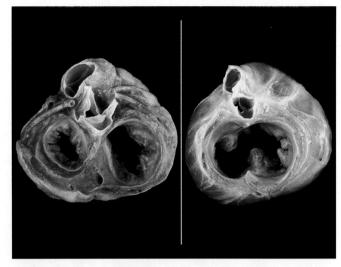

FIGURE 7.4. Unwedged aortic valve. Left: Normal pathologic specimen cut in short axis at the base demonstrating where the atrioventricular junction has a "figure of eight" configuration. **Right:** Similar projection in a heart with an atrioventricular septal defect (AVSD) where the atrioventricular junction is "unwedged." The aortic valve between the atrioventricular valve annuli is anteriorly displaced (instead of being wedged). This elongates the left ventricular outflow tract (LVOT) in AVSDs.

consists of five leaflets, and the two that span across the ventricular septum are known as the anterior and posterior bridging leaflets. Conceptually, the anterior bridging leaflet corresponds to the superior half of the anterior mitral leaflet, and the posterior bridging leaflet represents fusion of the septal tricuspid leaflets and the inferior portion of the anterior mitral leaflet. No tongue of tissue separates the AV valve into right and left components, and the space between the anterior and posterior bridging leaflets is analogous to the cleft in the anterior mitral leaflet in partial AVSDs.

Clockwise Rotation of the Left Ventricular Papillary Muscles

In all forms of AVSD, the LV papillary muscles are rotated counterclockwise compared with normal. In the parasternal short-axis projection, normal mitral papillary muscles are located at the "4 o'clock and 8 o'clock" positions. In AVSD, LV papillary muscles are rotated toward the "3 o'clock and 7 o'clock" positions. This causes the anterior mitral leaflet (or anterior bridging leaflet) to be more anteriorly located and contributes to narrowing of the LVOT.

ECHOCARDIOGRAPHIC EVALUATION OF ATRIOVENTRICULAR SEPTAL DEFECTS

Primum Atrial Septal Defects

Echocardiography is the diagnostic modality of choice for delineation of all anatomic features of AVSDs Figures (7.7–7.10). The best transducer position to define the number and size of ASDs is the subcostal view as the plane of sound is perpendicular to the atrial septum. Both the subcostal four-chamber and sagittal (bicaval) views are helpful in that regard. Color Doppler delineates the shunt. The primum ASD in partial AVSD is typically large and easily visualized in the subcostal, parasternal, and apical four-chamber projections. The transesophageal echocardiographic four-chamber view readily demonstrates a primum ASD and the insertion of the tricuspid and mitral valves onto the crest of the septum.

Mitral Valve Abnormalities

The cleft of the anterior mitral leaflet is best appreciated from subcostal and parasternal short-axis views (Fig. 7.11A). The cleft changes the appearance of the mitral valve from the usual "fish-mouth" to a triangular configuration. In patients with AVSD, the mitral valve cleft is directed toward the ventricular septum; in contrast, in patients with "isolated cleft of the mitral valve," it is directed toward the LVOT. The cleft causes mitral regurgitation due to improper leaflet coaptation in that area. This regurgitation is usually progressive as the patient ages. The cleft is closed at the time of repair.

Several other abnormalities may occur in the mitral valve or the left component of the common AV valve. Left AV valve abnormalities occur much more commonly in partial than in complete AVSD. A tongue of tissue may divide the mitral valve into two orifices, creating what is known as a "double-orifice" mitral valve. This has been described in approximately 3% to 5% of AVSDs. The effective combined area of the two orifices is always smaller than (Fig. 7.11B) the total area of the undivided orifice. Therefore, a double-orifice mitral valve is generally associated with stenosis. The leaflets are thickened and exhibit limited diastolic excursion.

Parachute deformity of the mitral valve has also been described in AVSDs. As the name suggests, mitral chordae attach to only one papillary muscle, creating the appearance of a parachute. This is also associated with valve stenosis. Due to the presence of one predominant papillary muscle, the left mural leaflet is underdeveloped or absent. The parasternal short-axis view best assesses the number of

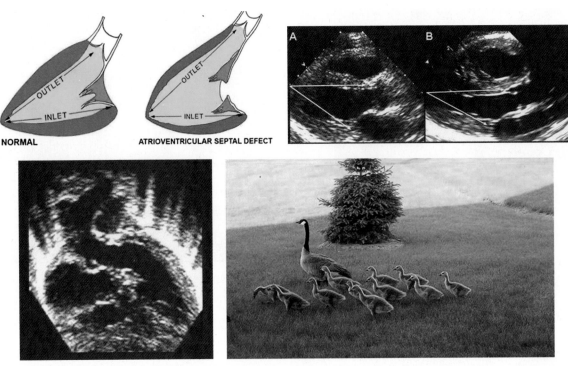

FIGURE 7.5. Left ventricular outflow elongation in atrioventricular septal defects (AVSD): The two diagrams in the upper left illustrate the LV inlet and outlet lengths in the normal heart (left) and one with an AVSD (right). In patients with AVSD, the outflow is much longer than the inflow. Due to deficiency of the ventricular component of the atrioventricular septum and the "unwedged" aortic valve, the distance from the LV apex to the posterior left atrioventricular valve annulus is 20% to 25% shorter than the distance from the apex to the aortic annulus. **Upper right:** Parasternal long-axis views in (a) a normal heart and (b) a heart with AVSD. These images demonstrate the changes in relative inlet/outlet length that were outlined by the diagrams. As a result, the distance from the LV apex to the aortic annulus is notably longer than the distance from the apex to the mitral annulus in AVSD, as opposed to nearly equal distances in the normal heart. **Lower left:** Apical five-chamber view demonstrating the elongated LVOT typical of AVSD. It has been described as a "goose neck." **Lower right:** Minnesota pediatric and adult "goose necks." (upper left, With permission from Robert Anderson, MD.)

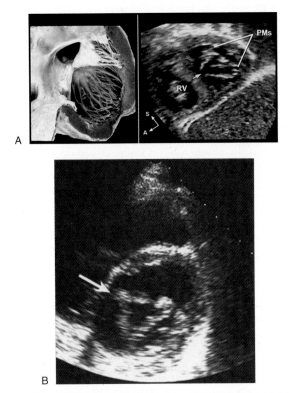

FIGURE 7.6. Cleft left atrioventricular valve. A: Left: In atrioventricular septal defect (AVSD), the cleft in the anterior leaflet of the left atrioventricular valve is typically oriented toward the mid-portion of the ventricular septum (*arrow*) along the anterior-inferior rim of the septal defect. **Right**: Subcostal sagittal image demonstrating the septal orientation of the cleft. **B:** The cleft (*arrow*) in the anterior leaflet gives the valve a trileaflet appearance as seen in this parasternal short-axis image.

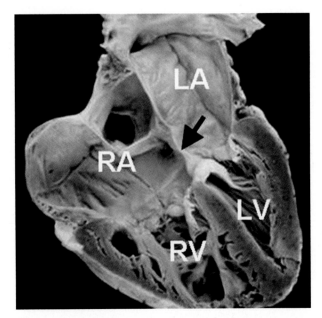

FIGURE 7.7. Partial atrioventricular septal defect (AVSD); anatomic specimen. This heart has been cut in a plane simulating the apical four chamber view and demonstrates the classic anatomy of a partial AVSD. The large primum atrial septal defect is highlighted by the arrow. Right atrial and right ventricular dilation are present. LA, left atrium; LV, left ventricle; RA, right atrium; RV, right ventricle.

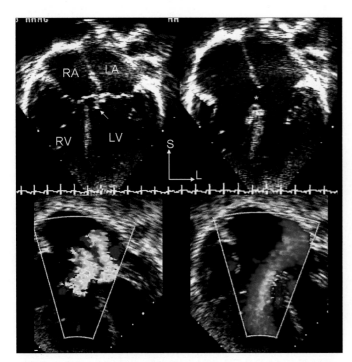

FIGURE 7.8. Partial atrioventricular septal defect (AVSD): Echocardiographic anatomy. Top/right: The four-chamber echocardiographic images in the two upper panels correspond to the anatomic plane shown in Figure 7.7. The upper left image was captured in systole and illustrates how the septal components of the two atrioventricular (AV) valves are at the same level. The potential VSD has been sealed by chordal attachments (arrow). The upper left panel was captured in diastole, it more clearly demonstrates the presence of a large primum ASD (*) and the distinctly separate right and left AV valve orifices. The two color Doppler images in the bottom panels are paired with the 2-dimensional images above them. The systolic frame on the left demonstrates regurgitation of both AV valves. The diastolic frame on the right, shows a low velocity, but large, left atrial to right atrial/ventricular shunt crossing the ASD. LA, left atrium; LV, left ventricle; RA, right atrium; RV, right ventricle.

papillary muscles and determines the presence of a two-orifice mitral valve. The mitral inflow gradient is typically evaluated by spectral Doppler from the apical four-chamber projection. However, in the setting of a large ASD, this measurement underestimates the severity of the stenosis because the ASD "decompresses" the left atrium.

Left Ventricular Outflow Tract Obstruction

In AVSD, the LVOT is elongate and narrow (Fig. 7.12). LVOT obstruction may be present preoperatively but more commonly develops postoperatively. LVOT obstruction is more common in partial AVSD than in complete AVSD. An explanation for this may be the fixation of the mitral valve leaflets to the crest of the ventricular septum.

Other factors that contribute to LVOT obstruction are accessory chordal attachments to the septum and anterior displacement of the papillary muscles.

THE CONCEPT OF BALANCE

Both partial and complete AVSD can be either "balanced" or "unbalanced" based on how the AV junction is shared by the ventricles. If the AV inlet is more or less equally shared by the two ventricular chambers, then this is consistent with a balanced AVSD. In an unbalanced AVSD, one ventricle is typically hypoplastic compared with the other. The larger ventricle is termed the "dominant" ventricle. For example, unbalanced AVSD with right ventricular (RV) dominance has a hypoplastic left ventricle with more than half of the AV junction committed to the right ventricle. This can occur in any form of AVSD and typically associated with severe coarctation of the aorta and arch anomalies. On the other hand, unbalanced AVSD with LV dominance has a hypoplastic right ventricle and is associated with pulmonary stenosis or atresia. Unbalanced AVSD occurs in 10% to 15% of AVSDs; two-thirds are RV dominant (Fig. 7.13).

Relative size of the ventricles is best appreciated from the apical four-chamber view. This view also allows visualization of malalignment between the atrial and ventricular septa in complete AVSD, another clue to an unbalanced AVSD. The subcostal en face view of the AV valves gives an estimate of the proportion of AV valve area committed to each ventricle. Determining balance with echo is important as it forms the basis for deciding on single-ventricle versus biventricular surgical pathway. Modest degrees of RV hypoplasia may also be addressed with a 1.5-ventricle repair. This includes closure of intracardiac shunts and "unloading" the right ventricle by performing a bidirectional cavopulmonary anastomosis.

Cohen and colleagues (Fig. 7.13) proposed a quantitative approach using the en face subcostal view to delineate cases with significant LV hypoplasia that may be better repaired by a single-ventricle approach. These authors measured the area of the AV valve apportioned over each ventricle and calculated an AV valve index (AVVI) as a left/right valve area ratio. The AVVI may be used as the basis for an algorithm to stratify patients into a single-ventricle or biventricular pathway. Those with AVVI less than 0.67 who have a large VSD would be considered for a single-ventricle path. A retrospective study by Walter and colleagues suggested that outcome was improved in patients with small left ventricles undergoing biventricular repair if the long-axis ratio of left ventricle to right ventricle measured by angiography was greater than 0.65.

One has to be aware of several caveats that may make interpretation of balance less straightforward. For example, the severity of valve malalignment may not necessarily correlate with the degree of ventricular hypoplasia. Moreover, pulmonary venous blood preferentially flows across the ASD, causing underfilling of the left ventricle. Finally, the presence of a large left-to-right shunt may cause severe RV enlargement with bowing of the septum to the left, lending a hypoplastic appearance to the left ventricle. van Son et al. have attempted to estimate the "potential volume" of the

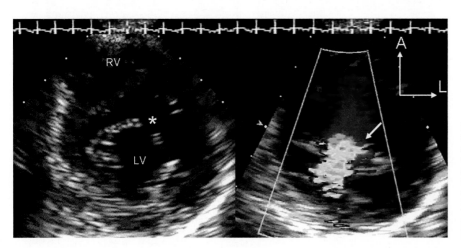

FIGURE 7.9. Cleft Mitral Valve associated with Partial atrioventricular septal defect (AVSD): These two parasternal short-axis scans are focused on the anterior mitral valve leaflet in the left ventricular inflow tract. The image on the left is taken in diastole and demonstrates the division of the anterior leaflet into two separate components. This division creates a triangular (three leaflet) appearance to the diastolic orifice of the mitral valve. The gap between the two components is referred to as the "cleft" (asterisk). The image on the right is a systolic color Doppler map demonstrating mitral regurgitation associated with the cleft. LV, left ventricle, RV, right ventricle.

FIGURE 7.10. Partial atrioventricular septal defect (AVSD): Transesophageal Echocardiographic (TEE) anatomy. This diastolic four-chamber TEE image demonstrates a large primum ASD (*) with insertion of both tricuspid and mitral valve leaflets to the crest of the ventricular septum. Marked RA and RV dilation are also evident, consistent with a large left to right shunt. LA, left atrium; LV, left ventricle; RA, right atrium; RV, right ventricle.

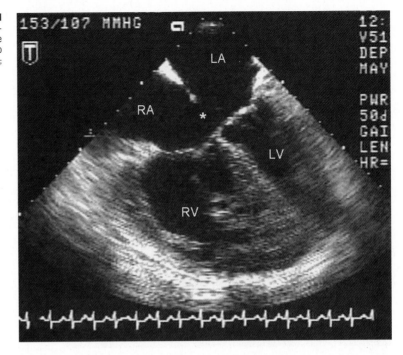

FIGURE 7.11. Cleft mitral valve (MV) and double-orifice atrioventricular valve. Left: Cleft MV. The anterior leaflet of the MV has a characteristic break (*asterisk*) that represents a cleft in the anterior leaflet. This feature is common to both partial and complete forms of atrioventricular septal defects (AVSDs). **Right:** Double-orifice atrioventricular valve. Each papillary muscle receives a separate atrioventricular valve orifice (*arrows*). The combined mitral orifice is less than the sum of both orifices and results in mitral stenosis. LV, left ventricle; RV, right ventricle; VS, ventricular septum. (Modified from Seward JB, Tajik AJ, Edwards WD, et al. *Two-Dimensional Echocardiographic Atlas. Vol. 1. Congenital Heart Disease.* New York: Springer-Verlag, 1987:270–292.)

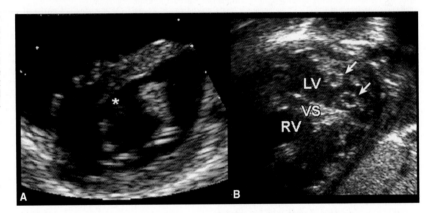

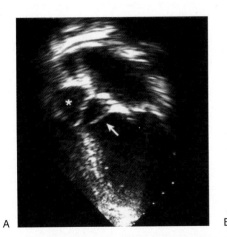
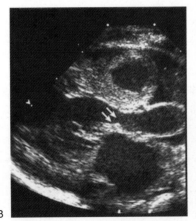
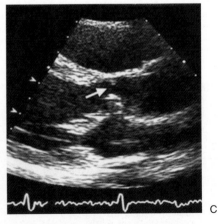

FIGURE 7.12. Left ventricular outflow tract (LVOT). A: Accessory mitral chordal attachments to the LVOT demonstrated on apical long-axis view. Note the relationship of the aortic valve (*asterisk*) and accessory chordal attachments (*arrow*), which can potentially contribute to LVOT obstruction. **B:** Parasternal long-axis view in a neonate with complete atrioventricular septal defect (AVSD) demonstrating tunnel-like LVOT obstruction and a discrete subaortic ridge (*arrows*). **C:** Parasternal long-axis view demonstrating LVOT obstruction in a 17-year-old after repair of partial AVSD at age 15 months. LVOT obstruction (*arrow*) is usually progressive and may be undetected at time of initial repair. Ten percent of patients with AVSD may require reoperation to relieve LVOT obstruction. Progressive LVOT obstruction is more common in partial than in complete AVSD. Mechanisms of LVOT obstruction include attachments of superior bridging leaflet to ventricular septum, extension of the anterolateral papillary muscle into the LVOT, discrete fibrous subaortic stenosis, and tissue from an aneurysm of the membranous septum bowing into the LVOT.

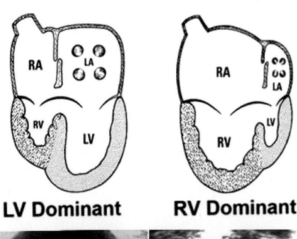

LV Dominant   RV Dominant

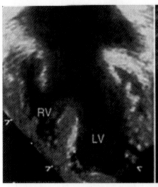 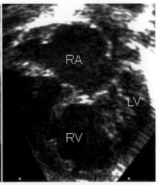

A

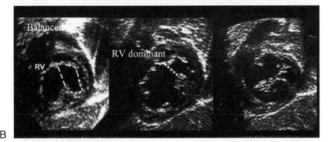

B

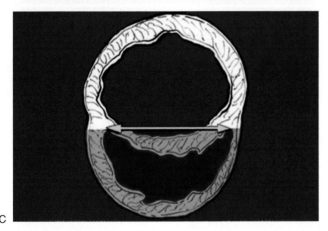

C

FIGURE 7.13. The four upper panels show examples of complete unbalanced atrioventricular septal defect (AVSD) with (*left*) left ventricular (LV) dominance and (*right*) right ventricular (RV) dominance. The plane of the ventricular septum is indicated with the dashed line. In the LV dominant form, the commonatrioventricular (AV) valve opens predominantly to the left ventricle, as opposed to the RV dominant form where the AV valve orifice opens predominantly to the right ventricle. **B:** Subcostal sagittal images demonstrating a variety of relative AV valve areas for use in evaluating ventricular dominance in AVSD. **C:** Diagram illustrating the concept of septal displacement in AVSD and its relative effect on ventricular dominance in AVSD. (**B,** Technique described by Cohen MS, Jacobs ML, Weinberg PM, et al. Morphometric analysis of unbalanced common atrioventricular canal using two-dimensional echocardiography. *J Am Coll Cardiol.* 1996;28:1017–1023. **C,** As described by van Son JA, Phoon CK, Silverman NH, et al. Predicting feasibility of biventricular repair of right-dominant unbalanced atrioventricular canal. *Ann Thorac Surg.* 1997;63:1657–1663.)

left ventricle preoperatively by using a theoretical model that calculates the relative areas of the left ventricle and right ventricle in short axis after assuming normal septal configuration (Fig. 7.13).

RASTELLI CLASSIFICATION OF THE COMMON ATRIOVENTRICULAR VALVE

Evaluation of common AV valve morphology is crucial to identify mechanism of regurgitation, commitment to RV and LV masses, attachments, and the existence of possible anomalies such as double-orifice left AV valve (Fig. 7.14 and 7.15). The best view that visualizes the anatomy of the valve is the "en face" view obtained from the subcostal window by rotating the transducer clockwise from the four-chamber view. Once the valve is seen "en face," the transducer is then tilted slowly inferiorly and superiorly to obtain multiple short-axis views of the valve from the inferior margin of the atrial septum to the superior margin of the ventricular septum. Classifying the common AV valve into Rastelli Type A, B, or C is often made from this plane (Table 7.3).

The Rastelli classification of the common AV valve was published in 1966 and is applicable only to patients with complete AVSD. The three types of common AV valve described by Rastelli and his colleagues are illustrated in Figure 7.14. The classification originally had prognostic implications. Currently, it is of historical interest and is helpful when communicating with surgeons. However, description of the details of the valve morphology should be the primary focus of the echocardiographer rather than purely labeling diverse anatomic features with an imperfect scheme. The classification is based on attachment and the degree of bridging of the anterior bridging leaflet. The spectrum of common AV valve anatomy seen in complete AVSD is illustrated in Figures 7.14 and 7.15 Type A complete AVSD has an anterior bridging leaflet that is evenly divided between the two ventricular inlets. Chordae anchor the center of the right and left components of the anterior bridging leaflet to the anterosuperior ventricular septum. The "commissure" between these components overlies the septum and VSD. In cases with Type B morphology, the anterior bridging leaflet is unevenly divided and its "commissure" and papillary muscle attachments lie within the RV. The anterior bridging leaflet in patients with Type C morphology is completely undivided with no central commissure. The chordal/papillary muscle attachments are evenly divided between the two ventricular cavities, but there are no attachments to the anterosuperior septum. As a result, this leaflet has been described as "free-floating".

ASSOCIATED LESIONS

A major anomaly described in association with AVSDs is tetralogy of Fallot (ToF). The association of RV outflow tract abnormalities with AVSDs is most common in Type C complete AVSD. Other anomalies are: pulmonary valve atresia, double-outlet right ventricle, and anomalous pulmonary venous connections. All occur more commonly with complete AVSD.

	RASTELLI CLASSIFICATION SCHEME FOR DIFFERENTIATING THE FORMS OF COMPLETE ATRIOVENTRICULAR SEPTAL DEFECT	
Table 7.3		
Rastelli Type	**Superior bridging leaflet and chordal attachments**	
A	Divided and attached to crest of ventricular septum (multiple chordae)	
B	Partly divided into 2 components, but not attached to crest of septum. Chordae from superior leaflet attached to papillary muscle in RV on septal surface	
C	Undivided and unattached to ventricular septal crest ("free-floating"); attachments to papillary muscle on RV free wall	

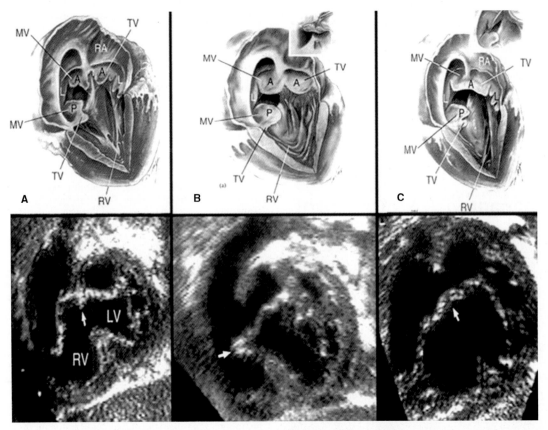

FIGURE 7.14. Rastelli Classification of Common Atrioventricular Valves in Complete Atrioventricular Septal Defects. A (left upper and lower panels): Rastelli Type A defects are characterized by insertion of the atrioventricular valves to the crest of the ventricular septum (VS). Central upper and lower panels: Type B defects are characterized by dominant insertion of the anterior leaflets into papillary muscles in the right ventricle (RV). In this example, the anterior bridging leaflet inserts onto the crest of the ventricular septum, as well as onto a large ventricular papillary muscle (P). Right upper and lower panels: Type C. The anterior leaflet is unattached (*small arrows*) and overrides the crest of the ventricular septum. The undivided, free- floating anterior leaflet does not insert onto the ventricular septum. I, inferior; L, left; LA, left atrium; LV, left ventricle; RA, right atrium; S, superior (Modified from Seward JB, Tajik AJ, Edwards WD, et al. *Two-Dimensional Echocardiographic Atlas. Vol. 1. Congenital Heart Disease.* New York: Springer-Verlag, 1987:270–292)

Abnormalities of sidedness (situs) can also occur in association with AVSDs. Most cases of right atrial isomerism are associated with complex forms of AVSD, typically with a common atrium and unbalanced ventricles (Fig. 7.13).

DOWN SYNDROME AND ATRIOVENTRICULAR SEPTAL DEFECTS

A clear association exists between AVSD and Down syndrome. About 40% of individuals with Down syndrome have an underlying congenital heart disease, and approximately 40% of those have an AVSD. Conversely, approximately half the patients afflicted with an AVSD have Down syndrome. Type A is the most common subtype of complete AVSD seen in Down syndrome. The combination of ToF with AVSD occurs much more commonly in patients with Down syndrome than in patients with normal karyotype. Heterotaxy is rare in Down syndrome patients. Also, patients with Down syndrome are less likely to have associated LVOT obstruction, LV hypoplasia, coarctation of the aorta, or additional muscular VSDs. In the 1960s–1970s, patients with Down syndrome reportedly had a worse prognosis after surgical repair of AVSD than did patients with normal karyotype. Currently, surgical outcome is excellent for all patients with AVSD.

FETAL ECHOCARDIOGRAPHY

AVSD is readily identified with fetal echocardiography, and is often detected during routine obstetrical four-chamber ultrasonography (Fig. 7.16). In a population-based study, Allen and colleagues from the United Kingdom found that AVSD was one of the most common

forms of congenital heart disease detected by fetal echocardiography. The ratio of the atrial-to-ventricular septal length (AVL) may assist in evaluation of fetal AVSD. This is based on the fact that the length of the atrial septum is not affected in AVSD. However, the "scooped-out" ventricular septum (measured from the level of AV valve insertion to LV apex in four-chamber view) is much shorter than normal. The mean AVL was found to be 0.47 in normal fetuses, versus 0.77 in AVSD. A cutoff value of AVL ratio of 0.6 is characteristic of AVSD. If used routinely, this measurement may be useful to increase the yield of obstetrical ultrasonography in detecting AVSD.

Antenatal detection of AVSD should also prompt the search for other associated cardiac anomalies as well as fetal karyotype testing. Up to 45% of cases of prenatally detected AVSD have heterotaxy syndromes; most have left atrial isomerism. Heart block has been described in 10% to 15% of fetal cases of AVSD and is more common in those with left atrial isomerism. An association of trisomy 21, AVSD, and complete heart block has also been described. Prognosis for fetuses with structural cardiac disease and complete heart block remains poor.

SURGICAL REPAIR AND POSTOPERATIVE ECHOCARDIOGRAPHY

Partial Atrioventricular Septal Defect

Major advancements have been made in the surgical management of partial AVSD, with significant reduction of morbidity and mortality over the past few decades. The aim of surgery in partial AVSD is to close the interatrial communication and restore mitral valve competence while avoiding creation of a stenotic valve and inadvertent damage to conduction tissue. The mitral valve cleft is typically

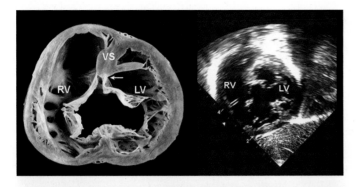

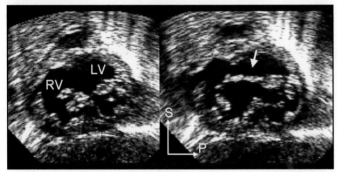

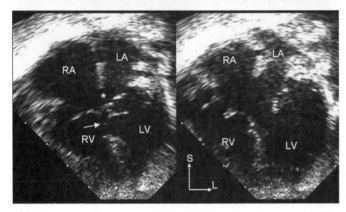

FIGURE 7.15. Anatomic and Echocardiographic Examples of Common Atrioventricular Valves: The image in the upper left panel is an anatomic specimen, dissected in a plane simulating a short axis view of the ventricles and common atrioventricular valve. This valve has Type A morphology with an evenly divided anterior bridging leaflet and central attachments to the ventricular septum (*arrow*). The echocardiographic (subcostal) image on the upper right shows similar findings in a different patient. The middle panels show a common AV valve with Type C morphology. The systolic (**left**) and diastolic (**right**) subcostal sagittal frames demonstrate a "free-floating," unattached anterior bridging leaflet (arrow). *Imaging note:* The subcostal sagittal view is the most helpful for the determination of the Rastelli classification of AVSD. The bottom panels show apical four-chamber echocardiographs from a patient with complete AVSD in systole (**left**) and diastole (**right**). *Imaging note:* The apical four chamber scanning plane is posterior to the anterior bridging leaflet and does not adequately evaluate its attachments. The posterior bridging leaflet can be seen and typically appears "attached" to the septum in all forms of AVSD. LA, left atrium; LV, left ventricle; RA, right atrium; RV, right ventricle; VS, ventricular septum.

closed. Sometimes the tricuspid valve also requires repair. Surgery for repair of partial AVSD is usually performed after 18 months of age. Transcatheter device closure of the primum ASD is not an option because of its proximity to the AV valves and AV node. Early surgical mortality has decreased to less than 3% in the current era and complete heart block is rare.

Complete Atrioventricular Septal Defect

Complete AVSD is generally repaired between 3 and 6 months of age. Early repair is desirable to avoid the development of pulmonary vascular disease. Operative mortality is usually less than 3%.

Despite these advancements, the need for reoperation remains a problem: 10% to 15% of patients require reoperation for left AV valve issues or development of progressive LVOT obstruction.

The aim of surgical repair in uncomplicated complete AVSD is to close any intracardiac shunts and divide the common AV valve into competent right and left orifices. In complete AVSD, the primum ASD and inlet VSD are contiguous, so they can be closed using a single-patch or a double-patch technique. The former technique has been modified from its original "classic" description and currently involves direct suturing of the common AV valve leaflets to the crest of the ventricular septum, then using a single patch for closing the defect above the AV valve and separating it into two orifices. The classic single-patch technique consists of dividing the AV valve into right and left components, placement of a single patch across the ASD and VSD, and then reattaching the two "halves" of the AV valve to the mid-portion of the patch. As the name implies, a double-patch technique uses two patches: a pericardial patch for closure of the ASD and a GORE-TEX or Dacron patch to closure the VSD. Both of these techniques have been used in clinical practice, each with its own advocates and opponents. Theoretical concerns with the single-patch technique include crowding of the LVOT, providing a setup for obstruction, higher incidence of residual VSD, and increased AV valve regurgitation due to shifting of the AV valve hinge-point to a "nonphysiologic" height. In contrast, the use of two patches is thought to result in "more" normal anatomy, as one of the patches serves to reconstruct the deficient portion of the inlet septum. Further studies are needed to elucidate these differences.

Patients with AVSD with associated ToF ("Tet canal") were traditionally repaired using a two-stage approach using a systemic-to-pulmonary shunt followed by complete repair later in childhood. More recently, multiple centers have reported primary repair in infancy with good results.

Transesophageal echocardiography is a useful tool in the operating room during the repair of AVSD. Transesophageal echocardiography before cardiopulmonary bypass further delineates the exact anatomy of the AV valves. After cessation of cardiopulmonary bypass, assessment of ventricular function, residual intracardiac shunts, and AV valve stenosis and regurgitation can occur.

ECHOCARDIOGRAPHIC EVALUATION: POSTOPERATIVE FOLLOW-UP

Postoperative echocardiography is used to assess AV valve regurgitation or stenosis, residual atrial or ventricular septal defects, LVOT obstruction, pulmonary hypertension, and ventricular dysfunction (Fig. 7.17).

Left AV valve regurgitation is the most common problem encountered after the repair of AVSD, and it is the most common reason for reoperation. Severe left AV regurgitation is present in approximately 20% of patients immediately postoperatively. However, approximately 25% of those patients show normalization of their left AV valve competence over time. Ultimately, 10% to 15% of all patients require reoperation for left AV valve regurgitation. The main predictor of the development of postoperative severe left AV valve regurgitation is the presence of severe regurgitation preoperatively. Other risk factors include the presence of significant regurgitation intraoperatively, dysplasia of the left AV valve, and, in some reports, failure to close the cleft at the time of surgery. Stenosis is more likely to develop in the hypoplastic, dysplastic, double-orifice, or parachute mitral valves and is further "unmasked" postoperatively once the ASD is closed.

In a recent review from our institution, Stulak and colleagues described the Mayo Clinic's 35-year experience with reoperation for patients with complete AVSD. Fifty patients underwent reoperation after having had successful repair of AVSD at a median age of 1 year. Forty of the 50 (80%) patients required reoperation due to left AV valve regurgitation. Half of these patients underwent left AV valve repair and half had valve replacement. These results are encouraging because traditionally, most patients have anticipated left AV valve replacement during the reintervention surgery. Fifteen-year survival after reoperation for complete AVSD was 86%.

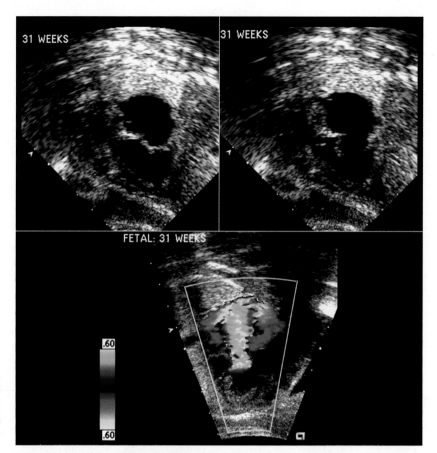

FIGURE 7.16. Prenatal common atrioventricular valve regurgitation: These images were taken during an examination of a 31-week gestation fetus. They revealed severe common atrioventricular valve regurgitation. The upper right panel was taken in diastole, the upper left in systole, and the lower panel in a systolic image with color Doppler. All demonstrate a common atrium, common atrioventricular valve, and common ventricle. Color flow outlined a broad regurgitant jet in this case.

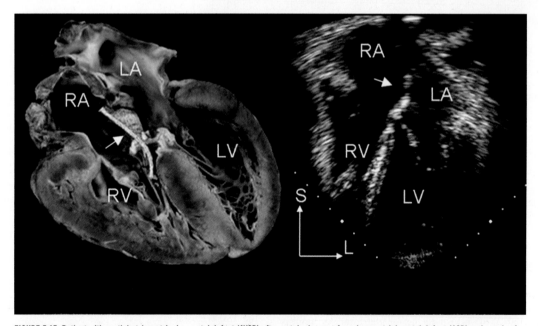

FIGURE 7.17. Patient with partial atrioventricular septal defect (AVSD) after patch closure of a primum atrial septal defect (ASD) and repair of a cleft mitral valve. Left: Four-chamber anatomic specimen. The patch (*arrow*) is attached to the right side of the atrial septum and the right AV valve to avoid damage to the conduction tissue and left AV valve. Right: Corresponding apical four-chamber echocardiograph.

Doppler interrogation of right and left AV valve stenosis or regurgitation is warranted. A search for residual shunts should also be performed. Doppler evaluation of the velocity profiles across a ventricular level shunt and right AV valve regurgitation can provide accurate determination of RV systolic pressure. However, in the setting of a residual VSD, the VSD jet may contaminate the right AV valve regurgitation signal and preclude accurate quantification of RV systolic pressure. In that setting, the echocardiographer needs to use indirect techniques such as assessment of ventricular septal flattening or bowing, RV size and function, and Doppler interrogation of the pulmonary regurgitation velocity to assess pulmonary artery diastolic pressure.

Progressive LVOT obstruction occurs in up to 15% of patients after repair of partial AVSD. It is more frequent in partial than complete AVSD. The "goose neck deformity" described earlier serves as the substrate for the development of obstruction. The rate of reoperation for LVOT obstruction is about 5% to 10% and appears higher for patients with partial AVSD. One approach to repair LVOT obstruction is resection of any discrete areas of obstruction due to muscle ridges or accessory chordal tissue and, when necessary, peeling of fibrous tissue from the anterior surface of the mitral valve. A septal myectomy may also decrease the likelihood of recurrence. Because of the persistent risk for the development or progression of LVOT obstruction years after the repair, lifelong follow-up is warranted.

 ## SUMMARY

Echocardiography is the imaging modality of choice for diagnosis and management of all forms of AVSDs. Meticulous assessment of progressive left AV valve regurgitation or stenosis and progression of LVOT obstruction is required during serial postoperative echocardiographic evaluations. Despite the need for reoperation in a subset of these patients, long-term survival is excellent.

SUGGESTED READINGS

Al-hay AA, MacNeill SJ, Yacoub M, et al. Complete atrioventricular septal defect, Down syndrome, and surgical outcome: Risk factors. *Ann Thorac Surg.* 2003;75:412–421.

Anderson RH, Webb S, Brown NA, et al. Development of the heart: (2) Septation of the atriums and ventricles. *Heart.* 2003;89:949–958

Backer CL, Stewart RD, Bailliard F, et al. Complete atrioventricular canal: Comparison of modified single-patch technique with two-patch technique. *Ann Thorac Surg.* 2007;84:2038–2046.

Cetta F, Minich LL, Edwards WD, et al. Atrioventricular septal defects. In: Allen HD, Driscoll DJ, Shaddy RE, Feltes TF, eds. *Moss and Adams' Heart Disease in Infants, Children, and Adolescents (Including the Fetus and Young Adult).* Philadelphia, Pa: Williams & Wilkins, 2008:646–667.

Chiu IS, How SW, Wang JK, et al. Clinical implications of atrial isomerism. *Br Heart J.* 1988;60:72–77.

Cohen GA, Stevenson JG. Intraoperative echocardiography for atrioventricular canal: Decision-making for surgeons. *Semin Thorac Cardiovasc Surg Pediatr Card Surg Annu.* 2007:47–50.

Cohen MS, Jacobs ML, Weinberg PM, et al. Morphometric analysis of unbalanced common atrioventricular canal using two-dimensional echocardiography. *J Am Coll Cardiol.* 1996;28:1017–1023.

Craig B. Atrioventricular septal defect: From fetus to adult. *Heart.* 2006;92:1879–1885.

Delmo Walter EM, Ewert P, et al. Biventricular repair in children with complete atrioventricular septal defect and a small left ventricle. *Eur J Cardiothorac Surg.* 2008;33:40–47.

Fesslova V, Villa L, Nava S, et al. Spectrum and outcome of atrioventricular septal defect in fetal life. *Cardiol Young.* 2002;12:18–26.

Geva T, Ayres NA, Pignatelli RH, et al. Echocardiographic evaluation of common atrioventricular canal defects: A study of 206 consecutive patients. *Echocardiography.* 1996;13:387–400.

Gutgesell HP, Huhta JC. Cardiac septation in atrioventricular canal defect. *J Am Coll Cardiol.* 1986;8:1421–1440.

Machlitt A, Heling KS, Chaoui R. Increased cardiac atrial-to-ventricular length ratio in the fetal four-chamber view: A new marker for atrioventricular septal defects. *Ultrasound Obstet Gynecol.* 2004;24:618–622.

Monteiro AJ, Canale LS, Rangel I, et al. Surgical treatment of complete atrioventricular septal defect with the two-patch technique: Early-to-mid follow-up. *Interact Cardiovasc Thorac Surg.* 2007;6:737–740.

Morris CD, Magilke D, Reller M. Down's syndrome affects results of surgical correction of complete atrioventricular canal. *Pediatr Cardiol.* 1992;13:80–84.

Smallhorn JF, de Leval M, Stark J, et al. Isolated anterior mitral cleft. Two dimensional echocardiographic assessment and differentiation from "clefts" associated with atrioventricular septal defect. *Br Heart J.* 1982;48:109–116.

Snider AR, Serwer GA, Ritter, SB. Defects in cardiac septation. In *Echocardiography in Pediatric Heart Disease.* St. Louis, Mo: Mosby-Year Book, 1997:235–296.

Stulak JM, Burkhart HM, Dearani JA, et al. Reoperations after initial repair of complete atrioventricular septal defect. *Annals of Thoracic Surgery.* 87(6):1872–1877; discussion 1877–1878, 2009 Jun.

Tandon R, Moller JH, Edwards JE. Tetralogy of Fallot associated with persistent common atrioventricular canal (endocardial cushion defect). *Br Heart J.* 1974;36:197–206.

Ten Harkel AD, Cromme-Dijkhuis AH, Heinerman BC, et al. Development of left atrioventricular valve regurgitation after correction of atrioventricular septal defect. *Ann Thorac Surg.* 2005;79:607–612.

Towbin R, Schwartz D. Endocardial cushion defects: Embryology, anatomy, and angiography. *AJR Am J Roentgenol.* 1981;136:157–162.

van Son JA, Phoon CK, Silverman NH, et al. Predicting feasibility of biventricular repair of right-dominant unbalanced atrioventricular canal. *Ann Thorac Surg.* 1997;63:1657–1663.

Warnes C, Somerville J. Double mitral valve orifice in atrioventricular defects. *Br Heart J.* 1983;49:59–64.

Wetter J, Sinzobahamvya N, Blaschczok C, et al. Closure of the zone of apposition at correction of complete atrioventricular septal defect improves outcome. *Eur J Cardiothorac Surg.* 2000;17:146.

Chapter 8
Ebstein's Malformation and Tricuspid Valve Diseases

Patrick W. O'Leary

The most common congenital malformations involving the tricuspid valve are Ebstein's malformation and tricuspid valvar dysplasia. This chapter will primarily consider Ebstein's malformation with concordant atrioventricular connections and biventricular circulation. Ebstein-like deformation of the morphologically tricuspid valve in association with atrioventricular discordance is discussed in Chapter 10. Isolated dysplasia of the tricuspid valvar leaflets, traumatic tricuspid regurgitation, and other right ventricular abnormalities will be briefly described, and the differences between these disorders and Ebstein's malformation are highlighted. Echocardiography has become the procedure of choice for both the diagnosis and long-term assessment of patients with Ebstein's malformation. In the 1980s, cross-sectional echocardiography replaced M-mode as the clinical standard. As early as 1984, cross-sectional imaging was considered sufficiently comprehensive that angiography was no longer necessary to diagnose Ebstein's malformation.

ON THE NAMING OF THE TRICUSPID VALVAR APPARATUS

We have chosen to adopt an anatomically unambiguous system of names to describe the components of the tricuspid valvar apparatus. This will create some differences between the descriptions contained within this chapter and in many previous publications. It seems best to concretely define this system to avoid potential confusion. The three valvar leaflets will be referred to as the *anterior,* the *septal,* and the *inferior* leaflets (Fig. 8.1). The designations of the anterior and septal leaflets are clear. The inferior leaflet has often been called the "posterior" leaflet. This designation is anatomically incorrect. This leaflet is positioned inferiorly within the

ventricular cavity, lying adjacent to the diaphragm in the normal heart. We recognize that abnormal valves often display rotation of their components away from the normal position. However, the inferior tricuspid leaflet is always associated with the ventricular free wall and is never in a posterior position. The posterior aspect of the right ventricle is the interventricular septum, not the free wall adjacent to the diaphragm. Therefore, in the human heart, it would be inappropriate to refer to the tricuspid valve leaflet nearest the free wall as being "posterior," when it is not. This leaflet is always positioned inferior to the anterior and septal leaflet, even in the most severely distorted valves, leading to our preference for the name "inferior" leaflet of the tricuspid valve.

Ebstein's Malformation

Ebstein's malformation has an extremely variable natural history. The clinical course depends on the degree of abnormality manifested by the right ventricle and the tricuspid valvar apparatus. These abnormalities can range from minimal to severe. If the deformity of the tricuspid valve is severe, it may result in profound congestive heart failure in the neonatal period, or even in intrauterine death. At the other end of the spectrum, patients with a mild degree of displacement and dysfunction may remain asymptomatic until late adult life.

DEFINITION AND ANATOMIC FEATURES OF EBSTEIN'S MALFORMATION

Ebstein's malformation is often thought of as a primary disorder of the tricuspid valve. In reality, it is a manifestation of a more global aberration in myocardial development. Those afflicted

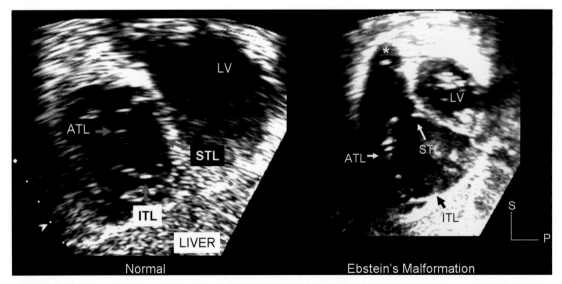

FIGURE 8.1. These subcostal, sagittal plane images demonstrate the anatomic relationships of the three tricuspid valve leaflets. Left: Normal tricuspid valve. The septal tricuspid leaflet (STL) lies parallel to the ventricular septum, and the anterior tricuspid leaflet (ATL) is positioned parallel to the anterior free wall of the right ventricle and separates the posterior inlet from the anterior outlet of the ventricle. The inferior tricuspid leaflet (ITL) is parallel to the diaphragmatic surface of the right ventricle and lies in the most inferior portion of the ventricle. This leaflet has often been referred to as the "posterior" leaflet, which is anatomically incorrect. **Right:** From an examination of the patient with Ebstein's malformation. The ATL remains parallel to the anterior free wall. The STL and ITL are more difficult to recognize in this diastolic image because they are adherent to the myocardium of the septum and right ventricular inferior wall. Only a small segment of the STL is seen separated from the ventricular septum near the right ventricular outflow tract (*arrow*). LV, left ventricle; P, posterior; S, superior.

with Ebstein's malformation invariably display abnormalities in both myocardial structure and function, as well as the characteristic valvar deformities. The right ventricle and tricuspid valve are universally involved, while changes in the left heart are less common.

The hallmark of Ebstein's malformation is displacement of the annular attachments (hinges) of the septal and inferior leaflets, away from the atrioventricular junction (Fig. 8.2). This results from failure of these leaflets fully to separate from the underlying ventricular wall during cardiac development. The normal separation process is referred to as "delamination" (Fig. 8.3). Delamination begins at the tips of the embryonic leaflets and proceeds "back" toward the atrioventricular junction. A completely delaminated leaflet will have a hinge point at (or very near) the anatomic tricuspid valvar annulus.

This failure of delamination results in the leaflets remaining variably adherent to the underlying right ventricular and septal myocardium (Fig. 8.4). This adherence creates the characteristic displacement of the annular attachments of the valve and rotates its functional orifice away from the normal position within the right ventricular inlet. It is now appreciated that the concept of apical displacement of the tricuspid valve in Ebstein's malformation was not anatomically precise. The displacement seen in Ebstein's malformation is *not* simply a linear shift of the tricuspid valve toward the cardiac apex. The displacement is actually rotational or spiral in nature, following the contours of the right ventricular cavity. The primary orientation of the rotation is in an anterior direction, toward the right ventricular outflow tract, and only to a lesser extent toward the apex. This spiral shift in the tricuspid valve apparatus moves the functional valvar orifice to the junction of the trabecular and outlet zones of the ventricle (Figs. 8.5 and 8.6). In the most severe cases, the functional leaflets may be positioned within the

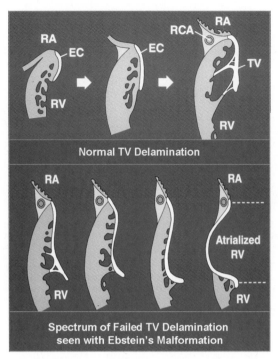

FIGURE 8.3. Delamination. Normal delamination process that gives rise to the tricuspid valve leaflets (**top**). During embryonic valve formation, the inner layer of endomyocardium separates (delaminates) from the underlying cardiac muscle and gradually loses its myocardial components. As development progresses (**left to right**), we begin to recognize the supportive chordal structures and leaflet of the mature valve. When a failure of delamination occurs (**bottom**), it results in adherence of the "tricuspid valve" tissues to the right ventricular myocardium. This is the hallmark of Ebstein's malformation. The four diagrams (**bottom**), progressing from mild to severe (**left to right**), demonstrate the spectrum of abnormality that can be associated with failed delamination. EC, endomyocardial layer; RA, right atrium; RCA, right coronary artery; RV, right ventricle; TV, tricuspid valve.

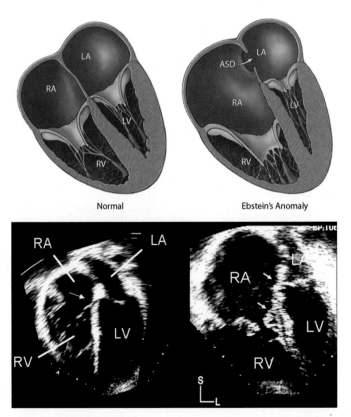

FIGURE 8.2. Apical four-chamber plane of a normal heart (left) and a heart afflicted with Ebstein's malformation (right). The hinge point (septal insertion) of the normal septal tricuspid leaflet is positioned slightly more toward the cardiac apex, compared with the septal hinge point of the anterior mitral leaflet (**bottom left**, *arrow*). This displacement is exaggerated in hearts with Ebstein's malformation, as shown by the diagram (**top right**) and the arrows in the echocardiographic image (**bottom right**). It should be noted that the valvar leaflets are also abnormal in Ebstein's malformation. In the case shown (**bottom right**), the leaflets are thickened and moderately dysplastic. ASD, atrial septal defect; L, left; LA, left atrium; LV, left ventricle; RA, right atrium; RV, right ventricle; S, superior.

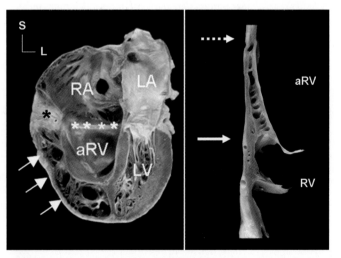

FIGURE 8.4. Anatomic specimen from a patient with a severe case of Ebstein's malformation (left) and a segment of right ventricular wall from a patient with Ebstein's malformation (right). The anatomic atrioventricular junction is marked (***). The failure of the tricuspid valve to delaminate in the specimen not only displaced the valve away from the junction but also produced extensive adherence of the valve tissue to the ventricular myocardium (**left**, *arrows*). No mobile segments of valve are appreciated within the right ventricular inlet. The remnant of tricuspid valve tissue (**right**) is also nearly completely adherent to the underlying myocardium. Only a small tag of tissue shows any separation from the wall (near the *solid arrow*). The segment of "valve" between the *dashed* and *solid arrows* is seen as the dense, white inner lining of the cavity (clearly different from normal endocardial tissue, which can be seen below the level of the *solid arrow*). The adherence of the tricuspid valve creates a zone of the right ventricular cavity that is "atrialized." This zone has walls composed of ventricular myocardium, but its cavity is proximal to the tricuspid valvar orifice. aRV, atrialized right ventricle; LA, left atrium; LV, left ventricle; RV, right ventricle; TV, tricuspid valve.

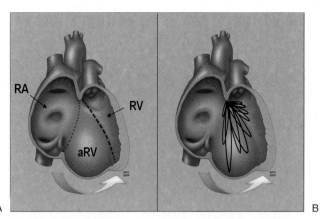

FIGURE 8.5. Rotation of the functional tricuspid orifice in Ebstein anomaly. Rotational shift of the functional tricuspid orifice away from the atrioventricular junction to the plane that divides the trabecular and outlet zones of the ventricle (**A**, *heavy dashed line*). The observed planes of the effective valvar orifices of the hearts with Ebstein's malformation studied by Schreiber and colleagues are shown (**B**, *ovals*). The effective displacement of the functional tricuspid valve (*heavy dashed line*) away from the atrioventricular junction (marked by the *dotted line*) is rotational, not linear. This rotation is spiral in nature and is directed both toward the apex and, more important, anteriorly toward the outflow tract. aRV, atrialized right ventricle; RA, right atrium; RV, right ventricle.

outlet itself. The adherent portions of the valvar leaflets usually have little or no motion. This typically leads to tricuspid regurgitation or, more rarely, to stenosis.

In hearts with Ebstein's malformation, the septal and inferior leaflets are most dramatically involved and show the largest change in the anatomic position of their hinge points. In contrast, the anterior leaflet forms at a different developmental stage. As a result, its junctional hinge usually retains a normal position near the atrioventricular groove and it can become very large and "sail-like." Mild cases can be encountered in which only the hinge of the septal leaflet is displaced away from the atrioventricular junction. Such cases are found most frequently in the setting of pulmonary atresia with an intact ventricular septum. In the absence of pulmonary atresia, it is unlikely that such minimal changes would produce the typical, if indeed any, symptomatology.

Clinically, it is important to distinguish pathologic displacement of the septal leaflet from the typical valvar off-setting found in the normal heart (Fig. 8.2). It is in making this distinction that the apical component of the displacement associated with Ebstein's malformation is most useful. The normal tricuspid septal leaflet hinges at a point on the ventricular septum that is slightly apical to the hinge point of the anterior mitral leaflet, when both are displayed in the apical four-chamber view. Although the two septal hinges are offset, this does not represent displacement of the

tricuspid valve. When the septal leaflet is abnormally adherent to the myocardium, as in Ebstein's malformation, the distance separating the two septal valvar hinge points becomes exaggerated. This exaggerated separation can be quantitated by measuring the linear distance between the two septal hinges in the four-chamber plane. (See discussion of the apical displacement index later in this chapter.)

The abnormalities associated with Ebstein's malformation also cause the leaflets to adopt a "bileaflet" configuration, with a plane of closure at the junction of the trabecular and the outlet components of the right ventricle (Figs. 8.6, 8.7, and 8.8).

The keys to understanding this malformation and its anatomic consequences are appreciating the developmental etiology of failed delamination and recognizing that the abnormal, displaced location of the valve represents a complex rotational or spiral deformity (Figs. 8.5 and 8.6), rather than the more simplistic linear "apical" displacement that has received attention in the past.

 ## CLINICAL PRESENTATION OF EBSTEIN'S MALFORMATION

Patients with Ebstein's malformation may present at any age. The most severe cases present prenatally or as newborns. Prenatal diagnosis is dependent on ultrasonic screening examinations. Fetal presentation is accompanied by increased heart size, a significant incidence of fetal hydrops, and, in the most severe cases, pulmonary parenchymal hypoplasia secondary to marked cardiac enlargement. Prenatal arrhythmia is not common. Newborns most often present with cyanosis, while slightly older infants present with a combination of desaturation and symptoms of cardiac failure. Murmurs and arrhythmias are more frequently encountered as presenting complaints in older patients. Although some patients remain asymptomatic, most will have some cardiovascular symptoms. Beyond infancy, the majority will display abnormal fatigueability, dyspnea, palpitations, or cyanosis with exertion. Palpitations in a cyanotic child should raise the possibility of Ebstein's malformation (Table 8.1).

Echocardiography has significantly influenced the age at which patients with Ebstein's malformation are diagnosed. In 1979, Guiliani and colleagues found that just under one third of patients were diagnosed before 4 years of age. Another two fifths were diagnosed before the age of 19, with the remainder presenting in adulthood, some at 80 years of age. In contrast, in the experience reported by Celermajer et al. in 1994 (Table 8.1), three-fifths came to clinical attention before the age of 1 year, with half diagnosed prenatally or as newborns. One tenth presented between 1 and 12 months of age, with only three tenths presenting as children or adolescents. Despite the increased availability of echocardiographic examination in this more recent cohort, one tenth remained undiagnosed until adulthood.

Table 8.1	MAJOR FEATURES OF EBSTEIN'S MALFORMATION IN 220 SUBJECTS AT PRESENTATION						
	Prenatal (n = 21)	Neonate (n = 88)	Infant (n = 23)	Child (n = 50)	Adolescent (n = 15)	Adult (n = 23)	Total (%)
Cyanosis	0	65	8	7	2	1	83 (38)
Heart failure	0	9	10	4	2	6	31 (14)
Murmur	0	8	3	33	5	3	52 (24)
Arrhythmia	1	5	1	6	6	10	29 (13)
Abnormal US	18	0	0	0	0	0	18 (8)

Definitions of age groups: neonate, 0–1 month; infant, 1 month–2 years; child, 2–10 years; adolescent, 10–18 years; and adult, >18 years. US, prenatal ultrasound. (Adapted from Celermajer DS, Bull C, Till JA, et al. Ebstein's anomaly: presentation and outcome from fetus to adult. *J Am Coll Cardiol.* 1994;23:170–176.)

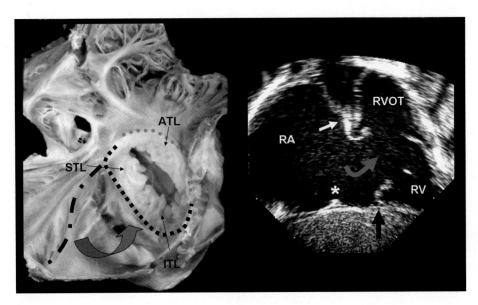

FIGURE 8.6. Patient with Ebstein's malformation. Left: Anatomic specimen shows the atrial aspect of the deformed valve. It illustrates how the anterior leaflet retains its normal attachment at the atrioventricular junction (*light blue dotted line*), but the conjoined septal and inferior leaflets have their hingepoints attached well away from the atrioventricular junction (compare the *dark blue dashed* and *black dotted lines*). The separation of the inferior and septal hinge points from the true annulus is also highlighted by the *curved red arrow*. The portion of the right ventricle between the *darker blue* and *black lines* is said to be "atrialized" and in this case has a very thin wall. Note that the leaflets of the deformed valve will close in "bileaflet" fashion. **Right:** Subcostal, coronal echocardiographic image displays some of the same features. Remnants of the anterior (near the *white arrow*) and the inferior tricuspid leaflets (*black arrow*) are seen. The hinge point of anterior leaflet (*white arrow*) retains a normal position, while the insertion of the inferior leaflet is displaced into the ventricular cavity away from the anatomic atrioventricular junction, which is marked (*). Similar to the anatomic image on the **left,** this echocardiogram confirms that the displacement of the tricuspid apparatus associated with Ebstein's malformation actually rotates the valve anteriorly, as well as apically (*curved red arrows*). ATL, anterior tricuspid leaflet; ITL, inferior tricuspid leaflet; RA, right atrium; RV, right ventricle; RVOT, right ventricular outflow tract; STL, septal tricuspid leaflet.

 ## ASSOCIATED CARDIOVASCULAR ABNORMALITIES

Nearly all patients with Ebstein's malformation will have an interatrial communication, with the most frequent being a patent foramen ovale or secundum atrial septal defect. Venosus and partial atrioven-tricular septal defects do coexist with Ebstein's malformation but are much less common. A large spectrum of other lesions has been described, including ventricular septal defects, tetralogy of Fallot, aortic coarctation, noncompaction of the left ventricular myocardium, and patency of the ductus arteriosus. The most common nonatrial cardiac abnormality is pulmonary stenosis or atresia, which is found in up to one third of those presenting in infancy. Obstruction of the right ventricular outflow tract is commonly associated with Ebstein's

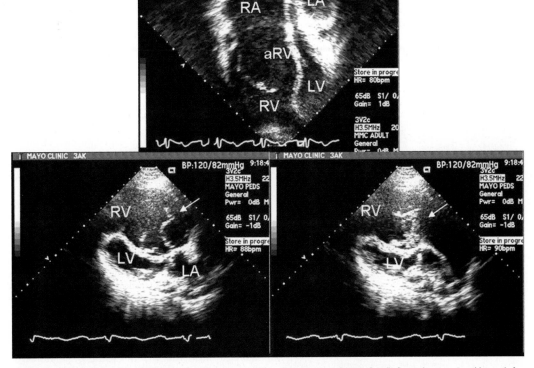

FIGURE 8.7. Patient with Ebstein's malformation. Top: Four-chamber echocardigraphic image. Bottom: Systolic frames in a parasternal long-axis format. The tricuspid valve's functional orifice does not lie in the "four-chamber" plane but rather has been rotated anteriorly and apically. A cross section of the orifice, as the valve closes, can be appreciated in the long-axis images (*arrows*). These frames highlight the bileaflet nature of the functional tricuspid valve in Ebstein's malformation. There is just a single, vertically oriented, line of closure between the functional segments of valve tissue. **Bottom right:** Coaptation gap that allows regurgitant flow. aRV, atrialized right ventricle; LA, left atrium; LV, left ventricle; RA, right atrium; RV, right ventricle.

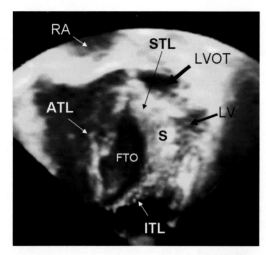

FIGURE 8.8. Three-dimensional echocardiographic image, from a transthoracic examination, has been cropped to show a view analogous to an apical long-axis image. It is focused on the abnormally positioned, functional tricuspid orifice (FTO) within the right ventricle. This valve not only shows how the functional orifice is rotated anteriorly in Ebstein's malformation but also is a good example of the "bileaflet" configuration of the functioning valve leaflets seen in this disorder. The large anterior leaflet (ATL) functions as one part of the coaptation mechanism, while the remnants of the inferior and septal leaflets (ITL and STL) combine with the ventricular septum to provide the surface against which the ATL can close (or attempt to close). Ao, aorta; LV, left ventricle; RA, right atrium; S, septum.

malformation when diagnosed in fetal life. In this setting, it may be difficult to distinguish stuctural from functional pulmonary valve atresia using echocardiography, especially in the presence of severe tricuspid regurgitation. When there is no systolic flow from the right ventricle to the pulmonary artery, the presence of pulmonary regurgitation is the most reliable marker of functional pulmonary atresia (Fig. 8.9). The regurgitant flow can be detected by either color flow or spectral Doppler echocardiography. Doppler detectable pulmonary regurgitaiton has been reported in more than 80% of series with ductal-dependent neonatal Ebstein's malformation. In the setting of anatomic pulmonary valve atresia, there no flow detectable during either phase of the cardiac cycle. In cases of Ebstein's malformation with either stenosis or atresia, the pulmonary valvar abnormality is probably secondary to the malformation of the tricuspid

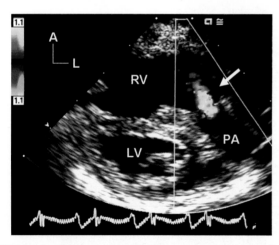

FIGURE 8.9. Functional pulmonary valve atresia. This parasternal color flow echocardiographic image is focused on the right ventricular outflow tract, pulmonary valve, and main pulmonary artery (PA). It was taken during the examination of a newborn with severe Ebstein's malformation. No systolic forward flow, crossing the pulmonary valve, could be demonstrated. However, this diastolic frame clearly shows a jet of pulmonary regurgitation (*arrow*). This transvalvar flow reveals that the pulmonary valve is patent, not atretic in an anatomic sense. The lack of forward flow is due to the inability of the right ventricle to generate a systolic pressure greater than the systolic pressure in the pulmonary artery. Such echocardiographic confirmation of pulmonary valve patency is critical to therapeutic planning. A, anterior; L, left; LV, left ventricle; RV, right ventricle.

valve, with hypoplasia of the outflow tract resulting from reduced anterograde flow through the right heart. When severe Ebstein's malformation is associated with fetal and neonatal distress, or death, both lungs are usually hypoplastic. The markedly enlarged heart compresses the lungs leading to the pulmonary hypoplasia seen in these cases.

ECHOCARDIOGRAPHIC RECOGNITION AND EVALUATION OF EBSTEIN'S MALFORMATION

Imaging of the internal cardiac crux, the components of the abnormal tricuspid valve, and the right ventricular myocardium reveals several features that are reliably used to identify patients with Ebstein's malformation. The single most sensitive and specific diagnostic feature is the displacement of the annular hinge of the septal leaflet. This displacement is most easily appreciated by comparison to the annular hinge of the mitral leaflet as seen in the apical four-chamber view. One must recall that the normal septal tricuspid leaflet inserts at a position that is slightly apical to the insertion of the anterior mitral valve leaflet. In patients with Ebstein's malformation, this displacement is exaggerated. The distance between the valvar hinge points can easily be measured in systole (Fig. 8.10, left) This distance, when divided by the body surface area in square meters, is known as the displacement index. In a heart with evidence of failed delamination, an index value greater than 8 mm/m^2 reliably distinguishes those with Ebstein's malformation from both normals and from patients with other disorders associated with enlargement of the right ventricle. In cases with severely adherent and displaced septal leaflets, the hinge of the septal tricuspid leaflet may not be seen in the 4 chamber plane. In these cases, the first septal structure seen on the right ventricular septal surface (apical to the insertion of the anterior mitral leaflet) will be the moderator band (Fig. 8.10, right panel). The apical displacement index is essentially infinite in these hearts, and recognition of the presence of Ebstein's malformation is straightforward.

Occasionally, it can be difficult to assess the offset between the valvar hinges at the internal crux. In these unusual situations, other echocardiographic features that can assist in making an accurate diagnosis include; elongation of the anterior leaflet, tethering of any of the leaflets to the underlying myocardium, shortened chordal supports, attachment of the leading edge of the anterior leaflet to the right ventricular myocardium, displacement of the annular attachment of the anterior leaflet, absence of the septal or inferior leaflets, congenital fenestration of the leaflets, and enlargement of the valvar annulus.

Echocardiography is also used to define suitability for valvar repair, associated cardiovascular abnormalities, and myocardial function. There are several anatomic features of the valvar apparatus that indicate potential success of the monoleaflet repair described by Danielson. The most important feature predictive of a durable monoleaflet repair is the mobility of the anterior leaflet. It is critical for approximately one half of the leaflet to be mobile, free of major tethering to the myocardium, and to have a leading edge that moves freely within the inlet of the right ventricle. This assessment must be made in the apical four-chamber view (Fig. 8.11). Extensive adherence of more than half of the anterior leaflet to the ventricular myocardium (Fig. 8.10, right) makes a successful repair unlikely. A single central jet of regurgitation (Fig. 8.12) is more easily eliminated than are multiple regurgitant orifices (Fig. 8.13). Even when there is a significant amount of leaflet tissue present, direct muscular insertions from the ventricular free wall into the body of the anterior leaflet can make monoleaflet repair impossible (Fig. 8.14). The presence of leaflet tissue adjacent to the pulmonary valve in a short-axis view indicates severe displacement and makes successful monoleaflet repair less likely. Additional delamination of the septal and/or inferior leaflets provides a more promising situation for successful repair. Figures 8.15 and 8.16 demonstrate the results of successful monoleaflet repairs.

Although the monoleaflet repair has been the surgical standard for many years, the recent addition of the "cone reconstruction" to the surgical options for Ebstein's malformation has increased the number of patients for whom valve repair is a possibility. A simplistic description of this complex repair is provided by Figure

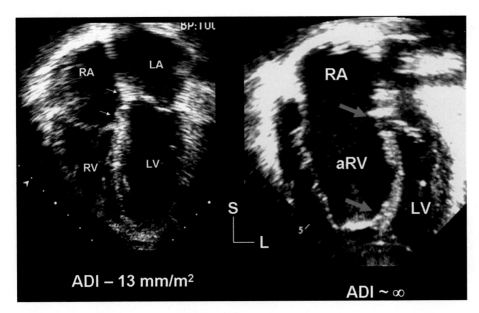

FIGURE 8.10. Four-chamber, systolic images obtained from two different patients with Ebstein's malformation. Left: Modest displacement of the tricuspid valve apparatus and excellent mobility of the valve leaflets. Both the anterior and septal leaflets remain visible in this plane because the degree of anterior rotation in this heart was minimal. The *small white arrows* highlight the separation between the septal insertions of the anterior mitral and septal tricuspid leaflets. The absolute distance between the insertions was 13 mm. Patient's body surface area was 1.0 m². Therefore, the displacement index in this case was equal to 13 mm/m². **Right:** A more severe example of Ebstein's malformation. The remnant of the septal leaflet (and its hinge point) was found near the right ventricular outflow tract, far anterior to the plane demonstrated in this image. The anterior leaflet is significantly tethered and was immobile in this plane; it remains parallel to the right ventricular free wall, even though this frame was taken at peak systole. Apically, it was also adherent to the moderator band (*apical red arrow*). In this situation, the apical displacement index is clearly large but cannot be accurately measured because no septal leaflet tissue is visualized in this plane. Nonetheless, the exaggerated separation between the septal insertion of the anterior mitral leaflet and the displaced tricuspid septal remnant clearly identifies this is a case of Ebstein's malformation. ADI, apical displacement index; aRV, atrialized right ventricle; L, left; LA, left atrium; LV, left ventricle; RA, right atrium; RV, right ventricle; S, superior.

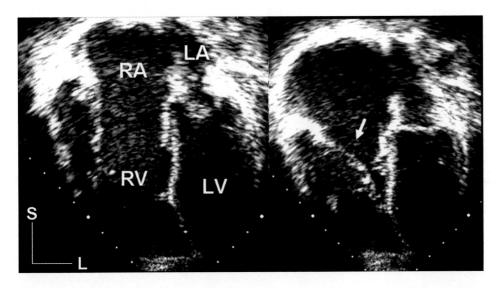

FIGURE 8.11. Apical four-chamber inflow images demonstrate a case of Ebstein's malformation with excellent anterior leaflet mobility. Left: Mid-diastole. **Right:** Peak systole. Features that suggest favorable anatomy for monoleaflet repair are that the anterior leaflet in this patient is freely mobile, including its leading edge. There are no muscular insertions that limit or distort the motion of the valve. The regurgitant jet originated only from the gap in coaptation seen between the anterior leaflet and the remnant of the septal leaflet. The leading edge of the valve reaches a point near enough to the septum that, given the degree of annular dilation, an annuloplasty can "advance" it to a position where it will coapt with the septum and the vestiges of the septal leaflet. L, left; LA, left atrium; LV, left ventricle; RA, right atrium; RV, right ventricle; S, superior.

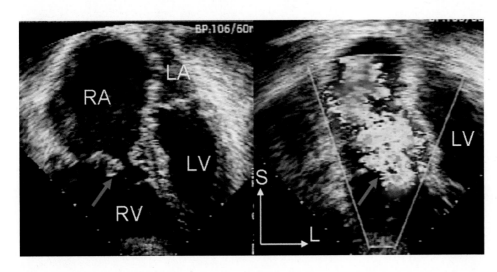

FIGURE 8.12. Severe Tricuspid Regurgitation in Ebstein Malformation. The anterior leaflet of this tricuspid valve is freely mobile (left) and color flow mapping (right) revealed that there was only a single, central jet of regurgitation (red arrow on the left panel). There is a coaptation gap between the anterior leaflet and the remnant of the septal leaflet in this case (right panel, red arrow). The vena contracta of the tricuspid regurgitant jet was greater than 50% of the normal tricuspid annulus diameter, consistent with very severe regurgitation. This patient subsequently had a successful monoleaflet repair, with only mild residual tricuspid regurgitation and no stenosis. L, left; LA, left atrium; LV, left ventricle; RA, right atrium; RV, right ventricle; S, superior.

FIGURE 8.13. Large muscular insertion to the middle of the anterior leaflet (left) and multiple fenestrations and associated jets of regurgitation (right). The tethering and multiple origins of regurgitant flow dramatically decrease the chance for successful monoleaflet repair, and a tricuspid valve replacement was performed. Although a monoleaflet repair was not possible, if this patient presented today the amount of leaflet tissue present suggests that a cone reconstruction would be possible, although each individual fenestration would need to be closed as a part of the repair. L, left; LA, left atrium; LV, left ventricle; RA, right atrium; RV, right ventricle; S, superior.

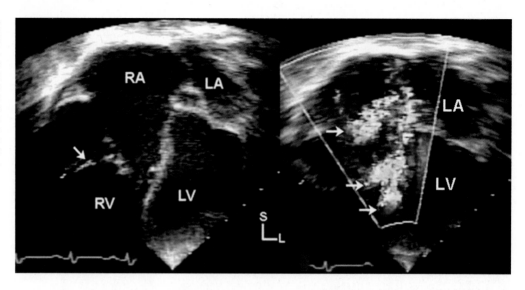

8.17. Unlike the monoleaflet repair, during a cone reconstruction the surgeon is able to recruit or "artificially delaminate" additional tricuspid valve tissue by dissecting the adherent components away from the underlying myocardium (Fig. 8.17, left). This increases the amount of mobile tissue available to assist in the reconstruction of the valve and results in a sheet of valve tissue separate from the myocardium and the atrioventricular junction (Fig. 8.17, center). Chordal support between the leading edge of this "surgically delaminated" valve tissue and the right ventricular walls must be preserved, or occasionally supplemented with Gore-Tex sutures. Fenestrations in the neo-tricuspid tissue must be closed. The tissue is then sutured into a "cone" and the base of the cone is anchored near the atrioventricular junction, avoiding the areas containing the conduction pathways (Fig. 8.17, right). Thus, a cone reconstruction not only decreases the amount of tricuspid regurgitation but also restores the hinge points of the repaired valve to a more normal position near the atrioventricular junction. Figure 8.18 shows an echocardiographic example of a cone reconstruction. It seems likely

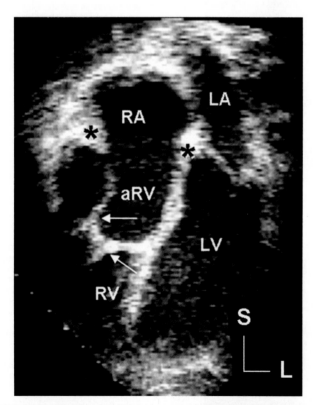

FIGURE 8.14. Apical four-chamber image showing (arrows) significant, direct muscular insertions from the right ventricular free wall into the mid-section of the anterior leaflet of the tricuspid valve. Even though this valve leaflet has separated from the underlying myocardium, its mobility was quite limited by these attachments to the ventricular free wall. Although a monoleaflet repair would not be possible, the surgical "delamination" that occurs during a cone reconstruction has made even this type of valve a candidate for repair. aRV, atrialized right ventricle; L, left; LA, left atrium; LV, left ventricle; RA, right atrium; RV, right ventricle; S, superior.

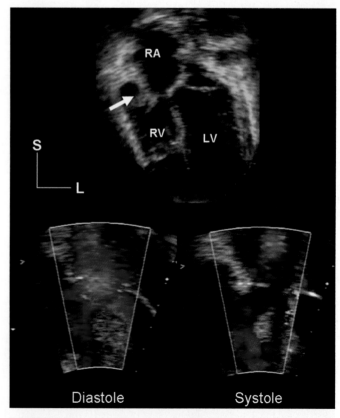

FIGURE 8.15. Postoperative examination of the patient shown in Figure 8.11. Top: Echocardiographic anatomy after a monoleaflet repair. The right ventricular cavity and right atrioventricular junction have been significantly reduced in size. This allows the anterior leaflet (*arrow*) to coapt with the ventricular septum in systole. **Bottom:** Magnified color flow images showing no stenosis or regurgitation. L, left; LV, left ventricle; RA, right atrium; RV, right ventricle; S, superior.

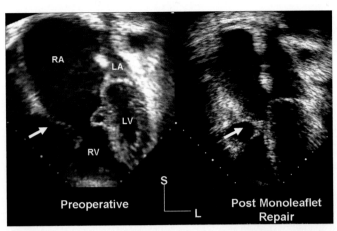

FIGURE 8.16. Two apical four-chamber images show the anatomy of a patient with Ebstein's malformation before and after a monoleaflet repair. The anterior leaflet (*arrow*) was successfully advanced to coapt with the ventricular septum and the remnant of the tricuspid septal leaflet, eliminating the tricuspid regurgitation. L, left; LA, left atrium; LV, left ventricle; RA, right atrium; RV, right ventricle; S, superior.

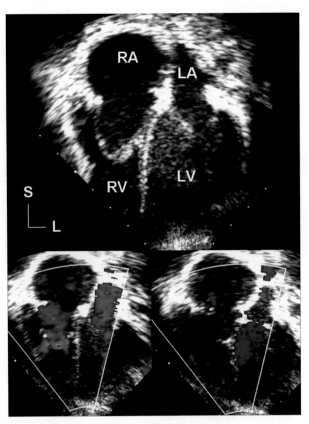

FIGURE 8.18. Apical four-chamber images taken 1 year after cone reconstruction for Ebstein's malformation. Top: Two-dimensional anatomy of the reconstructed tricuspid valve in diastole. Both the septal and lateral hinge points are now near the anatomic atrioventricular junction. **Bottom:** Color flow images in diastole (**left**) and systole (**right**). The reconstructed valve shows no signs of stenosis and minimal regurgitation with virtually no color flow disturbance during either phase of the cardiac cycle. L, left; LA, left atrium; LV, left ventricle; R, right; RA, right atrium; RV, right ventricle.

that valves such as those shown in Figure 8.10 (left), 8.13, and 8.14 would now be candidates for cone reconstructions, if they had presented after its introduction. Additional experience with and follow-up after the cone reconstruction of the tricuspid valve are needed before we can confidently define the anatomic features associated with favorable results from this procedure. Early impressions suggest that the amount of mobility in the native anterior leaflet and its leading edge will have an influence on the success and durability of these repairs. However, valves with even major degrees of tethering have been successfully repaired using this approach (Fig. 8.19). The presence of septal leaflet tissue within the right ventricular inlet also seems to relate to better function of the "cone" postoperatively.

Regardless of the patient's operative status (preoperative or postoperative) or even the type of valve (native, repaired, or prosthetic), the functional impact of the malformation on overall cardiac performance should be determined. Anatomical and functional severities are usually similar, but they are not always the same. For example, a patient can have a severe anatomic displacement with Ebstein's malformation but only mild functional impairment. This can occur if the myocardium is only mildly dysfunctional, the

interatrial communication is small, and the displaced valve leaflets allow little transvalvar regurgitation. Both anatomic and functional aspects of severity play an important role in determining functional state, prognosis, and, to a certain extent, the reparability of the tricuspid valve.

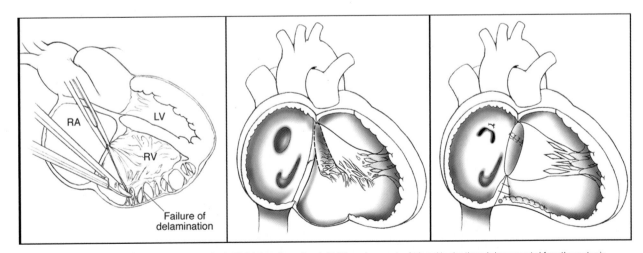

FIGURE 8.17. Concept of the cone reconstruction in Ebstein's malformation. Left: Adherent segments of tricuspid valve tissue being separated from the anatomic annulus and the underlying right ventricular myocardium. **Middle:** Sheet of tricuspid of tissue after it has been released. This tissue is used to create a cone, often attaching the anterior leaflet to the remnants of the septal leaflet (see suture line, **right**). Once the cone is created, the base is attached to the atrioventricular junction, restoring the hinge points to a nondisplaced position (**right**). When dilated, thin, or significantly dyskinetic, the atrialized right ventricle can be reduced in size by either elliptical resection or plication (**right**). The annuloplasty reduces the size of the intraventricular junction to what is appropriate to the size of the reconstructed cone.

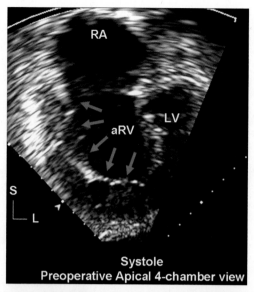

Systole
Preoperative Apical 4-chamber view

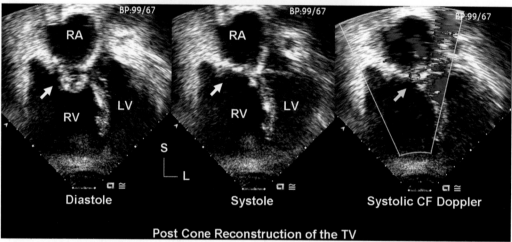

Post Cone Reconstruction of the TV

FIGURE 8.19. Series of apical four-chamber images from examinations of a 3-year-old girl with Ebstein's malformation. Top: Preoperative examination, demonstrating no remnants of tricuspid septal leaflet tissue within the anatomic right ventricular inlet. The anterior leaflet is severely tethered by multiple attachments to the right ventricular free wall. *Red arrows* outline the anterior leaflet. Even though this is a frame from peak systole, the leaflet tissue remains parallel to and very near the right ventricular free wall. The patient underwent a cone reconstruction of her tricuspid valve a short time later. **Bottom:** Postoperative, predischarge echocardiogram. **Left** and **middle:** Reconstructed valve in diastole and systole, respectively. By attaching the "annulus" of the reconstructed "cone" to a plane near the anatomic atrioventricular junction, the surgeon has completely eliminated the large atrialized portion of the right ventricle, as well as the regurgitation. Despite the severe deformity of the native valve, the color flow image in the postreconstruction echocardiogram **(right)** showed only mild tricuspid regurgitation. There was no obstruction (mean gradient = 4 mm Hg). aRV, atrialized right ventricle; L, left; LA, left atrium; LV, left ventricle; R, right; RA, right atrium; RV, right ventricle.

The degree of right atrial and ventricular enlargement and functional state of the right ventricular myocardium should be specifically defined. The largest right-sided chambers are associated with the most functional impairment and have less satisfactory clinical, as well as surgical, outcomes. Other important features include the degree of dilation of the right ventricular outflow tract, the presence and size of any atrial septal defect, and the degree of transvalvar regurgitation. Tricuspid regurgitation should not only be described but also quantified. The most common scheme used to grade tricuspid regurgitation is trivial (grade 0), mild (grade 1), moderate (grade 2), moderate-severe (grade 3), or severe (grade 4). The left ventricular myocardium has also been described as being abnormal in a significant fraction of the patients with Ebstein's malformation. Noncompacted segments of left ventricular myocardium can be seen in 10% to 20% of cases. Therefore, quantitative evaluation of left ventricular performance (as described in chapter 3) should also be a routine component of the echocardiographic evaluation of the patient with Ebstein's malformation. When ventricular septal defects and/or pulmonary stenosis coexist with Ebstein's malforma-

tion, standard echocardiographic assessments are required to define their impact on the patient's physiology.

The techniques used to assess tricuspid regurgitation and right ventricular function deserve some additional discussion. Tricuspid regurgitation, in particular, can be difficult to accurately assess in Ebstein's malformation. This is due to the rotational displacement of the functional valvar orifice away from the expected position within the right ventricular inlet. As a result, the origin of the transvalvar regurgitation is often not visualized in the usual views and can be oriented in unusual directions (Fig. 8.20). In these cases, the plane of sound must be angled more anteriorly toward the functional valvar orifice, typically at the junction of the body and outlet of the right ventricle (Fig. 8.6). The subcostal acoustic window often provides the optimal visualization of this area in young patients. In older patients, either transthoracic parasternal short-axis, anteriorly angled apical views, or transgastric transesophageal imaging planes can provide similar information.

In cases with a single regurgitant orifice, the width of the regurgitant jet at its origin is often the best quantitative indicator of the

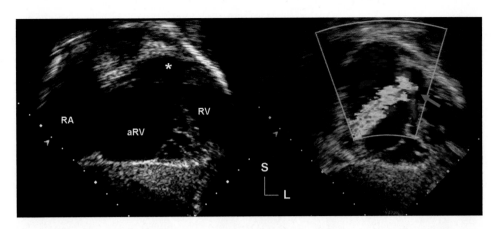

FIGURE 8.20. Subcostal position during examination of an infant with severe Ebstein's malformation displaying the right atrium (RA), atrialized right ventricle (aRV), and the trabecular right ventricle (RV) beyond the functional tricuspid valvar orifice (*). The functional orifice is also the origin of a single broad jet of regurgitation (**right**, *red arrow*). This jet begins near the right ventricular outflow tract and is oriented in inferiorly and toward the diaphragm, near the inferior vena cava–right atrial connection. aRV, atrialized right ventricle; L, left; RA, right atrium; RV, right ventricle; S, superior.

regurgitant volume (Figs. 8.21, 8.22, and 8.23). The diameter of the vena contracta provides a convenient and reproducible method for defining this width. In the adult, with only one tricuspid regurgitation jet present, a vena contracta width of less than 3 mm is associated with mild regurgitation. A single diameter of 8 to 10 mm represents severe transvalvar regurgitation. The combination of multiple jets is more difficult to assess. In this situation, the examiner must mentally combine the size of the regurgitant orifices in order to determine the overall degree of tricuspid regurgitation. The vena contracta guidelines listed for single jets can only be used in a general way when assessing multiple regurgitant orifices. One must remember that simply adding the jet diameters together will slightly overstate the amount of regurgitant volume.

These adult guidelines cannot be directly applied to smaller patients. However, given the large annular diameters associated with Ebstein's malformation, these cutpoints are useful even in the school-aged child. To avoid underestimating the degree of regurgitation in an infant or small child, the vena contracta diameter should be compared with the patient's expected normal diameter of the tricuspid valve. Vena contracta diameters that are less than 10% of the normal annulus would usually be considered mild. Jet origins measuring more than 25% to 30% of the normal annular dimension would be classified as severe. The density of the tricuspid regurgitant signal when examined by continuous-wave Doppler can also provide a semiquantitative marker of regurgitant severity. A very dense, easily obtained signal suggests a larger regurgitant volume than a faint signal.

The large and compliant right atrium often absorbs even tremendously large regurgitant volumes. Therefore, analysis of systemic venous flow reversals is less helpful in Ebstein's malformation than in patients with a normal right atrium and ventricle. The evaluation of tricuspid regurgitation must, therefore, focus more heavily on direct visualization of the color flow disturbance caused by the systolic flow, as described earlier. Qualitatively, the size of the right atrial chamber also reflects the degree of regurgitation. However, right atrial size is of limited utility, because it is also strongly influenced by the presence of right ventricular dysfunction and the ineffective contractions of the atrial component of the right ventricle.

The anatomy of the tricuspid valvar apparatus in the area of the regurgitant origin must be carefully assessed. Accurate definition of the leaflet deficiencies leading to transvalvar regurgitation simplifies surgical planning tremendously. High-quality two-dimensional surface and transesophageal images are required. Real-time three-dimensional imaging, especially during transesophageal echocardiography, can provide even more insight into the mechanisms underlying valvar dysfunction (Fig. 8.24).

Virtually no patient with Ebstein's malformation has truly normal right ventricular performance. Quantitative assessment of right ventricular systolic function is a challenge in all forms of congenital heart disease, and Ebstein's malformation is no exception. It is often difficult to visualize the entire right ventricle in one imaging plane. When evaluating right ventricular systolic performance qualitatively, one compares the systolic area occupied by the ventricular cavity with a diastolic area in that same plane. Better systolic function is associated with a smaller systolic cavity relative to the diastolic "starting point." Experienced observers can generally classify these ventricles into groups displaying mild, moderate, or severe dysfunction, but interobserver variable can be significant.

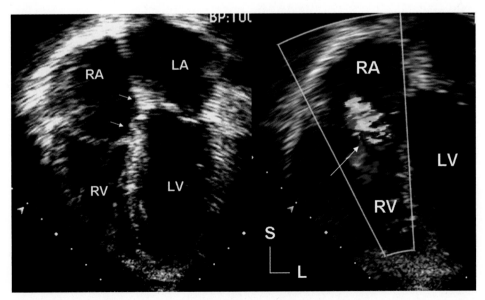

FIGURE 8.21. Echocardiographic images examination of an 8-year-old patient with relatively mild Ebstein's malformation. Left: Characteristic displacement of the septal insertion of the tricuspid valve (*two arrows*). **Right:** Color flow disturbance caused by the resulting tricuspid regurgitation (*arrow*). The vena contracta (VC) measured 4 mm. In an adult, this would be consistent with relatively mild regurgitation, but in this young child, it represented a moderate degree of regurgitation. In addition to the absolute VC diameter, the diameter should be compared to the patient's expected normal diameter of the tricuspid valve to avoid underestimating the degree of regurgitation in pediatric patients. L, left; LA, left atrium; LV, left ventricle; RA, right atrium; RV, right ventricle; S, superior.

FIGURE 8.22. Apical four-chamber echocardiographic images from the examination of a 21-year-old, displaying features consistent with severe Ebstein's malformation, as well as severe tricuspid regurgitation. **Left:** Components of the tricuspid valve do not coapt in systole. **Right:** Color flow image confirms the presence of severe tricuspid regurgitation (*arrow*). The vena contracta diameter was 21 mm. L, left; LA, left atrium; LV, left ventricle; RA, right atrium; RV, right ventricle; S, superior.

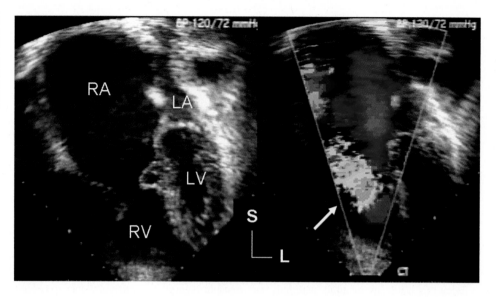

It is often helpful to add a quantitative component to the assessment of right ventricular function in these patients. The can be done by obtaining an ejection fraction with magnetic resonance scanning or in the echocardiographic laboratory by determining the fractional area change (FAC) of the right ventricle. FAC can be determined by either a monoplane or biplane technique. Because right ventricular shortening is primarily a longitudinal process; the apical four-chamber view must be included as one of the planes. Systolic and diastolic areas are traced in the apical four-chamber view or, more optimally, from the apical and one other orthogonal plane. Parasternal or subcostal short-axis views at the mid-ventricular level complement the apical view well. FAC is then calculated by subtracting the systolic area from the diastolic area and dividing the result by the original diastolic area ([Diastolic ventricular area – Systolic ventricular area]/Diastolic ventricular area). If more than one plane of imaging is used, two resulting FAC values are averaged. This measurement (FAC) is analogous to calculating ventricular shortening fraction, but it uses two-dimensional rather than M-mode data. In our laboratory, normal right ventricles show FACs equal to or greater than 40%. Other non-geometrically based methods of assessing ventricular performance such as the myocardial performance index, annular tissue Doppler velocities, and myocardial deformation imaging have been applied to the right ventricle and may be helpful in following these patients over time.

Echocardiography also plays an important role intraoperatively and postoperatively in assessing the adequacy of tricuspid valvar repair or replacement (Fig. 8.25). The most important use of intraoperative echocardiography is in the immediate evaluation of the repaired valve. A repair that is not functioning can be revised, or else the valve can be replaced without a repeat operation. The postoperative examination must also be used to assess prosthetic valvar function, to determine changes in right and left ventricular function, and to exclude significant residual atrial level shunting. Transthoracic echocardiography remains important both early and late after surgical procedures. It is the primary diagnostic mortality used to assess the ongoing adequacy of a surgically repaired valve, to assess the function of a prosthetic valve, to exclude residual intracardiac shunts, to assess ventricular performance, and to exclude less common postoperative complications, such as effusions and intracardiac thrombi.

The degree of residual tricuspid regurgitation and tricuspid stenosis should be determined during every examination after a tricuspid valve repair or replacement. Regurgitation of a prosthesis or a repaired valve would be evaluated as described previously. The mean Doppler inflow gradient provides the most satisfactory assessment of tricuspid stenosis. Due to the prominence of respiratory variation in right ventricular filling signals, multiple consecutive cycles should always be measured and the results averaged. Most

FIGURE 8.23. Apical four-chamber echocardiographic images from the examination of a 5-year-old, displaying features consistent with extremely severe Ebstein's malformation and severe tricuspid regurgitation. **Left:** Anterior leaflet has limited mobility and remains parallel to the ventricular septum in systole. No remnant of the septal leaflet can be seen. The components of the tricuspid valve do not coapt in systole. **Right:** Color flow image confirms the presence of massive tricuspid regurgitation (*arrow*). The marked tethering of the tricuspid valve in this case produced a nearly unguarded tricuspid valve orifice. The vena contracta diameter was 20 mm, similar to that in the case presented in Figure 8.17 but representing even more regurgitation given the patient's younger age and smaller body size. L, left; LA, left atrium; LV, left ventricle; RA, right atrium; RV, right ventricle; S, superior.

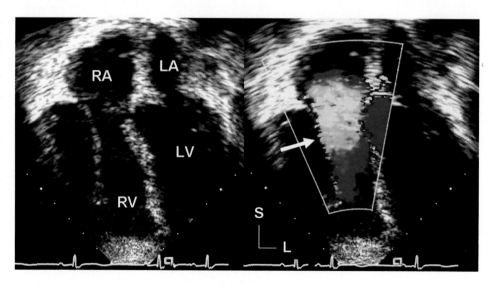

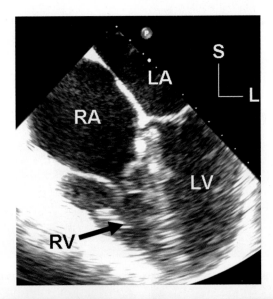

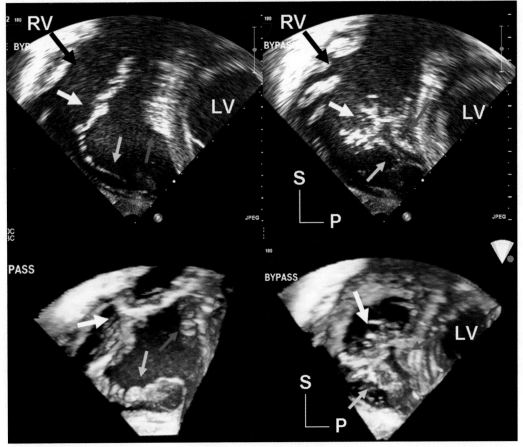

FIGURE 8.24. Preoperative transesophageal echocardiographic examination of a 16-year-old boy. Top: Two-dimensional, four-chamber view demonstrating features typical of Ebstein's malformation. **Middle:** Transgastric images oriented in a short-axis plane at the mid-ventricular level: diastolic image (**left**) and the systolic position of the valve leaflets (**right**). In this case, the septal leaflet (*red arrow*) is rudimentary. The inferior leaflet (*blue arrow*) is unusually large and mobile. Despite this, there is a large coaptation gap visible in the systolic frame (**right**), between the *red* and *blue arrows*. **Bottom:** Three-dimensional images from the same examination that are focused on the right ventricular cavity and tricuspid valve. The volumes were cropped so that the resulting images would correspond to those shown in the **middle**. The tricuspid valve is displayed as if the examiner is standing in the apex of the right ventricle looking toward the right atrium. The leaflet texture, thickening of the leading edges, and a direct muscular insertion into the middle of the anterior leaflet (**bottom left,** *white arrow*) were more easily appreciated in the three-dimensional scan. A coaptation gap was also easily appreciated three-dimensionally (**bottom right,** between the *red* and *blue arrows*). The abnormal papillary muscle attachment to the anterior leaflet and the rudimentary nature of the septal leaflet combined to create a single, posterior regurgitant orifice in this case. L, left; LA, left atrium; LV, left ventricle; P, posterior; RA, right atrium; RV, right ventricle; S, superior.

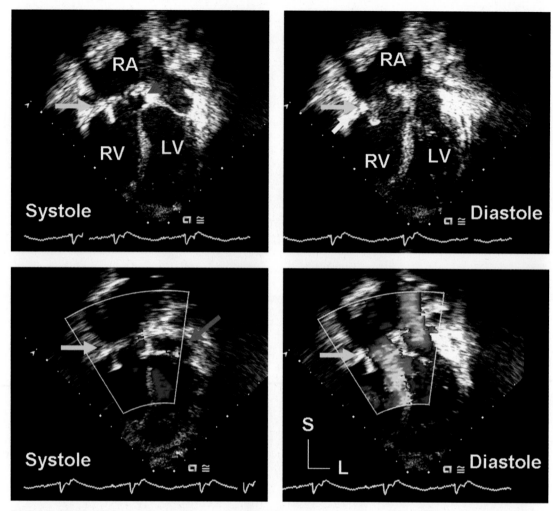

FIGURE 8.25. Ebstein's malformation after tricuspid valve replacement. A 29-mm porcine bioprosthesis can be seen in the tricuspid valve position (*yellow arrow*). **Top:** Two-dimensional images show that sewing ring of the valve has been placed at an angle to the anatomic atrioventricular junction. This was done to avoid injury to the conduction system. As a result, the coronary sinus orifice is on the ventricular side of the prosthesis (*red arrowhead*). This seems to be well tolerated in patients with Ebstein's malformation, probably due to the relatively low ventricular pressures, which are usually present. **Top:** Normal excursion of the prosthetic leaflets, becoming parallel to the supporting struts in diastole (**right**). The lower color flow Doppler images show no evidence of regurgitation (**bottom left**; note the trivial mitral regurgitation [*red arrow*] confirming that this is a systolic frame). The diastolic color "wavefront" fills the prosthetic annulus with little evidence of turbulence. The average mean Doppler gradient was 3 mm Hg. L, left; LV, left ventricle; RA, right atrium; RV, right ventricle; S, superior.

tricuspid valve bioprostheses will display a small pressure gradient. Normal bioprosthetic valves have mean gradients that are usually less than 6 mm Hg. An average mean gradient greater than 10 mm Hg generally indicates significant valve dysfunction. If a large volume of regurgitation is present or a residual left–to–right atrial shunt exists, the excess volume crossing the tricuspid annulus will artificially increase the gradient measured. These confounding conditions must be accounted for in the final assessment of the valve. Rarely, right coronary flow can be compromised by manipulation of the right atrioventricular groove by tricuspid annuloplasty or right ventricular plication. Therefore, both global and regional assessments of wall motion and function play an important role in the immediate postoperative evaluation of these patients.

 ## PRENATAL DETECTION OF EBSTEIN'S MALFORMATION

Echocardiography can accurately define the features of Ebstein's malformation in the fetus. Characteristics that have been associated with early neonatal mortality include marked enlargement of the right heart, severe tethering of the anterior leaflet, left ventricular

compression, and associated lesions such as pulmonary atresia. Pulmonary hypoplasia develops secondary to severe cardiomegaly (Fig. 8.26) and hydrops with pleural and pericardial effusions. Definition of the fetal cardiac rhythm should occur routinely because, although uncommon in the prenatal patient with Ebstein's malformation, tachyarrhythmias can contribute to the development of hydrops. Finding the ratio of the combined right atrial and atrialized ventricular area compared with the combined area of the functional right ventricle and left heart (Celermajer index) to be greater than 1 was shown to be associated with very poor fetal or neonatal outcome. Other fetal or neonatal findings that were associated with increased risk of mortality were a larger atrial septal defect, functional or anatomic pulmonary atresia, or reduced left ventricular function.

Other Tricuspid Valve Disorders

Ebstein's malformation is not the only congenital disorder that afflicts the right ventricle and tricuspid valve. Apart from Ebstein's malformation, **congenital dysplasia** of the tricuspid valve leaflets is the most common abnormality leading to congenital tricuspid regurgitation. There is no displacement of the annular hinge points in these valves. Rather the leaflet tissue is thickened and the chordal supports shortened, causing significant gaps in systolic coaptation

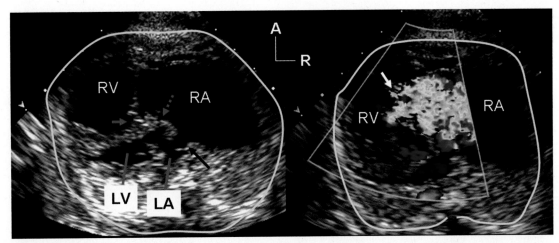

FIGURE 8.26. Two horizontal plane images of the thorax from a fetal echocardiogram performed at a gestational age of 26 weeks. Left: Two-dimensional image shows not only massive cardiac enlargement but also an exaggerated offset between the tricuspid (*solid red arrow*) and mitral (*dashed arrow*) valves. The outer boundary of the fetal thorax has been defined by the *yellow line*, highlighting the tremendous degree of cardiac enlargement present in this fetus. The entire heart is shifted, with the right atrium and right ventricle "pushing" the left ventricle posteriorly, away from its normal position. The cardiac apex is actually posterior to the mid-axillary line on the **left.** The *black arrow* indicated the position of the atrial septum, which has also been shifted posteriorly and to the left. The heart in this case occupies the majority of the thoracic volume and also compresses the lung tissue posteriorly. This resulted in significant pulmonary hypoplasia and contributes to the extremely poor prognosis associated with a prenatal presentation of severe Ebstein's malformation. **Right:** Color flow disturbance (*white arrow*) consistent with severe tricuspid regurgitation. LA, left atrium; LV, left ventricle; R, right; RA, right atrium; RV, right ventricle; S, superior.

(Fig. 8.27). The degree of tricuspid regurgitation is often severe, but the right ventricular myocardium is relatively normal, especially in contrast to patients with Ebstein's malformation. Surgical annuloplasty for symptomatic young patients can improve valvar function. Unfortunately, the improvements achieved are often temporary, leading to eventual tricuspid valve replacement later in life. Tricuspid **annular dilation** secondary to other congenital heart diseases, like tetralogy of Fallot or atrial septal defects, is a common cause of tricuspid regurgitation evaluated in the congenital echocardiographic laboratory. When intervention is required, this type of regurgitation is almost always amenable to surgical repair. When chordal support to the tricuspid valvar leaflets is interrupted or insufficient, the unsupported segment will **"flail"** past the plane of the atrioventricular junction and into the right atrium and systole (Fig. 8.28). This is a common manifestation of traumatic rupture of a tricuspid valve papillary muscle. The regurgitation caused by such flail segments is nearly always severe but may not produce symptoms for decades. This long presymptomatic natural history is a consequence of the fact that these hearts were normal with normal pulmonary pressure and resistance prior to the trauma that induced the regurgitation. The low-pressure volume load associated with isolated tricuspid regurgitation is tolerated reasonably well in the setting of normal myocardial function. The injury that led to **traumatic tricuspid regurgitation** is often in the distant past and sometimes can be difficult to clearly identify. As with annular dilatation, regurgitation due to chordal rupture can be successfully repaired in most patients.

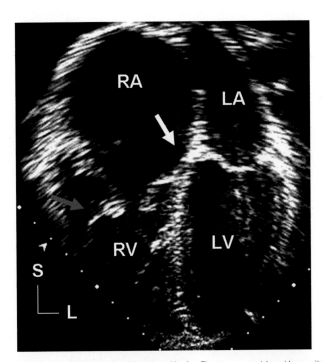

FIGURE 8.27. Congenital dysplasia of the tricuspid valve. There was severe tricuspid regurgitation and a large central gap in coaptation. The tricuspid leaflets are thickened and chordae are shorter than normal (*red arrow*), restricting the motion of all three leaflets. Despite the restricted mobility, these leaflets are not adherent to the underlying myocardium and the apical displacement index, representing the offset of the mitral and tricuspid valve septal insertions (*white arrow*), with only 6 mm/m². These features confirm the fact that this was not a case of Ebstein's malformation. L, left; LA, left atrium; LV, left ventricle; RA, right atrium; RV, right ventricle; S, superior.

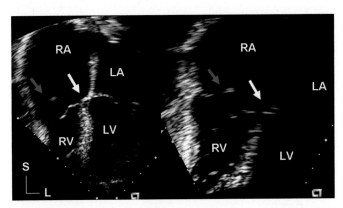

FIGURE 8.28. Traumatic tricuspid regurgitation. The patient was 40 years old at the time of this examination and had been involved in a motor vehicle accident as a teenager. Subsequent to the accident, he was described as having a heart murmur, but no further investigation was pursued until he complained of palpitations and exercise limitation at age 39. The echocardiogram showed severe tricuspid regurgitation due to rupture of several chordal supports to the anterior tricuspid leaflet. As a result, a significant segment of the anterior leaflet "flailed" into the right atrium during systole (*red arrows*). This valve was completely delaminated as evidenced by the normal relationship between the tricuspid and mitral septal insertions (*white arrows*). L, left; LA, left atrium; LV, left ventricle; RA, right atrium; RV, right ventricle; S, superior.

All of these causes of tricuspid regurgitation are reliably distinguished from Ebstein's malformation using the anatomic criteria and the apical displacement index described earlier in this chapter.

Acknowledgments

I gratefully acknowledge the mentorship and guidance provided by Drs. Gordon K. Danielson, Joseph A. Dearani, William D. Edwards, and James B. Seward, as well as Professor Robert H. Anderson in our studies of patients with Ebstein's malformation. Professor Anderson, Dr. Dearani, and Dr. Edwards have also generously contributed images to better illustrate this chapter (RHA Figures 8.5 and 8.6; JAD Figures 8.3, 8.5, and 8.17, and WDE Figure 8.4). Thank you all very much.

SUGGESTED READING

Attenhofer Jost C, Connolly H, O'Leary P, et al. Occurence of left ventricular myocardial dysplasia/noncompaction in patients with Ebstein's anomoly. *Mayo Clin Proc.* 2005;80:361–368.

Brown ML, Dearani JA, Danielson GK, et al. The outcomes of operations for 539 patients with Ebstein anomaly. *J Thoracic Cardiovasc Surg.* 2008; 135:1120–1136.

Celermajer D, et al. Ebstein's anomoly: Presentation and outcome from fetus to adult. *J Am Coll Cardiol.* 1994;23:170.

Celermajer D, Cullen S, Sullivan I, et al. Outcome in neonates with Ebstein's anomaly. *J Am Coll Cardiol.* 1992;19:1041–1046.

Connolly H, Warnes C. Ebstein's anomaly: Outcome of pregnancy. *J Am Coll Cardiol.* 1994;23:1194–1198.

Da Silva J, Baumgratz J, da Fonseca L, et al. The cone reconstruction of the tricuspid valve in Ebstein's anomaly. The operation: Early and midterm results. *J Thorac Cardiovasc Surg.* 2007;133:215–223.

Danielson GK, Maloney JD, Devloo RAE. Surgical repair of Ebstein's anomaly. *Mayo Clin Proc.* 1979;54:185–192.

Dearani JD, et al. Surgical management of Ebstein's anomaly in the adult. *Semin Thorac Cardiovasc Surg.* 2005;17:148–154.

Dearani J, O'Leary P, Danielson G. Surgical treatment of Ebstein's malformation: state of the art in 2006. *Cardiol Young.* 2006;16(Suppl)3:4–11.

Ebstein W. Ober einen sehr seltenen Fall von Insufficienz der Valvula tricuspidalis, bedingt durch elne angeborene hochgradige Missbildung derslben. *Arch Anat Physiol Wissensch Med.* 1866;33:238–254.

Eidem B, Tei C, O'Leary P, et al. Nongeometric quantitative assessment of right and left ventricular function: myocardial performance index in normal children and patients with Ebstein anomaly. *J Am Soc Echocardiogr.* 1998;11:849–856.

Giuliani E, Fuster V, Brandenburg R, et al. Ebstein's anomaly:The clinical features and natural history of Ebstein's anomaly of the tricuspid valve. *Mayo Clinic Proc.* 1979;54:163–173.

Gussenhoven E, Stewart P, Becker A. "Offsetting" of the septal tricuspid lealfet in normal hearts and in hearts with Ebstein anomaly: Anatomic and echographic correlation. *Am J Cardiol.* 1984;54:172–176.

Hagler D. Echocardiographic assessment of Ebstein's anomaly. *Prog Pediatr Cardiol.* 1993;2:28–37.

Knott-Craig C, Goldberg S. Management of neonatal Ebstein's anomaly. *Semin Thorac Cardiovasc Surg Pediatr Card Surg Annu.* 2007:112–16.

Quinonez L, Dearani J, Puga F, et al. Results of 1.5-ventricle repair for Ebstein anomaly and the failing right ventricle. *J Thorac Cardiovasc Surg.* 2007;133:1303–1310.

Roberson D, Silverman N. Ebstein's anomaly: Echocardiographic and clinical features in the fetus and neonate. *J Am Coll Cardiol.* 1989;14:1300–1307.

Schrieber C, Cook A, Ho S, et al. Morphology of Ebstein's malformation: revisitation relative to surgical repair. *J Thorac Cardiovasc Surg.* 1999; 117:148–155.

Seward J. Ebstein's anomaly: Ultrasound imaging and haemodynamic evaluation. *Echocardiography.* 1993;10:641–664.

Watson H. Natural history of Ebstein's anomaly of tricuspid valve in childhood and adolescence: An international co-operative study of 505 cases. *Br Heart J.* 1974;36:417–427.

Yetman A, Freedom R, McCrindle B. Outcome of cyanotic neonates with Ebstein's anomaly. *Am J Cardiol.* 1998;81:749–754.

Chapter 9
Echocardiographic Assessment of Mitral Valve Abnormalities

Jeffrey F. Smallhorn

This chapter details the echocardiographic assessment of congenital mitral valve abnormalities that might be encountered during the evaluation of primary or, more frequently, mitral valve pathology in association with other forms of congenital heart disease. It must be stated that congenital mitral valve abnormalities are rare, unlike their rheumatic counterpart. Also, when assessing a patient with suspected mitral valve pathology, it is important to pay attention to associated hemodynamic abnormalities that influence the interpretation of Doppler physiology.

With the recent advent of three-dimensional techniques, our understanding of mitral valve morphology and function as assessed by echocardiography is fundamentally changing. This technique in conjunction with its two-dimensional counterpart is currently becoming the reference standard for surgical or medical intervention.

This chapter will address both the two- and three-dimensional approach to the assessment of mitral valve abnormalities and their hemodynamic consequence.

MITRAL VALVE DEVELOPMENT

The atrioventricular junction comes into prominence following rightward looping of the heart tube after the 25th day of gestation. By the end of the fifth week, the developing ventricles are visible, with the future left ventricle supporting a large portion of the atrioventricular canal. The lumen of the atrioventricular canal is occupied by the inferior and superior endocardial cushions. Initially unfused, these cushions eventually fuse during the sixth week and form the right and left atrioventricular junctions, to which the developing leaflets of the mitral valve will be anchored. Parts of these fused cushions remain on the left side of the septal crest and form the aortic leaflet, often referred to as the anterior leaflet, of the mitral valve.

Formation of the normal mitral valve can only proceed when the aorta becomes committed to the left ventricle, resulting in fibrous continuity between the two leaflets; hence, the name the aortic leaflet is given, which distinguishes it from its mural counterpart, often referred to as the posterior leaflet. Initially, there is still a cleft at the parietal margins of the fusion of the superior and inferior cushions. The mural leaflet of the mitral valve develops from the lateral cushion tissue of the atrioventricular canal myocardium that protrudes into the ventricular lumen. The myocardium disappears via apoptosis, and therefore the entire leaflets are derived from cushion mesenchyme that is endocardial in origin. This provides an explanation as to why persistence of the myocardium results in the mitral arcade. Although the tricuspid septal leaflet delaminates from the ventricular myocardium, the aortic leaflet is never attached to or supported by the myocardium, except at its cranial and caudal margins, which represent chordal and papillary muscle attachments. Expansion of the inferior quadrants of the left atrioventricular junction involves growth of the parietal wall of the left ventricle, with comparable growth of the lateral cushion. This eventually results in the lateral cushion occupying two-thirds of the circumference of the developing mitral valve.

This expanded crescent, which represents the developing mitral valve, is associated with compacting columns in the spongy layer of the ventricular muscle, which eventually form the papillary muscles. Excessive or abnormal compaction of the trabecular layer of the developing ventricular myocardium is responsible for the parachute mitral valve. Failure of the formation of the tendinous chords from the myocardial primordiums results in the mitral arcade lesion, with muscle extending from the tips of the leaflets to the papillary muscles. When Ebstein's malformation of the mitral valve occurs, it is the mural leaflet that is involved as this is the leaflet that excavates from the parietal ventricular wall.

GENETICS OF MITRAL VALVE DEVELOPMENT

Reciprocal signaling between the endocardial and myocardial cell layers in the cushion is mediated in part by transforming growth factor (TGF)- family members and induces a transformation of endocardial cells into mesenchymal cells. *Sox9* is activated when myocardial cells undergo mesenchymal transforamtion and *Sox9*-deficient mesenchymal cells fail to express ErbB3, which is required for cushion cell proliferation. The mesenchymal cells migrate into the cushions and differentiate into the fibrous tissue of the valves. Several genes play a role in heart valve formation including calcineurin with signalling and downstream activation of NFAT (nuclear factor of activated T cells) family of transcription factors, with an absence of these resulting in fatal defects of valve formation.

ANATOMY OF THE MITRAL VALVE

About two-thirds of the annulus of the mitral valve is supported by a fibroaerolar junction, which serves also to separate the parietal portion of the left atrial myocardium from the ventricular myocardium. The remaining third of the ring is part of an extensive sheet of fibrous continuity with the leaflets of the aortic valve, strengthened at its ends by the left and right fibrous trigones. There are two so-called commissural areas within the valve, corresponding more or less to the areas of the fibrous trigones. The zone of apposition between these areas delineates the two primary valvar leaflets. The more extensive leaflet is attached to the parietal part of the annulus. It is more accurate to describe this as the mural leaflet, rather than posterior. It has relatively little depth; consequently, when the valve is closed, it is seen as a long rectangular structure that is usually divided into scallops. There are usually three scallops, with a large central and then smaller lateral and medial structures. The second major leaflet of the valve is attached along the area of aortomitral fibrous continuity. Although its overall shape is semicircular, it is much squarer and more boxlike than the long, rectangular mural leaflet. Often termed the 'anterior' leaflet, it is not strictly anterior in position. That is why we prefer to describe it as the aortic leaflet.

The tension apparatus of the valve consists of the tendinous cords and the papillary muscles. The important cords are those supporting the free edge of the leaflets (notably the commissural fan-shaped cords) and those supporting the rough zone (particularly the thick strut cords) of the aortic leaflet and the basal cords. The cords supporting the free edge are much more significant in support of the mural leaflet. In contrast, the rough zone and strut cords are more significant in support of the aortic leaflet. A study by Becker and de Wit showed considerable variation of the free edge chords in normal hearts. The papillary muscles of the mitral valve are relatively constant in position, although they, too, show marked variation in their detailed anatomy. They are sited beneath the ends of the zone of apposition between the leaflets in posteromedial and anterolateral position and have a typical paired appearance. The axis of opening of the valve subtends a considerable angle relative to the inlet septum. Unlike the septal leaflet of the tricuspid valve, the leaflets are never attached by tendinous cords directly to the inlet component of the muscular ventricular septum.

Mitral Annular Shape and Function

The shape of the mitral annulus was initially thought to be planar, which resulted in a gross overdiagnosis of mitral valve prolapse. With the advent of three-dimensional echocardiography, this was recognized as being incorrect, as the mitral annulus has both high

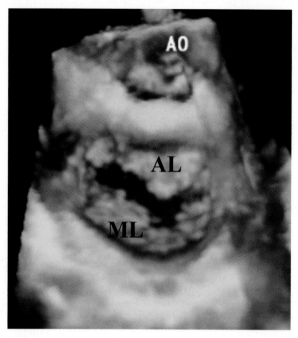

FIGURE 9.1. Three-dimensional image of the mitral annulus, as seen from the left atrium. Note the annular shape. The aortic and mural leaflets can be seen. AO, aorta; AL, aortic leaflet; ML, mural leaflet.

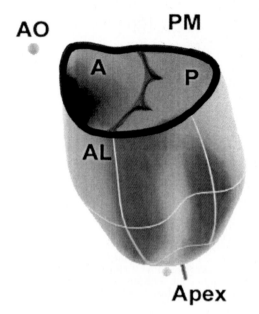

FIGURE 9.2. Mitral annular shape in the normal heart. Note the high points at the anterior and posterior parts of the annulus. The maximum bending of the annulus occurs along the commissures between the aortic and mural leaflets. A, anterior; AL, anterolateral; P, posterior; PM, posteromedial.

and low points, appearing with a shape like a saddle (Figs. 9.1 and 9.2). The anterior and posterior aspects represent the high points, while the medial and lateral represent the low points. Therefore, unless severe, mitral valve prolapse should be confidently diagnosed only in the long-axis view.

The saddle shape of the valve is most likely responsible for reducing leaflet stress, which is important when designing prosthetic valve rings or performing other surgical procedures that have an impact on normal annular function.

Previous animal and human studies demonstrated that mitral annular motion is very heterogeneous. The reported expansion of anterior mitral annulus and aortic root during ventricular systole corresponds with segmental diameter changes observed from previous data. The commissure-to-commissure (C-C) direction of the mitral annulus, which is muscular on both sides, moves dynamically throughout the cardiac cycle; however, the anteroposterior direction moves differently due to the sites of fibrous continuity with the aortic valve. In early systole, the mitral annular segments in the C-C direction start to contract, followed by diameter reduction in the anteroposterior direction with a slight expansion in the C-C direction in mid systole, which continues on during late systole. This shape change is thought to permit maximal expansion of the aortic root to facilitate ejection and good coaptation of the mitral valve leaflets.

Left atrial contraction contributes to area reduction of the mitral annulus before the ejection phase, contributing to 89% of area reduction in adult sheep. The contribution of atrial contraction to annular diameter reduction is most prominent in the anterolateral-posteromedial direction (i.e., the C-C direction for mitral valve) in children. This result was different from data in adult sheep for the mitral annulus, which showed a more prominent diameter reduction in the anteroposterior direction during atrial contraction. This difference might be due to the difference in species, maturity of myocardial tissue, and the fact that the human control subjects were not under general anesthesia.

When measured as C-C, the mitral annulus starts to bend in mid-systole, becoming most acute during the isovolumic relaxation phase of the mitral annulus (Fig. 9.3). After this, the annulus flattens, which may have a role in early diastolic filling. There appears to be a positive correlation between the bending angle of the mitral annulus and global left ventricular systolic function, which corresponds with the finding that the mitral annulus becomes planar after myocardial ischemia.

Mitral Valve Leaflets

It is generally accepted that the mitral leaflets move closer together, after opening widely at the beginning of the E wave, with leaflet separation being maximal at the second left atrial/left ventricular pressure cross-over, a pattern that corresponds exactly to the E wave as described with the use of Doppler echocardiography.

The line of closure of the mitral valve is on the atrial aspect of the valve and is about one-third of the distance from the free edge of the leaflets to their annular attachment. It is important to note, therefore, that the valve does not close at its free edge. This aspect of valve closure is much better appreciated by three-, rather than two-, dimensional echocardiography (Fig. 9.4).

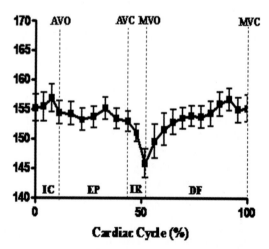

FIGURE 9.3. Graph demonstrating the bending angle in the normal mitral annulus in a pediatric case. Note the annulus starts to bend in late systole, becoming maximal during isovolumic relaxation, and subsequently becomes flatter. AVO, aortic valve opening; AVC, aortic valve closure; DF, diastolic phase; EF, ejection phase; MVC, mitral valve closure; IC, isovolumic contraction; IR, isovolumic relaxation; MVO, mitral valve opening,

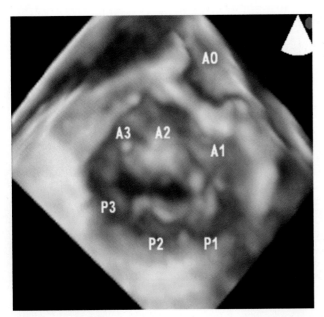

FIGURE 9.4. Mitral valve leaflets as seen by three-dimensional echocardiography, with the view being taken from below. Note the individual components of the leaflets. A1–3 represent the current nomenclature used to describe the aortic leaflet. P1–3 is the same for the mural leaflet.

Papillary Muscle Location

It is well accepted that in patients with ischemic mitral regurgitation, leaflet tethering due to papillary muscle displacement is responsible for restricted diastolic excursion that is independent of inflow volume. In addition, this mechanism is responsible for poor

systolic coaptation and the ensuing regurgitation. Therefore, there is an important and definite relationship between the mitral valve papillary muscles, leaflets, and supporting chordae to maintain normal valve function. Three-dimensional echocardiography provides a unique opportunity to image these relationships (Fig. 9.5), providing views that cannot be obtained with two-dimensional echocardiography.

It is also possible to see the chordal apparatus in three dimensions, which may have future implications with regard to their importance in mitral valve tethering (Fig. 9.6).

 ## INCIDENCE OF CONGENITAL MITRAL VALVE ABNORMALITIES

Congenital deformities of the mitral valve are rare, with mitral stenosis occurring in 0.6% of postmortem studies and in 0.21% to 0.42% of clinical series. Congenital mitral incompetence is rarer. There is a male-to-female ratio of around 1.5:1 to 2.2:1. The fully developed syndrome of "Shone syndrome" includes four obstructions within the left heart; the valvar lesion itself, supravalvar mitral ring, subaortic stenosis, and aortic coarctation. Any of these obstructions may coexist with any congenital lesion afflicting the mitral valve, particularly coarctation. Annular hypoplasia of the mitral valve is almost always associated with hypoplasia of the left ventricle and aortic stenosis or atresia. This may also be seen in association with ventricular septal defect or double-outlet right ventricle and tetralogy of Fallot. When the mitral valve is imperforate, left ventricular hypoplasia is inevitable unless there is an associated ventricular septal defect.

SPECIFIC MITRAL VALVE PATHOLOGY

At the outset, it should be stated that although in some cases there is pure mitral valve stenosis or regurgitation, in many other cases there is a combination.

FIGURE 9.5. Three-dimensional image of a normal mitral valve. **Top left:** Aortic leaflet, which is inserted into the anterior papillary muscle. **Top right:** Posterior papillary muscle. **Bottom left:** Two papillary muscles. **Bottom right:** Apex of the left ventricle. APM, anterior papillary muscle; LA, left atrium; LV, left ventricle; PPM, posterior papillary muscle.

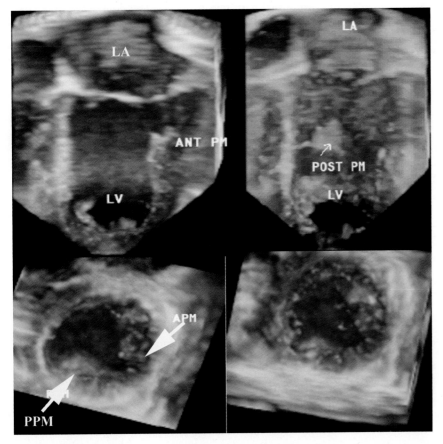

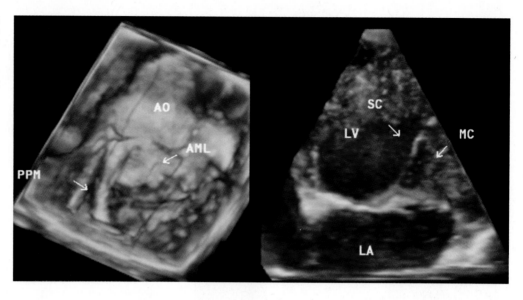

FIGURE 9.6. Three-dimensional images of the mitral chordal apparatus. Left: Mitral valve from above. *Left arrow* points to a strut chordae inserting into the aortic leaflet. **Right:** Strut and marginal chordae. AO, aorta; AOL, aortic leaflet; LA, left atrium; LV, left ventricle; MC, marginal chord; PPM, posterior papillary muscle; SC, strut chord.

Mitral Valve Dysplasia and Hypoplasia

With mitral valve dysplasia, the leaflets are thickened, the interchordal spaces often are obliterated, and the papillary muscles are deformed, the last frequently extending as muscular strands directly into the leaflets. Usually such a valve shows global hypoplasia and is the most common lesion associated with isolated congenital mitral stenosis. When the free edges of the dysplastic leaflets are thickened and rolled, the valve may be incompetent as well as stenotic. This appearance can be appreciated in the parasternal long-axis, short-axis, and four-chamber views by two-dimensional echocardiography, with evidence of thickened leaflets and reduced mobility (Fig. 9.7). Of note, it is often difficult to differentiate between the edge of the leaflets, the chordal apparatus, and the papillary muscles.

Color flow Doppler demonstrates the flow acceleration just proximal to the mitral annulus, followed by variance as the blood exits the restrictive orifice. In many cases, there are multiple exits due to the fused nature of the chordal apparatus (Fig. 9.8). In some cases, there is laminar flow through the orifice into the center of the valve, with more distal exits (Fig. 9.9).

Three-dimensional echocardiography provides an enface view of the mitral valve. The valve can be seen from the left ventricular aspect providing detailed anatomical details of the valve. The advantage of the 'looking up' view from the left ventricular cavity is that exquisite detail regarding the commissures can be appreciated (Fig. 9.7B). Although the surgical en face view is good, it is often difficult to appreciate the commissural detail due to the normal curved closure line of the mitral valve. To overcome this, it is possible to provide a slightly lower cut plane, which allows visualization of the commissures as well as the valve-supporting apparatus. It is also possible to remove the front of the left ventricle, such that the anterior aspect of the mitral valve and its tension apparatus can be seen. Three-dimensional color flow Doppler remains at a somewhat primitive stage and at present does not provide much added diagnostic information in congenital mitral valve stenosis (Fig. 9.8). Part of the problem is that, unlike rheumatic mitral valve stenosis, there are frequently multiple small eccentric jets, which make vena contracta summation difficult.

Occasionally, mitral stenosis may occur when the valve is miniaturized in its entirety but does not show dysplastic features. Of more significance is the arrangement when only part of the valve is hypoplastic. This is typically seen when one papillary muscle, usually the anterolateral muscle, is grossly reduced in size or even totally absent. Then the anterolateral commissure either inserts directly on to the left ventricular free wall or is supported on the wall by a small papillary muscle (Fig. 9.10).

The tension apparatus then has a grossly eccentric appearance, effectively inserting into a solitary papillary muscle. This arrangement

was illustrated by Shone and colleagues as a 'parachute mitral valve.' This is different from those cases where the two papillary muscles are fused into a solid solitary structure that supports the tension apparatus from the entire valve. In addition, an echocardiographic/morphologic correlation noted that many patients with aortic coarctation have altered positions of the left ventricular papillary muscles and narrowing of the interpapillary valley.

Supravalvar stenosing ring was described by Shone and his colleagues as part of the complex including the parachute valve. The supravalvar ring in this setting was a concentric thickening of the left atrial endocardium immediately above the atrioventricular junction. In the clinical setting, in contrast, it seems that the so-called stenosing supravalvar ring is formed on the atrial aspect of the valvar leaflets (Fig. 9.11). This is best seen in the parasternal long-axis view by two-dimensional echocardiography, as the beam is perpendicular to the ring in the axial plane where the resolution is best. Although it can be imaged in the four-chamber view, depth and lateral resolution may make differentiation from the annulus and leaflets difficult. Color flow Doppler is very helpful in this setting, as the flow accelaration seen proximal to the stenosis occurs well above the mitral annulus with the variance seen at the annular level (Fig. 9.8).

One of the advantages of three-dimensional echocardiography is that the ring can be seen in its entirety, unlike that seen by two-dimensional echocardiography. In the majority of cases the supravalvar ring does not occur in isolation but is seen in association with valve dysplasia. In some instances, there is the appearance of a membrane-like structure below the annulus that traverses the orifice of the valve. Whether this represents a component of valve dysplasia or is related to the supravalvar ring is unclear.

Anomalies of the Mitral Valve Leaflets

The most extreme anomaly is an imperforate mitral valve. An imperforate mitral valve usually coexists with aortic atresia, forming part of the 'hypoplastic left heart syndrome.' An imperforate mitral valve can also be found without aortic atresia and is then part of the combination termed 'mitral atresia with patent aortic root.' Often, the ventriculoarterial connection is double-outlet right ventricle; however, in a signficant number of cases, the patent aorta arises from a good-sized left ventricle that is connected via a ventricular septal defect. The ventricular septal defect can be of varying morphology.

Ebstein's malformation can rarely affect the morphologically mitral valve. The characteristic feature of Ebstein's malformation of the mitral valve is that the mural leaflet is plastered down onto the ventricular wall; consequently, its hinge is below the atrioventricular junction but there is no thinning of the atrialized inlet portion as is

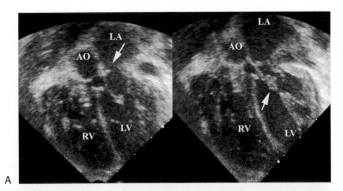

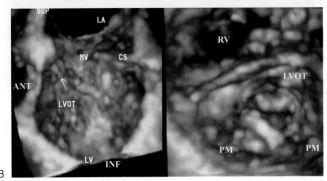

FIGURE 9.7. Patient with dysplastic mitral valve stenosis. A. Two dimensional four chamber view showing a small associated mitral valve ring (left) and the thickened mitral leaflets and subvalvar apparatus (right). AO, aorta; LA, left atrium; LV, left ventricle; RV, right ventricle. **B.** Three-dimensional echocardiogram from the same patient as in A. **Left:** Images from above the mitral valve. The supramitral ring is well seen. **Right:** Thickened mitral valve leaflets as well as tethering of the mural leaflet. ANT, anterior; INF, inferior; LA, left atrium; LVOT, left ventricular outflow tract; MV, mitral valve; PM, papillary muscle; RV, right ventricle; SUP, superior.

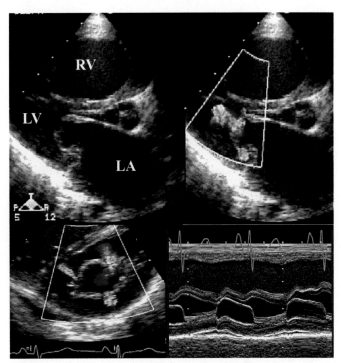

FIGURE 9.9. Mitral valve stenosis with multiple exit points and laminar flow centrally. Note in both the short- and long-axis views, there is no flow acceleration centrally. The M-mode shows a prolonged E-F slope. LA, left atrium; LV, left ventricle; RV, right ventricle.

usually seen when it is the morphologically tricuspid valve that is involved.

An isolated cleft of the mitral valve is also an anomaly confined to the leaflet, and one that primarily produces mitral incompetence. The affected leaflet tends to be dysplastic, and its edges are usually rolled and thickened. It is important to distinguish an isolated cleft of the aortic leaflet of the mitral valve in hearts with a separate atrioventricular junction from a "cleft" in the left valve of atrioventricular septal defects with a common atrioventricular junction. The isolated cleft "points" into the aortic outflow tract, often in association with a ventricular septal defect and the aortic leaflet is readily reconstituted by suture of its edges (Fig. 9.12).

In contrast, the so-called cleft in atrioventricular septal defects points to the septum and represents the space between the bridging leaflets. Closure of the bridging leaflets cannot produce a left atrioventricular valve that, in any way, resembles a normal mitral valve. These features, as well as differentiation from the cleft of an atrioventricular septal defect are well appreciated by both two- and three-dimensional echocardiography. One advantage of the latter technique is that the precise length of the cleft can be appreciated and measured (Figs. 9.13, 9.14).

In addition, the location and extent of the regurgitation are better appreciated with three-dimensional echocardiography. A significant problem with imaging color flow jets by two-dimensional echocardiography is that it is frequently difficult to appreciate multiple jets when imaging in one plane. Jets change direction, which provides additional confusion when changing from one imaging plane to another. Likewise, the presence of central and lateral commissural jets is best seen with three-dimensional echocardiography (Fig. 9.15).

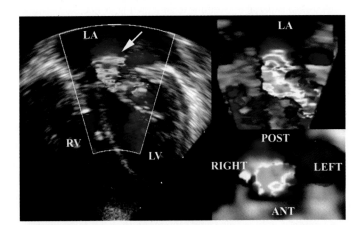

FIGURE 9.8. Color flow Doppler in the same patient as Figure 9.7. The two-dimensional color flow Doppler shows that the acceleration is occurring just above the annulus, which is consistent with the supramitral ring. Note the narrow inflow orifice. **Upper right:** Three-dimensional color flow data. **Bottom right:** En face view of the stenotic jet. LA, left atrium; LV, left ventricle; RV, right ventricle.

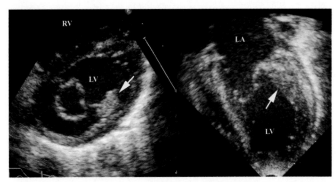

FIGURE 9.10. Two-dimensional image in a patient with a dominant anterior papillary muscle. LA, left atrium; LV, left ventricle; RV, right ventricle.

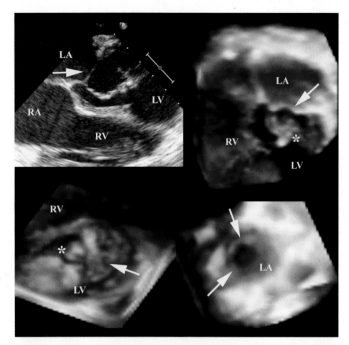

FIGURE 9.11. Two- and three-dimensional images from a patient with a supramital ring and an abnormal mitral valve. Bottom left: Three-dimensional image is a view of the mitral valve from below (left ventricular view). *Asterisk,* Mitral valve leaflets. *Arrow,* Single papillary muscle. **Right:** Three-dimensional images demonstrate the ring and its relationships shown with much greater clarity. LA, left atrium; LV, left ventricle; RA, right atrium; RV, right ventricle.

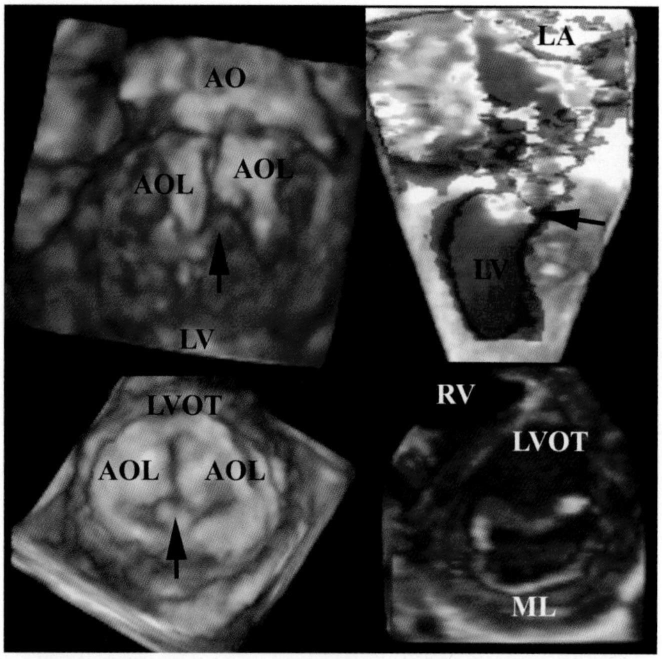

FIGURE 9.13. Three-dimensional data from the patient shown in Figure 9.12. Note that the cleft, as seen from a "looking up" view **(bottom left)** is complete and points toward the left ventricular outflow tract. This is also seen in the **top left,** which images the mitral valve with the front of the left ventricle removed. Also note the three-dimensional color flow jet **(top right).** AOL, aortic leaflet; LVOT, left ventricular outflow tract; LV, left ventricle; ML, mural leaflet; RV, right ventricle.

Double-Orifice Mitral Valve — The most common anatomical presentation is that in which a tongue of valvar tissue extends between the mural and aortic leaflets, dividing the valvar orifice into two components. Such an arrangement is frequently encountered in the left valve seen in an atrioventricular septal defect. The rarer variant, involving the otherwise normal mitral valve, shows duplication of the entire valvar structure. As a result, the left atrium is connected to the left ventricle by two valves, each with its own annulus, leaflets, cords, and papillary muscles (Fig. 9.16). This anomaly can exist in otherwise normal hearts where it is often discovered coincidentally, as well as in more complex anomalies such as tricuspid atresia or double-inlet ventricle.

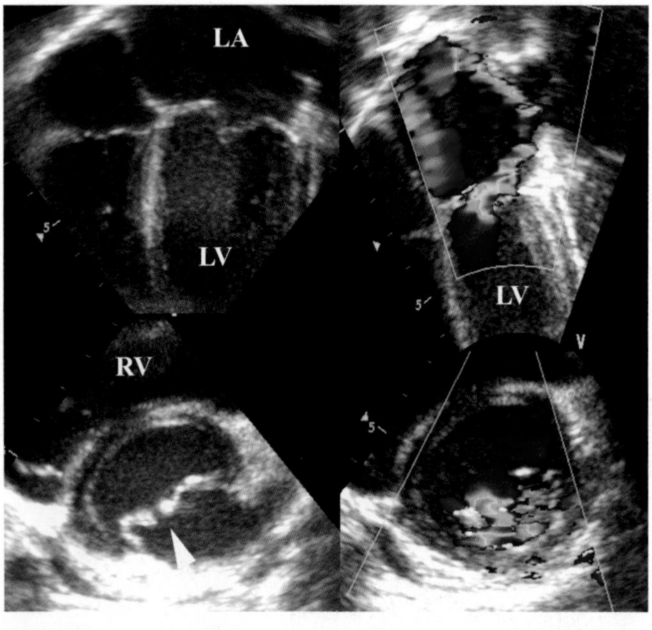

When a double-orifice mitral valve is associated with exact duplication of the leaflets, tension apparatus, and papillary muscles, it is readily appreciated with two-dimensional echocardiography, being best imaged in the parasternal long- and short-axis views (Fig. 9.16). Color flow Doppler usually demonstrates a competent valve, although occasionally stenosis and regurgitation are present. Three-dimensional echocardiography provides a more complete picture, as the whole valve from annulus to papillary muscle can be appreciated in one view. In addition, imaging the precise area of each orifice is possible with this technique (Fig. 9.17).

It is more difficult with two-dimensional echocardiography to appreciate a double orifice when seen in the setting of an atrioventricular septal defect, particular when there is a common atrioventricular valve. Although there are no studies available at present, there is the potential that three-dimensional echocardiography will overcome this limitation, mainly due to the ability of this modality to obtain a pereception of depth.

A rarer abnormality that can result in congenital mitral valve regurgitation is hypoplasia of the mural leaflet such that the valve leaflets cannot coapt normally during systole. This can be appreciated with two-dimensional echocardiography from the parasternal long-axis and apical four-chamber views, where the leaflet appears to be relatively splinted during systole (Fig. 9.18A).

Three-dimensional echocardiography permits the evaluation of the extent of leaflet immobility, which can be best seen from either the "looking up" or en face views (Fig. 9.18B). These views also allow a detailed assessment of the extent of the regurgitant jet. For example, if the whole valve is involved, then the regurgitant jet extends from commissure to commissure. This is helpful to the surgeon when planning mitral valve repair, invariably through the use of leaflet extension and annuloplasty.

FIGURE 9.12. Isolated cleft of the mitral valve with significant regurgitation. Note that the edges of the cleft are thickened and unsupported. LA, left atrium; LV, left ventricle; RV, right ventricle.

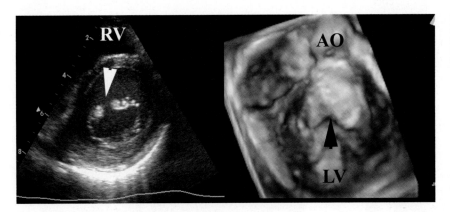

FIGURE 9.14. Cleft anterior mitral valve leaflet, which is only partial. Note that the two-dimensional appearance is similar to Figure 9.12, where the cleft extends toward the aortic valve. The three-dimensional image clearly demonstrates the extent of the cleft. AO, aortic valve; LV, left ventricle; RV, right ventricle.

Anomalies of the Tension Apparatus

Anomalies of the tension apparatus include the lesions variously referred to as *mitral arcade* or *hammock valve*. This abnormality is characterized by papillary muscles extending directly to the edges of the leaflets (Fig. 9.19). In the most severe form, the muscles fuse on the leading edge of the aortic leaflet, forming the muscular arcade observed by the pathologist or echocardiographer.

Straddling Mitral Valve – Mitral valve straddling occurs through an anterior ventricular septal defect, involving the anterior leaflet. It occurs more frequently in hearts where there is an abnormal ventriculoarterial connection, such as transposition with ventricular septal defect, or double-outlet right ventricle. There is invariably an associated cleft in the aortic leaflet, with the free edges being supported by the chordal apparatus. As a result, mitral valve regurgitation is uncommon, unlike the scenario of an isolated aortic cleft in the absence of a ventricular septal defect. The tension apparatus may be inserted into the crest of the interventricular septum, just to its right side, or to a major papillary muscle group situated more toward the apex of the right ventricle (Fig. 9.20). This entity is best appreciated in the parasternal long- and short-axis views, where the extent of the straddling and the associated cleft can be appreciated.

Mitral Valve Prolapse

Mitral valve prolapse is encountered less frequently in the pediatric age range in the absence of syndromes, such as Marfan syndrome. In the past, M-mode provided a gross overestimation of the true frequency, which was in part resolved by two-dimensional echocardiography. Even this did not completely resolve the issue, until three-dimensional techniques demonstrated that the mitral annulus was saddle shaped, with the four-chamber view again resulting in an overdiagnosis of this entity because it demonstrated the low points of the saddle. Therefore, mitral valve prolapse should be diagnosed only confidently in the long-axis view. Using such criteria, a report from the Framington study demonstrated an incidence of 2.4% in an adult population.

It is the mural leaflet that is most usually involved in floppy leaflets. The lesion may affect only one of its scallops, or the entire leaflet may be involved. It has been suggested that the mural leaflet of the mitral valve is less well supported at its free edges than its aortic counterpart, which may predispose it to prolapse.

The affected leaflets are grossly thickened with myxomatous transformation of their atrial aspect, with evidence of annular dilatation that is seen mostly on the atrial aspect of the leaflet. When studied microscopically, this is reflected by obvious myxomatous proliferation of the spongy layer of the leaflet. There is an increase

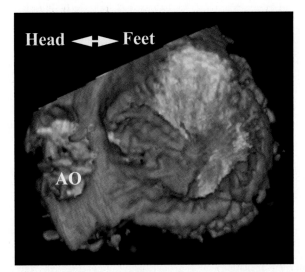

FIGURE 9.15. Three-dimensional color flow jet postoperative atrioventricular septal defect repair as seen from a surgical en face (left atrial) view. This image is from an older transesophageal three-dimensional rotation device. Note a larger jet of regurgitation from an area of leaflet deficiency, as well as another smaller jet along a commissure. AO, aorta.

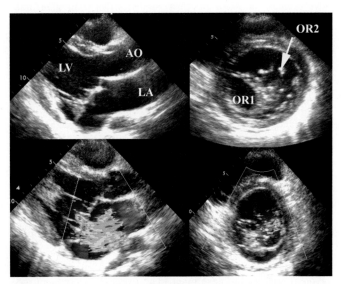

FIGURE 9.16. Two-dimensional echocardiogram in a double-orifice mitral valve. Note the smaller anterior orifice is regurgitant, unlike its larger counterpart. AO, aorta; LA, left atrium; LV, left ventricle; OR1, orifice 1; OR2, orifice 2.

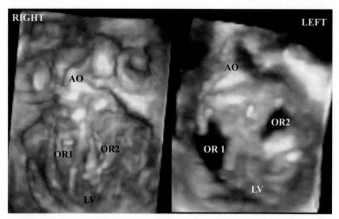

FIGURE 9.17. Three-dimensional echocardiographic images of the double-orifice mitral valve seen in Figure 9.16. The images are obtained by removing the front of the left ventricle, obtaining a view that looks down on top of the mitral valve. **Right:** Discrepancy in size of the two orifices. **Left:** Cut at a lower plane showing the supporting tension apparatus. AO, aorta; LV, left ventricle; OR1, orifice 1; OR2, orifice 2.

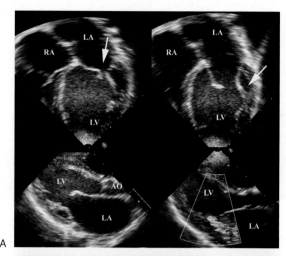

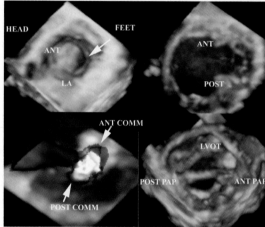

FIGURE 9.18. The upper four panels display two-dimensional echocardiographic images in the four-chamber and long axis projections from a patient with a tethered mural leaflet and significant mitral valve regurgitation. Note the relatively fixed position of the mural leaflet. The lower four panels are three-dimensional images of the mitral valve from the same case. **Bottom right:** The "looking up" view of the mitral valve as seen from the left ventricle. Note the tethering of the mural leaflet. **Bottom left:** Three-dimensional vena contracta, which extends from one commissure to the other. Note the improved visualization of the regurgitant jet, compared with the two-dimensional image. **Top left:** Surgical en face view, with the *arrow* pointing to the tethered mural leaflet. **Top right:** Two separate papillary muscles within the ventricular cavity. ANT, anterior; ANT COMM, anterior commissure; LA, left atrium; LV, left ventricle; LVOT, left ventricular outflow tract; POST COMM, posterior commissure; POST, posterior; POST PAP, posterior papillary muscle; RA, right atrium.

in the spongiosa layer including altered collagen and an increase in glycosaminoglycans and a disrupted fibrous backbone. Myxomatous valves show disorganized collagen and elastin fibers with pools of proteoglycans from the spongiosa layer present in the load-bearing fibrosa layer. Myxomatous chordae contain significantly more glycosaminoglycans than controls, specifically chondroitin dermatin-6-sulfate and hyaluroran, which binds more water, contributing to the enlarged gelatinous nature of chordae and leaflets. The end result is destruction of the fibrous core of the valve as the essence of the lesion.

Nonsyndromal mitral valve prolapse is most likely autosomal dominant with variable penetrance as there is clinical heterogeneity in families. It is well recognized that mitral valve prolapse is associated with Marfan syndrome. The recent ability to understand the three-dimensional nature of the mitral valve has provided greater diagnostic specifcity, which has aided in an improved understanding of the genetics of nonsyndromal mitral valve prolapse. Based on this new understanding, there has been a linkage of myxomatous mitral valve prolapse to chromosome 16 (MMVP1) in some families with an autosomal dominant form in others linked to MMVP2 on chromosome 11p15.4 and on 13q31.3-q32.1 in another. Some of the family studies have lead to a prodromal form with no actual mitral valve prolapse but with anteriorly shifted leaflet coaptation, indicating posterior leaflet elongation. Others have studied an X-linked valvular dystrophy that has been linked to filament A mutations. Therefore, mitral valve prolapse may be similar to hypertrophic cardiomyopathy with multiple genetic abnormalities responsible for a common phenotype.

Echocardiographic Assessment of Mitral Valve Prolapse –

Two-dimensional echocardiography enhances the diagnosis of prolapse by enhancing the spatial configuration of the valvar leaflets. During diastole, the leaflets of the normal valve lie widely open and are more-or-less parallel, as seen in long-axis sections. With the onset of systole, the two leaflets coapt to give a funnel-shaped appearance. As systole continues, the line of coaptation moves anteriorly and lags behind the aortic root. The entire valvar apparatus then moves anteriorly and inferiorly. Both leaflets frequently arch slightly toward each other and become more horizontal, but no part of the leaflets appears above the atrioventricular junction. Volume overload of the left ventricle from a ventricular septal defect results in an increase in the total excursion of the mitral valve and an even more horizontal position of the leaflets during ventricular systole.

In prolapsing valves, the mural or, less often, the aortic leaflet (or both) arch toward each other to an excessive degree and pass above the plane of the atrioventricular junction into the left atrium (Fig. 9.21). Either an individual component of the valve is involved, or there is pansystolic hammocking. If records of motion are made

from the body of the leaflets rather than from their free edges, about one in six normal patients will have pseudo-prolapse owing to holosystolic hammocking. Even mid-systolic buckling can be artefactually produced in patients with ventricular septal defect and normal mitral valves.

Transesophageal multiplane echocardiography has been a useful tool to identify specific leaflet prolapse. At 20 degrees, scallops A3–P1 are seen; at 60 degrees, scallops P3–A2–P1 are demonstrated; at 90 degrees, scallops P3–A1 are visualized; and at 120 to 160 degrees, scallops A2–P2 are seen. Even though this description has been helpful to the cardiologist and surgeon, this is being replaced by three-dimensional echocardiography to aid in the diagnosis and surgical planning of patients with mitral valve prolapse (Fig. 9.22). Indeed, en face surgical views can be obtained from either the transthoracic approach using either real-time three-dimensional echocardiography or, until recently, by transesophageal echocardiography using a rotational device. There is good evidence emerging that this technique is superior to either transthoracic or transesophageal two-dimensional echocardiography

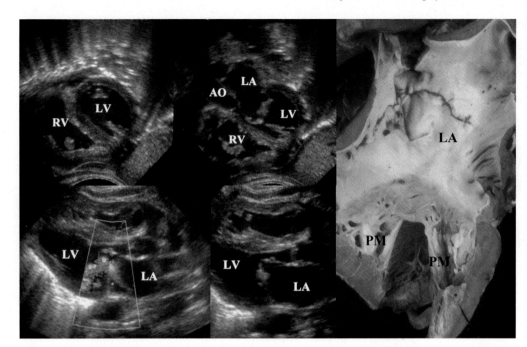

FIGURE 9.19. Two-dimensional echocardiogram and anatomic specimen (right) from the same patient with a form of mitral arcade. Note the complete fusion of the papillary muscles to the supporting tension apparatus and leaflets. This patient had severe mitral valve stenosis. AO, aorta; LA, left atrium; LV, left ventricle; PM, papillary muscle; RV, right ventricle.

with regard to specific leaflet pathology, as well as commissural abnormalities. There are little data on the use of three-dimensional echocardiography in the pediatric population. Recent reports, however, using the transesophageal rotation device have demonstrated additive value to standard two-dimensional assessment.

More recently, real-time three-dimensional tranesophageal echocardiography has become available, although its application is limited to older children and adults. Indeed, current real-time three-dimensional TEE probes are slightly larger than the standard biplane probes, which limits use to children who are about 18 kg and greater. Despite the size limitation, three-dimensional TEE provides superior images of the mitral valve. In a real-time mode it can be used to guide catheter interventions, although at the expense of frame rate.

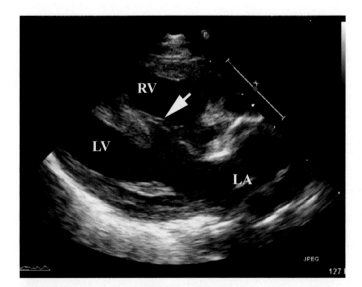

FIGURE 9.20. Parasternal long-axis view in a straddling mitral valve in the setting of ventriculo-arterial discordance and pulmonary outflow tract obstruction. Note the tension apparatus from the anterior leaflet that is inserted onto the right side of the interventricular septum (arrow).

ASSESSMENT OF STENOSIS AND REGURGITATION: QUALITATIVE OR QUANTITATIVE?

Mitral Valve Stenosis

A detailed assessment of mitral valve morphology is important, as this, in conjunction with the hemodynamic effects, determines not only the timing but also the type of intervention. For example, classic dysplastic mitral valve stenosis, without an associated supramitral ring, appears to respond more favorably to balloon dilatation. In adults, the pressure half-time provides an accurate assessment of mitral valve area, independent of cardiac output. This same technique can be applied to children, although absolute valve areas calculated in this way are of little value because of the wide variation in body surface area. Mean gradients across the mitral valve have traditionally been used in assessment of congenital heart disease, despite the limitation of its dependency on cardiac output (Fig. 9.23). Left atrial size is of value, although in some cases the presence of endocardial fribroelastosis of the left atrium prevents dilatation. In addition, the presence of an associated patent foramen ovale or atrial septal defect reduces the value of Doppler mitral inflow assessment. As congenital mitral valve stenosis rarely occurs in isolation, increased inflow from an associated left-to-right shunt at the ventricular or great vessel level provides additional confusion. An assessment of pulmonary arterial pressure, resulting from either tricuspid regurgitation or pulmonary insufficiency, is of value as invariably the greater the stenosis, the more likely there is to be associated pulmonary hypertension.

Mitral Valve Regurgitation

Left Atrial and Left Ventricular Size – In general, there is left atrial and ventricular enlargement in chronic mitral valve regurgitation. These are good indicators of the severity of regurgitation, and indeed both left ventricular end-systolic and end-diastolic dimensions are used to determine optimal timing for surgical intervention. In children, these measurements, as a true representation of the effect of the mitral regurgitation, are less subject to other variables that influence dimensions in an adult population. For example, diastolic dysfunction secondary to aging and ischemic regurgitation is rarely

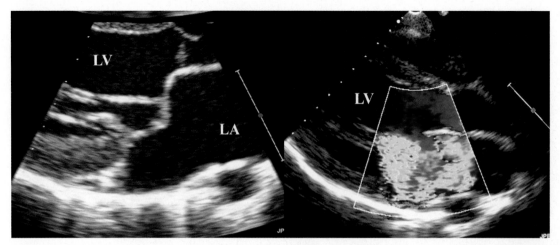

FIGURE 9.21. Parasternal long-axis view in mitral valve prolapse of the aortic leaflet. Note the significant regurgitation seen (**right**). LA, left atrium; LV, left ventricle.

an issue in the pediatric population. The one potential problem that might be encountered is in the patient with an underlying dilated cardiomyopathy who has associated mitral regurgitation.

Primary mitral valve regurgitation is uncommon in the infant and toddler and, if seen, the echocardiographer should pay particular attention to the status of the coronary arteries to exlclude an anomalous left coronary artery from the pulmonary artery. In this setting, the right coronary artery is usually dilated and provides an initial clue, with color Doppler permitting the identification of the abnormal origin, as well as the collateral flow.

Pulmonary Venous Doppler Flow Pattern – In general, systolic flow reversal in the pulmonary veins is a useful sign of significant mitral valve regurgitation. Care must be taken to sample all pulmonary veins, as a regurgitant jet may be directed toward one particular vein. Limitations of this technique relate to those patients with diastolic dysfunction, when the systolic pulmonary venous Doppler profile is blunted due to the raised left atrial pressure (Fig. 9.24).

Continuous Wave Doppler Regurgitant Jet Profile – In general, the more severe the regurgitation, the denser the continuous-wave Doppler profile (Fig. 9.24).

Mitral E Velocity Dominance – In general, patients with more severe regurgitation have a dominant Doppler E profile through the mitral valve (Fig. 9.24). Again, the main limitation here is in those cases with associated diastolic dysfunction.

Quantitative Assessment of Mitral Regurgitation by Doppler
PULSED DOPPLER ASSESSMENT OF REGURGITANT FRACTION, VOLUME, AND EFFECTIVE REGURGITANT ORIFICE AREA – This technique measures the stroke volume through the mitral valve and aorta, the difference of which represents the volume of regurgitation:

$$SV = CSA \times VTI = \pi d^2/4 \times VTI = 0.785 d^2 \times VTI$$

where SV is stroke volume, CSA is cross-sectional area, d is annular diameter and VTI is velocity-time integral. Therefore,

$$Regurgitant\ volume\ (mL) = SV_{MV} - SV_{LVOT}$$

$$Regurgitant\ fraction = (SV_{MV} - SV_{LVOT})/SV_{MV}$$

where MV is mitral valve and LVOT is left ventricular outlow tract. Limitations relate to cross-sectional area measurements, as any measurement errors are squared. Measurement errors can also

FIGURE 9.22. Three-dimensional echo viewed from the left ventricle. Note how A2 buckles back into the left atrium during systole, as seen by the indentation into the left atrium. A2, area of the aortic mitral leaflet; PAP, papillary muscle; RV, right ventricle.

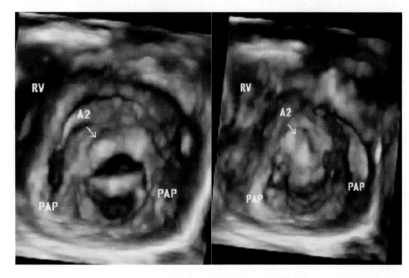

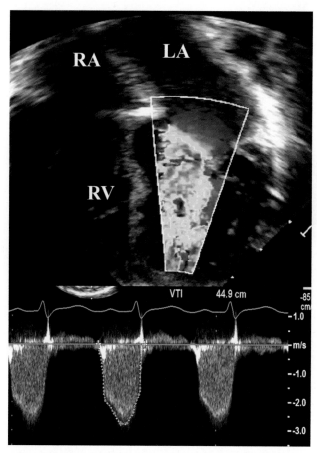

FIGURE 9.23. Continuous-wave and color Doppler in congenital mitral valve stenosis. Note that it is only possible to obtain a mean Doppler gradient and not a pressure half-time. LA, left atrium; RA, right atrium; RV, right ventricle.

be caused by poor Doppler alignment and failure to properly trace the modal velocity. Similar measurements can be made by calculating the left ventricular stroke volume with the use of biplane Simpson's rule and subtracting the left ventricular outflow stroke volume determined with Doppler. The main problem with this methodology relates to obtaining accurate and reprodicible stroke volume measurements by biplane Simpsons rule.

Contribution of Color Flow Doppler – Color Doppler is essential to identify the presence of mitral regurgitation and to pinpoint the site of insufficiency. This has been enhanced with the advent of three-dimensional echocardiography. It is important to understand some of the limitations of two-dimensional color flow mapping. Color flow mapping measures velocity and not volume, so it is very gain sensitive. In addition, it is affected by adjacent boundaries with the coanda affect having an impact on apparent jet size when the regurgitation is not central. For all these reasons, there has been a concerted effort to provide a volumetric assessment of regurgitation. Unlike its two-dimensional counterpart, this three-dimensional technique permits the construction of en face views, as seen by the surgeon, or 'looking up' views from the left ventricle, as seen by the echocardiographer. These permit a detailed assessment of the site of the regurgitant jet(s) (Fig. 9.15), as well as of the size of the vena contracta (the width of the jet origin). There is good evidence that the vena contracta size is an accurate representation of the volume of regurgitant flow (Figs. 9.8 and 9.18). Thus, by summating the vena contractas, a semiquantitatiive assessment of regurgitant volume can be assessed. This helps to overcome the limitations of color flow mapping by two-dimensional echocardiography. Although it is possible to measure vena contracta diameter by this method, it does not take shape into consideration. When imaged by three-dimensional echocardiography, it is clear that many vena contractas are irregular in shape hence, the potential for underestimation or overestimation of size. In addition, identifying multiple jets and those involving the commissures is problematic by two-dimensional echocardiography. At present, three-dimensional color flow Doppler is still somewhat crude, with gain dependency and some overlapping with tissues. Also, current vena contracta assessment is usually done during one phase of systole, which does not take the dynamic variation of regurgitation into consideration.

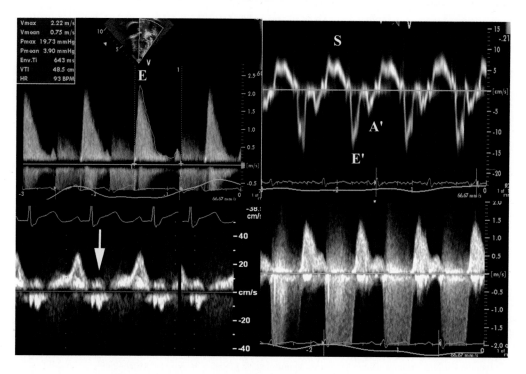

FIGURE 9.24. Doppler profiles from a child with significant mitral valve regurgitation. Top left: Dominant "E" wave. **Bottom left:** Blunted systolic forward flow in the pulmonary veins. **Top right:** Normal mitral annular tissue Doppler. **Bottom right:** Dense continuous-wave Doppler profile of mitral regurgitation.

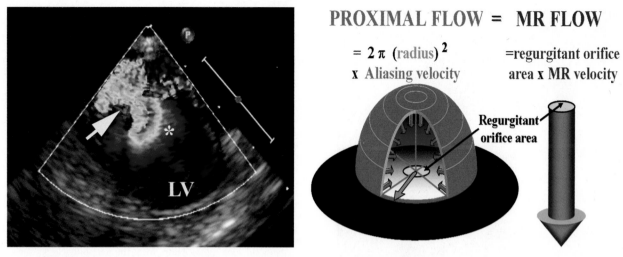

FIGURE 9.25. Proximal isovelocity surface area (PISA). A: Anatomy of a regurgitant color flow jet. Note the PISA (*asterisk*) and the vena contracta (outlined by *arrow*). LV, left ventricle. **B:** Cartoon demonstrating PISA and the measurements that are made in the PISA calculation. (**B**, Courtesy of Dr. Brian Sonnenberg.)

Proximal Isovelocity Surface Area or Flow Convergence

Proximal isovelocity surface area (PISA) is based on the principle that as blood approaches an orifice, it forms a series of concentric, roughly hemispheric shells that increase in velocity but decrease in area (Fig. 9.25A). In practical terms, the color Doppler Nyquist limit is set to a value at which aliasing occurs near the regurgitant orifice. From this the regurgitant flow is calculated as:

$$2\pi r^2 \times V_a$$

where r is radius of aliasing velocity and V_a is velocity at which aliasing occurs. From this, effective regurgitant orifice area (EROA) can be calculated as: Regurgitant flow/Peak velocity of regurgitation (Fig. 9.25B). Limitations of this technique are related to (a) the shape of the PISA shell, which may not be a hemisphere, (b) multiple jets, and (c) the effect of adjacent boundaries as well as in determining the precise location of the regurgitant orifice. A recent study comparing two-dimensional PISA calculation of regurgitant volume to that measured by real-time three-dimensional echocardiography showed that the former method significantly underestimated the true volume in comparison to actual volume.

Transesophageal Echocardiography

Transesophageal echocardiography has provided an additional tool for the evaluation of the congenitally abnormal mitral valve. Fortunately, apart from the older child or obese patient, this technique is unnecessary in the majority of cases. It is also apparent that transesophageal color flow mapping appears to be more sensitive than transthoracic assessment. Systematic overestimation of the severity of regurgitation is found when it is compared with standard transthoracic assessment.

FUTURE DIRECTIONS

What is needed to optimally assess mitral regurgitation is a true volumetric assessment of regurgitant volume by three-dimensional echocardiography. A first attempt at this using matrix array technology has provided encouraging results. Using broad-beam spectral Doppler on a matrix probe, it has been possible to measure a power velocity integral (PVI), which represents volume flow. The strength of this technique is that it takes into consideration variations of the regurgitant volume throughout systole. The current limitation is that

it is a prototype and still has a limited window; hence, it is applicable to single, more central jets.

TIMING OF INTERVENTION IN MITRAL REGURGITATION

It is currently unclear whether an increase in the size of the left ventricle represents a deterioration in ventricular function or just an alteration to accommodate an increase in regurgitant volume. The "Holy Grail" of echocardiography is to match reproducible and accurate volume changes with alterations in left ventricular function, which then predicts timing for intervention. Currently echocardiographers of the adult population struggle with this, so in the pediatric population, congenital echocardiographers are at even a greater disadvantage due to the smaller measurements that are being making.

What is probably safer is an extrapolation from adult data using an indexed end-systolic diameter of greater than 4.5 cm or an ejection fraction by volumetric assessment of less than 60% as echocardiographic indications for valve surgery in those with predominant mitral valve regurgitation. Of course, patient growth, symptoms, and pulmonary artery pressure have to be factored into the equation. In addition, it is unclear whether this extrapolation is an accurate one or whether the pediatric left ventricle is more robust than its "adult" counter part.

SUGGESTED READING

Agricols E, Oppizzi M, De Bonis M, et al. Multiplane transesophageal echocardiography performed according to the guidelines of the American Society of Echocardiography in patients with mitral valve prolapse, flail, and endocarditis: diagnostic accuracy in the identification of mitral regurgitant defects by correlation with surgical findings. *J Am Soc Echocardiogr.* 2003;16:61–66.

Arora R, Mukhopadhyay S, Yusuf J, et al. Technique, results, and follow-up of interventional treatment of rheumatic mitral stenosis in children. *Cardiol Young.* 2007;17: 3–11.

Asante-Korang A, O'Leary PO, Anderson RH. Anatomy and echo of the normal and abnormal mitral valve. *Cardiol Young.* 2006;16:27–34.

Banerjee A, Kohl T, Silverman NH. Echocardiographic evaluation of congenital mitral valve anomalies in children. *Am J Cardiol.* 1995;76: 1284–1291.

Barrea C, Levasseur S, Roman K, et al. Three-dimensional echocardiography improves the understanding of left atrioventricular valve morphology and function in atrioventricular septal defects undergoing patch augmentation. *J Thorac Cardiovasc Surg.* 2005;129:746–753.

Becker AE, de Wit APM. Mitral valve apparatus. A spectrum of normality relevant to mitral valve prolapse. *Br Heart J.* 1979;42:690.

Becker AE. Valve pathology in the paediatric age group. In: Anderson RH, MaCartney FJ, Shinebourne EA, Tynan M, eds. *Paediatric cardiology*, vol 5. Edinburgh: Churchill Livingstone; 1983:345–360.

Bini RM, Pellegrino PA, Mazzucco A, et al. Tricuspid atresia with double-outlet left atrium. *Chest.* 1980;78:109–111.

Bonow RO, Carabello BA, Chatterjee K, et al.; Writing Committee Members. ACC/AHA 2006 guidelines for the management of patients with valvular heart disease: executive summary. *J Am Coll Cardiol.* 2006;114:450–527.

Borer JS, Bonow RO. Contemporary approach to aortic and mitral regurgitation. *Circulation.* 2003;108:2432–2438.

Buck T, Plicht P, Hunold P, et al. Broad beam spectral Doppler sonification of the vena contracta using matrix-array technology. *J Am Coll Cardiol.* 2005;45:770–779.

Carlhall C, Wigstrom L, Heiberg E, et al. Contribution of mitral annular excursion and shape dynamics to total left ventricular volume change. *Am J Physiol Heart Circ Physiol.* 2004;287:H1836–H1841.

Carpentier A, Branchini B, Cour JC, et al. Congenital malformations of the mitral valve in children. Pathology and surgical treatment. *J Thorac Cardiovasc Surg.* 1976;72:854–866.

Castello R, Lenzen P, Aguire F, et al. Variability in the quantitation of mitral regurgitation by Doppler color flow mapping; comparison of transthoracic and transesophageal studies. *J Am Coll Cardiol.* 1992;20:433–438.

Chao K, Moises VA, Shandas R, et al. Influence of the Coanda effect on color Doppler jet area and color encoding. In vitro studies using color Doppler flow mapping. *Circulation.* 1992;85:333–341.

Cheitlin MD. Valvular heart disease: management and intervention. *Circulation.* 1991;84(suppl I):I-259–I-264.

Collins-Nakai RL, Rosenthal A, Castaneda AR, et al. Congenital mitral stenosis. A review of 20 years' experience. *Circulation.* 1977;56:1039–1046.

Coto EO, Jimenez MQ, Deverall PB, et al. Anomalous mitral 'cleft' with abnormal ventriculoarterial connection: anatomical findings and surgical implications. *Pediatr Cardiol.* 1984;5:1–6.

Daliento L, Thiene G, Chirillo F, et al. Congenital mitral valve malformations: clinical and morphological aspects. *Ital J Cardiol.* 1991;21:1205–1216.

de Lange FJ, Moorman AFM, Anderson RH, et al. Lineage and morphogenetic analysis of the cardiac valves. *Circ Res.* 2004;95:645–654.

Enriquez-Sarano M, Bailey KR, Seward JB, et al. Quantitative Doppler assessment of valvular regurgitation. *Circulation.* 1993;87:841–848.

Feigenbaum H. Echocardiography in the management of mitral valve prolapse. *Austral N Z J Med.* 1992;22:550–555.

Fernex M, Fernex C. La degenerescence mucoide des valvules mitrales. Ses repercussions functionelles. *Helv Med Acta.* 1958;25:694–705.

Freed LA, Levy D, Levine RA, et al. Prevalence and clinical outcome of mitral-valve prolapse. *N Engl J Med.* 1999;341:41–47.

García-Orta R, Moreno E, Vidal M, et al. Three-dimensional versus two-dimensional transesophageal echocardiography in mitral valve repair. *J Am Soc Echocardiogr.* 2007;20:4–12.

Glasson JR, Komeda M, Daughters GT, et al. Most ovine mitral annular three-dimensional size reduction occurs before ventricular systole and is abolished with ventricular pacing. *Circulation.* 1997;96(9 suppl):II-2.

Goldberg SJ, Gerlis LM, Ho SY, et al. Location of the left papillary muscles in juxtaductal aortic coarctation. *Am J Cardiol.* 1995;75:746–750.

Grande-Allen KJ, Griffin BP, Calabro A, et al. Myxomatous mitral valve chordae. II: Selective elevation of glycosaminoglycan content. *J Heart Valve Dis.* 2001;10:325–332; discussion 332–323.

Hatle L, Brubakk A, Tromsdal A, et al. Noninvasive assessment of pressure drop in mitral stenosis by Doppler ultrasound. *Br Heart J.* 1978;40:131–140.

Kanani M, Moorman AFM, Cook AC, et al. Development of the atrioventricular valves: clinicomorphologic correlations. *Ann Thorac Surg.* 2005;79:1797–1804.

Karlsson MO, Glasson JR, Bolger AF, et al. Mitral valve opening in the ovine heart. *Am J Physiol.* 1998;274(2 Pt 2):H552–H563.

Karr SS, Parness IA, Spevak PJ, et al. Diagnosis of anomalous left coronary artery by Doppler color flow mapping: distinction from other causes of dilated cardiomyopathy. *J Am Coll Cardiol.* 1992;19:1271–1275.

Kohl T, Silverman N. Comparison of cleft and papillary muscle position in cleft mitral valve and atrioventricular septal defect. *Am J Cardiol.* 1996;77:164–169.

Koike K, Musewe NM, Smallhorn JF, et al. Distinguishing between anomalous origin of the left coronary artery from the pulmonary trunk and dilated cardiomyopathy: role of echocardiographic measurement of the right coronary artery diameter. *Br Heart J.* 1989;61:192–197.

Kwan J, Qin JX, Popovic ZB, et al. Geometric changes of mitral annulus assessed by real-time 3-dimensional echocardiography: becoming enlarged and less nonplanar in the anteroposterior direction during systole in proportion to global left ventricular systolic function. *J Am Soc Echocardiogr.* 2004;17:1179–1184.

Levine RA, Slaugenhaupt SA. Molecular genetics of mitral valve prolapse. *Curr Opin Cardiol.* 2007;22:171–175.

Lansac E, Lim KH, Shomura Y, et al. Dynamic balance of the aortomitral junction. *J Thorac Cardiovasc Surg.* 2002;123:911–918.

Layman TE, Edwards JE. Anomalous mitral arcade. A type of congenital mitral insufficiency. *Circulation.* 1967;35:389–395.

Leung M, Rigby ML, Anderson RH, et al. Reversed offsetting of the septal attachments of the atrioventricular valves and Ebstein's malformation of the morphologically mitral valve. *Br Heart J.* 1987;57:184–187.

Levine RA, Triulzi MO, Harrigan P, et al. The relationship of mitral annular shape to the diagnosis of mitral valve prolapse. *Circulation.* 1987;75:756–767.

Little SH, Igo SR, Pirat B, et al. In vitro validation of real-time three-dimensional color Doppler echocardiography for direct measurement of proximal isovelocity surface area in mitral regurgitation. *Am J Cardiol.* 2007;99:1440–1447.

Malkowski MJ, Boudoulas H, Wooley CF, et al. Spectrum of structural abnormalities in floppy mitral valve echocardiographic evaluation. *Am Heart J.* 1996;132:145–151.

McElhinney DB, Sherwood MC, Keane JF, et al. Current management of severe congenital mitral stenosis, outcomes of transcatheter and surgical therapy in 108 infants and children. *Circulation.* 2005;112:707–714.

Mele D, Soukhomovskaia O, Pacchioni E, et al. Proximal flow convergence region as assessed by real-time three-dimensional echocardiography: challenging the hemispheric assumption. *J Am Soc Echocardiogr.* 2007;20:389–396.

Mickell JJ, Mathews RA, Anderson RH, et al. The anatomical heterogeneity of hearts lacking a patent communication between the left atrium and the ventricular mass ('mitral atresia') in presence of a patent aortic valve. *Eur Heart J.* 1983;4:477–486.

Moreno F, Quero M, Diaz LP. Mitral atresia with normal aortic valve. A study of eighteen cases and a review of the literature. *Circulation.* 1976;53:1004–1010.

Müller S, Müller L, Laufer G, et al. Comparison of three-dimensional imaging to transesophageal echocardiography for preoperative evaluation in mitral valve prolapse. *Am J Cardiol.* 2006;98:243–248.

Nii M, Roman KS, Macgowan CK, et al. Insight into normal mitral and tricuspid annular dynamics in pediatrics: a real-time three-dimensional echocardiographic study. *J Am Soc Echocardiogr.* 2006.

Oberhansli I, Baldovinos A, Beghetti M, et al. Hypoplasia of the posterior leaflet as a rare cause of congenital mitral insufficiency. *J Card Surg.* 1997;12:339–342.

Otsuji Y, Gilon D, Jiang L, et al. Restricted diastolic opening of the mitral leaflets in patients with left ventricular dysfunction: evidence for increased valve tethering. *J Am Coll Cardiol.* 1998;32:398–404.

Passafini A, Shiota T, Depp M, et al. Factors influencing pulmonary venous flow velocity patterns in mitral regurgitation: an in vitro study. *J Am Coll Cardiol.* 1995;26:1333–1339.

Patel V, Hsiung MC, Nanda NC, et al. Usefulness of live/real time three-dimensional transthoracic echocardiography in the identification of individual segment/scallop prolapse of the mitral valve. *Echocardiography.* 2006;23:513–518.

Pepi M, Tamborini G, Maltagliati A, et al. Head-to head comparison of two- and three-dimensional transthoracic and transesophageal echocardiography in the localization of mitral valve. *J Am Coll Cardiol.* 2006;48:2524–2530.

Ruckman RN, Van Praagh R. Anatomic types of congenital mitral stenosis: report of 49 autopsy cases with consideration of diagnosis and surgical implications. *Am J Cardiol.* 1978;42:592–601.

Salgo IS, Gorman JH 3rd, Gorman RC, et al. Effect of annular shape on leaflet curvature in reducing mitral leaflet stress. *Circulation.* 2002;106:711–717.

Shone JD, Sellers RD, Anderson RC, et al. The developmental complex of 'parachute mitral valve,' supravalvular ring of left atrium, subaortic stenosis, and coarctation of aorta. *Am J Cardiol.* 1963;11:714–725.

Sigfusson G, Ettedgui JA, Silverman NH, et al. Is a cleft in the anterior leaflet of an otherwise normal mitral valve an atrioventricular canal malformation? *J Am Coll Cardiol.* 1995;26:508–515.

Sittiwangkul R, Ma RY, McCrindle BW, et al. The echocardiographic assessment of obstructive lesions in atrioventricular septal defect. *J Am Coll Cardiol.* 2001;38:253–261.

Smallhorn JF, De Leval M, Stark J, et al. Isolated anterior mitral cleft. Two dimensional echocardiographic assessment and differentiation from 'clefts' associated with atrioventricular septal defect. *Br Heart J.* 1982;48:109–116.

Smallhorn JF, Sutherland GR, Anderson RH, et al. Cross-sectional echocardiographic assessment of conditions with atrioventricular valve leaflets attached to the atrial septum at the same level. *Br Heart J.* 1982;48:331–341.

Sugeng L, Shernan SK, Salgo IS, et al. Live three-dimensional transesophageal echocardiography: initial experience using a full-sampled matrix array probe. *J Am Coll Cardiol.* 2008;52:446–449.

Sugeng L, Shernan SK, Weinert L, et al. Real-time three-dimensional transesophageal echocardiography in valve disease: comparison with surgical findings and evaluation of prosthetic valves. *J Am Soc Echocardiogr.* 2008;21:1347–1354.

Sugeng L, Weinert BS, Lang RM. Real time three-dimensional color Doppler flow of mitral and tricuspid valve regurgitation: feasibility and initial quantitative comparison with 2-dimensional methods. *J Am Soc Echocardiogr.* 2007;20:1050–1057.

Sullivan ID, Robinson PJ, de Leval M, et al. Membranous supravalvular mitral stenosis: a treatable form of congenital heart disease. *J Am Coll Cardiol.* 1986;8:159–164.

Takahashi K, Guerra V, Roman KS, et al. Three-dimensional echocardiography improves the understanding of the mechanisms and site of left atrioventricular valve regurgitation in atrioventricular septal defect. *J Am Soc Echocardiogr.* 2006;19:1502–1510.

Tamura M, Menahem S, Brizard C. Clinical features and management of isolated cleft mitral valve in childhood. *J Am Coll Cardiol.* 2000;35:764–770.

Timòteo A, Galrinho A, Fiarresga A, et al. Isolated cleft of the anterior mitral valve leaflet. *Eur J Echocardiogr.* 2005;8:59–62.

Tsakiris AG, Von Bernuth G, Rastelli C, et al. Size and motion of the mitral valve annulus in anesthetized dog hearts. *J Appl Physiol.* 1971;30:611–618.

Van der Bel Kahn J, Duren DR, Becker AE. Isolated mitral valve prolapse: chordal architecture as an anatomic basis in older patients. *J Am Coll Cardiol.* 1985;5:1335–1340.

Watson DG, Rowe RD, Coren PE, et al. Mitral atresia with normal aortic valve. Report of 11 cases and review of the literature. *Pediatrics.* 1960;25:450–467.

Wenink ACG, Goot GD, Brom AG. Developmental considerations of mitral valve anomalies. *Int J Cardiol.* 1986;11:85–98.

Yellin EL, Peskin C, Yoran C, et al. Mechanisms of mitral valve motion during diastole. *Am J Physiol Heart Circ Physiol.* 1981;241:H389–H400.

Zoghbi WA, Enriquez-Sarano M, Foster E, et al. Recommendations for evaluation of the severity of native valvar regurgitation with two-dimensional and Doppler echocardiography. *J Am Soc Echocardiogr.* 2003;16:777–802.

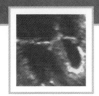

Chapter 10
Congenitally Corrected Transposition of the Great Arteries

Michael G. Earing • Nancy A. Ayres • Frank Cetta

Congenitally corrected transposition of the great arteries (CCTGA) is an uncommon cardiac anomaly. It is characterized by atrioventricular (AV) and ventriculoarterial (VA) discordance (Fig. 10.1). The discordance of both the AV and VA connections results in a situation where the systemic and pulmonary venous returns are appropriately directed to the pulmonary artery and aorta. However, the arrangement of the morphologic ventricles "between" the venous and arterial segments is the opposite of normal. The systemic venous return connects with the right atrium normally. The right atrium is then connected to the morphologic left ventricle (LV) via a mitral valve that is in turn connected to the pulmonary artery. There is no subpulmonary infundibulum because this is a morphologic LV and therefore there is mitral valve–pulmonary valve fibrous continuity. The pulmonary veins connect to the left atrium. The left atrium is then connected to the morphologic right ventricle (RV) via a tricuspid valve. The RV (systemic ventricle) is connected to the aorta. In CCTGA, the aorta is positioned anterior and leftward of the pulmonary artery with a well-developed subaortic infundibulum resulting in discontinuity between the tricuspid and aortic valves.

CCTGA is often referred to as "*l*" (*levo*)-transposition of the great arteries. This "*l*" refers to the leftward embryologic looping of the ventricles and not the spatial relationship of the great arteries. It is a confusing term given that many other complex conditions, including single ventricles, can have *l*-transposed (anterior and leftward) great arteries. Simply referring to CCTGA as "corrected transposition" is also inadequate since patients with complete or *d* (*dextro*)-TGA may have been "surgically corrected." For these reasons, the authors prefer the term "congenitally corrected transposition of the great arteries (CCTGA)" to describe patients with atrioventricular and ventriculoarterial discordance.

ECHOCARDIOGRAPHIC ASSESSMENT

Echocardiography is the imaging modality that provides the most robust diagnostic assessment of CCTGA. The unusual relationship between the two ventricles, ventricular septum, and the great arteries results in several unique echocardiographic features. These relationships make this malformation easily recognized by echocardiography. Similar to other forms of transposition of the great arteries, the initial (unbranched) segments of the great arteries run parallel to each other (Fig. 10.2). In addition, unlike the normal heart, the ventricles assume more of a side-by-side relationship, and as result, the ventricular septum is oriented in a straight anteroposterior plane (Fig. 10.3). In some cases, the ventricles are arranged in a superior-inferior manner with the morphologic RV being superior. The diagnosis of CCTGA is based on demonstrating discordance of both the AV and the VA connections [right atrium (RA) to morphologically left ventricle (mLV) to pulmonary artery (PA), and left atrium (LA) to morphologically right ventricle (mRV) to aorta]. The spatial relationship of the great arteries supports the diagnosis of CCTGA; however, it should not be considered the sole diagnostic criterion.

The subcostal and apical 4-chamber imaging planes are extremely useful in the examination of patients with CCTGA. The subcostal plane is used to define the atrial and visceral situs and the cardiac position. In 25% of cases, patients with CCTGA have dextrocardia or mesocardia (Fig. 10.4). The subcostal imaging planes also allow excellent imaging of the great arteries and their relationships of the ventricular chambers. From the subcostal coronal imaging plane, the parallel arrangement of the great arteries can be easily identified (Fig. 10.2). In addition, the unique relationship of the left ventricular outflow tract and the pulmonary artery can be seen with pulmonary outflow tract deeply wedged between the right and left atrioventricular valves (Fig. 10.5). Most important, in this imaging plane, the relationship of the atria, ventricles, and the great arteries can be defined. As described in previous chapters, a mRV can be defined by the presence of several unique anatomic features:

1. an apical position of the AV valve's septal attachment (relative to the contralateral AV valve's septal hinge),
2. presence of a trileaflet AV valve with chordal attachments to the ventricular septum,
3. presence of a moderator band,

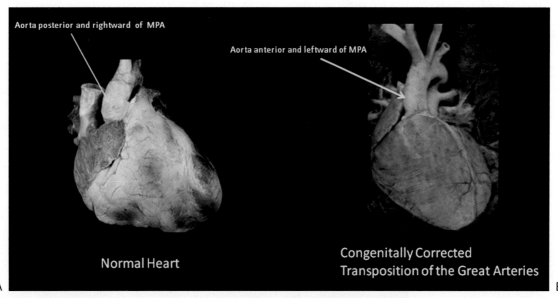

FIGURE 10.1. Pathology specimen. A: Normal relationship of great arteries to the ventricles (ventriculoatrial [VA] concordance) and normally related atrioventricular relationships (AV concordance). **B:** Congenitally corrected transposition of the great arteries with AV discordance and VA discordance. Aorta sits anterior and leftward to main pulmonary artery. (From the Dr. William Edwards collection, Mayo Clinic.)

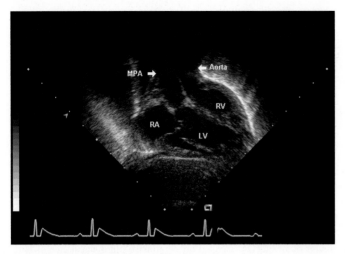

FIGURE 10.2. Subcostal imaging plane with transducer angulated anterior to demonstrate parallel relationship of great arteries.

4. an irregular (trabeculated) mural endocardial surface, and
5. a pyramidal (instead of elliptical) shape to the ventricular cavity (Fig. 10.3).

In the most common form of CCTGA (Fig. 10.6), the pulmonary veins will connect to the left-sided atrium (LA). The LA in turn connects to a morphologic RV via a tricuspid valve. The RV then connects to a great artery that arches and gives rise to coronary arteries, and is by definition the aorta. On the other side of the heart, the systemic veins connect to the right atrium (RA), which then connects to a morphologic LV. The LV connects to a great artery that bifurcates into two branches, and is by definition the pulmonary artery. In the young patient, these connections and relationships can be observed from the subcostal transducer position.

Similar to the subcostal coronal imaging plane, the apical four chamber imaging plane is extremely useful in the setting of CCTGA. In fact, the key anatomic feature of AV discordance is best visualized in the four chamber plane. In the four chamber image, the septal hinge points of the AV valves are readily appreciated (Figure 10.3). In concordant AV connections, the AV valve associated with the RA and RV will have a septal hinge that is positioned somewhat more toward the apex when compared to the contralateral valve. In CCTGA, due to the discordant connection, it is the left sided AV valve hinge point that is closer to the ventricular apex. Additional scans from the apical transducer position can define the anatomy of the atrioventricular valves, ventricular morphology, discordant atrioventricular connec-

tions, and ventriculoarterial relationships (Fig. 10.9A). In addition, atrioventricular valve abnormalities and outflow tract obstruction can be evaluated (Fig. 10.9B). In typical CCTGA, the apical four chamber view is useful to evaluate muscular VSDs.

Apical four chamber imaging is more challenging when the ventricles are positioned in a superior and inferior fashion. In these patients it will not be possible to image both atrioventricular valves in the same plane. In this setting, the transducer will need to be tilted inferiorly to see the right-sided morphologically mitral valve and superiorly to see the left-sided morphologically tricuspid valve. The septal hinge-point relationship can therefore be more difficult to appreciate. The diagnosis of CCTGA in these patients relies more on the other features which define ventricular morphology.

The side-by-side relationship of the ventricles, more vertical orientation of the ventricular septum, and side-by-side relationship of the great arteries all make the parasternal long-axis views in CCTGA confusing. Unlike in the normal heart, the long axis in CCTGA is more vertically oriented (Fig. 10.7). This allows easy confirmation of the parallel arrangement of the great arteries in CCTGA. However, because of the side by side relationship of the ventricles, when the transducer is placed in the standard long-axis imaging position, several long axis views can be obtained including a long-axis image through the morphologic LV and pulmonary artery on the right (Fig. 10.7A) and a long-axis image through the morphologic right ventricle and aorta on the left (Fig. 10.7B). Adding to the confusion, from the same standard long-axis imaging plane, it is also possible to obtain a long-axis image through the pulmonary valve and the left atrioventricular valve. The membranous septum is thin and often is shifted to the right, away from this plane. As a result, this plane can give the false impression that the left AV valve and the posteriorly positioned pulmonary valve are related to the same (left-sided) ventricle. A large ventricular septal defect (VSD) may make this plane of imaging even more challenging. In this setting, the pulmonary valve can seem to be related to either atrioventricular valve, creating the appearance of a single ventricle. Nevertheless, the long-axis imaging plane is useful for evaluating the great artery relationships and for detecting the presence of outflow tract obstruction.

The short-axis imaging plane in the setting of CCTGA is also very helpful. The ventricular septum in CCTGA is more horizontally oriented than it is in the normal heart (Fig. 10.8A). At the level of the aortic and pulmonary valve, the relationship of the great arteries can be confirmed. In the majority of cases, the aortic valve will be leftward, anterior, and superior to the pulmonary valve (Fig. 10.8B). With slight superior angulation from the level of the aortic valve, the coronary arteries can be identified (Fig. 10.8C). In 85% of cases, the coronary arteries will be inverted. The coronary artery that arises from the left posterior facing sinus has the epicardial distribution of a morphologically right coronary artery. Conversely, the coronary artery arising from right posterior facing sinus has the epicardial distribution of a morphologically left coronary artery, giving rise

FIGURE 10.3. Apical four-chamber view demonstrating anteroposterior relationship of ventricular septum resulting in more vertical orientation than usual of ventricular septum and side by side relationship of ventricles. Left-sided ventricle is morphologic right ventricle and right-sided ventricle is morphologic left ventricle.

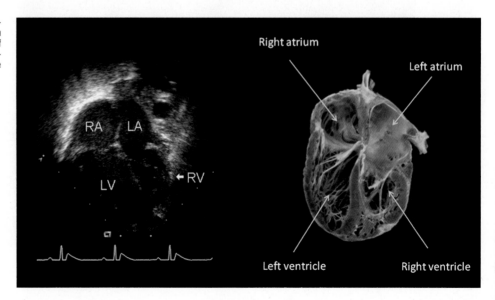

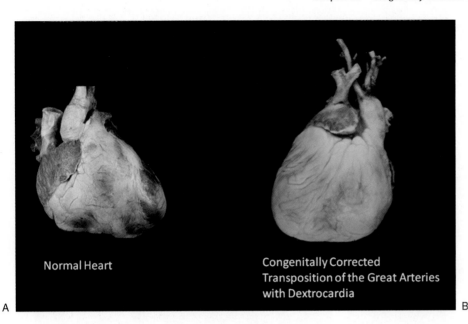

Normal Heart

A

Congenitally Corrected
Transposition of the Great Arteries
with Dextrocardia

B

FIGURE 10.4. Pathology specimens. A: Levocardia with normally related great vessels (ventriculoatrial [VA] concordance) and atrioventricular concordance. **B:** Congenitally corrected transposition of the great arteries with dextrocardia. (From the Dr. William Edwards collection, Mayo Clinic.)

to an anterior descending branch and a right-sided "circumflex" branch. Single coronary arteries are the most common coronary anomaly in CCTGA. With further superior angulation of the transducer, the bifurcation of the pulmonary artery can be identified. This image confirms the posterior position of the pulmonary artery and therefore TGA (Fig. 10.8D).

In CCTGA, it is often difficult to image the aortic arch from the standard suprasternal position. In CCTGA, the course of the ascending aorta is straight and leftward. It then arches with the descending aorta coursing downward on the left behind the ascending aorta. As a result, to image the aortic arch and a patent ductus arteriosus in the setting of CCTGA, the transducer needs to be placed in high left parasternal position, similar to the so-called ductal position. In this position, it is also important to delineate the branching pattern of the aortic arch given that a right aortic arch can occur in 18% of CCTGA.

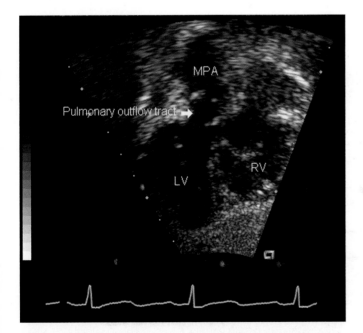

FIGURE 10.5. Subcostal imaging plane with transducer angulated anterior and superiorly. Demonstrates the unique anatomy of the left ventricular outflow tract with the pulmonary outflow tract deeply wedged between the right and left atrioventricular valves.

ASSOCIATED CARDIAC LESIONS

Tricuspid valve abnormalities are the most commonly associated abnormality in the setting of CCTGA, occurring in 90% of cases at autopsy. These features are best demonstrated in the apical four-chamber view but also can be seen in the subcostal coronal plane as well as a modified short axis. The most common and important underlying pathology is dysplasia of the valve, with or without displacement of the septal or posterior leaflets of the tricuspid valve. Most commonly, the degree of displacement is mild and does not meet criteria for Ebstein anomaly as described in a previous chapter (Fig. 10.10). When Ebstein anomaly does occur, typically the anterior leaflet is least affected, with severe involvement of both the septal and posterior leaflets. In the most severe form, there can be an unguarded tricuspid valve orifice with severe regurgitation (Fig. 10.11A–B). When significant Ebstein anomaly is present, there can be associated right ventricular hypoplasia with subaortic obstruction and possible coarctation of the aorta. This is rare, but it is always associated with an extremely abnormal tricuspid valve with severe systemic atrioventricular regurgitation and a disordered morphologic RV with marked thinning of the myocardium. Rarely, subaortic obstruction can occur with an intact ventricular septum. In these cases, the ascending aorta is usually very hypoplastic. The subcostal four-chamber and short-axis imaging planes are useful for evaluating right ventricular outflow tract obstruction. The high left parasternal view is useful for diagnosing coarctation of the aorta. Other associated left AV valve abnormalities include a supravalvular ring and in the setting of an inlet VSD, varying degrees of atrioventricular valve override and straddling.

A VSD occurs in 60% of patients with CCTGA. While these defects can occur anywhere in the septum, they most commonly are membranous with posterior extension into the inlet septum (Figures 10.12 and 10.13). The VSD in CCTGA is typically large but, because of the posterior position, may be partially occluded by the apically displaced septal leaflet of the tricuspid valve or by tissue that straddles through the defect into the right-sided morphologically LV (Fig. 10.14). The short-axis, apical four-chamber, and subcostal imaging planes are very useful for identifying these lesions. As a result of the VSD position, posterior straddling of the left atrioventricular valve is more common than straddling of the right atrioventricular valve.

Obstruction to the outflow tract of the morphologic LV (subpulmonary stenosis) is identified in 30% to 50% of patients with CCTGA. Such pulmonary outflow tract obstruction is uncommon in isolation and usually occurs in the setting of a large VSD. The

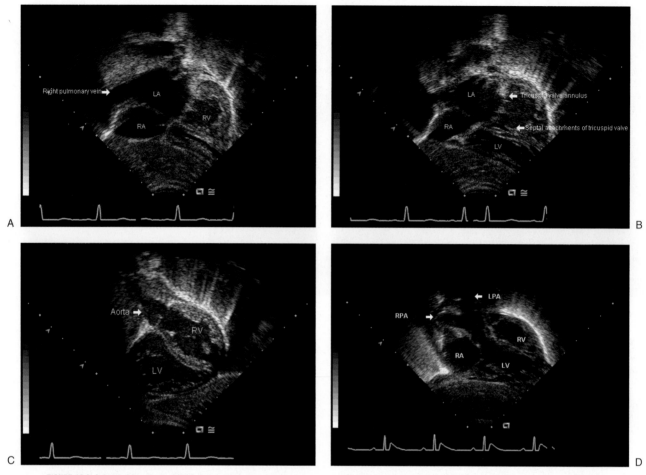

FIGURE 10.6. Subcostal Imaging in CCTGA. A: Subcostal coronal image demonstrating the most common form of congenitally corrected transposition of the great arteries (TGA) with the pulmonary veins connected to the left-sided atrium. **B:** Subcostal coronal imaging plane with transducer angulated anterior and superiorly demonstrating that the left atrium (LA) connects to a morphologic right ventricle (RV) and the septal attachments of the left-sided morphologically tricuspid valve. **C:** With the transducer angulated even more superiorly, the relationship of this ventricle to a great artery that arches and gives rise to coronary arteries (aorta) is identified. **D:** Subcostal coronal image demonstrating relationship of the right-sided structures. Right-sided atrium drains to morphologic left ventricle that then gives rise to an artery that branches, the main pulmonary artery.

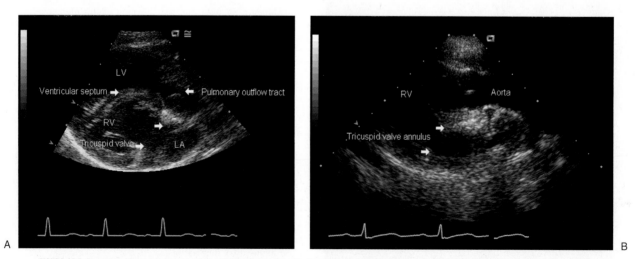

FIGURE 10.7. Parasternal long-axis images taken with transducer placed in the standard long-axis imaging position. Demonstrates the two separate long-axis views that can be obtained in congenitally corrected transposition of the great arteries with slight leftward or rightward angulation. **A:** Long-axis image through the morphologic left ventricle (LV) and pulmonary artery (right). **B:** Long-axis image through the morphologic right ventricle (RV) and aorta (left).

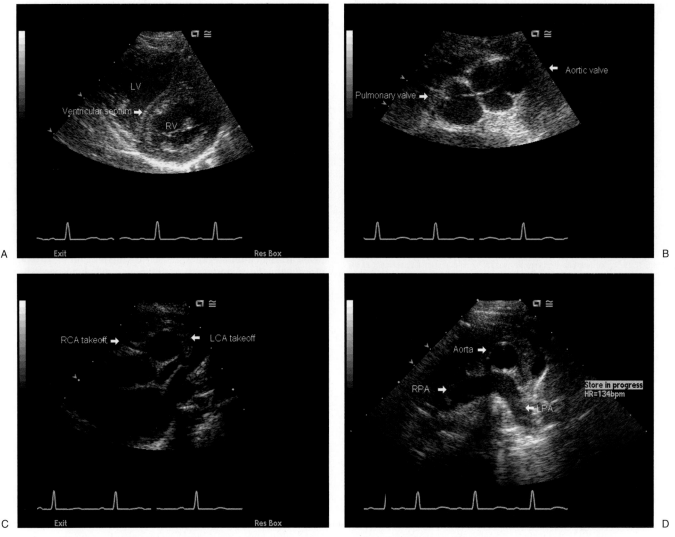

FIGURE 10.8. Parasternal Imaging in CCTGA. A: Short-axis imaging plane demonstrating that the septum in the setting of congenitally corrected transposition of the great arteries (CCTGA) is more horizontally oriented than usual. **B:** With superior angulation of the transducer, the level of the aortic and pulmonary valve can be imaged allowing confirmation of the relationship of the great arteries (aortic valve leftward, anterior, and superior to pulmonary valve). **C:** With further superior angulation from the level of the aortic valve, the coronary arteries can be identified. **D:** With further superior angulation of the transducer, the bifurcation of the pulmonary artery can be identified confirming the posterior position of the pulmonary artery and transposition of the great arteries.

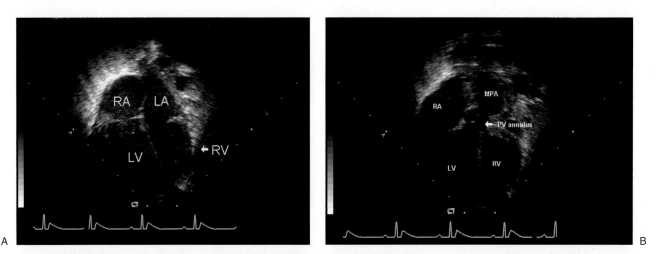

FIGURE 10.9. Apical Inflow and Outflow Images of CCTGA. A: Apical four-chamber view demonstrating atrioventricular relationships in the setting of congenitally corrected transposition of the great arteries. **B:** Apical four-chamber image with transducer angulated anterior and superiorly to demonstrate the pulmonary outflow tract.

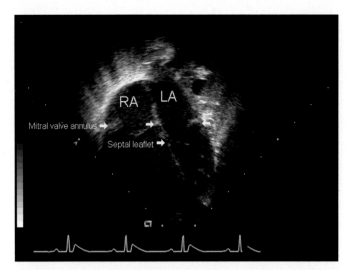

FIGURE 10.10. Apical four-chamber view demonstrating mild inferior displacement of the septal leaflet of the tricuspid valve in congenitally corrected transposition of the great arteries.

level of obstruction is typically at the subvalvular level secondary to wedging of the subpulmonary outflow tract between the infundibular septum and the ventricular free wall (Fig. 10.15A) or secondary to fibrous tissue from the membranous septum that protrudes into the subpulmonary area (Fig. 10.15B–C). Sometimes there can be tissue tags or abnormal chordal attachments from the mitral or tricuspid valve that exacerbate outflow obstruction. The pulmonary valve may also be dysplastic. Doppler interrogation from the subcostal coronal imaging plane, where flow is parallel to the beam of sound, allows for accurate quantitation of the gradient across the obstruction (Fig. 10.15D). However, given the close proximity to the atrioventricular valves and the presence of coexisting atrioventricular abnormalities, care must be taken not to confuse the systolic jet of atrioventricular regurgitation with pulmonary outflow tract obstruction.

In CCTGA, the atrioventricular node and the bundle of His have an unusual location and course and, as a result, are extremely fragile. While the sinus node is located normally, the atrioventricular node cannot give origin to the penetrating atrioventricular conduction bundle. As a result, an anomalous second atrioventricular node is present. It is located beneath the opening of the right atrial appendage at the lateral margin of the area between the pulmonary valve and mitral valve continuity. This second atrioventricular node is superficial and fragile. While this cannot be imaged directly by echocardiogra-

phy, over time many of these patients do develop complete heart block (1% to 2% per year), necessitating placement of transvenous pacemaker leads that can distort atrioventricular anatomy and lead to progressive mitral valve regurgitation (Fig. 10.16). If complete heart block occurs as a fetus, hyprops fetalis can develop and may come to the attention of the fetal sonographer. This situation is rare but the rhythm is readily demonstrated by fetal echocardiography. Figure 10.17A demonstrates the atrial rate in a fetus with complete heart block. In contrast, the simultaneous ventricular rate is much slower (Fig. 10.17B).

NATURAL HISTORY

Although there have been occasional reports of patients with isolated CCTGA having normal or near normal right ventricular function in their sixth and seventh decades, such a clinical course is extremely rare. In one of the largest series from Texas Children's Hospital, of 121 patients diagnosed with CCTGA at a median age of 1 month (range, 28 months to 48 years), 70% required surgery by a mean of 1.5 years (range, 1 day to 19 years). In this series, the mode of clinical presentation varied within patient age groups. Most neonates presented with cyanosis, whereas infants and older children presented with congestive heart failure and pulmonary overcirculation. Those patients who were asymptomatic had isolated CCTGA, a small VSD, or mild pulmonary outflow tract obstruction or were hemodynamically well balanced with a VSD and pulmonary outflow tract obstruction. In early childhood, required operations included systemic-to-pulmonary artery shunts, pulmonary artery banding, VSD closure with or without pulmonary valvotomy/resection, and tricuspid valve repair/replacement. Following initial surgical intervention, 80% of patients required reintervention, with tricuspid valve repair/replacement or LV–to–pulmonary artery conduit replacement. In both the operated and unoperated patient with CCTGA, the development of progressive systemic atrioventricular (tricuspid valve) regurgitation and right ventricular dysfunction remains the greatest long-term risks of morbidity.

The long-term risk for progressive right ventricular dysfunction and tricuspid regurgitation in CCTGA, has led some to promote the concept of an "anatomic repair" (double switch operation) that incorporates the LV into the systemic circulation. This therapeutic concept was first introduced in 1990. This anatomic repair is accomplished by using an atrial switch procedure (either Mustard or Senning), and a concurrent arterial switch procedure (Fig. 10.18). In those patients with pulmonary outflow tract obstruction and a VSD, the LV is tunneled through the VSD to the aorta by patch material and the RV is connected to the pulmonary artery by a valved conduit (a combination of Mustard- and Rastelli-type operations) (Fig. 10.19A). Another modification is to perform a bidirectional cavopulmonary connection in conjunction with a "hemi-Mustard" (inferior vena cava flow baffled to the left-sided tricuspid valve and an arterial switch) (Fig. 10.19B–C).

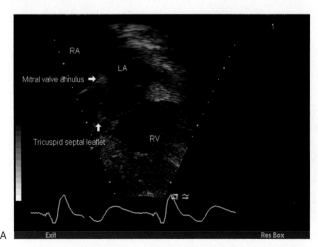
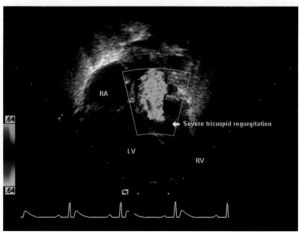

FIGURE 10.11. Ebstein-like Deformity of the Left AV Valve in CCTGA. A: Close-up image from the apical four-chamber view demonstrating severe displacement of the septal leaflet of the tricuspid valve (Ebstein's anomaly). B: Color image from the same plane demonstrating severe tricuspid valve regurgitation.

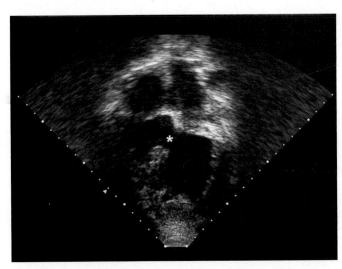

FIGURE 10.12. Apical four-chamber image demonstrating a large membranous ventricular septal defect (VSD) with extension into the inlet septum (*asterisk*).

In older patients, the LV has to be prepared to function as the systemic ventricle. In the absence of pulmonary outflow tract obstruction, this requires placement of a pulmonary artery band in an effort to raise the left ventricular pressure and induce hypertrophy. Echocardiographic assessment is a critical part of this process in the operating room to ensure proper band position and during the postoperative period to assess left ventricular preparation and remodeling. While initial promising results were published, the retraining of the LV has not been consistently effective except in young infants. Most centers have abandoned the "double switch" for older patients with unprepared LVs; however, it remains an attractive approach for young infants, especially when severe tricuspid valve dysplasia is present. The double switch provides an opportunity to remove the dyspastic tricuspid valve from the systemic circulation and restores the LV as the systemic pump.

In addition to trying to train the subpulmonic LV, placement of a pulmonary band in CCTGA has been performed as treatment for severe symptomatic tricuspid regurgitation. This technique is typically reserved for those patients with severe tricuspid regurgitation and severely reduced systemic right ventricular function, who are not surgical candidates other than for transplantation. This technique has resulted in varying results (Fig. 10.20A–B). In theory, placement of the pulmonary band increases the subpulmonic left

ventricular pressure, resulting in alteration of the ventricular septal position (septal shift) and improved tricuspid valve leaflet coaptation. Experience with this technique remains limited to only a few centers but does hold promise for patients with few other clinical options.

 ## ASSESSMENT OF THE SYSTEMIC RIGHT VENTRICLE

Many patients with CCTGA will develop right ventricular dysfunction and tricuspid valve regurgitation over time, making quantification of systemic right ventricular function and tricuspid regurgitation crucial components of the echocardiographic evaluation of these patients. Although the definition of "normal" systemic right ventricular ejection fraction remains debated, most authorities agree that an ejection fraction of 50% or greater is normal. Assessing the function of the morphologic RV, however, is challenging because of its complex anatomy. Difficulties are compounded by irregularities in the ventricular cavities and wall motion abnormalities in patients with congenital heart lesions. None of the geometric assumptions used to assess left ventricular function hold true for the systemic RV. Unlike the LV with both deep circumferential and longitudinal myocardial fibers, the majority of the right ventricular myocardial fibers originate at the apex of the heart and insert into the right atrioventricular junction, such that the bulk of the right ventricular myocardium is composed of longitudinally arranged fibers. This complex myocardial fiber arrangement and shape of the RV make quantification difficult. Thus, in clinical practice, most centers rely on visual estimation of right ventricular systolic function, which is then subject to variability because of incomplete visualization of the entire RV and the experience of the observer.

As a result of the difficulties with visual estimation of systemic right ventricular function, newer techniques for evaluating the systemic RV have gained growing acceptance in clinical practice. The myocardial performance index was first described by Tei and colleagues as a measure of combined systolic and diastolic function of the RV (Fig. 10.21). Since this first description, this index has been used to assess the systemic RV and in theory is independent of geometric assumptions. Preliminary data indicate a strong negative correlation between the right ventricular myocardial performance index and the calculated ejection fraction by cardiac MRI. In one of the few studies to evaluate this, the mean myocardial performance index for patients with normal systemic right ventricular function by cardiac MRI (ejection fraction 50% or greater) was 0.29 ± 0.08 (range, 0.21 to 0.43). This value is similar to the normal value for a systemic LV (0.34 to 0.40). As systemic right ventricular function decreases, several studies have demonstrated that the myocardial

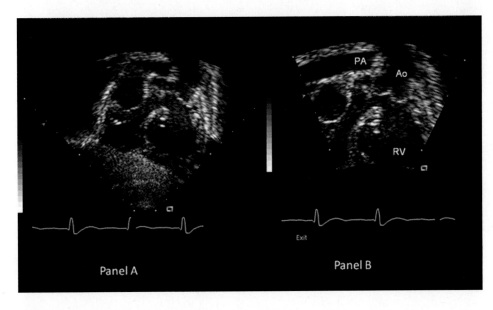

FIGURE 10.13. **Membranous VSD in CCTGA. A:** Subcostal imaging plane demonstrating large membranous ventricular septal defect extending into inlet septum in setting of congenitally corrected transposition of the great arteries. **B:** Close-up view demonstrating same anatomy.

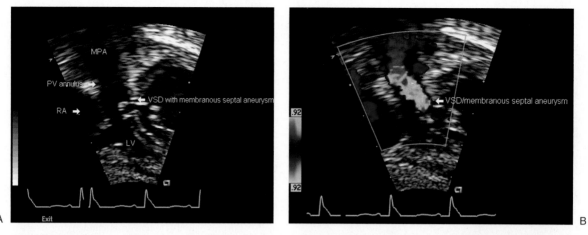

FIGURE 10.14. Membranous septal aneurysm and VSD in CCTGA. A: Subcostal image demonstrating membranous septal tissue protruding through ventricular septal defect into pulmonary outflow tract. **B:** Same subcostal image with color flow imaging demonstrating left-to-right shunting through ventricular septal defect into pulmonary outflow tract.

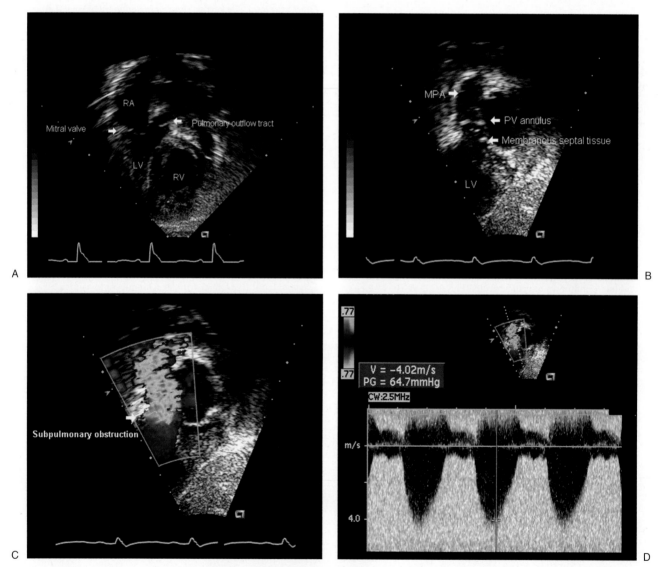

FIGURE 10.15. Pulmonary Outflow Tract and Subpulmonary Stenosis in CCTGA. A: Subcostal image demonstrating typical position of subpulmonary outflow tract deeply wedged between the right and left atrioventricular valves, in the setting of congenitally corrected transposition of the great arteries. **B:** Two-dimensional subcostal image demonstrating membranous septal tissue protruding into pulmonary outflow tract. **C:** Subcostal color flow image demonstrating aliasing of flow below valve at level of membranous septal tissue. **D:** Continuous-wave Doppler signal from same imaging plane, demonstrating significant fixed subpulmonary obstruction.

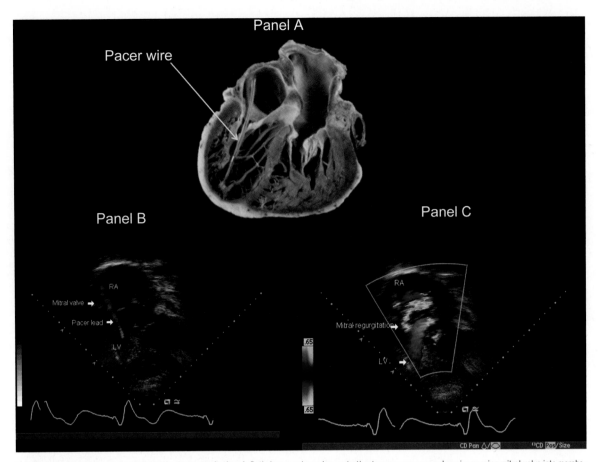

FIGURE 10.16. Pacemaker induced right AV valve regurgitation. A: Pathology specimen demonstrating transvenous pacemaker wire crossing mitral valve into morphologic left ventricle. **B:** Two-dimensional image from apical four-chamber imaging plane demonstrating pacer wire crossing mitral valve into morphologic left ventricle. **C:** Color flow image from same imaging plane demonstrating mitral regurgitation along entrance point of pacemaker lead across mitral valve. (**A**, From the Dr. William Edwards collection, Mayo Clinic.)

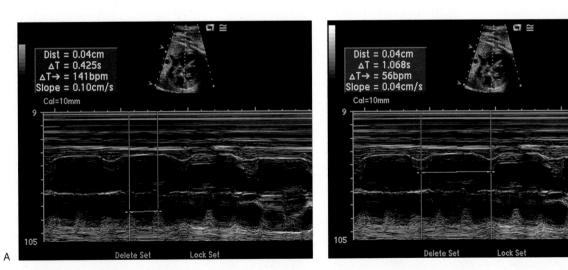

FIGURE 10.17. M-mode tracings of atrial and ventricular wall motion in a fetus with complete heart block. A: Determination of the Atrial rate. The A to A interval is 425 milliseconds (msec), predicting an atrial rate of 141 beats per minute (bpm). **B:** Determination of the ventricular rate. The V to V interval is 1068 msec, predicting a ventricular rate of only 56 bpm. The intervals are distinctly different, indicating electrical dissociation between the atrium and ventricles (complete heart block).

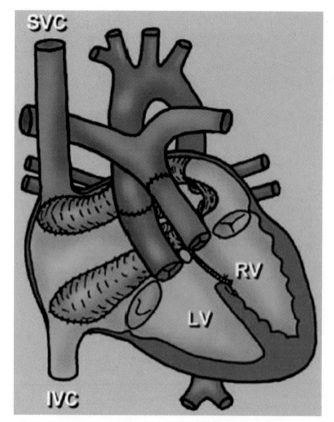

FIGURE 10.18. Diagram depicting a double switch operation for congenitally corrected transposition of the great arteries. This procedure incorporates elements of both an atrial switch operation (Mustard) and an arterial switch (Jatene). Printed with permission from DiBardino DJ, et al. The hemi-Mustard, bi-directional Glenn, and Rastelli operations used for correction of congenitally corrected transposition, achieving a "ventricle and a half" repair. *Cardiol Young* 2004; 14:330–2.

Quantifying systemic tricuspid valve regurgitation can also be a challenge. In general, techniques to quantify mitral regurgitation have been applied to the systemic tricuspid valve. Clinical correlation of these techniques in the setting of CCTGA is limited. Vena contracta width by color flow mapping appears to be one of the most reliable techniques with the majority of patients with severe regurgitation having a vena contracta width of 7 mm or greater. Other findings suggestive of severe systemic tricuspid regurgitation include (a) pulmonary vein systolic flow reversals, (b) color flow area of 40% of LA size or greater, (c) annulus dilation or inadequate cusp coaptation, (d) increased tricuspid valve Doppler inflow E velocity of 1.5 m/s or greater, (e) effective regurgitant orifice of 0.40 cm^2 or greater, (f) regurgitation fraction greater than 55%, and (g) regurgitation volume of 60 ml or greater.

Finally, because complete heart block is common in patients with CCTGA, many of these patients will have undergone placement of transvenous pacemaker systems. While this is often necessary to avoid complications associated with heart block, insertion of a pacemaker may precipitate deterioration in systemic ventricular function by altering the position of the septum leading to failure of tricuspid valve leaflet coaptation and worsening regurgitation. When systemic right ventricular dysfunction develops after placement of a transvenous system, many centers are now attempting to place biventricular pacing systems (cardiac resynchronization). The theory behind this maneuver is that biventricular pacing may help alleviate the ventricular mechanical dyssynchrony

performance index continues to increase with most patients having decreased ventricular function with significant tricuspid regurgitation having a right ventricular myocardial performance index score of greater than 0.72 ± 0.17.

Other techniques that have been used to evaluate systemic right ventricular function include measuring isovolumic myocardial acceleration (IVA) during isovolumic contraction using tissue Doppler imaging or velocity vector imaging (Fig. 10.22). IVA has been shown in several small studies to be a reliable technique to measure longitudinal systemic right ventricular function. Compared with subpulmonic RVs and systemic LVs, the IVA in systemic RVs is lower (mean: systemic RV, 1.0 ± 0.4; systemic LV, 1.4 ± 0.5; subpulmonic RV, 1.8 ± 0.6). Compared with other techniques, IVA may also provide the advantage of being less dependent on changes in preload and afterload.

Finally, because the bulk of the right ventricular myocardium is composed of longitudinal fibers, many researchers have proposed newer techniques to evaluate the longitudinal performance of the systemic RV. One of the earliest techniques was to measure the right ventricular total atrioventricular ring excursion using M-mode traces taken from the apical four-chamber view with the cursor positioned through the lateral angles of the tricuspid and mitral valves. Compared with systemic LVs and subpulmonic RVs, the total atrioventricular ring excursion has been shown to be lower in patients with CCTGA. Most recently, studies have focused on using strain, strain rate, and myocardial systolic and diastolic velocities to quantify longitudinal function. Preliminary data indicate that for both the systemic RV and the subpulmonic RV, the dominant myocardial motion is longitudinal. The greatest displacement, myocardial systolic and diastolic velocities, and strain to be measured are at the right ventricular basal septal and free walls with progressive declines as one moves toward the apex (Table 10.1).

Table 10.1	**VELOCITY VECTOR IMAGING OF THE SYSTEMIC RIGHT VENTRICLE COMPARED WITH THE NORMAL (SUBPULMONIC) RIGHT VENTRICLE**

Longitudinal Displacement(cm/s)

	Normal RV			Systemic RV	
	Free Wall	Septal Wall		Free Wall	Septal Wall
Basal	15.48	11.24	Basal	8.80	7.09
Mid	8.63	6.70	Mid	4.09	2.92
Apical	3.72	2.32	Apical	0.59	0.71

For both control and systemic RVs, the dominant myocardial motion was longitudinal.
Greatest displacement at basal free wall and septum.

Peak Systolic Velocity (cm/s)

	Normal RV			Systemic RV	
	Free Wall	Septal Wall		Free Wall	Septal Wall
Basal	7.60	6.18	Basal	3.27	3.51
Mid	5.52	4.06	Mid	2.99	1.58
Apical	2.85	1.37	Apical	1.37	0.90

Values for peak diastolic velocities similar decreasing from base to apex.

Peak Strain (%)

	Normal RV			Systemic RV	
	Free Wall	Septal Wall		Free Wall	Septal Wall
Basal	−36.17	−21.31	Basal	−18.16	−12.67
Mid	−27.21	−18.82	Mid	−11.30	−13.32
Apical	−12.75	−17.06	Apical	−13.18	−13.49

Values for strain also highest in basal free and septal wall for both normal and systemic RV cohort with progressive decrease moving toward apex.

Data adapted from abstract presented at the 2007 Midwest Pediatric Cardiology Scientific Session titled "Velocity Vector Imaging: A Novel Technique for the Assessment of Systemic RV Function in Patients with Transposition of the Great Arteries." **Top:** Longitudinal displacement measured by velocity vector imaging at the free and septal wall of the systemic right ventricle (RV) compared with the normal subpulmonic RV. **Middle:** Peak systolic velocity measured by velocity vector imaging at the free and septal wall of the systemic RV compared with the subpulmonic RV. **Bottom:** Peak strain measured by velocity vector imaging of the systemic RV compared with the subpulmonic RV.

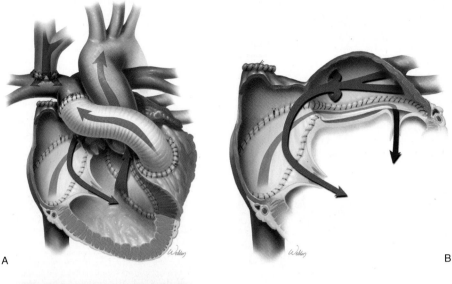

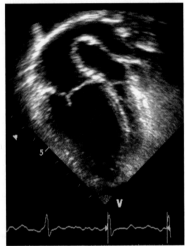

FIGURE 10.19. Double Switch Operation (Mustard-Rastelli type). A: Diagram depicting a modification of the double switch operation (Mustard-Rastelli type) used in patients with pulmonary/subpulmonary obstruction. Flow from the morphologic left ventricle (LV) is baffled via the ventricular septal defect (VSD) to the aorta. A conduit is placed to direct morphologic right ventricular (RV) blood to the pulmonary artery. An atrial switch operation is also performed. **B:** Diagram depicting a modification of the double switch operation (hemi-Mustard) in which only the inferior vena cava (IVC) flow is baffled to the morphologic right ventricle and tricuspid valve (TV). Superior vena cava (SVC) is diverted to the pulmonary artery via a bidirectional Glenn. Pulmonary venous blood passes behind the IVC baffle to enter the mitral valve (MV). An arterial switch is also performed. **C:** Apical four-chamber image in a child after a double switch operation. A widely patent pulmonary venous baffle is demonstrated. Printed with permission from DiBardino DJ, et al. The hemi-Mustard, bi-directional Glenn, and Rastelli operations used for correction of congenitally corrected transposition, achieving a "ventricle and a half" repair. *Cardiol Young* 2004; 14:330-2.

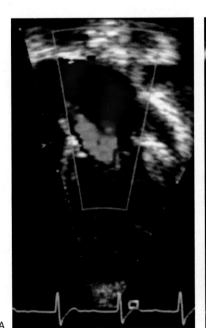
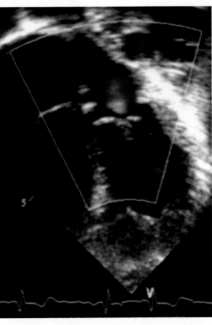

FIGURE 10.20. Pulmonary Artery Banding and its Impact on systemic Atrioventricular Valve Regurgitation in CCTGA. A: Before placement of a pulmonary artery band, this patient has severe tricuspid valve regurgitation. **B:** In the same patient, after pulmonary artery band placement, the morphologic LV pressure increase causes a leftward shift of the ventricular septum, thereby reducing the amount of tricuspid regurgitation.

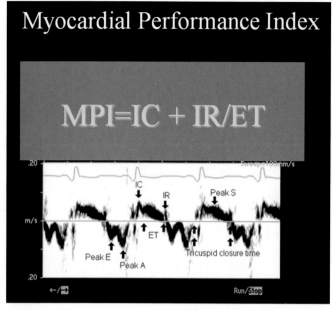

FIGURE 10.21. Tracing from the septal annulus of a patient using tissue Doppler imaging. Myocardial performance index (MPI) can be calculated by adding the measured isovolumic contraction time (IC) and isovolumic relaxation time (IR) and then dividing the total by the ventricular ejection time (ET).

and, as a result, improve regurgitation and ventricular function. The detection of mechanical dyssynchrony involves the use of Doppler tissue imaging, velocity vector imaging, or strain and strain imaging. Unfortunately, the experience of cardiac resynchronization in all congenital heart disease remains limited to case series and small experimental crossover studies in the acute postoperative setting. Access to the coronary sinus is important for placement of the biventricular pacing system. The echocardiographer may be called on to assist in identifying the orifice of the coronary sinus. In patients with systemic RVs, echocardiographers should routinely evaluate the location and course of the coronary sinus.

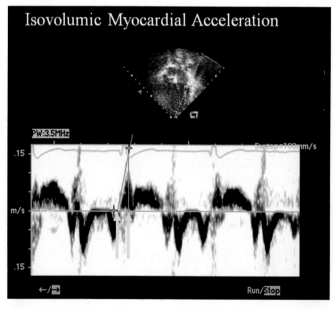

FIGURE 10.22. The isovolumic myocardial acceleration. This can be calculated by taking the difference between baseline and peak velocity (stars) during isovolumic contraction divided by their time interval (yellow arrows).

SUGGESTED READING

Beauchesne LM, Warnes CA, Connolly HM, et al. Outcome of the unoperated adult who presents with congenitally corrected transposition of the great arteries. *J Am Coll Cardiol.* 2002;40:285–290.

Benzaquen BS, Webb GD, Colmann JM, et al. Arterial switch operation after Mustard procedures in adult patients with transposition of the great arteries: Is it time to revise our strategy. *Am Heart J.* 2004;147:e8.

Celermajer DS, Cullen S, Deanfield JE, et al. Congenitally corrected transposition and Ebstein's anomaly of the systemic atrioventricular valve: Association with aortic arch obstruction. *J Am Coll Cardiol.* 1991;18:1056–1058.

Connelly MS, Liu PP, Williams WG, et al. Congenitally corrected transposition of the great arteries in the adult: Functional status and complications. *J Am Coll Cardiol.* 1996;27:1238–1243.

Derrick GP, Josen M, Vogel M, et al. Abnormalities of right ventricular long axis function after atrial repair of transposition of the great arteries. *Heart.* 2001;86:203–206.

Derrick GP, White PA, Tsang VT, et al. Pulmonary artery banding to retrain the subpulmonary ventricle: Optimization by intraoperative pressure volume analysis. *Circulation.* 2000;102(Suppl II):II-3164.

Eidem BW, O'Leary PW, Tei C, et al. Usefulness of myocardial performance index for assessing right ventricular function in congenital heart disease. *Am J Cardiol.* 2000;86:654–658.

Eyskens B, Weidemann F, Kowalski M, et al. Regional right and left ventricular function after the Senning operation: An ultrasonic study of strain rate and strain. *Cardiol Young.* 2004;14:255–264.

Freedom RM, Dyck JD, Atallah J. Congenitally correct transposition of the great arteries. In: Allen HD, Driscoll DJ, Shaddy RE, et al, eds. *Moss and Adam's Heart Disease in Infants, Children, and Adolescents.* Philadelphia, Pa: Lippincott Williams & Wilkins, 2008:1087–1099.

Freedom RM, Mawson JB, Yoo SJ, et al. Congenitally corrected transposition of the great arteries (atrioventricular and ventriculoarterial discordance). In: *Congenital Heart Disease: Textbook of Angiocardiography.* Armonk, NY: Futura Publishing, 1997:1071–1111.

Friedberg DZ, Nadas AS. Clinical profile of patients with congenitally corrected transposition of the great arteries. A study of 60 cases. *N Engl J Med.* 1970;282:1053–1059.

Graham TP, Bernard YD, Mellen BG, et al. Long-term outcome in congenitally corrected transposition of the great arteries: A multi-institutional study. *J Am Coll Cardiol.* 2000;36:255–261.

Graham TP. Congenitally corrected transposition. In: Gatzoulis MA, Webb GD, Daubeney PEF, eds. *Diagnosis and Management of Adult Congenital Heart Disease.* New York: Churchill Livingstone, 2003:379–387.

Han JK, Steendijk P, Khan H, et al. Acute effects of pulmonary artery banding in sheep on right ventricle pressure-volume relations: Relevance to arterial switch operation. *Acta Physiol Scand.* 2001;172:97–106.

Hornung TS, Bernard EJ, Celermajer DS, et al. Right ventricular dysfunction in congenitally corrected transposition of the great arteries. *Am J Cardiol.* 1999;84:1116–1119.

Hraska V, Duncan BW, Mayer JE Jr, et al. Long-term outcome of surgically treated patients with corrected transposition of the great arteries. *J Thorac Cardiovasc Surg.* 2005;129:182–191.

Ilbawi MN, DeLeon SY, Backer CL, et al. An alternative approach to the surgical management of physiologically corrected transposition with ventricular septal defect and pulmonary stenosis or atresia. *J Thorac Cardiovasc Surg.* 1990;100:410–415.

Ilbawi MN, Ocampo CB, Allen BS, et al. Intermediate results of the anatomic repair for congenitally corrected transposition. *J Thorac Cardiovasc Surg.* 2002;73:594–599.

Imamura M, Drummond-Webb JJ, Murphy DJ, et al. Results of the double switch operation in the current era. *Ann Thorac Surg.* 2000;70:100–105.

Khairy P, Fournier A, Thibault B, et al. Cardiac resynchronization therapy in congenital heart disease. *Int J Cardiol.* 2006;109:160–168.

Langley SM, Winlaw DS, Stumper O, et al. Midterm results after restoration of the morphologic left ventricle to the systemic circulation in patients with congenitally corrected transposition of the great arteries. *J Thorac Cardiovasc Surg.* 2003;125:1229–1241.

Lundstrom U, Bull C, Wyse RK, et al. The natural and unnatural history of congenitally corrected transposition. *Am J Cardiol.* 1990;65:1222–1229.

Penny DJ, Somerville J, Redington A, et al. Echocardiographic demonstration of important abnormalities of the mitral valve in congenitally corrected transposition. *Br Heart J.* 1992;686:498.

Pirat B, McCulloch ML, Zoghbi WA. Evaluation of global and regional right ventricular systolic function in patients with pulmonary hypertension using a novel speckle tracking method. *Am J Cardiol.* 2006;98:699–704.

Pislaru C, Abraham TP, Belohlavek M. Strain and strain rate echocardiography. *Curr Opin Cardiol.* 2002;17:443–454.

Poirier NC, Mee RB. Left ventricular reconditioning and anatomical correction for systemic right ventricular dysfunction. *Semin Thorac Cardiovasc Surg Pediatr Card Surg Annu.* 2000;3:198–215.

Prieto LR, Hordof AJ, Secic M, et al. Progressive tricuspid valve disease in patients with congenitally corrected transposition of the great arteries. *Circulation.* 1998;98:997–1005.

Rutledge JM, Nihill MR, Fraser CD, et al. Outcome of 121 patients with congenitally corrected transposition of the great arteries. *Pediatr Cardiol.* 2002;23:137–145.

Salehian O, Schwerzmann M, Merchant N, et al. Assessment of systemic right ventricular function in patients with transposition of the great arteries using the myocardial performance index: Comparison with cardiac magnetic resonance imaging. *Circulation.* 2004;110:3229–3233.

Snider RA, Serwer GA, Ritter SB. Abnormalities of ventriculoarterial connection. In: *Echocardiography in Pediatric Heart Disease.* St. Louis, Mo: Mosby–Year Book, 1990:317–323.

Tei C, Dujardin KS, Hodge DO, et al. Doppler echocardiographic index for assessment of global right ventricular function. *J Am Soc Echocardiogr.* 1996;9:838–847.

Tomasini JM, Earing MG, Bartz P, et al. Velocity vector imaging: A novel technique for the assessment of systemic RV function in patients with transposition of the great arteries. Proceedings of Midwest Pediatric Cardiology Society, 2007.

van der Zedde J, Oossterhof T, Tulevski II, et al. Comparison of segmental and global systemic ventricular function at rest and during dobutamine stress between patients with transposition and congenitally corrected transposition. *Cardiol Young.* 2005;15:148–153.

van Son JA, Danielson GK, Huhta JC, et al. Late results of systemic atrioventricular valve replacement in corrected transposition. *J Thorac Cardiovasc Surg.* 1995;109:642–652.

Vogel M, Derrick G, White PA, et al. Systemic ventricular function in patients with transposition of the great arteries after atrial repair: A tissue Doppler and conductance catheter study. *J Am Coll Cardiol.* 2004;43:100–106.

Warnes CA. Transposition of the great arteries. *Circulation.* 2006;114:2699–2709.

Williams RV, Ritter S, Tani LY, et al. Quantitative assessment of ventricular function in children with single ventricles using the Doppler myocardial performance index. *Am J Cardiol.* 2000;86:1106–1110.

Winlaw DS, McGuirk SP, Balmer C, et al. Intention-to-treat analysis of pulmonary artery banding in conditions with a morphologic right ventricle in the systemic circulation with a view to anatomic biventricular repair. *Circulation.* 2005;111:405–411.

Yeh T Jr, Connelly MS, Coles JG, et al. Atrioventricular discordance: Results of repair in 127 patients. *J Thorac Cardiovasc Surg.* 1999;117:1190–A

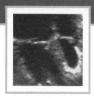

Chapter 11
Ventricular Septal Defects

Sarah Gelehrter • Gregory Ensing

Ventricular septal defect (VSD), the most common form of congenital heart disease, is frequently seen by both the adult and pediatric echocardiographer. Fifty percent of all children with congenital heart disease have an associated VSD, with 20% of cases being isolated VSDs. VSDs are an integral part in many forms of congenital heart disease, including tetralogy of Fallot, truncus arteriosus, and double-outlet right ventricle. The incidence of an isolated VSD in live births is 1.5 to 53 per 1000, with wide variation in reported incidence rates.

As in most congenital heart lesions, echocardiography has become the mainstay for clinical diagnosis, for direction of clinical care, and for determination of the approach to therapeutic intervention. Thus, while the presence of a VSD is often easily appreciated, ideal echocardiographic study and interpretation require that the echocardiographer have a detailed understanding of septal anatomy, relationships of VSDs to other intracardiac structures, and the impact of these VSDs on intracardiac hemodynamics.

ANATOMY OF THE VENTRICULAR SEPTUM

The normal ventricular septum is a curved structure extending from the posterior interventricular groove at its inferior and rightward aspect to the pulmonary outflow tract and anterior interventricular groove superiorly and leftward. The ventricular septum can be divided into four regions: the membranous, inlet, outlet, and trabecular septa (Fig. 11.1). The borders of these regions are determined by the tricuspid, pulmonary, and aortic valves, with subdivisions of the regions determined by the muscular bands in the right ventricle: the septal, parietal, and moderator bands. Of the muscular bands, only the moderator band is easily appreciated by standard two-dimensional echocardiography. This muscular bundle originates from the right ventricular (RV) side of the mid-septum at its apical third and crosses the RV chamber to the parietal wall. Also called the trabeculum septomarginalis, the septal band is difficult to appreciate echocardiographically. It is a muscular ridge extending along the RV side of the mid-septum from the insertion of the moderator band, toward the aortic outflow where it bifurcates into an anterior and posterior limb. Within this bifurcation are the membranous septum and the subpulmonary outlet septum.

The membranous septum is a small fibrous portion of the ventricular and atrioventricular (AV) septum located at the base of the heart, adjacent to the anteroseptal tricuspid commissure, the right posterior aortic valve commissure, and the anterior mitral valve leaflet. Because of the relative apical placement of the tricuspid valve compared with the mitral valve, a portion of the membranous septum, the membranous AV septum, separates the left ventricle (LV) from the right atrium.

The three other regions of the ventricular septum are all muscular; they radiate out from the membranous septum. The inlet septum is located between the AV valves inferior to the membranous septum with its apical border being the chordal attachments of the AV valves. The outlet septum makes up the most anterior and superior part of the ventricular septum and is located above an imaginary line between the membranous septum, the papillary muscle of the conus, and the anterior infundibular wall. The remainder of the ventricular septum is the trabecular septum, which is the largest region. The trabecular septum is broken into the subregions shown in Figure 11.2: posterior (sometimes called inlet muscular), anterior, mid-muscular, and apical. The posterior trabecular (or muscular) septum is posterior to the septal attachment of the tricuspid valve. The anterior trabecular septum is anterior to the septal band (or trabeculum septomarginalis). As the septal band is difficult to appreciate by echocardiography, the anterior trabecular septum is identified as anterior to the mid-septum and at, or superior to, the level of the moderator band. The mid-muscular septum is posterior to the septal band and superior to the moderator band. The apical septum is inferior to the moderator band and can be divided into an anterior or "infundibular" apex and posterior or "inflow" apex.

ANATOMY OF VENTRICULAR SEPTAL DEFECTS

VSDs can be divided into two fundamental types. In the first type, there may be adequate septal tissue, but there is malalignment of portions of the ventricular septum causing a "gap" or VSD. The malaligned septal components can be parallel but offset, can cross each other in oblique planes, or even can be perpendicular to each other. The second fundamental type of VSD is due to a deficiency

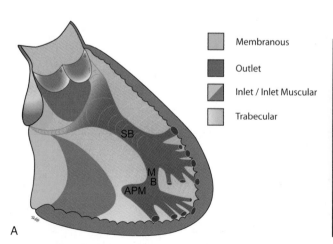

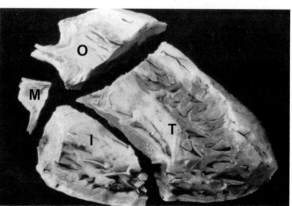

FIGURE 11.1. Diagrammatic (A) and pathologic (B) representations of the normal interventricular septum as viewed from the right ventricular aspect. APM, anterior papillary muscle of the tricuspid valve; I, inlet; M, membranous; MB, moderator band; O, outlet; SB, septal band; T, trabecular. (B, Reprinted with permission from Becker A, Anderson R. Anomalies of the ventricles. In: *Cardiac Pathology and Integrated Text and Colour Atlas*. New York: Raven Press, 1983:12.2.)

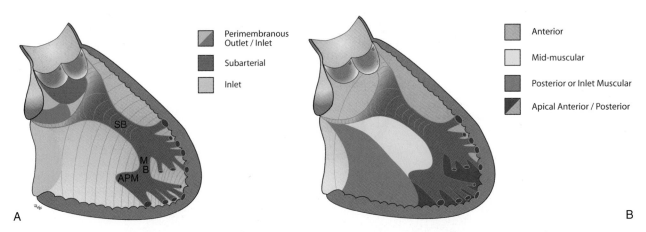

FIGURE 11.2. Location of ventricular septal defects (VSDs) within the ventricular septum as seen from the right ventricular aspect. **A:** Locations of perimembranous, subarterial, and inlet VSDs. **B:** Subtypes of muscular VSDs: anterior, mid-muscular, posterior, and apical (including VSDs of the posterior right ventricular [RV] inflow apex and the anterior infundibular apex). APM, anterior papillary muscle of the tricuspid valve; MB, moderator band; SB, septal band.

in septal tissue. This deficiency either can be congenital or can be acquired following myocardial infarction or trauma.

Several classification schemes to describe the location of VSDs are in common use. Thus, the nomenclature can be quite confusing. Efforts to synthesize the various naming systems have been made by the Congenital Heart Surgery Nomenclature and Database Project and subsequently by the International Working Group for Mapping and Coding of Nomenclatures for Paediatric and Congenital Heart Disease. The classification systems most commonly used are shown in Table 11.1. We use the Congenital Heart Surgery Nomenclature system in this chapter and have chosen to use the following names: perimembranous (including VSDs due to malalignment of the conal septum), subarterial, inlet, and muscular. Defects can occur entirely within a portion of the septum or can extend across portions of the septum (e.g., a perimembranous-to-inlet defect). Regardless of which naming system is used, it is most important is to be consistent so that accurate and clear communication can occur.

ECHOCARDIOGRAPHIC ASSESSMENT OF VENTRICULAR SEPTAL DEFECTS

A systematic echocardiographic assessment of VSDs involves a detailed anatomic and hemodynamic description. This includes description of the exact location of the defect in the ventricular septum with particular attention paid to (a) the relationship of the VSD to valves and valve attachments, (b) identification of location specific complicating factors, (c) description of the anatomic size of the defect, (d) estimation of right ventricular systolic pressures, and (e) estimation of overall shunt size.

The general imaging strategy used to identify and describe VSDs consists of sweeping the entire septum in both two-dimensional and color Doppler imaging from apex to base and from left to right. Imaging should be performed from the best acoustic window that shows the septum perpendicular to the ultrasound beam and the

flow across the defect parallel to the beam. Because of the curved nature of the ventricular septum, optimal imaging of a VSD can be from a subcostal, parasternal, apical, or right parasternal window.

Description of Ventricular Septal Defect Location

The exact location of the VSD can be identified echocardiographically and described using the categories described earlier (perimembranous, subarterial, inlet, or muscular). Figure 11.3 is a diagrammatic representation of the various types of defects and their location in standard echocardiographic views. Identification of the location of the major portion of the defect should be accompanied by descriptions of extension of the defect into adjacent portions of the ventricular septum and the direction of malalignment of the septum. Defects in larger regions, such as the trabecular septum, often need to be more precisely located by describing the relationship to adjacent cardiac structures. The presence or absence of specific complicating factors associated with each VSD location should also be evaluated and reported.

Perimembranous VSDs – Perimembranous defects are the most common type of VSD, comprising about 80% of VSDs. Perimembranous VSDs involve the membranous ventricular septum adjacent to the aortic and tricuspid valves. Perimembranous defects can be imaged from a parasternal, apical five-chamber, or subcostal window where they are seen immediately adjacent to both the tricuspid and aortic valves as demonstrated in Figure 11.4. When the VSD extends primarily toward the aortic valve, it is called a perimembranous outlet defect; when the defect is primarily adjacent to the tricuspid valve, it is called a perimembranous inlet defect.

A perimembranous VSD may be related to deficiency of tissue in the region of the membraneous septum or may be due to malalignment of the outlet septum with the muscular ventricular septum. The gap caused by malalignment of the outlet septum can be due to either anterior or posterior deviation of the outlet septum. Anterior deviation creates a VSD of the type seen in tetralogy of Fallot

CHS database	Van Praagh et al.	Anderson	Hagler et al.	Other
Perimembranous	Conoventricular	Perimembranous outlet	Membranous	Subaortic, infracristal, or paramembranous
Subarterial	Conal	Juxta-arterial	Infundibular or subarterial	Supracristal, subpulmonary, outlet, or doubly committed
Inlet	AV canal	Perimembranous inlet	AV Canal	
Muscular	Muscular	Muscular	Trabecular	

TABLE 11.1 VENTRICULAR SEPTAL DEFECT NOMENCLATURE SYSTEMS

AV, atrioventricular; CHS, Congenital Heart Surgery Nomenclature and Database Project.

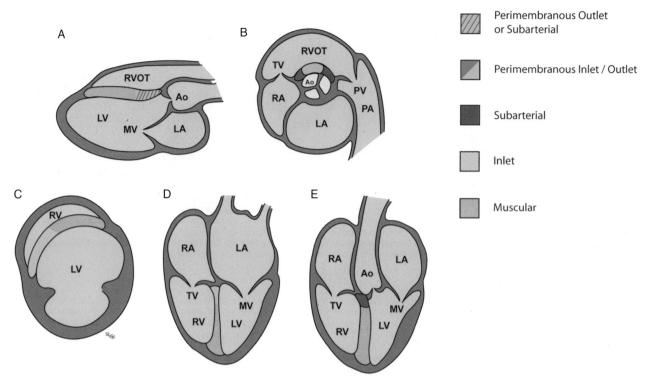

FIGURE 11.3. Diagrammatic representation of ventricular septal defect (VSDs) locations as seen in standard echocardiographic views. A: Parasternal long-axis view showing muscular, perimembranous outlet, and subarterial VSDs. **B:** Parasternal short-axis view at the base showing perimembranous and subarterial VSDs. **C:** Parasternal short-axis view at the level of the left ventricular (LV) papillary muscles showing muscular VSDs. **D:** Apical four-chamber view showing inlet and muscular VSDs. **E:** Apical five-chamber view showing muscular and perimembranous VSDs. Ao, aorta; LA, left atrium; MV, mitral valve; PA, pulmonary artery; PV, pulmonary valve; RA, right atrium; RV, right ventricle; TV, tricuspid valve.

(Fig. 11.5), with override of the aorta; this type of malalignment VSD can also be seen without associated pulmonary stenosis. Posterior deviation of the outlet septum creates a VSD of the type seen in association with interrupted aortic arch with muscular narrowing of the LV outflow tract (Fig. 11.6).

Because of their location adjacent to the tricuspid valve, perimembranous defects can be associated with tricuspid septal leaflet distortion and tricuspid regurgitation. Accessory tissue from the septal leaflet of the tricuspid valve, or a part of the septal leaflet itself, can partially or completely close the defect; this tissue is sometimes referred to as a ventricular septal aneurysm (Fig. 11.7). Occasionally, blood flow traverses through the VSD from the LV, through the aneurysmal tissue, and across tricuspid valve and enters right atrium resulting in LV–to–right atrial shunt. Misinterpretation of this high-velocity flow from this LV–to–right atrial shunt as tricuspid regurgitation can lead to an erroneous overestimation of RV pressure. A related, but distinct, type of LV–to–right atrial shunt is the Gerbode defect, which is an LV–to–right atrial connection created by a defect in the portion of the membranous ventricular septum separating the LV from the right atrium (Fig. 11.8).

As perimembranous VSDs are also adjacent to the aortic valve, this valve can also be affected. In about 10% of perimembranous VSDs, there is associated aortic valve prolapse, and in 6% to 8%, there is associated aortic regurgitation. Aortic valve prolapse into the VSD is identified echocardiographically by identification of the right or noncoronary aortic cusp protruding into the VSD; this is typically best seen in the parasternal long- and short-axis views. Because aortic cusp prolapse is more common with subarterial defects, it is discussed in detail below. Because of its importance in the development of aortic regurgitation, the presence or absence of aortic cusp prolapse should be reported with any defect located immediately adjacent to the aortic valve.

A subaortic ridge, with or without significant subaortic obstruction, is seen in 3% to 6% of cases of perimembranous VSDs. In most of these cases, the subaortic ridge or ring is fibromuscular and is located immediately at the inferior aspect of the VSD (VSD is

located distal to the ridge). In about half of these cases, there is an associated ventricular septal aneurysm. The subaortic ridge may develop with time; in a study by Eroglu, et al, three quarters of the patients developed a subaortic ridge after initial presentation. The subaortic ridge may also contribute to the development of aortic regurgitation.

Subarterial VSDs – Subarterial defects make up 5% to 10% of VSDs and are more common in the Asian population. These defects are located beneath both semilunar valves and result from a deficiency in the conal, or outlet, septum. Subarterial defects are seen by echocardiography to be immediately beneath the aortic valve in long-axis views and immediately adjacent to both the aortic and pulmonary valve in short-axis views (doubly committed VSD) (Fig. 11.9). These defects are sometimes referred to as supracristal, but there is controversy regarding the definition of the crista supraventricularis, which determines the location of a supracristal defect. There is agreement that the crista supraventricularis is the muscle mass separating the tricuspid and pulmonary valves, but its exact location in relation to the parietal band, infundibulum, and septal band is inconsistently defined in the literature. As it is typically difficult to appreciate these muscle bands by echocardiography, we believe that the term subarterial is a more precise echocardiographic description. With subarterial VSDs, there is typically an absence of muscular tissue between the semilunar valves. However, occasionally the defect can be completely surrounded by muscle.

Prolapse of the right coronary cusp of the aortic valve into the defect, with distortion of the aortic valve, is present in 60% to 70% of subarterial VSDs. Prolapse is demonstrated as a diastolic bulging of the right aortic cusp and portion of the sinus into the RV in the long- and short-axis views (Fig. 11.9). It can be mild and transient during early systole or severe, encompassing the entire cusp with tethering to the VSD throughout systole and diastole. The aortic cusp that is tethered into the defect will appear "beaked" and shortened in systole as compared to the uninvolved cusps. Because aortic prolapse can be

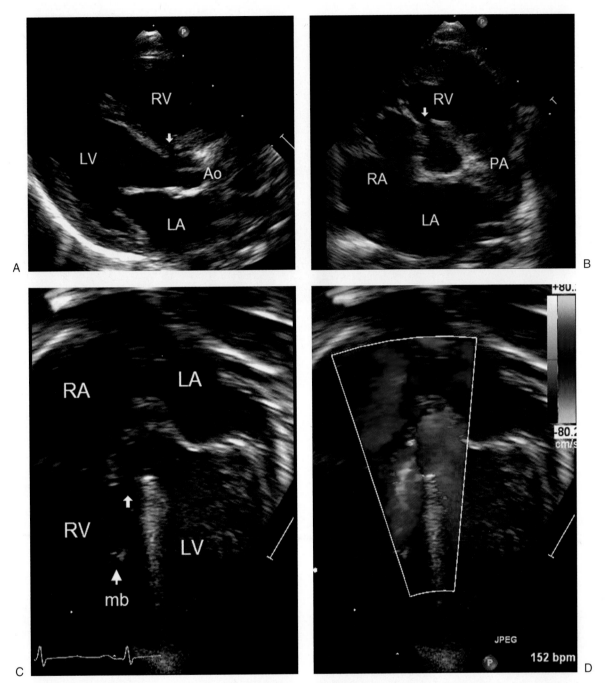

FIGURE 11.4. Perimembranous ventricular septal defect (VSD) (arrows). A: Parasternal long axis showing the VSD adjacent to the aortic valve. **B:** Parasternal short-axis image showing defect between aortic and tricuspid valves. Apical five-chamber view with two-dimensional **(C)** and color **(D)** images showing relationship of VSD to left ventricular (LV) outflow tract. Ao, aorta; LA, left atrium; LV, left ventricle; mb, moderator band; PA, pulmonary artery; RA, right atrium; RV, right ventricle.

associated with aortic regurgitation in up to one third of patients, the presence or absence of aortic cusp prolapse should be reported with any defect located immediately adjacent to the aortic valve. Because of the risk of aortic regurgitation, some cardiologists advocate surgical repair of all subarterial defects regardless of the size of the VSD. However, development of and progression of substantial aortic regurgitation in patients with aortic cusp prolapse into a subarterial VSD are not universal. Cheung, et al reported that in patients with mild to moderate aortic cusp prolapse, 92% had no change or improvement in their degree of aortic regurgitation following VSD closure; none progressed to moderate or severe aortic regurgitation. In contrast, moderate to severe aortic cusp prolapse was associated

with moderate to severe aortic regurgitation in most cases, and the degree of aortic regurgitation was unchanged or worsened following VSD closure with concomitant aortic valvuloplasty.

Inlet VSDs – Inlet VSDs are located posteriorly immediately adjacent to both AV valves. These defects are often best imaged from an apical four-chamber view or a parasternal short-axis view (Fig. 11.10). They most commonly occur as part of atrioventricular septal defects (AVSD) but can be isolated. Inlet VSDs should be distinguished from posterior muscular (also called inlet-muscular) VSDs, which are located near the inlet septum but are separated from the AV valves by a rim of muscle. Inlet VSDs may be formed by

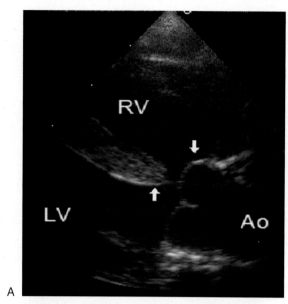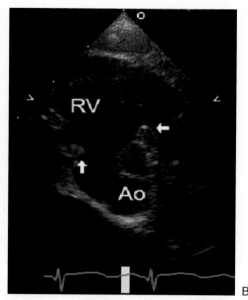

FIGURE 11.5. Anterior malalignment perimembranous ventricular septal defect in a patient with Tetralogy of Fallot as seen in parasternal long- (A) and short- (B) axis views. Anterior deviation and rotation of the outlet septum results in the ventricular septal defect, an enlarged aortic outflow overriding the main body of the ventricular septum, and narrowed subpulmonary outflow. Ao, aorta; LV, left ventricle; RV, right ventricle.

malalignment of the atrial and ventricular septa, resulting in some degree of AV valve override and not infrequently with straddling of AV valve chordal attachments.

AV valve override occurs when an AV valve is positioned over a VSD and relates to both ventricles. AV valve straddling occurs when chordal attachments from an AV valve cross the VSD to the opposite side of the ventricular septum or contralateral ventricle. An AV valve can override, straddle, or both. Tricuspid valve straddling with chordal attachments to the left ventricular side of the septum can be seen with inlet VSDs (Fig. 11.11). The mitral valve typically does not straddle an inlet VSD but more commonly may straddle an outlet or a perimembranous defect. Because of their surgical implications, straddling and overriding of either AV valve must be accurately identified and interpreted by the echocardiographer.

Other types of AV valve involvement are common with inlet VSDs, most often involving the tricuspid valve. The tricuspid valve

may be intrinsically abnormal with associated tricuspid regurgitation. The inlet defect may be partially or completely closed by redundant tricuspid septal leaflet tissue. When the VSD is associated with a partial AVSD, there is a cleft in the anterior leaflet of the mitral valve, which may result in regurgitation. Valve abnormalities associated with inlet VSDs should be identified as part of the complete echocardiographic evaluation.

Muscular VSDs – Muscular defects comprise 5% to 20% of VSDs. They can be described as being anterior, mid-muscular, posterior, or apical in location (Fig. 11.2). Anterior muscular defects are located anterior to the septal band (or trabeculum septomarginalis), which extends along the mid-septum from the insertion of the moderator band toward the membranous septum. The septal band bifurcates into an anterior and a posterior limb to surround the membranous septum and a portion of the outlet septum. The anterior muscular septum also includes anterior outlet defects which are located in the smooth walled outlet septum but separated by a muscular rim from the semilunar valves. Mid-muscular defects are posterior to the septal band, anterior to the septal attachment of the tricuspid valve, and superior to the moderator band. Posterior muscular defects are located posterior to the septal attachment of the tricuspid valve; posterior-inlet muscular defects are located immediately below the AV valves but separated from the valves by muscle tissue.

Apical muscular VSDs are located inferior to the moderator band and include defects of the RV inflow apex (which is located more posteriorly) and the more anterior "infundibular" apex. The two RV apices are divided by dense trabeculations that run from the septum to the RV free wall; the LV may connect with the infundibular apex (43% of cases), the RV inflow apex (45% of cases) or both RV apices. In LV-infundibular apical VSDs, there are usually multiple openings on the RV side of the septum. Hypertrophied RV apical trabeculations and the moderator band separate the infundibular apex and the VSD from the rest of the RV. Occasionally, closure of these defects, either by surgery or transcatheter device, results in placement of the device or patch among RV trabeculae rather than across the true septum. This may result in closing off the infundibular apex of the RV, thereby making it physiologically part of the LV.

The best imaging plane for muscular VSDs is dependent on the exact location of the defect within the muscular septum; the ideal plane will demonstrate the VSD in the axial resolution and the flow across it parallel to the ultrasound beam. Determining the precise location of a muscular VSD may require combining information

FIGURE 11.6. Posterior malalignment perimembranous ventricular septal defect in a patient with interrupted aortic arch. Posterior displacement of the outlet septum results in creation of the ventricular septal defect, narrowing of the left ventricular (LV) outflow tract, and enlargement of pulmonary outflow. Ao, aorta; LA, left atrium; LV, left ventricle; RV, right ventricle.

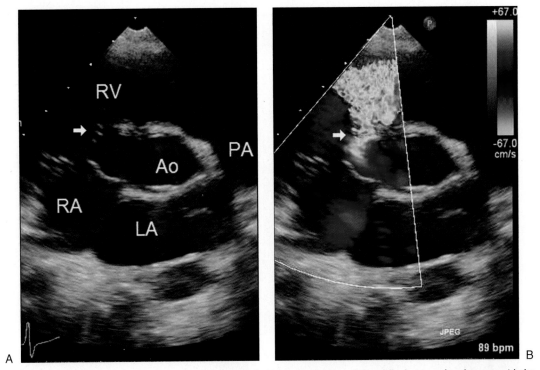

FIGURE 11.7. Ventricular septal aneurysm (arrow) made up of redundant tricuspid valve tissue that partially closes a perimembranous ventricular septal defect as seen in a parasternal short-axis view with two-dimensional and color Doppler. Ao, aorta; LA, left atrium; PA, pulmonary artery; RA, right atrium; RV, right ventricle.

gained from several imaging planes as shown in the example in Figure 11.12. Defining the particular subtype of muscular VSD can be difficult as, with the exception of the moderator band, the muscular bands of the RV that are used to define the subtypes of muscular VSD can be difficult or impossible to visualize by echocardiography. To help clarify the location of a muscular VSD, we recommend describing the defect in both the anterior/posterior location as well as an apical/basal location. In the example shown in Figure 11.12, the defect is located in the RV infundibular apex anterior to the position of an imaginary apical extension of the septal band. Figure 11.12 demonstrates a specific caveat of localization of VSDs using the apical four-chamber view. The apical four-chamber image plane demonstrates more posterior structures in the far field such as the atria and AV valves, but in the near field of the imaging plane it often displays a more anterior portion of the apical ventricular septum. The short-axis image in Figure 11.12 shows the more anterior location of this defect.

A patient may have multiple muscular VSDs, sometimes referred to as "Swiss cheese" septum, or may have a muscular VSD in addition to a VSD in another location (e.g., perimembranous or inlet). These additional defects can be easy to miss, especially when the first defect is large in size and there is equalization of pressures in both ventricles.

Special Considerations

Additional Abnormalities – As many as 60% of patients with VSDs have associated cardiac lesions. Some can be easily missed if not specifically looked for. Ventricular septal defects and aortic arch abnormalities keep close company. From 17% to 33% of patients with coarctation of the aorta have an associated VSD, as do nearly all patients with an interrupted aortic arch. The VSD is mid-muscular in almost half of these cases and perimembranous in almost a quarter of patients with coarctation and a VSD.

A patent ductus arteriosus is commonly coincident with a VSD. With a large VSD and associated pulmonary artery systolic hypertension, near equalization of aortic and pulmonary artery pressure often results in laminar (and difficult to appreciate) ductal flow. This same ductus may be easy to appreciate after VSD closure, when pulmonary artery pressure is decreased.

The association of subaortic stenosis with VSD has been described previously in this chapter. Subaortic stenosis associated with a perimembranous VSD is usually a fibromuscular ridge or ring with the VSD located distal to the obstruction. Muscular or tunnel-like subaortic stenosis can be created by posterior malalignment of the conal septum and is characteristically associated with aortic arch anomalies. In these cases, the VSD is located below the level of the LV outflow tract obstruction.

Double-chambered right ventricle (DCRV) has an associated VSD in 63% to 90% of patients. In DCRV, anomalous muscle bundles located below the infundibulum divide the RV into a high-pressure inlet chamber and a low-pressure outlet chamber (Fig. 11.13). The anomalous muscle bundles run from the ventricular septum to the RV anterior wall and can insert anywhere from the apex to the conoventricular junction. The VSD is most often perimembranous and connects to the high-pressure portion of the RV, but the VSD can be located anywhere. The relative locations of the anomalous muscle bundle and the VSD determine the RV chamber with which the VSD connects. When the VSD connects the LV to the low-pressure portion of the RV, it acts physiologically like an isolated VSD. When the VSD connects the LV to the high-pressure portion of the RV, it is physiologically like tetralogy of Fallot. If RV pressure is high, this can result in right-to-left shunt flow through the VSD. In natural history studies of VSD patients, 3% to 7% developed RV outflow tract stenosis, which tended to progress in severity over time. The separating RV muscle bundles are typically noted in the mid-RV. Flow disturbance across this region is poorly visualized from the parasternal transducer position as flow direction is perpendicular to the ultrasound beam. Because of their more anterior location, these bundles are poorly visualized using the apical transducer position, making the DCRV an easy lesion to miss by cursory examination. Images from the subcostal transducer position clearly demonstrate these obstructive muscle bundles and allow Doppler interrogation parallel to flow.

Traumatic VSDs – Traumatic VSDs occur most commonly in the muscular septum near the apex, but perimembranous defects have been reported associated with tricuspid valve injury. Multiple traumatic VSDs may also occur. A direct blow to the chest is the most common mechanism for creating this VSD. The trauma may cause septal rupture at the time of injury, or the development of the defect

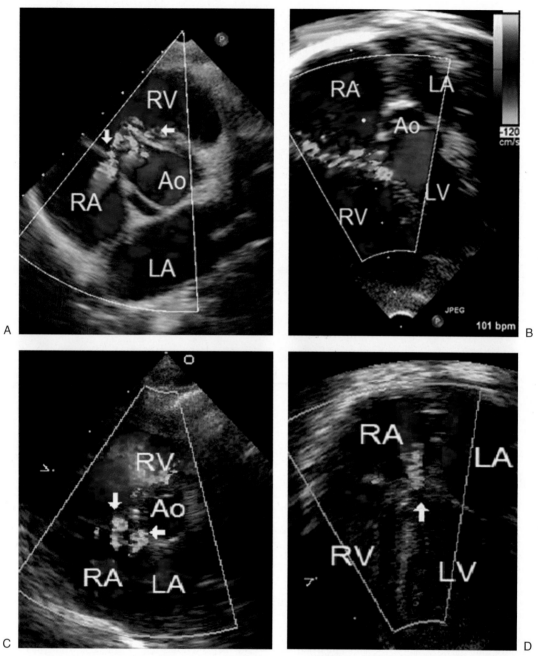

FIGURE 11.8. Left ventricular to right atrial shunts. A–B: Parasternal short-axis and apical images of a left ventricle–to–right atrial shunt (*arrows*) through tricuspid aneurysmal tissue closing a perimembranous ventricular septal defect. This shunt is of high velocity and may be confused with tricuspid regurgitation. **C–D:** Parasternal short-axis and apical four-chamber images of a defect in the membranous *atrioventricular* septum (Gerbode defect) with shunt flow directly from left ventricle to right atrium (*leftward arrow* in **C** and *upward arrow* in **D**). A second jet of tricuspid regurgitation is also present (*downward arrow* in **C**). Ao, aorta; LA, left atrium; LV, left ventricle; RA, right atrium; RV, right ventricle.

may be delayed for 2 to 6 days post injury. Delayed traumatic VSDs are thought to have arisen from areas of the septum where a myocardial contusion caused sufficient devascularization to lead to myocardial necrosis and perforation. Because traumatic VSDs can develop, or extend, in the days following the initial injury, serial echocardiograms are important even if a VSD is not seen on an initial study.

Assessment of Ventricular Septal Defect Size

Determining the size and significance of a VSD can be more complicated than it may seem. While small defects typically have large Doppler-measured pressure gradients between the ventricles and large defects have small pressure gradients, variations in pulmonary vascular resistance make this relationship far from universal. The infant with a delayed fall in pulmonary vascular resistance may have a minimal gradient across a small VSD or little left heart dilation with a large VSD. Similarly, the degree of left-to-right shunting in a moderate or large VSD with left heart overload often evolves over time. If pulmonary hypertension progresses, left-to-right shunt size, the degree of left heart dilation, and the VSD pressure gradient all regress. Eisenmenger syndrome results from the progression of pulmonary vascular obstruction with resultant development of right-to-left shunting at the VSD and progressive cyanosis. Thus, we recommend independent anatomic size and hemodynamic descriptions of VSDs.

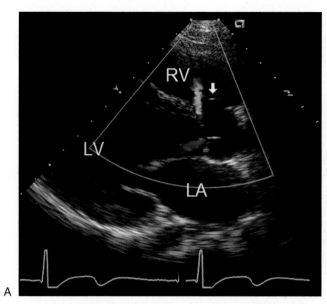
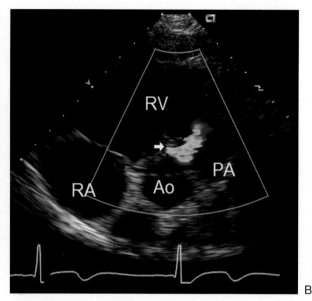

FIGURE 11.9. Parasternal long-axis (A) and parasternal short-axis (B) views of a subarterial ventricular septal defect (VSD) with prolapse of the right coronary cusp of the aortic valve (*arrows*) into the defect and mild aortic regurgitation. The subarterial defect is characterized by absence of muscular separation of the pulmonic valve from the VSD in the short axis view. Ao, aorta; LA, left atrium; LV, left ventricle; PA, pulmonary artery; RA, right atrium; RV, right ventricle.

Historically, the size of a VSD has been related to the size of the aortic annulus with a defect less than one third the diameter of the aortic annulus considered small, a defect one third to one half the size of the annulus considered moderate sized, and a large VSD being greater than one half to two thirds the size of the annulus. Measurement of the size of the VSD by measuring the largest diameter demonstrated by color flow mapping has been shown to closely reflect the measurements made by angiography and at surgery. However, this anatomic definition of VSD size can be limited as the defect may not be round and the size often varies throughout the cardiac cycle. Muscular defects, in particular, may have an oblique course through the ventricular septum and may have multiple openings on the RV side of the septum. Therefore, imaging the VSD in multiple planes is crucial to an accurate determination of VSD size. For irregularly shaped

defects, three-dimensional echocardiographic imaging may be particularly helpful.

HEMODYNAMIC DESCRIPTION OF VENTRICULAR SEPTAL DEFECTS

In addition to a detailed anatomic description of the VSD, echocardiography can provide a hemodynamic or "functional" description. As moderate and large VSDs are associated with dilation of the left heart chambers and/or pulmonary hypertension, the "functional" assessment would ideally include evaluation of right heart pressures and a quantification of the amount of shunt flow through the defect.

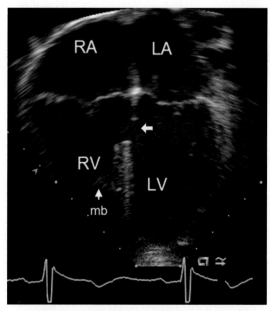
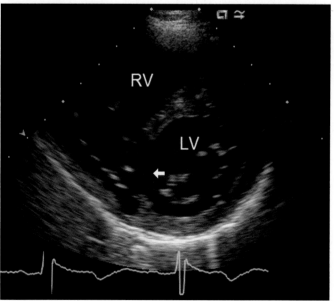

FIGURE 11.10. Inlet ventricular septal defect (*arrows*) imaged from apical four-chamber (A) and parasternal short-axis views (B). LA, left atrium; LV, left ventricle; mb, moderator band; RA, right atrium; RV, right ventricle.

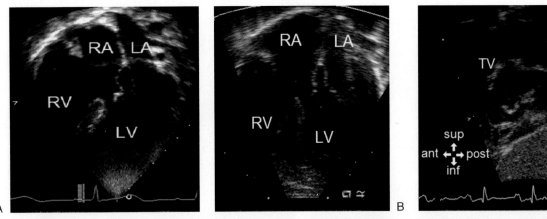

FIGURE 11.11. Apical four-chamber view (A) of the tricuspid valve overriding an inlet ventricular septal defect with tricuspid valve tissue partially closing the defect. Apical four-chamber **(B)** and supxiphoid oblique sagittal **(C)** en face views of a straddling tricuspid valve with attachments to the posteromedial papillary muscle of the left ventricle (LV) (*arrow in* **C**). ant, anterior; inf, inferior; LA, left atrium; MV, mitral valve; post, posterior; RA, right atrium; RV, right ventricle; sup, superior; TV, tricuspid valve.

Evaluation of Right Heart Pressures

The velocity of blood flow across the VSD as measured by spectral Doppler can be used to estimate right ventricular systolic pressure as long as the systolic blood pressure is known (Fig. 11.14). Using the modified Bernouli equation, the RV systolic pressure ($RVP_{systolic}$) is equal to 4 times the square of the peak VSD velocity (V_{VSD}^2) subtracted from the systolic blood pressure ($BP_{systolic}$) or

$$RVP_{systolic} = BP_{systolic} - 4V_{VSD}^2$$

The echocardiographic measurement of the peak VSD gradient works well in most cases, especially if the spectral Doppler tracing is plateau shaped. However, it will overestimate the LV-RV peak-to-peak gradient if the tracing peaks briefly in only a portion of systole. In these types of tracings, echo measurements of both the mean systolic gradient and the end-systolic gradient correlate well with invasive measures of the VSD gradient (Fig. 11.15).

The estimate of RV systolic pressure obtained using the VSD gradient can be validated by using the tricuspid regurgitation peak velocity. The RV systolic pressure is equal to 4 times the square of

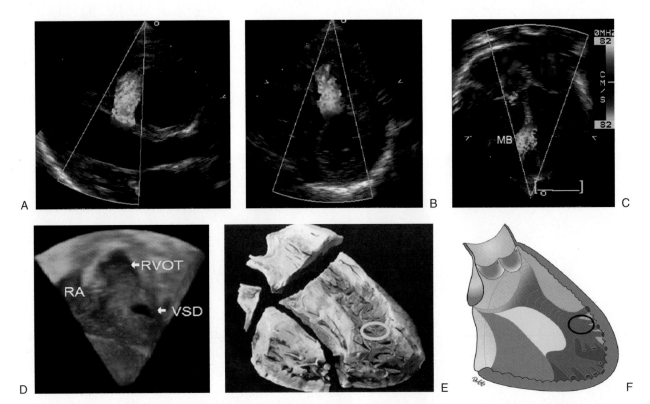

FIGURE 11.12. Localization of a muscular ventricular septal defect (VSD) near the right ventricular (RV) infundibular apex. Parasternal long-axis **(A)**, short-axis **(B)**, and apical four-chamber views **(C)** demonstrating localization of muscular VSD. **D:** Three-dimensional image acquired from a subxiphoid transducer position with the RV free wall cropped to show the entire septum from the RV aspect with localization of the defect in the anteroapical septum at the RV infundibular apex. Movie of this image demonstrates rotation of the septum with VSD imaged from left ventricular (LV) and RV aspects. **E:** Pathologic specimen showing the divisions of the ventricular septum as viewed from the RV aspect with the location of the muscular VSD circled. **F:** Representation of the subtypes of muscular VSDs with the location of the VSD seen in images **A–D** circled. MB, moderator band; RA, right atrium; RVOT, right ventricular outflow tract. (**E**, Reprinted and modified with permission from Becker A, Anderson R. Anomalies of the ventricles. In: *Cardiac Pathology and Integrated Text and Colour Atlas.* New York: Raven Press, 1983:12.2, Figure 12.1.)

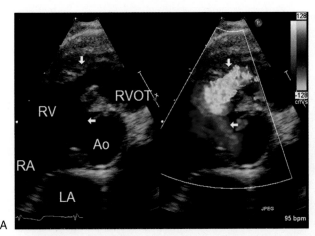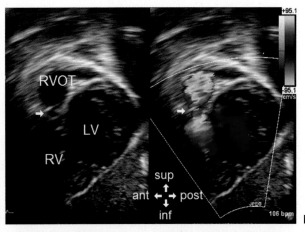

FIGURE 11.13. Large perimembranous ventricular septal defect (VSD) complicated by double-chambered right ventricle. Parasternal short-axis **(A)** and subcostal sagittal **(B)** views in two-dimensional and color flow mapping show the "napkin ring" of muscle bundles and flow disturbance (*arrow*) superior to the VSD. This VSD is on the "high pressure" side of the obstructing muscle bundles. ant, anterior; Ao, aorta; inf, inferior; LA, left atrium; LV, left ventricle; post, posterior; RA, right atrium; RV, right ventricle; RVOT, right ventricular outflow tract; sup, superior.

the tricuspid regurgitation velocity ($4V_{TR}^2$) plus the estimated or measured right atrial a-wave (RA) pressure:

$$RVP_{systolic} = 4V_{TR}^2 + RA\ pressure$$

Underestimation of RV pressure can occur due to a poor angle of Doppler interrogation or an incomplete TR signal. Overestimation of tricuspid regurgitation velocities may be due to contamination of the Doppler signal by an LV–to–right atrial shunt either through the tricuspid valve or a Gerbode defect. Estimation of RV systolic pressure by VSD gradient and tricuspid regurgitation velocities should give similar, if not identical, results. In the absence of pulmonary stenosis, the RV systolic pressure is equal to the pulmonary artery systolic pressure. Figure 11.14 gives an example of how VSD and tricuspid regurgitation velocities can be used to estimate right heart pressures noninvasively.

The pulmonary regurgitation velocity measured by spectral Doppler can be used to estimate mean and diastolic pulmonary artery pressures. This should be measured to serve as an additional validation of the hemodynamic assessment of a significant sized VSD. Elevated pulmonary regurgitation velocity should alert the echocardiographer to the presence of pulmonary artery diastolic hypertension, while normal pulmonary regurgitation velocities ensure the absence of substantial elevation of pulmonary artery diastolic pressure.

Quantification of Shunt Flow

VSD shunt volume is determined by the size of the VSD and the pulmonary vascular resistance. Quantification of the amount of shunt flow can be determined in several ways. Left heart chamber dilation is associated with pulmonary–to–systemic flow ratio (Q_p/Q_s) of greater than 1.5:1. Two Doppler-based methods can also be used to quantitate shunt flow and estimate Q_p/Q_s, although each method makes several assumptions. The first method uses pulsed-wave spectral Doppler across representative valves to quantify pulmonary and systemic flow (Fig. 11.16). Calculating systemic flow involves measuring the LV outflow tract pulsed-wave Doppler velocity-time integral (VTI) from an apical view and the LV outflow tract diameter

Echo Measures:
VSD velocity: 4.6 m/sec
Peak tricuspid regurgitation velocity: 2.5 m/sec
Peak LV to RA velocity: 5.0 m/sec

Other Measures:
Systolic blood pressure: 110 mmHg

LV systolic   = BP systolic

RVPsystolic   = BP sysolic- $4V_{VSD}^2$
            = $110 - 4\ (4.6)^2$
            = 25 mmHg

RVPsystolic   = $4V_{TR}^2$ + RA pressure
            = $4\ (2.5)^2 + 10$
            = 35 mmHg

RVPsystolic = PAsystolic ≈ 25-35 mmHg

Check
RA pressure = BP systolic - $4V_{LV-RA}^2$
              = $110 - 4(5.0)^2$
              = 10 mmHg

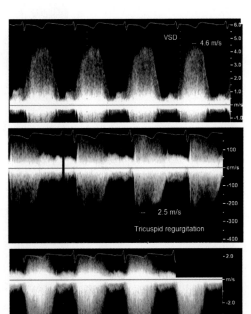

FIGURE 11.14. Noninvasive Doppler evaluation of right heart pressures. Spectral Doppler tracings of ventricular septal defect (VSD) are obtained from a left parasternal window, while tricuspid regurgitation and the left ventricular–to–right atrial shunt are both obtained from an apical window. BP, blood pressure; LV, left ventricle; PA, pulmonary artery; RA, right atrium; RV, right ventricle; TR, tricuspid regurgitation.

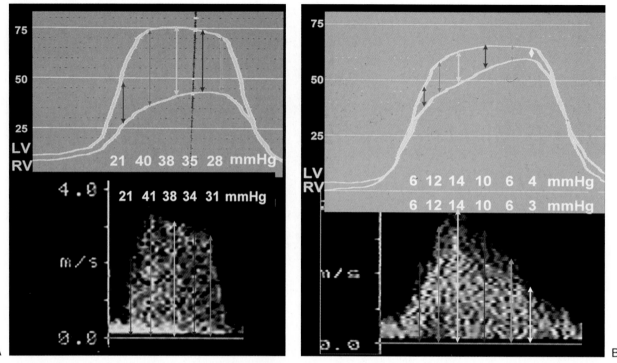

FIGURE 11.15. Simultaneous catheter measured intracardiac pressure tracings from the right ventricle (RV) and left ventricle (LV) with corresponding spectral Doppler tracing of velocities across ventricular septal defects (VSDs). **A:** VSD with a "plateau" shaped velocity tracing indicating holosystolic interventricular pressure gradient. **B:** "Spiky" tracing across a VSD with only transient early systolic interventricular pressure gradient.

Flow (l/min)
= (VTI x cross-sectional valve area x 60) / 1000

Qp:

RVOT diameter: 1.5 cm
RVOT area: 1.77 cm²
RVOT VTI: 21.2 cm/sec

Qp (l/min)
= (21.2 cm/sec x 1.77 cm² x 60 sec/min) / 1000cm³/liter
= 2.25 l/min

Qs:

LVOT diameter: 1.5 cm
LVOT area: 1.77 cm²
LVOT VTI: 16.7 cm/sec

Qs (l/min)
= (16.7 cm/sec x 1.77 cm² x 60 sec/min) / 1000cm³/liter
= 1.77 l/min

Qp/Qs = 1.3 : 1
Shunt Volume = 0.48 l/min

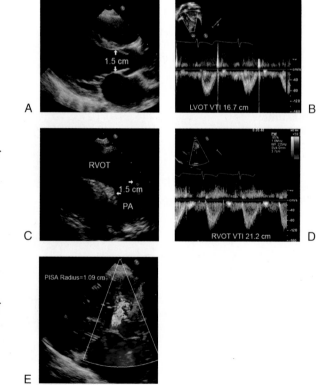

FIGURE 11.16. Doppler assessment of ventricular septal defect (VSD) shunt flow. **A–D:** Images and data necessary to calculate Qp/Qs include measurements of right and left ventricular outflow tract diameters and the velocity-time integral (VTI) of the spectral Doppler tracings of the right and left ventricular outflow tracts. **E:** Measurement of the distance (marked by calipers) from the VSD to the first aliasing velocity, which is used in the proximal isovelocity surface area (PISA) calculation of VSD shunt flow; in this patient, use of the PISA method resulted in overestimation of shunt flow as the flow toward the VSD did not accelerate in a hemispherical shape.

from a two-dimensional parasternal long-axis image. These values are then used in the following formula:

$$\text{Flow (L/min)} = (\text{VTI [cm/s]} \times \text{cross-sectional valve area [cm}^2]\\ \times 60 \text{ s/min})/1000 \text{ cm}^3/\text{L}$$

where the cross-sectional area of the aortic valve is $\pi \text{ (diameter/2)}^2$. Calculating the amount of pulmonary flow is more difficult. Accurate determination of VTI assumes laminar flow across the area in question; with VSDs, there is often turbulent flow across the pulmonary valve due to high flow volume, which may make the pulmonary outflow Doppler VTI unreliable in calculating the amount of pulmonary flow. In this case, mitral inflow Doppler VTI and mitral valve area can be used to calculate pulmonary flow. In the absence of a doming mitral valve, mitral valve area is based on two-dimensional measures of the mitral annulus in the four-chamber and/or parasternal long-axis views. Measurement of mitral valve flow volume is limited by the noncircular geometry of the mitral annulus. Several additional assumptions are made using this method of calculating systemic and pulmonary flows; these include the absence of significant semilunar valve regurgitation, the absence of other shunt lesions, and optimal Doppler angle alignment for measurement of VTI. Changes in the Doppler tracing with respiration can be minimized by averaging three consecutive heartbeats. In small children, there may be significant error in the measurement of flow volumes due to a proportionally greater error in the measurement of the diameter of flow regions. This diameter measure and its associated error are squared when calculating area for flow volumes. Because of these multiple, potential sources of error, this method of estimating systemic and pulmonary flow may not provide acceptable accuracy for decision making in many patients.

Another Doppler method for estimating the amount of shunt flow involves use of color Doppler and measures the proximal isovelocity surface area (PISA). The principle behind PISA is that blood flow crossing an orifice, such as a valve or VSD, speeds up as it approaches the orifice in a uniform, hemispherical pattern. By measuring the distance from the orifice to the point at which blood flow reaches a particular speed, the flow rate can be calculated. The location of the defined velocity can be determined by the Nyquist limit and the first line of aliasing color. This allows the following formula to be used:

$$\text{Flow rate (ml/s)} = 2\Pi(r)^2 \times \text{Nyquist limit (cm/s)}$$

where r is the distance from the VSD to the first aliasing velocity. Shunt volume across the VSD can then be calculated by multiplying the flow rate by the shunt duration time as determined by spectral Doppler across the VSD. This gives a final formula of:

$$\text{Shunt volume (L/min)} = [2\Pi(r)^2 \times \text{Nyquist limit (cm/s)} \times \text{shunt}\\ \text{duration (s)} \times \text{heart rate (beats/min)}]/\\ 1000 \text{ ml/s}$$

The PISA method requires several assumptions and has several important potential sources of error. One assumption is that the flow toward the VSD accelerates in a hemispherical shape. Second, all the flow that enters the area of aliasing velocity is assumed to cross the VSD. Precise localization of the VSD orifice can be difficult leading to errors in measurement of the distance from the VSD orifice to the first aliasing velocity (r). Finally, surface motion of the heart relative to the direction of VSD flow can cause additional errors in the measurement of the PISA radius (r). PISA has been reported to overestimate the Q_p/Q_s determined at catheterization but this method still may be helpful for serial assessment of shunt size over time in a subset of patients.

Closure of Ventricular Septal Defects

Many VSDs spontaneously close, or become significantly smaller, over time. Smaller defects are more likely to close spontaneously, but some large defects do close without intervention. In a study by Hornberger et al., all the VSDs that closed completely had an initial size, as measured by color flow mapping, of 4 mm or less. Even larger defects decreased in size with a frequency of 44% in defects less than 4 mm, 30% in defects of 4 to 6 mm, and 14% in defects greater than 6 mm in diameter. The most common mechanism of closure of perimembranous VSDs is by "anuerysmal transformation," in which redundant tricuspid valve tissue, or the tricuspid septal leaflet itself, closes the VSD (Fig. 11.7). Perimembranous

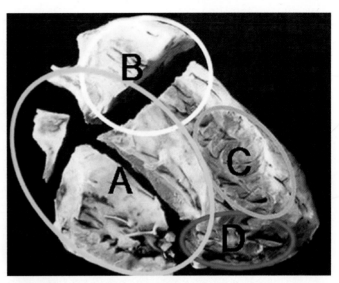

FIGURE 11.17. Potential surgical approaches to ventricular septal defect closure. A: Perimembranous, inlet, posterior muscular, and mid-muscular defects are typically closed by transatrial approach. **B:** Subarterial and some anterior muscular defects may be closed through the pulmonic valve. **C:** Anterior muscular defects inferior to the moderator band may require an anterior right ventriculotomy. **D:** Some surgeons use an apical left ventriculotomy to close posterior apical defects. (The pathologic specimen image is reprinted and modified with permission from Becker A, Anderson R. Anomalies of the ventricles. In: *Cardiac Pathology and Integrated Text and Colour Atlas.* New York: Raven Press, 1983:12.2, Figure 12.1.)

or subarterial VSDs can also be closed by prolapse of aortic valve leaflet tissue. Muscular VSDs close by ingrowth and hypertrophy of muscle; in infants this is thought to be a continuation of the in utero process of coalescence of sheets of muscle to close interventricular channels. Studies of muscular VSDs in newborns report spontaneous closure rates of 76% to 89% by 12 months of age.

Surgical Repair

Because no surgical approach allows visualization of the entire ventricular septum, a clear understanding of the number of defects, relative sizes, and exact location must be provided by the echocardiographer to facilitate a satisfactory surgical result. The surgical approach is determined by the expected defect location. Defects typically closed transatrially through the tricuspid valve include perimembranous, inlet, and some muscular defects. Subarterial defects are often best closed through the pulmonary valve. Muscular VSDs located below the moderator band and anterior to the septal band may be best approached with an anterior right ventriculotomy; an apical left ventriculotomy is occasionally used to approach posterior apical muscular defects (Fig. 11.17). The location of each defect must be presented clearly to the surgeon using the ultrasound images, mutually understood descriptors, and, often, diagrammatic presentation. Especially helpful descriptors include the distance and relationship to easily identifiable cardiac structures such as the moderator band, cardiac valves, and interventricular grooves. More detailed descriptions will result in a more brief surgical exploration, decrease trauma to adjacent myocardium or valves, and limit the potential for a significant residual intracardiac shunt.

Transcatheter Device Closure

More recently, transcatheter device closure and hybrid surgical and transcather approaches have developed as alternatives or adjuncts to surgical closure of VSDs. Currently, devices are available for closure of muscular and perimembranous defects. Prior to device closure, echocardiography should describe the size of the rims around the VSD in addition to information regarding the size and number of defects and their exact locations. For perimembranous defects, a rim of greater than 2 mm between the defect and aortic valve is required and the patient weight must be greater than 8 kg. Muscular VSD closure devices have been placed in infants as small as 3.2 kg. For both types of defects, the device is usually placed with

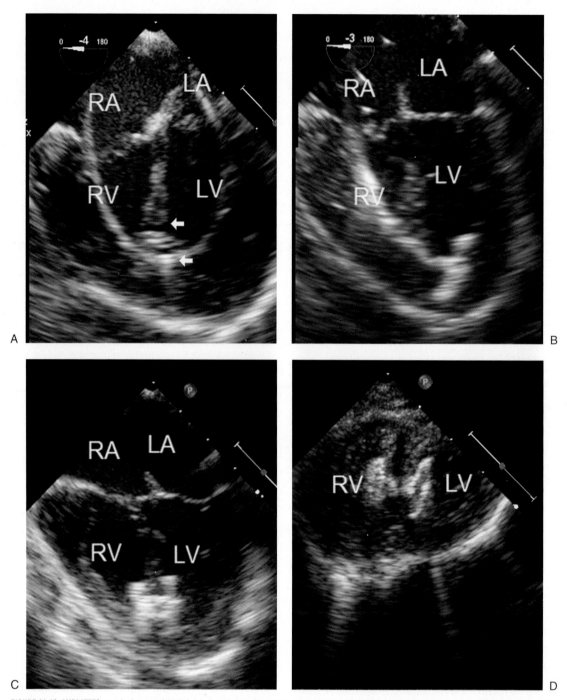

FIGURE 11.18. AMPLATZER ventricular septal occluder device closure of a muscular ventricular septal defect (VSD) in a patient with two apical muscular VSDs (arrows). A: Transesophageal four-chamber image of wire position across one of apical muscular VSDs. **B:** Transesophageal four-chamber image of the device still attached to the delivery cable but with the left ventricular disk delivered. **C:** Transesophageal four-chamber image of the AMPLATZER Septal Occluder (AGA Medical, Inc., Plymouth, Minn) device in its final position across the apical muscular VSD. **D:** Transesophageal short-axis image of the device in its final position. LA, left atrium; LV, left ventricle; RA, right atrium; RV, right ventricle.

transesophageal echocardiographic (TEE) guidance via either a percutaneous or perventricular approach. In a percutaneous approach, the location of the defect is identified by TEE and by angiography. The defect is sized at end diastole using a two-dimensional measurement. With a perventricular approach, TEE can guide the surgeon to indent the RV free wall progressively closer to the defect and identify a position to place the introducer sheath immediately over the defect and unobstructed by muscle bundles. In both the percutaneous and perventricular approaches, the sheath is advanced across

the VSD and an appropriate sized device is delivered. An example of transesophageal images obtained during VSD device placement via a percutaneous approach is shown in Figure 11.18.

In patients with multiple VSDs, device closure can be used in conjunction with surgical repair; this can be particularly helpful in cases where some, but not all, of the VSDs are positioned in locations that are difficult to approach surgically or when the defects are crossed by trabeculations, which can obscure visualization of the full extent of the defect. Complications of device closure that

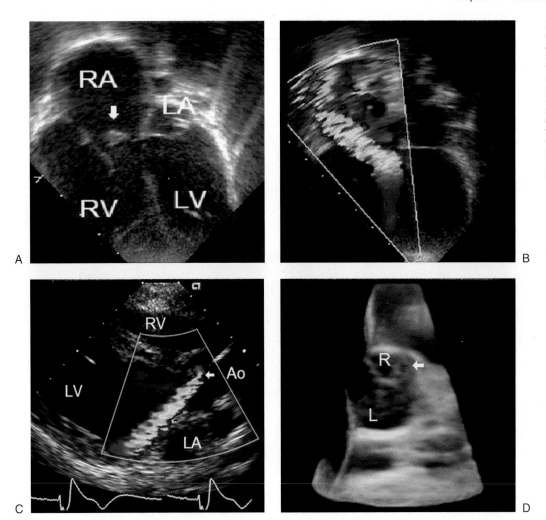

FIGURE 11.19. Complications of surgical closure of ventricular septal defects. **A–B:** Apical four-chamber view with two-dimensional and color Doppler of a flail septal leaflet of the tricuspid valve (*arrow*) due to disruption of septal attachments of the tricuspid valve. Parasternal long-axis **(C)** and three-dimensional short-axis **(D)** images showing perforation of the right coronary leaflet (*arrow* in **D**) of the aortic valve adjacent to the annulus with resultant aortic regurgitation (*arrow* in **C**). Ao, aorta; L, left; LA, left atrium; LV, left ventricle; R, right; RA, right atrium; RV, right ventricle.

can be identified echocardiographically include device embolization or migration, residual shunts, valve regurgitation (especially with perimembranous VSDs where the device is adjacent to the tricuspid and aortic valves), and pericardial effusion.

ECHOCARDIOGRAPHY OF POSTOPERATIVE VSDs

Echocardiography is commonly used in the postoperative evaluation following VSD closure. TEE or epicardial echocardiography can be used in the operating room to evaluate the surgical repair prior to chest closure. Ventricular dysfunction may occur immediately postoperatively or may develop later; possible etiologies include damage to the myocardium following ventriculotomy, acute volume unloading of the LV, and issues related to cardiopulmonary bypass. Other well-described complications include development of regurgitation of any of the valves adjacent to the VSD and residual or additional VSDs.

Surgical distortion of, or damage to, valves adjacent to the VSD most commonly effects the tricuspid and aortic valves. During repair of malalignment or perimembranous VSDs, the surgeon may sew the VSD patch to the annular edge of the tricuspid valve septal leaflet to avoid damage to the conduction system. Similarly, septal attachments of the tricuspid valve can be disrupted during patch closure. Substantial tricuspid regurgitation can develop from either prolapse or flail leaflet (Fig. 11.19A–B). The aortic valve can be affected following closure of any adjacent defect, typically perimembranous or subarterial. The development of aortic insufficiency may

be related to distortion of the aortic valve leaflet (most commonly the right aortic leaflet) by the VSD patch or from perforation of the valve leaflet due to inadvertent placement of a suture through the leaflet as the VSD patch is attached to the aortic valve annulus (Fig. 11.19C–D).

Residual or additional VSDs can be seen postoperatively. Additional VSDs that were not detected preoperatively are most common in patients where the identified defect was large, with equalization of right and left ventricular pressures and undisturbed flow. Once the large VSD has been closed, the smaller additional defects are easier to appreciate. Residual defects tend to occur along the margins of the VSD patch. Yang and colleagues reported residual VSDs less than 3 mm in size are generally well tolerated even in an infant. The coarse trabeculations of the RV wall make complete closure of some defects quite difficult as blood flow can continue to traverse the margins where the patch is sewn to trabeculae.

A subtype of residual defect is the "intramural" VSD, most commonly seen with the complex interventricular tunnel type of VSD patches used to repair double-outlet right ventricle, truncus arteriosus, or with a Rastelli-type repair of transposition of the great arteries. Intramural VSDs originate anteriorly, in the RV wall between the patch insertion and the aortic valve (Fig. 11.20), traversing the RV free wall trabeculae. They can be a particular challenge to image as the shunt flow percolating through RV trabeculae may appear to originate from the RV free wall, apparently away from the septum. Intramural VSDs are often not well seen from standard echocardiographic views and may require creative imaging strategies to allow careful interrogation of the RV anterior

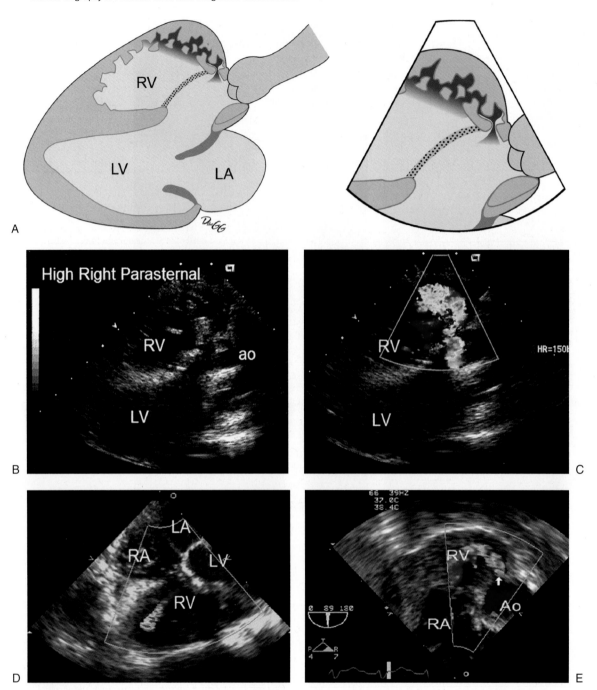

FIGURE 11.20. Intramural VSD. A: Diagrammatic representations of an intramural VSD. **B–C:** Transthoracic high right parasternal long-axis images with transducer over the anterior and rightward aorta. The ventricular septal defect (VSD) patch attaches to the trabeculae of the right ventricular (RV) free wall with percolation of flow through the trabeculae and along the RV free wall. **D:** Transesophageal anteriorly directed apical four-chamber view demonstrating transmyocardial entry of intramural VSD flow into the right ventricle. **E:** Transesophageal transverse plane image showing the intramural course of the VSD (*arrow*). Ao, aorta; LA, left atrium; LV, left ventricle; RA, right atrium; RV, right ventricle.

wall adjacent to the patch. Similarly, intramural defects are especially difficult to visualize by TEE. Imaging from the deep transgastric transducer position and careful short-axis sweeps may better define the defect.

Initially, these defects may be small, but they may enlarge as the channels in the RV trabeculae open up, resulting in significant left-to-right shunting. Intramural defects can be extremely difficult to repair surgically; improved understanding of these defects will likely result in greater success with operative repair.

Complications of VSD closure may also occur late after surgical repair. Endocarditis is especially common in the presence of

a residual shunt where the residual defect is adjacent to the site of a prosthetic patch and endothelialization may be inhibited. Subaortic obstruction can develop following either surgical or spontaneous VSD closure. In a study by Cicini, et al of postoperative VSD patients, 3.2% developed subaortic stenosis in the first 6 years postoperatively; the mechanism of subaortic narrowing was most often the development of a fibromuscular ridge or related to accessory mitral valve tissue. Other potential complications include development of a double-chambered RV, development or progression of pulmonary hypertension, and progressive aortic or tricuspid valve regurgitation.

SPECIAL STUDIES

Ventricular Septal Defect in the Fetus

Isolated VSDs make up 6% of congenital heart disease diagnosed in fetuses. Moderate to large muscular VSDs are the most common type of VSD diagnosed prenatally. Small, and even moderate sized, defects are rarely seen; defects less than 2 mm are near the limits of resolution of fetal ultrasound and the equalization of the ventricular pressures in utero makes flow across the defect laminar and more difficult to detect. As with transthoracic echocardiography, the best imaging plane is one in which the ventricular septum is perpendicular to the ultrasound beam with VSD flow parallel. This involves moving the transducer on the maternal abdomen until the appropriate imaging plane can be found. On fetal echocardiography, a VSD appears as an apparent dropout in the ventricular septum with bright margins of the defect. Color flow across the septum is bidirectional except in cases where there is associated outflow tract obstruction; the flow is of low velocity, usually between 40 and 70 cm/s.

Spontaneous closure of VSDs in utero is common. In a study by Paladini et al., one third of all defects closed spontaneously, with half of VSDs less than 3 mm closing in utero. The location of the VSD also affected the rate of spontaneous closure. Forty-four percent of perimembranous VSDs closed, but none of the outlet malalignment defects closed during gestation. All of the perimembranous VSDs that closed were less than 2 mm and closed by 30 weeks' gestation. Precise localization and sizing of VSDs by fetal echocardiography can allow the fetal cardiologist to provide accurate prognostic information to families.

Transesophageal Echocardiography

While occasionally used to evaluate VSDs preoperatively, transesophageal echocardiography (TEE) is more typically used intraoperatively to direct and evaluate surgical repair or to assist with device closure. While visualization of residual defects is often quite straightforward, transducer positions limited to the esophagus and transgastric windows may result in suboptimal Doppler interrogation angles. In addition, VSD patches and devices often have shadow artifacts, which limit visualization of VSD jets. However, careful assessment using standard and deep transgastric views can provide an accurate assessment of residual defects including identification of patients that require a return to cardiopulmonary bypass. In a series by Stevenson et al., 6.4% of patients with surgically closed VSDs underwent repeat bypass and additional closure based on TEE findings and intraoperative hemodynamics.

In a complete multiplane transesophageal examination, the ventricular septum should be swept along its entirety in short-axis, four-chamber, and long-axis planes with two-dimensional and color flow mapping. One systematic approach begins from a transgastric short-axis view at the apex, often with mild anteflexion, slight left lateral deflection, and approximately 20 degrees head rotation. The probe is gradually withdrawn until the entire septum has been traversed. When the transducer has been withdrawn superiorly to position behind and superior to the left atrium, the scope is retroflexed to a four-chamber view. From this position, anteflexion and retroflexion will scan the septum from the posterior to the anterior interventricular groove. Then, advancing to a low esophageal position with the transducer tip apical to the mitral annulus, the head is rotated to a long-axis plane (often 110 degrees). The ventricular septum is scanned in its long axis from its rightward and inlet portions to its leftward anterior and outlet portions. Finally, reimaging the septum from the RV aspect using a deep transgastric view is helpful to overcome shadowing artifact from a patch or device and to identify easily missed intramural VSDs.

The TEE examination in the patient after VSD closure should provide a detailed assessment of ventricular function; residual defects including their size, mechanism, and location; and any damage to valves adjacent to the defect. Small "patch leak" VSDs commonly observed in the operating room after VSD closure are of little significance and typically close postoperatively, or even after intraoperative administration of protamine. Yang et al. identified small VSD patch leaks in one third of intraoperative studies, two thirds of which closed spontaneously before hospital discharge. In this same study of 294 patients, 7 patients with no VSD or a small

residual VSD on intraoperative study had significant enlargement of the defect due to patch dehiscence or progressive enlargement of an intramural defect.

Three-dimensional Echocardiography

Assessment of VSD size and shape was identified as one of the earliest uses of three-dimensional (3D) and four-dimensional (3D in time) echocardiography. Still, difficulties with tissue thresholding "creating" nonexistent defects or seemingly "enlarging" existing defects have limited the application of 3D in the assessment of VSDs. With the advent of real-time transthoracic 3D echocardiography, improved mapping protocols, and higher-frequency pediatric transducers, the assessment of VSDs using 3D echocardiography has been increasingly reliable; it has been demonstrated to provide additional information to that provided by two-dimensional echocardiography. Specifically, the size of defects measured by 3D echocardiography better correlates with surgical measurements. Morphologic aspects of VSD aneurysm are better defined and the relationship of defects to important intracardiac structures is better assessed using 3D echoes. The irregular nature of many VSDs and their dynamic nature are understood to a much greater degree by 3D echocardiography as well.

While a standard approach to assessing VSDs using 3D echocardiography has not met with general use, a reasonable approach is suggested by an understanding of the physics of the image process. Ultrasound resolution is best in the axial (depth) plane and less in the two lateral planes. Image quality is progressively reduced in proportion to the number of reflectors between the transducer and the region of interest. The major limitation of 3D imaging of the interventricular septum has been false "fallout" of information, which "expands" or "creates" defects. Thus, it is especially important that the area of ventricular septum of interest is imaged in an axial plane while minimizing ultrasound reflectors between the transducer and this region of the septum, with a frequency and compression appropriate to create a solid-appearing myocardium and a translucent blood pool. Typically, this area of the septum is imaged obliquely with the transducer rotated to maintain the entire septum of interest within the data set. Because of the curved nature of the ventricular septum and variable quality of acoustic windows, an optimal transducer position may be subxiphoid, low parasternal, lateral to left parasternal, or periapical. Gain is increased until the blood pool appears solid and then reduced to the point where it just becomes translucent. The compression or opacity is then optimized.

After or during acquisition, the data set is "cropped." Removing portions of the LV and RV free wall allows an en face surgical view of the entire defect (Fig. 11.12D). An alternate method of cropping orients the data set in more standard echocardiographic plane such as a four-chamber or long-axis view and sets the cropping plane to course through the very edge of the defect (Fig. 11.21). Images are

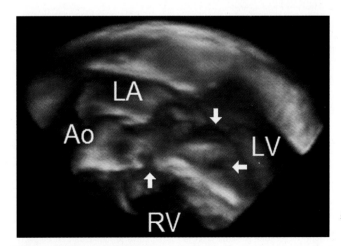

FIGURE 11.21. Three-dimensional image of inlet (*down arrow*), perimembranous (*up arrow*), and mid-muscular (*left arrow*) ventricular septal defects. The image is acquired from a low left parasternal transducer position and cropped in a pseudo–long-axis plane, allowing visualization of the membranous, inlet, and muscular septa from the left ventricular (LV) side. Ao, aorta; LA, left atrium; LV, left ventricle; RV, right ventricle.

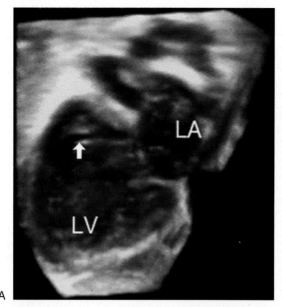
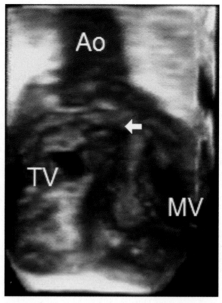

FIGURE 11.22. Three-dimensional echocardiogram of double outlet right ventricle with subaortic ventricular septal defect (VSD). Visualization of the septum en face from the left ventricular (LV) aspect **(A)** shows the subaortic VSD (*arrow*) and absence of the aorta exiting the LV. Video (see website) demonstrates rotation of this end-diastolic image with visualization of the VSD from RV to LV aspects. Cropping the dataset in a "short-axis" view **(B)** demonstrates the relationships of the tricuspid, mitral, and aortic valves to the defect. Videos (see website) demonstrate superior/inferior rotation of this mid-diastolic image to clarify intracardiac relationships. Ao, aorta; LA, left atrium; LV, left ventricle; MV, mitral valve; TV, tricuspid valve.

often displayed in the moving heart, but they may be more effectively understood if an end-diastolic still-frame is rotated through several planes to allow perspective.

Finally, as VSD anatomy and relationships become progressively more complicated, there is room for 3-D images to enhance understanding of intracardiac relationships. Relationships of AV valves to the defect, including straddling, as well as relationships of the defect to the great arteries can be optimally understood and presented using these images. Figure 11.22 clearly demonstrate the relationship of the VSD to the great arteries in this patient with double outlet right ventricle, subaortic VSD, and no AV valve straddling. It is clear that continued improvement of 3D imaging using both transthoracic and newly available real-time transesophageal transducers will allow understanding of complicated VSDs in detail not previously possible.

SUGGESTED READING

Anderson R, Becker A, Anomalies of the ventricles. In: Cardiac Pathology and Integrated Text and Colour Atlas. New York: Raven Press, 1983:12.2.

Allan L. Abnormalities of the ventricular septum. In: Allan L, Hornberger LK, Sharland G, eds. *Textbook of Fetal Cardiology*. London: Greenwich Medical Media, 2000:195–209.

Allan LD, Sharland GK, Milburn A, et al. Prospective diagnosis of 1,006 consecutive cases of congenital heart disease in the fetus. *J Am Coll Cardiol.* 1994;23:1452–1458.

Cheung, YF, Chiu CS, Yung TC, et al. Impact of preoperative aortic cusp prolapse on long-term outcome after surgical closure of subarterial ventricular septal defect. *Ann Thorac Surg.* 2002;73:622–627.

Cicini MP, Giannico S, Marino B, et al. "Acquired" subvalvular aortic stenosis after repair of a ventricular septal defect. *Chest.* 1992; 101:115–118.

Cil E, Saraclar M, Ozkutlu S, et al. Double-chambered right ventricle: experience with 52 cases. *Int J Cardiol.* 1995;50:19–29.

Corone P, Doyon F, Gaudeau S, et al. Natural history of ventricular septal defect. A study involving 790 cases. *Circulation.* 1977; 55 : 908–915.

Diab KA, Cao Q, Mora BN, et al. ZM. Device closure of muscular ventricular septal defects in infants less than one year of age using the Amplatzer device. *Cathet Cardiovasc Interv.* 2007; 70:90–97.

Eroglu AG, Oztunc F, Saltik L, et al. Aortic valve prolapse and aortic regurgitation in patients with ventricular septal defect. *Pediatr Cardiol.* 2003; 24;36–39.

Eroglu AG, Oztunc F, Saltik L, et al. Evolution of ventricular septal defect with deptal reference to spontaneous closure rate, subaortic ridge and aortic valve prolapse. *Pediatr Cardiol.* 2003; 24;31–35.

Ge Z, Zhang Y, Kang W, et al. Noninvasive evaluation of interventricular pressure gradient across ventricular septal defect: A simultaneous study of Doppler echocardiography and cardiac catheterization. *Am Heart J.* 1992;124:176–182.

Hagler DJ, Edwards WD, Seward JB, et al. Standardized nomenclature of the ventricular septum and ventricular septal defects, with applications for two-dimensional echocardiography. *Mayo Clinic Proc.* 1985;60:741–752.

Hijazi Z. Device closure of ventricular septal defects. *Cathet Cardiovasc Interv.* 2003; 60:107–114.

Hiraishi S, Agata Y, Nowatari M, et al. Incidence and natural course of trabecular ventricular septal defect: Two-dimensional echocardiography and color Doppler flow imaging study. *J Pediatr.* 1992;120:409–415.

Hornberger LK, Sahn DJ, Krabill KA, et al. Elucidation of the natural history of ventricular septal defects by serial Doppler color flow mapping studies. *J Am Coll Cardiol.* 1989;13:1111–1118.

Hsu JH, Wu JR, Dai ZK, et al. Real-time three-dimensional echocardiography provides novel and useful anatomic insights of perimembranous ventricular septal aneurysm. *Int J Cardiol.* 2007;118:326–331.

Jacobs JP, Burke RP, Quintessenza JA, et al. Congenital Heart Surgery Nomenclature and Database Project: Ventricular septal defect. *Ann Thorac Surg.* 2000;69(4 Suppl):S25–S35.

Kardon RE, Cao QL, Masani N, et al. New insights and observations in three-dimensional echocardiographic visualization of ventricular septal defects: Experimental and clinical studies. *Circulation.* 1998;98:1307-1314.

Kearney DL, Titus JL. Cardiovascular anatomy. In: Garson A, Bricker JT, Fisher DJ, et al, eds. *The Science and Practice of Pediatric Cardiology.* 2nd ed. Baltimore, Md: Williams & Wilkins, 1998:127–153.

Kumar K, Lock JE, Geva T. Apical muscular ventricular septal defects between the left ventricle and the right ventricular infundibulum. *Circulation.* 1997;95:1207–1213.

Latson LA, Prieto LR. Pulmonary stenosis. In: Allen HD, Gutgesell HP, Clark EB, et al, eds. *Moss and Adams' Heart Disease in Infants, Children, and Adolescents.* 6th ed. Philadelphia, Pa: Lippincott William & Wilkins, 2001:820–844.

Marx GR, Allen HD, Goldberg SJ. Doppler echocardiographic estimation of systolic pulmonary artery pressure in pediatric patients with interventricular communications. *J Am Coll Cardiol.* 1985;6:1132–1137.

McDaniel NL, Gutgesell HP. Ventricular septal defects. In: Allen HD, Gutgesell HP, Clark EB, et al, eds. *Moss and Adams' Heart Disease in Infants, Children, and Adolescents* 6th ed. Philadelphia, Pa: Lippincott William & Wilkins, 2001:636–651.

Mercer-Rosa L, Seliem MA, Fedec A, et al. Illustration of the additional value of real-time 3-dimensional echocardiography to conventional transthoracic and transesophageal 2-dimensional echocardiography in imaging muscular ventricular septal defects: Does this have any impact on individual patient treatment? *J Am Soc Echocardiogr.* 2006;19:1511–1519.

Moene RJ, Gittenberger-de Groot AC, Oppenheimer-Dekker A, et al. Anatomic characteristics of ventricular septal defect associated with coarctation of the aorta. *Am J Cadiol.*1987;59:952–955.

Moises VA, Maciel BC, Hornberger LK, et al. A new method for noninvasive estimation of ventricular septal defect shunt flow by Doppler color flow mapping: Imaging of the laminar flow convergence region on the left septal surface. *J Am Coll Cardiol.* 1991;18:824–832.

Mori K, Matsuoka S, Tartara K, et al. Echocardiography evaluation of the development of aortic valve prolapse in supracristal ventricular septal defect. *Eur J Pediatr.* 1995;154: 176–181.

Murphy DJ Jr, Ludomirsky A, Huhta JC. Continuous-wave Doppler in children with ventricular septal defect: Noninvasive estimation of interventricular pressure gradient. *Am J Cardiol.* 1986;57:428–432.

Ohye RG, Bove EL. Current topics in congenital heart surgery. In: Allen HD, Gutgesell HP, Clark EB, et al, eds. *Moss and Adams' Heart Disease in Infants, Children, and Adolescents.* 6th ed. Philadelphia, Pa: Lippincott William & Wilkins, 2001:382–394.

Ooshima A, Fukushige J, Ueda K. Incidence of structural cardiac disorders in neonates: An evaluation by color Doppler echocardiography and the results of a 1-year follow-up. *Cardiology.* 1995;86:402–406

Paladini D, Palmieri S, Lamberti A, et al. Characterization and natural history of ventricular septal defects in the fetus. *Ultrasound Obstet Gynecol.* 2000;16:118–122.

Preminger TJ, Sanders SP, van der Velde ME, et al. "Intramural" residual interventricular defects after repair of conotruncal malformations. *Circulation.* 1994;89:236–242.

Roberson DA, Muhiudeen IA, Cahalan MK, et al. Intraoperative transesophageal echocardiography of ventricular septal defect. *Echocardiography.* 1991;8:687–697.

Roguin N, Du ZD, Barak M, et al. High prevalence of muscular ventricular septal defect in neonates. *J Am Coll Cardiol.* 1995;26:1545–1548.

Rollins MD, Koehler RP, Stevens MH, et al. Traumatic ventricular septal defect: Case report and review for the English literature since 1970. *J Trauma.* 2005; 58:175–180.

Schamberger MS, Farrell AG, Darragh RK, et al. Use of peak Doppler gradient across ventricular septal defects leads to underestimation of right-sided pressures in patients with "sloped" Doppler signals. *J Am Soc Echocardiogr.* 2001;14: 1197–1202.

Singh M, Agarwala MK, Grover A, et al. Clinical, echocardiographic, and angiographic profile of patients with double chambered right ventricle: Experience with 48 cases. *Angiology.* 1999;50:223–231.

Snider AR, Serwer GA, Ritter SB. Abnormalities of ventricular outflow. In: *Echocardiography in Pediatric Heart Disease.* 2nd ed. St. Louis, Mo: Mosby, 1997:408–422.

Snider AR, Serwer GA, Ritter SB. Defects in cardiac septation. In: *Echocardiography in Pediatric Heart Disease.* 2nd ed. St. Louis, Mo: Mosby, 1997:246–277.

Soto B, Becker AE, Moulaert AJ, et al. Classification of ventricular septal defects. *Br Heart J.* 1980;43:332–343.

Stevenson JG, Sorensen GK, Gartman DM, et al. Transesophageal echocardiography during repair of congenital cardiac defects: Identification of residual problems necessitating reoperation. *J Am Soc Echocardiogr.* 1993;6:356–365.

Tantengco MV, Bates JR, Ryan T, et al. Dynamic three-dimensional echocardiographic reconstruction of congenital cardiac septation defects. *Pediatr Cardiol.* 1997;18:184–190.

The International Working Group for Mapping and Coding of Nomenclatures for Paediatric and Congenital Heart Disease. Available at www.ipccc.net.

Tohyama K, Satomi G, Momma K. Aortic valve prolapse and aortic regurgitation associated with subpulmonic ventricular septal defect. *Am J Cardiol.* 1997;79:1285–1289.

van den Bosch AE, Ten Harkel DJ, McGhie JS, et al. Feasibility and accuracy of real-time 3-dimensional echocardiographic assessment of ventricular septal defects. *J Am Soc Echocardiogr.* 2006;19:7–13.

van der Velde ME, Sanders SP, Keane JF, et al. Transesophageal echocardiographic guidance of transcatheter ventricular septal defect closure. *J Am Coll Cardiol.* 1994;23:1660–1665.

Van Praagh R, Geva AT, Kreutzer J. Ventricular septal defects: How shall we describe, name and classify them? *J Am Coll Cardiol.* 1989; 14:1298–1299.

van Praagh R, Plett JA, van Praagh S. Single ventricle. Pathology, embryology, terminology and classification. *Herz.* 1979;4:113–150.

Vogel M, Freedom RM, Brand A, et al. Ventricular septal defect and subaortic stenosis: An analysis of 41 patients. *Am J Cardiol.* 1983; 52: 1258–1263.

Weidman WH, Blount SG, DuShane JW, et al. Clinical course in ventricular septal defect. *Circulation.* 1977;56(1 Suppl):I56–I69.

Wienecke M, Fyfe DA, Kline CH, et al. Comparison of intraoperative transesophageal echocardiography to epicardial imaging in children undergoing ventricular septal defect repair. *J Am Soc Echocardiogr.* 1991;4:607–614.

Wilson W, Taubert K, Gewitz M, et al. Prevention of infective endocarditis. Guidelines from the American Heart Association. A guideline from the American Heart Association Rheumatic Fever, Endocarditis, and Kawasaki Disease Committee, Council on Cardiovascular Disease in the Young, and the Council on Clinical Cardiology, Council on Cardiovascular Surgery and Anesthesia, and the Quality of Care and Outcomes Research Interdisciplinary Working Group. *Circulation.* 2007;115. [Epub ahead of print].

Wu MH, Wu JM, Chang CL, et al. Implication of aneurysmal transformation in isolated perimembranous ventricular septal defect. *Am J Cardiol.* 1993; 72:596–601.

Yang SG, Novello R, Nicolson S, et al. Evaluation of ventricular septal defect repair using intraoperative transesophageal echocardiography: Frequency and significance of residual defects in infants and children. *Echocardiography.* 2000; 17:681–684.

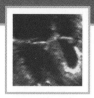

Chapter 12
Univentricular Atrioventricular Connections

Shaji C. Menon • Allison K. Cabalka

Patients with only one ventricle (i.e., "functional single ventricle," or the functionally univentricular heart) comprise a very heterogeneous group. With the Fontan operation as preferred definitive palliation in patients with a univentricular heart, it remains important to determine if a given ventricular chamber is inadequate for support of either systemic or pulmonary circulation. Often, the atrioventricular (AV) connection is the determining factor.

Nomenclature and classification of the univentricular heart have long been a subject of debate and controversy, with terms such as "single ventricle," "univentricular heart," "univentricular atrioventricular connection," and "double-inlet ventricle" being used over the years. Van Praagh and colleagues originally defined a univentricular heart as one ventricular chamber that receives both tricuspid and mitral valves or a common AV valve; hearts with one absent AV valve (including mitral and tricuspid atresia) were not included in this original review. Van Praagh et al. also pointed out that although these patients have a functionally univentricular heart, there are usually two ventricular chambers; thus, a "true" univentricular heart is exceedingly rare. Anderson and colleagues introduced the term "univentricular atrioventricular connection" and applied this to hearts where the AV connection was committed to one ventricle. They subsequently proposed that "univentricular heart of left ventricular type" be applied to hearts where the dominant ventricle was a morphologic left ventricle (LV) and "univentricular heart of right ventricular type" be applied to the dominant right ventricle (RV). Further characterization of the ventricular mass as consisting of three regions (inlet, trabecular, and outlet regions) was included. Assessment of a ventricle in this way could aid in the determination of the adequacy of a given ventricle, that is, whether a ventricle was complete or incomplete. However, the hypoplastic ventricle with all three components present does exist. In more recent publications on nomenclature, Jacobs and Anderson simply refer to the "functionally univentricular heart," wherein the emphasis was placed on the inadequacy of one or the other ventricle to support the pulmonary or systemic circulation. Regardless of the preferred nomenclature, a segmental approach to echocardiographic evaluation is necessary in all cases, defining connections and relationships to provide the clinician with relevant information.

This chapter will cover the three main types of univentricular AV connection that produce a functionally univentricular heart: tricuspid atresia, mitral atresia (or hypoplastic left heart syndrome), and double-inlet LV (DILV). A brief review of the hypoplastic LV or mitral stenosis in the setting of multiple left-sided obstructive lesions is included. Typically, all of these conditions are the result of an absent, hypoplastic, or atretic AV connection.

All patients with a functionally univentricular heart require careful anatomic assessment to plan for a staged surgical approach that will provide definitive palliation. Although nomenclature may be debated, it is important that there is consensus regarding such nomenclature at the institutional level so that clinicians understand each other and are able to communicate clearly about the nature of complex congenital heart disease. A complete description of segmental anatomy and physiology, which inherently lends itself to clinical application and decision making, is most useful for the broadest audience.

 ## TRICUSPID ATRESIA

Tricuspid atresia is the third most common form of cyanotic congenital heart disease, with a prevalence of 0.3% to 3.7%, and is characterized by absence of a direct communication between the right atrium (RA) and the RV (Fig. 12.1). There is a univentricular AV connection with the dominant ventricle having left ventricular morphology. The anatomic form of atresia is most commonly fibromuscular; less

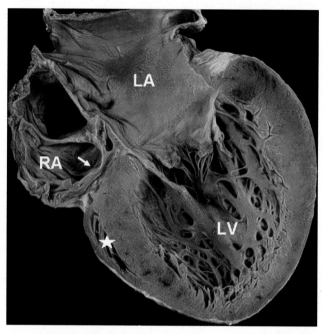

FIGURE 12.1. Pathologic specimen in tricuspid atresia showing the atretic fibrofatty tricuspid valve (*arrow*). The left atrium (LA) and left ventricle (LV) are enlarged. The right ventricle is extremely hypoplastic and appears as a "slit-like" space (*asterisk*). RA, right atrium.

commonly, it is membranous, valvar, or Ebstein-like with valvar atresia. In the majority of patients, the floor of the RA is entirely muscular with separation from the hypoplastic RV by fibrofatty tissue.

Historically, based on the great artery relationship, tricuspid atresia is classified into three types, with subclassification based on the anatomy of the ventricular septal defect (VSD) and pulmonary valve (Table 12.1). However, to avoid miscommunication, the echocardiographer should describe the anatomy and physiology in detail.

Table 12.1	CLASSIFICATION OF TRICUSPID ATRESIA	
Type	Description	Relative frequency, %
I	Normally related great arteries	69
I-A	Pulmonary atresia, no VSD	9
I-B	Pulmonary stenosis, Restrictive VSD	51
I-C	No pulmonary stenosis, Large VSD	9
II	D-transposed great arteries	28
II-A	Pulmonary atresia, VSD	2
II-B	Pulmonary stenosis, VSD	8
II-C	No pulmonary stenosis , VSD	18
III	L-transposed great arteries	3

Associated Anomalies

An opening in the atrial septum, either a patent foramen ovale or a secundum atrial septal defect (ASD), is obligatory for survival. Occasionally, the atrial septum is restrictive. Rarely, a primum ASD may be present. Thirty percent of patients with tricuspid atresia will have additional associated cardiac anomalies, including left superior vena cava (SVC) (16%), juxtaposed atrial appendages (more common with transposed great arteries), and coarctation of the aorta (8%). Associated cardiovascular anomalies are more common with transposed great arteries (63%) compared with normally related great arteries (18%). Also, approximately 20% of patients will have extracardiac anomalies including gastrointestinal and neurologic defects.

Clinical History

The majority of patients with tricuspid atresia present with cyanosis. Patients with tricuspid atresia and normally related great arteries (ventriculoarterial concordance) have a high incidence of subvalvular or valvular pulmonary stenosis (less commonly, atresia). Clinical presentation depends on the amount of pulmonary blood flow, which is proportional to the size of the VSD and the degree of pulmonary valvar/subvalvular stenosis. If there is no significant pulmonary stenosis or restriction of the VSD, these patients may present between 4 and 8 weeks of age with signs and symptoms of pulmonary overcirculation (similar to the infant with a large VSD) and only mild hypoxemia due to the large amount of pulmonary blood flow. If not recognized early, these infants are at risk for longer-term complications from hypoxemic pulmonary overcirculation and elevated vascular resistance. In the presence of pulmonary atresia or critical pulmonary stenosis, closure

of the ductus arteriosus results in severe cyanosis, hypoxemia, and acidosis, and, if not treated promptly, may result in death. Patients with transposed great arteries (ventriculoarterial discordance) typically have unobstructed pulmonary blood flow; as pulmonary vascular resistance drops in the neonatal period, these infants may also present with signs of congestive heart failure and pulmonary edema. However, if there is significant aortic arch obstruction or critical restriction of the VSD (supplying systemic output), once the ductus arteriosus closes, cardiovascular collapse and shock will develop.

Echocardiographic Examination of Tricuspid Atresia

Echocardiography in the neonate with tricuspid atresia provides comprehensive diagnostic information. Diagnostic cardiac catheterization is rarely needed. Careful attention to the absent right AV connection, the arrangement of the great arteries, the nature of the communication between the LV and hypoplastic RV, and the presence of aortic arch or pulmonary artery (PA) obstruction should provide the clinician with complete diagnostic assessment, allowing for accurate planning of staged surgical palliation.

Subcostal Views

SUBCOSTAL FOUR-CHAMBER (CORONAL) VIEW – Subcostal examination begins with a determination of abdominal viscera and atrial situs in all patients. Subcostal four-chamber (coronal) views will show dilation of the RA with absence of the connection to the RV (Fig. 12.2A). As foreshortening of the RV may occur in this plane, short-axis (sagittal) plane imaging is useful for "three-dimensional" assessment of right ventricular size. The atrial septum is best visualized from

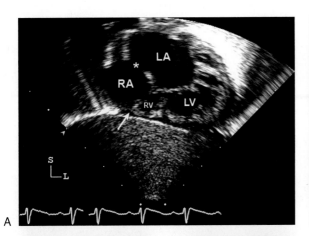

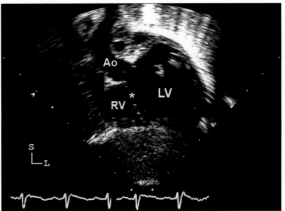

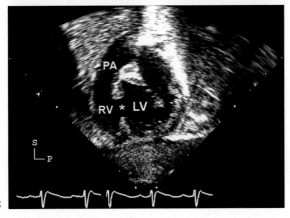

FIGURE 12.2. Tricuspid atresia with normally related great arteries; subcostal views. A: "Four-chamber" (coronal) view showing moderate-sized secundum atrial septal defect (*asterisk*), atretic tricuspid valve (*arrow*), hypoplastic right ventricle (RV), and dilated left ventricle (LV). **B:** Four-chamber view, angled anteriorly, illustrating the large ventricular septal defect (*asterisk*). Aortic (Ao) origin from LV in normally related great arteries. **C:** Short-axis (sagittal) view showing anterior RV, posterior LV, and muscular ventricular septal defect (*asterisk*). In normally related great arteries, the pulmonary artery (PA) arises anteriorly from the RV and bifurcates early. LA, left atrium; RA, right atrium.

subcostal imaging planes, and characterization of the ASD should be performed. Prominent eustachian valve tissue may be present but typically does not contribute to obstruction. Color Doppler will show a right-to-left shunt from the RA to the left atrium (LA) and no flow from the RA to the RV. It is unusual for the ASD to be restrictive, but pulsed-wave Doppler interrogation should be used to evaluate the RA-to-LA gradient, tracing the signal over three cardiac cycles to determine a mean gradient. An atrial shunt is obligatory for survival; therefore, a restrictive ASD may result in severe hemodynamic compromise requiring urgent septostomy. Evaluation of the great arteries from multiple imaging planes to determine ventriculoarterial connections is important (Fig. 12.2B–C). An enlarged, posterior great artery (PA) that bifurcates early is consistent with transposed great arteries (ventriculoarterial discordance) (Fig. 12.3A–B). Examination of the ventricular septum may provide information on the size and location of the VSD, but orthogonal views will be needed. The mitral valve and left ventricular function can be assessed initially from the four-chamber subcostal plane.

A left-juxtaposed right atrial appendage is visualized in the subcostal four-chamber scan plane. Both atrial appendages are located more leftward than normal. Echocardiographers should be alert to a left juxtaposed right atrial appendage when visualizing an abnormal convexity of the atrial septum to the left or a transverse orientation of the septum when imaging posteriorly from the subcostal four-chamber plane. Further anterior angulation of the probe will reveal the connection of the RA to the leftward right atrial appendage. Juxtaposition of the appendages should not be confused with an ASD.

SUBCOSTAL SHORT-AXIS (SAGITTAL) VIEW – Subcostal short-axis views demonstrate the absent connection between the floor of the RA and the hypoplastic RV. Orthogonal views are very useful for evaluation of the atrial septal anatomy. Again, the right-to-left shunt should be unrestricted in the setting of an adequate interatrial communication. Rightward angulation of the transducer facilitates evaluation of the absent communication between the RA and the hypoplastic RV, and the size of the RV is more easily assessed in the subcostal short-axis view than in the four-chamber imaging plane (Figs. 12.2C and 3C–D). Evaluation of the size of the VSD between the LV and hypoplastic anterior RV is important for documenting sites of obstruction to arterial outflow. Careful sweeps from right to left are important to obtain complete information about the location and degree of right ventricular outflow obstruction. Assessment of the ventriculoarterial connection is performed from the short-axis view; again, the proximal bifurcation of the PA should be assessed. The presence of parallel great arteries suggests transposition (ventriculoarterial discordance). A small anterior aorta should prompt a careful evaluation for coarctation of the aorta from additional views.

Parasternal View
PARASTERNAL LONG AXIS – Parasternal long-axis scans typically demonstrate a small anterior RV and a large posterior LV (Fig. 12.4A). This scan plane also provides excellent views of the ventricular septum. The size and position of the VSD should be noted (Fig. 12.4A). The position and origin of the great arteries are confirmed. In the presence of transposed great arteries, the arteries

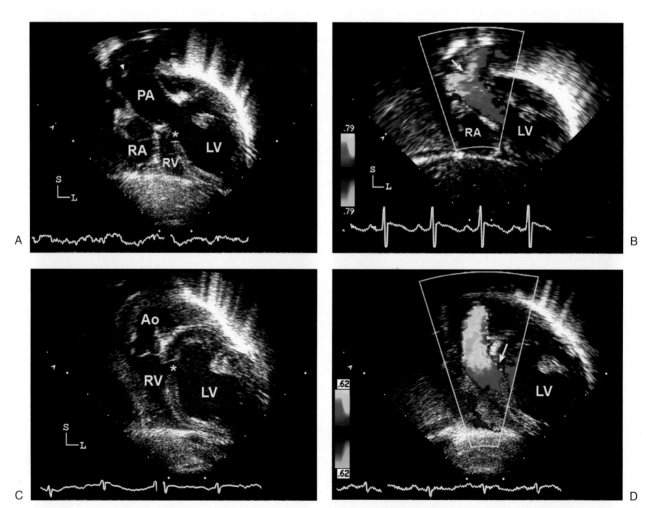

FIGURE 12.3. Tricuspid atresia with transposed great arteries; subcostal long-axis (coronal) views. A: Dilated left ventricle (LV), hypoplastic right ventricle (RV), and a small muscular ventricular septal defect (*asterisk*). Note the pulmonary artery (PA) arising from the LV with early bifurcation (*arrowhead*). **B:** Color Doppler imaging in the same patient demonstrating flow in the PA bifurcation (arrow). **C:** Slight anterior angulation of the transducer demonstrates the LV, hypoplastic RV, and the restrictive ventricular septal defect (*asterisk*). The anterior aorta (Ao) arises from the hypoplastic RV. **D:** Color Doppler demonstrating the flow across the small ventricular septal defect (*arrow*), antegrade into the aorta.

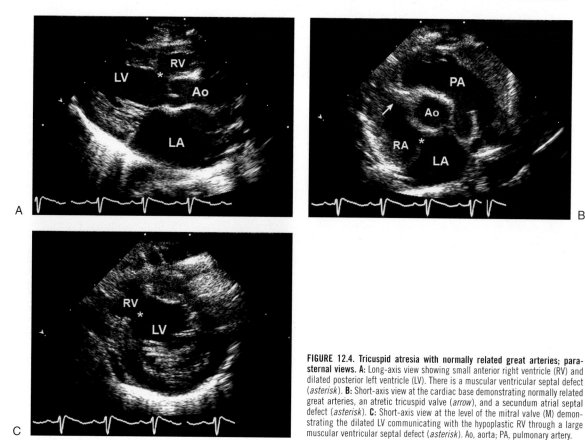

FIGURE 12.4. Tricuspid atresia with normally related great arteries; parasternal views. A: Long-axis view showing small anterior right ventricle (RV) and dilated posterior left ventricle (LV). There is a muscular ventricular septal defect (*asterisk*). **B:** Short-axis view at the cardiac base demonstrating normally related great arteries, an atretic tricuspid valve (*arrow*), and a secundum atrial septal defect (*asterisk*). **C:** Short-axis view at the level of the mitral valve (M) demonstrating the dilated LV communicating with the hypoplastic RV through a large muscular ventricular septal defect (*asterisk*). Ao, aorta; PA, pulmonary artery.

appear parallel in their proximal course from the ventricles; with the posterior vessel (PA) bifurcating early (Fig. 12.5A). If the VSD is present in the outlet portion of the septum, anterior deviation of the septum (seen most commonly with normally related great arteries) may produce subpulmonary obstruction. Posterior deviation is seen more often with transposed great arteries. Muscular ridges or membranes can also cause ventricular outflow obstruction and should be evaluated from multiple imaging planes. Anterior angulation of the transducer toward the patient's left shoulder may bring the right ventricular outflow tract (RVOT) into view. Doppler and color Doppler evaluation of the gradient from the LV to RV and into the RVOT should be used to provide information about the degree of restriction, either to the PA (for an estimation of the PA pressure) or to the anterior aorta in transposition.

Visualization of the atrial septum in a perpendicular orientation from the long-axis view may be consistent with a left-juxtaposed right atrial appendage. A dilated coronary sinus should alert the echocardiographer to the possibility of a left SVC returning to the coronary sinus (which has implications in planning for the bidirectional cavopulmonary shunt as palliation).

PARASTERNAL SHORT-AXIS VIEW – The parasternal short-axis view is useful for further characterization of the hypoplastic RV and VSD and position of the great arteries (Figs 12.4B and 5B). Left ventricular function should be evaluated. Scanning apically from the base of the heart toward the midventricular level, the right ventricle is seen in front of the dominant, large LV (Fig. 12.4C). In addition to orthogonal subcostal views, the size of the RV and the anatomy of

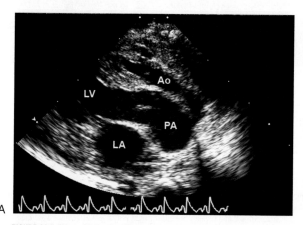

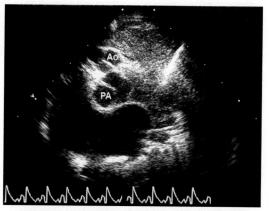

FIGURE 12.5. Tricuspid atresia with transposed great arteries; parasternal views. A: Long-axis view showing the parallel orientation of the great arteries classically seen in transposition, with an anterior aorta (Ao); posterior pulmonary artery (PA) originating from the dilated left ventricle (LV). **B:** Short-axis view at the cardiac base showing both semilunar valves in short axis at the same level, again consistent with transposition of the great arteries. The aortic valve (Ao) is hypoplastic and located anterior and slightly rightward, whereas the pulmonary valve (PA) is dilated and located posterior and leftward. LA, left atrium.

the VSD can be assessed in the short-axis plane (Fig. 12.4C). The presence of additional VSDs should be assessed with both imaging and color Doppler. Pulsed-wave Doppler interrogation can provide an estimation of the gradient between the LV and RV as well as aid in assessing the restrictive VSD. Scanning superiorly toward the base of the heart to the level of the great arteries will again confirm their arrangement. If transposed, both great vessels are seen in short axis, represented by two semilunar valves seen in the same imaging plane (Fig. 12.5B). In transposition, one can evaluate whether the anterior aorta is located rightward (*d*-transposition, more common) or leftward (*l*-transposition, less common).

It is necessary to evaluate the degree of restriction of the RVOT in the short-axis view. Color Doppler and pulsed-wave Doppler should be used in this assessment. With normally related great arteries, the presence of a large PA suggests that adequate or generous pulmonary blood flow is present. If the PA is very small or diminutive, it is necessary to confirm the presence of antegrade flow from the RV to the PA. Rarely, pulmonary atresia coexists with tricuspid atresia, a ductal-dependent critical condition. The ductus arteriosus should be assessed fully. Typically, a trifurcation view of the ductus, left PA, and right PA can be obtained in a high left parasternal plane.

Apical Views – An apical four-chamber view provides excellent definition of the absent right AV connection (Fig. 12.6A). Angling the transducer posteriorly demonstrates the muscular atresia of the tricuspid valve appearing as an echo-dense plate of tissue in the floor of the RA. Again, assessment of the hypoplastic RV and its communication from the LV (VSD) is important. In the presence of juxtaposed atrial appendages, one can again see an abnormal atrial septal configuration. Mitral valve morphology and function are well visualized from the apical approach. Angling the transducer anteriorly facilitates development of a "five-chamber view," providing further assessment of the outflow tracts and sites of potential obstruction (Fig. 12.6B–6C). The origin, size, and position of the great arteries and outflow tracts again are assessed in light of information obtained from all of the previous views. The size of the VSD and any evidence of obstruction are evaluated with both pulsed-wave and color Doppler, attempting to align the transducer beam in a parallel fashion with the VSD or outflow tracts. Para-apical imaging, directing the transducer more anteriorly toward the anterior great artery, can also facilitate assessment of obstruction and gradients.

Suprasternal Notch Views – Beginning with the long-axis view of the aortic arch, careful evaluation for evidence of arch obstruction is very important. In the setting of transposition of the great arteries, coarctation is more common, particularly when the VSD is restrictive and the aorta is small (Fig. 12.7A–B). Critical coarctation in the neonate requires immediate recognition so ductal patency can be maintained appropriately until surgical intervention can be performed. Doppler interrogation of the coarctation gradient is unreliable due to the ductal flow distal to the site of coarctation (Fig. 12.7C). In the setting of coarctation of the aorta, a large ductal arch is present (this can be visualized from multiple views, in addition to suprasternal notch imaging). The native, diminutive aorta may insert "end-on-side" onto the large ductal arch (Fig. 12.7A). Typical Doppler interrogation of the ductus will show bidirectional shunting with right-to-left flow in systole and reversal of flow into the PA branches in diastole. The amount of left-to-right diastolic flow is proportional to the pulmonary vascular resistance, with more flow seen with lower resistance. In normally related great arteries, the ductus is usually longer and narrower, as fetal flow patterns are predominantly from the aorta into the PA. If there is critical obstruction to PA flow from the RV, the ductus may be quite tortuous.

Short-axis suprasternal notch imaging demonstrates the branching pattern of brachiocephalic arteries and the sidedness of the aortic arch. The PA bifurcation is also seen from short-axis imaging, with branch sizes measured. The absence of an innominate vein should raise the possibility of a left SVC. A typical "crab view" should demonstrate normal pulmonary venous connections.

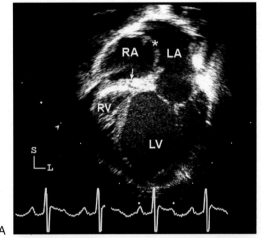

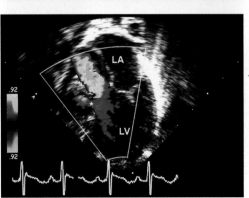

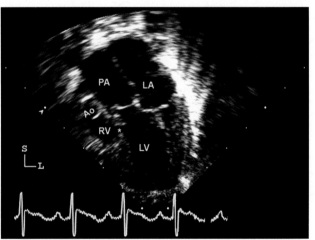

FIGURE 12.6. Tricuspid atresia with transposed great arteries; apical views in same patient in Figure 12.4. A: Four-chamber view demonstrating the dilated left ventricle (LV), atretic tricuspid valve (*arrow*), and severely hypoplastic right ventricle (RV). There is a secundum atrial septal defect (*asterisk*). **B:** Slight anterior angulation of the transducer from the four-chamber view shows the aorta (Ao) arising from the hypoplastic RV and the dilated pulmonary artery (PA) from the LV. **C:** Color Doppler imaging demonstrates antegrade flow into the PA with a small amount flow into the restrictive ventricular septal defect (*asterisk*). LA, left atrium.

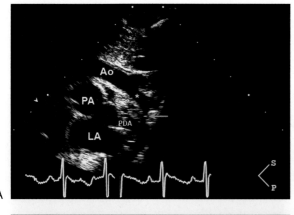

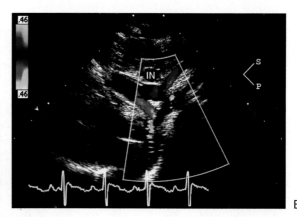

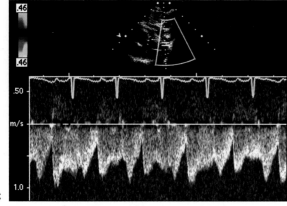

FIGURE 12.7. Tricuspid atresia with transposed great arteries and restrictive ventricular septal defect; suprasternal notch views. A: Long-axis (sagittal) view in the same patient described in Figures 12.4 and 12.5 showing the hypoplastic transverse aortic arch (*asterisk*) and coarctation of the aorta (*arrow*). **B:** Color Doppler imaging shows antegrade flow in the area of coarctation. **C:** Pulsed-wave Doppler interrogation of the coarctation in the presence of a large patent ductus arteriosus shows low-velocity flow; Doppler in this setting is unreliable in predicting the true severity of coarctation. Two-dimensional anatomic assessment is critical. Ao, aorta; IN, innominate vein; LA, left atrium; PDA, patent ductus arteriosus.

 ## HYPOPLASTIC LEFT HEART SYNDROME

Hypoplastic left heart syndrome (HLHS) is the fourth most common congenital cardiac anomaly of infancy, with a reported prevalence of 0.016% to 0.036% of live births, and occurs twice as often in boys as in girls.

Anatomy

HLHS encompasses a heterogeneous group of cardiac malformations characterized by normally related great arteries and varying degrees of underdevelopment of the left heart–aorta complex, resulting in obstruction to systemic cardiac output and the inability of the left heart to support the systemic circulation. The spectrum of anomalies includes mitral stenosis (Fig. 12.8A) or atresia, hypoplasia of the LV, aortic stenosis or atresia (Fig. 12.8B), and hypoplastic aortic arch. At the most severe end of the spectrum are mitral and aortic atresia, with a severely hypoplastic or "slit-like" LV. In milder forms, there is hypoplasia of the aortic and mitral valves and a varying degree of left ventricular hypoplasia. The ventricular septum is usually intact; a VSD, if present, is usually small. In rare cases of a large VSD with mitral atresia, the LV is usually well developed.

In HLHS, the systemic circulation is dependent on the RV and the ductus arteriosus for systemic circulation. The aortic arch, ascending aorta, and coronary arteries are perfused by retrograde flow. Coarctation of the aorta is typically present.

The presence of an intact or highly restrictive atrial septum has been recognized as a predictor of poor outcome among patients with HLHS. An intact atrial septum is present in approximately 6% of patients with HLHS; however, clinically deleterious restriction to flow at the level of the atrial septum can occur in as many as 22% of patients. During fetal life, a severely restricted atrial septum may be associated with nonimmune fetal hydrops and pulmonary lymphangiectasia. In the presence of an intact atrial septum and mitral atresia, the only egress of blood from the LA may be a levoatriocardinal

vein, a pulmonary-systemic connection that provides an alternative route for pulmonary venous blood to enter the systemic venous circulation. In the majority of patients, this vein connects the LA to the innominate vein. However, it may drain to other sites, including the left SVC or jugular venous system.

Clinical Presentation

The majority of fetuses with HLHS tolerate this cardiac anomaly well, with the majority of infants born at full-term, initially healthy in appearance. However, acute hemodynamic collapse follows closure of the ductus arteriosus (which may occur after discharge from newborn nursery). If ductal patency is not restored promptly, poor systemic perfusion results in hypoxemia, acidosis, shock, and eventual death. On examination, the infant appears poorly perfused, tachypneic, and pale, with diffusely diminished pulses. There may be only a nonspecific cardiac murmur, but an S_3 gallop is very common. The second heart sound is loud and single. There is often hepatomegaly. Echocardiographic identification of HLHS should prompt immediate intervention with infusion of prostaglandin E_1 to maintain or improve ductal patency.

Infants with HLHS and nearly intact atrial septum present with severe pulmonary venous hypertension and are even more critically ill with severe respiratory distress. These patients often present with cardiogenic shock and profound cyanosis at birth, needing immediate catheter-based septostomy/cutting balloon dilation of the atrial septum for survival to a palliative surgical procedure.

Echocardiography in Hypoplastic Left Heart Syndrome

The overall approach to imaging in HLHS is to provide complete diagnostic and hemodynamic information. Cardiac catheterization is reserved only for the patient requiring emergent intervention (usually for enlargement of the ASD). An assessment of right ventricular and tricuspid valve function, ductal physiology, and atrial septal anatomy is crucial for clinical management.

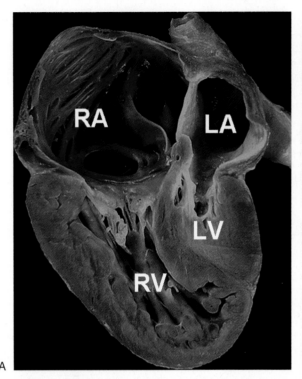
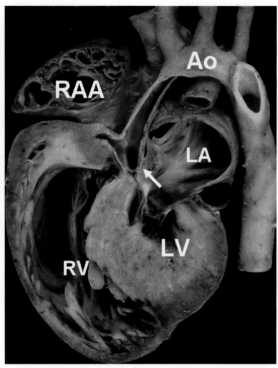

FIGURE 12.8. Pathologic specimen from a patient with hypoplastic left heart syndrome (HLHS). A: Four-chamber view showing severely hypoplastic left ventricle (LV), hypoplastic mitral valve, and a small left atrium (LA). The right ventricle (RV) and right atrium (RA) are dilated. **B:** Long-axis outflow view demonstrates the atretic aortic valve (*arrow*) and hypoplastic aorta (Ao).

Systemic and pulmonary flow ratios are dependent on the difference in resistance between the two respective vascular beds. A large, nonrestrictive interatrial communication in the setting of low pulmonary resistance promotes preferential flow into the pulmonary vascular bed at the expense of the systemic circulation. Pulmonary overcirculation and imbalance in the pulmonary/systemic vascular resistance ratio contribute to hemodynamic instability in infants with HLHS. Conversely, a restrictive ASD in the presence of severely elevated PA pressure and resistance produces preferential right-to-left ductal shunting and restricted pulmonary blood flow at the expense of the patient's oxygenation. Intervention to relieve severe obstruction may be needed before definitive surgical palliation. Thus, in patients with HLHS, clinical presentation can be variable. Immediate echocardiographic assessment of the underlying physiology is critical for management of the patient before palliative surgery is planned and undertaken.

Subcostal Four-Chamber (Coronal) View – The subcostal four-chamber view typically demonstrates a dilated RA and RV. When angling the transducer posteriorly and imaging toward the base of the LA, the LV either appears very small or is not visualized (Fig. 12.9A). It should be immediately apparent when the LV is diminutive or "slit-like" that a significant discrepancy in the size of the RV compared with the LV is present. Once this view is obtained, the echocardiographer should evaluate the mitral valve and the great arteries very carefully. Anterior angulation of the transducer typically shows the dilated RVOT and main PA (MPA), but the very tiny aorta may be difficult to visualize in coronal plane imaging. A large patent ductus arteriosus (PDA) may be seen, essentially a continuation of the MPA as the ductal arch, but this is better visualized in subcostal short-axis views. In the setting of cardiovascular collapse, right ventricular function may also be reduced, sometimes significantly so. Tricuspid regurgitation is usually present in this clinical setting.

The atrial septum should be carefully evaluated from the subcostal windows. The size, number, and location of communications from LA to RA should be assessed (Fig. 12.9A–B). Bulging of the atrial septum from the LA into the RA is suggestive of restriction to egress from the LA. Also, in the presence of a restrictive or intact

atrial septum, the atrial septum is usually thick and the pulmonary veins are dilated (if normally connected). Color Doppler aids in mapping of the defects with the shunt typically occurring from left to right (Fig. 12.9B). Alignment of the Doppler cursor parallel with the defect allows estimation of the mean transeptal gradient by tracing the Doppler signal across three cardiac cycles.

Bidirectional shunting is very unusual but may be seen in presence of severe tricuspid regurgitation or anomalous venous connections. The echocardiographer should be alert to the possibility of anomalous connection and drainage of the pulmonary veins. While present in a minority of patients with HLHS, this should be suspected particularly if venous return into the diminutive LA cannot be seen from subcostal imaging.

Subcostal Short-Axis (Sagittal) Views – Orthogonal plane imaging provides confirmation of the cardiac anatomy. Subcostal short-axis views are excellent for interrogation of the atrial septum. The presence/location of atrial communications should be determined and color Doppler mapping of atrial shunting should be performed. The relative size of the very hypoplastic aorta posteriorly and dilated PA anteriorly is evaluated. Again, by angling the transducer rightward, the continuation of the dilated MPA as the ductal arch is easily demonstrated. Color Doppler interrogation may show bidirectional PDA shunting (typically right-to-left in systole with left-to-right shunting in diastole depending on pulmonary resistance characteristics). The entire aortic arch may be visualized in this view (with definitive imaging obtained from suprasternal notch imaging). Scanning toward the mid-ventricular level shows the enlarged anterior RV and hypoplastic, posterior LV (Fig. 12.9C). Right ventricular function and tricuspid regurgitation should be assessed.

Parasternal View

PARASTERNAL LONG-AXIS VIEW – Parasternal long-axis views confirm the size discrepancy between the large RV anteriorly and the diminutive or small LV posteriorly (Fig. 12.10A). Careful examination for the slit-like, muscle-bound LV confirms that the anterior ventricle is the RV. The ventricular septum is most often intact. Right ventricular systolic function can be evaluated from the long-axis view, although angling the transducer inferiorly toward the tricuspid

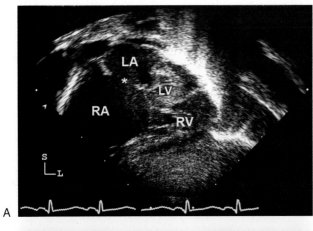

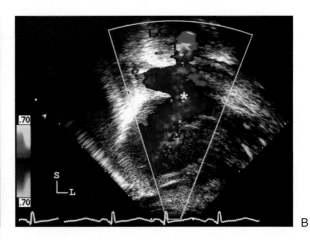

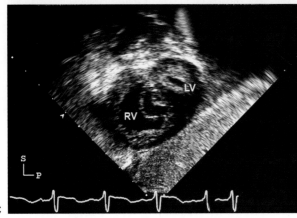

FIGURE 12.9. Hypoplastic left heart syndrome (HLHS); subcostal views. A: Long-axis (coronal) image showing very dilated right atrium (RA) and small left atrium. The secundum atrial septal defect (*asterisk*) is large and unrestrictive. The right ventricle (RV) is hypertrophied, and the left ventricle (LV) and mitral valve are severely hypoplastic. **B:** Color Doppler imaging demonstrating nonrestrictive laminar flow across the atrial septal defect. **C:** Short-axis (sagittal) view in the same patient, angled toward the mid-ventricular level showing the anterior, hypertrophied RV. Note the echo-bright LV endocardium often seen in HLHS.

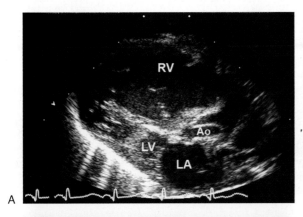

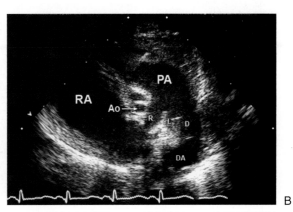

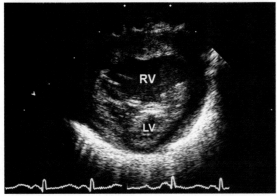

FIGURE 12.10. Hypoplastic left heart syndrome; parasternal views. A: Long-axis view showing severely hypoplastic left ventricle (LV), severe mitral valve stenosis, and aortic atresia. The right ventricle (RV) is severely dilated. The ascending aorta (Ao) is diminutive, serving primarily as a conduit for retrograde coronary perfusion. **B:** Short-axis view at the cardiac base demonstrating the diminutive ascending Ao (*arrow*) and dilated pulmonary artery (PA) with trifurcation of branches into the right (R) and left (L) branch pulmonary arteries and large ductus arteriosus (D). The ductal arch continues into the descending aorta (DA). **C:** Short-axis view at mid-ventricular level showing the enlarged, hypertrophied RV with severely hypoplastic LV. LA, left atrium; RA, right atrium.

inflow is usually required. Left ventricular systolic function is usually severely decreased if a cavity is present. In this instance, the left ventricular endocardium and papillary muscles may be echo-bright, suggesting the presence of endocardial fibroelastosis secondary to long-term subendocardial ischemia. Mitral and aortic valve leaflets should be examined for mobility or patency. The mitral annulus is characteristically hypoplastic with the mitral valve and its subvalvular apparatus appearing abnormal. If patent, the valve may be thickened and doming, with shortened chordae. A supravalvar mitral ring may also be present. The aortic valve is usually completely atretic but may be thickened and doming. Subaortic obstruction may be present. The size of the hypoplastic aortic annulus and ascending aorta (usually an internal diameter of less than 5 mm) is more easily measured in the parasternal long-axis view (Fig. 12.10A).

The transducer is angled anteriorly and superiorly to evaluate the RVOT, the dilated MPA, and ductal arch. Typically, the ductus is very large. With Doppler interrogation, the PDA shunt is right-to-left during systole, while the amount of left-to-right shunt during diastole being dependent on pulmonary vascular resistance. Moving the transducer to a high left parasternal window may bring the large ductus/ductal arch into view more easily. Pulsed-wave Doppler is used to evaluate a ductal gradient in the setting of early ductal constriction as typically indicated by an increased systolic Doppler flow velocity through the PDA (greater than 2.5 m/s).

From parasternal long-axis imaging, the LA is usually small. However, the LA can be dilated in the presence of a nearly intact atrial septum.

PARASTERNAL SHORT-AXIS VIEW – In the parasternal short-axis view, there is a large anterior RV and small posterior LV (Fig. 12.10B). This view is also useful in the assessment of ventricular function, mitral valve size and morphology, and mitral papillary apparatus number and position. The mitral valve may be "parachute" in nature with a single papillary muscle group. Short-axis scans at the base of heart allow assessment of the ascending aortic size in cross section and further evaluation of aortic valve morphology.

The great arteries are normally related with the severely hypoplastic aorta in the center. The coronary artery origins are most often normal and may appear as extensions of the diminutive aorta (Fig. 12.10C). The MPA is usually very dilated and the PDA is prominent (Fig. 12.10C). The branch PAs should be assessed in this view, with slightly higher positioning of the probe on the patient's chest to obtain the trifurcation view (Fig. 12.10C). Again, with color Doppler and pulsed-wave Doppler examination, the PDA flow is most typically bidirectional. A systolic gradient should be assessed for early ductal constriction (particularly if the prostaglandin infusion has not been initiated).

Apical Views – An apical four-chamber view provides comparison of the relative sizes of the ventricles. The RV is typically dilated and hypertrophied. The LV is small, muscle bound, and non–apex forming (Fig. 12.11A). The mitral valve annulus is usually hypoplastic with either an atretic opening or severely stenotic leaflets. If flow is present, one should assess of the degree of stenosis from this view (taking into account that a larger interatrial communication may reduce the measured gradient). Furthermore, the mitral leaflet excursion may be limited in the presence of critical aortic stenosis or atresia, secondary to severely elevated left ventricular end-diastolic pressure. The transmitral gradient may also be artificially reduced in this setting. Spectral and color Doppler flow may be used to evaluate mitral inflow, mitral regurgitation, and aortic outflow (if the valve is patent). Tricuspid valve function should be assessed carefully; significant tricuspid regurgitation is a poor prognostic indicator (Fig. 12.11B–C). Anterior angulation of the probe to a para-apical view will show the dilated MPA and color Doppler assessment of pulmonary valve regurgitation should be performed.

Suprasternal Notch Views – Suprasternal notch long-axis scans provide an excellent view of the ascending aorta, aortic arch, and upper descending aorta. The ascending aortic size may range from mild to severely hypoplastic (Fig. 12.12); however, the caliber of the aorta is much larger at the level of the innominate artery and

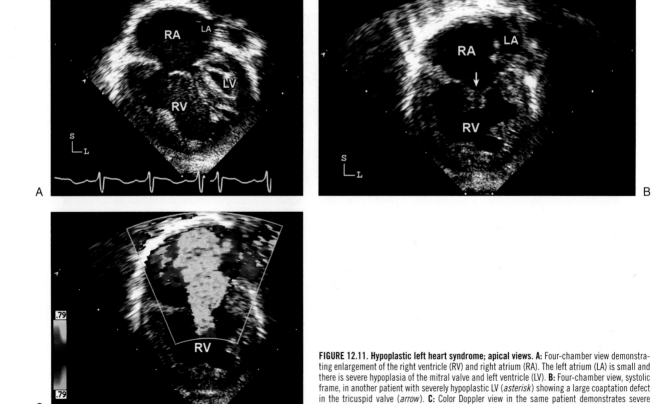

FIGURE 12.11. Hypoplastic left heart syndrome; apical views. A: Four-chamber view demonstrating enlargement of the right ventricle (RV) and right atrium (RA). The left atrium (LA) is small and there is severe hypoplasia of the mitral valve and left ventricle (LV). **B:** Four-chamber view, systolic frame, in another patient with severely hypoplastic LV (*asterisk*) showing a large coaptation defect in the tricuspid valve (*arrow*). **C:** Color Doppler view in the same patient demonstrates severe tricuspid valve regurgitation (*arrow*).

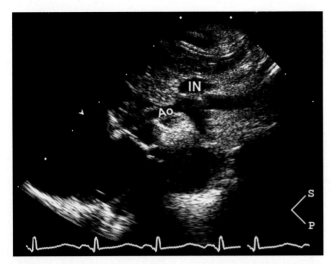

FIGURE 12.12. Hypoplastic left heart syndrome; suprasternal notch view. Long-axis view showing the severely hypoplastic ascending aorta (Ao). IN, innominate vein.

beyond. Coarctation of the aorta is usually present (Fig. 12.13A). In the presence of a severe coarctation, there is a juxtaductal posterior ledge and increased distance between left common carotid and subclavian artery. The presence of coarctation may be difficult to assess due to a severely dilated ductus arteriosus. An anterior ledge is common where the dilated ductus enters the descending aorta. Using color Doppler, the flow in the transverse aortic arch and ascending aorta is retrograde in the presence of critical aortic stenosis or atresia. A transient forward flow in the aortic arch in systole may be secondary to movement of the atretic aortic valve during systole

(Fig. 12.13B–C). Confirmation of ductal shunt physiology is also performed from this view. Anomalous pulmonary venous drainage to a vertical vein or a levoatriocardinal vein draining the pulmonary venous system needs to be assessed from comprehensive suprasternal notch imaging. Color flow in the venous system toward the transducer in the suprasternal notch should prompt a thorough evaluation of pulmonary venous connections.

Borderline Left Ventricle

One of the key questions in the management of patients with mitral and aortic stenosis is determining the ability of the hypoplastic LV to sustain a systemic circulation. Investigators have suggested numerous echocardiographic parameters that might be used to predict outcome following attempted biventricular or univentricular repair. However, it is important to recognize that these factors are lesion specific and may not always be generalized. That is, the criteria used for univentricular versus biventricular repair in aortic stenosis may not be generalized or applied to mitral stenosis in the setting of a hypoplastic LV.

In aortic stenosis, based on an extensive retrospective analysis, Rhodes and colleagues showed the following echocardiographic parameters correlated with increased risk for hospital death: left ventricular long axis–to–heart long axis ratio less than 0.8, indexed aortic root diameter less than 3.5 cm/m^2, indexed mitral valve area less than 4.75 cm^2/m^2, and left ventricular mass index less than 35 g/m^2. The authors of this study proposed a scoring system called the "score of Rhodes." Data for the Rhodes score were based on retrospective data from a small group (65 patients) with critical aortic stenosis who were preselected for biventricular repair. The scoring system was based on the following equation:

$$14.0 \, (BSA) + 0.943 \, (iROOT) + 4.78 \, (LAR) + 0.157 \, (iMVA) - 12.03$$

where BSA is body surface area, iROOT is indexed aortic root dimension, LAR is the ratio of the long-axis dimension of the LV to

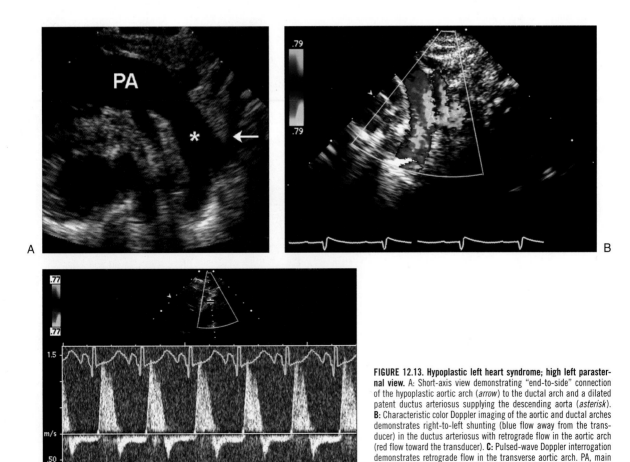

FIGURE 12.13. Hypoplastic left heart syndrome; high left parasternal view. A: Short-axis view demonstrating "end-to-side" connection of the hypoplastic aortic arch (*arrow*) to the ductal arch and a dilated patent ductus arteriosus supplying the descending aorta (*asterisk*). B: Characteristic color Doppler imaging of the aortic and ductal arches demonstrates right-to-left shunting (blue flow away from the transducer) in the ductus arteriosus with retrograde flow in the aortic arch (red flow toward the transducer). C: Pulsed-wave Doppler interrogation demonstrates retrograde flow in the transverse aortic arch. PA, main pulmonary artery.

the long-axis dimension of the heart, and iMVA is the indexed mitral valve area.

A score of less than 0.35 was predictive of mortality after biventricular repair. Subsequent reports have shown poor predictive capability of the Rhodes score, especially in lesions other than aortic stenosis.

Additional authors have proposed that other factors lead to an increased mortality following biventricular repair in HLHS (Table 12.2). The Congenital Heart Surgeon's Society of North America has also proposed a "Critical Aortic Stenosis Calculator" that uses demographic and echocardiographic parameters. This equation is designed to predict the optimal surgical strategy (biventricular versus univentricular approach) in patients with aortic stenosis. Ongoing discussion of these different morphologic, demographic, and echocardiographic parameters by numerous investigators is an indication that there are inherent flaws in any rigid assessment system. Ongoing review of surgical results and assessment of echo parameters may continue to provide further information in the future. In conclusion, for patients with multiple left heart obstructive lesions and a borderline LV, there are no clear-cut guidelines. It is important to remember that univentricular palliation following attempted biventricular repair (crossover) is associated with higher mortality. Furthermore, a complicated biventricular repair with significant residual lesions may be worse than a successful univentricular palliation. None of these scores take into account the long-term functional and quality of life outcomes. Risk factors will keep changing and evolving with newer surgical techniques. A combination of the above-mentioned parameters and clinical/surgical experience will likely dictate the preference of an individual institution.

 ## DOUBLE INLET LEFT VENTRICLE

Double inlet left ventricle (DILV), first described by Holmes in 1824 and named by De La Cruz and Miller in 1968, comprises 1% of all congenital heart malformations. DILV exists when the greater part of both AV junctions is supported by the same ventricular chamber. If mitral and tricuspid atresia are excluded, DILV is the most common form of univentricular AV connection. This malformation likely originates embryologically from a partial or complete block in the left-to-right expansion process of the AV canal, resulting in connection of both atria to the primitive ventricle, which then forms the LV and a hypoplastic RV. In DILV, the hypoplastic RV lacks the inlet portion and has either bipartite (trabecular and outlet) or monopartite (trabecular) morphology. Typically, both left and right AV valves have mitral valve morphology with deeper anterior leaflets and shallower posterior leaflets. Both AV valves lie posteriorly in fibrous continuity with a semilunar valve.

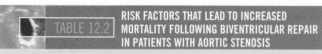

TABLE 12.2	RISK FACTORS THAT LEAD TO INCREASED MORTALITY FOLLOWING BIVENTRICULAR REPAIR IN PATIENTS WITH AORTIC STENOSIS

- Cardiac apex not formed by the LV
- Presence of endocardial fibroelastosis
- Lower aortic annular Z-scores
- Lack of antegrade flow in the ascending aorta and aortic arch
- Prematurity
- Low birth weight
- Presence of chromosomal anomalies
- Reduced left ventricular end diastolic volume (<60% of normal)
- Mitral valve Annulus <9 mm
- Left ventricular inflow dimensions <25 mm
- Diameter of the ventriculo-aortic junction <5 mm
- Left ventricular cross-sectional area <2.0 cm^2
- Indexed left ventricular end diastolic volume< 20 mL/m^2

Anatomy of Double Inlet Left Ventricle

Typically, the AV connections are committed to the dominant posterior LV (Fig. 12.14). The inlet septum is absent and both AV valves are in close proximity to each other, posterior to the trabecular septum. Less commonly seen is a hypoplastic, or atretic, AV valve. An ASD must be present in this situation to provide communication from one atrium to the other.

Double Inlet Left Ventricle With Transposed Great Arteries (Hypoplastic Subaortic Right Ventricle)

When there is a dominant LV and a hypoplastic RV, the ventriculoarterial connections are usually discordant. In this form of DILV, the aorta arises from the rudimentary RV or outlet chamber. This chamber is connected with the LV through a VSD, which is the embryologic remnant of the bulboventricular foramen. This is seen in approximately 85% of DILV cases. The aorta is usually leftward and anterior in position, with *l*-looping of the right ventricular outlet chamber. Alternatively, with *d*-looping of the right ventricular chamber, the aorta is anterior and rightward to the PA. There may be obstruction of the bulboventricular foramen and it may be associated with coarctation of aorta.

Double Inlet Left Ventricle With Normally Related Great Arteries

Concordant ventriculoarterial connection, or normally related great arteries, is less common (15%) in DILV. This arrangement is called the "Holmes heart." The bulboventricular foramen is frequently quite stenotic and results in subpulmonary stenosis.

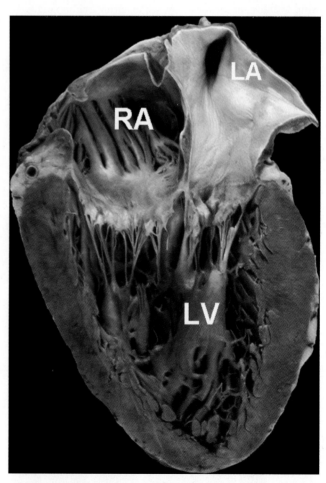

FIGURE 12.14. Pathologic specimen from a patient with double inlet left ventricle. Long-axis inflow view showing both right atrium (RA) and left atrium (LA) emptying in to left ventricle (LV).

Clinical Presentation

Infants with DILV typically present within the first few weeks of life. For those with restricted pulmonary blood flow, as the ductus arteriosus constricts, the presenting symptom will be cyanosis. Those with severe aortic obstruction (restrictive bulboventricular foramen or aortic arch) will typically present with poor peripheral perfusion and signs of low cardiac output as the ductus constricts. On clinical examination, the infant with restricted pulmonary blood flow will have cyanosis and a harsh systolic ejection murmur over the precordium; not unlike the infant with tetralogy of Fallot. Those infants with restricted systemic output will appear tachypneic and pale and have poor pulses throughout. The cardiac examination demonstrates precordial overactivity, a single second heart sound, a gallop, and a pulmonary flow murmur. Institution of prostaglandin E_1 therapy is life-saving after the diagnosis of DILV with ductal-dependent physiology (either systemic or pulmonary circulation) is confirmed by echocardiography.

Patients with unobstructed pulmonary blood flow and no significant subaortic obstruction may present a few weeks later with signs of congestive heart failure and pulmonary overcirculation as pulmonary vascular resistance falls. Infants with pulmonary overcirculation will have significant tachypnea and very mild desaturation (which may be evident only on pulse oximetry). In this setting, the clinical examination is much like that for the patient with a large VSD.

Echocardiographic Evaluation of Double Inlet Left Ventricle

Echocardiography plays a critical role in the early diagnosis and management of univentricular AV connection. Once again, the key to evaluation of complex univentricular anatomy and physiology is to use the segmental anatomic approach. As an initial approach to diagnosis, the apical and subcostal four-chamber scan planes provide excellent views of the two closely placed AV valves without an intervening ventricular septum, providing the echocardiographer with the initial impression of a univentricular AV connection. Further imaging to evaluate the cardiac anatomy in detail should be conducted in a segmental approach as outlined later.

Subcostal Views

SUBCOSTAL FOUR-CHAMBER (CORONAL) VIEW – Abdominal and atrial situs should be determined in this view. In DILV, atrial situs is predominantly solitus, followed by right or left isomerism. The long-axis, or four-chamber, view reveals the dominant left ventricle with both AV valves entering this chamber; one must angle the transducer *anteriorly* to see the rudimentary outlet chamber and great arteries. The number, size, and location of defects in the atrial septum should be assessed. Assessment of the atrial septum is particularly important in the setting of a restrictive or atretic AV valve component. The origin and orientation of the two great arteries should be assessed. Ventriculoarterial connections

are usually discordant with the aorta anterior and to the left of the PA, so that echocardiographic similarities to transposition exist. Both great arteries are parallel in their course, with the posterior PA bifurcating. The size of the bulboventricular foramen, the communication between the LV and the outlet chamber, should be evaluated in orthogonal views to rule out potential restriction. In the presence of a restrictive bulboventricular foramen, color Doppler flow appears aliased with increased velocity seen on spectral Doppler interrogation.

SUBCOSTAL SHORT-AXIS (SAGITTAL) VIEW – The subcostal short-axis view is useful for evaluation of atrial septal anatomy, visualization of the posterior LV receiving two AV valves, examination of the bulboventricular foramen, and confirmation of the arrangement of the great arteries. The two AV valves appear as two circles in the short-axis view; the leaflets touch each other when open in diastole if there is no stenosis. There is an anterior trabecular chamber that is not connected to the atrium. The communication of this anterior chamber with the LV is via the bulboventricular foramen, which is examined in this orthogonal plane to determine its size. In the presence of transposed great arteries, as is most common, the arteries have a parallel course at the base of the heart, with the posterior PA bifurcating. If the great arteries are normally related, the bulboventricular foramen is usually quite restrictive.

Parasternal View

PARASTERNAL LONG-AXIS VIEW – Parasternal long-axis imaging in DILV will demonstrate the posterior LV. With rightward/leftward angling of the transducer, it is seen that both AV valves enter this posterior left ventricular chamber. One must be careful to not confuse this anatomy with a VSD and enlarged LV, as typically only one AV connection is seen at a time (rotation to parasternal short axis makes this apparent) (Fig. 12.15A). In DILV, one great artery will typically originate from the main ventricular chamber and the other great artery is seen more anteriorly, arising from the rudimentary outlet chamber. The bulboventricular foramen should be evaluated for anatomic size and evidence of restriction, again from multiple imaging planes with two-dimensional, spectral, and color Doppler interrogation.

PARASTERNAL SHORT-AXIS VIEW – Imaging from the parasternal short axis shows both AV valves posterior to the trabecular septum (Fig. 12.15B), which is oriented in a horizontal plane. In DILV, the hypoplastic right ventricular outlet chamber is usually positioned anterosuperior and leftward to the morphologic LV. However, it can occasionally be rightward; one must angle the transducer toward the base of the heart to visualize this relationship. A Doppler gradient is obtained in a parallel plane to the flow directed anteriorly through the bulboventricular foramen. Typically, the mean gradient will reflect the amount of obstruction more closely than the peak instantaneous gradient, as the obstruction is not typically dynamic.

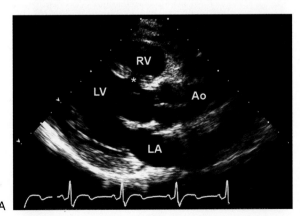
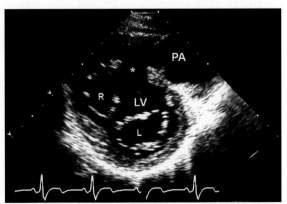

FIGURE 12.15. Double-inlet left ventricle with normally related great arteries; parasternal views. A: Long-axis view showing the anterior hypoplastic right ventricle (RV), enlarged left ventricle (LV), and a muscular ventricular septal defect (*asterisk*). The LV gives rise to the aorta (Ao). **B:** Short-axis view at the level of atrioventricular valves showing classic appearance of both the right (R) and left (L) atrioventricular valves committed to the LV posterior to the large ventricular septal defect (*asterisk*). LA, left atrium; PA, pulmonary artery.

Angling further toward the base of the heart should bring the great arteries into view, seen as two circles in the short-axis view when transposed, due to their parallel course. The relative leftward/rightward position of the anterior aorta in relation to the PA should be noted. With normally related great arteries (Holmes heart), the relationship of the great arteries is similar to that seen in a normal heart, with the aorta seen in cross section and the PA in a more longitudinal plane. The PA confluence should be evaluated. Imaging from a higher left parasternal plane may bring the PA "trifurcation" into view in the patient with normally related great arteries, also showing the PDA.

Apical Four-Chamber View

The apical four-chamber scan plane provides the best view of the crux of the heart. In DILV, the dominant LV has fine apical trabeculations, two main papillary muscle groups, and a smooth "septal" surface with no chordal attachments and receives two AV valves. These two separate AV valves guard the AV junction; both typically have mitral morphology and are in continuity with the posterior great artery (Fig. 12.16A–B). The function of both AV valves, including whether there is stenosis or atresia, should be assessed in this view. Ventricular systolic function and AV valve regurgitation can also be evaluated.

Angling anteriorly, the origin, relationship, and size of the great arteries can be evaluated. When the great arteries are transposed, the PA typically originates from the main left ventricular cavity with the anterior (usually leftward) aorta arising from the rudimentary outlet right ventricular chamber. One should also assess the size of the bulboventricular foramen from this plane, using spectral and color flow Doppler.

Suprasternal Notch Views – The longitudinal suprasternal notch view demonstrates the aortic arch anatomy and the presence/absence of coarctation. If there is significant bulboventricular foramen obstruction, one should suspect arch obstruction—either coarctation or interruption of aorta. In the neonate, a ductus arteriosus may be present, and if the arch is critically obstructed, patency is needed. The PA confluence and bilateral branch sizes can be evaluated in the short-axis imaging plane, as can pulmonary venous connections ("crab" view).

Interventricular Communication in Double Inlet Left Ventricle

Many different terms have been used to define the connection between the dominant and rudimentary ventricle in univentricular AV connections, including "VSD," "bulboventricular foramen," and "the outlet foramen." We prefer to use the term "bulboventricular foramen." The bulboventricular foramen is a common site of outflow tract (subvalvular) obstruction. This communication is not circular but tends to be more elliptical. As a result, the area of the bulboventricular foramen should be measured in two orthogonal planes (long and short axis) by two-dimensional echocardiography. The area is calculated as follows:

$$\text{Area} = [\text{diameter (1)} \times \text{diameter (2)}] \times \pi/4$$

and is indexed to body surface area.

An individual with bulboventricular foramen area less than $2 \text{ cm}^2/\text{m}^2$ is at higher risk for developing late obstruction. In addition, the Doppler gradient should be interrogated from multiple views to obtain the best alignment of the beam to the angle of flow acceleration. One should remember that the gradient may be inaccurate in presence of a large PDA or with suboptimal Doppler angle of interrogation.

In addition, it is critical to assess the bulboventricular foramen size and rule out potential obstruction before the Fontan operation is carried out. Obstruction at the bulboventricular foramen may complicate the course of patients with single ventricle, resulting in pressure overload, which leads to ventricular hypertrophy, fibrosis, and dysfunction (both systolic and diastolic). Such obstruction should be addressed at the time of surgery.

It is controversial whether PA banding accelerates the process of bulboventricular foramen obstruction or it is a de novo event. In a study of 28 neonates, all patients with an initial bulboventricular foramen area index of less than $2 \text{ cm}^2/\text{m}^2$, who did *not* undergo early bulboventricular foramen bypass, developed late obstruction. The rate of development of bulboventricular stenosis did not differ in patients with and without PA banding, but smaller size of the bulboventricular foramen correlated with the presence of aortic arch obstruction.

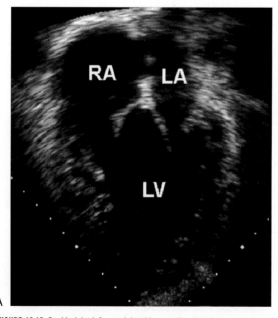
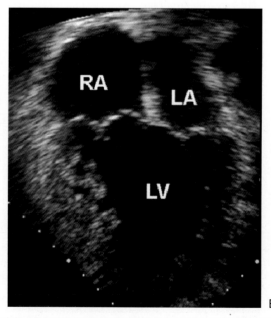

FIGURE 12.16. Double-inlet left ventricle with normally related great arteries; apical views. A: Diastolic frame, showing both left atrium (LA) and right atrium (RA) emptying into the left ventricle (LV) through the left and right atrioventricular valves. **B:** Systolic frame in the same patient.

In the future, routine use of three-dimensional echocardiography may provide a more accurate assessment of the area of the bulboventricular foramen in DILV, identifying patients with subaortic stenosis caused by a restrictive defect, or potentially identifying those at risk for future obstruction.

APPROACH TO THE PATIENT WITH UNIVENTRICULAR ATRIOVENTRICULAR CONNECTION: SURGICAL PLANNING

In all patients with univentricular AV connection (excluding those who had a 1.5- or even 2-ventricle repair), the final common pathway for surgical palliation is that of the modified Fontan procedure, wherein systemic venous return flows passively into the pulmonary circulation. The critical factor in surgical planning for all infants with univentricular physiology is to perform palliation in a timely fashion and in a way that will reduce the risk for later successful completion of the modified Fontan procedure. Thus, looking forward, one must keep in mind that the best candidates for the Fontan procedure will have the following: (a) preserved ventricular function without significant AV valve regurgitation, (b) low PA pressure and resistance, (c) normal pulmonary branch architecture, (d) absence of obstruction to the systemic circulation, and (e) an unrestrictive ASD. In the initial evaluation of the patient with single-ventricle physiology, the plan for initial palliation and eventual surgical approach should be directed toward optimization of all of these factors.

The Neonate With Excessive Pulmonary Blood Flow

For those patients with tricuspid atresia or DILV, initial management is guided by the presenting physiology and amount of pulmonary blood flow. In a patient with tricuspid atresia with normally related great arteries, the degree of restriction of the VSD and pulmonary outflow tract will dictate the initial approach. Infants with unrestrictive pulmonary blood flow will typically require a palliative PA band procedure between 4 and 8 weeks of age to protect the pulmonary bed from exposure to systemic pressure, which, if not addressed, will lead to irreversible pulmonary hypertension and vascular disease. The band serves two purposes: to decrease the downstream PA pressure in preparation for second- and third-stage surgery and to restrict the pulmonary blood flow.

The timing of the PA banding procedure will depend on the infant's clinical course, as placement of a band is usually delayed until the pulmonary resistance declines (as manifested by increased left-to-right shunting) so that the surgeon may judge the adequacy of the band more easily. Echocardiographic follow-up during this time in the patient with tricuspid atresia/normally related great arteries may reveal signs of pulmonary overcirculation with increased flow in the PA, dilation of the LA and LV, and low-velocity VSD/RVOT Doppler signals indicative of persistent PA hypertension.

Echocardiographic Evaluation of Pulmonary Artery Band

The echocardiogram following PA banding should evaluate both the position of the band and the gradient across the band (Fig. 12.17A–B). Confirmation of band position, branch PA anatomy, and Doppler gradient by echocardiography is warranted before hospital dismissal, so that comparison is possible with serial echocardiographic examinations. Over time, a band may migrate distally and cause distortion of the branch PAs (typically the right PA) (Fig. 12.17C–D). A PA band may also distort the MPA resulting in varying degrees of pulmonary valve regurgitation.

The gradient across the PA band will help in estimation of distal PA pressure (Fig. 12.17B). Peak instantaneous and mean gradients should be recorded for serial examinations. Optimal Doppler alignment with the band positioned in the mid-MPA can be achieved from parasternal short-axis or subcostal views. Over time, the band gradient should increase, as the band is "outgrown." A progressive decrease in the trans-PA band gradient should raise the possibility of increasing distal PA pressure. Elevation in distal pressure may be

secondary to a loose band and resultant inadequate protection of distal PA bed, resulting in pulmonary vascular obstructive disease, or due to elevation of distal pressure (perhaps in a situation where the band was placed relatively late).

In a patient with transposition of the great arteries or subaortic stenosis, PA banding may result in accelerated narrowing of the VSD or progression of the subaortic stenosis, resulting in obstruction to both great arteries. In this situation, echocardiography plays a critical role in following patients for the development of subaortic stenosis, which produces ventricular hypertrophy and potential ventricular dysfunction, all of which complicate future palliation.

The Neonate With Restricted Pulmonary Blood Flow

Infants with tricuspid atresia/normally related great arteries and a restrictive VSD or pulmonary stenosis, or the infant with DILV and normally related great arteries, will usually have cyanosis at presentation. As the VSD becomes more restrictive, the echocardiogram will show the reduced flow through the VSD or pulmonary outflow tract with increased Doppler gradient if proper alignment can be achieved. In this setting, a modified Blalock-Taussig (BT) shunt is the most commonly performed systemic-to-PA shunt for initial palliation to provide a stable source of pulmonary blood flow. The modified BT shunt is generally a 3- to 4-mm nonvalved polytetrafluoroethylene conduit connecting the subclavian or innominate artery and the right branch PA (Fig. 12.18A). Postoperative echocardiographic assessment of a BT shunt should include the evaluation of shunt patency and flow pattern. The BT shunt is best visualized from the suprasternal notch in a short-axis view. Additional off-axis views may be needed depending on the course and length of the shunt. Color Doppler imaging will facilitate mapping of the shunt course and entry into the PA (Fig. 12.18A). It is important to recognize that a continuous-wave Doppler gradient across the BT shunt and other shunts made of prosthetic material will not be accurate, as the long tubular nature of the shunt interferes with accurate determination of pressure drop (Fig. 12.18B). However, an increasing gradient on serial exams may help identify shunt stenosis. The echocardiographer should evaluate the size and relative flow patterns in each PA (right and left) to rule out important branch stenosis.

"The Balanced Infant"

The infant with DILV and pulmonary stenosis, or tricuspid atresia and pulmonary stenosis, will have a balanced circulation and a protected pulmonary bed (no exposure to increased pressure), adequate oxygen saturation, and no significant clinical signs or symptoms of heart failure or excessive cyanosis. In this situation, very early neonatal palliation may not be necessary and the initial palliative procedure may be delayed until the time of the bidirectional cavopulmonary anastomosis (usually between 3 and 6 months of age).

The Neonate With Restricted Systemic Blood Flow

In neonates with HLHS or severe left-sided obstruction with a small LV, a modified Norwood operation is the first-stage surgical procedure. The modified Norwood approach, first introduced for patients with HLHS, has been applied to a heterogeneous group of cardiac defects characterized by the presence of a functional single ventricle with systemic outflow tract obstruction, including patients with tricuspid atresia and transposed great arteries with restrictive VSD and arch obstruction. In the neonate with DILV and aortic arch obstruction, the initial approach likely includes modifications of the Norwood or Damus-Kaye-Stansel operation.

Modified Norwood Procedure

The modified Norwood procedure is designed (a) to provide unobstructed systemic output, including relief of aortic arch obstruction, (b) to maintain the functional single ventricle as the systemic ventricle, and (c) to provide a stable source of pulmonary blood supply. The Norwood procedure consists of surgical reconstruction and augmentation of the ascending aorta and aortic arch, an atrial septectomy, and a systemic-to-pulmonary shunt. Important aspects of the initial procedure include successful relief of arch obstruction and creation of an unrestrictive ASD. The two means of providing pulmonary blood flow in these patients are either a modified BT

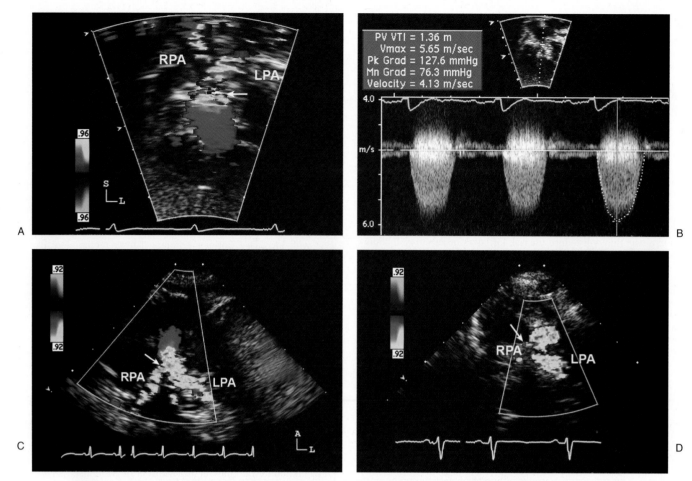

FIGURE 12.17. Pulmonary artery band (PAB). A: Modified para-apical view with the transducer angled anteriorly to image the pulmonary artery. Color Doppler imaging with aliased flow through the PAB (*arrow*). **B:** Continuous-wave Doppler interrogation of the PAB demonstrating high-velocity systolic flow with a maximum instantaneous gradient of 127 mm Hg and a mean gradient of 76 mm Hg. **C:** High left parasternal short-axis image in different patient with PAB; Color Doppler interrogation of branch pulmonary arteries demonstrates potential distal migration of the band with early impingement of flow (*arrow*) into the right pulmonary artery (RPA). Note normal flow in the left pulmonary artery (LPA). **D:** On subsequent follow-up in the patient in C, further compression of the proximal RPA (*arrow*) results in almost complete occlusion with little flow demonstrated.

shunt or an RV-to-PA conduit (also known as a Sano shunt). The latter has the potential advantage of a stable immediate postoperative hemodynamic status by preventing diastolic runoff. However, many experienced centers have shown no significant survival advantage of Sano shunt over a traditional BT shunt. Moreover, the long-term effects of a ventriculotomy-related scar on right ventricular function and arrhythmia potential remains to be seen. The operative risk factors for the Stage 1 Norwood procedure include low birth weight, prematurity, associated chromosomal and noncardiac congenital anomalies, pulmonary venous obstruction, tricuspid valve regurgitation, smaller caliber of ascending aorta, and increased circulatory arrest time.

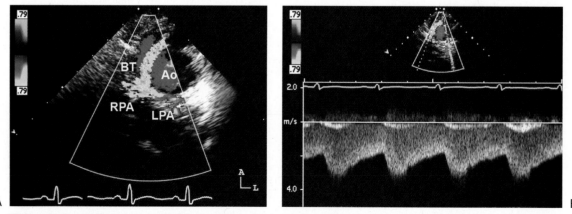

FIGURE 12.18. Right Modified Blalock-Taussig (BT) shunt. A: Suprasternal short-axis imaging with color Doppler mapping to aid in visualization of shunt. **B:** Continuous-wave Doppler in the shunt demonstrates high-velocity continuous flow throughout the cardiac cycle. Ao, aorta; LPA, left pulmonary artery; RPA, right pulmonary artery.

Echocardiographic Evaluation Following Stage 1 Norwood Procedure

Apart from the usual postoperative echocardiographic evaluation, patients undergoing a Norwood procedure should be carefully evaluated for restriction of the ASD, residual or recurrent aortic arch obstruction, and PA branch stenosis or distortion. Evaluation of the BT shunt is as discussed earlier. The atrial septal gradient will depend on the size of systemic-to-PA shunt/conduit and amount of pulmonary blood flow. If restriction is present, color Doppler will show aliased flow and an elevated mean gradient from LA to RA (Fig. 12.19A–C).

Echocardiography plays a key role in evaluation of reconstructed aortic arch following Stage 1 Norwood palliation (Fig. 12.20A–B). The systemic RV in HLHS patients does not tolerate aortic arch obstruction. Accordingly, one of the earliest clues that should direct the echocardiographer to suspect aortic arch obstruction is the development of tricuspid regurgitation and reduced right ventricular function. Suprasternal notch views are optimal for aortic arch imaging. Due to the relatively larger size of the "neoaorta," there will be a change in caliber of the aorta at the usual site of recurrent coarctation, which also makes the diagnosis challenging (Fig. 12.21A–C). Mild flow acceleration at the junction of the reconstructed aorta and native descending aorta is a common finding secondary to the size discrepancy between the two segments (Fig. 12.20B). Significant anatomic obstruction in the neoaortic arch will typically occur at the distal anastomosis. A significant gradient, a discrete posterior shelf, and significant narrowing compared with the abdominal aorta at the level of the diaphragm are all indicative of recoarctation. An abnormal abdominal Doppler flow pattern with blunted upstroke and continued diastolic forward flow (rather than brief early diastolic reversal) is also consistent with coarctation (Fig. 12.21D). Recoarctation occurs in the majority of patients within the first 6 months following the procedure, usually within the first 3 months.

In the patient with the Sano shunt modification, the ventriculotomy is typically on the anterior surface of the RV, approximately 1 cm below the native pulmonary valve (now the "neoaortic") annulus (Fig. 12.22A–B). Over time, the right ventricular connection may become severely obstructed secondary to muscular hypertrophy and dynamic obstruction. The sternum may also compress the conduit anteriorly. The origin of the Sano conduit is visualized from the parasternal long-axis view angled toward the right (Fig. 12.22A). The subcostal sagittal or the parasternal long-axis view may be used to obtain the conduit gradient. As the conduit travels to the PA, it takes an abrupt posterior angulation. The PA end of the conduit is best imaged in a high suprasternal short-axis view (Fig. 12.22C–D). Depending on the surgical technique, the conduit may arch to the right or left of the neoaorta, connecting to the PA confluence, or proximal right PA or left PA. An optimal Doppler gradient at the distal anastomosis may also be obtained from a suprasternal notch short-axis view, but, as with the BT shunt, gradients are unreliable for absolute determination of distal pressure. However, pulmonary hypertension is uncommon.

As is true with the right ventricular end of the Sano, the pulmonary insertion of conduit may also be prone to stenosis. Distortion or stenosis of the PAs is somewhat common. The Sano shunt is valveless, so there is "free" regurgitation and diastolic Doppler flow reversal may be seen in the branch PAs. The Doppler signal appears as a "to-and-fro" signal with the highest velocity in systole. Diastolic velocities are typically low and taper to the baseline very rapidly (Fig. 12.22E). In contrast to patients with a modified BT shunt, there is an absence of diastolic runoff in the aorta.

Echocardiographic Evaluation of the Bidirectional Cavopulmonary (Glenn) Anastomosis

The second stage in the management of patients with a univentricular AV connection is a bidirectional cavopulmonary anastomosis (or modified bidirectional Glenn shunt) where the right SVC

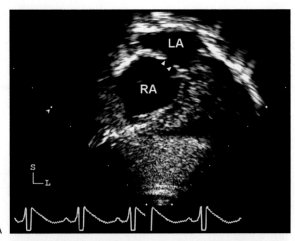

A

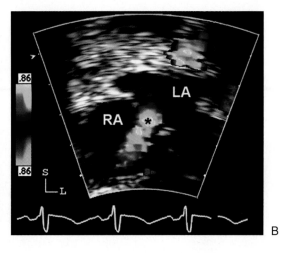

B

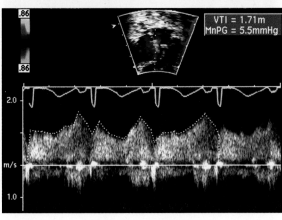

C

FIGURE 12.19. **Hypoplastic left heart syndrome; postoperative Stage I Norwood with restriction of the atrial septal defect (ASD). A:** Subcostal long-axis (coronal) view showing restriction of surgically created ASD (*arrowheads*) with thickened tissue rims. **B:** Color Doppler flow demonstrating aliased signal through the narrowed ASD (*asterisk*). **C:** Continuous-wave Doppler interrogation with the gradient (5 to 6 mm Hg) determined by tracing the Doppler flow over two or three cardiac cycles. LA, left atrium; RA, right atrium.

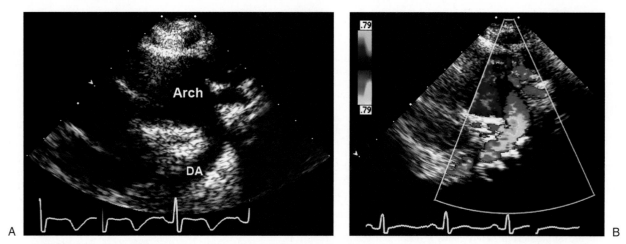

FIGURE 12.20. Hypoplastic left heart syndrome; postoperative evaluation of normal aortic arch. A: Suprasternal long-axis imaging following Norwood Stage I palliation, demonstrating size discrepancy between the dilated proximal reconstructed neoaorta and the normal-caliber descending aorta. **B:** Color Doppler flow in the reconstructed aortic arch following Norwood procedure demonstrating mild flow acceleration in this anatomic transition zone secondary to the size discrepancy.

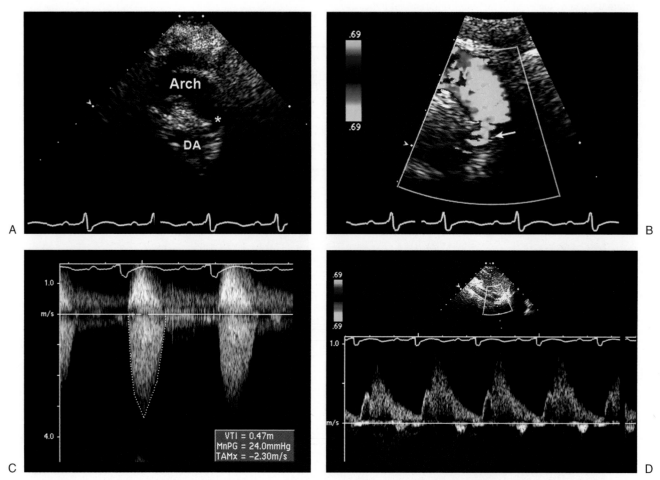

FIGURE 12.21. Hypoplastic left heart syndrome; Stage I Norwood with postoperative recurrent coarctation of the aorta. A: Suprasternal long-axis view of arch reconstruction showing recoarctation (*asterisk*) of aorta at the junction of reconstructed aorta and native descending aorta (DA). Note the more significant size discrepancy than illustrated in normal arch in Figure 12.20. **B:** Color Doppler interrogation of the aortic arch demonstrating the area of coarctation (*arrow*). **C:** Continuous-wave Doppler interrogation of aortic arch using nonimaging probe demonstrating recoarctation of aorta with a mean gradient of 24 mm Hg. **D:** Pulsed-wave Doppler interrogation of the abdominal aorta in the same patient demonstrates delayed upstroke with continued antegrade flow into diastole (and the absence of diastolic flow reversal) suggestive of significant recoarctation.

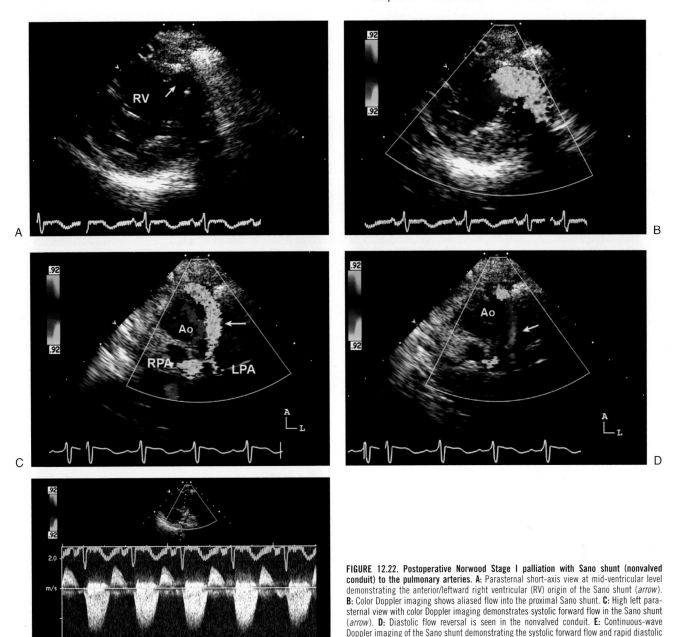

FIGURE 12.22. Postoperative Norwood Stage I palliation with Sano shunt (nonvalved conduit) to the pulmonary arteries. A: Parasternal short-axis view at mid-ventricular level demonstrating the anterior/leftward right ventricular (RV) origin of the Sano shunt (*arrow*). **B:** Color Doppler imaging shows aliased flow into the proximal Sano shunt. **C:** High left parasternal view with color Doppler imaging demonstrates systolic forward flow in the Sano shunt (*arrow*). **D:** Diastolic flow reversal is seen in the nonvalved conduit. **E:** Continuous-wave Doppler imaging of the Sano shunt demonstrating the systolic forward flow and rapid diastolic reversal suggestive of unrestricted conduit regurgitation. LPA, left pulmonary artery; RPA, right pulmonary artery.

is connected directly to the right PA. In a patient with bilateral SVCs, these anastomoses are performed to both the right PA and left PA. A cavopulmonary shunt is typically performed between the ages of 3 and 6 months. If no other source of pulmonary blood is present, the volume load on the heart is significantly decreased once the cavopulmonary shunt is constructed, which is of particular benefit to the patient with a systemic RV. The right cavopulmonary anastomosis is best visualized from the suprasternal short-axis view. In this view, the entire length of SVC and anastomosis to the right PA can be seen (Fig. 12.23A–B). With color Doppler interrogation, this is laminar venous flow (Fig. 12.23C). The Nyquist limit should be lowered to appreciate the low-velocity flow, Doppler interrogation over multiple cardiac cycles will show variation with respiration. In the absence of any additional blood flow, pulsed-wave Doppler interrogation of SVC or branch PA will show biphasic, low-velocity forward flow with significant accentuation of flow with inspiration. Continuous flow at mildly elevated

velocities that does not return to the Doppler baseline is very suggestive of obstruction. If present, tracing the mean gradient over three cardiac cycles will likely show a gradient of more than 3 mm Hg; in the venous system, such a gradient may be clinically significant. Noting the presence of a dilated azygous vein (if it was not surgically ligated) warrants a careful evaluation for obstruction in the cavopulmonary anastomosis. One should also be vigilant in looking for PA stenosis or distortion at site of the previous BT or Sano shunt, including evaluating the caliber of branch PAs by two-dimensional imaging.

Echocardiographic Evaluation of the Fontan Circulation

The evaluation of a patient following completion of the modified Fontan procedure will be covered elsewhere in the text.

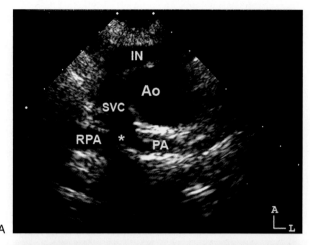

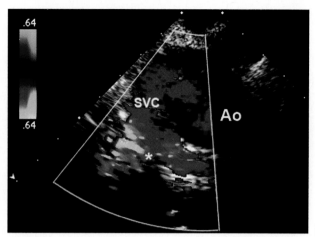

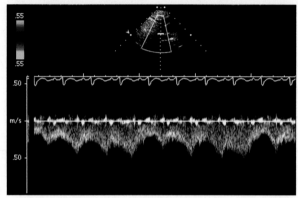

FIGURE 12.23. Right bidirectional Glenn shunt (cavopulmonary anastomosis). A: Suprasternal notch short-axis view of the widely patent anastomosis (*asterisk*) between the right superior vena cava (SVC) and right pulmonary artery (RPA). **B:** Color Doppler imaging of the Glenn shunt (*asterisk*) showing low-velocity laminar flow from SVC to the pulmonary artery. Note the use of a low Nyquist limit to document laminar venous flow. **C:** Pulsed wave Doppler interrogation demonstrating normal phasic flow with accentuation during atrial contraction and ventricular diastole. Ao, aorta; IN, innominate vein; PA, pulmonary artery.

 SUMMARY

In conclusion, echocardiographic evaluation of the neonate with univentricular AV connection is critical for diagnosis, early management, and planning the approach to initial palliation.

SUGGESTED READING

Alwi M. Management algorithm in pulmonary atresia with intact ventricular septum. *Cathet Cardiovasc Interv.* 2006;67(5):679–686.

Anderson RH, Becker AE, Wilkinson JL. Proceedings: Morphogenesis and nomenclature of univentricular hearts. *Br Heart J.* 1975;37(7):781–782.

Baffa JM, Chen SL, Guttenberg ME, et al. Coronary artery abnormalities and right ventricular histology in hypoplastic left heart syndrome. *J Am Coll Cardiol.* 1992;20(2):350–358.

Bharati S, McAllister HA Jr, Tatooles CJ, et al. Anatomic variations in underdeveloped right ventricle related to tricuspid atresia and stenosis. *J Thorac Cardiovasc Surg.* 1976;72(3):383–400.

Cardis BM, Fyfe DA, Ketchum D, et al. Echocardiographic features and complications of the modified Norwood operation using the right ventricle to pulmonary artery conduit. *J Am Soc Echocardiogr.* 2005;18(6):660–665.

Checchia PA, McGuire JK, Morrow S, et al. A risk assessment scoring system predicts survival following the Norwood procedure. *Pediatr Cardiol.* 2006;27(1):62–66.

Cook AC, Anderson RH. The anatomy of hearts with double inlet ventricle. *Cardiol Young.* 2006;16(Suppl 1):22–26.

Cook AC, Anderson RH. The functionally univentricular circulation: anatomic substrates as related to function. *Cardiol Young.* 2005;15(Suppl 3):7–16.

Corno AF. Borderline left ventricle. *Eur J Cardiothorac Surg.* 2005;27(1):67–73.

Daubeney PE, Wang D, Delany DJ, et al. Pulmonary atresia with intact ventricular septum: predictors of early and medium-term outcome in a population-based study. *J Thorac Cardiovasc Surg.* 2005;130(4):1071.

Daubeney PEF, Delany DJ, Anderson RH, et al. Pulmonary atresia with intact ventricular septum: range of morphology in a population-based study. *J Am Coll Cardiol.* 2002;39(10):1670–1679.

De La Cruz MV, Miller BL. Double inlet left ventricle. *Circulation.* 1968;37: 249–260.

Driscoll D. Tricuspid atresia. In: Garson A, et al. eds. *Science and practice of pediatric cardiology.* Philadelphia, Pa: Lea & Febiger; 1990:1118–1126.

Edwards J, Burchell HB. Congenital tricuspid atresia; a classification. *Med Clin North Am.* 1949;33:1177–1196.

Fraisse A, Colan SD, Jonas RA, et al. Accuracy of echocardiography for detection of aortic arch obstruction after Stage I Norwood procedure. *Am Heart J.* 1998;135(2 Pt 1):230–236.

Freedom RM, Benson LN, Smallhorn JF, et al. Subaortic stenosis, the univentricular heart, and banding of the pulmonary artery: an analysis of the courses of 43 patients with univentricular heart palliated by pulmonary artery banding. *Circulation.* 1986;73(4):758–764.

Freedom RM, Nykanen DG. Pulmonary atresia and intact ventricular septum. In: Allen HD, Gutgesell HP, Clark EB, et al. eds. *Moss and Adams' Heart disease in infants, children, and adolescents.* New York: Lippincott Williams & Wilkins; 2000:845–863.

Fyfe DA, Edwards WD, Driscoll DJ. Myocardial ischemia in patients with pulmonary atresia and intact ventricular septum. *J Am Coll Cardiol.* 1986;8(2):402–406.

Fyler D. Report of the New England Regional Infant Cardiac Program. *Pediatrics.* 1980;65:375–461.

Gaynor JW, Mahle WT, Cohen MI, et al. Risk factors for mortality after the Norwood procedure. *Eur J Cardiothorac Surg.* 2002;22(1):82–89.

Gewillig M, Boshoff DE, Dens J, et al. Stenting the neonatal arterial duct in duct-dependent pulmonary circulation: new techniques, better results. *J Am Coll Cardiol.* 2004;43(1):107–112.

Gundry SR, Behrendt DM. Prognostic factors in valvotomy for critical aortic stenosis in infancy. *J Thorac Cardiovasc Surg.* 1986;92(4):747–754.

Hanley FL, Sade RM, Blackstone EH, et al. Outcomes in neonatal pulmonary atresia with intact ventricular septum. A multiinstitutional study. *J Thorac Cardiovasc Surg.* 1993;105(3):406–423.

Hijazi ZM, Patel H, Cao QL, et al. Transcatheter retrograde radio-frequency perforation of the pulmonic valve in pulmonary atresia with intact ventricular septum, using a 2 French catheter. *Cathet Cardiovasc Diagn.* 1998;45(2):151–154.

Holmes AF. Case of malformation of the heart. *Trans Med-chir Soc Edinb.* 1824;1:252–259.

Humpl T, Soderberg B, McCrindle BW, et al. Percutaneous balloon valvotomy in pulmonary atresia with intact ventricular septum: impact on patient care. *Circulation.* 2003;108(7):826–832.

Jacobs ML, Anderson RH. Nomenclature of the functionally univentricular heart. *Cardiol Young.* 2006;16(Suppl 1):3–8.

Jacobs ML, Mayer JE Jr. Congenital Heart Surgery Nomenclature and Database Project: single ventricle. *Ann Thorac Surg.* 2000;69(Suppl 4):S197–S204.

Khairy P, Poirier N, Mercier LA. Univentricular heart. *Circulation.* 2007;115(6):800–812.

Kleinman CS. The echocardiographic assessment of pulmonary atresia with intact ventricular septum. *Cathet Cardiovasc Interv.* 2006;68(1):131–135.

Lofland GK, McCrindle BW, Williams WG, et al. Critical aortic stenosis in the neonate: a multi-institutional study of management, outcomes, and risk factors. Congenital Heart Surgeons Society. *J Thorac Cardiovasc Surg.* 2001;121(1):10–27.

Marin-Garcia J, Tandon R, Moller JH, et al. Common (single) ventricle with normally related great vessels. *Circulation.* 1974;49(3):565–573.

Marshall AC, van der Velde ME, Tworetzky W, et al. Creation of an atrial septal defect in utero for fetuses with hypoplastic left heart syndrome and intact or highly restrictive atrial septum. *Circulation.* 2004;110(3):253–258.

Matitiau A, Geva T, Colan SD, et al. Bulboventricular foramen size in infants with double-inlet left ventricle or tricuspid atresia with transposed great arteries: influence on initial palliative operation and rate of growth. *J Am Coll Cardiol.* 1992;19(1):142–148.

McCaffrey FM, Leatherbury L, Moore HV. Pulmonary atresia and intact ventricular septum. *J Thorac Cardiovasc Surg.* 1991;102:617–623.

Minich LL, Tani LY, Ritter S, et al. Usefulness of the preoperative tricuspid/mitral valve ratio for predicting outcome in pulmonary atresia with intact ventricular septum. *Am J Cardiol.* 2000;85(11):1325–1328.

Miyaji K, Shimada M, Sekiguchi A, et al. Pulmonary atresia with intact ventricular septum: long-term results of "one and a half ventricular repair." *Ann Thorac Surg.* 1995;60(6):1762–1764.

Morris CD, Outcalt J, Menashe VD. Hypoplastic left heart syndrome: natural history in a geographically defined population. *Pediatrics.* 1990;85(6):977-983.

Munoz-Castellanos L, Espinola-Zavaleta N, Keirns C. Anatomoechocardiographic correlation double inlet left ventricle. *J Am Soc Echocardiogr.* 2005;18(3):237–243.

Norwood WI, Lang P, Hansen DD. Physiologic repair of aortic atresia-hypoplastic left heart syndrome. *N Engl J Med.* 1983;308(1):23–26.

Pizarro C, Malec E, Maher KO, et al. Right ventricle to pulmonary artery conduit improves outcome after stage I Norwood for hypoplastic left heart syndrome. *Circulation.* 2003;108(Suppl 1):II-155–II-160.

Rao PS. A unified classification for tricuspid atresia. *Am Heart J.* 1980;99(6):799-804.

Rao PS. Tricuspid atresia. *Curr Treat Options Cardiovasc Med.* 2000;2(6):507–520.

Reemtsen BL, Pike NA, Starnes VA. Stage I palliation for hypoplastic left heart syndrome: Norwood versus Sano modification. *Curr Opin Cardiol.* 2007;22(2):60–65.

Rhodes LA, Colan SD, Perry SB, et al. Predictors of survival in neonates with critical aortic stenosis [erratum appears in *Circulation.* 1995;92(7):2005]. *Circulation.* 1991;84(6):2325–2335.

Rigby ML, Anderson RH, Gibson D, et al. Two dimensional echocardiographic categorisation of the univentricular heart. Ventricular morphology, type, and mode of atrioventricular connection. *Br Heart J.* 1981;46(6):603–612.

Rychik J, Gullquist SD, Jacobs ML, et al. Doppler echocardiographic analysis of flow in the ductus arteriosus of infants with hypoplastic left heart syndrome: relationship of flow patterns to systemic oxygenation and size of interatrial communication. *J Am Soc Echocardiogr.* 1996;9(2):166–173.

Rychik J, Rome JJ, Collins MH, et al. The hypoplastic left heart syndrome with intact atrial septum: atrial morphology, pulmonary vascular histopathology and outcome. *J Am Coll Cardiol.* 1999;34(2):554–560.

Salvin JW, McElhinney DB, Colan SD, et al. Fetal tricuspid valve size and growth as predictors of outcome in pulmonary atresia with intact ventricular septum. *Pediatrics.* 2006;118(2):e415–e420.

Samanek M, Slavik Z, Zborilova B, et al. Prevalence, treatment, and outcome of heart disease in live-born children: a prospective analysis of 91,823 live-born children. *Pediatr Cardiol.* 1989;10(4):205–211.

Satou GM, Perry SB, Gauvreau K, et al. Echocardiographic predictors of coronary artery pathology in pulmonary atresia with intact ventricular septum. *Am J Cardiol.* 2000;85(11):1319–1324.

Seliem MA, Chin AJ, Norwood WI. Patterns of anomalous pulmonary venous connection/drainage in hypoplastic left heart syndrome: diagnostic role of Doppler color flow mapping and surgical implications. *J Am Coll Cardiol.* 1992;19(1):135–141.

Seward JB, Tajik AJ, Hagler DJ, et al. Echocardiographic spectrum of tricuspid atresia. *Mayo Clin Proc.* 1978;53(2):100–112.

Simsic JM, Bradley SM, Stroud MR, et al. Risk factors for interstage death after the Norwood procedure. *Pediatr Cardiol.* 2005;26(4):400–403.

Snider R, Serwer G, Ritter S. Ventricular hypoplasia. In: Snider R, Ritter S, eds. *Echocardiography in pediatric heart disease.* 2nd ed. St. Louis, Mo: Mosby; 1997:343–384.

Starnes VA, Griffin ML, Pitlick PT, et al. Current approach to hypoplastic left heart syndrome. Palliation, transplantation, or both? *J Thorac Cardiovasc Surg.* 1992;104(1):189–194; discussion 94–95.

Stasik CN, Gelehrter S, Goldberg CS, et al. Current outcomes and risk factors for the Norwood procedure [erratum appears in *J Thorac Cardiovasc Surg.* 2007 Mar;133(3):602 (note: Gelehrter, S added]. *J Thorac Cardiovasc Surg.* 2006;131(2):412–417.

Tandon R, Edwards JE. Tricuspid atresia. A re-evaluation and classification. *J Thorac Cardiovasc Surg.* 1974;67(4):530–542.

Ueda K, Saito A, Nakano H, et al. Absence of proximal coronary arteries associated with pulmonary atresia. *Am Heart J.* 1983;106(3):596–598.

Van Praagh R, Ongley PA, Swan HJ. Anatomic types of single or common ventricle in man. Morphologic and geometric aspects of 60 necropsied cases. *Am J Cardiol.* 1964;13:367–386.

Weinberg PM. Anatomy of tricuspid atresia and its relevance to current forms of surgical therapy. *Ann Thorac Surg.* 1980;29(4):306–311.

Zuberbuhler JR, Anderson RH. Morphological variations in pulmonary atresia with intact ventricular septum. *Br Heart J.* 1979;41(3):281–288.

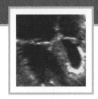

Chapter 13
Abnormalities of Right Ventricular Outflow

Erik C. Michelfelder • William L. Border

 VALVAR PULMONARY STENOSIS

Background

Clinical Presentation – In the vast majority of cases, stenosis of the pulmonary valve represents a primary, congenital abnormality. In children, acquired pulmonary valve stenosis (PS) is very rare and typically would occur as a sequela of rheumatic carditis. Regardless of etiology, the clinical presentation of valvar PS can be variable. In most cases, however, patients are asymptomatic in the face of mild and even moderate PS. With more severe degrees of PS, symptoms may vary from mild dyspnea and fatigue with exertion to cyanosis with or without overt symptoms of right heart failure. In most cases, symptoms arise from the decreased ability of the right ventricle to provide cardiac output across the stenotic valve. Signs of heart failure such as low output, hepatomegaly, and edema can be seen in the setting of high central venous pressure due to right ventricular (RV) failure in patients with severe pulmonary valve obstruction. Hypoxemia and cyanosis are classic findings in infants with critical pulmonary valve stenosis. Rarely, patients with severe PS may present with syncope on exertion due to limited right heart output. As most patients with PS are asymptomatic, clinical presentation frequently occurs during auscultation of a systolic murmur. The murmur of valvar PS is typically a systolic ejection murmur, heard best at the upper left sternal border. The murmur often radiates into the lung fields and is frequently more prominent in the left posterior lung field than the in right. A murmur is often accompanied by a variable systolic ejection click. Electrocardiographic findings typically feature variable degrees of right-axis deviation and findings of RV hypertrophy.

Anatomy and Physiology – The pulmonary valve is typically thickened and doming with restricted movement in systole. The valve is often bicuspid. In children and young adults, the pulmonary valve annulus, pulmonary root, sinotubular junction, and main pulmonary artery segment are often normal in size. However, poststenotic dilation of the main pulmonary artery can often be noted. In neonates and young infants, severe pulmonary valve stenosis, along a spectrum of critical PS, can also be associated with a small pulmonary valve annulus and pulmonary artery segment. In some cases, a very thickened, dysplastic, myxomatous pulmonary valve can present with severe stenosis and hypoplasia of the main pulmonary artery segment.

Physiologically, contraction of the right ventricle against a fixed obstruction results in RV systolic hypertension. As a result, varying degrees of RV hypertrophy will develop relative to the degree of outflow tract obstruction. As RV hypertrophy progresses, diastolic dysfunction can develop. Impairment of RV relaxation occurs relatively early during the process of hypertrophy; as the right ventricle thickens it becomes less compliant. RV filling pressures can increase and right atrial pressure may be elevated.

Complications – In patients with mild to moderate PS, symptoms and cardiovascular sequelae may be minimal. In the more severe forms of PS, chronic RV pressure overload may result in biventricular systolic dysfunction with the development of signs and symptoms of right heart failure. Subsequent dilation of the right ventricle in the face of pressure overload can result in development of tricuspid regurgitation. Chronic RV diastolic dysfunction can result in significant elevations of right heart filling pressures with right atrial dilation. In addition, when atrial level shunts are present, elevation of right atrial pressure can produce right-to-left shunting at the atrial level producing hypoxemia and cyanosis.

Principles of Echocardiographic Anatomy and Imaging

Classic Two-dimensional Echocardiographic Anatomy and Hemodynamics – Two-dimensional imaging of the pulmonary valve can be performed in several imaging planes. In the parasternal window, the pulmonary valve can be visualized in the long-axis view by sweeping the plane of sound to the left and anteriorly from the standard view. In the parasternal short-axis view, the RV outflow tract (RVOT) is typically imaged by sweeping the plane of sound superiorly toward the base of the heart. In the apical four-chamber view, it is often possible to sweep the plane of sound anteriorly to image the subvalvar infundibulum and pulmonary valve, particularly in infants and younger children. The pulmonary valve can also be imaged in the subcostal window in both the coronal and sagittal planes.

On initial inspection, the stenotic pulmonary valve leaflets will appear to be variably thickened. The valve typically domes during systole due to incomplete leaflet opening. The pulmonary artery root and main pulmonary artery segment are typically normal in size. In many cases, there can be poststenotic dilation of the main pulmonary artery segment (Fig. 13.1). The degree of poststenotic dilation in the main pulmonary artery segment does not typically correlate with the degree of PS and therefore can be seen even in the setting of mild to moderate stenosis. The subvalvar infundibulum is typically widely patent and normal in caliber, although with significant RV hypertrophy, mild narrowing of the infundibulum may result (Fig. 13.2).

Careful inspection of the supravalvar portion of the main pulmonary artery in the area of the sinotubular junction should be performed specifically to look for evidence of supravalvar narrowing (Fig. 13.3). The supravalvar area is typically well seen in the parasternal long- and short-axis windows but can also be visualized in subcostal windows and on anterior sweeps the apical window. As the stenotic pulmonary valve typically domes at the level of the sinotubular junction, coexistent supravalvar PS may be missed on two-dimensional imaging unless this area is examined carefully. Although the pulmonary valve annulus is usually normal in size, it is often useful to measure the pulmonary valve annulus by two-dimensional imaging. Comparison of the annulus dimension to the sinotubular junction will reveal whether the supravalvar area is significantly smaller than the annulus dimension (Fig. 13.3); in the normal heart, the sizes of the two areas are typically equal. The pulmonary valve annulus is typically measured in either the parasternal long- or short-axis views, although the annulus may also be adequately measured in subcostal views. Although isolated subvalvar PS is rare, discrete fibromuscular narrowing of the proximal infundibulum (Fig. 13.4) should be distinguished by both two-dimensional and Doppler echocardiography from valvar PS.

Hemodynamic assessment is centered on direct estimation of the pressure gradient across the stenotic pulmonary valve and the sequelae of valve stenosis. Doppler interrogation of the flow across the stenotic pulmonary valve is performed by pulsed-wave and/or continuous-wave Doppler (Fig. 13.5A). In our experience, accurate alignment of the Doppler interrogation beam with the flow jet is best obtained in either the parasternal short-axis or subcostal windows. In the parasternal short-axis view, it will often be evident that flow across the pulmonary valve is often directed more anteriorly than usual. This somewhat atypical location for the pulmonary flow jet will often correlate with the area of poststenotic dilation seen in the main pulmonary artery (Fig. 13.1). The angle of Doppler interrogation should therefore be modified in this instance to achieve better alignment with the anteriorly directed flow jet. The peak gradient across the stenotic pulmonary valve can be estimated using the modified

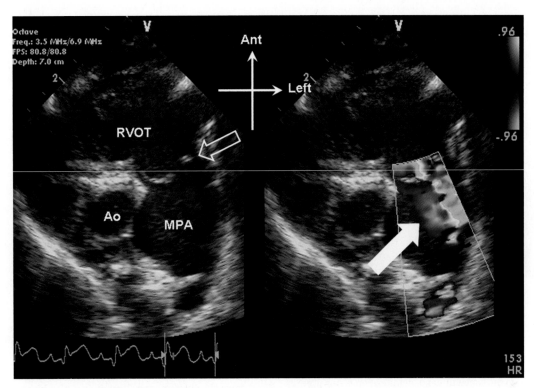

FIGURE 13.1. Parasternal short-axis view of the right ventricular outflow tract (RVOT). The pulmonary valve (*open arrow*) domes in systole. Note the anterior, leftward orientation of the stenotic outflow jet, with swirling of flow (*white arrow*) seen within the dilated main pulmonary artery (MPA). Ao, aorta.

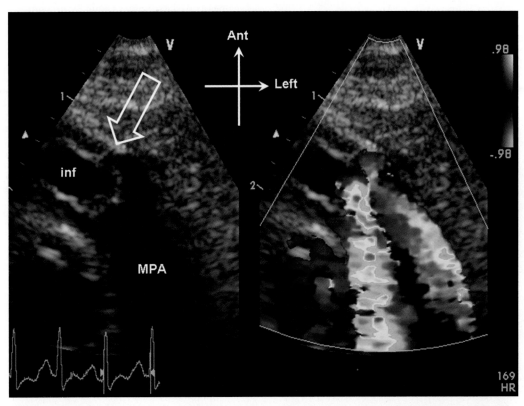

FIGURE 13.2. Parasternal short-axis view of the right ventricular outflow tract. The pulmonary valve domes in systole, and the annulus dimension is slightly small (*arrow*). The infundibulum (inf) is hypertrophied and appears slightly narrowed in systole. Note the stenotic flow jet in the main pulmonary artery (MPA) is directed posteriorly.

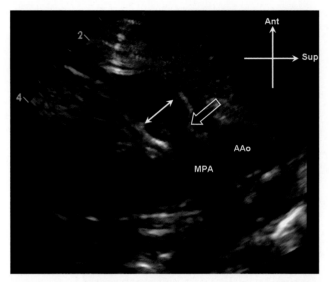

FIGURE 13.3. Supravalvar pulmonary stenosis. Parasternal long-axis view of the main pulmonary artery (MPA). There is discrete narrowing of the sinotubular junction (*open arrow*), which is significantly smaller in comparison to the pulmonary valve annulus (*white arrows*). AAo, ascending aorta.

Bernoulli equation. Color flow Doppler imaging also allows localization of the gradient to the leaflet tips and identification of any preexisting pulmonary regurgitation due to the anatomic valve abnormality.

Variable degrees of RV hypertension will result due to the pulmonary valve obstruction. RV pressure should be estimated, when possible, by measuring tricuspid regurgitant jet velocities using either pulsed-wave or continuous-wave Doppler. Using the peak tricuspid regurgitant jet velocity, the RV–to–right atrial systolic gradient can be estimated by the modified Bernoulli equation, and by adding an assumed central venous pressure, one can solve for estimated RV pressure. Estimates of central venous pressure between 6 and 10 mm Hg are typically used to perform this quantitation. In the absence of tricuspid regurgitation, indirect evidence of RV hypertension should be assessed. RV hypertrophy can be quantified as RV anterior wall thickness (by either

M-mode or two-dimensional imaging); however, the degree of RV hypertrophy does not correlate well with the gradient across the pulmonary valve, particularly postintervention. Flattening of the interventricular septum can be seen when RV pressure equals the pressure in the left ventricle; when RV pressure is suprasystemic, the interventricular septum will bow leftward into the left ventricle (Fig. 13.6).

Variations on Classic Anatomy

CRITICAL PULMONARY STENOSIS – In this group of patients, the pulmonary valve typically consists of a thickened, domed, and often dysplastic pulmonary valve. In addition, the pulmonary valve annulus is often variably hypoplastic. The degree of pulmonary valvar stenosis is typically severe. The subvalvar infundibulum is often short and muscle bound due to prominent RV hypertrophy. In addition, the right ventricle is often globally hypertrophied with reduced cavitary size. Critical PS typically presents in the newborn period with hypoxemia and cyanosis due to the severity of the RVOT obstruction. This leads to elevated right heart pressures and right-to-left shunting at the foramen ovale.

Critical PS belongs to a spectrum of anatomy that includes severe valvar PS with normal RV size to pulmonary valve atresia with intact ventricular septum and severe RV hypoplasia (see "Pulmonary Atresia with Intact Ventricular Septum"). Patients with this condition can have varying degrees of pulmonary valve, RV cavity, and tricuspid valve hypoplasia (Fig. 13.7). It is therefore important on a two-dimensional echocardiographic evaluation to quantify tricuspid valve annular dimension and pulmonary valve annular dimension and to evaluate the degree of RV hypoplasia.

In addition to tricuspid valve annular hypoplasia, abnormalities of tricuspid anatomy and function can also be seen. On two-dimensional imaging, severe PS can be associated with echogenic areas of endocardial sclerosis that may involve the tricuspid valve papillary muscles (Fig. 13.8). Tricuspid valve function can be abnormal with significant degrees of tricuspid regurgitation (Fig. 13.9). Tricuspid regurgitation may be due, in part, to anatomic abnormalities involving the tricuspid valve chordal apparatus and papillary muscle function, as well as suprasystemic RV pressure secondary to severe RVOT obstruction. In addition to assessing the severity of tricuspid regurgitation, RV pressure estimates can be obtained using the tricuspid regurgitant jet velocity by applying the Bernoulli equation (Fig. 13.9).

Additional physiologic information that should be obtained include the presence or absence of a ductus arteriosus, the pattern of shunting across the foramen ovale (typically right to left), and the presence or absence of a gradient across the pulmonary valve. In the neonate, the presence of a widely patent ductus arteriosus as well as the presence of elevated pulmonary vascular resistance may result in an observed pulmonary valve gradient that is relatively low, and not reflective of the degree of anatomic stenosis (Fig. 13.10). Therefore, demonstration of suprasystemic RV pressure by either tricuspid regurgitant jet velocity (Fig. 13.9) or two-dimensional evidence of prominent interventricular septal bowing into the left ventricle in the parasternal short-axis scan (Fig. 13.6) can often be the most useful physiologic evidence of the severity of the pulmonary valve stenosis. In the setting of pulmonary valve atresia, the frequency and degree of RV hypoplasia, tricuspid valve hypoplasia, and associated anomalies become much higher.

DYSPLASTIC PULMONARY VALVE

Occasionally, pulmonary valve stenosis can be associated with severe dysplasia of the pulmonary valve leaflets. This is most typically seen in association with Noonan syndrome. In these patients, the pulmonary valve leaflets are typically very thickened and myxomatous (Fig. 13.11). Often, it is very difficult to demonstrate normal valve motion on two-dimensional imaging. In addition to the pulmonary valve abnormality, the pulmonary valve annulus is often hypoplastic and the main pulmonary artery segment beyond the pulmonary valve is also often quite small. Overall, the frequency of pulmonary valve stenosis is approximately 25%, with pulmonary valve dysplasia occurring in approximately 7% of cases (Burch, 1993). Therapeutically, these valves typically do not respond well to balloon angioplasty. This is due both to the annular hypoplasia and to the severe thickening and dysplasia of the pulmonary valve leaflets.

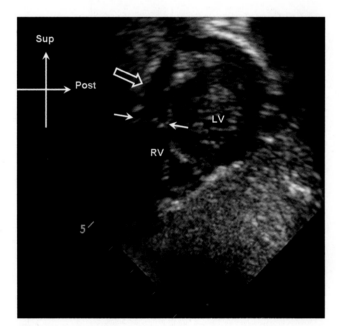

FIGURE 13.4. Subcostal sagittal view demonstrating a discrete subpulmonary membrane (*white arrows*) in the proximal right ventricular (RV) outflow tract (*white arrows*). Note the position of the membrane relative to the pulmonary valve annulus (*open arrow*). LV, left ventricle.

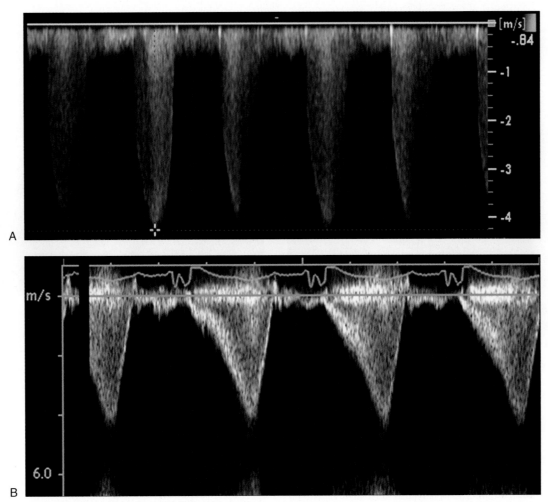

FIGURE 13.5. Doppler evaluation of pulmonary stenosis. A: Continuous-wave Doppler profile is consistent with fixed obstruction across a stenotic pulmonary valve. The peak instantaneous gradient across the valve = 4(4.25 m/s)² = 72 mm Hg. **B:** Continuous-wave Doppler flow profile is consistent with a dynamic obstruction and predicts a peak instantaneous gradient of about 70 mm Hg.

Common Associated Lesions and Findings – Common lesions associated with valvar PS are summarized in Table 13.1.

Interventional and Postinterventional Imaging – Cardiac catheterization with balloon valvuloplasty is the treatment of choice when the pulmonary valve annulus is adequate in size and there are no concerns regarding RV or tricuspid valve hypoplasia. Following balloon valvuloplasty, echocardiographic evaluation should be performed to determine the residual PS gradient and degree of postvalvuloplasty regurgitation as well as to assess RV function and pressure post intervention. Occasionally, postintervention subvalvar PS can be observed. In this setting—the "suicide right ventricle"—a typical dynamic pattern of obstruction can be observed (Fig. 13.5B).

Isolated surgical pulmonary valvotomy is seldom performed in the current era. However, when the pulmonary valve annulus is hypoplastic, pulmonary valvotomy with a transannular RVOT patch is typically performed to increase the size of the RVOT and relieve valvar obstruction. Following transannular patch placement, it is typical to see moderate or greater degrees of pulmonary regurgitation, unless the transannular patching was quite limited or the surgical technique included some form of pulmonic valve prosthesis. In the setting of significant pulmonary regurgitation, it is important to follow RV size and function by serial echocardiographic studies. Long-standing significant pulmonary regurgitation can be associated with RV dilation and dysfunction.

In the setting of severe pulmonary valve stenosis or atresia with associated hypoplasia of the right ventricle, single ventricular palliation may be undertaken. Postoperative evaluation of the hypoplastic right ventricle after single ventricular surgical palliation will be discussed in the section on pulmonary atresia with intact ventricular septum.

SUBVALVAR PULMONARY STENOSIS

Background

Clinical Presentation – The clinical presentation in patients with subvalvar PS and intact ventricular septum closely resembles that of isolated valvar PS. Anomalous muscle bundles in the RV infundibulum (i.e., "double-chamber right ventricle") are often seen in association with a ventricular septal defect. In this setting, the ventricular septal defect may produce the most prominent clinical findings. As with isolated valvar PS, when the degree of subvalvar obstruction is mild to moderate, most patients will be asymptomatic. When

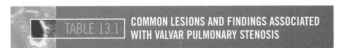

TABLE 13.1	COMMON LESIONS AND FINDINGS ASSOCIATED WITH VALVAR PULMONARY STENOSIS

- Poststenotic dilation of main and branch pulmonary arteries
- Right ventricular hypertrophy
- Tricuspid regurgitation
- Dysplastic pulmonary valve

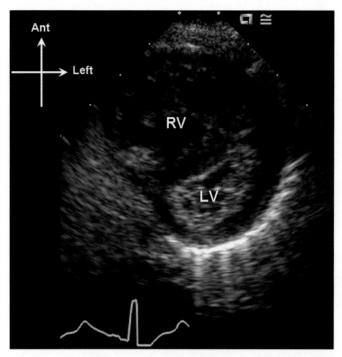

FIGURE 13.6. Parasternal short-axis image of the right (RV) and left (LV) ventricles. Note that the interventricular septum bows into the LV in late systole, consistent with suprasystemic RV systolic pressure.

obstruction is severe and/or long-standing, RV hypertrophy and failure may result, with the accompanying clinical findings of right heart failure. These are outlined in more detail in the section on valvar PS. On physical examination, the murmur of subvalvar stenosis is typically a long, pansystolic crescendo-decrescendo murmur that is heard at the upper left sternal border. The murmur is often heard lower down the sternal border than is typical in isolated valvar stenosis. Subvalvar PS is often associated with a palpable thrill along the left sternal border. The pulmonary component of the second heart sound may be more normal than expected—in comparison to valvar PS—for the degree of murmur on auscultation. A systolic ejection click should not be appreciated. Electrocardiographic findings typically feature variable degrees of right-axis deviation and

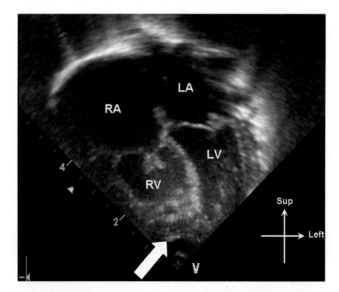

FIGURE 13.7. Apical four-chamber view in an infant with critical pulmonary stenosis. Note the mild hypoplasia of the right ventricle (RV), which is not apex-forming (*white arrow*). The tricuspid valve leaflets are also thickened with incomplete leaflet coaptation. LA, left atrium; LV, left ventricle; RA, right atrium.

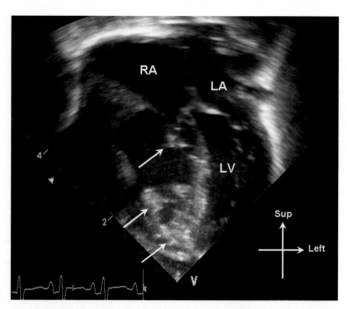

FIGURE 13.8. Apical four-chamber view in an infant with critical pulmonary valve stenosis. Note multiple areas of increased echogenicity (*arrows*) involving the right ventricular endocardium, moderator band, and tricuspid valve apparatus, consistent with endocardial sclerosis. LA, left atrium; LV, left ventricle; RA, right atrium.

RV hypertrophy, although these will not allow one to distinguish between subvalvar or valvar PS.

Anatomy and Physiology – The most common form of subvalvar PS consists of anomalous muscle bundles narrowing the proximal RV infundibulum. This malformation is also known as "double-chamber right ventricle." Pathologically, the two "chambers" in double-chamber right ventricle consist of the RV sinus and inflow portions, which are upstream of the obstructive muscle bundles, and the RV infundibulum and apical trabecular right ventricle, which lay downstream of the obstructive bundles. The muscular bundles themselves appear to consist, most frequently, of hypertrophied septoparietal muscle bands that course anteriorly from the septal band on the ventricular septum to the RV free wall. Some reports have suggested that the muscular obstruction is due to abnormal, anterosuperior positioning of the moderator band. It is likely that the nature of the muscular obstruction can vary and that no single mechanism accounts for all cases. One consistent finding in double-chamber right ventricle is that the downstream chamber includes both RV infundibulum and some portion of the apical trabecular right ventricle.

Primary fibromuscular infundibular stenoses can also produce subpulmonary obstruction. However, these types of obstruction are more rare than double-chamber right ventricle. In one type, a discreet fibromuscular band separates the main RV cavity from the infundibular chamber. Alternatively, there can be infundibular narrowing due to prominent muscular hypertrophy of the infundibular wall, producing either short- or long-segment subvalvar PS.

Regardless of the anatomic type of subvalvar stenosis, the physiology is similar. The obstruction will produce elevated pressure in the upstream portion of the right ventricle. As these lesions often consist of a muscular narrowing, there can be a dynamic component with progressive obstruction during ventricular contraction. These findings can be exaggerated during exercise. RV hypertension is accompanied by a varying degree of compensatory hypertrophy as in other forms of RVOT obstruction.

Complications – Complications relating to RVOT obstruction are indistinguishable from those described for valvar PS and are discussed in detail earlier. In patients with mild to moderate outflow tract obstruction, symptoms and cardiovascular sequelae may be minimal. When severe, chronic RV pressure overload may result in systolic RV dysfunction with the development of signs and symptoms of right heart failure. RV diastolic dysfunction can result in significant elevations of right heart filling pressures with right atrial dilation.

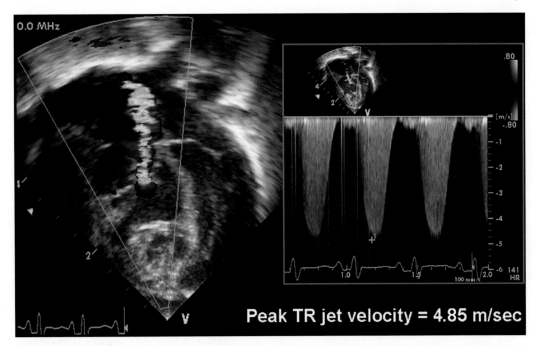

FIGURE 13.9. Color flow Doppler evaluation of tricuspid valve regurgitation in an infant with critical pulmonary valve stenosis. There is moderate tricuspid regurgitation. Continuous-wave Doppler evaluation of the regurgitant jet velocity (4.85 m/s) predicts a right ventricular pressure–right atrial gradient of $4(4.85)^2 = 94$ mm Hg. The estimated right ventricular pressure is therefore 94 mm Hg + central venous pressure, or approximately 100 to 104 mm Hg.

Principles of Echocardiographic Anatomy and Imaging

Classic Two-dimensional Echocardiographic Anatomy and Hemodynamics – Subpulmonary obstruction is often most clearly demonstrated in subcostal coronal and sagittal images, particularly in infants and young children. However, subcostal imaging often becomes technically difficult in older children, adolescents, and adults. In the subcostal window, imaging of the RV sinus and the RVOT can be used to demonstrate both double-chamber right ventricle (Fig. 13.12A–B) and the more uncommon subpulmonary ridge or membrane (Figs. 13.13 and 13.14). In double-chamber right ventricle, prominent muscle bundles can be seen traversing the proximal RVOT obliquely on coronal or sagittal imaging (Fig. 13.12A). Color-flow Doppler imaging in this area will demonstrate

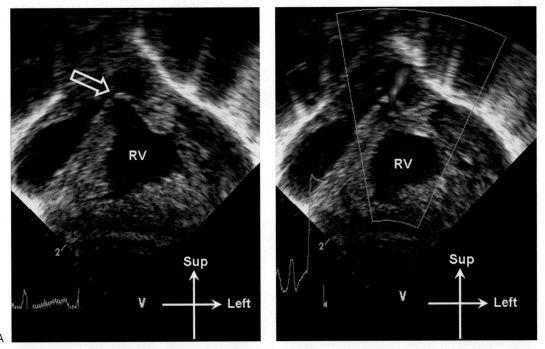

FIGURE 13.10. Subcostal coronal image of the right ventricle (RV) in a neonate with critical pulmonary valve stenosis. A: RV is markedly hypertrophied. The pulmonary valve is thickened and doming (*open arrow*). **B:** Narrow jet of transvalvar antegrade flow is demonstrated. Note the lack of color flow aliasing; the flow velocity is low due to the presence of a large patent ductus arteriosus (not pictured).

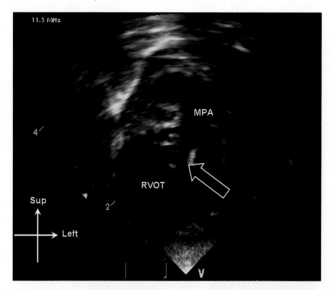

FIGURE 13.11. Dysplastic pulmonary valve (*open arrow*) **seen on anterior sweep from standard apical window.** The valve leaflets are thickened and myxomatous. Note also the poststenotic dilation of the main pulmonary artery (MPA). RVOT, right ventricular outflow tract.

plane of sound can be swept anteriorly into the RVOT, and both two-dimensional and color-flow Doppler are used to diagnose and localize subvalvar PS.

As double-chamber right ventricle often occurs in the setting of a perimembranous-outlet ventricular septal defect, care must be taken during two-dimensional imaging to distinguish double-chamber right ventricle with VSD from an anteriorly deviated conal septum in the setting of tetralogy of Fallot. In cases where the pulmonary valve annulus and distal infundibulum are relatively normal in size, "mild" tetralogy of Fallot can be difficult to differentiate from a double-chamber right ventricle. Lack of aortic valve override, normal aortic root size, and prominent RV muscle bundles on the anterior free wall that contribute to the obstruction should help distinguish double-chamber right ventricle from tetralogy of Fallot.

Hemodynamic assessment should focus on the assessment of stenosis severity and estimation of RV pressure. Doppler interrogation of the flow across the RVOT is performed by pulsed-wave and/or continuous-wave Doppler. In our experience, accurate alignment of the Doppler angle of insonation with the subvalar flow jet is best obtained in either the subcostal or apical windows. The Doppler *pattern* of flow should also be noted, to distinguish between dynamic and fixed obstruction (Fig. 13.5). The peak gradient across the RVOT can be estimated using the modified Bernoulli equation.

Variable degrees of RV hypertension are present due to the subpulmonary obstruction. RV pressure should be estimated, when possible, by measuring tricuspid regurgitant jet velocities using either pulsed-wave or continuous-wave Doppler. Using the peak tricuspid regurgitant jet velocity, the RV–to–right atrial systolic gradient can be estimated by the modified Bernoulli equation, and by adding an assumed central venous pressure, one can estimate RV pressure. In the absence of tricuspid regurgitation, indirect evidence of RV hypertension should be assessed. RV hypertrophy can be quantified as RV anterior wall thickness (by either M-mode or two-dimensional imaging); however, the degree of RV hypertrophy does not correlate well with the gradient across the pulmonary valve, particularly post intervention. Flattening of the interventricular septum can be seen when RV pressure equals the pressure in the left ventricle; when RV pressure is suprasystemic, the interventricular septum will bow leftward into the left ventricle (Fig. 13.6).

turbulent flow originating at the level of the RV muscle bundles (Fig. 13.15).

In the subcostal sagittal view, two-dimensional imaging will again demonstrate the RV muscle bundles in the proximal infundibulum, coursing from the anterior RV free wall to the interventricular septal surface (Fig. 13.12B). Imaging of the RVOT in parasternal long- and short-axis views can often be used to demonstrate subpulmonary obstruction. In double-chamber right ventricle, the parasternal window can also be used to screen for perimembranous ventricular septal defects often associated with subpulmonary obstruction. In the apical window, particularly in infants and young children, the

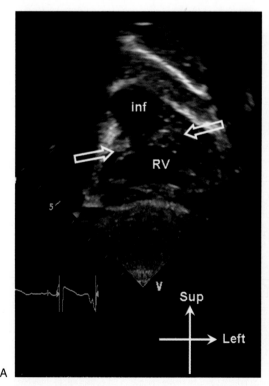

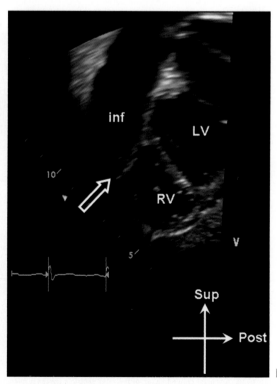

FIGURE 13.12. Subcostal imaging in double-chambered right ventricle (RV). A: Coronal image demonstrating oblique muscle bundles (*open arrows*) between the body of the RV and the infundibulum (inf). **B:** Sagittal image demonstrating muscle bundle (*open arrow*). LV, left ventricle.

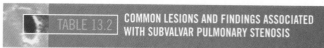

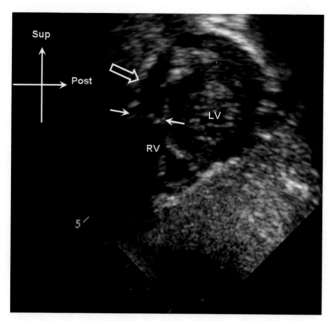

TABLE 13.2 COMMON LESIONS AND FINDINGS ASSOCIATED WITH SUBVALVAR PULMONARY STENOSIS

- Ventricular septal defect, typically perimembranous-outlet
- Subaortic membrane (with ventricular septal defect and double-chamber right ventricle)
- Right ventricular hypertrophy
- Tricuspid regurgitation

FIGURE 13.13. Subcostal sagittal image demonstrating discrete membranous obstruction (*white arrows*) in the proximal right ventricular (RV) outflow tract. Note the position of the membrane relative to the pulmonary valve annulus (*open arrow*). LV, left ventricle.

Variations on Classic Anatomy – Hypertrophic cardiomyopathy can occasionally result in subpulmonary obstruction due to septal hypertrophy impinging on the RVOT. This can also be the case in infiltrative diseases of the myocardium, such as glycogen storage diseases. Intracardiac tumors such as rhabdomyomata, particularly when large, can produce subpulmonary obstruction.

Common Associated Lesions and Findings – Common lesions associated with pulmonary regurgitation are summarized in Table 13.2.

Interventional and Postinterventional Imaging – Following surgical resection of a subpulmonary membrane or muscle bundles, the echocardiographic evaluation should focus on the assessment of residual RVOT obstruction. When there is significant RV hypertrophy in association with obstruction, there is often some degree of

dynamic RVOT obstruction (Fig. 13.5) despite an adequate surgical resection. Postintervention, RV pressure estimates can also be used to quantify the success of the intervention. Occasionally, aggressive resection of RV muscle bundles can produce coronary-RV cameral fistulas, which can be demonstrated with color flow Doppler imaging along the interventricular septum in the region of muscle resection.

SUPRAVALVAR PULMONARY STENOSIS

Background

Clinical Presentation – The clinical presentation of supravalvar PS is similar to that of valvar PS and is dependent on the severity of the pulmonary arterial obstruction. As with valvar PS, patients with mild to moderate degrees of unilateral or bilateral pulmonary artery stenosis are typically asymptomatic. With more severe degrees of arterial stenosis, symptoms may include dyspnea on exertion, exercise intolerance, fatigability, and evidence of RV failure. On examination, auscultatory findings may help differentiate pulmonary arterial stenoses from valvar pulmonic stenosis. A systolic ejection click, typically a feature of valvar PS, is absent. The second heart sound is typically split, and the pulmonary component may be loud, particularly in the setting of multiple severe branch pulmonary arterial obstructions. With severe peripheral obstruction, prominent systolic or continuous murmurs may be heard over the lung fields and in the back. The electrocardiogram typically features the same findings as in valvar PS.

Anatomy and Physiology – Supravalvar PS can occur in numerous forms, ranging from isolated supravalvar narrowing of the main pulmonary artery to diffuse distal pulmonary arterial stenoses. The various patterns of peripheral pulmonary artery stenosis have been classified angiographically (Gay et al., 1963). In approximately two thirds of cases, pulmonary artery stenoses are localized to the main

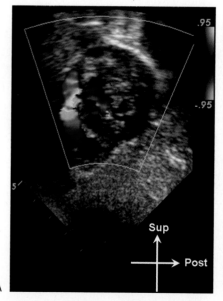

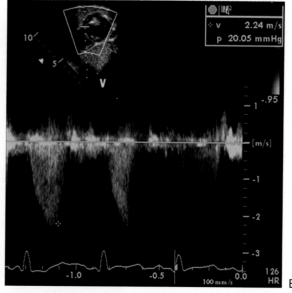

FIGURE 13.14. Color flow Doppler evaluation of subpulmonary membrane seen in Figure 13-13. Note the discrete acceleration at the level of the membrane (A). **B:** Peak gradient across the membrane is 20 mm Hg.

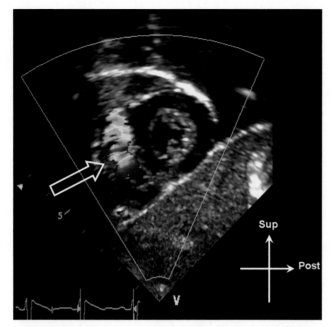

FIGURE 13.15. Color flow Doppler evaluation of the right ventricular outflow tract in double-chamber right ventricle. Note the midcavitary flow acceleration (*open arrow*) produced by the right ventricular muscle bundle.

pulmonary artery trunk, the pulmonary artery bifurcation, or the proximal right and left branch pulmonary arteries. Peripheral and main pulmonary artery stenoses are commonly seen in association with other types of congenital heart disease, notably tetralogy of Fallot (particularly with pulmonary atresia), and in PS associated with ventricular septal defect. It has been our experience that discrete stenosis of the proximal left pulmonary artery is more common in the setting of a reverse-oriented (tortuous) ductus arteriosus seen in conjunction with conotruncal defects featuring pulmonary outflow tract stenosis. Peripheral pulmonary artery stenoses can also be seen in association with supravalvar aortic stenosis typically seen in Williams syndrome. It may also be seen in association with Noonan

syndrome, Alagille syndrome, and congenital Rubella syndrome. In these settings, diffuse pulmonary artery hypoplasia is usually the case. In addition to the more common congenital causes of branch pulmonary artery stenosis, acquired forms of pulmonary artery stenosis can also exist. For example, branch pulmonary artery stenosis can occur following a surgical Waterston shunt (right pulmonary artery–to–ascending aortic anastomosis), Pott's shunting (left pulmonary artery–to–descending aortic anastomosis), unifocalization procedures for pulmonary atresia with VSD, left pulmonary artery reimplantation following pulmonary sling repair, and in transposition of the great arteries following a Lecompte maneuver.

As with valvar PS, physiologic sequelae stem from RV hypertension that results from contraction of the right ventricle against a fixed downstream obstruction. The degree of RV hypertrophy develops relative to the degree of outflow tract obstruction in RV hypertension. Diastolic dysfunction, increased RV filling pressures, and RV failure can ultimately result as the severity of the lesion increases.

Complications – Sequelae of supravalvar PS are the same as those for valvar PS. In patients with mild to moderate stenosis, symptoms and cardiovascular sequelae may be minimal. With more severe forms of stenosis, chronic RV pressure overload may result in ventricular systolic dysfunction and right heart failure. Dilation of the right ventricle in the face of pressure overload can result in development of tricuspid regurgitation. Chronic RV diastolic dysfunction can result in significant elevations of right heart filling pressures with right atrial dilation. When an atrial level shunt is present, elevation of right atrial pressures can result in right-to-left interatrial shunting, producing hypoxemia and cyanosis.

Principles of Echocardiographic Anatomy and Imaging

Classic Two-dimensional Echocardiographic Anatomy and Hemodynamics – Two-dimensional imaging of the main and branch pulmonary arteries can be performed in several imaging planes (discussed elsewhere in this text).

Careful inspection of the supravalvar portion of the main pulmonary artery in the area of the sinotubular junction should be performed specifically to look for evidence of supravalvar narrowing. The supravalvar area is typically well seen in the parasternal long- and short-axis windows (Figs. 13.16 and 13.17), but can also

FIGURE 13.16. Supravalvar pulmonary stenosis. Parasternal long-axis image of the pulmonary valve and main pulmonary artery (MPA). Note the narrowed caliber of the supravalvar ridge (*open arrow*) relative to the size of the pulmonary valve annulus (*white arrows*). AAo, ascending aorta.

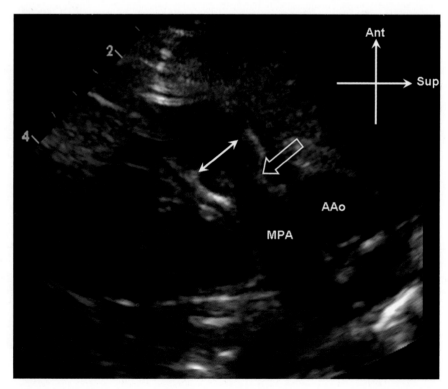

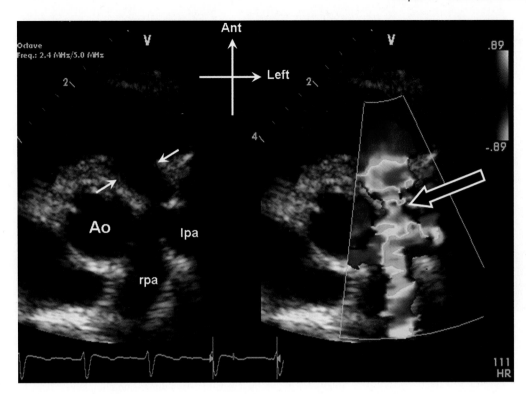

FIGURE 13.17. Parasternal short-axis imaging of supravalvar pulmonary stenosis. On two-dimensional imaging (left), there is discrete supravalvar narrowing. This area is substantially smaller that the pulmonary valve annulus (*white arrows*). On color flow Doppler imaging (**right**), there is a discrete flow acceleration at the supravalvar ridge (*open arrow*). Ao, aorta; lpa, left pulmonary artery; rpa, right pulmonary artery.

be visualized in subcostal windows and on anterior sweeps from the apical window. Comparison of the pulmonary valve annulus to the sinotubular junction dimension will reveal whether the supravalvar area is significantly smaller than the annulus dimension; the sizes of the two areas are normally about equal.

Examination of the branch pulmonary arteries should be focused on identification of branch pulmonary artery narrowing. This may occur as either a discrete, focal narrowing (Fig. 13.18) or diffuse hypoplasia of either branch pulmonary artery (Fig. 13.19). Two-dimensional measurements of both proximal and more distal pulmonary artery dimensions can be compared with published normal values. These measurements are typically best made in either suprasternal notch short-axis (particularly for the right pulmonary artery) or high parasternal short-axis images. When 2D imaging of the branch pulmonary arteries is difficult, color flow Doppler can be used to improve visualization and identify stenoses (Figures 13.19 and 13.20). Some investigators have demonstrated that color flow Doppler imaging can be used to quantify branch pulmonary artery size and has shown good correlation with angiographic studies (Hiraishi et al., 1994). Magnetic resonance imaging (MRI; see later) may be necessary when echocardiographic imaging is inadequate to demonstrate branch pulmonary artery anatomy, particularly if more distal stenoses are suspected.

Pressure gradient estimates in branch pulmonary artery stenosis generally correlate poorly to catheter-derived measurements. Therefore, hemodynamic assessment should be centered on estimation of RV pressure in this setting. Pressure gradients across discrete supravalvar PS are more reliably estimated. Doppler interrogation of the flow across the area of narrowing is performed by pulsed-wave and/or continuous-wave Doppler, with the minimum possible angle of insonation during Doppler interrogation. Although absolute pressure gradient estimation in branch pulmonary artery stenosis can be limited, a characteristic "sawtooth" flow pattern—with continuous forward flow during diastole—can be seen when obstruction is significant, particularly in the setting of discrete stenoses (Fig. 13.21).

RV pressure should be estimated, when possible, by measuring tricuspid regurgitant jet velocities using either pulsed-wave or continuous-wave Doppler. In the absence of tricuspid regurgitation, indirect evidence of RV hypertension should be assessed. RV hypertrophy can be quantified as RV anterior wall thickness (by either M-mode or

two-dimensional imaging); however, the degree of RV hypertrophy does not correlate well to the gradient across the pulmonary valve, particularly postintervention. Flattening of the interventricular septum can be seen when RV pressure equals the pressure in the left ventricle; when RV pressure is suprasystemic, the interventricular septum will bow leftward into the left ventricle.

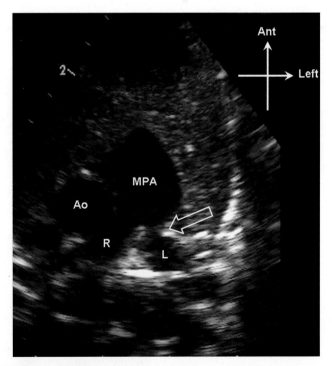

FIGURE 13.18. Parasternal short-axis imaging of proximal left (L) pulmonary artery stenosis (*open arrow*). Note the discrete reduction in vessel lumen in comparison to the size of the proximal right (R) pulmonary artery. Ao, aorta; MPA, main pulmonary artery.

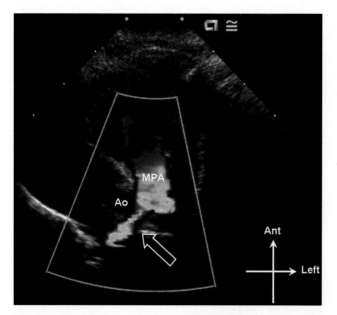

FIGURE 13.19. Color Doppler demonstration of proximal right pulmonary artery hypoplasia (*open arrow*). Parasternal short-axis view at the base of the heart demonstrating ascending aorta (Ao), main pulmonary artery (MPA), and proximal stenosis of the right pulmonary artery.

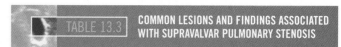

TABLE 13.3 COMMON LESIONS AND FINDINGS ASSOCIATED WITH SUPRAVALVAR PULMONARY STENOSIS

- Right ventricular hypertrophy
- Tricuspid regurgitation
- Dysplastic pulmonary valve (with Noonan syndrome)
- Supravalvar aortic stenosis (with Williams syndrome, familial elastin gene abnormalities)
- Valvar pulmonary stenosis
- Ventricular septal defect
- Patent ductus arteriosus
- Atrial septal defect (especially with congenital rubella syndrome)

multiple stenoses, catheter-based techniques are usually the therapy of choice. Catheter-based techniques include balloon angioplasty (either in the catheterization laboratory or intraoperative setting) or use of balloon-expandable endovascular stents. More recently, "cutting" balloons have been used to dilate difficult stenoses.

Following intervention, echocardiographic imaging is used to assess efficacy of the intervention, as well as to screen for sequelae. Postintervention estimation of RV pressure is the best means of documenting a clinically effective intervention, either through direct estimation by tricuspid regurgitation velocity or through indirect means. As in the preintervention setting, estimates of pressure gradients are generally unreliable. Two-dimensional imaging is used to document improvements in vessel caliber, as well as to rule out the presence of pulmonary artery aneurysms related to the intervention. Patency of stented pulmonary arteries may be demonstrated by two-dimensional imaging, but due to interference with sound waves by the stent itself, color flow Doppler is often required to confirm patency. Occasionally, contraction of the vessel along suture lines (post patch angioplasty) will result in narrowing of the vessel lumen in the mid to long term, despite adequate relief of the stenosis in the short term.

Common Associated Lesions and Findings – Common lesions associated with pulmonary regurgitation are summarized in Table 13.3.

Interventional and Postinterventional Imaging – When supravalvar PS involves the main pulmonary artery, surgical patch arterioplasty is usually performed. With branch pulmonary artery stenosis, surgical patching techniques may be used for proximal pulmonary artery stenosis, as well. However, when there are more distal, or

FIGURE 13.20. High left parasternal short-axis image. Diffuse left pulmonary artery hypoplasia (*open arrow*) by two-dimensional (*left*) and color flow Doppler (*right*) imaging. MPA, main pulmonary artery; RPA, right pulmonary artery.

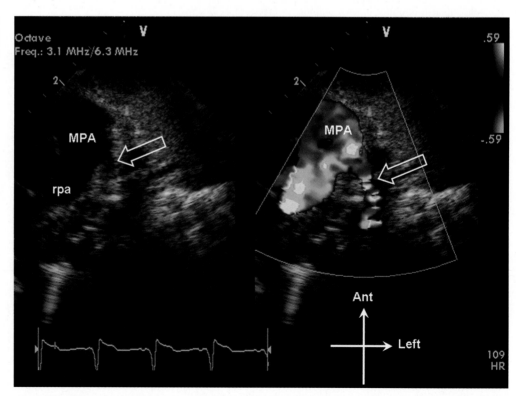

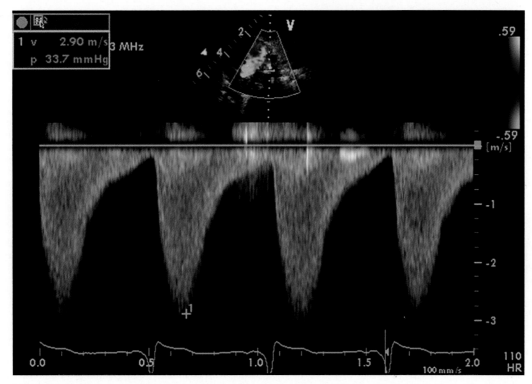

FIGURE 13.21. Continuous-wave Doppler evaluation of proximal left pulmonary artery stenosis in Figure 13.20. There is a high peak Doppler velocity (2.9 m/s) with a continuous diastolic flow gradient producing a "sawtooth" flow pattern.

 PULMONARY REGURGITATION

Background

Clinical Presentation – In children and young adults, trivial to mild degrees of pulmonary regurgitation on routine echocardiography are relatively common, occurring in approximately 75% of subjects. The observation that pulmonary regurgitation is more common in children than in adults may be related to higher sensitivity due to better echocardiographic image resolution in the young patients. Hemodynamically significant, primary pulmonary regurgitation is very uncommon in the pediatric age range. More commonly, significant pulmonary regurgitation is seen following intervention for RVOT obstruction or valvar PS, such as following tetralogy of Fallot repair/RVOT patching or pulmonary valvotomy. Given these considerations, the clinical presentation of pulmonary regurgitation in children often consists of pulmonary regurgitation noted as an incidental finding on echocardiography performed for other indications. When more significant, pulmonary regurgitation can present as a diastolic decrescendo murmur heard best at the left upper and mid-sternal border. Much less commonly, pulmonary regurgitation can present with symptoms related to RV volume overload and right heart failure. This is much more common in the setting of long-standing pulmonary regurgitation, particularly following RVOT palliative surgery such as tetralogy of Fallot repair. When symptomatic, patients typically develop exercise intolerance and, in severe cases, can present with symptoms of right heart failure, such as hepatomegaly, peripheral edema, and shortness of breath.

Anatomy and Physiology – The regurgitant pulmonary valve is often seen in conjunction with a stenotic valve. The valve may therefore feature variable degrees of thickening and doming in systole with cusp fusion or, less commonly, a bicuspid pulmonic valve. Prolapse of the pulmonic valve or incomplete leaflet coaptation may be seen. The degree of pulmonary regurgitation will determine the degree of RV volume overload. Pulmonary regurgitation will be impacted by multiple factors. The size of the pulmonary regurgitant orifice will have a direct impact on lesion severity. The diastolic compliance

of the right ventricle will affect RV diastolic pressure, and thus the magnitude of the pressure gradient favoring pulmonary artery–to–RV regurgitant flow across the pulmonary valve. Pulmonary arterial impedance will influence the propensity for forward versus reverse flow in the pulmonary artery. Finally, high impedance, such as anatomic pulmonary artery stenoses or high pulmonary vascular resistance, will favor retrograde flow through the regurgitant pulmonary valve.

Complications – The primary sequela of pulmonary regurgitation is RV volume overload. In mild to moderate pulmonary regurgitation, the degree of RV volume overload is often modest and often well tolerated. As the degree of regurgitation becomes more severe, RV volume overload increases, and the risk of developing RV dysfunction increases. RV dysfunction may progress even more rapidly in the setting of severe regurgitation and residual PS, although this is a much more common scenario in lesions such as repaired tetralogy of Fallot.

Principles of Echocardiographic Anatomy and Imaging

Classic Two-dimensional Echocardiographic Anatomy and Hemodynamics – Imaging planes and sweeps for the imaging of the pulmonary valve are outlined in the previous discussion of pulmonary valve stenosis. The regurgitant pulmonary valve is often seen in association with stenosis, so careful assessment for both is necessary. In the setting of primary pulmonary regurgitation, two-dimensional imaging should be focused on the presence of valve leaflet prolapse or incomplete leaflet coaptation. The pulmonary valve annulus and main pulmonary artery can be dilated, particularly in the setting of connective tissue disease. Two-dimensional measurement of the pulmonary valve annulus, sinotubular junction, and main pulmonary artery should be performed and compared with normal values. These measurements, particularly of the annulus, may be important not only in identifying pathologic enlargement but also in planning valve replacement surgery, should it become necessary. Imaging of the right and left branch pulmonary arteries should also be performed to rule out stenoses that may exacerbate the degree of regurgitation. Severe, long-standing pulmonary regurgitation may be associated with significant tricuspid regurgitation related to RV and tricuspid annular dilation; thus, color flow Doppler evaluation of tricuspid regurgitation should also be performed.

In theory, techniques used to evaluate aortic regurgitation can also be used to quantify the severity of pulmonic regurgitation. However, there are multiple reasons why these techniques have not been used clinically in the pediatric population. Any method requiring two-dimensional estimation of RV volumes would be limited by the significant difficulty in reliably estimating RV volumes by cross-sectional echocardiography. In addition, hemodynamically significant isolated pulmonary regurgitation is rare. Significant pulmonary regurgitation is an important issue following transannular RVOT patching in postoperative tetralogy of Fallot; however, reliable measurement of the surgically altered RVOT and transected pulmonary valve annulus makes reliable estimation of transpulmonary flow difficult. For all of these reasons, the severity of pulmonary regurgitation is largely assessed by semiquantitative assessment of RV dimensions (assessing the degree of volume loading of the right ventricle), qualitative impressions of the size of the regurgitant jet by color flow Doppler imaging and by color or pulsed-wave Doppler assessment of retrograde flow in the branch pulmonary arteries. In general, the presence of significant flow reversals in the distal portions of the branch pulmonary arteries is consistent with 3-4+ pulmonary regurgitation. Recently, reappraisal of Doppler methods characterizing the profile of the pulmonary regurgitant spectral display has suggested that short duration of the pulmonary regurgitant flow relative to the total diastolic time may be associated with greater degrees of pulmonary regurgitation as seen by angiography and as estimated by MRI methods (Lei, 1995; Li, 2004).

Although not related to the assessment of pulmonary regurgitant volume, it is useful to note that the pulmonary regurgitant spectral display can be utilized to estimate pulmonary artery end-diastolic pressure. By using an assumed RV end-diastolic pressure, the pulmonary artery end-diastolic pressure (PAP$_{ed}$) can be estimated by measuring the peak end-diastolic gradient between the pulmonary artery and right ventricle (Fig. 13.22):

$$PAP_{ed} = \Delta P_{PA-RV} + 10 \text{ mm Hg}$$

where ΔP_{PA-RV} is the estimated pressure gradient between pulmonary artery and right ventricle in end-diastole, and 10 mm Hg represents an assumed RV end-diastolic pressure. In addition, quantitation of the peak diastolic gradient between pulmonary artery and right ventricle has been shown to correlate well with mean pulmonary artery pressure at catheterization (Masuyama et al., 1986).

Color flow Doppler imaging can be useful in demonstrating the width of the pulmonary regurgitant jet and reversal of flow in the main and branch pulmonary arteries. Reversal of flow in the main pulmonary artery due to valvar regurgitation should be distinguished from "swirling" of flow in the main pulmonary artery (Figs. 13.1 and 13.2) as well as flow into the pulmonary artery from a patent ductus arteriosus, both of which can produce flow in the same direction as regurgitation. In both cases, flow from distal to proximal main pulmonary artery will occur in systole, occurring in later systole in the case of swirling main pulmonary artery flow, and typically during both systole and diastole in the case of a patent ductus arteriosus.

Variations on Classic Anatomy – As previously discussed, isolated pulmonary regurgitation is rare and is most frequently seen in children following repair of tetralogy of Fallot or in the setting of tetralogy of Fallot with absent pulmonary valve. Isolated dysplasia of the pulmonary valve can rarely present predominantly as regurgitation. Variants of pulmonary valve dysplasia/absent pulmonary valve can be seen in the setting of intact ventricular septum, often in conjunction with tricuspid valve anomalies such as membranous atresia or Ebstein malformation.

Common Associated Lesions and Findings – Common lesions associated with pulmonary regurgitation are summarized in Table 13.4.

Interventional and Postinterventional Imaging – Pulmonary regurgitation is commonly seen following valvotomy for pulmonary valve stenosis. Alternatively, when the pulmonary valve annulus is hypoplastic, pulmonary valvotomy with a transannular RVOT patch is typically performed. In either case, it is typical to see moderate or greater degrees of pulmonary regurgitation. In the setting of significant pulmonary regurgitation, it is important to follow RV size and function by serial echocardiographic study. Long-standing,

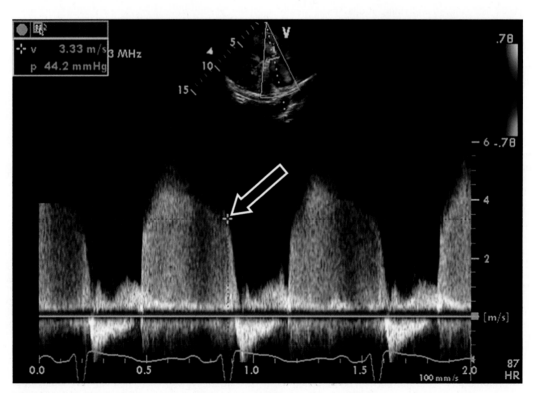

FIGURE 13.22. Continuous-wave Doppler evaluation of pulmonary regurgitation. The end-diastolic velocity (*open arrow*) is high and predicts an end-diastolic gradient of 44 mm Hg between pulmonary artery and right ventricle, consistent with high pulmonary artery diastolic pressure.

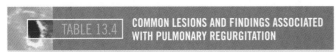

TABLE 13.4   COMMON LESIONS AND FINDINGS ASSOCIATED WITH PULMONARY REGURGITATION

- Right ventricular dilation
- Right ventricular dysfunction
- Pulmonary artery dilation
- Pulmonary valve stenosis
- Tetralogy of Fallot (with absent pulmonary valve)

significant pulmonary regurgitation can be associated with RV dilation and dysfunction.

Intervention for pulmonary regurgitation itself most frequently consists of surgical valve replacement with a bioprosthesis, such as a pulmonary homograft or porcine xenograft. Although not widely available, particularly in the United States, stent-mounted valves can now be placed in the pulmonary position. Echocardiographic evaluation in these settings should be focused on ongoing valve competence and/or the development of graft valve stenosis, which can often be the result of calcification. Surgical implantation of valved conduits can also be associated with distal main or branch pulmonary artery distortion/obstruction; imaging of the distal and branch pulmonary arteries should be performed in this setting.

PULMONARY ATRESIA WITH INTACT VENTRICULAR SEPTUM

Background

Clinical Presentation – Pulmonary atresia with intact ventricular septum (PA-IVS) is a rare form of complex congenital heart disease, occurring in approximately 0.0045 to 0.085 per 1000 live births. It is characterized by complete obstruction to RV outflow, an intact ventricular septum, and varying degrees of hypoplasia of the tricuspid valve and right ventricle.

Typically, these infants are cyanotic at birth. The clinical examination usually reveals a single second heart sound, and there is frequently a systolic murmur (from tricuspid regurgitation). The electrocardiogram characteristically shows left ventricular (LV) dominance with diminished RV forces and LV hypertrophy. On chest radiography, the lung fields are oligemic with a normal heart size (unless there is severe tricuspid regurgitation resulting in right atrial enlargement).

In the current era, many of these infants are detected prenatally. Investigators have examined a variety of echo-derived measures in the fetus that help to predict outcome. These have included such measures as fetal tricuspid valve annulus z-score, the RV/LV length ratio, the tricuspid valve/mitral valve ratio, tricuspid valve inflow duration, and the presence of RV sinusoids. Fetal detection allows for prenatal counseling and ensures the institution of prostaglandin infusion for stabilization at the time of delivery.

Anatomy and Physiology – The hallmark of PA-IVS is an atretic pulmonary valve; however, in reality, it reflects a wide spectrum of morphologic abnormalities that variably affect the tricuspid valve, the right ventricle, the RVOT, the branch pulmonary arteries, and the coronary arteries.

The United Kingdom and Ireland Collaborative Study of PA-IVS (Daubeney et al., 2002) is a population-based study describing 183 infants born with PA-IVS, and it provides helpful data regarding the prevalence of the various abnormalities. Eight percent had significant RV dilation, and this was associated with moderate to severe tricuspid regurgitation in all cases, with a very thin-walled right ventricle in half of them; in the remainder, the right ventricle was normal sized or hypoplastic, associated with significant myocardial hypertrophy. In most cases, the right ventricle was tripartite (consisting of inlet, trabecular, and outlet portions); however, bipartite ventricles and unipartite ventricles did occur, with a frequency of 34% and 8%, respectively. The median tricuspid valve z-score was –5.2. Ebstein malformation coexisted in 18 of 183 cases. Pulmonary atresia was

valvar/membranous in 75% and muscular/infundibular in 25%. The branch pulmonary arteries are typically confluent and normal sized.

Coronary artery abnormalities have been well described in PA-IVS, and they significantly affect outcomes. Ventriculocoronary arterial connections, stenotic or interrupted coronaries, and abnormalities of coronary origin or distribution have been described. Myocardial sinusoids (distinguished from ventriculocoronary fistulas because they traverse a capillary bed) can also occur. Daubeney et al. (2002) found normal coronary arteries in 54% and fistulous connections between the right ventricle and the coronaries in 46%. Ten cases (8%) were thought to have truly RV-dependent coronary circulation with associated coronary stenosis, interruption, or severe ectasia.

Complications – The critical decision-point for neonates with PA-IVS is deciding which patient is suitable for a biventricular versus a univentricular repair. In general, a biventricular repair is favored when the right ventricle is tripartite, the tricuspid valve z-score is adequate (greater than –2.4) and the pulmonary valve obstruction is membranous, since this allows for membrane perforation and dilation in the cardiac catheterization laboratory. However, this RV decompression does place the neonate at risk for myocardial ischemia in the setting of RV-dependent coronary artery circulation. However, even in neonates where a univentricular approach is favored, development of coronary insufficiency due to the presence of these underlying coronary abnormalities can occur. The role and timing of catheterization remain somewhat contentious; however, most clinicians support the practice of obtaining an early catheterization to detect the presence of coronary stenoses or interruptions (which cannot be clearly delineated by echocardiography alone).

Principles of Echocardiographic Anatomy and Imaging

Classic Two-dimensional Echocardiographic Anatomy and Hemodynamics – The first objective when initially imaging a patient with PA-IVS is to confirm anatomical pulmonary atresia and determine whether it is membranous (suitable for perforation and balloon dilation) or muscular (unsuitable for catheter intervention). Imaging of the RVOT in the parasternal long-axis, parasternal short-axis, and subcostal views is most helpful. Careful anterior sweeps in the subcostal coronal view can clearly demonstrate the morphologic type of atresia in most cases. The RV cavity usually narrows and ends before visualization of the pulmonary trunk in muscular atresia (Fig. 13.23), whereas the membranous type can often mimic normal valve function (Fig. 13.24). It is imperative to use color and pulsed-wave Doppler to differentiate whether the valve/membrane is perforate or not.

The second main objective is to evaluate whether the cardiac anatomy and physiology are consistent with biventricular or univentricular repair. This involves evaluation of the size of the right ventricle and determining whether the right ventricle is tripartite, bipartite, or unipartite (Fig. 13.25). RV volume calculations are typically inaccurate; however, unipartite morphology has been shown to be an independent risk factor for death in these patients (Daubeney et al., 2005). The subcostal coronal and sagittal views are helpful for evaluating whether the right ventricle has an inlet, outlet, and/or trabecular portion. Careful evaluation of the tricuspid valve with two-dimensional and color Doppler should be done to evaluate its morphology and function. In addition, a careful measurement of the tricuspid valve annulus should be performed in the apical four-chamber view and the z-score calculated. The relative dimensions of both tricuspid and mitral valve annuli should be compared, because Minich et al. (2000) showed that a tricuspid/mitral ratio greater than 0.5 was a good predictor of biventricular repair.

The third main objective is to assess the coronary arteries and detect the presence of significant ventriculocoronary arterial connections, which result in RV-dependent coronary circulation. These fistulous connections are usually not seen directly; however, the presence of dilated, tortuous proximal coronary arteries suggests their presence (Figs. 13.26 and 13.27). Coronary sinusoids (which traverse a capillary bed) can be seen using low-scale color Doppler (Fig. 13.28). However, their presence does not necessarily confirm or negate the presence of RV-dependent coronary circulation. The determination of RV dependence typically requires

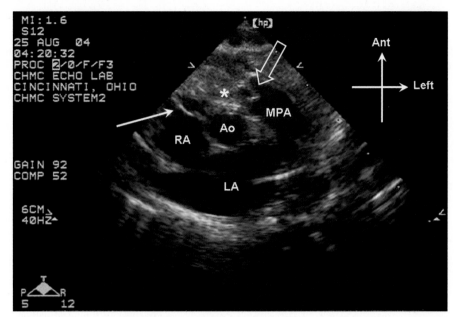

FIGURE 13.23. Parasternal short-axis image in a patient with pulmonary atresia with intact ventricular septum. There is an atretic pulmonary valve (*open arrow*), as well as muscular atresia of the right ventricular outflow tract (*asterisk*) between the tricuspid valve (*white arrow*) and pulmonary valve. Ao, aorta; LA, left atrium; MPA, main pulmonary artery; RA, right atrium.

angiography to assess for potential RV steal, coronary stenoses, or potential isolation of distal coronary artery flow with RV decompression. Satou et al. showed that a Tricuspid Value (TV) z-score of –2.5 or less predicted the presence of coronary artery fistulas with a high degree of sensitivity. Imaging in the standard coronary artery planes (especially parasternal short axis) will help to delineate these abnormalities.

Additional objectives are to evaluate the confluence and size of the branch pulmonary arteries (usually confluent and normal sized) from right parasternal images; delineate the size and course of the PDA (usually from suprasternal notch long axis and right parasternal axis; measure the atrial septal defect size and gradient from subcostal views; and obtain an RV pressure estimate from the tricuspid regurgitant jet velocity in the apical four-chamber view.

Common Associated Lesions and Findings – Major associated findings are outlined in Table 13.5. In the series reported by Daubeney et al. (2002), the most common associated findings in PA-IVS were Ebstein malformation of the tricuspid valve (10%) (Fig. 13.29), hypoplastic pulmonary arteries (9%), LV and LV outflow tract abnormalities including LV noncompaction, bicuspid aortic valve and dysplastic mitral valve (8%), tiny ventricular septal defect (6%), and persistent left superior vena cava (3%).

Interventional and Postinterventional Imaging – If a pulmonary valvotomy alone is performed, then the following postinterventional aspects are important to delineate when imaging: (a) tricuspid regurgitant velocity for RV pressure estimate; (b) transpulmonary flow velocity for RV obstruction; (c) RV size and volume;

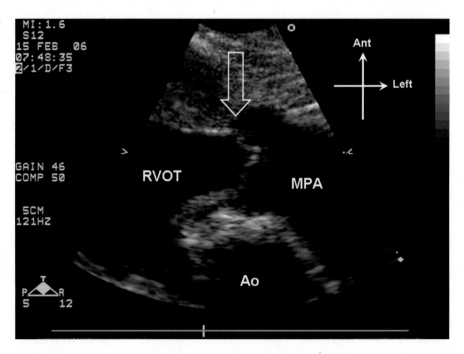

FIGURE 13.24. Membranous pulmonary atresia. The right ventricular outflow tract (RVOT) is patent, but the pulmonary valve (*open arrow*) is imperforate. Ao, aorta; MPA, main pulmonary artery.

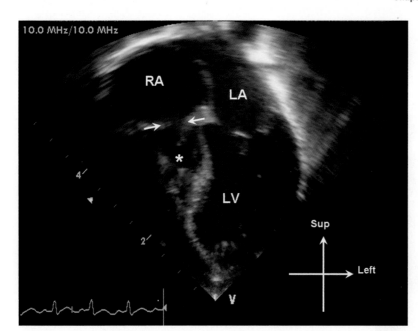

FIGURE 13.25. Pulmonary atresia with intact ventricular septum. Apical four-chamber view demonstrating severe hypoplasia of the right ventricular cavity (*asterisk*). The tricuspid valve annulus (*white arrows*) is also hypoplastic. LA, left atrium; LV, left ventricle; RA, right atrium.

(d) trans–tricuspid valve velocity, annulus, and z-score; and (e) direction of atrial level shunting. If a systemic–to–pulmonary artery shunt is placed, the following aspects are important to assess postintervention: (a) assess shunt flow; (b) assess LV and left atrial sizes; (c) tricuspid regurgitant velocity for RV pressure; and (d) pulmonary artery size in preparation for bidirectional Glenn operation. As an alternative to aortopulmonary shunting, some centers may stent the ductus arteriosus (Fig. 13.30). Occasionally the decision is made to have a "one-and-a-half" ventricle repair. This is when a bidirectional Glenn operation is performed together with either closed or open relief of RVOT obstruction.

POTENTIAL ROLES FOR ALTERNATIVE IMAGING MODALITIES IN RIGHT VENTRICULAR OUTFLOW TRACT ABNORMALITIES

The primary reasons to consider alternative imaging modalities in the assessment of RVOT abnormalities are related to limitations in either echocardiographic image quality or the limited ability to

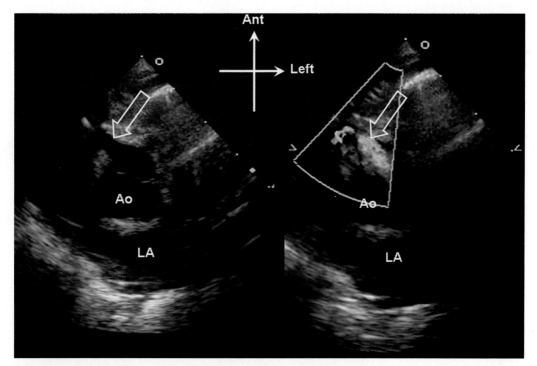

FIGURE 13.26. Coronary artery abnormalities in pulmonary atresia with intact ventricular septum. Parasternal short-axis image demonstrating dilation of the proximal right coronary artery (*open arrow*) on two-dimensional imaging (left). Color flow Doppler imaging (**right**) demonstrates retrograde filling of the right coronary artery (*open arrow*) with flow coursing toward the aortic root (Ao).

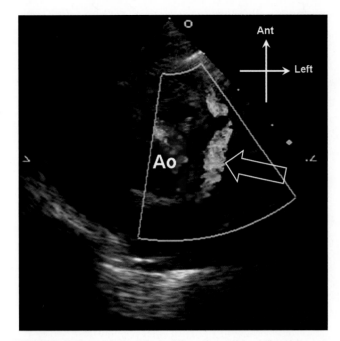

FIGURE 13.27. Parasternal short-axis image of the aortic root (Ao) and dilated left coronary artery (*open arrow*) in an infant with pulmonary atresia, intact ventricular septum, and right ventricular–dependent coronary artery circulation. Color flow Doppler imaging reveals that the dilated left coronary artery fills retrograde.

TABLE 13.5	COMMON LESIONS AND FINDINGS ASSOCIATED WITH PULMONARY ATRESIA/INTACT VENTRICULAR SEPTUM

- Hypoplastic right ventricle
- Hypoplastic tricuspid valve annulus
- Tricuspid valve abnormalities (e.g., Ebstein malformation)
- Tricuspid regurgitation
- Coronary artery sinusoids

on geometric models. In addition, imaging of the right ventricle in older patients, or in patients following multiple surgical procedures, is often limited by marginal acoustic windows. For these reasons, alternative imaging modalities for assessment of RV size and function may be considered. In the current era, MRI is gaining increasing application as a means of quantifying RV size and function, primarily by estimation of RV volumes and ejection fraction. Particularly in older patients, MRI can be performed without sedation and can produce excellent image quality with simple breath holding and gating to the heart rate. Alternatively, catheterization and angiography can be performed to evaluate RV size and function, particularly when physiologic information is also desired. Catheterization has the obvious limitations of being relatively invasive, as well as exposing the patient to fluoroscopy and intravenous contrast. Estimates of RV size and volume on angiography are again limited by the geometric models used to estimate RV volume on biplane images.

Physiologic Measures

Determination of RV pressure in the setting of RVOT obstruction is important to determine lesion severity and the indication for intervention. Often, RV pressure cannot be estimated echocardiographically due to an inadequate tricuspid regurgitant Doppler profile. Other indirect measures of RV pressure overload, such as hypertrophy or interventricular septal position, are inadequately sensitive to discriminate significant RV hypertension. Hemodynamic assessment during catheterization is the most reliable means of determining RV pressure. Catheterization has the additional advantage of facilitating RV angiography as well as angiography of the branch pulmonary arteries should there be questions regarding RV size, function, or branch pulmonary artery anatomy (see later).

obtain desired physiologic information echocardiographically. In patients with RVOT abnormalities, the most frequent indications for alternative imaging are (a) assessment of RV size and function, (b) quantitation of RV pressure, (c) estimation of pulmonary regurgitant fraction, and (d) imaging of the branch pulmonary arteries.

Right Ventricular Size and Function

Quantitative estimation of RV size and function by echocardiography has been a long-standing challenge. The irregular shape of the right ventricle, particularly in the setting of pathologic anatomy, limits the reliability of estimates of RV volume based

FIGURE 13.28. Apical four-chamber view of the right ventricle and left ventricle (LV) at the level of the coronary sinus (*open arrow*). Multiple coronary sinusoidal channels within the right ventricular myocardium (*white arrows*) are demonstrated by color flow Doppler imaging. RA, right atrium.

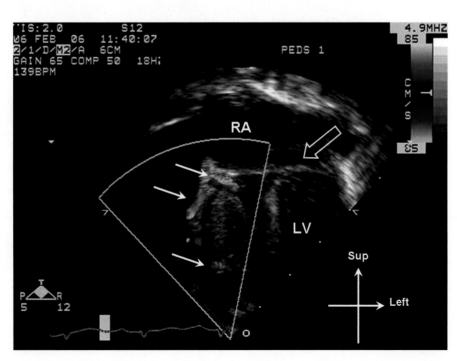

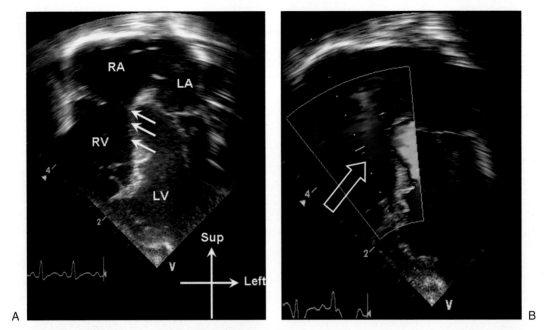

FIGURE 13-29. Apical four-chamber view in an infant with pulmonary atresia with intact ventricular septum. A: Tricuspid valve septal leaflet tissue is absent (*white arrows*), suggesting a severe variant of Ebstein anomaly. The right ventricular (RV) cavity is also hypoplastic. **B:** Color flow Doppler imaging demonstrates severe, laminar tricuspid regurgitation. LA, left atrium; LV, left ventricle; RA, right atrium.

Estimation of pulmonary regurgitant volume by two-dimensional and Doppler methods is problematic, as discussed earlier. Regurgitant flows are quite readily obtained by phase contrast MRI. This technique allows estimation of both forward and regurgitant pulmonary artery flow. Pulmonary regurgitant fraction can then be derived. Flow into the individual branch pulmonary arteries can also be determined using this technique.

Imaging of Pulmonary Artery Anatomy

There are several alternative modalities with which to image the main and branch pulmonary arteries. In addition to angiography during catheterization, both MRI and computed tomography (CT) can be used to evaluate the branch pulmonary arteries. Both techniques allow for tomographic imaging of the pulmonary arteries in a myriad

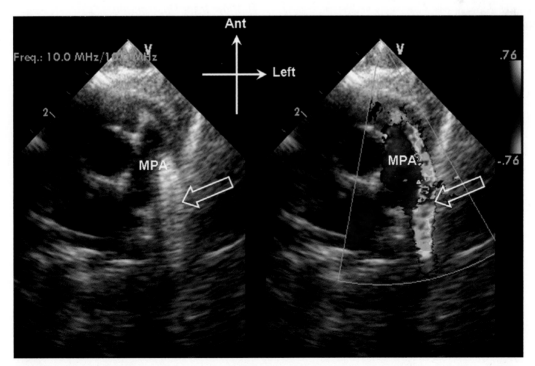

FIGURE 13.30. Parasternal short-axis image in an infant with pulmonary atresia with intact ventricular septum. A stent (*open arrow*) has been placed across the ductus arteriosus to create a stable source of pulmonary blood flow. Patency of the ductus arteriosus and stent can be confirmed by color flow Doppler (*right*). MPA, main pulmonary artery.

of imaging planes. In addition, processing of both MR and CT images will allow three-dimensional image reconstruction, which can supplement anatomic characterization of pulmonary artery anatomy.

Acknowledgment

The authors would like to thank Stacy Meredith, RDCS, for her assistance in preparing images and figures for use in this chapter.

SUGGESTED READING

Valvar Pulmonary Stenosis

Burch M, Sharland M, Shinebourne E, et al. Cardiologic abnormalities in Noonan syndrome: phenotypic diagnosis and echocardiographic assessment of 118 patients. *J Am Coll Cardiol.* 1993;22:1189–1192.

Lima OC, Sahn DJ, Valdes-Cruz LM, et al. Noninvasive prediction of transvalvular pressure gradient in patients with pulmonary stenosis by quantitative two-dimensional echocardiographic Doppler studies. *Circulation.* 1983;67:866–871.

Trowitzsch E, Colan SD, Sanders SP. Two-dimensional echocardiographic evaluation of right ventricular size and function in newborns with severe right ventricular outflow tract obstruction. *J Am Coll Cardiol.* 1985;6:388–393.

Weyman AE, Hurwitz RA, Girod DA, et al. Cross-sectional echocardiographic visualization of the stenotic pulmonary valve. *Circulation.* 1977;56:769–774.

Subvalvar Pulmonary Stenosis

Alva C, Ho SY, Lincoln CR, et al. The nature of the obstructive muscular bundles in double-chambered right ventricle. *J Thorac Cardiovasc Surg.* 1999;117:1180–1189.

Wong PC, Sanders SP, Jonas RA, et al. Pulmonary valve-moderator band distance and association with development of double-chambered right ventricle. *Am J Cardiol.* 1991;68:1681–1686.

Supravalvar Pulmonary Stenosis

Frank DU, Minich LL, Shaddy RE, et al. Is Doppler an accurate predictor of catheterization gradients for postoperative branch pulmonary stenosis? *J Am Soc Echocardiogr.* 2002;15:1140–1144.

Gay BB Jr, French RH, Shuford WH, et al. The roentgenologic features of single and multiple coarctations of the pulmonary artery and branches. *Am J Roentgenol Radium Ther Nucl Med.* 1963;90:599–613.

Hiraishi S, Misawa H, Hirota H, et al. Noninvasive quantitative evaluation of the morphology of the major pulmonary artery branches in cyanotic congenital heart disease. Angiocardiographic and echocardiographic correlative study. *Circulation.* 1994;89:1306–1316.

Kim YM, Yoo SJ, Choi JY, et al. Natural course of supravalvar aortic stenosis and peripheral pulmonary arterial stenosis in Williams' syndrome. *Cardiol Young.* 1999;9:37–41.

Rein AJ, Preminger TJ, Perry SB, et al. Generalized arteriopathy in Williams' syndrome: an intravascular ultrasound study. *J Am Coll Cardiol.* 1993;21:1727–1730.

Pulmonary Regurgitation

Lei MH, Chen JJ, Ko YL, et al. Reappraisal of quantitative evaluation of pulmonary regurgitation and estimation of pulmonary artery pressure by continuous-wave Doppler echocardiography. *Cardiology.* 1995;86:249–256.

Li W, Davlouros PA, Kilner PJ, et al. Doppler echocardiographic assessment of pulmonary regurgitation in adults with repaired tetralogy of Fallot: comparison with cardiovascular magnetic resonance imaging. *Am Heart J.* 2004;147:165–172.

Masuyama T, Kodama K, Kitabatake A, et al. Continuous-wave Doppler echocardiographic detection of pulmonary regurgitation and its application to noninvasive estimation of pulmonary artery pressure. *Circulation.* 1986;74:484–492.

Puchalski MD, Askovich B, Sower CT, et al. Pulmonary regurgitation: determining severity by echocardiography and magnetic resonance imaging. *Congenit Heart Dis.* 2008;3:168–175.

Pulmonary Atresia with Intact Ventricular Septum

Daubeney PEF, Delany DJ, Anderson RH, et al. Pulmonary atresia with intact ventricular septum: range of morphology in a population-based study. *J Am Coll Cardiol.* 2002;39:1670–1679.

Daubeney PEF, Wang D, Delany DJ, et al. Pulmonary atresia with intact ventricular septum: predictors of early and medium-term outcome in a population-based study. *J Thorac Cardiovasc Surg.* 2005;130:1071–1078.

Minich LL, Tani LY, Ritter S, et al. Usefulness of the preoperative tricuspid/mitral valve ratio for predicting outcome in pulmonary atresia with intact ventricular septum. *Am J Cardiol.* 2000;85:1325–1328.

Roman KS, Fouron JC, Nii M, et al. Determinants of outcome in fetal pulmonary valve stenosis or atresia with intact ventricular septum. *Am J Cardiol.* 2007;99:699–703.

Salvin JW, McElhinney DB, Colan SD, et al. Fetal tricuspid valve size and growth as predictors of outcome in pulmonary atresia with intact ventricular septum. *Pediatrics.* 2006;118:e415–e420.

Satou GM, Perry SB, Gauvreau K, et al. Echocardiographic predictors of coronary artery pathology in pulmonary atresia with intact ventricular septum. *Am J Cardiol.* 2000;85:1319–1324.

Zuberbuhler JR, Anderson RH. Morphologic variations in pulmonary atresia with intact ventricular septum. *Br Heart J.* 1979;41:281–288.

Alternative Imaging Modalities in Right Ventricular Outflow Tract Obstruction

Greenberg SB, Crisci KL, Koenig P, et al. Magnetic resonance imaging compared with echocardiography in the evaluation of pulmonary artery abnormalities in children with tetralogy of Fallot following palliative and corrective surgery. *Pediatr Radiol.* 1997;27:932–935.

Chapter 14
Abnormalities of Left Ventricular Outflow

Leo Lopez

Morphologic abnormalities of the left ventricular (LV) outflow tract generally result in one or more of the following pathophysiologic states: obstruction, regurgitation, and aneurysmal dilation of the proximal aorta. Obstruction is the most prevalent problem, whereas the other two are rare in children. Known generally as aortic stenosis (AS), LV outflow tract obstruction occurs in approximately 5 per 10,000 live births, represents 5% to 8% of all congenital heart diseases, and usually ranks as the sixth or seventh most common lesion. Among all patients with LV outflow tract obstruction, valvar AS is the most common subgroup (with a frequency of 60% to 75%), followed by subvalvar AS (8% to 30%) and supravalvar AS (1% to 2%). In addition, a bicuspid aortic valve (AoV) with or without stenosis occurs in up to 2% of the general population, thereby representing the most common congenital heart lesion.

CLINICAL PRESENTATION

LV outflow tract obstruction is associated with a pressure-overloaded left ventricle, often accompanied by progressive LV hypertrophy. Patients with LV outflow tract obstruction generally present with a systolic murmur whose frequency and intensity are determined by the degree of obstruction. Occasionally, a systolic click is heard in the setting of an abnormal AoV. Symptoms in children with LV outflow tract obstruction are rare, although severe obstruction can be associated with syncope, chest pain, and/or exercise intolerance. Very rarely, older children with significant obstruction will present with signs of congestive heart failure as severe LV hypertrophy results in progressive diastolic and systolic dysfunction. Many patients with the rare subgroup of supravalvar AS also have Williams syndrome with its characteristic features of infantile hypercalcemia, failure to thrive, elfin-like facial abnormalities, and mental retardation. The electrocardiogram may show increased left-sided voltages with ST-T wave changes consistent with LV hypertrophy. The heart is generally normal in size on the chest radiograph, although the ascending aorta may be dilated.

Significant LV outflow tract obstruction in the newborn period often involves severe LV dysfunction, mitral regurgitation, and increased left-to-right shunting across the foramen ovale, all contributing to compromised cardiac output. These infants generally present with signs and symptoms of congestive heart failure and shock. In cases of critical AS, cardiac output across the LV outflow tract is inadequate, and ductal patency must be maintained with prostaglandin E_1 infusion so that the right-to-left flow across the ductus augments cardiac output for sufficient tissue oxygen delivery. The electrocardiogram may show increased right-sided and/or left-sided voltages with ST-T wave changes. The heart is usually enlarged on the chest radiograph, and pulmonary edema may be present.

Aortic regurgitation (AR) is associated with a volume-overloaded left ventricle. In contrast to the ventricular hypertrophy, which results from pressure overload, volume overload results in ventricular dilation with compensatory hypertrophy (compensated AR). However, the heart's ability to sustain hypertrophy eventually fails (decompensated AR) and LV wall stress increases, eventually leading to irreversible ventricular dysfunction and poor contractility. A diastolic murmur is generally heard on physical examination. Significant AR is usually associated with a hyperdynamic LV impulse and prominent peripheral pulses. These patients may begin to show signs and symptoms of congestive heart failure. The electrocardiogram will usually show increased left-sided voltages with ST-T wave changes, and cardiomegaly may be seen on the chest radiograph.

Aneurysmal dilation of the aortic root and/or ascending aorta is generally discovered because its association with a genetic syndrome or a specific disease prompts a clinician to perform an echocardiogram or another diagnostic study. Rarely, an individual with aneurysmal dilation of the ascending aorta has an aortic dissection or rupture and presents with acute chest or abdominal pain, shock, or sudden death. Occasionally, a sinus of Valsalva aneurysm can rupture without catastrophic results, resulting primarily in a significant left-to-right shunt from the aorta into a right-sided chamber with consequent congestive heart failure. The chest radiograph generally shows the enlarged aortic root or ascending aorta, and cardiomegaly may be present in the setting of significant left-to-right shunting.

NORMAL ANATOMY

The normal LV outflow tract can be divided into three anatomic segments: the subaortic region, the AoV, and the proximal aorta (Fig. 14.1). In utero, the conus or infundibulum represents the subarterial muscular chamber separating the atrioventricular valve from

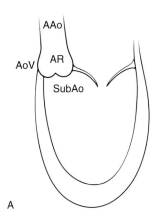
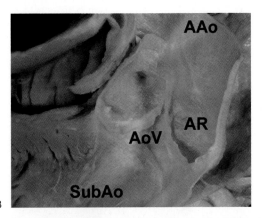
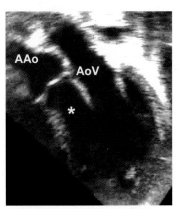

FIGURE 14.1. The anatomic segments of the left ventricular outflow tract. Includes the subaortic region (SubAo, *asterisk*), the aortic valve (AoV), and the ascending aorta (AAo), as depicted in (**A**) an illustration, (**B**) a pathology specimen, and (**C**) an apical two-chamber view. AR, aortic root. (**B**, With permission from Prof. Robert H. Anderson, Institute of Child Health, London, United Kingdom.)

FIGURE 14.2. Fibrous continuity between the mitral valve and the aortic valve. A: Pathology specimen showing the anatomic ventriculoarterial junction (*star*). **B:** Parasternal long-axis view. AML, anterior mitral leaflet; AoV, aortic valve; IVS, interventricular septum; LA, left atrium; LV, left ventricle. (**A,** With permission from Prof. Robert H. Anderson, Institute of Child Health, London, United Kingdom.)

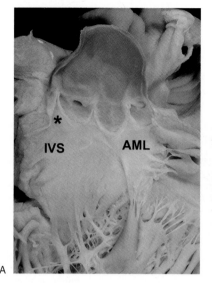
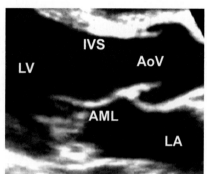

the corresponding semilunar valve in both the right ventricular (RV) and LV outflow tracts. In normal fetal hearts, the subaortic conus regresses, resulting in varying degrees of fibrous continuity between the mitral valve (MV) and the AoV (Fig. 14.2). The area of fibrous continuity is often referred to as the mitral-aortic intervalvular fibrosa, a structure that originates from the primordial left ventriculoinfundibular fold and can be elongated in cases of subvalvar AS and tetralogy of Fallot. It is usually measured as the shortest distance from the anterior mitral leaflet to the base of the noncoronary or left coronary leaflet of the AoV. Within the LV outflow tract, the anterior mitral leaflet represents the posterior boundary of the subaortic region and the muscular ventricular septum represents the anterior boundary (Fig. 14.2).

The normal AoV is a three-dimensional structure that involves three leaflets attached to the aortic root and supporting ventricular muscle in a semilunar or crown-like fashion (Figs. 14-1B and 14-2A). The leaflets are separated by three commissures, which are lines of apposition between the leaflets extending from the center of the valve to the periphery (Fig. 14.3) and from the area of the ventriculoarterial junction to the sinotubular junction (the junction between the aortic root and proximal ascending aorta). An important and somewhat problematic issue in AoV morphology is the concept of the "aortic annulus," a diagnostician construct that does not correspond to a true anatomic structure. Although an anatomic ventriculoarterial junction can usually be identified pathologically, the basal attachments of the semilunar leaflets actually extend beyond this ring into the supporting ventricular muscle (Fig. 14.2), thereby confounding the use of the most proximal or basal attachment of the semilunar valve leaflets to define the "aortic annulus" (Fig. 14.4). In other words, the "aortic annulus" is not synonymous with the

anatomic ventriculoarterial junction along the LV outflow tract. In addition, this ventriculoarterial ring does not fully support the AoV because the leaflets are attached or hinged within the entire aortic root up to the level of the sinotubular junction.

The components of the proximal aorta include the aortic root and ascending aorta, structures that meet at the sinotubular junction (Fig. 14.4). Because the sinotubular junction represents the most distal attachments of the AoV leaflets within the aortic root, it may be somewhat confusing to label an anomaly at the sinotubular junction a supravalvar anomaly because it often involves the distal segment of the AoV. Nevertheless, the walls of the aortic root and the ascending aorta are composed primarily of vascular smooth muscle cells and extracellular matrix proteins secreted by the cells. The most common component of the aortic wall is elastin, a protein that now appears to play a significant role in the morphogenesis and homeostasis of the arterial vessel walls. In addition, it appears to be involved in the development of supravalvar obstruction and aneurysmal dilation of the proximal aorta.

ABNORMAL ANATOMY AND COMMON ASSOCIATIONS

Valvar Aortic Stenosis

Etiologies for valvar AS are listed in Table 14.1. The most common abnormality of AoV morphology is the bicuspid AoV, in which two of the three leaflets are fused or one of the commissures between adjacent leaflets is underdeveloped (also known as a raphé) (Fig. 14.5).

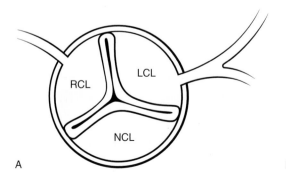
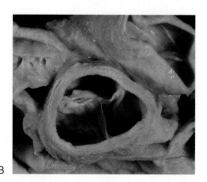
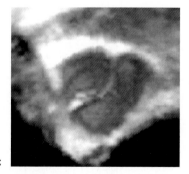

FIGURE 14.3. Cross-sectional view of the aortic valve with three leaflets separated by three commissures. Depicted in (**A**) an illustration, (**B**) a pathology specimen, and (**C**) a three-dimensional echocardiographic image. LCL, left coronary leaflet; NCL, noncoronary leaflet; PV, pulmonary valve; RCL, right coronary leaflet. (**B**, With permission from Prof. Robert H. Anderson, Institute of Child Health, London, United Kingdom.)

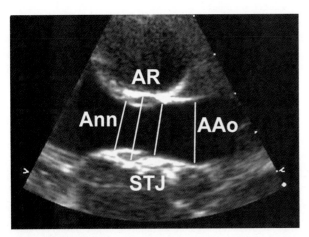

FIGURE 14.4. Parasternal long-axis view of the proximal aorta. Diameters are measured at the levels of the aortic "annulus" (Ann), aortic root (AR), sinotubular junction (STJ), and ascending aorta (AAo).

A true bicuspid AoV with only two leaflets is a rare phenomenon. In most cases of a bicuspid AoV, the size of the combined leaflet (secondary to fusion or underdevelopment of a commissure) is larger than the unaffected leaflet, although it is rarely exactly twice the size of the unaffected leaflet. This latter finding suggests that the lesion is a developmental problem of the entire valve rather than simple fusion of two of the three leaflets. Among all patients with a bicuspid AoV, fusion or underdevelopment occurs most commonly at the intercoronary commissure between the right and left coronary leaflets (with a frequency of 70% to 86%) followed by the commissure between the right and noncoronary leaflets (12% to 28%) and the commissure between the left and noncoronary leaflets (very rare) (Fig. 14.6). In addition, the rate of AS progression appears to be higher with underdevelopment of the intercoronary commissure. Common associations with a bicuspid AoV include aortic coarctation (which occurs more frequently with intercoronary commissural underdevelopment) or interrupted aortic arch, subvalvar AS, ventricular septal defect (VSD), coronary anomalies (such as a displaced coronary ostium or a shortened left coronary artery), Turner syndrome, aortic dilation or aneurysm formation (with the increased risk for aortic dissection and rupture) (Fig. 14.7), and endocarditis (Fig. 14.8, Table 14.2).

The most common AoV morphology in neonatal valvar AS is a unicuspid unicommissural AoV where the only open commissure is located between the left and noncoronary leaflets; in addition, a small eccentric valvar orifice is seen (Fig. 14.9). Occasionally, the leaflets are thickened and poorly formed with decreased mobility (Fig. 14.10). These cases are often associated with a small aortic root and ascending aorta. The left ventricle may be small and hypertrophied with endocardial fibroelastosis, or it may be dilated with poor systolic function, mitral regurgitation, and left atrial dilation.

Subvalvar Aortic Stenosis

Because subvalvar AS is rarely diagnosed in utero or in the newborn period, many have suggested that this lesion is an acquired heart disease rather than a congenital one. Nevertheless, it is a progressive disease whose postoperative recurrence rate is as high as 33%. The mechanisms for the development of subvalvar AS, as suggested by Cape and colleagues, are listed in Table 14.3. The associated LV outflow tract morphologic abnormalities include a small aortic annulus and root, a steep aortoseptal angle, abnormal LV muscle bundles, a prominent anterolateral muscle bundle of Moulaert, elongation of the mitral-aortic intervalvular fibrosa, MV pathology, and protrusion of aneurysmal tricuspid valve tissue or membranous septum into the LV outflow tract. Subvalvar AS can occur in isolation or with several common associations (Table 14.4).

In the absence of a VSD or other cardiac associations, subvalvar AS most frequently presents as a discrete fibrous or fibromuscular shelf extending from the ventricular septum just below the AoV (Fig. 14.11). Occasionally, the shelf extends to the anterior mitral leaflet in a diaphragmatic fashion (Fig. 14.12). Rarely the muscular component is so extensive that it creates a tunnel-like LV outflow tract with significant subaortic obstruction (Fig. 14.13). This is, of course, distinct from the more diffusely hypertrophied ventricular septum and dynamic subaortic obstruction associated with hypertrophic cardiomyopathy.

In the presence of a VSD, the most significant type of subaortic obstruction results from posterior deviation of the conal or infundibular septum (Fig. 14.14). This lesion is often associated with aortic coarctation or an interrupted aortic arch. Another type of potential subvalvar AS with a VSD involves the presence of endocardial folds or fibromuscular ridges at the crest of the muscular septum (Fig. 14.15). Last, abnormal MV attachments to the ventricular septum, particularly in the setting of unrepaired or repaired atrioventricular canal defects, can also cause subaortic obstruction (Fig. 14.16).

An important and not uncommon association with subvalvar AS involves the development of AR, which can progress in children and result in the need for early surgical intervention (Fig. 14.17). The mechanism for AR presumably involves AoV damage secondary to the high-velocity jet coursing through the subaortic region. In addition, the abnormal fibromuscular tissue in subvalvar AS may be continuous with the base of the AoV, potentially disrupting the normal support for the AoV leaflets. It is important to note, however, that AR associated with subvalvar AS in adults is not usually a progressive problem and does not necessarily suggest a need for surgical intervention.

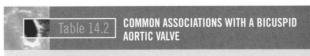

Table 14.2	COMMON ASSOCIATIONS WITH A BICUSPID AORTIC VALVE

Aortic coarctation or interrupted aortic arch
Subvalvar aortic stenosis
Ventricular septal defect
Coronary anomalies
  Displaced coronary ostium
  Shortened left coronary artery
Turner syndrome
Aortic dilation or aneurysm formation
Endocarditis

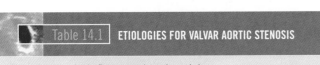

Table 14.1	ETIOLOGIES FOR VALVAR AORTIC STENOSIS

Abnormal aortic valve leaflet or commissural morphology
  Bicuspid or bicommissural aortic valve
  Unicuspid acommissural aortic valve
  Unicuspid unicommissural aortic valve
  Quadricuspid aortic valve
Dysplastic tricuspid aortic valve with thickened leaflets and decreased mobility
Aortic "annular" hypoplasia

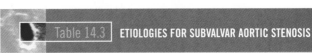

Table 14.3	ETIOLOGIES FOR SUBVALVAR AORTIC STENOSIS

- Abnormal left ventricular outflow tract morphology
- Increased septal shear stress secondary to the abnormal morphology
- Genetic predisposition
- Cellular proliferation secondary to the increased septal shear stress

From Cape EG, Vanauker MD, Sigfusson G, et al. Potential role of mechanical stress in the etiology of pediatric heart disease: septal shear stress in subaortic stenosis. *J Am Coll Cardiol.* 1997;30:247–254.

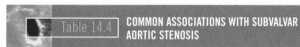
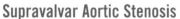

Table 14.4   COMMON ASSOCIATIONS WITH SUBVALVAR AORTIC STENOSIS

- Ventricular septal Defect
- Bicuspid aortic valve
- Double-chamber or divided right ventricle
- Aortic coarctation or interrupted aortic arch
- Atrioventricular canal defect

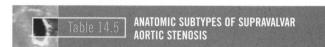

Table 14.5   ANATOMIC SUBTYPES OF SUPRAVALVAR AORTIC STENOSIS

- Hourglass type
- Diaphragmatic or membranous type
- Tubular type

Supravalvar Aortic Stenosis

Although supravalvar AS is usually associated with Williams syndrome, it can also present as an autosomal dominant lesion in a familial form or as a sporadic idiopathic disorder. Supravalvar AS is in fact an elastin arteriopathy resulting from the mutation or deletion of the *elastin* gene on chromosome 7. There are three anatomic subtypes of supravalvar AS: the hourglass type, which is the most common subtype and frequently involves dilation of the aortic root and the ascending aorta distal to the narrowing (Fig. 14.18); the diaphragmatic or membranous type; and the tubular type, which is quite rare and involves diffuse hypoplasia of the ascending aorta (Table 14.5). Common associations include abnormalities of the AoV, the coronary arteries (e.g., coronary artery dilation, intrinsic coronary thickening and ostial stenosis, and ostial occlusion or entrapment by a tethered AoV leaflet) (Fig. 14.19), aortic arch branches, and branch pulmonary arteries (Table 14.6).

Aortic Regurgitation

Aortic regurgitation (AR), defined somewhat loosely as diastolic flow from the aorta into the left ventricle, is rare in childhood, especially in isolation. Congenital etiologies for functional AR include a stenotic or nonstenotic bicuspid AoV (Fig. 14.20); other abnormalities of AoV leaflet or commissural morphology; an aortico-LV tunnel (Fig. 14.21); absence of one or more AoV leaflets; a fibrous band between an AoV leaflet and the aortic root wall; a coronary-cameral fistula into the left ventricle; and a ruptured left sinus of Valsalva aneurysm into the left ventricle (Table 14.7). Other associations with AR include a membranous VSD or a doubly committed subarterial VSD with AoV prolapse into the defect secondary to the Venturi phenomenon (Fig. 14.22), subvalvar AS, neonatal Marfan syndrome with concurrent aortic root dilation, repaired truncus arteriosus, and tetralogy of Fallot (Table 14.8). In addition, AR occurs commonly with a ruptured sinus of Valsalva aneurysm, secondary to disruption of the normal AoV leaflet support within the aortic root (Fig. 14.23). Acquired etiologies include endocarditis (Fig. 14.24), rheumatic fever, and surgical valvotomy or transcatheter balloon valvotomy for valvar AS (Fig. 14.25, Table 14.9).

Aneurysm of the Proximal Aorta

Most aortic root aneurysms involve the right sinus of Valsalva, followed by the noncoronary sinus and then the left sinus (Fig. 14.26). Aneurysm formation in the aortic root and aneurysmal dilation of the ascending aorta (Fig. 14.7) occur when structural weakness and thinning of the aortic wall result from smooth muscle cell loss and extracellular matrix disruption. Elastin production and maintenance appear to be as important in the development of aortic aneurysms as in the arteriopathy associated with supravalvar AS. For example, Marfan syndrome results from mutations in the *fibrillin* gene on chromosome 15. The fibrillin protein is necessary in the formation of elastin and other components of the extracellular matrix. In addition, it may inhibit the availability and effects of the cytokine transforming growth factor-β and endogenous matrix metalloproteinases, both of which are thought to be involved in the degradation of elastin and other components of the extracellular matrix. Common associations with aneurysmal dilation of the proximal aorta include Marfan syndrome, Loeys-Dietz syndrome, Ehlers-Danlös syndrome, Turner syndrome, a bicuspid AoV, systemic hypertension, and coarctation (Table 14.10). It is important to recognize that the term "poststenotic dilation" of the aorta is no longer appropriate in light of the intrinsic aortopathy associated with valvar AS. In addition, the degree of aortic dilation does not usually correlate to the severity of the stenosis.

APPROACH TO TRANSTHORACIC ECHOCARDIOGRAPHY

Valvar Aortic Stenosis

The transthoracic echocardiogram of a patient with valvar AS must include evaluation of the following features (Table 14.11).

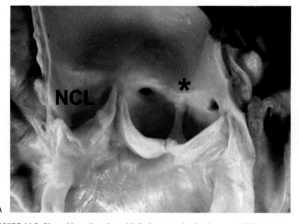
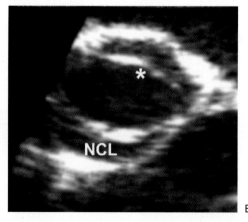

FIGURE 14.5. Bicuspid aortic valve with fusion or underdevelopment of the intercoronary commissure (star). Depicted in (**A**) a pathology specimen and (**B**) a parasternal short-axis view. NCL, noncoronary leaflet. (**A**, With permission from Prof. Robert H. Anderson, Institute of Child Health, London, United Kingdom.)

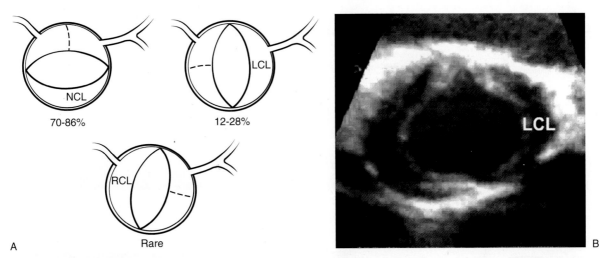

FIGURE 14.6. Bicuspid aortic valve. A: Illustration of the three subtypes of a bicuspid aortic valve and their relative frequencies. **B:** Parasternal short-axis view of a bicuspid aortic valve with fusion or underdevelopment of the commissure between the right coronary and noncoronary leaflets. LCL, left coronary leaflet; NCL, noncoronary leaflet; RCL, right coronary leaflet.

Leaflet and Commissural Morphology – The number and relative sizes of the leaflets and commissures are best evaluated with cross-sectional views of the AoV in parasternal short-axis views. The raphé of a fused or underdeveloped commissure is usually difficult to distinguish from a normal commissure when the AoV is viewed in its closed position during diastole. However, during systole when the AoV is open, the affected commissure remains visible as an echogenic line from the leaflet edge to the aortic wall. Occasionally, there is only partial underdevelopment of a commissure such that the separation between two leaflets occurs but does not extend to the aortic wall (Fig. 14.27). When fusion or underdevelopment occurs at the intercoronary commissure in a bicuspid AoV, the AoV opening during systole has a horizontal orientation in parasternal short-axis views (Fig. 14.5B). In contrast, fusion or underdevelopment of the commissure between the right and noncoronary leaflets results in a more vertical orientation of the AoV opening in the same views (Fig. 14.6B). In a unicuspid unicommissural AoV, the opening is usually slit-like in appearance and almost always located at the commissure between the left and noncoronary leaflets (Fig. 14.9). Acommissural valves usually have a more centrally located orifice. Apical two-chamber and parasternal long-axis views are very useful

in characterizing the AoV leaflets. They may be thickened, and the degree of thickening may vary along the length of the leaflet with thicker edges giving it a "lumpy" appearance (Figs. 14-9D and 10A). In addition, the leaflets usually dome in systole, secondary to the restrictive lateral mobility caused by incomplete commissural separation along the distal zone of apposition (which is located more distally near the sinotubular junction).

Degree of Obstruction – Continuous-wave Doppler interrogation across the AoV is best performed in apical, right sternal border, and suprasternal notch views and can provide information regarding the maximum instantaneous gradient and the mean gradient across the AoV. Every effort should be made to align the Doppler beam with the high-velocity jet across the stenotic AoV. It is well known that discrepancies usually occur between the maximum instantaneous gradient measured by echocardiography and the peak-to-peak gradient measured by catheterization, with the former measurement almost always higher than the latter one. These discrepancies result partly from a phenomenon called pressure recovery. Echocardiographic assessment of maximum instantaneous gradients occurs at the vena contracta, the volume of space in the aorta immediately distal to a stenotic AoV where blood flow velocity, kinetic energy, and the pressure drop are highest (Fig. 14.28). The flow velocity normally decreases farther downstream as kinetic energy is converted back to potential energy and pressure is recovered (thereby decreasing the pressure difference between the subaortic region and the more distal ascending aorta). Because the peak-to-peak gradient involves direct pressure measurement more distally in the ascending aorta, pressure recovery may or may not play a role in the arterial pressure. In cases of severe stenosis, the high-velocity jet extends farther into the ascending aorta, and pressure recovery is less influential;

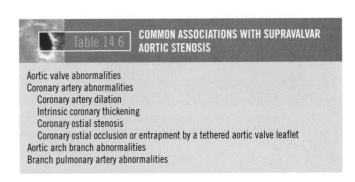

FIGURE 14.7. Parasternal long-axis view of a bicuspid aortic valve with a dilated ascending aorta. AAo, ascending aorta; BAV, bicuspid aortic valve.

Table 14.6	COMMON ASSOCIATIONS WITH SUPRAVALVAR AORTIC STENOSIS

Aortic valve abnormalities
Coronary artery abnormalities
   Coronary artery dilation
   Intrinsic coronary thickening
   Coronary ostial stenosis
   Coronary ostial occlusion or entrapment by a tethered aortic valve leaflet
Aortic arch branch abnormalities
Branch pulmonary artery abnormalities

FIGURE 14-8. Bicuspid aortic valve with endocarditis involving a vegetation adherent to the valve (*star*) as well as a leftward posterior aortic root abscess (*hashed*). Depicted in (**A**) a parasternal long-axis view and (**B**) a three-dimensional echocardiographic short-axis view. AR, aortic root; LV, left ventricle.

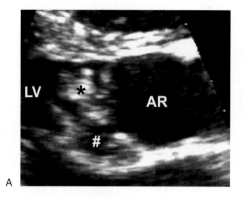
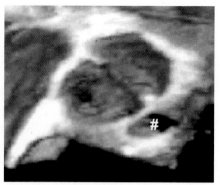

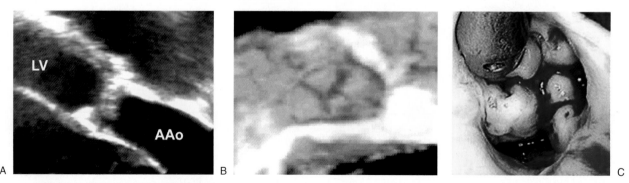

FIGURE 14.9. Unicuspid unicommissural aortic valve. The only open commissure is located between the left coronary and noncoronary leaflets (*star*); the aortic valve leaflets are abnormally thickened; and the left ventricle is small with endocardial fibroelastosis, as depicted in (**A**) a cross-sectional illustration of the aortic valve, (**B**) a pathology specimen, (**C**) a parasternal short-axis view, (**D**) a parasternal long-axis view, and (**E**) an apical four-chamber view. Ao, aorta; LA, left atrium; LV, left ventricle; RV, right ventricle. (**B**, With permission from Prof. Robert H. Anderson, Institute of Child Health, London, United Kingdom.)

FIGURE 14.10. Thickened and dysplastic aortic valve leaflets. Depicted in (**A**) a transesophageal view along a plane oriented at approximately 120 degrees, (**B**) a three-dimensional short-axis view, and (**C**) an intraoperative photograph.

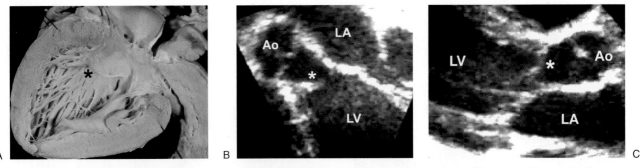

FIGURE 14.11. Subaortic fibromuscular ridge (*star*). Depicted in (**A**) a pathology specimen, (**B**) an apical two-chamber view, and (**C**) a parasternal long-axis view. Ao, aorta; LA, left atrium; LV, left ventricle. (**A,** With permission from Prof. Robert H. Anderson, Institute of Child Health, London, United Kingdom.)

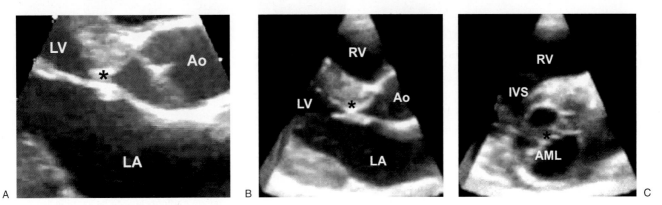

FIGURE 14-12. Subaortic fibromuscular shelf extending to the anterior mitral leaflet (*star*). Depicted in (**A**) a parasternal long-axis view, (**B**) a three-dimensional long-axis view, and (**C**) a three-dimensional short-axis view with display of the crescentic shelf adjacent to the anterior mitral leaflet and the diaphragm-like obstruction along the subaortic region. AML, anterior mitral leaflet; Ao, aorta; IVS, interventricular septum; LA, left atrium; LV, left ventricle; RV, right ventricle.

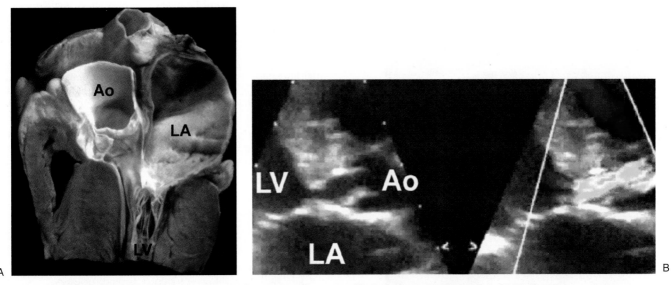

FIGURE 14.13. Marked septal hypertrophy along the left ventricular outflow tract resulting in significant subaortic stenosis. Depicted in (**A**) a pathology specimen and (**B**) a parasternal long-axis view. Ao, aorta; LA, left atrium; LV, left ventricle. (**A,** With permission from Prof. Robert H. Anderson, Institute of Child Health, London, United Kingdom.)

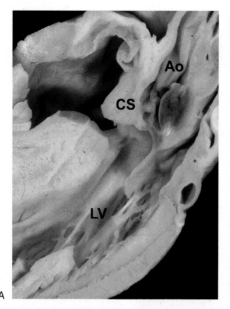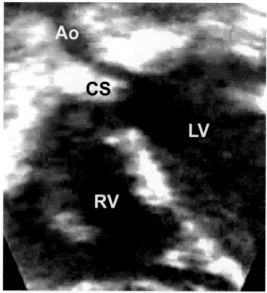

FIGURE 14.14. Conoventricular septal defect and posterior deviation of the conal septum into the subaortic region. Depicted in (A) a pathology specimen and (B) an apical two-chamber view. Ao, aorta; CS, conal septum; LV, left ventricle; RV, right ventricle. (A, With permission from Prof. Robert H. Anderson, Institute of Child Health, London, United Kingdom.)

in this situation, the discrepancies are less pronounced. On the contrary, the extent of the high-velocity jet is relatively short and pressure recovery occurs more proximally in the ascending aorta with mild stenosis, and the discrepancies in this situation become more apparent. Because determination of the degree of valvar AS and the thresholds for intervention are based primarily on catheterization data using peak-to-peak gradients, these discrepancies have confounded the use of echocardiographic data in clinical decision making for these patients. Many prefer the use of Doppler mean gradients to classify valvar AS because these values correlate more closely with catheterization-derived mean gradients. Others accept the limitations associated with using maximum instantaneous gradients, and they use thresholds of 25 to 30 mm Hg to distinguish mild from moderate stenosis and 50 to 60 mm Hg to distinguish

moderate from severe stenosis. An important determinant of the measured AoV gradient is the amount of transvalvar flow. Cases of significant valvar AS are often associated with severe LV dysfunction, which in turn results in decreased cardiac output, decreased transvalvar flow, and a decreased maximum instantaneous gradient across the AoV despite the severity of the obstruction. In these situations, Doppler mean gradients tend to be less affected by transvalvar flow than maximum instantaneous gradients.

Degree of Left Ventricular Hypertrophy – LV hypertrophy suggests significant obstruction in these patients, thereby providing an index for the degree of obstruction. M-mode measurements of LV wall thickness at the septum and along the free wall in parasternal short-axis views can be compared to measurements from normal children with the same age and body surface area (z-score calculations) to determine the degree of LV hypertrophy. LV mass is often used to determine the degree of LV hypertrophy and can be calculated from M-mode measurements of LV thickness or from LV volumetric calculations using various standard methods.

Endocardial Fibroelastosis – Echocardiography presents endocardial fibroelastosis (EFE) as abnormally bright and thick LV endocardium (Fig. 14.29). The Congenital Heart Surgeons' Society has provided a system to grade EFE in the setting of valvar AS in the newborn (Table 14.12).

Ascending Aortic Size – As discussed previously, a bicuspid AoV is often associated with intrinsic ascending aorta dilation (Fig. 14.7). Therefore, measurement of the aortic annulus and root, sinotubular

FIGURE 14.15. Apical two-chamber view. Ventricular septal defect (VSD), a fibrous ridge at the crest of the ventricular septum (*star*), and peginificant aortic overriding. Ao, aorta; LV, left ventricle; RV, right ventricle.

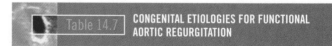

Table 14.7 CONGENITAL ETIOLOGIES FOR FUNCTIONAL AORTIC REGURGITATION

- Stenotic or nonstenotic bicuspid aortic valve
- Other abnormalities of aortic valve leaflet or commissural morphology
- Aortico–left ventricular tunnel
- Absent aortic valve leaflet
- Fibrous band between an aortic valve leaflet and the aortic root wall
- Coronary-cameral fistula into the left ventricle
- Ruptured left sinus of Valsalva aneurysm into the left ventricle

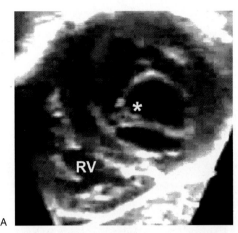 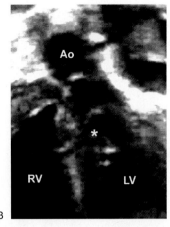 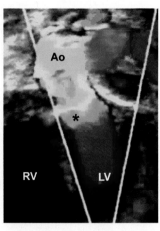

FIGURE 14.16. Repaired transitional atrioventricular canal defect. Residual cleft mitral valve and subaortic stenosis secondary to the septal attachments of the cleft mitral valve (*star*), as depicted in (**A**) a subcostal short-axis view, (**B**) an apical two-chamber view, and (**C**) an apical two-chamber view with color mapping. Ao, aorta; LV, left ventricle; RV, right ventricle.

junction, and ascending aorta in parasternal long-axis views should always be performed.

Left Atrial Dilation – As the LV diastolic function decreases with progressive LV hypertrophy, left atrial dilation becomes more apparent in subcostal and apical views. Occasionally, restrictive left-to-right flow is seen across a patent foramen ovale, consistent with the increased LV diastolic pressure and left atrial pressure associated with LV diastolic dysfunction.

Neonatal Critical Valvar Aortic Stenosis

Because the left ventricle is often small in neonates with critical valvar AS, an important early decision in their management involves the choice between biventricular repair and univentricular pallia-

tion. Echocardiographic assessments have not revealed a single feature that can predict survival with either management approach. In an important study published in 1991 by Rhodes and colleagues, a retrospective multivariate analysis was performed on a group of neonates with critical valvar AS to identify the independent predictors of outcome after biventricular repair. The parameters evaluated in their analysis included LV volumes, LV mass, LV long-axis measurements, Doppler gradient, aortic annular diameter, aortic root diameter, transverse aortic arch diameter, MV annular diameter and area, tricuspid valve annular diameter and area, and ejection fraction. They derived an equation to calculate a discriminant score that predicts survival after biventricular repair:

$$(14.0 \times \text{body surface area}) + (0.943 \times \text{aortic root diameter indexed to body surface area}) + (4.78 \times \text{LV long axis–to–heart long axis ratio}) + (0.157 \times \text{MV area indexed to body surface area}) - 12.03$$

Scores below –0.35 predicted death after a biventricular repair with 90% accuracy. They also identified four risk factors that predicted 100% mortality after biventricular repair if more than one risk factor was present, and these risk factors included LV long axis–to–heart long axis ratio of 0.8 or less (Fig. 14.30); aortic root diameter indexed to body surface area of 3.5 cm^2/m^2 or less (Fig. 14.4); MV area indexed to body surface area of 4.75 cm^2/m^2 or less; and LV mass indexed to body surface area of 35 g/m^2 or less (Table 14.13). In addition to the morphometric predictors of survival after biventricular repair for this group of patients, Kovalchin and colleagues identified an important hemodynamic predictor, namely the presence of predominant or total antegrade flow in the ascending aorta and transverse aortic arch by color mapping and Doppler interrogation (Fig. 14.31).

In 2001, the Congenital Heart Surgeons' Society conducted a multicenter study of this group of patients and identified several risk factors for mortality 5 years after biventricular repair, and these include a high EFE grade, a low aortic root diameter z-score, and a young age at presentation. Risk factors for mortality 5 years after

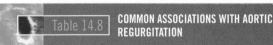

Table 14.8	COMMON ASSOCIATIONS WITH AORTIC REGURGITATION

- Aortic valve prolapse into a membranous or doubly committed subarterial Ventricular septal defect
- Subvalvar aortic stenosis
- Neonatal Marfan syndrome
- Truncus arteriosus
- Tetralogy of Fallot
- Ruptured sinus of Valsalva aneurysm

FIGURE 14.17. Apical two-chamber view. Color mapping of the patient in Figure 14.16 showing mild aortic regurgitation. Septal attachments of the cleft mitral valve (*star*). Ao, aorta; LV, left ventricle.

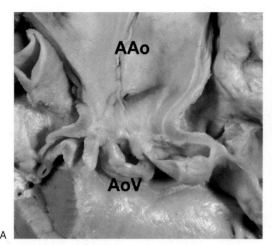
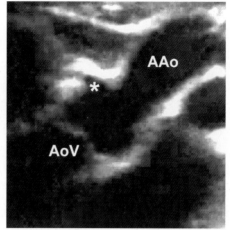

FIGURE 14.18. Hourglass type of supravalvar aortic stenosis. Somewhat high origin of the right coronary artery (*star*), as depicted in (**A**) a pathology specimen and (**B**) a right sternal border long-axis view. AAo, ascending aorta; AoV, aortic valve. (**A,** With permission from Prof. Robert H. Anderson, Institute of Child Health, London, United Kingdom.)

univentricular palliation included a small ascending aorta diameter and moderate or severe tricuspid regurgitation. Risk factors associated with differential survival between the two management approaches included all of the above as well as a low LV length z-score (Table 14.14).

More recently in 2006, Colan and colleagues evaluated the efficacy of the Rhodes score and the Congenital Heart Surgeons' Society model in predicting outcomes in a larger group of patients undergoing biventricular repair. In this analysis, the Rhodes score predicted outcome accurately in only 76% of the patients. In addition, the Congenital Heart Surgeons' Society model predicted a survival advantage with univentricular palliation in 58% of these patients. However, over half of this group actually survived a biventricular repair, suggesting that the model may be biased in favor of univentricular palliation for this patient population. The new analysis derived an equation to predict survival after biventricular repair where the discriminant score is equal to (10.98 × body surface area) + (0.56 × AoV annular z-score) + (5.89 × LV long axis–to–heart long axis ratio) – 0.79 (if EFE grade ≥2) – 6.78

(Table 14.13). A threshold score of –0.65 predicted the outcome accurately in 90% of the study patients. Unlike the original Rhodes score, MV area did not play a significant role in this analysis, presumably because all patients with critical valvar AS and MV area z-scores less than –2 underwent univentricular palliation and were therefore not included in the analysis.

In response to the bias that a high-risk biventricular repair may be better than a low-risk univentricular palliation, the Congenital Heart Surgeons' Society, in turn, refined their approach to this group of patients in a paper published in 2007. In this new analysis, the risk factors for mortality 5 years after biventricular repair included a small minimum LV outflow tract diameter indexed to body surface area, LV dysfunction, a high EFE grade, and a small mid-aortic arch diameter indexed to body surface area. Risk factors for mortality 5 years after univentricular palliation included moderate or severe tricuspid regurgitation, a large VSD, a small MV annular z-score, and a small dominant ventricular length indexed to body surface area (Table 14.14).

Subvalvar Aortic Stenosis

The transthoracic echocardiogram in a patient with subvalvar AS must include evaluation of the following features (Table 14.15).

Mechanism of Obstruction – The mechanism of the subaortic obstruction is best evaluated in apical and parasternal long-axis views, particularly if the stenosis results from a fibromuscular ridge (Fig. 14.11), an endocardial fold at the crest of the muscular septum (Fig. 14.15), or diffuse muscular narrowing along the LV outflow tract (Fig. 14.13). These views are also useful when the conal septum is deviated into the subaortic region (Fig. 14.14) or if the MV is involved (Fig. 14.16), although subcostal long-axis and short-axis views are also quite informative. Parasternal short-axis views can be useful in characterizing fibromuscular ridges that extend to the anterior mitral leaflet, although three-dimensional echocardiography may provide a better representation of this type of subvalvar AS (Fig. 14.12C).

FIGURE 14.19. Transesophageal view along a plane oriented at approximately 120 degrees of supravalvar aortic stenosis. Entrapment of the right coronary artery (RCA) by the aortic valve (AoV). AAo, ascending aorta; LV, left ventricle.

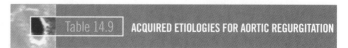

	ACQUIRED ETIOLOGIES FOR AORTIC REGURGITATION
Table 14.9	

- Endocarditis
- Rheumatic fever
- Surgical or transcatheter balloon valvotomy for valvar aortic stenosis

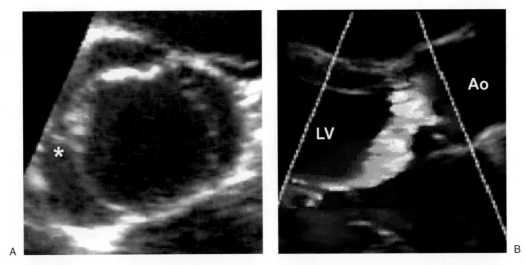

FIGURE 14.20. Bicuspid aortic valve. (A) Parasternal short-axis view of a bicuspid aortic valve involving fusion or underdevelopment of the commissure between the right coronary and noncoronary leaflets (*star*). **(B)** Parasternal long-axis view with color mapping showing moderate aortic regurgitation. Ao, aorta; LV, left ventricle.

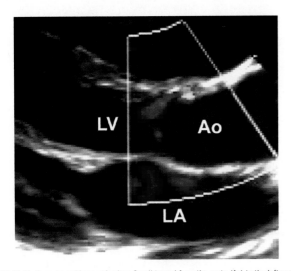

FIGURE 14.21. Parasternal long-axis view. Small tunnel from the aorta (Ao) to the left ventricle (LV) causing mild functional aortic regurgitation. LA, left atrium.

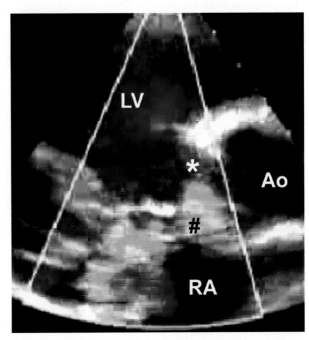

FIGURE 14.23. Parasternal long-axis view of a ruptured sinus of Valsalva aneurysm into the right atrium (*hashed*). Associated mild aortic regurgitation (*star*). Ao, aorta; LV, left ventricle; RA, right atrium.

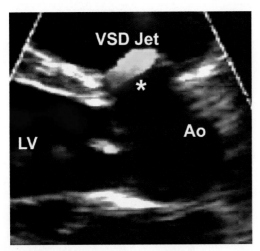

FIGURE 14.22. Parasternal long-axis view of aortic valve prolapse into a ventricular septal defect (*star*). Shows some distortion of the aortic valve in the area of the defect and mild aortic regurgitation. Ao, aorta; LV, left ventricle; VSD, ventricular septal defect.

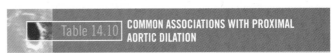

Table 14.10	COMMON ASSOCIATIONS WITH PROXIMAL AORTIC DILATION

- Marfan syndrome
- Loeys-Dietz syndrome
- Ehlers-Danlös syndrome
- Turner syndrome
- Bicuspid aortic valve
- Systemic hypertension
- Aortic coarctation

FIGURE 14.24. Bicuspid aortic valve with endocarditis resulting in a flail aortic valve segment. (A) Parasternal long-axis view. (B) Color mapping in the same view showing significant aortic regurgitation (*star*) associated with the flail aortic valve segment. AAo, ascending aorta; LV, left ventricle.

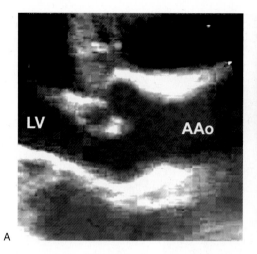
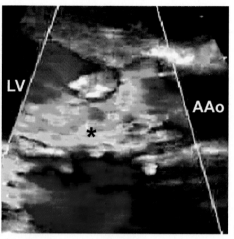

FIGURE 14.25. Valvar aortic stenosis after transcatheter balloon valvotomy with thickened aortic valve leaflets. (A) Apical two-chamber view. (B) Color mapping in the same view showing moderate aortic regurgitation. Ao, aorta; LV, left ventricle; RV, right ventricle.

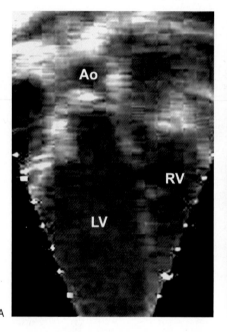
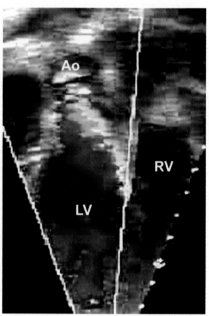

FIGURE 14.26. Unruptured aneurysm of the right sinus of Valsalva into the right ventricle (*star*). Depicted in (A) a parasternal long-axis view and (B) a parasternal short-axis view. AAo, ascending aorta; LA, left atrium; LSV, left sinus of Valsalva; LV, left ventricle; RA, right atrium; RV, right ventricle.

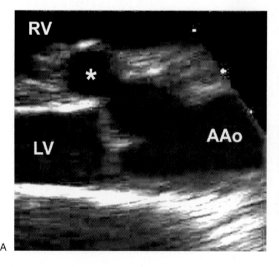
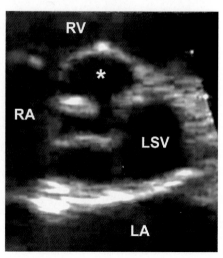

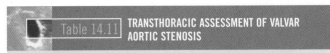

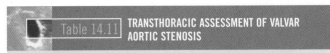 Table 14.11	TRANSTHORACIC ASSESSMENT OF VALVAR AORTIC STENOSIS

- Leaflet and commissural morphology
- Degree of obstruction
- Degree of left ventricular hypertrophy
- Endocardial fibroelastosis
- Ascending aorta size
- Left atrial dilation

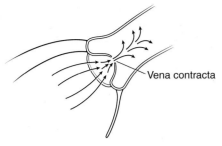

FIGURE 14-28. Illustration of the vena contracta, the narrowest segment of the high-velocity jet coursing across a stenotic aortic valve during ventricular contraction. AAo, ascending aorta; LV, left ventricle.

Location of Obstruction – The distance from the fibromuscular ridge to the AoV leaflets can usually be measured in parasternal long-axis and apical views (Fig. 14.11). It is especially important to evaluate any continuity between the fibromuscular ridge and the AoV leaflets because surgical resection may involve disruption of the normal supporting structures of the AoV.

Degree of Obstruction – The Doppler-derived maximum instantaneous gradient across the LV outflow tract is best measured in apical, right sternal border, and suprasternal notch views. Thresholds for surgical intervention for subvalvar AS are generally lower than those for valvar AS because of the progressive nature of this anomaly. In fact, the degree of obstruction along the subaortic region may increase fairly quickly over a short period of time in children, thereby necessitating periodic echocardiographic follow-up of the gradient every 6 to 12 months in some patients. Beyond adolescence, however, patients with mild subvalvar AS usually do not develop worsening obstruction.

Aortic Regurgitation – Similar to the progression of the degree of obstruction along the LV outflow tract, AR can appear suddenly and worsen fairly quickly in children with subvalvar AS. In contrast, AR is not usually a progressive association in adults with subvalvar AS.

Associated Abnormalities – The initial echocardiogram of any patient with subvalvar AS should always exclude the presence of a VSD, an MV anomaly, and partial or complete obstruction along the aortic arch. Because a double-chamber or divided right ventricle can develop in the setting of subvalvar AS and a VSD, the right ventricular outflow tract should always be evaluated in the follow-up echocardiograms of this group of patients.

Several reports have been published identifying morphometric and hemodynamic parameters related to the development and progression of subvalvar AS. In 1993, Kleinert et al. compared patients with isolated subvalvar AS as well as patients with a VSD or aortic coarctation who developed subvalvar AS after their initial presentation to a normal control population. In their analysis, they identified several morphometric predictors of the development of fixed subvalvar AS, and these include a wide mitral-aortic separation (elongated intervalvular fibrosa), exaggerated aortic override (Fig. 14.15), and a steep aortoseptal angle (Fig. 14.32, Table 14.16). In the same year, Tal Geva and colleagues looked specifically at patients with an interrupted aortic arch and VSD, a group of patients whose LV outflow tract is often small. Because of the left-to-right flow across the VSD and the right-to-left flow across the patent ductus arteriosus, there is often decreased flow across the LV outflow tract, and turbulence may not be seen along this area despite the presence of significant subvalvar AS (Fig. 14.33). Their analysis revealed that the best predictor of the development of postoperative subvalvar AS in these patients is the LV outflow tract cross-sectional area, with a threshold value of 0.7 cm^2/m^2. In 1998, Bezold and colleagues performed a multivariate analysis of patients with simple discrete subvalvar AS for whom echocardiographic follow-up was available 1 year or longer after presentation. They found that the best predictors of significantly progressive subvalvar AS included the distance from the fibromuscular ridge to the AoV indexed to the square root of the body surface area, involvement of the anterior MV leaflet, and the initial Doppler gradient (Table 14.17). More recently in 2007, Geva and colleagues identified several independent predictors of reoperation after surgical resection of discrete subvalvar AS, and these

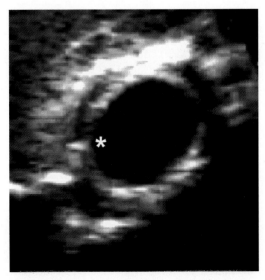

FIGURE 14.27. Parasternal short-axis view of partial fusion or underdevelopment of the commissure between the right coronary and noncoronary leaflets (*star*).

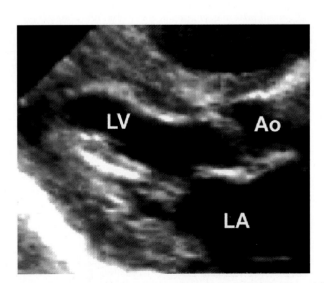

FIGURE 14-29. Parasternal long-axis view of endocardial fibroelastosis involving a left ventricular papillary muscle group and some left ventricular endocardial segments (Grade 2). Ao, aorta; LA, left atrium; LV, left ventricle.

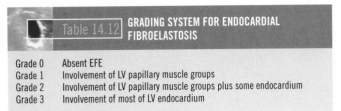

Table 14.12 GRADING SYSTEM FOR ENDOCARDIAL FIBROELASTOSIS

Grade 0	Absent EFE
Grade 1	Involvement of LV papillary muscle groups
Grade 2	Involvement of LV papillary muscle groups plus some endocardium
Grade 3	Involvement of most of LV endocardium

EFE, endocardial fibroelastosis; LV, left ventricular.
From CHSS, Congenital Heart Surgeons' Society (2001).

include a distance between the fibromuscular ridge and the AoV less than 6 mm, a maximum Doppler gradient of 60 mm Hg or greater, and involvement of the AoV or MV with the need for surgical peeling (Table 14.18).

Supravalvar Aortic Stenosis

In the setting of supravalvar AS, the aortic root and ascending aorta are best evaluated in apical, parasternal long-axis, and right sternal border views (Fig. 14.18). The diameters at the levels of the aortic annulus, aortic root, sinotubular junction, and ascending aorta should be measured in parasternal long-axis views (Fig. 14.4), and z-scores should be calculated. Echocardiographic assessment of the hourglass type of supravalvar AS usually reveals a z-score discrepancy between the sinotubular junction and ascending aorta diameters, often with values less than −2 for the former. The rare tubular supravalvar AS is usually associated with low concordant z-score values for both the sinotubular junction and ascending aorta diameters. The AoV morphology should be carefully evaluated because AoV disease along with diffuse tubular hypoplasia of the ascending aorta correlate strongly with death and reoperations in these patients. Continuous wave Doppler interrogation to calculate the maximum instantaneous gradient along the aortic outflow tract should be performed in apical, right sternal border, and suprasternal notch views. Because obstruction can occur at more than one level in patients with supravalvar AS, pulsed-wave Doppler interrogation should also be performed along the various segments of the aortic outflow tract. Spontaneous improvement rarely occurs and the degree of obstruction often worsens over time, so patients with supravalvar AS should be evaluated by echocardiography every year.

The coronary arteries (including the coronary ostia) should be carefully assessed in parasternal short-axis views, especially given the higher incidence of coronary artery dilation, ostial stenosis, and coronary entrapment in patients with supravalvar AS (Figs. 14.18 and 14-19). The aortic arch should be carefully evaluated in suprasternal notch long-axis and short-axis views because aortic coarctation and proximal stenosis of aortic arch branches may occur, particularly in the setting of Williams syndrome. Peripheral pulmonary artery stenosis is also frequently seen in Williams syndrome, although spontaneous improvement of the obstruction along the branch pulmonary arteries can occur. The branch pulmonary arteries are usually best evaluated in parasternal short-axis views, although occasionally suprasternal notch short-axis and apical views

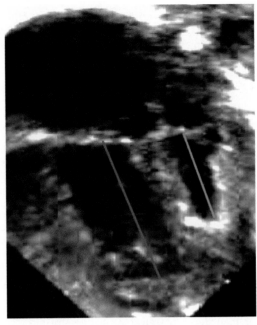

FIGURE 14.30. Apical four-chamber view of critical aortic stenosis with mild left ventricular hypoplasia depicting the left ventricular long-axis length (*yellow line*) and the heart long-axis length (*red line*).

can delineate the stenotic segments along the branch pulmonary arteries.

Aortic Regurgitation

When AR is present, echocardiography should determine the etiology and identify any of the common associations. AoV morphology is best evaluated in parasternal short-axis and long-axis views. An aortico-LV tunnel or a ruptured sinus of Valsalva aneurysm is best seen in subcostal, apical, and parasternal views (Fig. 14.21). These views are also useful when the AoV prolapses into a VSD, although the parasternal long-axis view usually provides the best display of the AoV leaflet distortion in the area of the VSD flow (Fig. 14.22). As discussed previously, subvalvar AS is best evaluated in apical and parasternal views, and color mapping can sometimes depict exactly how the high-velocity jet across the subaortic region can damage the AoV (Fig. 14.17).

Echocardiographic determination of the severity of AR usually involves characterization of the regurgitant jet, measurement of

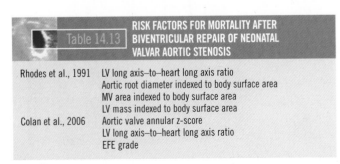

Table 14.13 RISK FACTORS FOR MORTALITY AFTER BIVENTRICULAR REPAIR OF NEONATAL VALVAR AORTIC STENOSIS

Rhodes et al., 1991	LV long axis–to–heart long axis ratio
	Aortic root diameter indexed to body surface area
	MV area indexed to body surface area
	LV mass indexed to body surface area
Colan et al., 2006	Aortic valve annular z-score
	LV long axis–to–heart long axis ratio
	EFE grade

EFE, endocardial fibroelastosis; LV, left ventricular; MV, mitral valve.
From Rhodes & Colan.

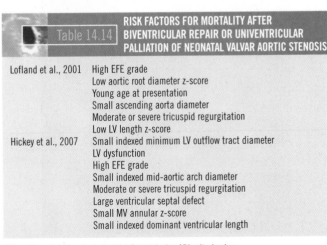

Table 14.14 RISK FACTORS FOR MORTALITY AFTER BIVENTRICULAR REPAIR OR UNIVENTRICULAR PALLIATION OF NEONATAL VALVAR AORTIC STENOSIS

Lofland et al., 2001	High EFE grade
	Low aortic root diameter z-score
	Young age at presentation
	Small ascending aorta diameter
	Moderate or severe tricuspid regurgitation
	Low LV length z-score
Hickey et al., 2007	Small indexed minimum LV outflow tract diameter
	LV dysfunction
	High EFE grade
	Small indexed mid-aortic arch diameter
	Moderate or severe tricuspid regurgitation
	Large ventricular septal defect
	Small MV annular z-score
	Small indexed dominant ventricular length

EFE, endocardial fibroelastosis; LV, left ventricular; MV, mitral valve.
From Lofland & Hickey

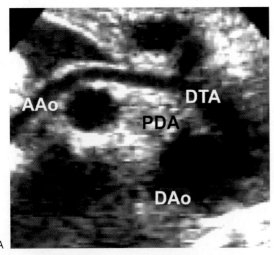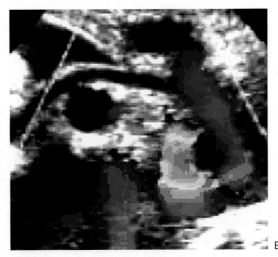

FIGURE 14.31. Critical aortic stenosis with hypoplasia of the ascending aorta and a large patent ductus arteriosus. (A) Suprasternal long-axis view. **(B)** Color mapping in the same view depicting reversal of flow in the transverse aortic arch. AAo, ascending aorta; Dao, descending aorta; DTA, distal transverse aortic arch; PDA, patent ductus arteriosus.

Doppler-derived parameters, and assessment of LV size and function (Table 14.19).

Regurgitant Jet – The length and area of the regurgitant jet as characterized by color mapping in apical views have been proposed as indices for AR severity. However, these measurements generally do not correlate well with the severity of the AR, particularly because the Coanda effect tends to alter the shape and extent of a regurgitant jet when it courses along a surface such as the ventricular septum or anterior mitral leaflet. As in valvar AS, the vena contracta in AR represents the smallest area of the regurgitant jet at or below the AoV. The width or diameter of the vena contracta measured in parasternal long-axis views may correlate better with AR severity in adults (Fig. 14.34), though the ratio of the vena contracta diameter to the LV outflow tract diameter (also measured in parasternal long-axis views) may be a more appropriate index for children. According to a 2003 report from the American Society of Echocardiography Task Force on Valvular Regurgitation, a vena contracta width greater than 6 mm and a ratio greater than 65% correspond to severe AR. Others have suggested using the area of the vena contracta or proximal regurgitant jet as measured in parasternal short-axis views as a more accurate determinant of severity, particularly because the regurgitant orifice is frequently not circular. Another method that calculates the effective regurgitant orifice area by using the proximal isovelocity surface areas (PISA) is quite complicated and therefore rarely used.

Doppler Indices – Abnormal diastolic reversal of flow in the abdominal aortic Doppler pattern is often used as a simple indicator of moderate AR, with pan-diastolic reversal representing severe AR (Fig. 14.35). A more accurate assessment may be obtained by

calculating the ratio of the velocity time integrals of the diastolic reverse flow and the systolic forward flow, and ratios greater than 35% generally represent severe AR. Continuous-wave Doppler assessment of the AR jet deceleration over time also provides some measures for AR severity. The most commonly used indices include deceleration rate (calculated as the slope from the peak regurgitant velocity to the velocity at end diastole) and pressure half-time (defined as the time from peak regurgitant velocity to half the peak value) (Fig. 14.36). A deceleration rate greater than 3.5 m/s^2 and a pressure half-time less than 250 ms generally represent severe AR. However, both indices can be significantly affected by abnormal systemic vascular resistance and LV compliance. For example, a stiff left ventricle will have a higher deceleration rate and a lower pressure half-time than a more compliant left ventricle with the same degree of AR. In addition, the higher heart rates in children tend to decrease the reproducibility and reliability of these measurements. Other Doppler-derived indices for regurgitant volume or regurgitant fraction as calculated from the total forward flow across the AoV and the MV are also quite complicated and therefore rarely used.

Left Ventricular Size and Function – According to a 2006 report from the American College of Cardiology and American Heart Association Task Force on Practice Guidelines, the recommended LV size thresholds for intervention in asymptomatic adults with significant AR include an end-diastolic diameter of 75 mm and an end-systolic diameter of 55 mm. There are, however, no significant data showing that end-diastolic diameter is an independent risk factor for irreversible LV dysfunction in patients with severe AR. On the other hand, the preoperative LV end-systolic diameter has been shown to predict LV recovery after surgical intervention, and a LV end-systolic diameter z-score greater than> 4.5 appears to increase the risk for postoperative problems, persistent LV dysfunction, and death. Because the goal is to intervene before irreversible LV dysfunction ensues, an under-

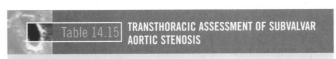

Table 14.15 TRANSTHORACIC ASSESSMENT OF SUBVALVAR AORTIC STENOSIS

Mechanism of obstruction
Location of obstruction
Degree of obstruction
Aortic regurgitation
Associated abnormalities
   Ventricular septal defect
   Mitral valve anomaly
   Aortic coarctation or interrupted aortic arch
   Double-chamber or divided right ventricle

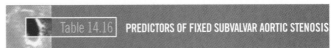

Table 14.16 PREDICTORS OF FIXED SUBVALVAR AORTIC STENOSIS

- Wide mitral-aortic separation (elongated intervalvular fibrosa)
- Exaggerated aortic override
- Steep aortoseptal angle

From Kleinert S, Geva T. Echocardiographic morphometry and geometry of the left ventricular outflow tract in fixed subaortic stenosis. *J Am Coll Cardiol.* 1993;22:1501–1508.

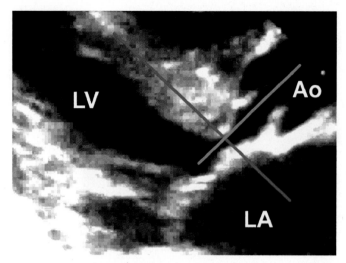

FIGURE 14.32. Parasternal long-axis view of significant muscular subaortic stenosis depicting a steep aortoseptal angle. Ao, aorta; LA, left atrium; LV, left ventricle.

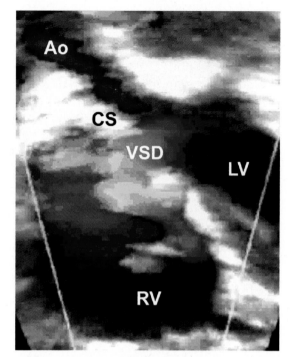

FIGURE 14.33. Color mapping in an apical two-chamber view of a ventricular septal defect and posterior deviation of the conal septum into the subaortic region. Depicting laminar flow along the subaortic region despite significant subaortic obstruction. Ao, aorta; CS, conal septum; LV, left ventricle; RV, right ventricle; VSD, ventricular septal defect.

standing of myocardial mechanics may provide some insight into the development of LV dysfunction in these patients. Decompensated AR occurs when there is inadequate hypertrophy with a consequent increase in peak systolic and end-systolic wall stress, a measure of afterload. This, in turn, affects load-dependent indices of LV function such as shortening fraction and ejection fraction, initially without any significant effect on intrinsic myocardial contractility. It appears that irreversible LV dysfunction occurs after myocardial contractility diminishes, suggesting that echocardiographic measures of contractility or afterload-adjusted ejection fraction might provide better guidelines for the timing of intervention.

Aneurysm of the Proximal Aorta

The aortic root and ascending aorta diameters are usually measured in parasternal long-axis views (Fig. 14.4), and calculation of the corresponding z-scores provides an easy index to identify aneurysmal dilation of these structures. Occasionally, aneurysmal dilation of the aortic root results in a windsock deformity of one of the sinuses of Valsalva, although sinus of Valsalva aneurysms may also be present sporadically without preexisting aortic root dilation (Fig. 14.26). Parasternal long-axis and short-axis images usually present the best views for evaluating the extent and effects of these aneurysms. If an aneurysm does not rupture, it can extend into one of the right or left heart chambers, sometimes causing problems such as right ventricular outflow tract obstruction or disruption of the tricuspid or mitral valve. Color flow mapping in most views will depict the associated problems with a ruptured sinus of Valsalva aneurysm (Fig. 14.37), including the effective left-to-right shunt resulting from a ruptured aneurysm into a right heart chamber or pulmonary artery, the functional AR resulting from a ruptured aneurysm into the left ventricle, and the continuous high-velocity jet resulting from a ruptured aneurysm into the left atrium.

Rarely, aneurysmal dilation of the ascending aorta resulting from the intrinsic aortopathy of diseases such as Marfan syndrome, Loeys-Dietz syndrome, and Turner syndrome is associated with aortic dissection and catastrophic rupture. Parasternal, right sternal border, and suprasternal notch views may display the characteristic parallel lines of the dissection along the ascending aorta wall, and occasionally color mapping will show the connection between the dissection and the aortic lumen (Fig. 14.38). Because dissection generally occurs in adolescents or adults with poor echocardiographic windows, transthoracic imaging may be inadequate. In addition, artifacts may falsely suggest the presence of a dissection in patients at risk (Fig.14.39). In these cases, transesophageal echocardiography or computed tomography may be necessary to make or confirm the diagnosis.

FETAL ECHOCARDIOGRAPHY

Although aortic atresia is the most common LV outflow tract abnormality seen in utero by echocardiography, this lesion will not be discussed because it usually results in a hypoplastic left heart syndrome or some variation thereof and requires a staged univentricular surgical approach. Among 2136 fetal cardiac diagnoses reported

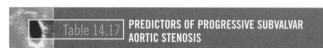

Table 14.17 PREDICTORS OF PROGRESSIVE SUBVALVAR AORTIC STENOSIS

- Indexed distance from the fibromuscular ridge to the aortic valve
- Anterior mitral valve leaflet involvement
- Initial Doppler gradient

From Bezold LI, Smith EO, Kelly K, et al. Development and validation of an echocardiographic model for predicting progression of discrete subaortic stenosis in children. *Am J Cardiol.* 1998;81:314–320.

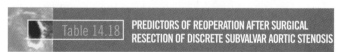

Table 14.18 PREDICTORS OF REOPERATION AFTER SURGICAL RESECTION OF DISCRETE SUBVALVAR AORTIC STENOSIS

- Distance between the fibromuscular ridge and the aortic valve <6 mm
- Maximum Doppler gradient ≥60 mm Hg
- Involvement of the aortic valve or mitral valve with the need for surgical peeling

From Geva A, McMahon CJ, Gauvreau K, et al. Risk factors for reoperation after repair of discrete subaortic stenosis in children. *J Am Coll Cardiol.* 2007;50:1498–1504.

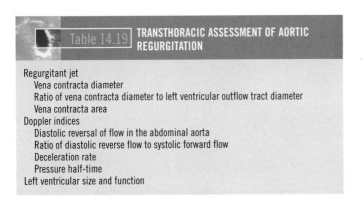

Table 14.19 TRANSTHORACIC ASSESSMENT OF AORTIC REGURGITATION

Regurgitant jet
    Vena contracta diameter
    Ratio of vena contracta diameter to left ventricular outflow tract diameter
    Vena contracta area
Doppler indices
    Diastolic reversal of flow in the abdominal aorta
    Ratio of diastolic reverse flow to systolic forward flow
    Deceleration rate
    Pressure half-time
Left ventricular size and function

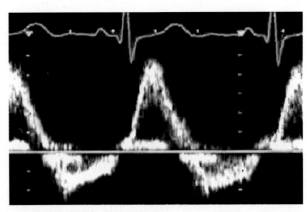

FIGURE 14.35. Pan-diastolic reversal of flow in the abdominal aortic Doppler pattern of severe aortic regurgitation.

by Sharland and Allan in 2000, valvar AS represented almost 3% of the group, ranking as the 11th most common diagnosis. Subvalvar AS, supravalvar AS, and isolated AR are extremely rare diagnoses. Occasionally a fetus that appears to have significant AR actually has an aortico-LV tunnel, and this lesion is usually associated with LV dilation, LV dysfunction, and aortic root dilation.

Some of the echocardiographic features of a fetus with significant or critical valvar AS include a left-to-right shunt across the patent foramen ovale (in contrast to the usual right-to-left shunt seen in normal fetuses) (Fig. 14.40); significant mitral regurgitation (Fig. 14.41); a dilated left ventricle with poor systolic function (Fig. 14.42); echogenic LV papillary muscle groups and endocardium; thickened AoV leaflets with turbulent flow (if the LV function is still preserved); hypoplasia of the ascending aorta; and retrograde flow along the aortic arch (Fig. 14.43, Table 14.20). The altered hemodynamics in fetuses with significant LV outflow tract obstruction involves abnormal redistribution of blood flow to the right atrium and right ventricle, which, in turn, can reduce the growth rate of left heart structures such as the left ventricle and aorta. Consequently, a fetus with significant valvar AS may develop hypoplastic left heart syndrome wherein the left ventricle is unable to support the systemic circulation (Fig. 14.44).

Several studies have attempted to identify the predictors of LV hypoplasia in fetuses with critical valvar AS. In 1995, Hornberger and colleagues identified several predictors of postnatal LV hypoplasia, and these include a mid-trimester MV diameter z-score, a mid-

trimester ascending aorta diameter z-score, and decreased growth rate of left heart structures (Table 14.21). In 2002, Rychik and colleagues demonstrated that a ratio of LV length to right ventricular length greater than 0.75 predicted LV adequacy for a biventricular circulation after birth. More recently in 2006, Mäkikallio and colleagues evaluated 43 fetuses that were diagnosed with valvar AS at less than 30 weeks' gestation and had normal LV size at presentation. In their analysis, the best predictors of progression to hypoplastic left heart syndrome included retrograde flow along the aortic arch, left-to-right shunt across the patent foramen ovale, a monophasic MV inflow Doppler pattern, and LV dysfunction (Table 14.21). These studies have become especially relevant with the advent of fetal cardiac interventions such as transcatheter balloon aortic valvotomy for fetal valvar AS. The strategy involves in utero relief of the LV outflow tract obstruction to restore nearly normal distribution of blood between the right and left sides of the heart, thereby preventing growth retardation of the left ventricle and progression to hypoplastic left heart syndrome. In 2004, Tworetzky and colleagues reported technically successful balloon valvotomy for 14 of 20 fetuses that had valvar AS and a potential risk for developing LV hypoplasia. More recently in 2007, Selamet Tierney and colleagues reported that technically successful balloon valvotomy improved LV systolic function and left heart Doppler characteristics.

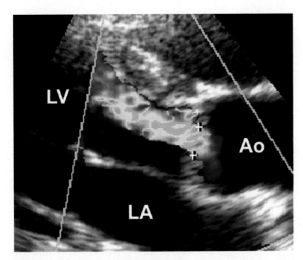

FIGURE 14.34. Color mapping in a parasternal long-axis view of moderate aortic regurgitation depicting measurement of the width of the vena contracta. Ao, aorta; LA, left atrium; LV, left ventricle.

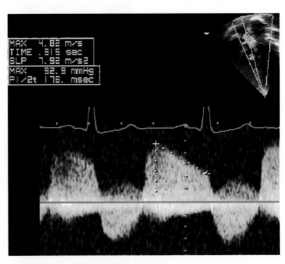

FIGURE 14.36. Measurement of the deceleration rate and pressure half-time by continuous wave Doppler interrogation for severe aortic regurgitation.

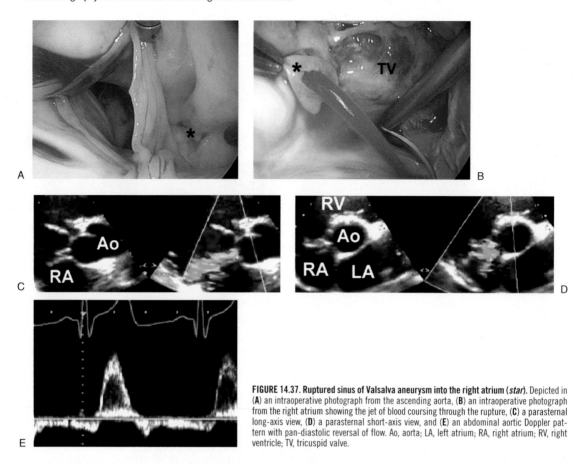

FIGURE 14.37. Ruptured sinus of Valsalva aneurysm into the right atrium (*star*). Depicted in (**A**) an intraoperative photograph from the ascending aorta, (**B**) an intraoperative photograph from the right atrium showing the jet of blood coursing through the rupture, (**C**) a parasternal long-axis view, (**D**) a parasternal short-axis view, and (**E**) an abdominal aortic Doppler pattern with pan-diastolic reversal of flow. Ao, aorta; LA, left atrium; RA, right atrium; RV, right ventricle; TV, tricuspid valve.

FIGURE 14.38. Aortic dissection along the posterior aspect of the aortic root and ascending aorta in a Marfan patient with marked aortic dilation. A: Parasternal long-axis view. **B:** Parasternal short-axis view. AAO, ascending aorta; Ao, aorta; LA, left atrium; LV, left ventricle.

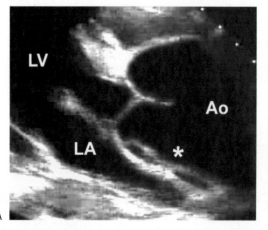
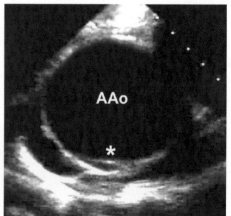

FIGURE 14.39. Marfan patient with marked aortic dilation and chest pain showing possible dissection (*star*). A: Parasternal long-axis view. **B:** Subcostal long-axis view. Computed tomography did not reveal any aortic dissection. AAo, ascending aorta; Dao, descending aorta.

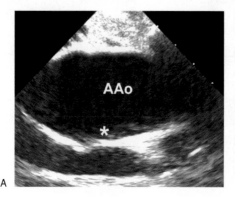
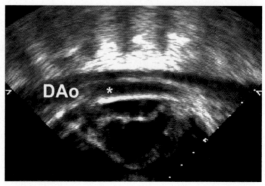

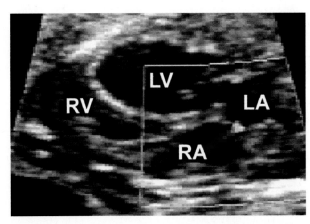

FIGURE 14.40. Four-chamber view of fetal aortic stenosis with a left-to-right shunt across the patent foramen ovale. LA, left atrium; LV, left ventricle; RA, right atrium; RV, right ventricle.

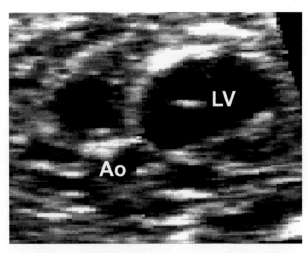

FIGURE 14.42. Left ventricular outflow tract view of fetal aortic stenosis at 22 weeks' gestation with significant left ventricular dilation and dysfunction. Ao, aorta; LV, left ventricle.

 ## TRANSESOPHAGEAL ECHOCARDIOGRAPHY

Because few patients with LV outflow tract abnormalities undergo surgical intervention during infancy or early childhood, many of these patients have limited transthoracic windows at the time of their operation. Transesophageal echocardiography can be quite useful in further delineating the abnormal anatomy associated with LV outflow tract obstructive lesions, AR or its functional variants, and diseases of the aortic root and ascending aorta, thereby providing the surgeon and cardiologist increased information in the operating room. Some of the anatomic features for which transesophageal echocardiography can provide improved images are listed in Table 14.22. Although multiple gastroesophageal locations and image planes should be used during a transesophageal study to evaluate these features, several views are particularly useful in patients with LV outflow tract abnormalities: high and mid-level transesophageal views in a horizontal plane (at 0 degrees) can provide useful information regarding the AoV morphology; low transesophageal and transgastric views in a horizontal plane can provide information regarding MV morphology as well as LV function before and after the operation; a mid-level transesophageal view at approximately 120-degree image plane usually provides long-axis images of the subaortic region and its relationship to the aorta, similar to the parasternal long-axis view in transthoracic imaging (Figs. 14.10A and 14.19); and a transgastric view in a vertical plane (at 90 degrees) often provides an accurate means to measure the degree of LV outflow tract obstruction by continuous-wave Doppler interrogation (Fig. 14.45).

 ## POSTOPERATIVE AND POSTINTERVENTIONAL ECHOCARDIOGRAPHY

Techniques in postoperative and postinterventional echocardiography are similar to preoperative approaches and should include assessment of the following parameters (Table 14.23).

Residual Left Ventricular Outflow Tract Obstruction

Valvar AS, particularly when it presents in the first year of life, is a chronic problem that usually requires multiple "palliative" interventions during the individual's lifetime. The absence of a residual gradient immediately after a surgical or transcatheter valvotomy does not necessarily preclude recurrence and progression of residual valvar AS in the future. Therefore, follow-up echocardiograms should be performed yearly for these patients. Because subvalvar AS is a progressive disease, recurrence after surgical resection is also

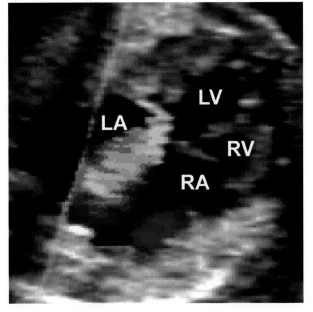

FIGURE 14.41. Four-chamber view of fetal aortic stenosis with significant mitral regurgitation. LA, left atrium; LV, left ventricle; RA, right atrium; RV, right ventricle.

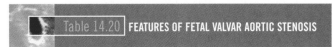

Table 14.20 **FEATURES OF FETAL VALVAR AORTIC STENOSIS**

- Left-to-right shunt across the patent foramen ovale
- Significant mitral regurgitation
- Dilated left ventricle with poor systolic function
- Echogenic left ventricular papillary muscle groups and endocardium
- Thickened aortic valve leaflets with turbulent flow
- Hypoplastic ascending aorta
- Retrograde flow along the aortic arch

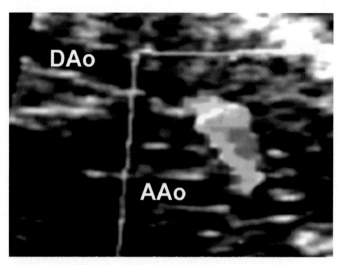

FIGURE 14.43. Arch view of fetal aortic stenosis with retrograde flow in the transverse aortic arch by color mapping. AAo, ascending aorta; Dao, descending aorta.

common, particularly because resection may not correct the intrinsic abnormality in LV outflow tract morphology and the genetic predisposition that are believed to cause subvalvar AS. Yearly follow-up echocardiograms should also be performed for these patients, regardless of the absence of postoperative subaortic obstruction.

Residual or Postintervention Aortic Regurgitation

AR is seen frequently in patients who have undergone surgical or transcatheter valvotomy for valvar AS, and these patients should undergo follow-up echocardiograms yearly. In a 2007 report by Pasquali and colleagues, patients with valvar AS who have undergone the Ross procedure (which involves aortic valve and root replacement with the patient's native pulmonary valve and root and placement of a homograft from the right ventricle to the pulmonary artery) are at risk for progressive neo-AR, particularly if the patient previously underwent a VSD repair or an AoV replacement. If the AoV has been significantly damaged by the high-velocity jet associated with subvalvar AS or because of chronic prolapse into a VSD, significant residual AR may be present postoperatively, and the clinical and echocardiographic guidelines for future intervention apply to these patients.

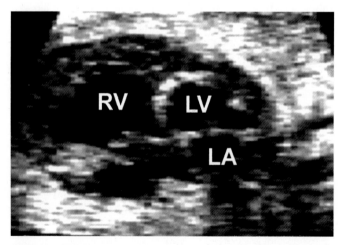

FIGURE 14.44. Four-chamber view of the same fetal aortic stenosis as shown in Figure 14-42 at 33 weeks' gestation, now with left ventricular hypoplasia. LA, left atrium; LV, left ventricle; RV, right ventricle.

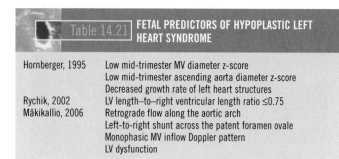

Table 14.21	FETAL PREDICTORS OF HYPOPLASTIC LEFT HEART SYNDROME
Hornberger, 1995	Low mid-trimester MV diameter z-score
	Low mid-trimester ascending aorta diameter z-score
	Decreased growth rate of left heart structures
Rychik, 2002	LV length–to–right ventricular length ratio ≤0.75
Mäkikallio, 2006	Retrograde flow along the aortic arch
	Left-to-right shunt across the patent foramen ovale
	Monophasic MV inflow Doppler pattern
	LV dysfunction

LV, left ventricular; MV, mitral valve.

Left Ventricular Size and Function

LV hypertrophy may persist after surgical or transcatheter valvotomy for valvar AS, especially if there is residual LV outflow tract obstruction. As discussed previously, LV dysfunction may or may not improve after surgical intervention for AR, depending on whether the intervention is undertaken before irreversible myocardial damage occurs. Therefore, the usual methods for assessing LV size and function should be included in the follow-up protocol for all patients who have undergone intervention for AS or AR.

Size of the Proximal Aorta

Aortic dilation may occur even after plication or size reduction of the proximal aorta because the etiology in most cases is an intrinsic aortopathy that can affect any remaining aortic tissue after surgery. Therefore, these patients should also undergo yearly follow-up echocardiograms. In addition, the 2007 paper by Pasquali and colleagues on mid-term follow-up after the Ross procedure also reported that the neoaortic root size in these patients increased significantly out of proportion to somatic growth.

Prosthetic Aortic Valve Function

Occasionally, the intervention for a patient with significant LV outflow tract obstruction or AR involves AoV replacement with a prosthetic AoV. The most commonly used prosthetic AoV in many centers is the St. Jude valve, a metallic valve ring to which two hemidisc leaflets are hinged at both ends of a bisecting line across the ring (blood flows through the ring on either side of this bisecting line). Echocardiographic follow-up is often difficult because the patients are usually older with poor transthoracic echocardiographic windows. In addition, acoustic interference from the

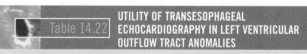

Table 14.22	UTILITY OF TRANSESOPHAGEAL ECHOCARDIOGRAPHY IN LEFT VENTRICULAR OUTFLOW TRACT ANOMALIES

- Aortic valve morphology
- Mechanism for valvar stenosis or regurgitation
- Location and mechanism for subvalvar obstruction
- Mechanism for supravalvar aortic stenosis
- Distortion of the aortic valve secondary to aortic valve prolapse into a Ventricular septal defect
- Ruptured sinus of Valsalva aneurysm
- Aortic root abscess formation
- Dissection along the ascending aorta
- Abnormalities of the proximal coronary arteries
- Abnormalities of mitral valve morphology
- Preoperative and postoperative left ventricular function
- Postoperative function of a prosthetic aortic valve

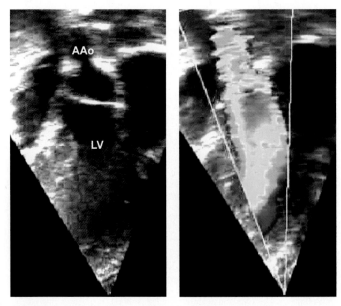

FIGURE 14.45. Long-axis transesophageal view from the transgastric position of supravalvar aortic stenosis. This provides an acceptable angle for Doppler interrogation to assess the degree of obstruction. AAo, ascending aorta; LV, left ventricle.

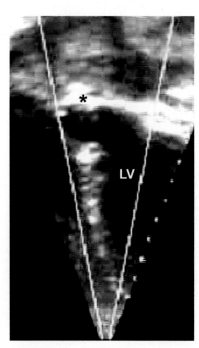

FIGURE 14.47. Color mapping in a long-axis transgastric view of a prosthetic aortic valve showing normal trivial intravalvar regurgitation (*star*) that is not localized outside the prosthetic valve ring. LV, left ventricle.

prosthetic valve ring can obscure assessment of the hemidisc leaflets as well as any structure on the other side of the ring from the echocardiographic probe. Nevertheless, every effort should be made to assure full symmetric mobility of the prosthetic hemidisc leaflets. Occasionally transesophageal echocardiography may be used if no information is available by transthoracic echocardiography (Fig. 14.46). Doppler interrogation of the flow across a prosthetic valve almost always results in a maximum instantaneous gradient that overestimates the peak-to-peak gradients measured in the catheterization laboratory because the pressure recovery effects are significantly increased with prosthetic valves, especially for the smaller ones used in children. For example,

the normal maximum instantaneous gradient across a 19-mm St. Jude prosthesis in the aortic position may be as high as 30 to 50 mm Hg by continuous-wave Doppler interrogation without significant obstruction across the prosthetic valve. Color flow mapping will usually show trivial AR associated with the hemidisc leaflets, a normal finding for a St. Jude prosthetic valve (Fig. 14.47).

Echocardiographic assessment should distinguish this finding from the pathologic paravalvar leaks, which are localized outside the prosthetic valve ring and usually represent disruption of the normal connection between the prosthetic valve ring and the surrounding tissue.

ALTERNATIVE IMAGING MODALITIES

Because of poor echocardiographic windows in older children and young adults, computed tomography and magnetic resonance imaging can be useful in assessing the caliber of the aortic root and ascending aorta as well as the coronary arteries. In addition, these modalities are quite valuable when aortic dissection is suspected. Magnetic resonance imaging also provides an accurate means to quantify LV size and function. When prosthetic valve dysfunction is suspected, fluoroscopy often provides information that cannot be gleaned from echocardiography because of the obscuring issues discussed previously.

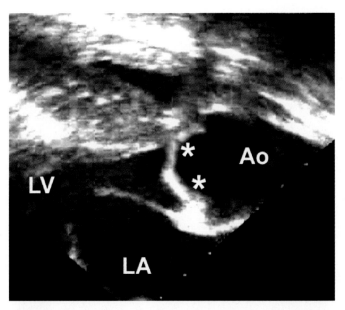

FIGURE 14.46. Long-axis transesophageal view of a prosthetic aortic valve with symmetric positioning of the prosthetic hemidisc leaflets (*stars*). Ao, aorta; LA, left atrium; LV, left ventricle.

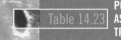

	POSTOPERATIVE AND POSTINTERVENTIONAL ASSESSMENT FOR LEFT VENTRICULAR OUTFLOW TRACT ANOMALIES
Table 14.23	

- Residual left ventricular outflow tract obstruction
- Aortic regurgitation
- Left ventricular size and function
- Proximal aorta size
- Prosthetic aortic valve function

SUGGESTED READING

Bezold LI, Smith EO, Kelly K, et al. Development and validation of an echocardiographic model for predicting progression of discrete subaortic stenosis in children. *Am J Cardiol.* 1998;81:314–320.

Bonow RO, Carabello BA, Chatterjee K, et al. ACC/AHA 2006 guidelines for the management of patients with valvular heart disease: a report of the American College of Cardiology/American Heart Association Task Force on Practice Guidelines (Writing Committee to Revise the 1998 Guidelines for the Management of Patients With Valvular Heart Disease). *J Am Coll Cardiol.* 2006;48:1–148.

Cape EG, Vanauker MD, Sigfusson G, et al. Potential role of mechanical stress in the etiology of pediatric heart disease: septal shear stress in subaortic stenosis. *J Am Coll Cardiol.* 1997;30:247–254.

Colan SD, McElhinney DB, Crawford EC, et al. Validation and re-evaluation of a discriminant model predicting anatomic suitability for biventricular repair in neonates with aortic stenosis. *J Am Coll Cardiol.* 2006;47:1858–1865.

Fedak PWM, David TE, Borger M, et al. Bicuspid aortic valve disease: recent insights in pathophysiology and treatment. *Expert Rev Cardiovasc Ther.* 2005;3:295–308.

Fernandes SM, Sanders SP, Khairy P, et al. Morphology of bicuspid aortic valve in children and adolescents. *J Am Coll Cardiol.* 2004;44:1648–1651.

Freedom RM, Yoo SJ, Mikailian H, et al, eds. *The natural and modified history of congenital heart disease.* Toronto: Blackwell Publishing, Futura Division; 2004.

Freedom RM, Yoo SJ, Russell J, et al. Thoughts about fixed subaortic stenosis in man and dog. *Cardiol Young.* 2005;15:186–205.

Geva A, McMahon CJ, Gauvreau K, et al. Risk factors for reoperation after repair of discrete subaortic stenosis in children. *J Am Coll Cardiol.* 2007;50:1498–1504.

Hickey EJ, Caldarone CA, Blackstone EH, et al. Critical left ventricular outflow tract obstruction: the disproportionate impact of biventricular repair in borderline cases. *J Thorac Cardiovasc Surg.* 2007;134:1429–1436.

Kleinert S, Geva T. Echocardiographic morphometry and geometry of the left ventricular outflow tract in fixed subaortic stenosis. *J Am Coll Cardiol.* 1993;22:1501–1508.

Lacro RV, Dietz HC, Wruck LM, et al. Rationale and design of a randomized clinical trial of beta-blocker therapy (atenolol) versus angiotensin II receptor blocker therapy (losartan) in individuals with Marfan syndrome. *Am Heart J.* 2007;154:624–631.

Lofland GK, McCrindle BW, Williams WG, et al. Critical aortic stenosis in the neonate: a multi-institutional study of management, outcomes, and risk factors. *J Thorac Cardiovasc Surg.* 2001;121:10–27.

Mäkikallio K, McElhinney DB, Levine JC, et al. Fetal aortic valve stenosis and the evolution of hypoplastic left heart syndrome: patient selection for fetal intervention. *Circulation.* 2006;113:1401–1405.

Pasquali SK, Cohen MS, Shera D, et al. The relationship between neo-aortic dilation, insufficiency, and reintervention following the Ross procedure in infants, children, and young adults. *J Am Coll Cardiol.* 2007;49:1806–1812

Rhodes LA, Colan SD, Perry SB, et al. Predictors of survival in neonates with critical aortic stenosis. Circulation. 1991;84:2325–2335.

Sharland G. Aortic valve abnormalities. In: Allan L, Hornberger L, Sharland G, eds. *Textbook of fetal cardiology.* London: Greenwich Medical Media; 2000:213–232.

Tworetzky W, Wilkins-Haug L, Jennings RW, et al. Balloon dilation of severe aortic stenosis in the fetus: potential for prevention of hypoplastic left heart syndrome: candidate selection, technique, and results of successful intervention. *Circulation.* 2004;110:2125–2131.

Vlahos AP, Marx GR, McElhinney DB, et al. Clinical utility of Doppler echocardiography in assessing aortic stenosis severity and predicting need for intervention in children. *Pediatr Cardiol.* 2007(online).

Wilcox BR, Cook AC, Anderson RH. Surgical anatomy of the heart, 3rd ed. Cambridge, UK: Cambridge University Press; 2004.

Zoghbi WA, Enriquez-Sarano M, Foster E, et al. Recommendations for evaluation of the severity of native valvular regurgitation with two-dimensional and Doppler echocardiography: a report from the American Society of Echocardiography's Nomenclature and Standards Committee and the Task Force on Valvular Regurgitation. *J Am Soc Echocardiogr.* 2003; 16:777–802.

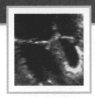

Chapter 15
Tetralogy of Fallot

Himesh Vyas • Benjamin W. Eidem

Tetralogy of Fallot (TOF) is a morphologic diagnosis whose essential features include a large unrestrictive ventricular septal defect (VSD), right ventricular (RV) outflow tract (RVOT) obstruction, an overriding aorta, and RV hypertrophy (RVH) (Fig. 15.1). Although four seemingly disparate features are described, the syndrome actually results from a single morphologic abnormality—namely, anterior deviation or malalignment of the conal septum. All of the four cardinal features in TOF are a manifestation of this malalignment. This condition was first described by Stensen as early as 1672. However, it was Fallot in 1888 who provided the clinical-pathologic correlation of this malformation and termed it *la maladie bleue*.

The clinical features of TOF are very diverse and depend on the degree of RVOT obstruction. In this chapter, we will describe the echocardiographic morphology of this malformation in detail as well as the key features of the postoperative examination. We will also describe the morphologic aspects of TOF with absent pulmonary valve syndrome. Pulmonary atresia with VSD has similar intracardiac anatomy to TOF; however, the morphology and blood supply of the pulmonary arteries are so variable that this condition is considered separately.

When describing the anatomic and echocardiographic morphology of TOF, a segmental approach should be used.

VENOUS CONNECTIONS

There is situs solitus in most cases of TOF. About 10% of patients may have a left superior vena cava (L-SVC) draining to the right atrium via the coronary sinus. This can be visualized in multiple echocardiographic scan planes. The parasternal long-axis view typically demonstrates a dilated coronary sinus—a finding that should prompt the echocardiographer to suspect an L-SVC. However, it should be noted that the coronary sinus is not always dilated in patients with an L-SVC, particularly in the following circumstances:

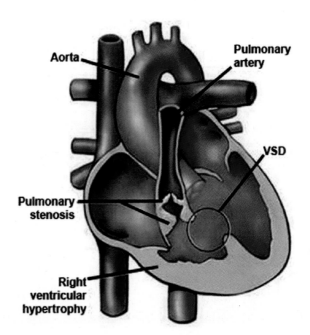

FIGURE 15.1. Anatomical components of tetralogy of Fallot. Anterior malalignment ventricular septal defect, pulmonary stenosis, overriding aorta, and right ventricular hypertrophy.

- Small L-SVC with prominent bridging innominate vein
- Elevated left atrial pressure, such as in patients with a predominant left-to-right shunt physiology ("pink tetralogy")
- Termination of the L-SVC in the left atrium rather than the coronary sinus

In the parasternal short-axis view, a prominent venous structure is identified anterior to the left pulmonary artery. Slight clockwise rotation of the transducer will typically display the entire course of the left SVC in its long axis with drainage to the coronary sinus along the posterior aspect of the heart. Color flow mapping and pulsed-wave Doppler confirm that this blood vessel is venous and demonstrates low-velocity phasic systolic and diastolic flow toward the heart. Other vascular structures in this area that may be confused with an L-SVC include the following:

- Ascending vertical vein (anomalous pulmonary venous connection) in which venous flow is away from the heart
- The left upper pulmonary vein as it crosses the left pulmonary artery may be confused with an L-SVC, particularly when a long length of this vein can be visualized (as in infants). However, this vein can be tracked distally to the hilum of the left lung to define its origin.
- Levo-atrial cardinal vein: this venous structure is a connection from the left atrium to a systemic vein and thus has flow away from the heart. Almost all cases of levo-atrial cardinal vein are associated with left-sided obstructive lesions, particularly left atrial outlet obstruction. This vein generally courses posterior to the left pulmonary artery (unlike the anterior course of the L-SVC).

ATRIAL SEPTUM

Approximately one-third of patients with unrepaired TOF have an ASD. Many additional patients have a small patent foramen ovale. Defects in the atrial septum are best imaged from the subcostal scan planes because the atrial septum is perpendicular to this imaging plane. The atrial septum can be visualized in orthogonal subcostal planes (coronal and sagittal) to optimally define the ASD. A subcostal sagittal (short-axis) view provides excellent visualization of the inferior vena cava (IVC) and SVC connections and the ASD. Patients without significant RVH and without severe RVOT obstruction will have a predominant left-to-right shunt at the atrial level. Conversely, those with significant RVH or RVOT obstruction will have a bidirectional or predominantly right-to-left atrial level shunt.

It is important to remember that for color flow mapping of right-to-left atrial level shunt (generally displayed blue), the Nyquist limit must be reduced to as low as 30 to 50 cm/s to optimally demonstrate the shunt. A predominant right-to-left shunt at the atrial level is generally considered an indication for surgical intervention in patients with TOF.

ATRIOVENTRICULAR CONNECTIONS

Most cases of tetralogy of Fallot have concordant atrioventricular connections. The tricuspid and mitral valves are usually structurally normal. Significant atrioventricular valve pathology is uncommon. However, in approximately 2% of patients with TOF, a complete atrioventricular septal defect may be present—particularly in patients with Down syndrome. In such cases, the apical four-chamber view demonstrates a typical image of a large primum atrial defect and a large inlet VSD. Many of these common AV valves are Rastelli Type C (i.e., free floating—without chordal attachments of the anterior bridging leaflet to the interventricular septum).

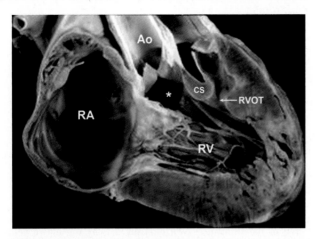

FIGURE 15.2. Pathologic specimen of tetralogy of Fallot. Anterior deviation of the conal septum (CS) into the right ventricular outflow tract (RVOT) results in a large malalignment ventricular septal defect *(asterisk)* with aortic override (Ao) as well as significant RVOT obstruction and RV hypertrophy. RA, right atrium; RV, right ventricle. (Photograph courtesy of Dr. William Edwards.)

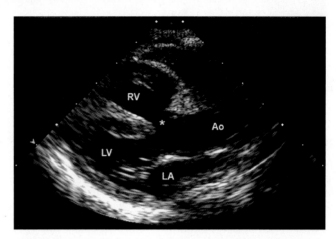

FIGURE 15.4. Parasternal long-axis view in tetralogy of Fallot. Note the large ventricular septal defect (VSD; *asterisk*) with approximately 50% aortic override (Ao) of the VSD.

 VENTRICULAR SEPTAL DEFECT

The typical VSD in patients with TOF is an anterior malalignment type of outlet VSD. The conal/infundibular septum is deviated anteriorly from the muscular septum (Fig. 15.2). This single malformation results in RVOT obstruction (by encroaching on the RVOT), RVH (secondary to RVOT obstruction), and aortic override (due to the malaligned conal septum) (Fig. 15.3). In other words, the four components of TOF are in reality the result of a single malformation—anterior malalignment of the conal septum.

This anteriorly malaligned VSD occurs in the vast majority of patients with TOF; however, other anatomic types of VSD may occur. A description of the anatomical and echocardiographic assessment of the different types of VSD in patients with TOF is listed next:

- **Anteriorly malaligned VSD (74%):** This represents a large subaortic defect that extends from the right and noncoronary cusps of the aortic valve superiorly to the membranous septum inferiorly. The defect is well seen in the parasternal long-axis view (Fig. 15.4). The anterior malalignment of the conal septum with an overriding aorta is obvious from this view. However, this image is not pathognomonic of TOF because this malaligned VSD with an overriding aorta may be seen in patients with pulmonary atresia with VSD and in those with truncus arteriosus. Hence, it is critical to define the morphology of the pulmonary valve and RVOT.

By rotating the transducer clockwise, a parasternal short-axis view at the base of the heart is obtained. The extent of the VSD is well seen in this view extending from the area of aortic-tricuspid continuity (membranous septum) often up to the crista supraventricularis ("12 o'clock" position in the parasternal short-axis view) (Fig. 15.5). A prominent "knuckle" of the anteriorly malaligned conal septum is often evident in this view leading to the os infundibulum where the RVOT obstruction typically begins (Fig. 15.6A–B). The demonstration of a pulmonary valve in this view with antegrade flow across it excludes the possibilities of pulmonary atresia with VSD and truncus arteriosus.

The direction of the VSD shunt flow should be visualized by color flow Doppler as well as by pulsed-wave and continuous-wave Doppler. Patients with mild to moderate degrees of RVOT obstruction will have predominant left-to-right shunting, while more severe degrees of RVOT obstruction often lead to bidirectional and, later, predominantly right-to-left shunting.

- **Perimembranous VSD without aortic-tricuspid fibrous continuity due to a muscular rim (18%)**
- **Atrioventricular septal defect in continuity with the subaortic defect (2%)**
- **Inlet VSD with straddling tricuspid valve (1%)**
- **Doubly committed subarterial defect (5%):** In this setting, there is a complete lack of conal septum. In the parasternal short-axis view, the VSD is noted to extend beyond the crista supraventricularis ("12 o'clock position") up to the pulmonary valve. This VSD is usually separated from the tricuspid valve by a muscular rim. RVOT obstruction is most commonly due to pulmonary valve stenosis and concomitant annular hypoplasia and not due to infundibular stenosis.

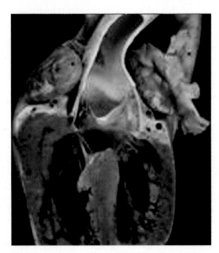

FIGURE 15.3. Pathologic specimen of tetralogy of Fallot. Anatomic four-chamber view demonstrating large ventricular septal defect with aortic override. (Photograph courtesy of Dr. William Edwards.)

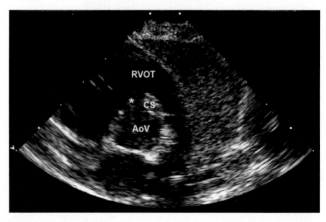

FIGURE 15.5. Parasternal short-axis view in tetralogy of Fallot. Note the large ventricular septal defect *(asterisk)* with anterior deviation of the conal septum (CS) into the right ventricular outflow tract (RVOT). Ao, aorta.

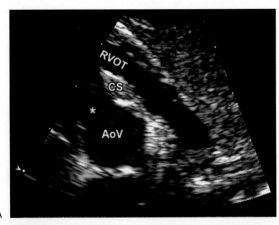
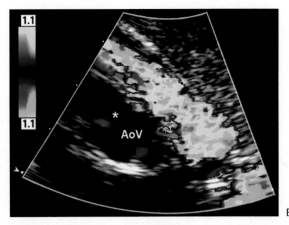

FIGURE 15.6. Parasternal short-axis view in tetralogy of Fallot. A: Note the prominent deviation of the conal septum (CS) into the right ventricular outflow tract (RVOT), resulting in significant narrowing. **B:** Color Doppler. Note that obstruction, represented by a mosaic pattern in the color flow Doppler signal, begins within the RVOT and extends into the pulmonary artery. *Ventricular septal defect. AoV, aortic valve.

In general, all of these types of VSD in TOF are unrestrictive. Restrictive VSDs are rare in the setting of TOF but can occur (approximately 1%). The reason for restriction is generally the presence of accessory tricuspid tissue within the VSD. Rarely, a hypertrophied septal band may also contribute to a restrictive VSD.

Physiologic Assessment

Spectral Doppler analysis and color flow mapping of the VSD provide a wealth of physiologic information. In patients with mild RVOT obstruction, the predominant interventricular shunting will be left to right. Such patients have a physiology consistent with a large VSD and are at risk of developing congestive heart failure and pulmonary hypertension. These patients are generally referred to as having "pink tetralogy." With increasing degrees of RVOT obstruction, the VSD shunt may be bidirectional (Fig. 15.7A–B). Eventually, with severe RVOT obstruction, the ventricular level shunt is predominantly right to left. These patients are cyanotic and may be at risk of developing hypercyanotic spells ("tet spells"). Flow across the VSD is almost always laminar when the VSD is unrestrictive.

Ventriculoarterial Connections

The ventriculoarterial connections in TOF are typically concordant. However, the aorta does characteristically override the ventricular septum. This override is best demonstrated in the parasternal long-

axis view (Fig. 15.4) but is also obvious in other views including the apical four-chamber view (Fig. 15.8). It must be pointed out that even in normal individuals, there can be some degree of aortic override. A spectrum exists in the setting of this anomaly from less than 50% override in patients with TOF to greater than 50% aortic override (predominant RV origin of the aorta) in patients with double-outlet right ventricle. It is also important to understand that the position of the transducer on the chest wall can affect the visual impression of aortic override.

The Right Ventricular Outflow Tract

Assessment of the RVOT is critically important in patients with TOF. Anterior and cephalad deviation of the conal septum leads to characteristic narrowing of the RVOT. This muscular obstruction often begins at the crista supraventricularis and extends to the pulmonary valve annulus. The RVOT can be visualized in multiple echocardiographic views. The subcostal 4-chamber (coronal) and short-axis (sagittal) views are useful to delineate the morphology of the RVOT and define obstructive muscle bundles (Fig. 15.9A–D). The parasternal short-axis view helps to differentiate TOF from other congenital heart lesions including truncus arteriosus and pulmonary atresia with VSD, all of which may have a similar echocardiographic appearance in the parasternal long-axis view (Fig. 15.4). In TOF, the parasternal short-axis view demonstrates a patent RVOT and pulmonary valve (Figs. 15.5 and 15.6A–B).

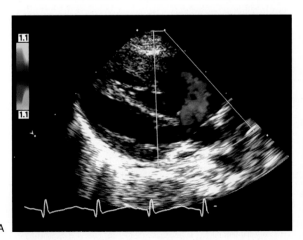
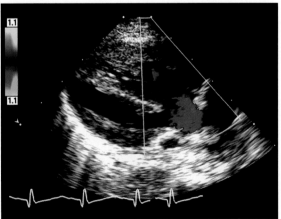

FIGURE 15.7. Parasternal long-axis view in tetralogy of Fallot. Color Doppler demonstrates left-to-right shunting (red flow) in systole (A) and right-to-left shunting (blue flow) in diastole (B).

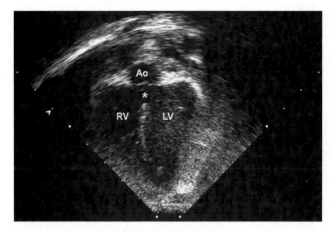

FIGURE 15.8. Apical view in tetralogy of Fallot. Note the aortic override (Ao) of the ventricular septal defect *(asterisk)*. RV, right ventricle; LV, left ventricle.

FIGURE 15.10. Pathologic specimens of the pulmonary valve in tetralogy of Fallot. Anatomical variability of the pulmonary valve in tetralogy of Fallot, including acommissural, unicommissural, bicommissural, and dysplastic tricommissural valves.

Pulmonary Valve

The pulmonary annulus is often hypoplastic and the pulmonary valve may be acommissural, unicommissural, bicommissural, or tricommissural with thickening/dysplasia (Fig. 15.10). Accurate measurement of the pulmonary annulus is important and may determine the necessity for transannular patch repair if significant hypoplasia exists. Z-score of the pulmonary valve annulus should be recorded. In general, a pulmonary annular z-score of less than –2 is likely to indicate the need for a transannular surgical approach. In the extreme form, the pulmonary valve may be completely atretic. However, because the clinical and surgical management and anatomical variations of this anomaly are very different from TOF, the entity of pulmonary atresia with VSD is considered separately. The presence and severity of pulmonary valve regurgitation should also be noted (Fig. 15.11A–C).

Great Arteries

Often, there is supravalvar stenosis noted in the main pulmonary artery. Typically, this is located at the tips of the open pulmonary valve in systole and the valve may have attachments in this region.

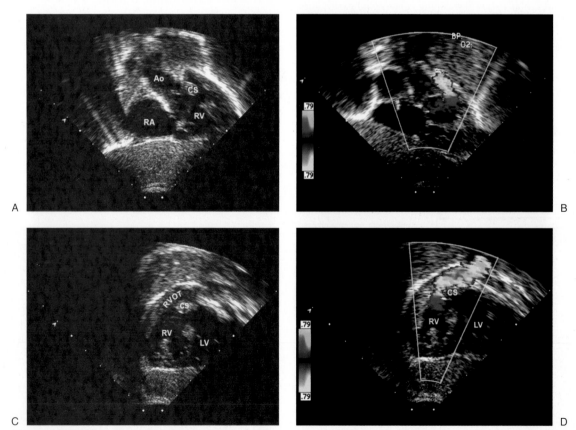

FIGURE 15.9. Subcostal four-chamber (coronal) and short-axis (sagittal) views in tetralogy of Fallot. A: Note the prominent deviation of the conal septum (CS) into the right ventricular outflow tract (RVOT) in this subcostal four-chamber view. B: Aliasing of color flow Doppler in this subcostal four-chamber view demonstrates obstruction within the RVOT. C: Subcostal short-axis view demonstrating deviation of CS into RVOT. D: Subcostal short-axis view with color Doppler aliasing within the RVOT demonstrating region of obstruction within RVOT.

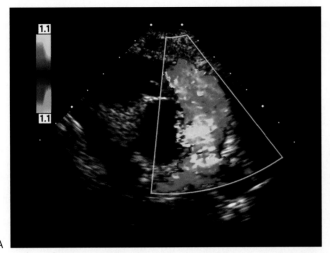
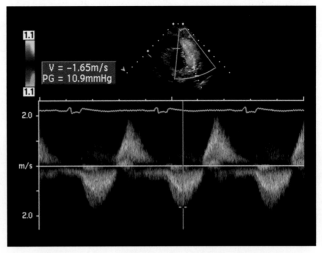

FIGURE 15.11. Severe pulmonary regurgitation in postoperative tetralogy of Fallot. A: Color Doppler demonstrating broad jet of pulmonary regurgitation extending into the branch pulmonary arteries consistent with severe ("free") regurgitation. **B:** Continuous-wave Doppler demonstrating return of the pulmonary regurgitant signal to the Doppler baseline consistent with equalization of right ventricular (RV) and pulmonary arterial pressure. Systolic Doppler velocity of 1.6 m/s confirms a widely patent RV outflow tract (RVOT) without significant residual obstruction.

Recognition of this narrowing is important because patch angioplasty of the main pulmonary artery may be needed to relieve this obstruction during surgical repair. This abnormality is well visualized in the high left parasagittal view. The anatomy of the branch pulmonary arteries is important to define. These pulmonary artery branches are best visualized in the parasternal short-axis view as well as the high left parasternal and suprasternal short-axis views (Fig. 15.12). In fact, measurements of the right pulmonary artery from the suprasternal short-axis view correlate better with angiography-derived measurements than those from parasternal views. Branch pulmonary artery z-scores should be calculated and focal stenoses should be identified. Severe branch pulmonary artery hypoplasia may make complete repair difficult. Staged palliation with a primary systemic-pulmonary artery shunt may be necessary.

It is also important to document additional sources of pulmonary arterial blood supply. Pulmonary blood flow may be provided entirely by antegrade flow across the pulmonary valve, via the ductus arteriosus (occasionally bilateral ductal arteries) or via multiple aortopulmonary collateral vessels. With a left aortic arch, the ductus arteriosus generally arises from the upper descending aorta, whereas with a right aortic arch, the ductus remains left sided but

arises from the base of the (left) innominate artery. The ductus arteriosus is best visualized in the high left parasagittal view and suprasternal long-axis view (Fig. 15.13). Color flow mapping and Doppler evaluation are invaluable in accurately determining the ductal physiology. A continuous left-to-right ductal shunt is suggestive of severe RVOT obstruction, particularly if significant antegrade flow is not demonstrated. Continuous multiple tortuous channels of systemic-to-pulmonary artery flow are typical of aortopulmonary collaterals and are far more common with pulmonary atresia with VSD rather than in TOF.

Assessment of the degree of RVOT obstruction requires a comprehensive echocardiographic approach including two-dimensional evaluation of anatomic features, color flow mapping, and spectral Doppler analysis. Aliasing may be noted in the subvalvar region with color flow mapping (Fig. 15.14A, 15.14B). Pulsed-wave Doppler is helpful to delineate the area of maximal obstruction, while continuous-wave Doppler should be used to determine the maximal instantaneous and mean systolic gradient (Fig. 15.15A–C). Although the maximal instantaneous RVOT gradient is often reported, the mean gradient often correlates better with the peak-to-peak gradient measured at cardiac catheterization. To avoid underestimation of the RVOT gradient, it is important to remember to use lower-frequency

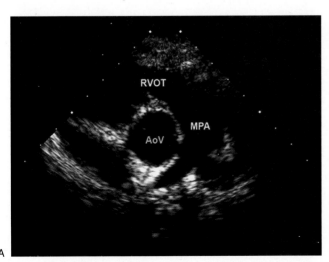
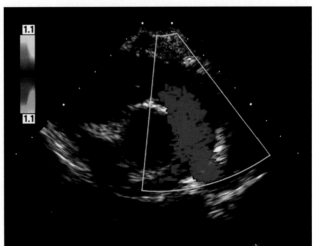

FIGURE 15.12. Branch pulmonary arteries in tetralogy of Fallot (TOF). A: Parasternal short-axis scan demonstrating right ventricular outflow tract (RVOT), main pulmonary artery (MPA), and branch pulmonary arteries after TOF repair. **B:** Laminar color flow Doppler across the RVOT into the pulmonary arteries.

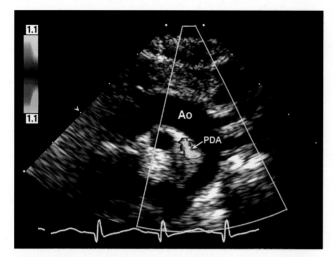

FIGURE 15.13. Suprasternal long-axis scan demonstrating origin of a patent ductus arteriosus (PDA) from the proximal descending aorta in tetralogy of Fallot. The aortic arch was left sided in this patient. Ao, aorta.

probes and particularly the nonimaging probe for high-quality Doppler analysis. It should also be noted that in the presence of a large patent ductus arteriosus, the RVOT gradient may be underestimated. Similarly, the gradient is sometimes low in the neonatal period despite significant obstruction due to elevated "downstream" pulmonary arteriolar resistance.

Finally, the side of the aortic arch must be defined. Up to 25% to 30% of patients with TOF have a right-sided aortic arch, usually with mirror image branching. A right aortic arch is more common with increasing degrees of RVOT obstruction. The suprasternal short-axis sweep will optimally define this anomaly. In patients with a right aortic arch, the first brachiocephalic branch travels to the left and bifurcates into the left common carotid and left subclavian arteries (if there is mirror-image branching). In addition, the tracheal air column can often be identified and the arch can be noted to extend to the right of the tracheal air-column.

Coronary Arteries

Up to 10% of patients with TOF have coronary artery anomalies that may potentially affect surgical management. The unifying feature of important coronary artery anomalies is the presence of a coronary artery crossing the RVOT (Fig. 15.16A–B). A prominent conal branch is frequently seen arising from the right coronary artery that supplies

the infundibulum. More important, the anterior descending coronary artery may arise from the right coronary artery. There may be paired anterior descending coronary arteries; one from the right coronary artery and one from the left coronary artery. A prominent conal branch can be differentiated from an anterior descending artery in that a conal branch terminates in the infundibulum, while an anterior descending coronary artery will occupy the interventricular groove.

TETRALOGY OF FALLOT WITH ABSENT PULMONARY VALVE SYNDROME

A small subset of patients with TOF have an "absent pulmonary valve" in which the pulmonary valve annulus is represented by dysplastic tissue. This dysplastic tissue is often obstructive but is always regurgitant. Severe pulmonary regurgitation is present, even in the fetus, leading to RV dilation. The pulmonary arteries are characteristically aneurysmally dilated, and this severe dilation often negatively affects pulmonary development. The ductus arteriosus is frequently absent. It has been hypothesized that during gestation, in the absence of the normal pulmonary valve, aortic outflow returns back through the ductus arteriosus to the right ventricle and then returns to the left ventricle through the VSD, thus creating the pathophysiology of severe aortic regurgitation. This "circular shunt" may be incompatible with fetal life. Clinically, postnatal respiratory symptoms are often more severe than cardiac symptoms. The echocardiographic examination demonstrates intracardiac anatomy very similar to TOF with pulmonary stenosis; however, the pulmonary annulus is represented by dysplastic remnants of tissue and the main and branch pulmonary arteries are massively dilated. The surgical repair of this condition involves restoration of pulmonary valve competency using a valved conduit, often a pulmonary homograft. The pulmonary arteries characteristically need reduction arterioplasty.

SURGICAL MANAGEMENT OF TETRALOGY OF FALLOT

TOF was one of the first congenital heart lesions to undergo surgical correction. However, high mortality was reported in this early surgical era that was related to many factors including difficulties with cardiopulmonary bypass techniques. This led to the widespread adoption of a two-stage repair strategy including an initial palliative systemic-to-pulmonary artery shunt performed early in infancy and a subsequent complete repair performed later in infancy or childhood. Introduction of systemic to pulmonary artery shunts, such as the Blalock-Taussig shunt in 1945, was devised as a method of providing palliation to severely affected patients. Subsequently, the Potts (1946) and Waterston (1962) shunts were introduced. Both of

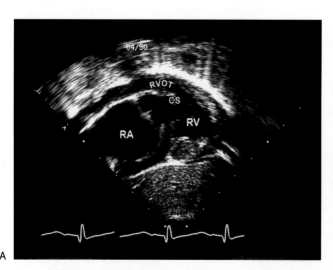
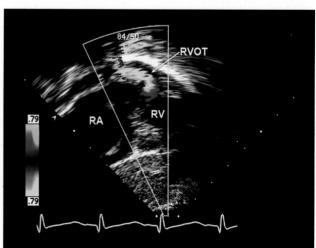

FIGURE 15.14. Modified subcostal four-chamber view in tetralogy of Fallot. A: Anterior deviation of the conal septum (CS) into the right ventricular outflow tract (RVOT). B: Color Doppler demonstrates aliased flow in the RVOT. RV, right ventricle; RA, right atrium.

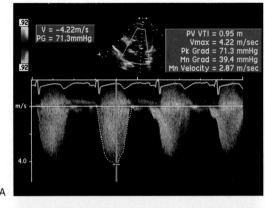

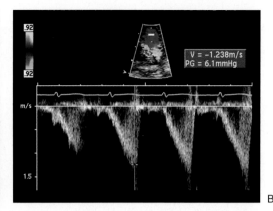

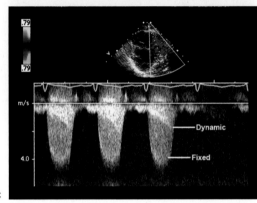

FIGURE 15.15. Evaluation of right ventricular outflow tract (RVOT) obstruction in tetralogy of Fallot. A: Continuous-wave Doppler interrogation across the RVOT and pulmonary artery from a parasternal short-axis orientation. Note both the peak gradient and mean gradient are assessed. **B:** Pulsed-wave Doppler in the RVOT proximal to the pulmonary valve demonstrates a late peaking Doppler profile consistent with mild dynamic RVOT obstruction. **C:** Continuous-wave Doppler demonstrating both Doppler profiles (dynamic and fixed RVOT obstruction) within the same signal.

these palliations were subsequently found to have a high incidence of pulmonary arterial hypertension and pulmonary arterial distortion. Subsequently, the classic Blalock-Taussig shunt was gradually replaced by the modified Blalock-Taussig shunt using a GORE-TEX interposition graft. This graft was naturally restrictive, thus providing controlled pulmonary blood flow and a lower risk of pulmonary artery distortion.

The surgical approach for complete repair of TOF continues to evolve. The initial intracardiac repair for TOF was performed by Lillehei and colleagues in 1954 using controlled cross-circulation, while the first successful repair using a heart-lung machine was made by Kirklin and colleagues in 1955. With improving surgical results, the age at complete repair has been gradually decreasing and presently surgery is routinely done in early infancy. The emphasis in this early surgical area had been complete relief of RVOT obstruction, even at the cost of creating free pulmonary regurgitation. It is now well recognized that severe pulmonary regurgitation is not well tolerated in the long term. Late postoperative sequelae of cardiac arrhythmias, RV dysfunction, tricuspid valve insufficiency, and sudden cardiac death tend to be more frequent with greater

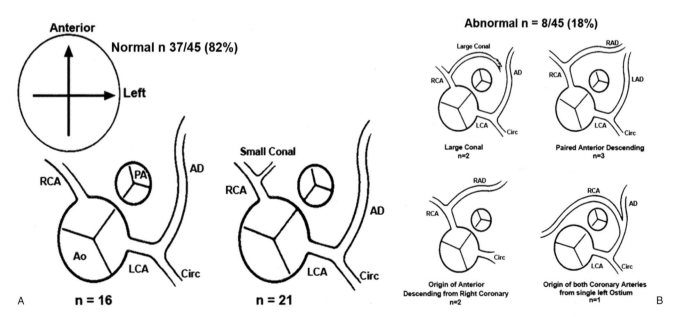

FIGURE 15.16. Tetralogy of Fallot. A: Normal coronary arterial patterns in tetralogy of Fallot. **B:** Major coronary artery anomalies in tetralogy of Fallot. (Adapted with permission from Jureidini SB, Appleton RS, Nouri S. Detection of coronary artery abnormalities in tetralogy of Fallot by two-dimensional echocardiography. *J Am Coll Cardiol.* 1989;14:960–967.)

severity of pulmonary regurgitation and RV dilation. Thus, the surgical emphasis has changed from complete relief of RVOT obstruction to preservation of a competent pulmonary valve, if possible, even at the expense of mild residual RVOT obstruction.

While this may represent an oversimplification of a complex surgical decision-making process, the major surgical repair goals remain the same: closure of the VSD, relief of RVOT obstruction, and, if possible, preservation of pulmonary valve competency. A patent foramen ovale or small ASD may, at times, be intentionally left to act as a "pop-off" valve for the right ventricle, particularly if there is significant RV hypertrophy. This may facilitate the postoperative management by augmenting systemic cardiac output at the expense of mild arterial desaturation. If there is a patent ductus arteriosus, it is generally ligated.

SURGICAL REPAIR OF TETRALOGY OF FALLOT

1. **Systemic-pulmonary artery shunt:** A modified Blalock-Taussig shunt may be performed either through a left thoracotomy or via a midline sternotomy. Currently, this staging palliation is less commonly performed due to excellent surgical outcomes following complete repair of TOF in infancy. However, if the neonate is premature or of low birth weight with significant cyanosis or hypercyanotic spells, a palliative Blalock-Taussig shunt may be considered. Contraindications to cardiopulmonary bypass may also lead to consideration of a palliative systemic-pulmonary shunt. The presence of coronary artery anomalies that require an RV–pulmonary artery conduit placement may also be an indication for a primary shunt procedure to allow an eventual larger right ventricle–to–pulmonary artery conduit.

2. **Right ventricular outflow tract patch:** In patients who have an adequate sized pulmonary annulus, VSD closure is performed followed by resection of muscle from within the RVOT. Augmentation with an RVOT patch that does not include incision across the pulmonary annulus (to preserve pulmonary valve competency) may also be performed. A concomitant pulmonary valvotomy may be performed to relieve valvar stenosis. This is generally the method of choice when pulmonary valve annular z-score is greater than –2 SD.

3. **Transannular RVOT patch:** In patients with significant pulmonary annular hypoplasia, a transannular extension of the RVOT patch repair may be needed. This involves incising the pulmonary valve annulus in addition to the RVOT with placement of an onlaid patch. This often effectively relieves RVOT obstruction but leaves the patient with severe regurgitation, likely necessitating future pulmonary valve replacement. This approach is generally used in patients with a pulmonary valve annular z-score of –2 SD or less. More recently, some surgeons have advocated the placement of a monocusp valve (using a very thin patch of GORE-TEX) within the outer transannular patch to function as a temporary "valve" due to its redundancy. Although these monocusp valves tend to degenerate in the early postoperative period, the absence of free pulmonary regurgitation following surgical repair is thought to aid the immediate postoperative course.

4. **Right ventricle–to–pulmonary artery conduit repair:** In simple anatomical variants of TOF, a RV–pulmonary artery conduit repair is uncommon, except in the presence of an anomalous coronary artery that crosses the infundibulum and precludes an incision in the RVOT. Rarely, complex multilevel obstruction may exist including chordal attachments or complex subvalvar stenosis that may be best managed by RV–pulmonary artery conduit placement.

POSTOPERATIVE ECHOCARDIOGRAPHIC EXAMINATION

With continually improving surgical outcomes after TOF repair, there is an ever-increasing number of patients who present for postoperative evaluation. The key areas of interest in the postoperative period include evaluation for residual intracardiac shunts (Fig. 15.17A–D) (atrial or ventricular), the presence of a pericardial effusion (early

postoperative examination), detailed anatomical assessment of the RVOT, and serial quantitative evaluation of ventricular size and function.

Residual Shunts

Residual VSDs are often identified at the margins of the VSD patch and, unless they are large, are not well seen with two-dimensional imaging alone. Color flow Doppler typically demonstrates a left-to-right shunt (because the RVOT obstruction is largely relieved). Continuous-wave Doppler interrogation of the late systolic VSD jet provides an estimation of the left ventricle–to–right ventricle pressure gradient. The early systolic gradient is generally unreliable due to delayed activation of the right ventricle with concomitant postoperative right bundle branch block. These small VSD patch defects often resolve over a period of several months due to endothelialization of the VSD patch. It is also important to recognize the presence of additional muscular defects that may be identified for the first time after surgical VSD closure. These small muscular defects are often missed before surgical repair due to equal ventricular pressures. Parasternal long- and short-axis views as well as the apical five-chamber view are optimal for identifying these residual defects and for Doppler interrogation. Coronary artery fistulas may also be seen after RVOT muscle resection and are characterized by continuous or predominantly diastolic Doppler flow signals into the right ventricle. The atrial septum should be interrogated to determine if an atrial level shunt persists. The direction of atrial shunting should also be assessed.

Assessment of the Right Ventricular Outflow Tract

There may be persistent RVOT obstruction after surgical repair of TOF. It is important to optimally define the location(s) of this obstruction at the subvalvar, valvar, or supravalvar level(s). Assessment of the peak and mean outflow gradient should be assessed by continuous-wave Doppler interrogation. If there is sufficient tricuspid regurgitation, the estimated RV systolic pressure serves as a validation to corroborate the measured RVOT gradient (Fig. 15.18A–B). In case of discrepancy, it is important to remember that the derived RV pressure estimate by tricuspid regurgitation is usually more accurate.

Assessment of the branch pulmonary arteries is important since there can be distal stenoses. Although the visualization of branch pulmonary artery anatomy may be problematic in the older postoperative patient, a combination of parasternal short-axis, high left and right parasternal, and suprasternal views may allow adequate noninvasive assessment of this anatomy. With increasing frequency, centers have begun to use computed tomography (CT) or magnetic resonance imaging (MRI) to delineate more accurately the presence and severity of distal pulmonary arterial branch obstruction in patients with limited postoperative echocardiographic windows.

The assessment of pulmonary regurgitation is a critical part of the serial noninvasive evaluation of the postoperative TOF patient (Fig. 15.11A–B). The key echocardiographic features of severe pulmonary regurgitation include the following:

- Laminar, low-velocity regurgitant flow by color Doppler
- Diastolic flow reversal in the branch pulmonary arteries (Fig. 15.11A)
- The pulsed-wave Doppler signal of pulmonary regurgitation demonstrates a rapid return to baseline (Fig. 15.11B). Physiologically, this implies that the pulmonary artery pressure is equal to RV pressure early in diastole.

It is important to exclude "downstream" obstruction, such as pulmonary artery branch stenosis, that can exacerbate the severity of pulmonary regurgitation. With severe pulmonary regurgitation, there is often an increased systolic outflow Doppler velocity across the RVOT and pulmonary valve in the absence of obstruction secondary to the increased RV stroke volume. Typically, this Doppler velocity does not exceed 2.5 m/s.

Assessment of Right Ventricular Systolic Function

The anatomical and hemodynamic consequences of severe pulmonary valve regurgitation over a prolonged period of time include RV dilation (Fig. 15.19A–C), hypertrophy, and dysfunction. Accurate

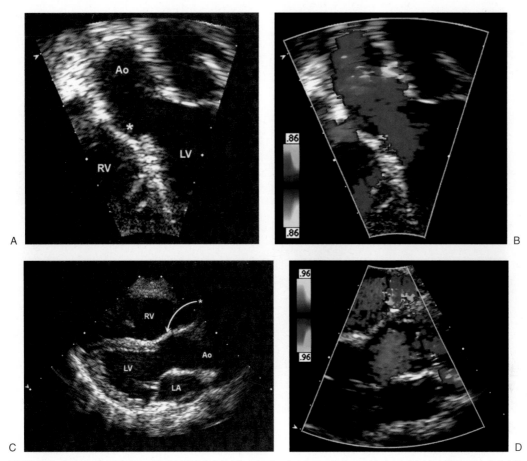

FIGURE 15.17. Postoperative tetralogy of Fallot (TOF). A: Apical five-chamber view demonstrating ventricular septal defect (VSD) patch *(asterisk)* repair in TOF. **B:** Color Doppler interrogation reveals and intact VSD patch without residual intracardiac shunting. **C:** Parasternal long-axis scan in same patient demonstrating the VSD patch repair. **D:** Color Doppler interrogation again reveals no evidence of residual shunting around the VSD patch. Ao, aorta; RV, right ventricle; LV, left ventricle.

assessment of RV size and function remains important. This is particularly important because indications for pulmonary valve replacement following TOF repair include the development of RV dysfunction or progressive RV dilation. However, unlike the left ventricle, there are many inherent limitations in the ability to assess the right ventricle by two-dimensional echocardiography. These limitations include the following:

- The shape of the right ventricle is complex and precludes geometric assumptions that are used in calculating LV systolic function.

- Due to the proximity of the right ventricle to the anterior chest wall, there is an inherent limitation in image resolution due to near-field effects. This limited resolution particularly affects evaluation of the anterior wall of the right ventricle.
- The three parts of the right ventricle namely, the inlet, the body, and the outlet (infundibulum) are typically not imaged together in any one echocardiographic plane. Thus, two-dimensional assessment has to include multiple echocardiographic planes, which are often limited following surgical repair and in older individuals.

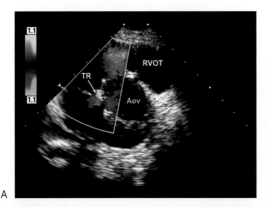
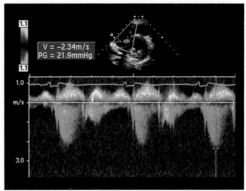

FIGURE 15.18. Tricuspid regurgitation in postoperative tetralogy of Fallot (TOF). A: Parasternal short-axis scan demonstrating eccentric tricuspid regurgitation (TR) along the site of ventricular septal defect (VSD) repair *(asterisk)*. TR should not be confused with a residual intracardiac shunt. **B:** Continuous-wave Doppler interrogation of TR predicting normal right ventricular pressure post TOF repair (22 mm Hg + right atrial pressure). AoV, aortic valve; RVOT, right ventricular outflow tract.

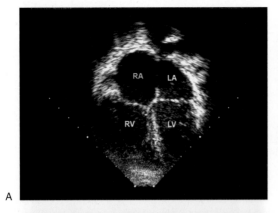

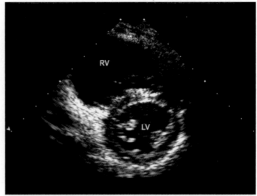

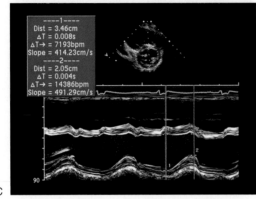

FIGURE 15.19. Right ventricular (RV) dilatation after tetralogy of Fallot repair. A: Apical four-chamber view demonstrating significant RV enlargement. **B:** Parasternal short-axis scan demonstrating RV dilatation. **C:** M-mode demonstrating paradoxical septal wall motion secondary to RV volume overload. RA, right atrium; RV, right ventricle; LA, left atrium; LV, left ventricle.

Due to these issues, there have been a multitude of parameters that have been suggested to quantify systolic function of the right ventricle. Some of these methodologies are presented next.

Fractional Area Change

Fractional area change (FAC) is measured by planimetry of the area of the right ventricle, typically in the apical four-chamber view. FAC has been shown to correlate with MRI-derived ejection fraction. Limitations of this methodology include the need to visualize the entire endocardial border, which may be difficult in some patients, and the lack of inclusion of the RV infundibular region in the functional assessment. Also, FAC in the parasternal short-axis view has not been adequately validated and likely has low reproducibility because the exact level at which FAC is determined may differ between studies and between examiners. Using FAC also assumes uniformity of function throughout the right ventricle, which may not be the case. In addition, it is not uncommon to see discrepant results between FAC in the apical four-chamber view and the parasternal short-axis view, because the two represent contraction in different echocardiographic planes. Normal FAC in the apical four-chamber view ranges from 32% to 60%.

Tricuspid Annular Systolic Plane Excursion

Because the fibers of the right ventricle are predominantly longitudinal in orientation (unlike the left ventricle, which has primarily circumferential fibers), systolic shortening in the RV occurs primarily in the ventricular long axis. Tricuspid annular systolic plane excursion (TASPE) has been used as an index of RV function. In adults, normal TASPE determined by M-mode echocardiography is approximately 1.5 to 2.0 cm. TAPSE has not been extensively validated in pediatric studies.

Myocardial Performance Index

The myocardial performance index (MPI), also termed the Tei index, is a Doppler-derived measure of combined systolic and diastolic ventricular function. This index can often be measured even if the anatomical two-dimensional images of the right ventricle are suboptimal. The MPI is calculated as follows:

$$MPI = \frac{ICT + IRT}{ET}$$

where ICT is isovolumic contraction time, IRT is isovolumic relaxation time, and ET is ejection time.

In practice, ICT + IRT + ET is equal to atrioventricular (AV) valve closure to opening time, which is easily measured from the pulsed-wave Doppler inflow signal (tricuspid inflow for the right ventricle, mitral inflow for the left ventricle). The ejection time is measured from the pulsed-wave Doppler signal across the semilunar valve (pulmonary valve for the right ventricle, aortic valve for the left ventricle). The equation can be simplified to:

$$MPI = \frac{[AV \text{ valve closure to opening time}] - [\text{ejection time}]}{\text{Ejection time}}$$

In general, a MPI greater than 0.35 ± 0.05 is abnormal for either ventricle.

Tissue Doppler Imaging

Tissue Doppler echocardiography involves the measurement of myocardial velocities during different phases of the cardiac cycle. Signals from the blood pool are filtered out and only signals from myocardial motion are analyzed. Three distinct waves are generally recognized: the systolic (s') wave, the early diastolic wave (e'), and the late diastolic (a') wave. Higher velocities generally correlate with better ventricular function. Normative values have been established for pediatric and adult populations. In addition, the isovolumic acceleration (IVA) can also be calculated by dividing the peak isovolumic velocity by the time to peak velocity. IVA has been proposed as a relatively load-independent index of ventricular function and can be applied to both left ventricular and RV functional assessment.

Strain and Strain Rate Imaging

Strain and strain rate imaging are relatively new tools that measure myocardial deformation. *Strain* is the change in the length of an object (e.g., the myocardium) with respect to its original length, while the rate of change is termed *strain rate*. These indices are used as a measure of regional myocardial function. Strain can be derived by both Doppler technology and tissue tracking technology, which has the advantage of being angle independent (unlike Doppler-derived strain). Commercially available software is now readily available to analyze strain and strain rate. Relatively small studies have established normal values of strain and strain rate in children and adolescents. Abnormalities of strain and strain rate have been demonstrated in patients after repair of TOF.

Three-dimensional Echocardiography

The use of three-dimensional echocardiography in the assessment of RV volume and function is now well established. Studies have shown good correlation between three-dimensional echo–derived ejection fraction and cardiac MRI. Software for the analysis of RV volumes is now commercially available.

In clinical practice, echocardiographers use a variety of methodologies to determine RV size and function. More recently, cardiac MRI and CT have been shown to provide accurate quantitative assessment of RV volume and function. These evaluations are most commonly performed before planned surgical intervention to corroborate the findings of echocardiography. MRI and CT do not have inherent limitations such as poor echocardiographic windows and do not depend on geometric assumptions to calculate ventricular volumes and function.

Assessment of right ventricular diastolic function

The quantitative assessment of RV diastolic function in patients with TOF also is challenging from an echocardiographic perspective. Evidence of restrictive RV filling can be demonstrated by pulsed-wave Doppler interrogation within the RVOT and proximal main pulmonary artery (Fig. 15.20). The presence of antegrade flow into the main pulmonary artery with atrial contraction is the Doppler hallmark of a "stiff" noncompliant RV. Tissue Doppler echocardiography has also been shown to demonstrate abnormalities of RV diastolic function in patients after TOF repair.

 ## CONCLUSION

TOF is one of the most common cyanotic congenital heart defects. Accurate anatomical and physiologic delineation is mandatory before

surgical repair, and with high-quality echocardiographic evaluation, the need for angiography and cardiac catheterization can be largely avoided. Careful postoperative surveillance after repair of TOF is critical. Timing of late postoperative pulmonary valve replacement remains a matter of controversy and is discussed later in this text.

SUGGESTED READING

Anderson RH, Weinberg PM. The clinical anatomy of tetralogy of fallot. *Cardiol Young.* 2005;15(Suppl 1):38–47.
Berry JM Jr, Einzig S, Krabill KA, et al. Evaluation of coronary artery anatomy in patients with tetralogy of Fallot by two-dimensional echocardiography. *Circulation.* 1988;78:149–156.
Blalock A, Taussig HB. The surgical treatment of malformations of the heart in which there is pulmonary stenosis or pulmonary atresia. *JAMA.* 1945;128:189–202.
Dabizzi RP, Caprioli G, Aiazzi L, et al. Distribution and anomalies of coronary arteries in tetralogy of Fallot. *Circulation.* 1980;61:95–102.
D'Hooge J, Heimdal A, Jamal F, et al. Regional strain and strain rate measurements by cardiac ultrasound: principles, implementation and limitations [erratum appears in *Eur J Echocardiogr.* 2000;1:295–299]. *Eur J Echocardiogr.* 2000;1:154–170.
Eidem BW, McMahon CJ, Cohen RR, et al. Impact of cardiac growth on Doppler tissue imaging velocities: a study in healthy children. *J Am Soc Echocardiogr.* 2004;17:212–221.
Ettedgui JA, Sharland GK, Chita SK, et al. Absent pulmonary valve syndrome with ventricular septal defect: role of the arterial duct. *Am J Cardiol.* 1990;66:233–234.
Fellows KE, Freed MD, Keane JF, et al. Results of routine preoperative coronary angiography in tetralogy of Fallot. *Circulation.* 1975;51:561–566.
Gatzoulis MA, Balaji S, Webber SA, et al. Risk factors for arrhythmia and sudden cardiac death late after repair of tetralogy of Fallot: a multicentre study. *Lancet.* 2000;356:975–981.
Gladman G, McCrindle BW, Williams WG, et al. The modified Blalock-Taussig shunt: clinical impact and morbidity in Fallot's tetralogy in the current era. *J. Thorac Cardiovasc Surg.* 1997;114:25–30.
Harada K, Toyono M, Yamamoto F. Assessment of right ventricular function during exercise with quantitative Doppler tissue imaging in children late after repair of tetralogy of Fallot. *J Am Soc Echocardiogr.* 2004;17:863–869.
Hui W, Abd El Rahman MY, Dsebissowa F, et al. Comparison of modified short axis view and apical four chamber view in evaluating right ventricular function after repair of tetralogy of Fallot. *Int J Cardiol.* 2005;105:256–261.
Jonas RA. Tetralogy of Fallot with pulmonary stenosis. In: Jonas RA, ed. *Comprehensive surgical management of congenital heart disease.* London: Arnold; 2004:279–300.
Kirklin JW, Blackstone EH, Pacifico AD, et al. Routine primary repair vs two-stage repair of tetralogy of Fallot. *Circulation.* 1979;60:373–386.
Kirklin JW, DuShane JW, Patrick RT, et al. Intracardiac surgery with the aid of a mechanical pump-oxygenator system (Gibbon type): report of eight cases. *Proc Mayo Clin.* 1955;30:201.
Lang RM, Bierig M, Devereux RB, et al. Recommendations for chamber quantification: a report from the American Society of Echocardiography's Guidelines and Standards Committee and the Chamber Quantification Writing Group, developed in conjunction with the European Association of Echocardiography, a branch of the European Society of Cardiology. *J Am Soc Echocardiogr.* 2005;18:1440–1463.
Lillehei CW, Cohen M, Warden HE, et al. Direct vision intracardiac surgical correction of the tetralogy of Fallot, pentalogy of Fallot, and pulmonary atresia defects; report of first ten cases. *Ann Surg.* 1955;142:418–442.
Morris DC, Felner JM, Schlant RC, et al. Echocardiographic diagnosis of tetralogy of Fallot. *Am J Cardiol.* 1975;36:908–913.
Murphy JG, Gersh BJ, Mair DD, et al. Long-term outcome in patients undergoing surgical repair of tetralogy of Fallot. *N Engl J Med.* 1993;329:593–599.
Papavassiliou DP, Parks WJ, Hopkins KL, et al. Three-dimensional echocardiographic measurement of right ventricular volume in children with congenital heart disease validated by magnetic resonance imaging. *J Am Soc Echocardiogr.* 1998;11:770–777.
Pigula FA, Khalil PN, Mayer JE, et al. Repair of tetralogy of Fallot in neonates and young infants. *Circulation.* 1999;100(19 Suppl):II157–II161.
Potts WJ, Smith S, Gibson S. Anastomosis of the ascending aorta to a pulmonary artery. *JAMA.* 1946;132:627–631.
Reddy VM, Liddicoat JR, McElhinney DB, et al. Routine primary repair of tetralogy of Fallot in neonates and infants less than three months of age. *Ann Thorac Surg.* 1995;60(6 Suppl):S592–S596.
Schwerzmann M, Samman AM, Salehian O, et al. Comparison of echocardiographic and cardiac magnetic resonance imaging for assessing right ventricular function in adults with repaired tetralogy of Fallot. *Am J Cardiol.* 2007;99:1593–1597.
Silvilairat S, Cabalka AK, Cetta F, et al. Echocardiographic assessment of isolated pulmonary valve stenosis: which outpatient Doppler gradient has the most clinical validity? *J Am Soc Echocardiogr.* 2005;18:1137–1142.

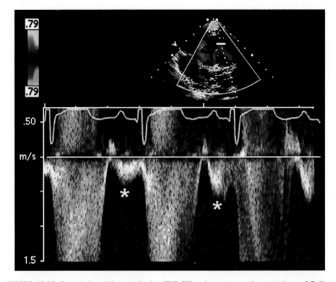

FIGURE 15.20. Restrictive right ventricular (RV) filling in postoperative tetralogy of Fallot. Parasternal short-axis scan with pulsed-wave Doppler interrogation in the main pulmonary artery. Note the antegrade forward flow *(asterisk)* into the pulmonary artery with atrial contraction. This Doppler pattern is consistent with decreased RV compliance.

Silvilairat S, Cabalka AK, Cetta F, et al. Outpatient echocardiographic assessment of complex pulmonary outflow stenosis: Doppler mean gradient is superior to the maximum instantaneous gradient. *J Am Soc Echocardiogr.* 2005;18:1143–1148.

Siwik ES, Patel CR, Zahka KG. Epidemiology and genetics [by Goldmuntz E]. In: Allen HD, Gutgesell HP, Clark EB, et al, eds. *Heart disease in infants, children and adolescents.* 6th ed. Philadelphia: Lippincott Williams & Wilkins, 2001:880–902.

Snider RA, Serwer GA, Ritter SB. *Echocardiography in pediatric heart disease.* 2nd ed. St. Louis: Mosby; 1997.

Therrien J, Provost Y, Merchant N, et al. Optimal timing for pulmonary valve replacement in adults after tetralogy of Fallot repair. *Am J Cardiol.* 2005;95:779–782.

Uretzky G, Puga FJ, Danielson GK, et al. Complete atrioventricular canal associated with tetralogy of Fallot. Morphologic and surgical considerations. *J Thorac Cardiovasc Surg.* 1984;87:756–766.

van Straten A, Vliegen HW, Lamb HJ, et al. Time course of diastolic and systolic function improvement after pulmonary valve replacement in adult patients with tetralogy of Fallot. *J Am Coll Cardiol.* 2005;46:1559–1564.

Vick GW 3rd, Serwer GA. Echocardiographic evaluation of the postoperative tetralogy of Fallot patient. *Circulation.* 1978;58:842–849.

Vogel M, Cheung MM, Li J, et al. Noninvasive assessment of left ventricular force-frequency relationships using tissue Doppler-derived isovolumic acceleration: validation in an animal model. *Circulation.* 2003;107:1647–1652.

Waterston DJ, Stark J, Ashcraft KW. Ascending aorta-to-right pulmonary artery shunts: experience with 100 patients. Surgery. 1972;72:897–904.

Weidemann F, Eyskens B, Jamal F, et al. Quantification of regional left and right ventricular radial and longitudinal function in healthy children using ultrasound-based strain rate and strain imaging. *J Am Soc Echocardiogr.* 2002;15:20–28.

Weidemann F, Eyskens B, Mertens L, et al. Quantification of regional right and left ventricular function by ultrasonic strain rate and strain indexes after surgical repair of tetralogy of Fallot. *Am J Cardiol.* 2002;90:133–138.

Zilberman MV, Khoury PR, Kimball RT. Two-dimensional echocardiographic valve measurements in healthy children: gender-specific differences. *Pediatr Cardiol.* 2005;26:356–360.

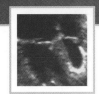

Chapter 16
d-Transposition of the Great Arteries

Amy H. Schultz • Mark B. Lewin

CLINICAL PRESENTATION

d-Transposition of the great arteries (*d*-TGA) is one of the two most common forms of cyanotic congenital heart disease, with tetralogy of Fallot having comparable incidence. In a population-based series, the incidence of *d*-TGA is 20 to 22 per 100,000 live births. Typically, neonates with *d*-TGA present in the first day or two of life with cyanosis without significant respiratory distress. Frequently no cardiac murmur is present, particularly in the absence of a ventricular septal defect (VSD). The electrocardiogram and chest radiograph can also appear normal. If a VSD or outflow tract obstruction is present, a murmur characteristic of these associated lesions may be present.

Maintenance of a compensated clinical state is dependent on adequate mixing between the pulmonary and systemic circuits. Neonates with an intact atrial septum or very restrictive patent foramen ovale can present with profound cyanosis and findings consistent with low cardiac output in the delivery room. Those whose intercirculatory mixing is initially augmented by a patent ductus arteriosus (PDA) can develop worsening cyanosis and low cardiac output as the ductus constricts. Uncommonly, neonates with *d*-TGA who have good intercirculatory mixing escape notice in the first few days of life and may present later with signs of heart failure, typically accompanied by a murmur originating from either excessive flow across the left ventricular outflow tract or across a VSD.

Diagnosis by fetal echocardiography is another mode of presentation, generally prompted by abnormal findings on a routine obstetric screening ultrasound. Prenatal detection of *d*-TGA by echocardiography requires examination of the outflow tracts, as examining only the number and size of cardiac chambers will not detect this anomaly (Figs 16.1 to 16.4). The frequency of antenatal diagnosis of *d*-TGA varies considerably.

ANATOMY AND PHYSIOLOGY

In *d*-TGA, the atrial situs, atrioventricular alignments, and ventricular looping are all normal. TGA is present, meaning that the aorta

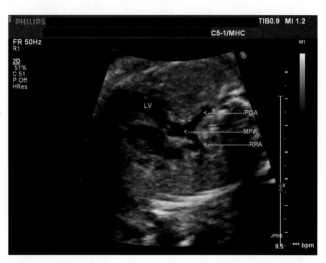

FIGURE 16.2. Fetal *d*-transposition of the great arteries (*d*-TGA) at 20 weeks' gestation demonstrates a well developed pulmonary artery arising posteriorly from the left ventricular chamber. The patent ductus arteriosus is directed posteriorly toward the spine, and the right pulmonary artery branch is also seen.

arises from the right ventricle while the pulmonary artery arises from the left ventricle (Fig. 16.5). The designation *d*- refers to the relative positions of the aortic and pulmonary valves; *d*- (*dextro*-) indicates that the aortic valve is rightward of the pulmonary valve, in accordance with the convention established by Van Praagh. There may be other associated malformations, most commonly the presence of a VSD, which occurs in approximately 35% to 40% of cases and can be of various anatomical types.

The physiologic consequence of these anatomic relationships is that two parallel circulations are established. Systemic venous blood returns to the right atrium and then there passes to the right ventricle and aorta and back to the systemic arterial bed without being oxygenated. Pulmonary venous blood returns to the left atrium and

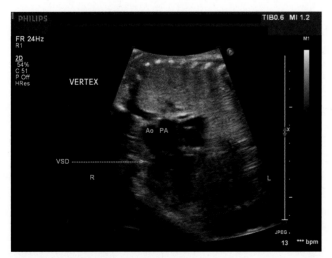

FIGURE 16.1. Fetal echocardiogram performed at 20 weeks' gestation. Imaging from the four-chamber view, directed anteriorly, demonstrates the parallel nature of the great arteries. The great vessels appear symmetrical with a large outlet ventricular septal defect positioned directly below the semilunar valves.

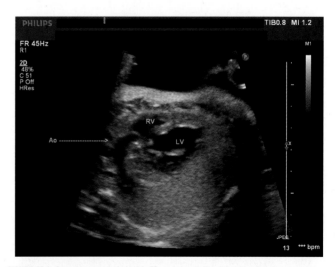

FIGURE 16.3. Scanning anteriorly in this 20 weeks gestation fetus, the anterior aorta is seen to arise from the right ventricle. Two head-and-neck vessels are seen originating from the transverse aortic arch, confirming this as the true aortic arch. A ventricular septal defect is noted in the region of the outlet septum.

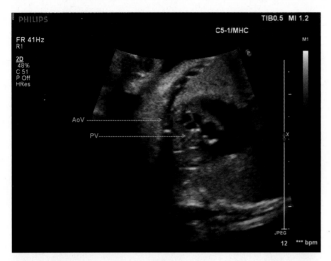

FIGURE 16.4. Short-axis view of the semilunar valves. The aortic valve is seen to be trileaflet and positioned anterior and rightward relative to the pulmonary valve.

thereafter passes to the left ventricle, pulmonary artery, and pulmonary arterial bed without any opportunity to deliver its oxygen cargo. This arrangement is only compatible with life if some intercirculatory mixing (bidirectional shunting) is present. Mixing can occur via an interatrial communication (patent foramen ovale or true atrial septal defect), VSD, or PDA but is most effective across an atrial septal defect.

 COMPLICATIONS

The preferred operative approach in the current era for management of *d*-TGA is the arterial switch operation (ASO). Thus, any anatomical feature that makes performing an ASO difficult or impossible is important for the echocardiographer to identify. In this operation,

both great vessels are transected, the branch pulmonary arteries are brought anterior to the neoaortic root (LeCompte maneuver), the coronary arteries are transferred from the native aortic root to the neoaortic root, and the great vessels are reanastomosed in the "switched" position (Fig. 16.6). Obstruction of either outflow tract, abnormalities of the pulmonary valve (which would function as the neoaortic valve after ASO), certain coronary patterns, nonfacing sinuses of the semilunar valves, and straddling of the tricuspid valve through a VSD are examples of such anatomical features that may preclude an ASO. Multiple muscular VSDs may be difficult to close and thus affect the management strategy. Aortic arch obstruction needs to be identified so that it can be appropriately addressed at surgery.

Late clinical presentations of *d*-TGA raise additional concerns that need to be addressed before proceeding with ASO. If the left ventricular systolic pressure is low, due to low pulmonary vascular resistance, the ability of the left ventricle to handle an acute transition to the pressure load of the systemic circulation must be assessed. Second, pulmonary vascular disease is known to develop at an accelerated rate in patients with *d*-TGA and should be a consideration in patients over several months of age.

The echocardiographer has an important role in evaluating patients who have previously undergone surgery for *d*-TGA. The ASO became the predominant surgical strategy at most institutions by the late 1980s, and thus the longest published longitudinal follow-up data available are at 15 to 20 years after ASO. As such data emerge, it has become apparent that important postoperative issues include coronary occlusion (symptomatic or asymptomatic) in 3% to 14%, stenosis at the great vessel anastomoses (supravalvar pulmonic stenosis being more common than supravalvar aortic stenosis [5% to 30% versus 2% to 5%]), neoaortic root dilation in about 50%, neoaortic insufficiency (trivial to mild, about 30%; moderate to severe, 1% to 7%), and uncommonly clinically significant bronchopulmonary collateral vessels. Rarely, patients who underwent ASO in the neonatal period present later with pulmonary arterial hypertension; the etiology of this phenomenon remains unclear.

Before the ASO era, patients were managed with an atrial level "switch," using either the Senning or Mustard technique. These two techniques involve rerouting systemic venous drainage to the mitral valve and pulmonary venous drainage to the tricuspid valve by way of intra-atrial baffles. The circulation is physiologically "corrected," but the right ventricle serves as the systemic ventricle while the left ventricle serves as the pulmonary ventricle. Late complications include sinus node dysfunction and other atrial arrhythmias (40% to 60%), baffle obstruction or leak (5% to 31%), right ventricular dysfunction (about 60% at 25-year follow-up), tricuspid regurgitation, and left ventricular outflow tract obstruction.

 BASICS OF ECHOCARDIOGRAPHIC ANATOMY AND IMAGING

Classic Two-dimensional Echocardiographic Anatomy and Hemodynamics

The diagnosis of *d*-TGA is established by demonstrating normal atrial situs, atrioventricular alignments, and ventricular looping, in association with ventriculoarterial discordance. The aorta arises from the right ventricle, while the pulmonary artery arises from the left ventricle. In most cases, the aortic valve is anterior and to the right of the pulmonary valve, and there is characteristically fibrous continuity between the pulmonary and mitral valve. With this fundamental anatomy established, the sonographer can then proceed to evaluate additional key anatomical features such as the presence or absence of VSD(s), coronary artery pattern, outflow tract and semilunar valve anatomy, and aortic arch anatomy.

Beginning with a two-dimensional subcostal frontal sweep allows the sonographer to establish atrioviscceral situs, atrioventricular alignments, and ventricular looping (Fig. 16.7). As the sweep is extended to the outflow tracts and great vessels, the more posterior semilunar valve arising from the left ventricle is seen to give rise to a great vessel that bifurcates, consistent with the pulmonary artery. The more anterior great vessel arises from the right

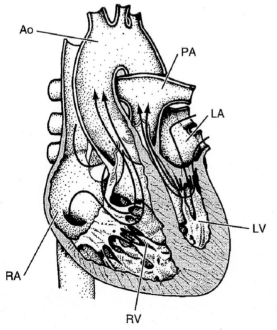

FIGURE 16.5. Schematic diagram of *d*-transposition of the great arteries (*d*-TGA). (Reprinted from Friedman WF, Silverman N: Congenital heart disease in infancy and childhood. In Braunwald E, Zipes DP, Libby P, eds. *Heart disease: a textbook of cardiovascular medicine*, 6th ed. Philadelphia: WB Saunders; 2001, with permission.)

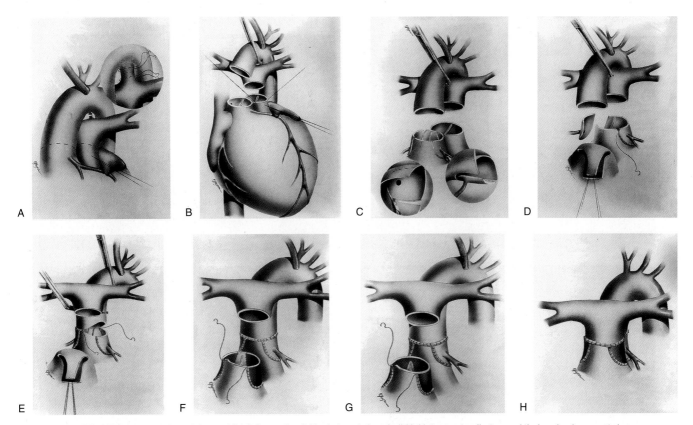

FIGURE 16.6. Surgical technique of the arterial switch operation. A: The ductus arteriosus is divided between suture ligatures and the branch pulmonary arteries are dissected out to the hilum to provide adequate mobility for anterior translocation. **B:** Transection of the great arteries. The left ventricular outflow tract, neoaortic valve, and coronary arteries are thoroughly inspected. **C:** The coronary arterial buttons are excised from the free edge of the aorta to the base of the sinus of Valsalva. **D:** The coronary buttons are anastomosed to V-shaped excisions made in the aorta. **E:** The pulmonary artery is brought anterior to the aorta (LeCompte maneuver). Anastomosis of the proximal neoaorta is shown. **F:** The coronary donor sites are filled with autologous pericardial patches. Two separate patches (F) or a single U-shaped patch (G) may be used. **G:** Anastomosis of the proximal neopulmonary artery and distal pulmonary artery. H: Completed anastomosis of the proximal neopulmonary artery and the distal pulmonary artery. (Reprinted from Wernovsky G. Transposition of the great arteries. In: Allen HD, Driscoll DJ, Shaddy RE, et al, eds. *Moss and Adams' Heart disease in infants, children, and adolescents.* 7th ed. Philadelphia: Lippincott Williams & Wilkins; 2008:1038–1087, with permission. Permission also obtained from the original source: Sabiston DC Jr, Spencer FC, eds. *Surgery of the chest.* Philadelphia: WB Saunders; 1990:1435–1446.)

ventricle and does not bifurcate, consistent with the aorta. This initial sweep also allows the sonographer to glean preliminary information about the size of the interatrial communication and the presence or absence of a VSD. Two-dimensional subcostal short-axis sweeps provide further opportunities to evaluate the atrial and ventricular septa and ventricular morphology and to visualize the parallel orientation of the great vessels (Fig. 16.8). The size of any interatrial communication or VSD should be measured. The coronary arteries may be visualized from various subcostal views. In particular, the subcostal frontal sweep is useful when the circumflex coronary artery arises from the right coronary artery and has a retropulmonary course (Fig. 16.9). Information about coronary arterial anatomy from subcostal views is usually complementary to that from the parasternal short-axis view. Color Doppler evaluation from subcostal views further defines shunting across an interatrial communication or VSD and provides information about atrioventricular and semilunar valve function (Fig. 16.10). Spectral Doppler interrogation of the PFO or ASD (with mean gradient) should be obtained from the subcostal frontal or short-axis view as well as spectral Doppler interrogation of the outflow tracts and semilunar valves.

For sonographers who start the study from a parasternal long-axis view, the characteristic parallel orientation of the two great vessels is readily apparent (Fig. 16.11), although this view does not provide as ready assessment of the normalcy of other aspects of the anatomy as the subcostal approach does. Pulmonary–mitral valve fibrous continuity is usually present in this view. From the parasternal long-axis view, the aortic and pulmonary annuli should

be measured in systole; the pulmonary valve annulus is normally slightly larger than the aortic valve annulus. Any abnormalities of the semilunar valve structure or function should be noted. Outflow tract obstruction or a malalignment-type VSD should be readily apparent. Color Doppler evaluation of all four cardiac valves should be performed.

Turning to the parasternal short-axis view, one notes the relative position of the aortic and pulmonary valves (Fig. 16.12). Typically, the aortic valve is anterior and slightly rightward of the pulmonary valve annulus, although the positions can range along a continuum from the aortic valve directly anterior to the pulmonary valve, to side-by-side great vessels (aortic valve rightward) to even an anterior leftward aortic valve position in a minority of cases. Again, any structural abnormality of the aortic or pulmonary valve should be noted. The intercoronary commissure of the aortic valve is most commonly directly aligned with the commissure of the pulmonary valve. If this is not the case, this should be communicated to the surgeon as it may complicate the coronary transfer.

The parasternal short-axis view is also the primary view from which the coronary arterial pattern is determined. This information is of paramount importance for surgical planning as certain coronary artery patterns may add significantly to the technical difficulty of the operation (see also "Key Findings that Alter Management" later). Several nomenclature schemes have been developed to describe coronary artery patterns in *d*-TGA; the most commonly used nomenclatures are the Leiden convention (Table 16.1) and the descriptive approach popularized by Children's Hospital Boston (Table 16.2,

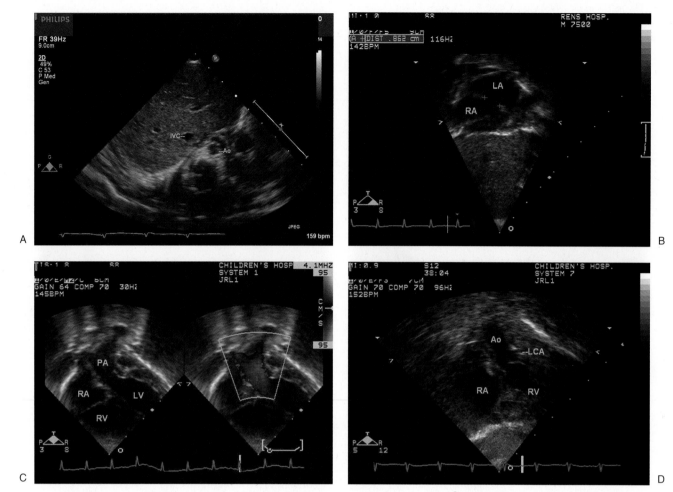

FIGURE 16.7. Subcostal four-chamber view. A: Transverse view through the liver demonstrates normal visceral situs with normal position of the inferior vena cava and aorta. **B:** View of the atria demonstrates the atrial situs and the atrial septal defect. In this case, a large communication after balloon atrial septostomy is demonstrated. **C:** With continued anterior angulation, the left ventricle is seen to give rise to the pulmonary artery. **D:** With extreme anterior angulation, the right ventricle is seen to give rise to the aorta, which courses superiorly and does not bifurcate.

Fig. 16.13). Yacoub and Radley-Smith also developed a nomenclature scheme in the 1970s (Types A through F), but this scheme is not comprehensive and is not further described in this text. The most common coronary artery patterns are shown in Figures 16.13, 16.14 and 16.15. Table 16.3 gives the relative frequencies of the most common coronary patterns. If coronary arterial anatomy is difficult to resolve, moving up one or two interspaces from the usual parasternal short-axis view ("high parasternal" view) may be helpful. The parasternal long-axis view, apical view, and subcostal views often add valuable complementary information (Figs. 16.9 and 16.16). Color Doppler with a low Nyquist value can be used to confirm the appropriate direction of flow within structures thought to be the coronary arteries.

A careful inspection of the ventricular septum for VSD(s) with two-dimensional imaging is also performed in the parasternal short-axis view (Fig. 16.17). If a VSD is present, its anatomical type is determined. Color Doppler interrogation of the ventricular septum confirms the presence or absence of VSD(s) as well as the direction of flow, which is frequently bidirectional in the neonate with *d*-TGA. If a VSD is present, spectral Doppler interrogation of the VSD jet allows estimation of the transventricular pressure gradient.

The apical views are most useful in *d*-TGA for assessing valvar function and ensuring normal ventricular sizes (Fig. 16.18). The great vessel arising from the left ventricle can be visualized to bifurcate, demonstrating that it is the pulmonary artery. The structure and function of the atrioventricular and semilunar valves are assessed with two-dimensional, color Doppler, and spectral Doppler

imaging. The apical view can also add some confirmatory information about coronary artery anatomy, particularly in the coronary variant in which the circumflex coronary artery arises from the right coronary artery and passes posterior to the pulmonary root. This course of the circumflex coronary artery can be seen on an apical sweep from posterior to anterior.

Long-axis suprasternal notch imaging provides the best view of the ductus arteriosus to assess its patency and size by two-dimensional imaging (Fig. 16.19). In addition, the aortic arch should be carefully inspected to rule out transverse arch hypoplasia or coarctation. Color flow Doppler demonstrates the direction of ductal flow as well as flow through the aortic arch. Pulsed-wave spectral Doppler interrogation within the ductus arteriosus further clarifies the pattern of shunting, which is typically predominantly from the aorta to pulmonary artery. Short-axis suprasternal notch imaging may be useful in clarifying coronary artery anatomy as well.

Generally, identification of *d*-TGA is straightforward for any sonographer who has at least some experience with congenital heart disease. Delineation of the coronary artery anatomy is much more challenging, given the small size and quite anterior location of the coronary arteries. Higher-frequency transducers with lower dynamic range settings may make the coronary arteries easier to visualize. At times, one sees linear, echo-free spaces in the vicinity of the semilunar valves, which are easily confused with the true coronary arteries. Confirmation that a structure truly represents a coronary artery can be made by demonstrating

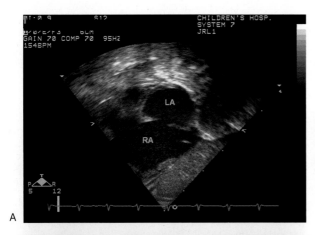

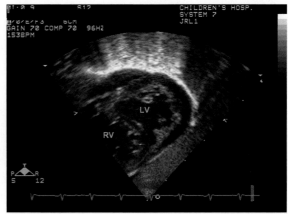

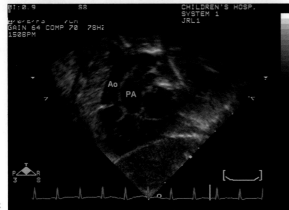

FIGURE 16.8. Subcostal short-axis view. A: The right and left atria and the atrial septal defect are well seen. **B:** Sweeping toward the apex, the ventricles are seen. The left ventricle has a characteristically smooth septal surface and two mitral valve papillary muscles are seen. **C:** The great vessels are seen in parallel with the aorta anterior and arising from the right ventricle.

color Doppler flow with appropriate direction within the space and acquiring confirmatory images from other views. Coronary arteries that arise higher than usual (at the sinotubular junction or above) will be difficult to visualize in the expected parasternal short-axis view but may be identified by sweeping more cranially in the parasternal short-axis view or from the parasternal long-axis view (Fig. 16.20).

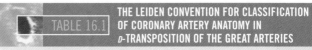

TABLE 16.1

THE LEIDEN CONVENTION FOR CLASSIFICATION OF CORONARY ARTERY ANATOMY IN *d*-TRANSPOSITION OF THE GREAT ARTERIES

- Symbolic notation using numbers, letters, and symbols
- Aortic sinuses are numbered from the perspective looking from aorta towards the pulmonary artery.
  - Sinus 1: adjacent to the pulmonary artery on the right hand side of observer
  - Sinus 2: adjacent to the pulmonary artery on the left hand side of observer
- Major coronaries artery branches are abbreviated as follows:
  - Right coronary artery (R)
  - Anterior descending artery (AD)
  - Circumflex artery (Cx)
- Symbols separating abbreviations:
  - Comma: major branches originate from common vessel
  - Semicolon: separate origins
- Supplemental terms also used to describe epicardial course and unusual origins
  - Anterior: a coronary artery branch passing anterior to the aorta
  - Posterior: a coronary artery branch passing posterior to the pulmonary artery
  - Between: a coronary branch passing between the great arteries (usually intramural)
  - Commissural: a coronary artery origin near an aortic commissure
  - Separate: separate origins of two coronary branches from the same aortic sinus
  - Remote or distal: origin of the circumflex artery and the posterior descending artery as a distal bifurcation of the right coronary artery
- Example: the most common coronary pattern is represented as: (1 AD, Cx; 2 R)

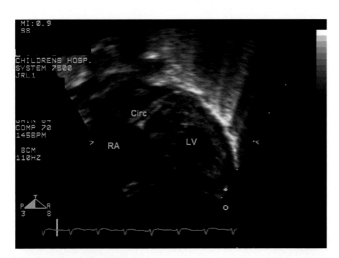

FIGURE 16.9. The circumflex coronary artery is well seen in this subcostal four-chamber view. Watching this entire imaging sweep allows one to identify that the circumflex courses posterior to the pulmonary artery.

Modified from Scheule AM, Jonas RA. Management of transposition of the great arteries with single coronary artery. *Semin Thorac Cardiovasc Surg.* 2001;4:34–57.

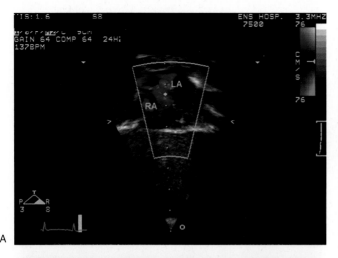

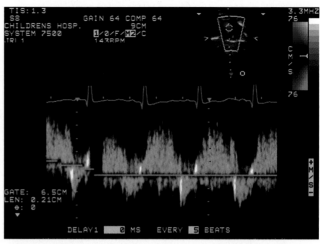

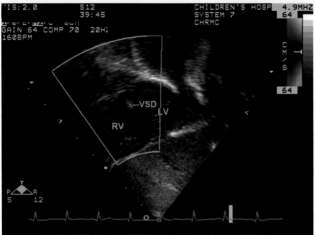

FIGURE 16.10. Subcostal views with the addition of color Doppler. A: Color flow Doppler across the atrial septal defect from the subcostal four chamber view demonstrates the direction of shunting, which at this moment in time is left to right. **B:** Spectral Doppler interrogation of the atrial septal defect demonstrates low velocity, bidirectional shunting. **C:** Color flow Doppler across the ventricular septum from the subcostal short-axis view demonstrates a small muscular ventricular septal defect.

Assessment of the degree of outflow tract obstruction or semi-lunar valve stenosis is critical to surgical management decisions. However, Doppler assessment of the severity of obstruction may be misleading. In the presence of a large PDA, great vessel pressures are equalized and the Doppler interrogation of either the outflow tracts or semilunar valves may underestimate the amount of obstruction present. In an older infant or child whose pulmo-nary vascular resistance has fallen and who has effective intercir-culatory mixing (with pulmonary blood flow significantly greater than systemic blood flow), the degree of left ventricular outflow tract obstruction or pulmonary valve stenosis may be overesti-mated by the Doppler gradient. In either instance, careful two-dimensional imaging can add valuable information about the de-gree of obstruction.

TABLE 16.2 — DESCRIPTIVE CLASSIFICATION OF CORONARY ARTERY ANATOMY IN *d*-TRANSPOSITION OF THE GREAT ARTERIES AS POPULARIZED BY CHILDREN'S HOSPITAL BOSTON

- Sinuses are described with words rather than numbered
  - First describe the relative positions of the aorta and pulmonary artery
  - Describe sinuses. Most typically coronary arteries arise from:
    - Rightward and posterior facing sinus
    - Leftward and posterior facing sinus
- Brief names have been developed for the 9 most common variants to allow for classification in studies (see Fig. 16.13):
  - Usual
  - Circumflex from RCA
  - Single LCA
  - Single RCA
  - Inverted
  - Inverted RCA and circumflex
  - Intramural LCA
  - Intramural LAD
  - Intramural RCA
- For more complex patterns, provide a detailed description in words.

LAD, left anterior descending coronary artery; LCA, left coronary artery; RCA, right coronary artery

TABLE 16.3 — FREQUENCY DISTRIBUTION OF THE CORONARY ARTERY PATTERNS IN *d*-TRANSPOSITION OF THE GREAT ARTERIES

Coronary pattern	Percent of cases
Usual	66.9
Circumflex from RCA	16.1
Single RCA	3.9
Single LCA	1.7
Inverted	2.4
Inverted circumflex/RCA	4.2
Intramural LCA	2.1
Intramural LAD	0.1
Intramural RCA	1.0
Other	1.6

LAD, left anterior descending coronary artery; LCA, left coronary artery; RCA, right coronary artery.
From Wernovsky G. Transposition of the great arteries. In: Allen HD, Driscoll DJ, Shaddy RE, et al, eds. *Moss and Adams' Heart disease in infants, children, and adolescents.* 7th ed. Philadelphia: Lippincott Williams & Wilkins; 2008:1038–1087

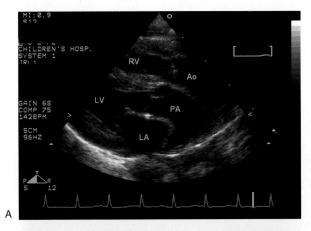

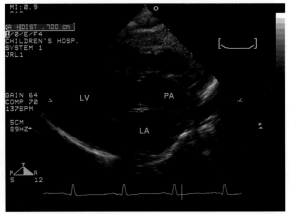

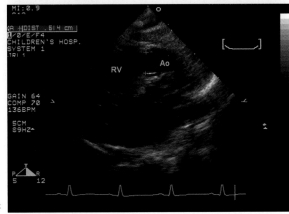

FIGURE 16.11 Parasternal long-axis view. A: The great vessels are seen in parallel. **B:** The pulmonary valve annulus measures 7 mm. **C:** The aortic valve annulus (6 mm) is normally slightly smaller than the pulmonary valve annulus.

 ## COMMON ASSOCIATED LESIONS AND FINDINGS

Key Findings that Alter Clinical Management

The basic approach to the management of *d*-TGA includes a balloon atrial septostomy followed by surgical intervention. The current era of cardiovascular surgery entails the performance of the arterial switch procedure. In the past era (pre-1980), the surgery of choice was the atrial switch (Senning or Mustard) but these procedures fell out of favor due to the nonphysiologic nature of the operation as well as the high risk of the development of late atrial arrhythmias. As with all cardiac malformations, center-to-center variability exists regarding alterations in management based on variations in cardiac anatomy. The following represents a range of management approaches that might be considered when a specific associated anomaly is detected that alters the basic underlying anatomy (Table 16.4):

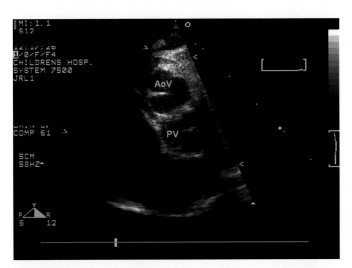

FIGURE 16.12. Parasternal short-axis view. Typical relative positions of the aortic and pulmonary valves, with the aortic valve anterior and slightly rightward. Note that the facing commissures of the two valves are aligned.

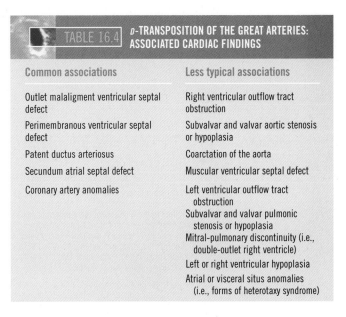

TABLE 16.4	*d*-TRANSPOSITION OF THE GREAT ARTERIES: ASSOCIATED CARDIAC FINDINGS
Common associations	**Less typical associations**
Outlet malalignment ventricular septal defect	Right ventricular outflow tract obstruction
Perimembranous ventricular septal defect	Subvalvar and valvar aortic stenosis or hypoplasia
Patent ductus arteriosus	Coarctation of the aorta
Secundum atrial septal defect	Muscular ventricular septal defect
Coronary artery anomalies	Left ventricular outflow tract obstruction
	Subvalvar and valvar pulmonic stenosis or hypoplasia
	Mitral-pulmonary discontinuity (i.e., double-outlet right ventricle)
	Left or right ventricular hypoplasia
	Atrial or visceral situs anomalies (i.e., forms of heterotaxy syndrome)

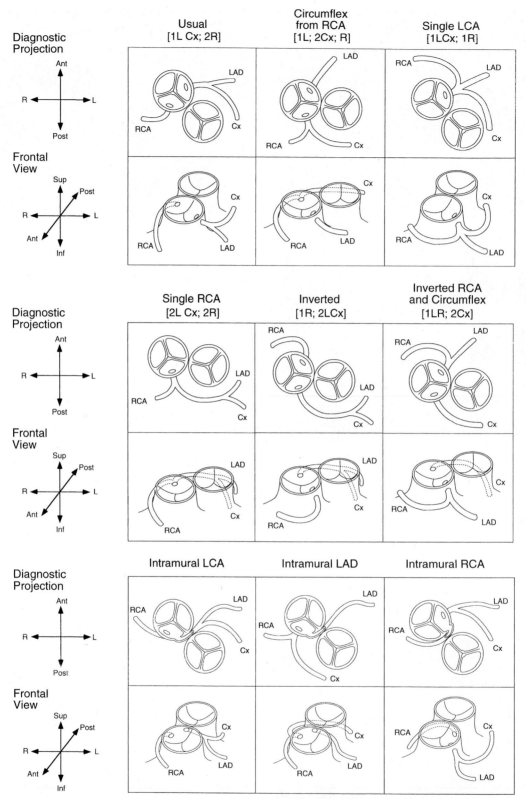

FIGURE 16.13. Coronary artery patterns in *d*-transposition of the great arteries (*d*-TGA). Nomenclature for each pattern (Children's Hospital Boston and Leiden conventions) is given in each set of images. **Top:** Diagnostic projection; diagram of the origin and proximal course as visualized by two-dimensional echocardiography and caudally angulated aortography. **Bottom:** Same coronary artery distribution as viewed anteriorly (surgeon's view, frontal projection). Note that the circumflex coronary artery, or even the entire left coronary artery system, is more likely to pursue a retropulmonary course when the great arteries are in a side-by-side relationship. Reprinted from Wernovsky G. Transposition of the great arteries. In: Allen HD, Driscoll DJ, Shaddy RE, et al, eds. *Moss and Adams' Heart disease in infants, children, and adolescents.* 7th ed. Philadelphia: Lippincott Williams & Wilkins; 2008:1038–1087, with permission. Permission also obtained from the original source: Wernovsky G, Sanders SP. *Coronary artery anatomy and transposition of the great arteries. Coron Artery Dis.* 1993;4:148–157.)

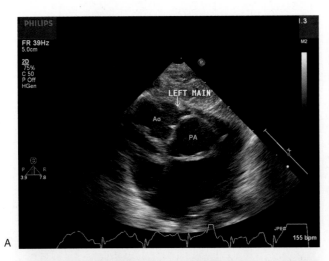

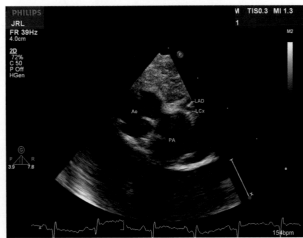

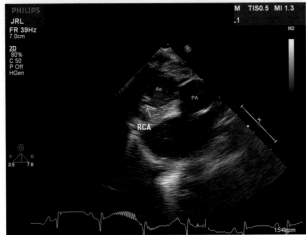

FIGURE 16.14. Two dimensional parasternal short-axis views of the most common coronary artery pattern, termed "usual" or by the Leiden classification [1 AD, Cx; 2 R]. **A:** The origin of the left coronary artery is from the leftward sinus that is adjacent to or "facing" the pulmonary valve. Slight angulation away from a standard parasternal short-axis view may be necessary to demonstrate the origin of the vessel. **B:** The bifurcation of the left coronary artery cannot be demonstrated in the same still frame as the origin but is well seen here. **C:** The origin of the right coronary artery is from the rightward sinus that is "facing" the pulmonary valve.

1. **Restrictive patent foramen ovale.** Most centers use balloon atrial septostomy in the majority of cases of *d*-TGA. During the initial baseline transthoracic echocardiogram, the identification of a restrictive atrial communication prompts performance of a septostomy. Restriction of the atrial septum is echocardiographically determined by two-dimensional imaging of a small foraminal flap in addition to color Doppler attenuation of the left-to-right flow pattern with associated pulsed Doppler interrogation identifying an obstructive pattern (elevated velocity and mean gradient). However, this assessment is complicated by changes in pulmonary artery pressure over the first hours and days of life; higher pulmonary resistance results in reduced left atrial venous return and a reduced flow volume across the atrial septum. This decrease in left-to-right shunting may be due to the atrial septal restriction itself or to the physiologic changes inherent in the perinatal transition period. Clinically, the neonate will manifest reduced oxygen saturation as an indicator of either elevated pulmonary vascular resistance or a restrictive atrial septum. In addition, a large VSD in the presence of a well-saturated neonate may prompt the care team to decide against balloon septostomy and to proceed directly to surgery. The rationale for the performance of the septostomy is to (a) decompress the left atrium and (b) improve mixing, thus resulting in improved oxygen saturation. The septostomy is typically performed via echocardiographic guidance (Figs. 16.21 and 16.22). Imaging is performed via an apical or a subcostal window, with interaction occurring between the interventional cardiologist and echocardiographer such that identification of balloon position as well as adequacy of the newly created atrial communication may be discussed.

2. **Muscular ventricular septal defect.** It is common to identify a perimembranous or malalignment VSD in the setting of *d*-TGA. However, occasionally a mid-muscular or apical VSD is identified. If the VSD is deemed to be of hemodynamic significance, the surgical approach is usually to attempt primary closure at the time of the arterial switch. But many of these VSDs will be inaccessible to the surgeon. In the neonate, this would prompt alternative management strategies. At our center, a pulmonary artery band would be considered at the time of the arterial switch, placed in such a way that eventually the patient might be a candidate for percutaneous balloon pulmonary angioplasty to relieve band restriction. If, at the time of band removal, the VSD is considered to be hemodynamically important, then concomitant performance of either a percutaneous VSD device implantation or surgical closure can be considered.

3. **Pulmonary valve stenosis or subpulmonic stenosis.** In the presence of pulmonary outflow tract obstruction, a number of surgical approaches can be considered. An arterial switch can be performed if the valve stenosis is mild or deemed amenable to repair and the semilunar valves are of similar size. Resection of subpulmonic conal tissue can also be considered, although residual left ventricular outflow tract narrowing may lead to a marked degree of systemic obstruction after the arterial switch. If these modifications to the arterial switch are considered to be of unacceptable risk and a large VSD is present, then a Rastelli-type repair can be considered with closure of the VSD to the aorta and placement of a right ventricle–to–pulmonary artery conduit (Figs. 16.23 and 16.24). More recently, the Nikaidoh procedure has been developed, which involves enlargement of the VSD, translocation of the aorta posteriorly, closure of the VSD, and reconstruction of the

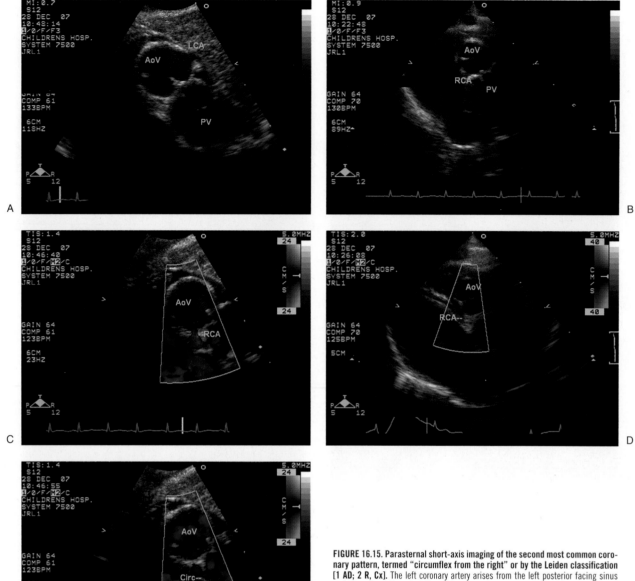

FIGURE 16.15. Parasternal short-axis imaging of the second most common coronary pattern, termed "circumflex from the right" or by the Leiden classification [1 AD; 2 R, Cx]. The left coronary artery arises from the left posterior facing sinus and gives rise only to the left anterior descending coronary artery. The right coronary artery arises from the right posterior facing sinus and gives rise to the right and circumflex coronary arteries. The circumflex courses posterior to the pulmonary root. **A:** The origin of the left coronary artery is seen. **B:** The origin of the right coronary artery is seen. **C:** Color confirmation of the origin of the right coronary artery. Note the low Nyquist limit necessary to visualize color flow in this structure. **D:** Two-dimensional and color flow imaging of the right coronary artery coursing towards the right atrioventricular groove. **E:** Color flow imaging of the circumflex coronary artery coursing posterior along the pulmonary root.

right ventricular outflow tract to the pulmonary artery. However, enlargement of a muscular VSD does carry a risk of atrioventricular conduction block. If there is no VSD, then choices would include atrial switch with left ventricle–to–pulmonary artery conduit or a single-ventricle palliation.

4. **Aortic valve stenosis or subaortic stenosis.** Right ventricular outflow tract obstruction is commonly found in association with an anterior malaligned VSD. If not severe, this anatomical variant is better tolerated than obstruction to pulmonary outflow in that the arterial switch will result in postoperative neopulmonary obstruction. Depending on the severity and extent of RVOT obstruction, this lesion can be palliated via valve repair, subvalvar muscular resection, transannular patch, or pulmonary conduit placement.

5. **Coarctation of the aorta.** Coarctation of the aorta may be difficult to identify early after birth in that these children are invariably

receiving prostaglandin E_1 and therefore a large patent ductus arteriosus is present. At the initial echocardiographic evaluation, secondary features may suggest the possibility of underlying aortic arch obstruction. These findings may include (a) a bicuspid aortic valve, (b) two-dimensional appearance of arch obstruction, (c) impingement to flow at the aortic isthmus, (d) right-to-left ductal shunting, (e) an abnormally extended distance from the left common carotid to the left subclavian artery (typically greater than 1 cm), or (f) blunted antegrade flow in the descending aorta with diastolic runoff. In addition, the finding of an anterior malalignment VSD may not only result in subaortic narrowing but may also predict the presence of coarctation. Subaortic narrowing associated with a malalignment VSD is best detected from the subcostal four-chamber imaging plane; aortic coarctation is best seen from a suprasternal long-axis view. In those neonates where prostaglandin is stopped and the ductus arteriosus is allowed to

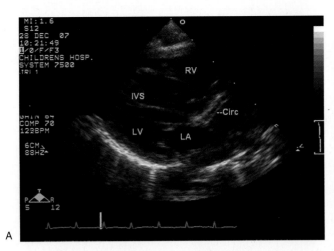
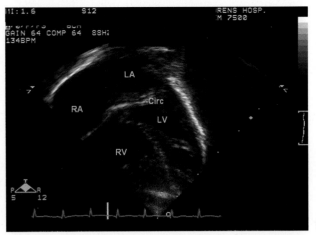

FIGURE 16.16. Supplemental coronary views from alternative windows in a patient with the coronary pattern of circumflex from the right coronary artery. **A:** Parasternal long-axis view of the circumflex coronary artery. Its posterior position relative to the pulmonary root is apparent when sweeping through the heart. **B:** Apical four-chamber view demonstrating the course of the circumflex coronary artery; anteroposterior sweeps demonstrate that it runs posterior of the pulmonary root.

close before the arterial switch, aortic arch obstruction should be unmasked. If a coarctation is identified, this is typically repaired at the time of the arterial switch.

6. **Coronary artery anomaly.** Coronary anatomy variants were reviewed earlier in this chapter. These variations are virtually always identified by echocardiographic assessment, but occasionally cardiac catheterization may be necessary. There are

several articles and textbook chapters stating unequivocally that there are no "unswitchable" coronary artery patterns. That being said, a single coronary from either the nonfacing (anterior) sinus or even the left or right facing sinuses if arising anteriorly within that sinus has been described to have very high operative risk for an ASO. Other patterns that carry higher surgical risk include intramural coronary arteries. In these situations,

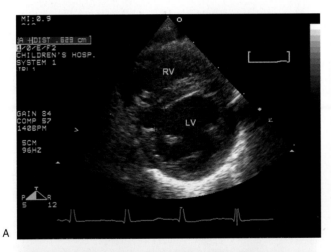
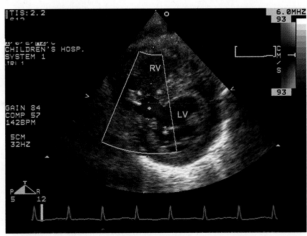
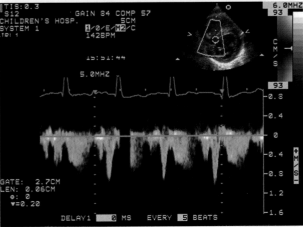

FIGURE 16.17. Parasternal short-axis views demonstrating a large posterior muscular ventricular septal defect in *d*-transposition of the great arteries (*d*-TGA). **A:** Two-dimensional imaging. **B:** Color flow imaging showing right ventricle–to–left ventricle shunting. **C:** Spectral Doppler display confirming low-velocity, right ventricle–to–left ventricle shunting.

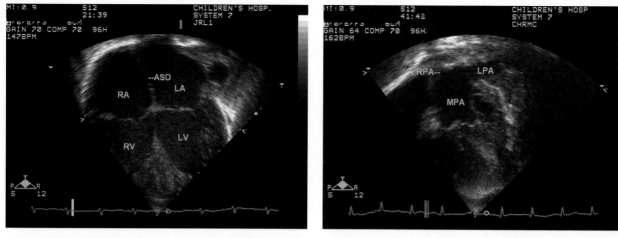

FIGURE 16.18. Apical views. A: Apical four chamber view in this patient who previously had a balloon atrial septostomy. The four chamber view shows normal cardiac chamber morphology and size. **B:** Anterior angulation from the apical four chamber view demonstrates the pulmonary artery arising from the left ventricle.

alternate surgical strategies may be considered, including the Damus-Kaye-Stansel procedure, which does not require coronary reimplantation (Fig. 16.25).

7. **Late diagnosis or complications that delay surgery.** Delay in the diagnosis of *d*-TGA beyond several weeks of life or the presence of noncardiac conditions that preclude a timely arterial switch procedure (e.g., prematurity, infection, noncardiac organ dysfunction) may necessitate staging of the ASO with an initial pulmonary artery band (frequently accompanied by an aortopulmonary shunt to maintain adequate oxygen saturations) until the left ventricle is deemed to be adequately "trained" to tolerate systemic pressure. This is only necessary in the neonate without a VSD of adequate size to maintain systemic left ventricular pressure. In this situation, serial assessment before

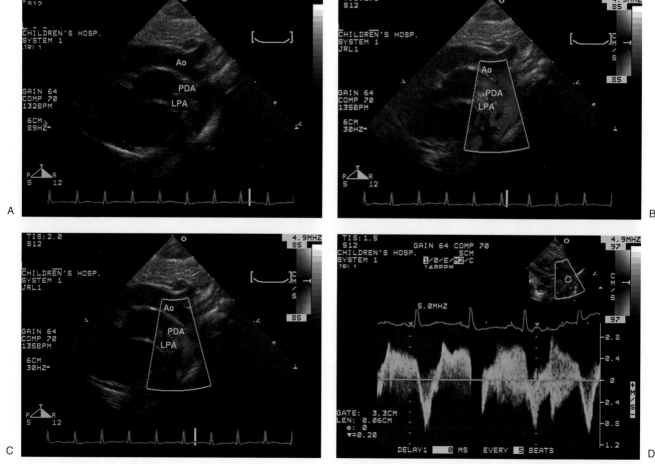

FIGURE 16.19. The patent ductus arteriosus is best visualized from the suprasternal long-axis view in *d*-transposition of the great arteries (*d*-TGA). A: Two-dimensional imaging. **B:** Color flow imaging in systole demonstrating pulmonary artery–to–aorta shunting. **C:** Color flow imaging in diastole demonstrating aorta–to–pulmonary artery shunting. **D:** Spectral Doppler display showing the typical bidirectional shunting pattern in a neonate with *d*-TGA and a patent ductus arteriosus.

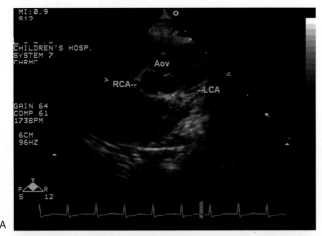

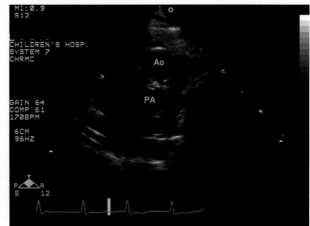

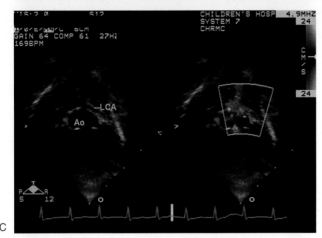

FIGURE 16.20. High arising left coronary artery. A: From the parasternal short-axis view, a normal right coronary origin is seen. A portion of the left coronary artery, although not its origin, is also visualized. Note that the aortic valve leaflets are easily seen in this frame. **B:** With more cranial angulation in the parasternal short-axis view, the left coronary origin is visualized. Note that the aortic valve leaflets are no longer seen in this plane. **C:** From a subcostal frontal view, anteriorly angulated to the aortic outflow, the origin of the left coronary artery can be seen arising above the sinotubular junction. This observation is confirmed by color flow Doppler.

definitive surgery includes the evaluation of left ventricular mass. Adequacy of the left ventricle for successful performance of the arterial switch is predicted by achievement of a mass index increase from approximately 40 to 80 g/m² (Fig. 16.26). In successful palliations, increased LV mass is also accompanied by increases in left ventricular end-diastolic internal diameter and assumption of a left ventricular "circular" shape on cross section with the interventricular septum contracting in synergy with the left ventricular mass. Postoperatively, left ventricular contractility may be impaired and at times the infant may require transient postoperative extracorporeal membrane oxygenation (ECMO) support. When there is failure of left ventricular training, choices include an atrial switch procedure or listing for cardiac transplantation.

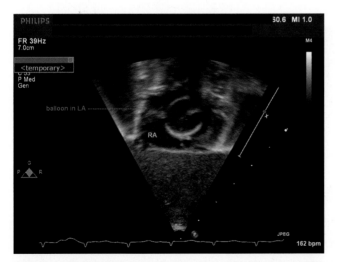

FIGURE 16.21. Subcostal long-axis view of the right and left atria with imaging performed during bedside balloon atrial septostomy. Echocardiographic guidance ensures optimal catheter and balloon position prior to the performance of the septostomy. The balloon is positioned against the atrial septum prior to the procedure, with positioning away from the pulmonary veins and mitral valve apparatus.

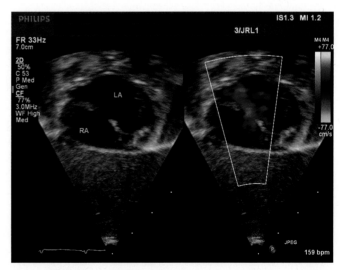

FIGURE 16.22. Subcostal long-axis imaging after balloon atrial septostomy confirms lack of restriction across a widely patent foramen flap. This should be accompanied by a prompt improvement in oxygen saturation.

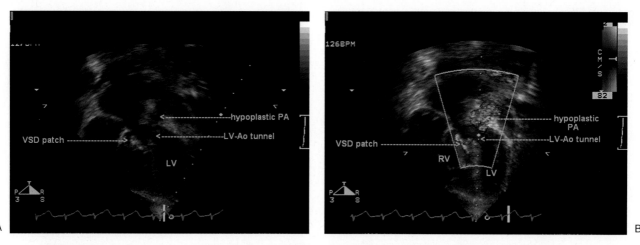

FIGURE 16.23. Four-chamber view from a patient with *d*-transposition of the great arteries (*d*-TGA), subpulmonic stenosis, and pulmonary valve hypoplasia. A: Two-dimensional imaging demonstrating the ventricular septal defect baffle repair creating a tunnel from the left ventricle to the anteriorly positioned aorta. **B:** Color Doppler interrogation demonstrates turbulent flow through the stenotic and hypoplastic pulmonary outflow tract, with laminar flow through the tunnel created by the ventricular septal defect patch directing flow to the aorta.

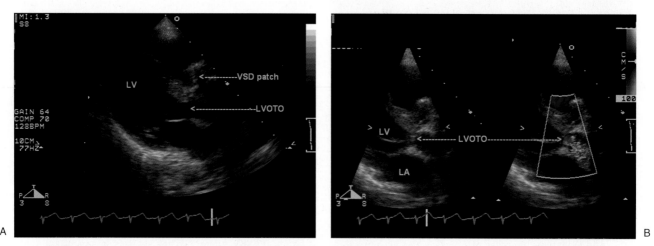

FIGURE 16.24. *d*-Transposition of the great arteries (*d*-TGA) with left ventricular outflow tract obstruction secondary to subvalvar and valvar pulmonary stenosis. A: Imaging from the parasternal long-axis imaging plane after Rastelli procedure (right ventricle [RV]–to–pulmonary artery [PA] conduit and ventricular septal defect patch baffle of left ventricular outflow to the aorta). **B:** Color Doppler demonstrates the site of subvalvar turbulence with flow directed anteriorly toward the aorta through the ventricular septal defect.

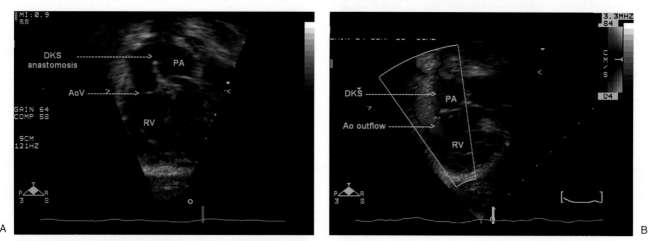

FIGURE 16.25. Patient with *d*-transposition of the great arteries (*d*-TGA) and a single anteriorly positioned coronary artery ostia necessitating the performance of a Damus-Kaye-Stansel (D-K-S) anastomosis. A: Subcostal short-axis imaging plane demonstrates the widely patent D-K-S connection between the posteriorly positioned pulmonary artery arising from the left ventricle and the anterior aorta arising from the right ventricle. **B:** Color Doppler interrogation demonstrates a lack of turbulence at the site of the D-K-S anastomosis with flow directed superiorly into the ascending aorta.

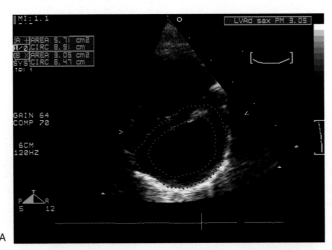
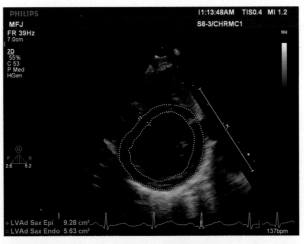

FIGURE 16.26. Three-month-old recently diagnosed with *d*-transposition of the great arteries (*d*-TGA) and an intact interventricular septum. A: The left ventricular (LV) systolic pressure is approximately 35 mm Hg based on the tricuspid regurgitant jet. The baseline LV mass index is 34 g/m². The patient underwent pulmonary artery banding and Blalock-Taussig shunt placement, with serial follow-up echocardiography performed to assess the "training" of the LV. **B:** Twenty days after placement of the pulmonary artery band, the arterial switch procedure is performed subsequent to echocardiographic confirmation of the development of adequate ventricular hypertrophy (LV mass index = 75 g/m²) as well as a more dilated and rounded LV cavity geometry.

INTERVENTIONAL AND POSTINTERVENTIONAL IMAGING

Preoperative Cardiac Catheterization

In the neonate with unoperated *d*-TGA, the most common use of transthoracic echocardiography in conjunction with cardiac catheterization involves the performance of a balloon atrial septostomy. The use of transthoracic imaging is crucial regardless of where the interventionalist is performing the procedure (i.e., at the bedside or in the catheterization laboratory). Before septostomy (after balloon inflation), an evaluation is made of balloon position within the left atrium, ensuring it is away from the pulmonary veins and mitral valve apparatus. After septostomy, the anatomy of the newly created atrial communication is assessed, and restriction to flow is determined by color and pulsed-wave Doppler. Postseptostomy, the infant will typically manifest a prompt improvement in oxygen saturation such that prostaglandin can be discontinued. At our center, prostaglandin infusion is discontinued after the oxygen saturation has improved and a repeat echocardiogram is performed in the subsequent 48 hours to reassess the adequacy of the atrial communication and to assess for ductal closure.

Angiography for coronary artery imaging may also be required to delineate the coronary arterial pattern. The need for this level of definition is surgeon specific, but the lack of identification of specific high-risk patterns has been associated with less-optimal surgical outcomes.

Intraoperative Imaging

Many pediatric centers currently use transesophageal echocardiography for all cases of *d*-TGA repair. Preoperative imaging typically entails a complete reassessment of anatomy and physiology. This includes evaluation of the great artery relationships, VSD(s), atrial communication (native or created), valve anatomy and function, coronary artery anatomy, outflow tract obstruction, systemic and pulmonary venous anatomy, and ventricular chamber dimensions and contractility. Postoperative assessment begins during warming to assess for myocardial or intracardiac cavitations consistent with air. After separation from cardiopulmonary bypass, a thorough evaluation is undertaken to ensure that the repair is acceptable. After the arterial switch procedure, the following are important components of the examination: (a) resolution of atrial, ventricular, and ductal shunts, (b) flow into the coronary artery buttons, (c) relief or development of outflow tract obstruction, (d) valve function, (e) supravalvar aortic or pulmonary stenosis at the anastomotic sites, (f) estimate of pulmonary artery pressures, (g) evaluation of ventricular contractility, and (h) assessment of bilateral branch pulmonary artery anatomy and flow either by two-dimensional imaging, by color and pulsed-wave Doppler interrogation, or via secondary criteria based on confirmation of left- and right-sided pulmonary venous return.

Postoperative Imaging: Arterial Switch Operation

There is an occasional need for coronary artery imaging after the arterial switch procedure in the clinical situation where the patient has either (a) electrocardiographic changes suggestive of ischemia, (b) myocardial dysfunction suggestive of reduced coronary perfusion, or (c) concerning clinical symptoms (chest pain and syncope being the most common). While echocardiographic assessment may suggest kinking or flow disturbance within a coronary artery, echocardiography rarely, if ever, is of acceptable precision for the surgeon to consider repair on these noninvasive data alone (Fig. 16.27).

Early in the history of the arterial switch procedure, mobilization of the pulmonary trunk and branches was less optimal. After introduction of the LeCompte procedure, the anterior movement of the pulmonary trunk resulted in the potential for tension (i.e., stretching) of the main and branch pulmonary arteries. The supravalvar pulmonary artery anastomosis is readily evaluated from either a parasternal short-axis imaging plane or a subcostal short-axis view (Fig. 16.28). Postoperative two-dimensional, color and spectral Doppler evaluation of the pulmonary artery branches as they straddle the aorta can be readily accomplished from the high parasternal short-axis imaging plane (Fig. 16.29). Catheter-based intervention, as necessary, can be performed via balloon angioplasty or percutaneous stent implantation with significant degrees of obstruction. In addition, echocardiographic assessment after the ASO includes evaluation for residual ASDs or VSDs, function of the atrioventricular valves, and detailed assessment of the neoaortic and neopulmonary valves (Fig. 16.30).

There are ample data identifying aortic root dilation after the arterial switch procedure. Hutter and colleagues demonstrated progressive aortic root dilation (z-score greater than 2 in 51 of 144 patients) at a median of 9 years postoperatively. Significant degrees of aortic stenosis and insufficiency were uncommon. Aortic dilation was more frequently associated with *d*-TGA with a VSD as opposed to those with an intact ventricular septum.

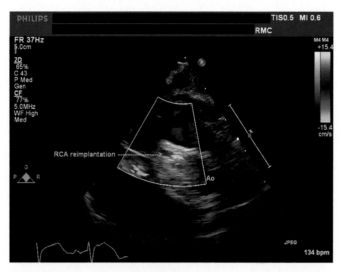

FIGURE 16.27. Parasternal short-axis imaging of the aortic root with color Doppler delineation of flow entering the reimplanted right coronary artery.

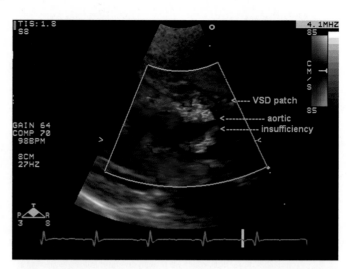

FIGURE 16.30. Parasternal long-axis view in a patient with *d*-transposition of the great arteries (*d*-TGA), perimembranous ventricular septal defect, and a bicuspid pulmonary valve. After the arterial switch operation (ASO), the neoaortic valve has two jets of insufficiency. The ventricular septal defect patch is noted to be intact.

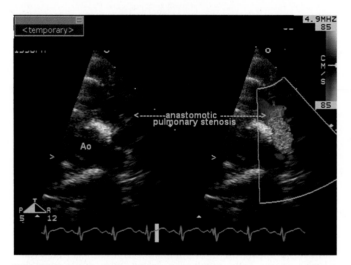

FIGURE 16.28. Parasternal short-axis view demonstrates narrowing at the supravalvar pulmonary artery anastomotic site after the arterial switch procedure. Color Doppler interrogation defines the site of obstruction, located distal to the valve leaflets.

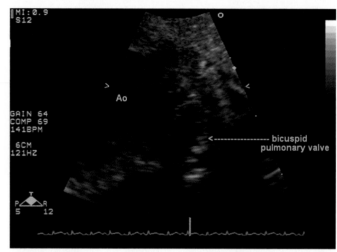

FIGURE 16.31. Posterior and leftward position of the pulmonary valve relative to the aortic valve from the parasternal short-axis view. The bicuspid pulmonary valve is hypoplastic with thickened leaflets.

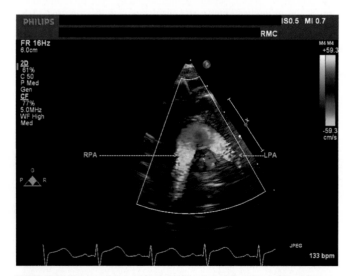

FIGURE 16.29. High parasternal short-axis imaging plane status post arterial switch procedure with Lecompte procedure. The branch pulmonary arteries straddle the aortic root. Color Doppler interrogation demonstrates laminar flow in both branches.

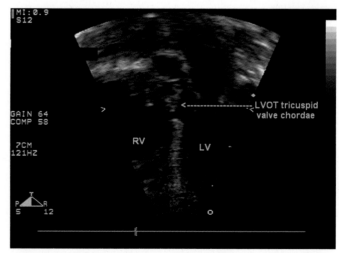

FIGURE 16.32. Apical four-chamber view with anterior angulation in a patient with *d*-transposition of the great arteries (*d*-TGA) and left ventricular outflow tract (LVOT) obstruction. The tricuspid valve septal leaflet is seen to billow into the subpulmonic region resulting in a narrowed LVOT.

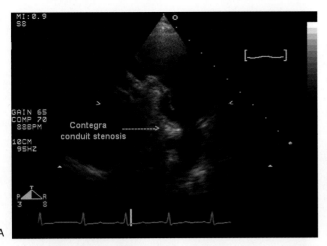
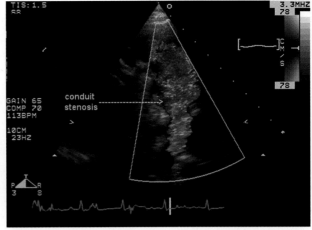

FIGURE 16.33. Parasternal short-axis view in a patient with *d*-transposition of the great arteries (*d*-TGA) and left ventricular outflow tract obstruction, status post Rastelli right ventricle (RV)–to–pulmonary artery (PA) conduit repair using a Contegra bovine jugular vein conduit. A: The RV-to-PA conduit is narrowed at the distal aspect proximal to the PA branches. **B:** Color Doppler interrogation demonstrates obstruction at the site of narrowing.

Postoperative Imaging: Rastelli Procedure

A range of etiologies exist for the development of left ventricular outflow tract obstruction in *d*-TGA and include a posterior malalignment VSD, a subpulmonic fibromuscular ridge, valvar pulmonic stenosis (Fig. 16.23), a bicuspid pulmonary valve (Fig. 16.31), and atrioventricular valve accessory tissue prolapsing into the left ventricular outflow tract (Fig. 16.32). Regardless of the etiology of left ventricular outflow tract obstruction, one of the more common surgical methods of ameliorating this complication of *d*-TGA is the performance of the Rastelli procedure with VSD closure to the anterior aorta and placement of a right ventricle–to–pulmonary artery conduit. Echocardiographic imaging after the Rastelli procedure entails two-dimensional, color, and pulsed Doppler interrogation. The channel from left ventricle to aorta is best visualized from the apical four-chamber or subcostal imaging window. The right ventricle–to–pulmonary artery conduit is best imaged from the parasternal or subcostal windows (Fig. 16.33). However, Doppler interrogation may not accurately delineate the actual degree of stenosis in that the simplified Bernoulli equation may not be valid in long-segment obstructive processes. Therefore, whenever possible, right ventricular pressure (and the degree of right ventricular outflow tract obstruction) should be validated by assessment of the tricuspid regurgitant jet velocity. If a discrepancy is found between direct and indirect pressure assessments, it is also crucial to take into account the impact of concomitant branch pulmonary artery stenosis, which will result in a lower velocity across the conduit as compared with the tricuspid regurgitant velocity.

Postoperative Imaging: Atrial Switch Operation (Mustard or Senning Procedure)

Echocardiographic imaging is routinely performed status post atrial switch to assess the systemic and pulmonary venous baffles (Figs. 16.34 through 16.37). The atrial switch procedure may result in narrowing of either the systemic venous or pulmonary venous baffles. Transthoracic imaging of these pathways may identify blunted pulsed Doppler venous flow patterns, turbulence by color Doppler interrogation, flow reversal with atrial contraction into the inferior or superior vena cava, or anatomical baffle narrowing by two-dimensional imaging. Given that it has been decades since the atrial switch was common surgical practice in *d*-TGA, many of these individuals are now adults,

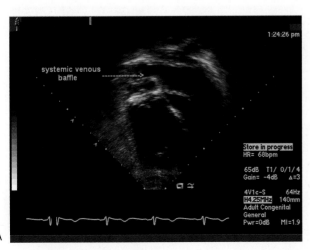
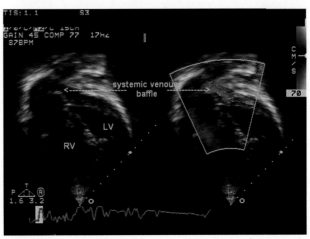

FIGURE 16.34. *d*-Transposition of the great arteries (*d*-TGA) status post Mustard procedure. A: Apical four-chamber view just anterior to the pulmonary venous baffle demonstrates the position of the systemic venous baffle directing blood from the inferior and superior venae cavae to the left ventricle (LV). **B:** Unobstructed systemic venous flow pattern directed towards the mitral valve is demonstrated with color Doppler.

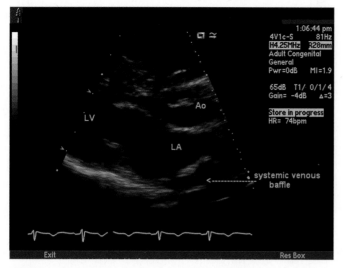

FIGURE 16.35. Parasternal long-axis view shows the left atrial aspect of the systemic venous baffle in a patient status post Mustard procedure for *d*-transposition of the great arteries (*d*-TGA).

FIGURE 16.37. *d*-Transposition of the great arteries (*d*-TGA) status post Mustard procedure. Apical four-chamber view directed posteriorly to image the pulmonary venous baffle. The right ventricle is dilated and hypertrophied.

often with poor transthoracic windows. In these patients, transesophageal echocardiography may be necessary to delineate the obstructive process. In addition, subsequent catheter-based intervention to ameliorate the obstruction is often best accomplished with associated TEE guidance.

Post atrial switch procedure baffle leak may also occur. This can also be detected by echocardiographic imaging, with color or pulsed Doppler interrogation identifying the leak between the systemic venous baffle and the right atrium, or between the pulmonary venous baffle and the left atrium. Systemic baffle leaks can also be readily identified via saline contrast injection. If contrast injection into a peripheral arm vein traverses the baffle and enters into the nonbaffle portion of the right atrium or into the right ventricle, this provides good evidence for a systemic venous baffle leak. Tandem imaging with angiography and transesophageal echocardiography can then be used to place an occlusion device or covered stent across the baffle leak (Fig. 16.38).

POTENTIAL ROLES OF ALTERNATIVE IMAGING MODALITIES

Echocardiography remains the gold standard for the evaluation of cardiac anatomy and physiology in the vast majority of cases of *d*-TGA. The most common reason that additional imaging modalities are used involves clarification of coronary artery anatomy. When there is uncertainty, most centers rely on cardiac catheterization to provide definitive delineation of the coronary arteries.

In the patient after the ASO, symptoms or findings may arise that raise concerns regarding the adequacy of the coronary artery circulation due to either kinking of these reimplanted vessels or complications associated with their underlying anatomical arrangement (as described earlier). In most of these situations, cardiac catheterization may provide adequate information. However,

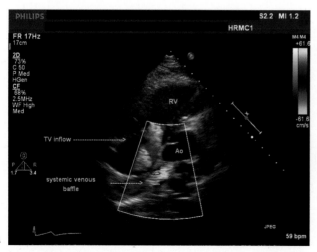
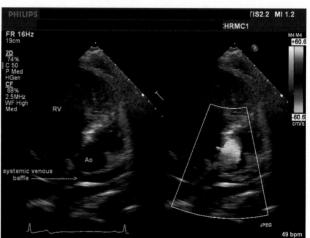

FIGURE 16.36. Parasternal short-axis view in patient status post Mustard procedure for *d*-transposition of the great arteries (*d*-TGA). **A:** Venous flow is noted through the systemic venous baffle into the left ventricle (LV). **B:** The systemic venous baffle is located just posterior to the aortic root.

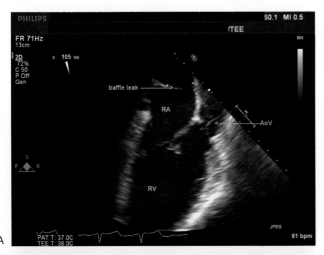

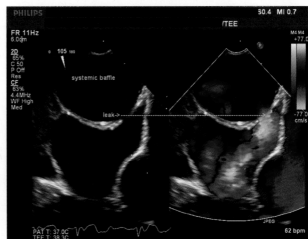

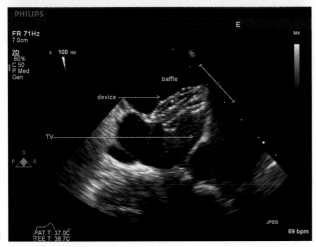

FIGURE 16.38. *d*-Transposition of the great arteries (*d*-TGA) status post Mustard procedure. **A:** Right heart imaging via transesophageal echocardiography (TEE) imaging demonstrates a systemic venous baffle leak. **B:** Color flow is noted from the systemic venous baffle through a large baffle leak. **C:** TEE directs placement of an AMPLAZER atrial septal defect occlusion device across the systemic venous baffle defect. The left and right atrial aspects of the device are well seated such that the venous channel is unobstructed and tricuspid valve apparatus function is preserved.

less-invasive modalities are also available. For larger patients with lower heart rates, computed tomography angiography can provide detailed anatomical definition of the coronary artery origins and branches. Often, this requires three-dimensional reconstructive techniques. In addition, there may be normal coronary circulation

[Figure 16.39 image]

FIGURE 16.39. *d*-Transposition of the great arteries (*d*-TGA) status post Mustard procedure. Parasternal short-axis imaging demonstrates flattening of the interventricular septum in response to systemic right ventricular pressure. The right ventricle is dilated and hypertrophied.

at rest with myocardial ischemia developing only with increases in myocardial demand. In this case, strategies that can be used include pharmacologic stress echocardiography (dobutamine is the most common agent) or nuclear medicine stress testing (with sestamibi, as well as other radioisotopes) to delineate myocardial perfusion. The difficulty with both of these techniques is the relative lack of expertise in data interpretation at many pediatric centers. In adult centers, stress echocardiography and nuclear medicine are used commonly, allowing providers to obtain adequate experience in data interpretation. This is not necessarily true in the pediatric center, especially in the patient population with complex heart disease. In this setting, difficulties can occur not only due to a lack of adequate expertise in interpreting data derived these modalities but also because prior surgical intervention may complicate data interpretation.

Three-dimensional echocardiographic imaging may prove useful, especially when there are complexities to the underlying anatomy. Specific instances where three-dimensional imaging may be helpful occur when complex outflow tract anomalies are present. This may allow the surgeon to better understand complex anatomical relationships and potential paths to successful reconstruction, which are more difficult to ascertain by two-dimensional imaging. In addition, three-dimensional imaging may be of benefit in volumetric rendering of the ventricular chambers.

After the atrial or arterial switch procedure, a variety of echocardiographic techniques may prove helpful where there are concerns regarding ventricular dysfunction (Fig. 16.39). These include the TEI index (myocardial performance index) to assess combined systolic and diastolic function and parameters of diastolic functional assessment, including tissue Doppler imaging, strain, and strain rate. The difficulty with all of these techniques is that only limited data are available delineating normal and abnormal parameters in this population. While some data are available regarding normal values in the presence of congenital cardiac lesions, *d*-TGA has not been thoroughly studied. Nevertheless, patients can potentially serve as their own controls. It is our practice to acquire functional data during every postoperative study so that changes occurring during serial assessment may point toward evolving functional disturbances.

SUGGESTED READING

Chin AJ, Yeager SB, Sanders SP, et al. Accuracy of prospective two dimensional echocardiographic evaluation of the left ventricular outflow tract in complete transposition of the great arteries. *Am J Cardiol.* 1985;55:759–764.

Gittenberger-de Groot AC, Sauer U, Quaegebeur J. Aortic intramural coronary artery in three hearts with transposition of the great arteries. *J Thorac Cardiovasc Surg.* 1986;91:566–571.

Gottlieb D, Schwartz ML, Bischoff K, et al. Predictors of outcome of arterial switch operation for complex D-transposition. *Ann Thorac Surg.* 2008;85:1698–1702.

Hutter P, et al. Fate of the aortic root after arterial switch operation. *Eur J Cardiothorac Surg.* 2001;20:82–88.

Iyer KS, et al. Serial echocardiography for decision making in rapid two-stage arterial switch operation. *Ann Thorac Surg.* 1995;60:658–664.

Losay J. Late outcome after arterial switch operation for transposition of the great arteries. *Circulation.* 2001;18(12 Suppl 1):I121–I126.

Pasquini L, Parness IA, Colan SD. Diagnosis of intramural coronary artery in transposition of the great arteries using two-dimensional echocardiography. *Circulation.* 1993;88:1136–1141.

Pasquini L, Sanders SP, Parness IA, et al. Coronary echocardiography in 406 patients with d-loop transposition of the great arteries. *J Am Coll Cardiol.* 1994;24:763–768.

Poerner TC, Goebel B, Figulla HR, et al. Diastolic biventricular impairment at long-term follow-up after atrial switch operation for complete transposition of the great arteries: an exercise tissue Doppler echocardiography study. *J Am Soc Echocardiogr.* 2007;20:1285–1293.

Prifti E, Crucean A, Bonacchi M, et al. Early and long term outcome of the arterial switch operation for transposition of the great arteries: predictors and functional evaluation. *Eur J Cardiothorac Surg.* 2002; 22:864–873.

Scheule AM, Jonas RA. Management of transposition of the great arteries with single coronary artery. *Semin Thorac Cardiovasc Surg.* 2001;4:34–57.

Takeuchi D, Nakanishi T, Tomimatsu H, et al. Evaluation of right ventricular performance long after the atrial switch operation for transposition of the great arteries using the Doppler Tei index. *Pediatr Cardiol.* 2006;27:783.

Wernovsky G, Sanders SP. Coronary artery anatomy and transposition of the great arteries. *Coron Artery Dis.* 1993;4:148–157.

Wong D, et al. Intraoperative coronary artery pulse Doppler patterns in patients with complete transposition of the great arteries undergoing the arterial switch operation. *Am Heart J.* 2008;156:466–472.

Yacoub MH, Radley-Smith R. Anatomy of the coronary arteries in transposition of the great arteries and methods for their transfer in anatomicalal correction. *Thorax.* 1978;33:418–424.

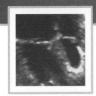

Chapter 17
Double-Outlet Right and Left Ventricles

Donald J. Hagler

TERMINOLOGY

The ventriculoarterial connection is considered "double-outlet" when more than 50% of each great artery arises from one ventricle. The origin of both great arteries from the right ventricle (RV) is termed *double-outlet right ventricle (DORV)*. Conversely, the origin of both great arteries from the left ventricle (LV) is termed *double-outlet left ventricle (DOLV)*.

DOUBLE-OUTLET RIGHT VENTRICLE

Basically recognized by the origin of both great arteries from the morphologic RV, DORV encompasses features of a variety of entities, ranging from simple ventricular septal defect (VSD) to tetralogy of Fallot (ToF) to transposition of the great arteries (TGA). This congenital malformation is a rare anomaly. Its frequency has been reported as approximately 0.09 per 1000 births and represents 1% to 1.5% of patients with congenital heart disease. No racial/ethnic or sexual predilection is evident.

There are 16 possible variations of DORV based on the great artery relationships and the location of the VSD. Figure 17.1 illustrates these variations but shows that only 9 types were observed clinically. However, this series includes only cases with situs solitus of the atria and viscera, atrioventricular (AV) concordance, and two well-developed ventricles and AV valves. The location of the VSD is described as subaortic, subpulmonary, doubly committed (below both great arteries), noncommitted, or remote. In addition, an intact ventricular septum (very rare) allows four other possible types of DORV, depending on the great artery relationships. Multiple other variations and combinations are possible if one also includes situs inversus and situs ambiguous as well as AV discordance.

Double-Outlet Right Ventricle With Side-by-Side Great Arteries and Subaortic Ventricular Septal Defect

This represents the most common and typical form of DORV. The presence of bilateral conus separates both semilunar valves from both AV valves. The VSD is the only outlet from the LV, and the

Relation of great arteries	Location of VSD (%)				Total
	Subaortic	Subpulmonary	Subaortic & Subpulmonary	Remote	
Normal	3%	0	0	0	3%
Side-by-side	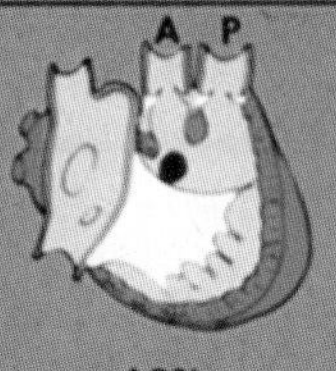 46%	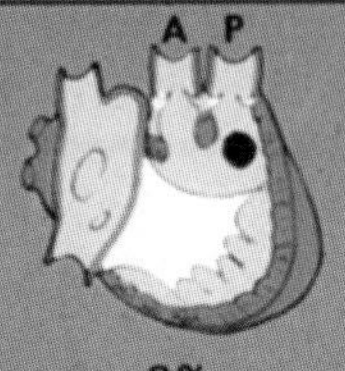 8%	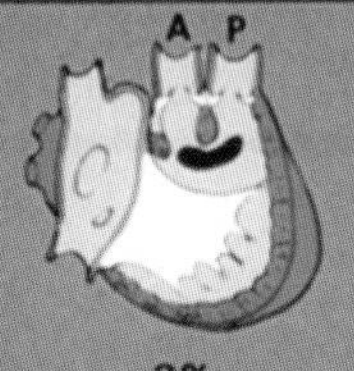 3%	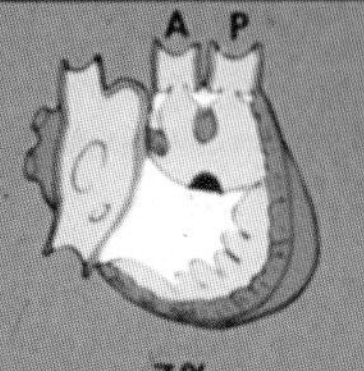 7%	64%
d – MGA	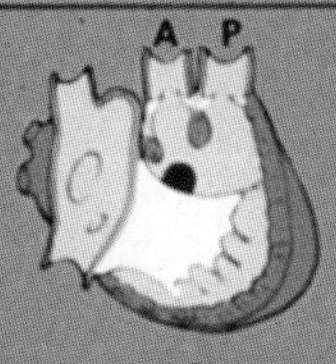 16%	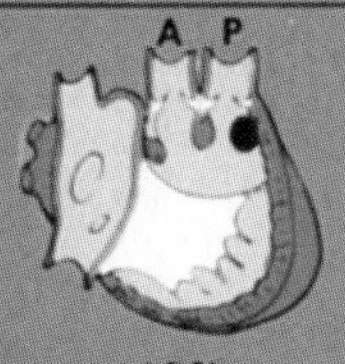 10%	0	0	26%
l – MGA	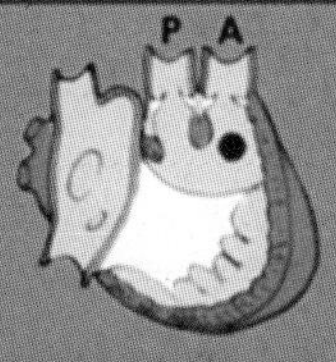 3%	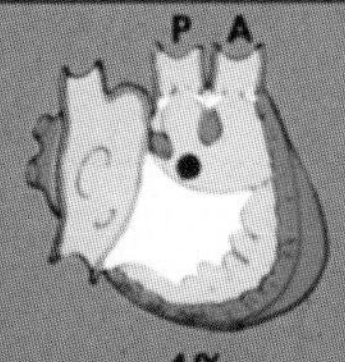 4%	0	0	7%
Total	68%	22%	3%	7%	

FIGURE 17.1. Relationships of the great arteries and locations of the ventricular septal defect (VSD) in 70 patients with double-outlet right ventricle (DORV). A, aorta; d-MGA, dextro-malposed great arteries; l-MGA, levo-malposed great arteries; P, pulmonary artery. (Reprinted with permission from Hagler DJ, Tajik AJ, Seward JB, et al. Double-outlet right ventricle: wide-angle two-dimensional echocardiographic observations. *Circulation.* 1981;63:419–428.)

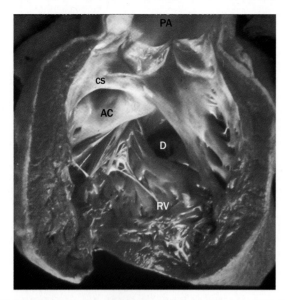

FIGURE 17.2. Pathologic specimen of double-outlet right ventricle. The right ventricle (RV) has been opened, demonstrating the origin of both great arteries from the RV. AC, aortic conus; CS, conus septum; D (defect ventricular septal defect [VSD]); PA, pulmonary artery.

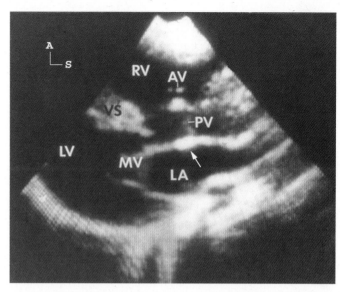

FIGURE 17.4. Parasternal long-axis scan in a patient with double-outlet right ventricle, with the aorta anterior and right of the pulmonary artery with a subpulmonary ventricular septal defect (VSD). There is a relatively small amount of conus tissue (*arrow*) separating the pulmonary valve (PV) from the mitral valve (MV). Both great arteries are entirely committed to the right ventricle (RV). LA, left atrium; LV, left ventricle.

aortic conus is a muscular structure between the aortic valve and the anterior leaflet of the mitral valve. Figure 17.2 illustrates the pathologic findings of this type of DORV. The RV has been opened illustrating both great arteries originating from the RV.

Two-dimensional echocardiographic findings for the diagnosis of DORV have been reported. Three observations were noted for the diagnosis: (a) origin of both great arteries from the anterior RV, (b) mitral–semilunar valve discontinuity, and (c) absence of left ventricular outflow other than the VSD. In a series of 36 patients studied by two-dimensional echocardiography, both great arteries were observed to originate predominantly from the anterior RV. If one great artery overrode the VSD, nearly exclusive or predominant commitment to the RV was required for diagnosis. Figures 17.3, 17.4, and 17.5 illustrate the most common forms of DORV with normally related, *d*-malposed great arteries, and *l*-malposed great arteries, respectively. In addition, Figure 17.5 illustrates

the associated finding of left juxtaposed atrial appendages. Most patients with DORV will have situs solitus of the atria and viscera, but situs ambiguous with bilateral right- or left-sidedness and situs inversus may be present. Most patients with DORV will have AV concordance, but less commonly AV discordance (ventricular inversion) may be present.

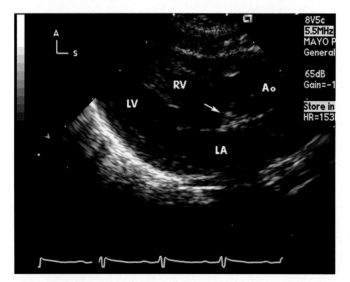

FIGURE 17.3. Parasternal long-axis scan in a neonate with double-outlet right ventricle, with side-by-side great arteries and subaortic ventricular septal defect (VSD). With the aorta (Ao) anterior and rightward, it is the only great artery observed in this scan. *Arrow*, subaortic conus separating the aortic valve from the mitral valve. LA, left atrium; LV, left ventricle; RV, right ventricle.

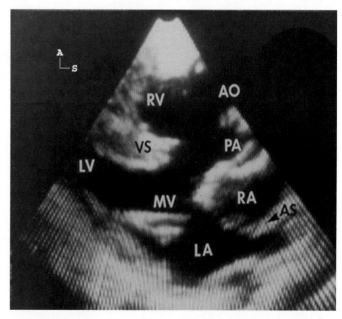

FIGURE 17.5. Parasternal long-axis scan in a patient with double-outlet right ventricle, with the aorta (Ao) anterior and to the left of the pulmonary artery (PA). Both great arteries are entirely committed to the right ventricular cavity and are observed in parallel orientation originating from the right ventricle (RV). In this standard long-axis scan, all four cardiac chambers and both great arteries are observed simultaneously. In this example, findings of left-juxtaposed atrial appendages are also evident. The right atrial (RA) appendage courses posterior to the great arteries to lie next to the left atrial appendage. The pulmonary valve appears slightly thickened and, in real time, the valve was dome shaped during systole, consistent with pulmonary stenosis. The mitral valve (MV) is markedly separated from the semilunar valves. AS, atrial septum; LA, left atrium; LV, left ventricle; TV, tricuspid valve; VS, ventricular septum. (Reprinted with permission from Hagler DJ, Tajik AJ, Seward JB, et al. Double-outlet right ventricle: wide-angle two-dimensional echocardiographic observations. *Circulation.* 1981;63:419–428.)

IMAGING NOTES

Position of the Great Arteries

In two-thirds of the cases, both great arteries can be observed simultaneously originating from the anterior RV. In the subcostal sagittal plane, both semilunar valves may not be visualized simultaneously. However, each semilunar valve may be demonstrated with slight right or left transducer angulation. The semilunar valves are positioned in a more anterior and superior location relative to the rest of the ventricle because of conus muscle beneath the valves. It is important to sweep in the short-axis scans from apex to base to demonstrate the commitment of each great artery to the right ventricular cavity (Fig. 17.6). With the use of a short-axis scan at the cardiac base, a double-circle appearance of the great arteries is consistent with a parallel orientation of the great arteries. A superior short-axis scan demonstrates the pulmonary artery bifurcation.

Parasternal long-axis scans are often obtained from a slightly more superior position at the left sternal edge. This view demonstrates the initial parallel course of the great arteries (Figs. 17.4

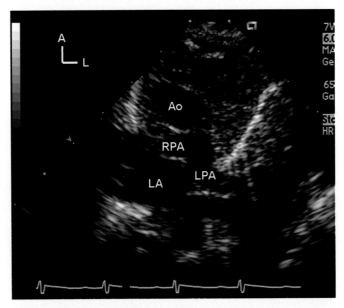

FIGURE 17.7. High parasternal short axis image of both great arteries in a neonate with double-outlet right ventricle (DORV) and right anterior aorta. The scan demonstrates the great artery location and the bifurcation of the left-sided artery to identify it as the pulmonary artery. A, anterior; Ao, aorta; L, left; LA, left atrium; LPA, left pulmonary artery; RPA, right pulmonary artery.

and 17.5). The pulmonary artery may be recognized by its posterior course to the lungs and by its bifurcation into the right and left pulmonary arteries, as noted with short-axis (Figs. 17.6 and 17.7) or subcostal scans. The more anterior and superior great artery is the aorta (Fig. 17.8). Parasternal long-axis scans demonstrate mitral–semilunar valve discontinuity with the presence of muscular conus separation (Figs. 17.2, 17.3, and 17.8). Mitral–semilunar valve discontinuity is demonstrated by two-dimensional echocardiography as a dense echo (fibromuscular) or muscular conus separating the two valves. As observed in Figure 17.3, the degree of separation is variable, but with high-resolution imaging (7- and 10-MHz transducers), it can be demonstrated even when 2 to 3 mm in size.

Position of the Ventricular Septal Defect

Two-dimensional echocardiography accurately predicts the position of the VSD in reference to the great arteries. In most patients, typical subaortic or subpulmonary defects can be demonstrated by parasternal and subcostal scans (Figs. 17.4, 17.5, 17.9, and 17.10A). Doubly committed defects appear nearly equally committed to both great arteries. Remote or noncommitted defects are usually complete AV septal defects, but there may also be isolated or multiple muscular VSDs. Figure 17.10B illustrates a remote posterior muscular VSD in DORV. Neither great artery is committed to the VSD. Similar complete AV septal defects are best recognized on apical four-chamber or subcostal views (Fig. 17.11).

Doppler echocardiography and color flow Doppler may be helpful adjuncts for demonstrating these abnormalities as well as associated muscular VSDs. Continuous-wave Doppler interrogation of the VSD may demonstrate a high-velocity jet consistent with an LV-to-RV pressure gradient from a restrictive VSD. Although some associated muscular VSDs may be appreciated with color flow imaging, many centers recommend complete angiographic assessment if multiple muscular ("Swiss cheese septum") VSDs are suspected.

DORV may be associated with a number of AV valve anomalies, including complete AV septal defect, isolated cleft of the anterior mitral leaflet, and overriding (atrial and ventricular septal malalignment) or straddling left or right AV valves. Apical and subcostal four-chamber views and short-axis scans easily demonstrate these AV valve abnormalities at the crux of the heart. It is particularly important to accurately delineate the location and points of insertion of the AV valve chordal apparatus. Abnormal chordal insertions of the tricuspid valve into the conus septum may prohibit surgical efforts to direct the left ventricular outflow anteriorly toward the

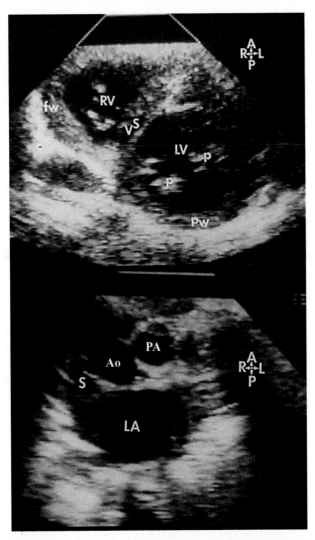

FIGURE 17.6. Short-axis scans of the heart from apex (top) to base (bottom) in a patient with double-outlet right ventricle. Top: Short-axis scan at the mid-ventricular level. This image illustrates the plane of the ventricular septum (VS) below the level of the ventricular septal defect (VSD). **Bottom:** Short-axis scan at the level of the great arteries. The great arteries are related normally. The superior vena cava (S) is to the right of the aorta (Ao). The pulmonary artery (PA) is to the left and anterior. Thus, the VSD is noted to be subaortic at the cardiac base. (Reprinted with permission from Hagler DJ, Tajik AJ, Seward JB, et al. Double-outlet right ventricle: wide-angle two-dimensional echocardiographic observations. *Circulation.* 1981;63:419–428.)

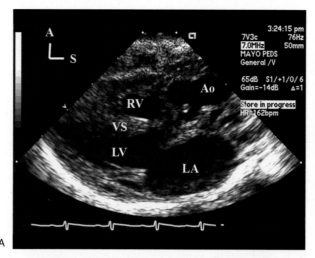 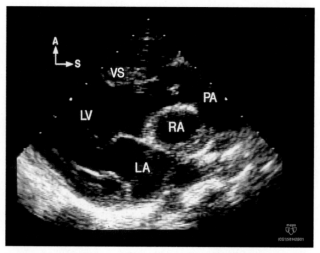

FIGURE 17.8. Neonate with double-outlet right ventricle (DORV) and right anterior aorta. A: Parasternal long-axis image in the same neonate as in Figure 17.7. The scan demonstrates commitment of the aorta (Ao) to the right ventricle (RV) and mitral aortic discontinuity. The ventricular septal defect (VSD) is subaortic in location. The aorta courses directly superior. **B:** Similar parasternal long-axis image in another patient with DORV and subpulmonary VSD. The pulmonary artery (PA) is recognized by its posterior course to the lungs. In addition, there is left juxtaposition of the right atrial (RA) appendage as it courses beneath the pulmonary annulus. The RA appendage also separates the pulmonary valve from the mitral valve. A, anterior; LA, left atrium; LV, left ventricle; S, superior; VS, ventricular septum.

aorta. Isolated clefts of the anterior mitral leaflet often have chordal attachments to the ventricular septum or attachments that straddle the ventricular septum into the RV. Associated anomalies with DORV include left-juxtaposed atrial appendage (Fig. 17.5), ASD, anomalous systemic (left SVC to coronary sinus) and pulmonary venous connections, and coarctation of the aorta. Multiple imaging planes must be used to exclude these associated anomalies.

 SURGICAL TREATMENT

Because of the complexity of intracardiac repair of these anomalies, it may be necessary to palliate some infants and small children who become symptomatic in the first year of life. Simple forms of DORV with subaortic VSD have been successfully repaired in infancy. For patients with DORV and subpulmonary VSD, the arterial switch operation appears to be the procedure of choice and can

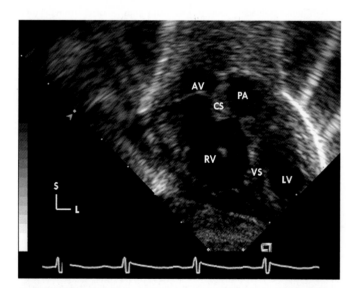

FIGURE 17.9. Subcostal scan in a neonate with double-outlet right ventricle (DORV) and right anterior aorta (Fig. 17.7). Illustrates the anterior location of the aorta and clear origin of both great arteries from the right ventricle (RV). Prominent conus septum (CS) separates the great arteries and is malaligned with the rest of the ventricular septum (VS). There is severe subpulmonary stenosis. Slightly more posterior images showed the ventricular septal defect to be subaortic in location. AV, aortic valve; LV, left ventricle; PA, pulmonary artery.

be performed in the neonatal period. Pulmonary arterial banding in DORV without PS will reduce pulmonary flow and protect the pulmonary arterioles from obstructive arteriopathy but may induce or aggravate subaortic stenosis due to hypertrophy of the subaortic conus. Pulmonary artery banding may be appropriate in the setting of DORV with multiple muscular VSDs or a remote VSD. Conversely, in patients with DORV and pulmonary stenosis (PS), pulmonary blood flow may need to be augmented. Systemic–to–pulmonary artery shunts will increase pulmonary flow and reduce cyanosis in patients with PS and complex associated anomalies. Forms of DORV that have large VSD physiology or tetralogy of Fallot physiology can be corrected in infancy.

Complete correction of DORV depends on the complexity of the intracardiac anatomy. In the surgical correction of DORV, the position of the VSD and its relationship to the great vessels are of paramount importance. The classic form of repair is possible only in those patients with a subaortic VSD. Ideally, in complex anatomy this may be attempted when the patient is about 2 years old or if an extracardiac conduit is anticipated.

The objectives of the operation are as follows.

1. **Establishment of LV-to-aorta continuity.** In general, this is accomplished by creating a tunnel between the VSD and the subaortic outflow tract by means of a patch. Care must be exercised to prevent obstruction of this connection. Some VSDs may need to be enlarged to avoid LVOT obstruction and care is needed to avoid injury to the conduction tissue.
2. **Establishment of RV–to–pulmonary artery continuity.** In the simple forms of the anomaly—with situs solitus and AV concordance in which PS is absent—this requires care in preventing the subaortic tunnel from encroaching on the subpulmonary outflow tract. But, in patients with PS, this may require pulmonary valvotomy, infundibular resection, patch enlargement of the RV outflow tract, or insertion of an extracardiac valved conduit to bring the RV into communication with the pulmonary artery.
3. **Repair of complex DORV.**
   3a: *Subpulmonary VSD:* When the defect is positioned at a distance from the aortic outflow tract, in the muscular septum posteriorly or below the pulmonary outflow tract, then tunneling from the VSD to the aortic outflow tract is not possible. Under these circumstances, other surgical solutions are required. In subpulmonary VSD, closure of the defect in such a manner as to divert LV blood to the pulmonary artery creates TGA, which is then corrected by an inflow procedure (Mustard or Senning) or by an outflow procedure (Jatene, Kaye-Damus-Stansel, or Aubert). In DORV with left anterior aorta, LV blood should be diverted to the subaortic outflow tract, establishing RV–to–pulmonary artery continuity.

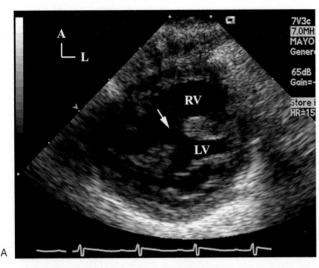 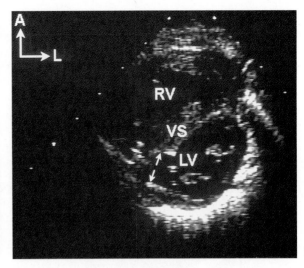

FIGURE 17.10. Double-outlet right ventricle (DORV). A: Parasternal short-axis image of neonate with DORV showing the ventricular septal defect (VSD; *arrow*) that is subaortic in location. Note that the aorta was right anterior in location in more superior short-axis scans. LV, left ventricle; RV, right ventricle. B: Parasternal short-axis image in another patient with DORV but with a remote or noncommitted VSD that is posterior in location (*arrows*). Neither great artery could be connected through the VSD to the left ventricle (LV). A, anterior; L, left; RV, right ventricle; VS, ventricular septum.

3b: *Straddling AV valves:* This complicates the anatomy of the VSD and septation may not be possible without replacement of the straddling valve. Alternatively, if the pulmonary pressure and resistance are low, definitive palliation (as opposed to correction) can be achieved by obliteration of the right-sided AV valve and closure of any ASD, interruption of ventriculo-pulmonary arterial continuity, and establishment of an cavopulmonary connection (bidirectional Glenn and modified Fontan procedures).

3c: *DORV with AV discordance* can be corrected by closure of the VSD, transection of the pulmonary artery, and establishment of morphologic LV–to–pulmonary artery continuity with an extracardiac conduit. In these patients, the RV remains as the systemic ventricle. Kiser et al. reported repair of dextrocardia, AV discordance, VSD, and DORV. More recently, efforts have been directed to establish continuity between the morphologic LV and the ascending aorta through the VSD to allow physiologic function of the LV as the systemic ventricle. However, this also requires a concomitant atrial switch procedure to direct the pulmonary venous blood to the morpho-

logic LV. Gomes et al. reported the results of complete repair of DORV without PS in 18 patients. The overall operative mortality rate was 22%; higher mortality was encountered in patients with elevated pulmonary arterial resistance and in those with associated lesions, especially AV septal defects. These researchers concluded that patients with DORV and no PS should have early operation before the onset of severe obstructive pulmonary arteriopathy. The same group reported on 22 patients with DORV and PS who underwent complete repair. The overall mortality rate was 32%, but in patients who had surgery after 1960, the mortality rate decreased to 16%. More recent reports of repair in the neonatal period have demonstrated surgical mortality rates of 4% to 8%. Patients with anomalies of coronary distribution, multiple VSDs, or residual PS are at higher risk. Extracardiac conduits may be necessary in cases with complex anatomy.

DOUBLE-OUTLET LEFT VENTRICLE

DOLV is a very rare anomaly most accurately defined as a malformation in which the aorta and the main pulmonary artery both arise predominantly from the morphologic LV. As a conotruncal anomaly, it has features that are very similar to those observed in DORV. As in DORV, the clinical and pathologic features described with DOLV also encompass features of a variety of entities: large VSD, ToF, or complete TGA. DOLV occurs far less frequently than DORV.

Van Praagh et al. provided a complete review of 109 cases of DOLV based on autopsy material, personal communications, and a literature review. This review pointed out the various anatomic conditions associated with DOLV and attempted a categorization of anatomic types of DOLV. It included associated cardiovascular and noncardiovascular anomalies. Similar to the classification scheme for DORV, in DOLV the relationship of the VSD (if present) to the great arteries was of primary importance. Associated anomalies included pulmonary stenosis, subaortic stenosis, and AV valve abnormalities.

DOLV with subaortic VSD was the most common and was observed in 52 (48%) cases, and in 73% of the cases with situs solitus and AV concordance. The patients with subaortic VSD were further categorized based on their great artery relationships as having a right anterior or a left anterior aorta. Figure 17.12 illustrates the most common form of DOLV with a subaortic VSD and right/anterior aorta. The second most frequent form of DOLV was characterized by a subaortic VSD, left/anterior aorta, and PS. The third most common form of DOLV in the Van Praagh et al. series occurred in 11 patients having a subpulmonary VSD (Fig. 17.13). The VSD in this subgroup of patients is described as a high

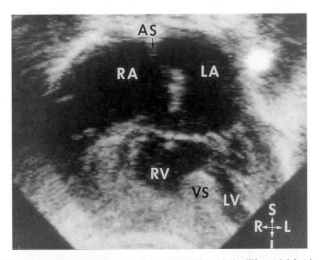

FIGURE 17.11. Apical four-chamber view of a complete atrioventricular (AV) septal defect in a patient with double-outlet right ventricle (DORV). In some patients, the common AV valve may be unbalanced favoring one or the other ventricular chamber. In conotruncal defects, the common AV valve is usually undivided and free floating as described with a Type C complete AV septal defect. The more posterior defect in complete AV septal defects may be too remote from the great arteries to allow patch direction of blood from the left ventricle (LV) to one of the great arteries. AS, atrial septum; I, inferior; L, left; LA, left atrium; R, right; RA, right atrium; RV, right ventricle; S, superior.

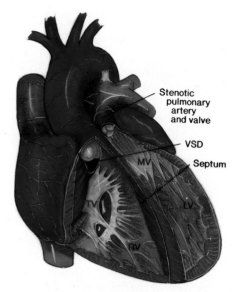

FIGURE 17.12. Double-outlet left ventricle (DOLV) with subaortic ventricular septal defect (VSD) and right anterior aorta. Schematic illustration of the VSD and great artery relationships. Note that the VSD involves the membranous and outlet septum. There is fibrous continuity between both semilunar valves and the mitral valve. In DOLV, patients with subaortic VSD and right anterior aorta, 83% had associated pulmonary stenosis. LV, left ventricle; MV, mitral valve; RV, right ventricle; TV, tricuspid valve.

and anterior type of VSD involving the outlet and, specifically, the conus septum. This VSD is in a typical supracristal location, allowing the pulmonary artery to override the ventricular septum and to have a varying degree of commitment to both RV and LV cavities. Because the VSD involves the conus septum, the subpulmonary conus is relatively deficient. In patients with a subpulmonary VSD, the great artery relationships were normal or had a right/anterior aorta (Fig. 17.14).

Malalignment of the aortic and pulmonary conus septum relative to the ventricular septum often results in narrowing of the outflow tract with associated aortic valve hypoplasia and stenosis (Fig. 17.15). Arch hypoplasia and coarctation of the aorta may also occur in these patients. Patients with a deficient subpulmonary conus associated with a supracristal type of VSD lack PS and present with typical clinical or hemodynamic findings of a large VSD. Rarely, the VSD in DOLV is doubly committed. As opposed to the rather striking conal development observed in patients with DORV and doubly committed VSD, patients described with a DOLV and doubly committed VSD have markedly underdeveloped subarterial conus, which allows aortic–mitral and pulmonary–mitral fibrous continuity. Absence of subarterial conal septum would be consistent with the embryologic explanation proposed by Van Praagh et al. in the morphologic development of DOLV. With a virtual absence of conus septum, none of these patients had PS. Unlike DORV, a remote or noncommitted VSD has been an unusual observation in patients with DOLV. In the Van Praagh et al. series, there were no patients with classic findings of complete AV septal defects and DOLV, nor were any described with muscular VSDs and DOLV.

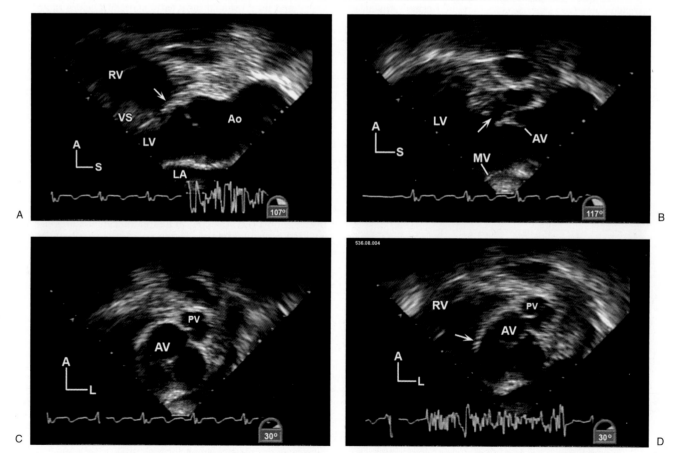

FIGURE 17.13. Transesophageal echocardiography images of double-outlet left ventricle (DOLV) with subaortic ventricular septal defect (VSD) and normally related great arteries. A: Scan in the left ventricular long axis showing aortic–mitral continuity and patch closure (arrow) of a large VSD. Ao, aorta; LA, left atrium; LV, left ventricle; RV, right ventricle; VS, ventricular septum. **B:** A slightly rotated leftward scan illustrating the anterior pulmonary outflow (arrow) also committed to the left ventricle (LV). AV, aortic valve; MV, mitral valve. **C:** Short-axis scans demonstrate the great artery relationship with the aorta posterior and to the right. The aortic valve (AV) and pulmonary valve (PV) are on the same level. **D:** Slightly lower short-axis scan also demonstrating the VSD patch position (arrow) in the membranous-to-outlet portion of the septum medial to the aortic valve (AV).

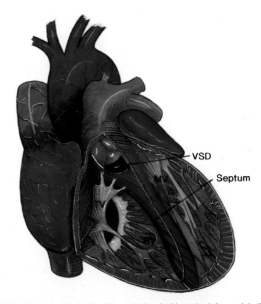

FIGURE 17.14. Schematic illustration demonstrating double-outlet left ventricle (DOLV) with subpulmonary ventricular septal defect (VSD) and right posterior aorta (normally related great arteries). The VSD is anterior or supracristal and involves the outlet conus septum. The pulmonary artery overrides the VSD but is predominantly committed to the left ventricle. Without pulmonary stenosis, it is evident that this defect would be hemodynamically similar to a large VSD with pulmonary hyperperfusion. MV, mitral valve; RV, right ventricle; TV, tricuspid valve.

As noted in the Van Praagh et al. series of DOLV, the vast majority of patients have situs solitus of the atria and viscera and with AV concordance. But, similar to DORV, DOLV has been observed with situs inversus and AV discordance. More commonly, tricuspid atresia or stenosis in association with hypoplastic RV was described in 20 cases of DOLV. These cases were associated with a subaortic VSD. Three patients with DOLV and VSD also had Ebstein anomaly of the tricuspid valve. Rarely, DOLV has been associated with the following: mitral atresia, double-inlet LV, situs ambiguous, or crisscross AV relationships in association with large doubly committed inlet-to-outlet VSDs.

Surgical Correction of Double-Outlet Left Ventricle

Early surgical reports by Sakakibara et al. and Pacifico et al. emphasized surgical correction of DOLV with two developed ventricles by VSD closure and placement of an RV–to–pulmonary artery conduit. Most patients with DOLV with two ventricles in association with situs solitus should be able to undergo a "two-ventricle" repair. Unlike DORV, the VSD may be simply closed regardless of its relationship to the great arteries. The major exception to this is in those patients with an anterior subpulmonary VSD involving the conal septum. In this example, all the patients who have been reported had a right lateral or right anterior aorta, and therefore patch closure of the VSD excluding the pulmonary artery from the LV, would represent those who received the easiest and most direct type of repair. However, this also may be altered by the presence of subaortic or aortic valvar stenosis. If severe subaortic stenosis cannot be relieved by resection, VSD closure leaving the pulmonary artery

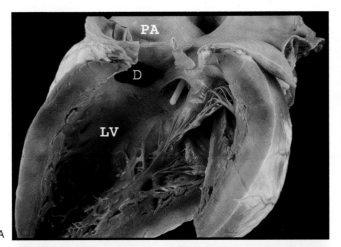

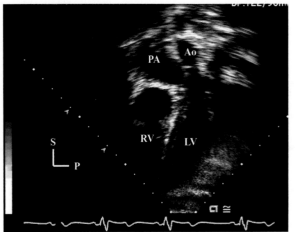

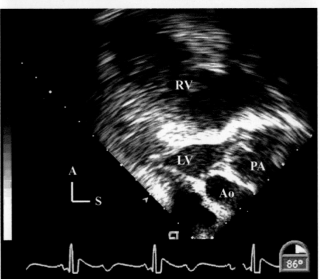

FIGURE 17.15. Double outlet LV (DOLV) with aortic stenosis. A: Pathologic example of DOLV with subpulmonary VSD with aortic stenosis and aortic annular hypoplasia. The white probe is exiting the aortic outflow tract and both outflow tracts are predominantly committed to the left ventricle. **B:** TTE image of a 12-year-old patient with features suggestive of DOLV and aortic stenosis. Although the pulmonary outflow overrides the ventricular septum in this subcostal image, the aortic outflow clearly exits the LV and is moderately hypoplastic. **C:** TEE image of the same patient at the time of RV conduit replacement shows a typical long-axis image. The pulmonary outflow again is noted to override the ventricular septum; however, the aortic outflow is committed to the LV and there is mitral–aortic continuity. There is severe aortic hypoplasia and subaortic stenosis. These images could also be classified as normally related great arteries with AS. A, anterior; Ao, aorta; D, defect; LV, left ventricle; P, posterior; PA, pulmonary artery; RV, right ventricle; S, superior.

to the LV with creation of an aortopulmonary window and place-ment of an RV–to–pulmonary artery conduit may be an option for repair. The reports by Pacifico et al. and others suggested that other forms could be repaired by VSD closure but that most also required closure of the native LV–to–pulmonary outflow and placement of an RV–to–pulmonary artery conduit. DeLeon et al. described pulmo-nary root translocation as an alternative for biventricular repair of DOLV. More complex forms of DOLV with functional single ventricle or AV valve atresia will require a Fontan type of correction.

SUGGESTED READING

Ciaravella JM Jr, McGoon DC, Hagler DJ, et al. Caplike double-horned dou-ble-outlet right ventricle: report of two cases. *J Thorac Cardiovasc Surg.* 1979;77:536–542.

Davachi F, Moller JH, Edwards JF. Origin of both great vessels from right ven-tricle with intact ventricular septum. *Am Heart J.* 1968;75:790–794.

DeLeon SY, Ow EP, Chiemmongkoltip P, et al. Alternatives in biventricular repair of double-outlet left ventricle. *Ann Thorac Surg.* 1995;60:213–216.

Gomes MMR, Weidman WH, McGoon DC, Danielson GK. Double-outlet right ventricle with pulmonic stenosis: surgical considerations and results of operation. *Circulation.* 1971;43:131–136.

Gomes MMR, Weidman WH, McGoon DC, et al. Double-outlet right ventricle with pulmonic stenosis: surgical considerations and results of operation. *Circulation.* 1971;43:889–894.

Goor DA, Edwards JE. The spectrum of transposition of the great arteries: with specific reference to developmental anatomy of the conus. *Circulation.* 1973;48:406–415.

Grant RP. The morphogenesis of transposition of the great vessels. *Circulation.* 1962;26:819–840.

Hagler DJ, Tajik AJ, Seward JB, et al. Double-outlet right ventricle: wide-angle two-dimensional echocardiographic observations. *Circulation.* 1981;63:419–428.

Hagler DJ, Tajik AJ, Seward JB, et al. Wide-angle two-dimensional echo-cardiographic profiles of conotruncal abnormalities. *Mayo Clin Proc.* 1980;55:73–82.

Judson JP, Danielson GK, Ritter DG, et al. Successful repair of co-existing double-outlet right ventricle and two-chamber right ventricle. *J Thorac Cardiovasc Surg.* 1982;84:113–121.

Kiser JC, Ongley PA, Kirklin JW, et al. Surgical treatment of dextrocardia with inversion of ventricles and double-outlet right ventricle. *J Thorac Cardiovasc Surg.* 1968;55:6–15.

Kleinert S, Sano T, Weintraub RB, et al. Anatomic features and surgical strate-gies in double-outlet right ventricle. *Circulation.* 1997;96:1233–1239.

Lev M, Bharati S, Meng L, et al. A concept of double-outlet right ventricle. *J Thorac Cardiovasc Surg.* 1972;64:271–281.

Manner J, Seidl W, Steding G. Embryological observations on the morphogen-esis of double-outlet right ventricle with subaortic ventricular septal defect and normal arrangement of the great arteries. *Thorac Cardiovasc Surg.* 1995;43:307–312.

Mitchell SC, Korones SB, Berendes HW. Congenital heart disease in 56,109 births: incidence and natural history. *Circulation.* 1971;43:323–332.

Neufeld HN, DuShane JW, Edwards JE. Origin of both great vessels from the right ventricle. II: With pulmonary stenosis. *Circulation.* 1961; 23:603.

Pacifico AD, Kirklin JW, Bargeron LM Jr. Complex congenital malformations: surgical treatment of double-outlet right ventricle and double-outlet left ventricle. In: Kirklin JW, ed. *Advanced cardiovascular surgery.* New York: Grune & Stratton; 1973:57.

Pacifico AD, Kirklin JW, Bargeron LM, et al. Surgical treatment of double-outlet LV. report of four cases. *Circulation.* 1973;48(suppl III):III19–III23.

Paul MH, Sinha SN, Muster AJ, et al. Double-outlet left ventricle with an intact ventricular septum: Clinical and autopsy diagnosis and developmental implications. *Circulation.* 1970;41:129–139.

Ruttenberg HD, Anderson RC, Elliott LP, et al. Origin of both great vessels from the arterial ventricle: a complex with ventricular inversion. *Br Heart J.* 1964;26:631–641.

Sakakibara S, Takao A, Arai T, et al. Both great vessels arising from the left ventricle (double-outlet left ventricle) (origin of both great vessels from the left ventricle). *Bull Heart Inst Jpn.* 1967:66.

Sridaromont S, Feldt RH, Ritter DG, et al. Double-outlet right ventricle: hemo-dynamic and anatomic correlations. *Am J Cardiol.* 1976;38:85–94.

Sridaromont S, Ritter DG, Feldt RH, et al. Double-outlet right ventricle: ana-tomic and angiocardiographic correlations. *Mayo Clin Proc.* 1978;53:555–577.

Stellin G, Ho SY, Anderson RH, et al. The surgical anatomy of double-outlet right ventricle with concordant atrioventricular connection and noncom-mitted ventricular septal defect. *J Thorac Cardiovasc Surg.* 1991;102:849–855.

Taussig HB, Bing RJ. Complete transposition of the aorta and a levoposition of the pulmonary artery: clinical, physiological and pathological findings. *Am Heart J.* 1949;37:551.

Uemura H, Yagihara T, Kawashima Y, et al. Coronary arterial anatomy in double-outlet right ventricle with subpulmonary VSD. *Ann Thorac Surg.* 1995;59:591–597.

Van Mierop LHS, Wiglesworth FW. Pathogenesis of transposition complexes. II: anomalies due to faulty transfer of the posterior great artery. *Am J Cardiol.* 1963;12:226–232.

Van Praagh R, Weinberg PM, Srebro JP. Double-outlet left ventricle. In: Adams FH, Emmanouilides GC, Riemenschneider JA, eds. *Moss' heart disease in infants, children, and adolescents,* 4th ed. Baltimore: Williams & Wilkins, 1989:461–485.

Van Praagh S, Davidoff A, Chin A, et al. Double-outlet right ventricle: ana-tomic types and developmental implications based on a study of 101 cases. *Coeur (Paris).* 1982;12:389–439.

Vierordt H. Die angeborenen herzkrankheiten (In: Nothnagel's Spez.) *Path Therapie.* 1898;15:244.

Wilcox BR, Ho SY, Macartney FJ, et al. Surgical anatomy of double-outlet right ventricle with situs solitus and atrioventricular concordance. *J Thorac Cardiovasc Surg.* 1981;82:405–417.

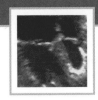

Chapter 18
Truncus Arteriosus

Frederick D. Jones • Bernadette Fenstermaker • John P. Kovalchin

Persistent truncus arteriosus is a rare congenital heart defect in which the aortic arch, pulmonary arteries, and coronary arteries arise from a common great artery originating from the base of the heart. It occurs in 1% to 4% of all cases of congenital heart disease. Truncus arteriosus is typically fatal without intervention in early infancy; however, with current surgical therapy most children with truncus arteriosus survive. Most cases are sent to surgery based on echocardiographic imaging alone. Accurate noninvasive imaging is critical to defining the cardiac anatomy, guiding appropriate surgical management, and following these patients in the long term.

 ## DEVELOPMENT AND ANATOMY

Truncus arteriosus occurs within the first 3 to 4 weeks of fetal life when there is failure of the aorticopulmonary septum to form and spiral within the embryonic truncus arteriosus, preventing a partition between the two great arteries. The anatomic description of truncus arteriosus consists of an outlet ventricular septal defect (VSD), a single semilunar valve, and a common great artery that overrides the VSD. Collett and Edwards first established four different anatomic classifications of truncus arteriosus based on the origin of the pulmonary arteries (Fig. 18.1). In type I, the main pulmonary artery arises from the truncal root and bifurcates into

a right and a left pulmonary artery. In type II, each pulmonary artery originates from a separate origin off the posterior aspect of the truncal root. In type III, each pulmonary artery arises independently from the lateral aspects of the truncal root. In type IV, no true pulmonary arteries are present and pulmonary blood flow is supplied via aortopulmonary collateral vessels. This type of truncus arteriousus is considered to be a form of pulmonary atresia with VSD. Van Praagh later developed a classification based on truncus patients with a VSD (group A) and those without (group B [very rare]). Among both groups A and B, the four subgroups are the same (Fig. 18.1). In the Van Praagh classification system, type III truncus arteriosus includes patients with origin of one pulmonary artery from the truncus. In this subset of patients, the other pulmonary artery is supplied via the ductus arteriosus or an aortopulmonary collateral vessel. In the Van Praagh classification system, type IV truncus arteriosus includes interruption of the aortic arch, with the descending aorta supplied by the patent ductus arteriosus. In cases of aortic arch interruption, type B is the most common form of interruption. A modified version of the Collett and Edwards classification was established by Konstantinov and colleagues. Fig. 18.2 represents variations of truncus arteriosus with interrupted aortic arch based on a multi-institutional study of 50 neonates in an effort to better define the morphology and characteristics of this particular anomaly.

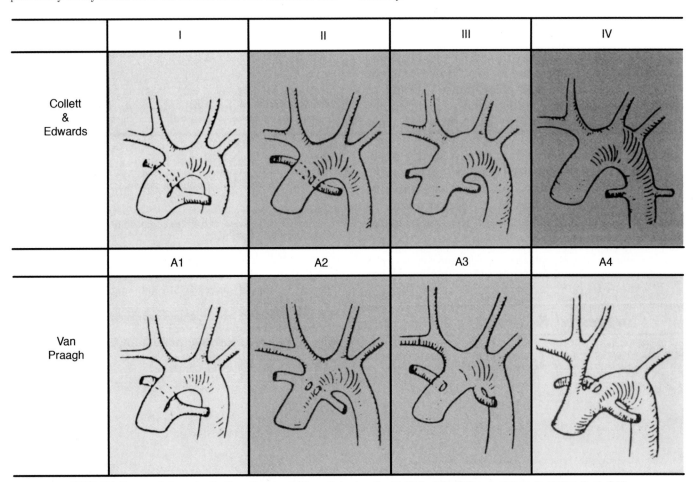

FIGURE 18.1. Truncus arteriosus classifications. (Reproduced with permission from Slesnick TC, Kovalchin JP. Truncus arteriosus. In: McMilan JA, ed. *Oski's pediatrics.* 4th ed. Philadelphia: Lippincott Williams & Wilkins; 2006:1540–1543.)

FIGURE 18.2. Truncus arteriosus with interrupted aortic arch classification. Ao, aorta, LSA, left subclavian artery. (Reproduced with permission from Konstantinov IE, Karamlou T, Blackstone EH, et al. Truncus arteriosus associated with interrupted aortic arch in 50 neonates: a congenital heart surgeons society study. *Ann Thorac Surg.* 2006;81:214–223, Elsevier.)

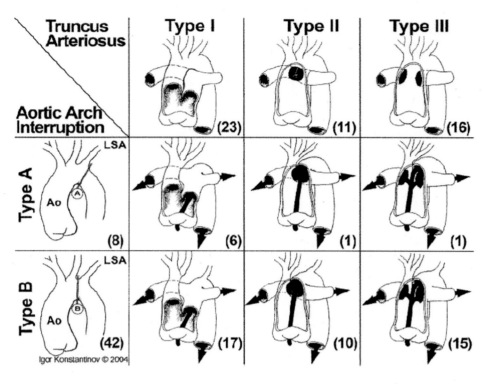

The truncal valve commonly overrides both ventricles but may be more committed to one ventricle than the other. Isolated truncal root origin from a ventricle is more common from the right ventricle than from the left ventricle. The truncal valve has a variable number of leaflets (one to six), and they are often morphologically thickened and dysplastic. Approximately two-thirds of all truncal valves are trileaflet, whereas almost one-quarter are quadricuspid. Less than 10% are found to be bicuspid. The truncal valve may be competent but is more commonly stenotic and/or regurgitant because of the valve's abnormal morphology.

CLINICAL PRESENTATION

Truncus arteriosus may be diagnosed prenatally with fetal echocardiography, although truncus arteriosus can be difficult to diagnose from obstetrical screening ultrasound four-chamber views. Patients not diagnosed prenatally with truncus arteriosus typically present during early infancy with tachypnea, feeding difficulty, failure to thrive, or other symptoms and signs related to pulmonary overcirculation as pulmonary vascular resistance falls. Patients with truncus and interrupted aortic arch typically present earlier because of decreased perfusion. The cardiac examination in patients with truncus arteriosus typically demonstrates a hyperactive precordium and a widened pulse pressure. There is characteristically a loud single S2, with a loud systolic murmur. Patients often have a click from the truncal valve and may have a diastolic murmur if there is significant truncal valve regurgitation. The chest radiograph demonstrates cardiomegaly and increased pulmonary vascularity because of an increase in pulmonary blood flow. The electrocardiogram typically shows biventricular hypertrophy.

ASSOCIATED CONDITIONS

Cardiac abnormalities commonly associated with truncus arteriosus include (a) coronary artery anomalies, with a single coronary artery and an intramural course having the most important surgical implications, (b) right aortic arch, (c) secundum atrial

septal defect, (d) left superior vena cava to coronary sinus, and (e) interrupted aortic arch (Table 18.1). Absence or atresia of the ductus arteriosus is usually expected with truncus arteriosus, the exception being truncus arteriosus with an interrupted aortic arch. Extracardiac anomalies include renal, skeletal, intestinal, and systemic defects. The association of truncus arteriosus with DiGeorge syndrome and chromosome 22 deletion is well recognized, with up to 35% of patients with truncus arteriosus having DiGeorge syndrome.

ECHOCARDIOGRAPHIC FEATURES

Two-dimensional Echocardiographic Examination

Echocardiography has evolved as the modality of choice for diagnosing the many anatomic variations of truncus arteriosus. The anatomic information obtained from two-dimensional and Doppler echocardiography is usually sufficient to send the patient for surgical repair without the need for further testing.

TABLE 18.1	ASSOCIATED FINDINGS
Finding	Percentage of Patients
Coronary artery anomalies	30–50%
Right aortic arch	30–40%
Atrial septal defect	10–20%
Interrupted aortic arch	10–20%
Left superior vena cava to coronary sinus	5–15%
Extracardiac anomalies	≤30%
DiGeorge syndrome	≤35%

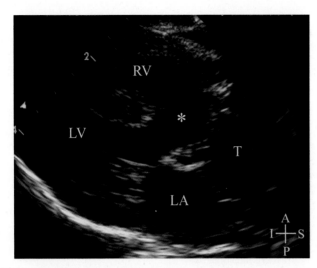

FIGURE 18.3. Parasternal long-axis view. Note the truncus arteriosus (T) overriding the large ventricular septal defect (*asterisk*). LA, left atrium; LV, left ventricle; RV, right ventricle.

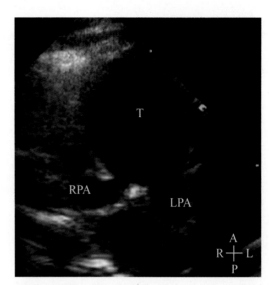

FIGURE 18.5. High parasternal short-axis view of a type II truncus arteriosus. Note the separate origins of the branch pulmonary arteries. LPA, left pulmonary artery; RPA, right pulmonary artery; T, truncus arteriosus.

In the parasternal long-axis view, the diagnosis of truncus arteriosus is suggested by a dilated single great artery, in continuity with the mitral valve, arising from the base of the heart, overriding the interventricular septum concomitant with a malalignment type VSD (Fig. 18.3). In truncus arteriosus type I, the short main pulmonary artery segment can frequently be seen arising from the truncal vessel posteriorly and leftward. In some cases of truncus arteriosus, sweeping from the right to the patient's left in the long axis demonstrates the deficiency of a separate pulmonary valve and the pulmonary arteries arising from the truncal vessel.

The parasternal short-axis view at the base of the heart is the preferred view for determining truncal valve morphology and number of leaflets (Fig. 18.4). It is an excellent window to view the VSD in the outlet septum. The pulmonary valve, main pulmonary artery, and branches are absent from their usual location. Visualization of the pulmonary arteries arising from the common truncus is a key finding in differentiating this anomaly from pulmonary atresia with VSD. The coronary artery origins and proximal courses are usually best imaged from the parasternal short-axis views, with the right coronary artery originating from the anterolateral aspect of the truncal root and the left coronary artery originating from the left posterolateral aspect of the truncal root. In truncus arteriosus type I, the truncal vessel can be seen in cross section with a short main pulmonary artery segment originating from the lateral aspect and bifurcating into the right and left pulmonary arteries. In truncus arteriosus type II, the pulmonary artery branches can be seen emerging posteriorly from the truncal root, originating from close but separate orifices (Fig. 18.5). In truncus arteriosus type III (Collett and Edwards), it is seldom possible to image both branch pulmonary arteries simultaneously in the parasternal short-axis view because both pulmonary arteries originate independently from widely separated origins off the truncal root.

The apical and subcostal views allow evaluation of the VSD, the degree of truncal override, the ventricular sizes, and the origin of the main and/or branch pulmonary arteries (Fig. 18.6). In truncus arteriosus type I, tilting the scan plane anteriorly in the apical four-chamber view allows the main pulmonary artery and branch pulmonary arteries to be visualized originating from the posterior

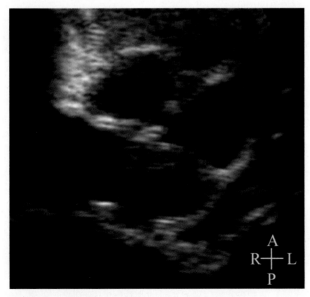

FIGURE 18.4. Parasternal short-axis view of a quadricuspid truncal valve.

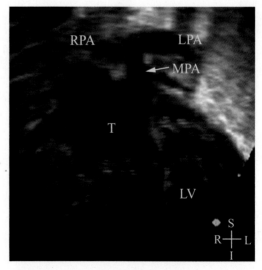

FIGURE 18.6. Subcostal coronal view demonstrating a type I truncus arteriosus. Note the main pulmonary artery (MPA) arising from the truncus arteriosus (T). LPA, left pulmonary artery; LV, left ventricle; RPA, right pulmonary artery.

aspect of the truncal root. The degree of truncal valve dysplasia may also be assessed from the apical and subcostal views, and these views typically provide for excellent Doppler evaluation of the truncal valve. Defects in the atrial septum are commonly present with truncus arteriosus and are optimally seen from the subcostal windows.

The suprasternal notch views are valuable for determining aortic arch sidedness, along with branch pulmonary artery anatomy and distribution. Aortic arch anomalies are common in patients with truncus arteriosus, with a right aortic arch being the most common. Truncus arteriosus with an interrupted aortic arch occurs in up to 20% of patients and is best diagnosed from the suprasternal notch views. From an echocardiographic standpoint, truncus arteriousus with interrupted aortic arch presents a unique challenge due the anatomic complexity and potential surgical implications. Defining the aortic arch branching pattern, and head and neck vessels is critical to correctly defining this anatomy (Fig. 18.7).

Doppler Echocardiographic Examination

The Doppler examination in truncus arteriosus should focus primarily on those factors that have the greatest influence on the patient's hemodynamic state—truncal valve stenosis/regurgitation and pulmonary artery blood flow. Color flow Doppler can provide a qualitative estimation of truncal valve insufficiency as well as identifing aliasing flow at the level of the truncal valve in cases of truncal valve stenosis (Fig. 18.8). The peak and mean gradients across the truncal valve can be estimated using continuous wave Doppler and the Bernoulli equation. Color flow Doppler is useful in delineating pulmonary artery anatomy as well as complex sources of pulmonary blood flow, particularly when pulmonary blood flow is supplied via aortopulmonary collaterals. Spectral Doppler is useful when interrogating the pulmonary arteries for the presence of stenosis, which can occur at any level but is most commonly at the takeoff from the truncal root.

In addition, color Doppler echocardiography can help to identify the origin and anatomic patterns of the coronary arteries. In cases of truncus arteriosus with interrupted aortic arch, color Doppler can greatly aid in the diagnosis and identification of the

arch vessel anatomy. Additional VSDs, not easily seen by two-dimensional echocardiography alone, can be identified using color flow Doppler.

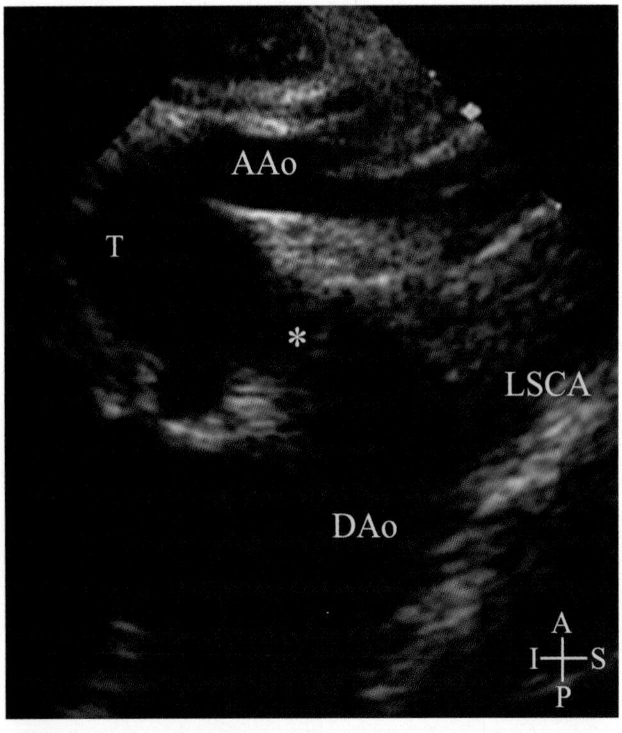

Preoperative Echocardiographic Evaluation of Truncus Arteriosus

The accurate preoperative assessment of truncus arteriosus can have a profound impact on clinical and surgical management. The preoperative two-dimensional and Doppler echocardiographic assessment should include an accurate description of the following:

1. Type of truncus arteriosus
2. Pulmonary artery anatomy and size
3. Coronary artery anatomy and distribution
4. Truncal valve morphology and degree of truncal override
    a. Severity of truncal valve stenosis—estimated by the peak and mean spectral Doppler gradients
    b. Severity of truncal valve regurgitation—estimated by the regurgitant jet characteristics and spectral Doppler velocity pressure half-time
5. Associated cardiac anomalies
    a. Right aortic arch
    b. VSD
    c. Atrial septal defect
    d. Persistent left superior vena cava to the coronary sinus
    e. Absence of the ductus arteriosus
    f. Interrupted aortic arch

Postoperative Echocardiographic Evaluation of Truncus Arteriosus

The surgical repair of truncus arteriosus consists of removing the pulmonary arteries from the truncal root, patch closure of the VSD, and usually placement of a valved conduit between the right ventricle and the pulmonary arteries (Fig. 18.9). When the truncal valve is significantly regurgitant or stenotic, repair or replacement with a homograft valve is typically performed. Intraoperative transesophageal echocardiography is often performed to evaluate the cardiac repair. Patients are followed longitudinally for evidence of right ventricle–to–pulmonary artery conduit stenosis and/or regurgitation, because these conduits typically require replacement over time and as the patient grows (Figs. 18.10 and 18.11). Patients may develop branch pulmonary artery stenosis, and some require intervention, such as pulmonary artery stenting (Figs. 18.12 to 18.14). Truncal (neoaortic) valve regurgitation should be moni-

FIGURE 18.7. Suprasternal notch view of truncus arteriosus with an interrupted aortic arch. AAo, ascending aorta; DAo, descending aorta; LSCA, left subclavian artery; T, truncus arteriosus, *asterisk*, patent ductus arteriosus.

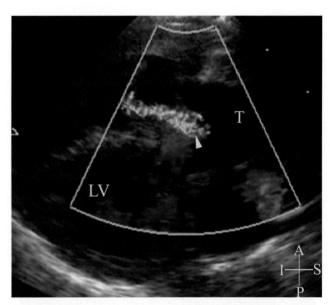

FIGURE 18.8. Parasternal long-axis view with truncal valve regurgitation (*arrow*) demonstrated by color Doppler. LV, left ventricle; T, truncus arteriosus.

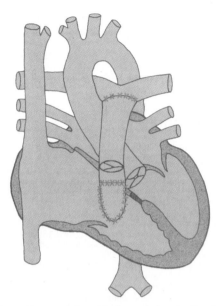

FIGURE 18.9. Figure of truncus arteriosus following surgical repair with patch closure of the ventricular septal defect and right ventricle to pulmonary artery conduit. (Reproduced with permission from Slesnick TC, Kovalchin JP. Truncus arteriosus. In: McMilan JA, ed. *Oski's pediatrics.* 4th ed. Philadelphia: Lippincott Williams & Wilkins; 2006:1540–1543.)

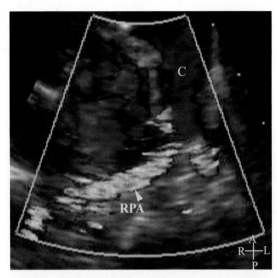

FIGURE 18.12. Parasternal short-axis view. Severe right pulmonary artery stenosis (RPA) following truncus arteriosus repair demonstrated by color Doppler. C, conduit; RPA, right pulmonary artery.

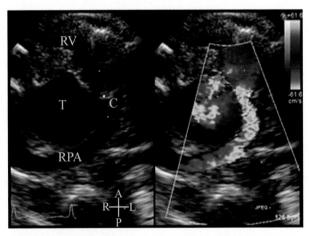

FIGURE 18.10. Parasternal short-axis view of the right ventricle (RV) to pulmonary conduit (C) following surgical repair. Note the turbulent Doppler flow representing conduit stenosis. RPA, right pulmonary artery; T, truncus.

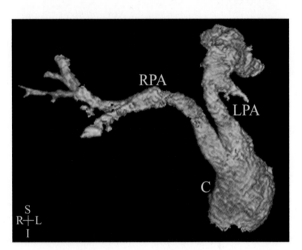

FIGURE 18.13. Cardiac computed tomography three-dimensional reconstruction demonstrating diffusely small branch pulmonary arteries following surgical repair. C, conduit; LPA, left pulmonary artery; RPA, right pulmonary artery.

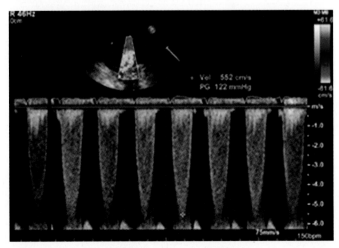

FIGURE 18.11. Continuous-wave Doppler demonstrating conduit stenosis.

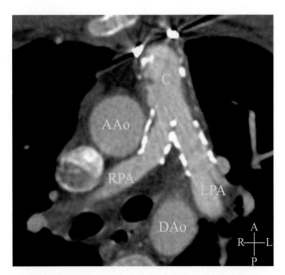

FIGURE 18.14. Cardiac computed tomography. Axial image demonstrating bilateral pulmonary artery stents for severe branch pulmonary artery stenosis following truncus arteriosus repair. AAo, ascending aorta; C, conduit; DAo, descending aorta; LPA, left pulmonary artery; RPA, right pulmonary artery.

tored serially, and some patients may require valvuloplasty or valve replacement. When echocardiography alone does not provide adequate information, then other imaging modalities may be used such as cardiac magnetic resonance imaging, computed tomography, or cardiac catheterization with angiography.

The postoperative two-dimensional and Doppler echocardiographic assessment should include an accurate assessment of the following:

1. Residual shunting across the VSD patch
2. Stenosis across the right ventricle–to–pulmonary artery conduit, including the peak spectral Doppler velocity and pressure gradient
3. Degree of pulmonary regurgitation
4. Branch pulmonary size and the presence of any stenosis or narrowing
5. Truncal valve stenosis and regurgitation
6. Left ventricular outflow tract patency
7. Right ventricular systolic pressure based on either the peak Doppler velocity of a residual VSD or tricuspid regurgitation jet, if available
8. Evaluation of the aortic arch
9. Right and left ventricular size and function

 ## SUMMARY

Truncus arteriosus is a rare form of congenital heart disease with several distinct variations. Echocardiography is the primary tool for preoperative assessment of cardiac anatomy and in determining

the surgical approach. Postoperative patients are followed serially by echocardiography to monitor for potential problems that may develop over time. Additional forms of noninvasive cardiac imaging such as magnetic resonance imaging or computed tomography become more important as these patients become older and echocardiographic imaging alone may not be sufficient.

SUGGESTED READING

Cabalka AK, Edwards WD, Dearani JA. Truncus arteriosus. In: Allen HD, Driscoll DJ, Shaddy RE, Feltes TF, eds. *Moss and Adams' heart disease in infants, children and adolescents: including the fetus and young adult.* 7th ed. Philadelphia: Lippincott Williams & Wilkins; 2008.

Collett RW, Edwards JE. Persistent truncus arteriosus: a classification according to anatomic types. *Surg Clin North Am.* 1949;29:1245.

Konstantinov IE, Karamlou T, Blackstone EH, et al. Truncus arteriosus associated with interrupted aortic arch in 50 neonates: a Congenital Heart Surgeons Society study. *Ann Thorac Surg.* 2006;81:214–223.

Reynolds T, ed. *The pediatric echocardiographer's pocket reference.* 3rd ed. Phoenix: Arizona Heart Institute; 2002.

Silverman NH. *Pediatric echocardiography*: Baltimore, MD: Williams & Wilkins; 1993.

Slesnick TC, Kovalchin JP. Truncus arteriosus. In: McMilan JA, ed. *Oski's pediatrics.* 4th ed. Philadelphia: Lippincott Williams & Wilkins; 2006:1540–1543.

Snider AR, Serwer GA, Ritter SB, eds. *Echocardiography in pediatric heart disease.* 2nd ed. St. Louis: Mosby–Year Book; 1997.

Van Praagh R, Van Praagh S: The anatomy of common aorticopulmonary trunk (truncus arteriosus communis) and its embryological implications. *Am J Cardiol.* 1965;16:406.

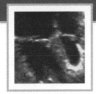

Chapter 19
Patent Ductus Arteriosus and Aortopulmonary Window

Ritu Sachdeva

 ## PATENT DUCTUS ARTERIOSUS

The ductus arteriosus is a normal fetal cardiac structure that functionally closes within the first days of life. However, it may remain patent either in isolation or in association with other congenital cardiac malformations. In premature infants, continued patency of the ductus arteriosus is common after birth and closure is dependent on maturation. The clinical significance of a patent ductus arteriosus (PDA) is determined by the magnitude and direction of shunting across it. Two-dimensional echocardiography is useful in delineating the morphologic features of the PDA, while Doppler echocardiography provides a noninvasive method for evaluating the shunt flow dynamics across it.

Two-dimensional Echocardiography

As an isolated lesion, a PDA is seen as a tubular structure connecting the superior junction of the main pulmonary artery and left pulmonary artery to the ventral aspect of the proximal descending aorta just beyond the origin of left subclavian artery. A PDA can be visualized from the parasternal short-axis, high-left parasternal short-axis, and suprasternal long-axis views.

In the parasternal short-axis view, the PDA is seen arising from the main pulmonary artery and connecting to the descending aorta. Angulating the transducer superiorly and leftward toward the pulmonary artery bifurcation provides images of the PDA (Fig. 19.1). A dropout between the main pulmonary artery and the descending aorta may occur in standard parasternal short-axis views. For optimal imaging of the PDA, avoiding any foreshortening or dropout, a high-parasternal short-axis view, also called the "ductal view," is used. To obtain this view, the transducer is positioned between the suprasternal notch and the standard parasternal region in the left infraclavicular region. The plane of transducer is directed similar to the suprasternal long-axis views through the left pulmonary artery. In this view, the PDA can be seen between the origin of left pulmonary artery and the descending aorta (Fig. 19.2). With slight rotation of the transducer to obtain the long-axis view of the aorta, the entire length of the PDA can be visualized. However, a small PDA may be unapparent in this view as it is positioned vertically within the scan plane and therefore imaged with the lateral resolution of the transducer. If the ductus is right-sided, similar views can be obtained by scanning from a right parasternal approach.

In the suprasternal long-axis views, a PDA is seen connecting the main pulmonary artery and the descending aorta, beyond the origin of the left subclavian artery. In this view, better imaging of the PDA can be obtained by tilting the imaging plane anteriorly toward the left pulmonary artery. The PDA is seen in this view, between the origin of the left pulmonary artery and the descending aorta.

Visualization of a PDA in the parasternal long-axis view may not be as optimal as it is from the parasternal short-axis views. To view the PDA in the parasternal long-axis view, the transducer is placed in the second or third intercostal space parallel to the sternum and then is rotated clockwise and directed inferiorly. In neonates, a similar view can be obtained from the right second intercostal space or subclavicular area with leftward and inferior angulation. In some older patients, one may have to rotate the transducer counterclockwise from the parasternal long-axis plane and then direct it leftward and superiorly. The PDA is then visualized above the left pulmonary artery–main pulmonary artery junction connecting to the descending aorta, which is seen in its longitudinal plane.

Morphologic Variations in Patent Ductus Arteriosus

The PDA in a normal heart runs in an oblique course, forming an obtuse angle with the descending aorta. This normal course of a PDA is altered in congenital heart diseases associated with right ventricular outflow tract obstruction, such as tetralogy of Fallot and pulmonary atresia. In these cases, the PDA has a nearly vertical

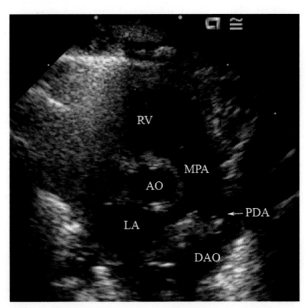

FIGURE 19.1. Parasternal short-axis view of the patent ductus arteriosus (PDA) connection between the main pulmonary artery (MPA) and descending aorta (DAO). Ao, aorta; LA, left atrium; RV, right ventricle.

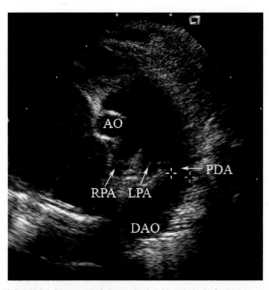

FIGURE 19.2. A high left parasternal short-axis view (ductal view) of a large patent ductus arteriosus (PDA) between the origin of left pulmonary artery (LPA) and descending aorta (DAO), in a patient with hypoplastic left heart syndrome. In this view, the right pulmonary artery (RPA), left pulmonary artery, and PDA are demonstrated from right to left of the image. Notice the small aorta (AO).

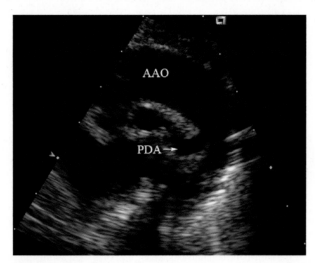

FIGURE 19.3. Suprasternal long-axis view of the aortic arch of a tortuous patent ductus arteriosus (PDA) in a patient with pulmonary atresia. AAO, ascending aorta.

orientation between distal aortic arch and the pulmonary artery and therefore is at an acute angle to the descending aorta. A PDA may also be long and tortuous in these patients (Fig. 19.3) and may be difficult to visualize in a single imaging plane. Occasionally, the PDA may originate from the base of the innominate artery on the left or the right side or bilaterally and consequently has an abnormal course. To image this ductus arising from the base of innominate artery, the transducer is rotated from the suprasternal or high paratsernal view into a frontal plane such that the aorta is seen in its short axis and the right pulmonary artery is seen in its long axis. From this position, the innominate artery can be visualized by angulating the transducer toward the right or left depending on the side of the aortic arch. The bifurcation of the innominate artery into the subclavian and carotid arteries along with origin of PDA at its base can be seen in this view. In the rare instance when there are bilateral PDAs, one ductus is seen in the usual position and the other may arise from the base of either the subclavian artery or the innominate artery on the contralateral side. In hypoplastic left heart syndrome as well as with an interrupted aortic arch, the PDA is almost always large when imaged soon after birth and is at an obtuse angle to the descending aorta. In fact, in the presence of an interrupted aortic arch, one should remember that the true aortic arch is superior to the continuum formed by the pulmonary artery, PDA, and the descending aorta.

Hemodynamic Consequences of a Patent Ductus Arteriosus

The hemodynamic consequence of a large left-to-right shunt across a PDA is volume overload of the left heart and hence dilatation of the left atrium and left ventricle. Historically, the left atrium–to–aortic root (LA/Ao) ratio on M-mode examination has been used for indirect quantification of PDA size. This ratio was popular before the introduction of two-dimensional and Doppler echocardiography. The LA/Ao ratio has been reported to be greater than 1.15 (mean, 1.38 ± 0.19) in neonates with a large left-to-right shunt across a PDA requiring surgical ligation. This M-mode assessment is obtained from the parasternal short-axis view measuring the anterior-posterior dimensions of the left atrium. Using this single dimension, measurement of the left atrium may result in inaccurate estimation of the left atrial size. If the LA/Ao ratio is used in isolation, it has a low specificity for diagnosing a significant-sized PDA. Thus, the usefulness of this ratio has decreased with the advent of two-dimensional and Doppler echocardiography, where one not only can assess the size and flow across the PDA but also can determine left heart enlargement through direct visualization. In addition to the finding of a dilated left atrium and left ventricle, the atrial septum can be seen bulging toward the right atrium. The left ventricular systolic function is often hyperdynamic. In the subcostal views, increased pulsatility of the descending aorta can be seen as a result of large diastolic runoff to the pulmonary arteries resulting in a widened pulse pressure.

Doppler Examination

A color-Doppler echocardiogram provides information regarding the direction and amount of shunt flow across a PDA. Color Doppler has markedly improved the ability of echocardiography to identify a PDA, especially if it is small. Color-Doppler also guides optimal alignment of the spectral Doppler beam. In addition, spectral Doppler interrogation of the PDA provides useful information regarding the shunt direction and pressure gradients throughout the cardiac cycle.

In a patient with an isolated large PDA with normal pulmonary artery pressure and a large left-to-right shunt, continuous red flow from the aorta into the pulmonary arteries will be seen with color Doppler from the parasternal short-axis view (Fig. 19.4). However, a small isolated PDA with normal pulmonary artery pressure will have a high-velocity turbulent jet across it extending to the lateral wall of the pulmonary artery with a color mosaic caused by aliasing (Fig. 19.5). As this jet approaches the pulmonary valve, it is deflected back along the medial wall of pulmonary artery, causing an antegrade diastolic flow pattern in the pulmonary artery. During systole, the normal antegrade flow across the pulmonary valve deflects this jet from the PDA toward the right pulmonary artery. As a result, the retrograde flow in the pulmonary artery is no longer seen. When the ductus is very large, the left-to-right shunt across it may completely fill the pulmonary artery, resulting in loss of secondary flow patterns in the pulmonary artery as described above. A variety of other conditions can produce diastolic flow in the pulmonary arteries that can be confused with a PDA. These include pulmonary insufficiency, a coronary fistula, anomalous origin of coronary artery from pulmonary artery, an aortopulmonary window, and surgically created systemic–to–pulmonary artery shunts.

Spectral Doppler interrogation of a PDA with left-to-right flow and normal pulmonary artery pressure will demonstrate continuous flow above the Doppler baseline with a peak in late systole (Fig. 19.6). Using the modified Bernoulli equation, one can calculate the peak gradient across the PDA using this late systolic peak velocity. This measure has been shown to closely correlate with the peak instantaneous gradient between the aorta and pulmonary artery at catheterization. If the systemic arterial systolic blood pressure is obtained simultaneous to Doppler interrogation across the PDA, one can derive the pulmonary artery systolic pressure by subtracting the peak gradient across the PDA from the systolic blood pressure. In assessing peak Doppler velocities across a PDA to obtain pressure gradients, it is important to remember that for a left-to-right shunt the sample volume should be positioned at the pulmonary end of the PDA. Conversely, for a right-to-left shunt, the sample volume should be positioned at the aortic end of the PDA. Doppler estimation of pulmonary artery pressure using the PDA velocity may not always be accurate and is limited by the position of the sample volume, interference from

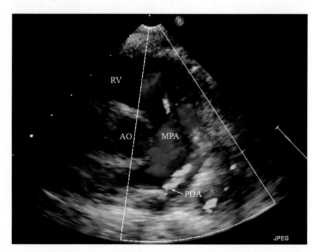

FIGURE 19.4. Parasternal short-axis view with color Doppler showing continuous flow (red) from the patent ductus arteriosus (PDA) into the main pulmonary artery (MPA). Ao, aorta; RV, right ventricle.

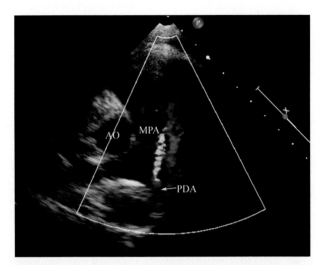

FIGURE 19.5. Color Doppler imaging in the parasternal short-axis view showing a high-velocity, turbulent jet across a small patent ductus arteriosus (PDA) into the main pulmonary artery (MPA) in a patient with normal pulmonary artery pressure. This high velocity Doppler flow is indicative of a large pressure gradient between the aorta and the pulmonary artery. Ao, aorta.

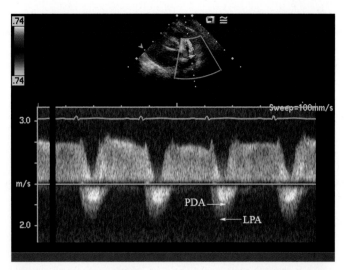

FIGURE 19.7. Continuous-wave Doppler tracing from a neonate with pulmonary artery hypertension. There is a bidirectional shunt across the patent ductus arteriosus (PDA) with a positive deflection from left-to-right shunting from the aorta to the pulmonary artery beginning in late systole and extending into late diastole. A negative deflection resulting from a right-to-left shunt is demonstrated from the pulmonary artery to aorta in mid-to-late systole. With continuous-wave Doppler, a negative deflection caused by flow within the left pulmonary artery (LPA) may interfere with that from a right-to-left shunt across a PDA. These signals can be differentiated in that Doppler flow from the LPA begins at the onset of systole and peaks early, while the right-to-left shunt across the PDA begins later in systole and peaks in mid to late systole.

signals from adjacent structures such as the left pulmonary artery, and the unusual shape and size of the PDA.

In the presence of severe pulmonary hypertension or in congenital cardiac malformations in which the systemic circulation is dependent on the PDA (i.e., critical aortic stenosis, critical coarctation, hypoplastic left heart syndrome, and interrupted aortic arch), there is a right-to-left shunt across the PDA. Color Doppler will demonstrate blue color flow in the PDA representing blood flow from the pulmonary artery into the descending aorta. A spectral Doppler interrogation of such a PDA shows continuous flow below the Doppler baseline with a peak Doppler velocity in early systole.

In normal neonates, a bidirectional shunt across the PDA is present for the first few hours of life but rapidly changes to a continuous left-to-right shunt before functional closure. A bidirectional shunt is present across a PDA with pulmonary hypertension. Color Doppler demonstrates a right-to-left shunt in systole (blue color flow) and a left-to-right shunt in diastole (red color flow). On spectral Doppler, a negative deflection arising from the right-to-left shunt signifies flow from the pulmonary artery to aorta in mid-to-late systole, whereas a positive deflection arising from left-to-right shunt represents flow

from the aorta to pulmonary artery in late systole with extension into late diastole (Fig. 19.7). One should be cautious to differentiate the negative deflection from a right-to-left ductal shunt from a negative deflection caused by flow within the left pulmonary artery. Spectral Doppler from the left pulmonary artery begins at the onset of systole and peaks early, while the right-to-left shunt across a PDA begins later in systole and peaks in mid to late systole.

Pulsed-wave Doppler allows assessment of flow disturbances on either side of the PDA. In a PDA with large left-to-right shunt, there is increased diastolic forward flow in the left pulmonary artery and retrograde diastolic flow in the postductal descending aorta. These retrograde diastolic flow signals are M-shaped, with peaks in early diastole and with atrial systole (Fig. 19.8). These phenomena are useful markers of a hemodynamically significant shunt across the PDA. In the presence of a large left-to-right ductal shunt, reversed diastolic flow

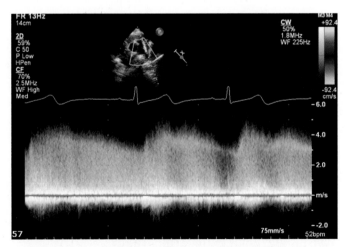

FIGURE 19.6. Continuous-wave Doppler tracing obtained from the parasternal short-axis view in a patient with a small patent ductus arteriosus (PDA) and normal pulmonary artery pressure. There is continuous left-to-right shunting across the PDA in systole and diastole, with a peak Doppler velocity obtained in late systole. The high-velocity of the jet (4 m/s) across the PDA indicates normal pulmonary artery pressure.

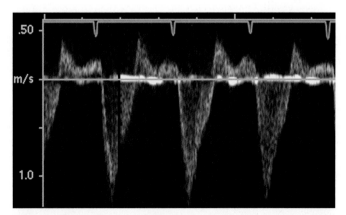

FIGURE 19.8. Pulsed-wave Doppler within the descending aorta from suprasternal imaging in a patient with a large left-to-right ductal shunt with the sample positioned at the origin of the patent ductus arteriosus (PDA). The positive deflection in diastole (M-shaped signal) reflects retrograde flow from the descending aorta into the PDA that peaks in early diastole and after atrial systole. The negative deflection results from forward flow in the descending aorta during systole.

may also be present in other systemic arteries, including the brachial, femoral, carotid, and cerebral arteries. It is important to remember that the finding of retrograde flow in descending aorta is not specific for a PDA but can be seen in any condition with significant diastolic runoff from the aorta, including aortic insufficiency, systemic–to–pulmonary artery shunts, and an aortopulmonary window.

The magnitude of shunt flow across a PDA can be calculated as the difference between the pulmonary and systemic blood flow. Because the shunting occurs distal to the pulmonary valve, calculation of flow across the pulmonary valve provides a measure of systemic flow, and not the pulmonary flow, which is the sum of systemic and ductal shunt flow. Therefore, the flow across the aortic valve represents the actual pulmonary flow. In children with a PDA, close correlation has been found between cardiac catheterization and the Doppler estimated pulmonary–to–systemic flow ratio. However, in neonates, this Doppler estimation is less reliable, because of possible errors in the measurement of the small vessels.

Transesophageal Echocardiogram

In adolescent or adult patients, it may be difficult to image the PDA using a transthoracic probe because of poor echocardiographic windows. In such cases, transesophageal echocardiography (TEE) provides improved imaging of the PDA and its shunt flow because of a closer spatial relationship between the PDA and the transducer within the esophagus. Multiplane TEE provides optimal imaging of a PDA and the color Doppler flow across it.

Ductal Aneurysm

Ductal aneurysms have been reported mostly in the fetus, neonate, and infant but can also occur in older children and adults. These aneurysms may spontaneously regress or may result in complications including compression of adjacent structures, thromboembolism, infection, and rupture. In the parasternal short-axis view, a ductal aneurysm is seen as a saccular dilation adjacent to the left of the main pulmonary artery that extends into the superior mediastinum and may rarely become gigantic (Fig. 19.9). The maximal diameter of the aneurysm is at the aortic end. With color Doppler interrogation, swirling of blood may be seen within the aneurysm. The aneurysm is typically closed at the pulmonary end, but in some cases the ductus may still be patent and can be easily recognized with color Doppler. Thrombus formation within the ductal aneurysm with extension into the branch pulmonary arteries can occasionally be seen on parasternal short-axis views. Normally, the PDA constricts at the pulmonary end first, but occasionally it may constrict along its entire length. If the PDA closes at either the aortic or pulmonary end in isolation, then a diverticulum can be seen, which should be differentiated from a ductal aneurysm.

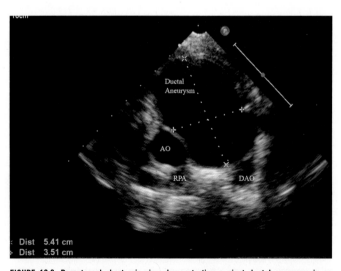

FIGURE 19.9. Parasternal short-axis view demonstrating a giant ductal aneurysm in an asymptomatic 4-year-old girl. The aneurysm is in communication with the descending aorta. A compressed proximal right pulmonary artery (RPA) is seen. AO, aorta.

Echocardiographic Limitations in Imaging the Patent Ductus Arteriosus

When the lumen of the PDA is smaller than the lateral resolution of the transducer, then the PDA cannot be visualized directly. Doppler interrogation can overcome this limitation. Patient size, on either extreme, may be a problem. In very small preterm neonates, especially with pulmonary disease or those on ventilators, it may be difficult to obtain optimal images. Similarly, in older children and adults, the ductal view may be more difficult to obtain. A dropout artifact may resemble a PDA, but this error can be avoided by interrogating the PDA along its entire length, rather than just at the aortic or pulmonary end.

Echocardiographic Evaluation After Device Closure or Surgical Ligation of Patent Ductus Arteriosus

In recent decades, significant advances have been made in the transcatheter approach to ductal closure. Various devices including the Portsmann plug, Rashkind device, Gianturco embolization coils, and, more recently, the Amplatzer ductal occluder device have been used for percutaneous closure of a PDA (Fig. 19.10). Residual shunting across the PDA may be present after percutaneous closure or surgical ligation. Color Doppler is a sensitive technique for detecting residual ductal shunting. When the ductal occlusion procedure has used a Rashkind prosthesis, residual shunting is characteristically seen at the superior margin of the device, whereas with an Amplatzer ductal occluder, residual shunting is most often central through the device. Color and spectral Doppler interrogation of the left pulmonary artery and descending aorta should be performed after both percutaneous PDA closure or surgical ligation because there is a risk for partial occlusion of these structures with either approach. In a multicenter USA Amplatzer PDA occlusion device trial, 89% of the 433 patients demonstrated complete closure on the day after the procedure and 99.7% at 1-year follow-up. In this report, two patients developed partial obstruction of the left pulmonary artery with a peak gradient greater than 20 mm Hg. Inadvertent surgical ligation of the left pulmonary artery instead of the PDA may occur in small infants or premature neonates.

 AORTOPULMONARY WINDOW

An aortopulmonary window is a communication between the ascending aorta and the pulmonary artery above the semilunar valves. Mori et al. proposed three types of aortopulmonary connections:

- Type I, proximal defect–This is the most common and is present midway between the semilunar valves and pulmonary bifurcation.

- Type II, distal defect–This is a communication between the left posterior wall of the ascending aorta and the junction of right pulmonary artery and main pulmonary artery. This type is commonly associated with aortic origin of the right pulmonary artery.
- Type III, total defect–This is a very large defect and involves the entire length of pulmonary trunk from immediately above the semilunar valves to the level of the pulmonary bifurcation and proximal portion of right pulmonary artery.

About half of the patients with an aortopulmonary window have other associated anomalies. These include type A interruption of the aortic arch, aortic origin of the right pulmonary artery (especially in those with distal or total defect), anomalous origin of one or both coronary arteries from pulmonary artery, tetralogy of Fallot, right aortic arch, ventricular septal defect, and transposition of the great arteries.

Two-dimensional Echocardiography

An aortopulmonary window can be seen as a defect between the ascending aorta and the pulmonary artery from the parasternal short-axis, subcostal, and suprasternal views (Fig. 19.11). With slight anterosuperior angulation in the parasternal short-axis view, one can recognize this defect and delineate its extent up to the bifurca-

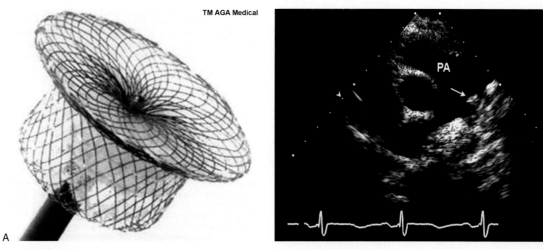

FIGURE 19.10. PDA occluder device. A: AGA medical Amplatzer ductal occluder device. **B:** Parasternal short-axis scan demonstrating Amplatzer device in PDA (*arrow*).

tion of the pulmonary arteries, including the origin of the right pulmonary artery from the aorta. This defect cannot typically be seen in parasternal long-axis views. In the subcostal long-axis view, the transducer should be rotated counterclockwise into a position where the ascending aorta is seen in its long axis with the pulmonary trunk crossing it. In this view, the wall separating the great arteries is aligned along the lateral resolution of the transducer. Therefore, a dropout seen in the region where the aorta and right pulmonary artery intersect can be mistaken for an aortopulmonary window. A "T"-artifact at the edge of the defect can help distinguish an actual defect from artifactual dropout. The subcostal view is especially useful for determining the proximity of the defect to the origin of the left coronary artery. In the suprasternal long-axis view, as the lower border of the ascending aorta is followed superiorly, instead of the usual circular pattern of the main pulmonary artery, an aortopulmonary window is seen as a semicircle.

Secondary effects of an aortopulmonary window result from the large left-to-right shunt across it. The left atrium and left ventricle are dilated, and so are the pulmonary arteries. The right ventricle may occasionally be hypertrophied.

Doppler Echocardiography

In contrast to a PDA, the jet of blood flow from the aorta enters the pulmonary artery perpendicular to its long axis and then rapidly expands. In a small restrictive aortopulmonary window, color Doppler

interrogation shows a continuous high-velocity turbulent jet from the aorta to the pulmonary artery. In larger defects with normal pulmonary vascular resistance, a continuous antegrade flow is seen in the pulmonary arteries distal to the anterior-posterior window as a result of a large left-to-right shunt from aorta to pulmonary artery. Abnormal retrograde diastolic flow is seen in the descending aorta during diastole caused by runoff from aorta into pulmonary arteries. The antegrade flow in distal MPA and branch pulmonary arteries distinguishes an aortopulmonary window from a PDA. In the presence of pulmonary hypertension, a low-velocity bidirectional flow will be present across the anterior-posterior window. Even though this is an extremely rare cardiac defect, appropriate diagnosis is possible with echocardiography.

Echocardiograpic Evaluation After Closure of an Aortopulmonary Window

A large aortopulmonary window with or without other associated with other cardiac malformations is closed surgically using a patch technique. A small aortopulmonary window or a residual surgical defect may be closed using transcatheter devices. Closure of the anterior-posterior window with either technique can be complicated by stenosis within the ascending aorta or pulmonary artery or a residual v defect. These can be best assessed using the two-dimensional and Doppler echocardiographic approach described earlier to locate the aortopulmoary window.

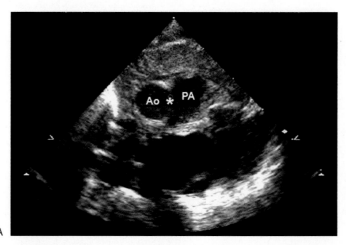
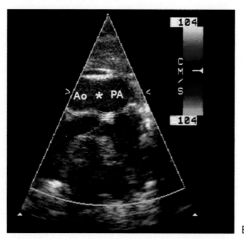

FIGURE 19.11. Aortopulmonary window. A: A high parasternal short axis scan demonstrating characteristic defect (*) between aorta (Ao) and main pulmonary artery (PA) **B:** Color Doppler demonstrating defect (*) and origin of branch pulmonary arteries.

SUGGESTED READING

Ali Khan MA, al Yousef S, Mullins CE, et al. Experience with 205 procedures of transcatheter closure of ductus arteriosus in 182 patients, with special reference to residual shunts and long-term follow-up. *J Thorac Cardiovasc Surg.* 1992;104:1721–1727.

Allen HD, Goldberg SJ, Valdes-Cruz LM, et al. Use of echocardiography in newborns with patent ductus arteriosus: a review. *Pediatr Cardiol.* 1982;3:65–70.

Alverson DC, Eldridge M, Aldrich M, et al. Effect of patent ductus arteriosus on lower extremity blood flow velocity patterns in preterm infants. *Am J Perinatol.* 1984;1:216–222.

Balaji S, Burch M, Sullivan ID. Accuracy of cross-sectional echocardiography in diagnosis of aortopulmonary window. *Am J Cardiol.* 1991;67:650–653.

Cloez JL, Isaaz K, Pernot C. Pulsed Doppler flow characteristics of ductus arteriosus in infants with associated congenital anomalies of the heart or great arteries. *Am J Cardiol.* 1986;57:845–851.

Dyamenahalli U, Smallhorn JF, Geva T, et al. Isolated ductus arteriosus aneurysm in the fetus and infant: a multi-institutional experience. *J AM Coll Cardio* 2000;36:262–269.

Ellison RC, Peckham GJ, Lang P, et al. Evaluation of the preterm infant for patent ductus arteriosus. *Pediatrics.* 1983;71:364–372.

Feldtman RW, Andrassy RJ, Alexander JA, et al. Doppler ultrasonic flow detection as an adjunct in the diagnosis of patent ductus arteriosus in premature infants. *J Thorac Cardiovasc Surg.* 1976;72:288–290.

Freedom RM, Moes CA, Pelech A, et al. Bilateral ductus arteriosus (or remnant): an analysis of 27 patients. *Am J Cardiol.* 1984;53:884–891.

Hiraishi S, Horiguchi Y, Misawa H, et al. Noninvasive Doppler echocardiographic evaluation of shunt flow dynamics of the ductus arteriosus. *Circulation.* 1987;75:1146–1153.

Huhta JC, Cohen M, Gutgesell HP. Patency of the ductus arteriosus in normal neonates: two-dimensional echocardiography versus Doppler assessment. *J Am Coll Cardiol.* 1984;4:561–564.

Krauss D, Weinert L, Lang RM. The role of multiplane transesophageal echocardiography in diagnosing PDA in an adult. *Echocardiography.* 1996;13:95–98.

Liao PK, Su WJ, Hung JS. Doppler echocardiographic flow characteristics of isolated patent ductus arteriosus: better delineation by Doppler color flow mapping. *J Am Coll Cardiol.* 1988;12:1285–1291.

Lund JT, Jensen MB, Hjelms E. Aneurysm of the ductus arteriosus. A review of the literature and the surgical implications. *Eur J Cardiothorac Surg.* 1991;5:566–570.

Martin CG, Snider AR, Katz SM, et al. Abnormal cerebral blood flow patterns in preterm infants with a large patent ductus arteriosus. *J Pediatr.* 1982;101:587–593.

Mori K, Ando M, Takao A, et al. Distal type of aortopulmonary window. Report of 4 cases. *Br Heart J.* 1978;40:681–689.

Musewe NN, Benson LN, Smallhorn JF, et al. Two-dimensional echocardiographic and color flow Doppler evaluation of ductal occlusion with the Rashkind prosthesis. *Circulation.* 1989;80:1706–1710.

Musewe NN, Poppe D, Smallhorn JF, et al. Doppler echocardiographic measurement of pulmonary artery pressure from ductal Doppler velocities in the newborn. *J Am Coll Cardiol.* 1990;15:446–456.

Musewe NN, Smallhorn JF, Benson LN, et al. Validation of Doppler-derived pulmonary arterial pressure in patients with ductus arteriosus under different hemodynamic states. *Circulation.* 1987;76:1081–1091.

Naik GD, Chandra VS, Shenoy A, et al. Transcatheter closure of aortopulmonary window using Amplatzer device. *Cathet Cardiovasc Interv.* 2003;59:402–405.

Pass RH, Hijazi Z, Hsu DT, et al. Multicenter USA Amplatzer patent ductus arteriosus occlusion device trial: initial and one-year results. *J Am Coll Cardiol.* 2004;44:513–519.

Perlman JM, Hill A, Volpe JJ. The effect of patent ductus arteriosus on flow velocity in the anterior cerebral arteries: ductal steal in the premature newborn infant. *J Pediatr.* 1981;99:767–771.

Sahn DJ, Allen HD. Real-time cross-sectional echocardiographic imaging and measurement of the patent ductus arteriosus in infants and children. *Circulation.* 1978;58:343–354.

Santos MA, Moll JN, Drumond C, et al. Development of the ductus arteriosus in right ventricular outflow tract obstruction. *Circulation.* 1980;62:818–822.

Seward JB, Khandheria BK, Freeman WK, et al. Multiplane transesophageal echocardiography: image orientation, examination technique, anatomic correlations, and clinical applications. *Mayo Clin Proc.* 1993;68:523–551.

Shiraishi H, Yanagisawa M. Bidirectional flow through the ductus arteriosus in normal newborns: evaluation by Doppler color flow imaging. *Pediatr Cardiol.* 1991;12:201–205.

Shyu KG, Lai LP, Lin SC, et al. Diagnostic accuracy of transesophageal echocardiography for detecting patent ductus arteriosus in adolescents and adults. *Chest.* 1995;108:1201–1205.

Silverman NH, Lewis AB, Heymann MA, et al. Echocardiographic assessment of ductus arteriosus shunt in premature infants. *Circulation.* 1974;50:821–825.

Smallhorn JF, Anderson RH, MaCartney FJ. Two dimensional echocardiographic assessment of communications between ascending aorta and pulmonary trunk or individual pulmonary arteries. *Br Heart J.* 1982;47:563–572.

Snider AR. The ductus arteriosus: a window for assessment of pulmonary artery pressures? *J Am Coll Cardiol.* 1990;15:457–458.

Sorensen KE, Kristensen B, Hansen OK. Frequency of occurrence of residual ductal flow after surgical ligation by color-flow mapping. *Am J Cardiol.* 1991;67:653–654.

Stamato T, Smallhorn JF, et al. Transcatheter closure of an aortopulmonary window with a modified double umbrella occluder system. *Cathet Cardiovasc Diagn.* 1995;35:165–167.

Stevenson JG, Kawabori I, Guntheroth WG. Noninvasive detection of pulmonary hypertension in patent ductus arteriosus by pulsed Doppler echocardiography. *Circulation.* 1979;60:355–359.

Swensson RE, Valdes-Cruz LM, Sahn DJ, et al. Real-time Doppler color flow mapping for detection of patent ductus arteriosus. *J Am Coll Cardiol.* 1986;8:1105–1112.

Vargas Barron J, Sahn DJ, Valdes-Cruz LM, et al. Clinical utility of two-dimensional Doppler echocardiographic techniques for estimating pulmonary to systemic blood flow ratios in children with left to right shunting atrial septal defect, ventricular septal defect or patent ductus arteriosus. *J Am Coll Cardiol.* 1984;3:169–178.

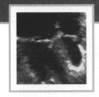

Chapter 20
Abnormalities of the Aortic Arch

Angira Patel • Luciana T. Young

Anomalies of the aortic arch represent a group of lesions that may occur in isolation or in conjunction with other cardiac defects. In this chapter, aortic arch anomalies will be described as they occur in isolation. Important associations with other cardiac defects will be acknowledged. Aortic arch anomalies to be discussed in this chapter include (a) brachiocephalic branching and vascular rings (including pulmonary artery sling), (b) coarctation of the aorta, and (c) interrupted aortic arch (IAA).

ABNORMALITIES OF BRACHIOCEPHALIC BRANCHING

During normal development, six pairs of arches form the primitive dorsal and ventral aortae (Fig. 20.1). Most portions of the first, second, and fifth arches regress. The carotid arteries are formed by the third arches. The ventral portion of the sixth arch contributes to formation of the pulmonary artery. The right dorsal sixth arch disappears, while the left dorsal portion of the sixth arch becomes the ductus arteriosus. The subclavian arteries are formed by the seven dorsal intersegmental arteries. Involution of the right fourth arch typically results in the usual left aortic arch arrangement. A right aortic arch forms when there is involution of the left fourth arch.

Echocardiographic Assessment of the Aortic Arch

Echocardiographic imaging of the aortic arch is best achieved from the suprasternal notch views. In patients with a left aortic arch, the ascending, transverse, and descending portions of the arch, including the origins of the three arch vessels can be imaged from the suprasternal long axis view with the sector plane extending anteriorly from the right nipple to the left scapula posteriorly (Fig. 20.2). If the descending portion of the aorta is not visible,

clockwise rotation with minimal angulation of the transducer to the right may identify the presence of a right aortic arch.

Cross-sectional imaging of the transverse aorta is obtained from the suprasternal short axis view. Anterior angulation of the transducer allows visualization of the first brachiocephalic vessel originating from the arch, which is the innominate artery. The direction in which this vessel courses cephalad is important for determining arch sidedness. The presence of a left aortic arch is confirmed when the innominate artery courses rightward (Fig. 20.3) and the aorta descends leftward. If the vessel courses leftward (Fig 20.4) and the aorta descends rightward, a right aortic arch is present. The innominate artery should be followed distally to its bifurcation into the carotid and subclavian arteries. Echocardiographic demonstration of the bifurcation of the first brachiocephalic vessel in either a left or right aortic arch confirms the absence of a vascular ring. Absence of this bifurcation in a left aortic arch suggests the presence of an aberrant right subclavian artery. A common vascular anomaly, an aberrant right subclavian artery, occurs in 0.5% of humans and carries little, if any, clinical significance (Fig. 20.5). On the other hand, absence of bifurcation of the innominate artery with a right aortic arch suggests the presence of an aberrant left subclavian artery, which has a retroesophageal course and may form a vascular ring in the presence of a left-sided ligamentum arteriosum or ductus arteriosus. Addition of color Doppler is helpful for confirming bifurcation of the first brachiocephalic vessel.

Posterior tilting of the imaging plane in the suprasternal short-axis view allows determination of whether the aorta remains on the same side of the spine as it descends within the thorax. The subcostal short-axis view is also helpful for determining which side of the spine the arch is on as it crosses below the diaphragm.

Another arch variant that deserves mentioning is the cervical aortic arch. Typically presenting as a pulsatile neck mass, the cervical arch extends farther into the neck than a normal arch and is best identified in the suprasternal long-axis view by moving the transducer out of the suprasternal notch and onto the neck.

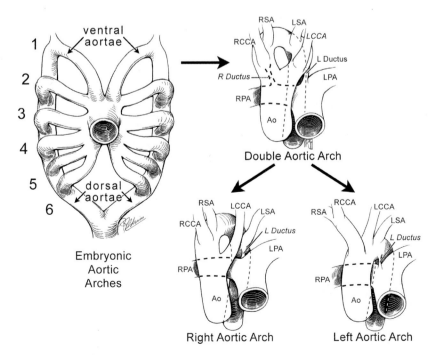

FIGURE 20.1. Embryology of the aortic arches LPA, left pulmonary artery; RPA, right pulmonary artery; RCCA, right common carotid artery; LCCA, left common carotid artery; RSA, right subclavian artery; LSA, left subclavian artery; Ao, aorta. (From Mavroudis and Backer. *Pediatric Cardiac Surgery*, 3rd ed. New York: Mosby; 2003. Used with permission.)

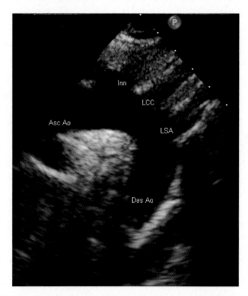

FIGURE 20.2. Suprasternal long-axis view of normal brachiocephalic branching in a left aortic arch. Asc Ao, ascending aorta; Des Ao, descending aorta; Inn, innominate artery; LCC, left common carotid artery; LSA, left subclavian artery.

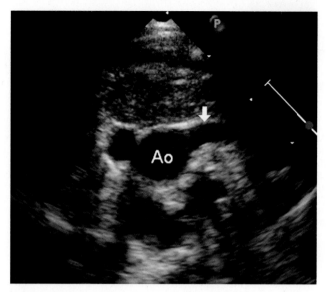

FIGURE 20.4. Right aortic arch. The first brachiocephalic branch off the aortic arch courses leftward (arrow).

 ## VASCULAR RINGS

Vascular rings represent a group of vascular anomalies that cause compression of the trachea, esophagus, or both. Development of a vascular ring depends on the preservation or deletion of specific portions of the rudimentary embryonic aortic arch and may in part be formed by a patent ductus arteriosus or ligamentum arteriosum (Fig. 20.6).

Most children with vascular rings develop symptoms early, usually within the first several weeks to months of life. Symptoms may include breathing difficulty, wheezing, stridor, cough, recurrent respiratory infections, and/or dysphagia. The severity of the clinical presentation depends primarily on the degree of compression by the abnormal vessel on the trachea, bronchus, or esophagus. Respiratory symptoms are often mild and may not be apparent during the newborn period. An infant may gain appropriate weight initially because they often tolerate liquid formula without difficulty. However, once they advance to solid food, their symptoms become more evident and may include apnea or cyanosis. Patients with a double aortic arch tend to present at an earlier age than those with

other types of vascular rings. Symptoms are often aggravated by crying, physical exertion, or the presence of a respiratory infection.

Left Aortic Arch With Aberrant Right Subclavian Artery

A left aortic arch with aberrant right subclavian artery is formed when there is regression of the right fourth arch, which lies between the subclavian and carotid arteries. In most cases, a left aortic arch with an aberrant right subclavian artery is not considered a clinically significant finding. However, when a right-sided ductus arteriosus or ligamentum arteriosus is present, a complete vascular ring can be formed (Fig. 20.7). Inability to visualize the bifurcation of the right innominate artery originating from a left aortic arch suggests the presence of a left arch with aberrant right subclavian artery. Complete sweeps of the aortic arch from the suprasternal long- and short-axis views demonstrate the origin of the aberrant right subclavian artery from the

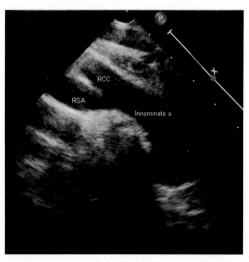

FIGURE 20.3. Left aortic arch. Bifurcation of the innominate artery into the right common carotid artery (RCC) and right subclavian artery (RSA). The left arch is confirmed when the innominate artery courses rightward.

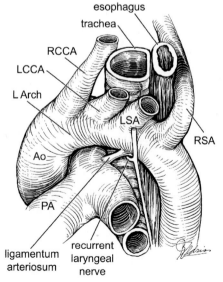

FIGURE 20.5. Left aortic arch with aberrant right subclavian artery (RSA) from the descending aorta. LCCA, left common carotid artery; RCCA, right common carotid artery; LSA, left subclavian artery. (From Mavroudis and Backer. *Pediatric Cardiac Surgery*, 3rd ed. New York: Mosby; 2003. Used with permission.)

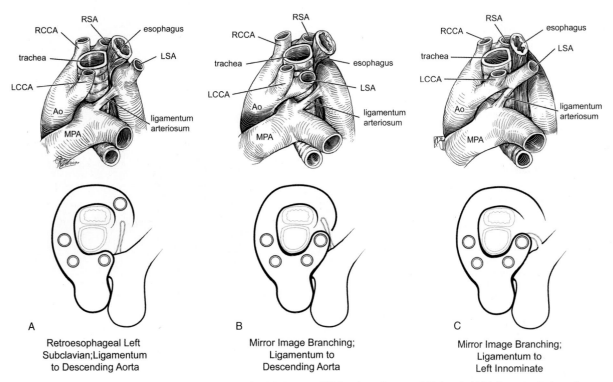

FIGURE 20.6. Right aortic arches. A. Right arch with aberrant left subclavian artery (LSA) from descending aorta. **B.** Right arch with left ligamentum to descending aorta. **C.** Right arch with left ligamentum to left subclavian artery (LSA). (From Mavroudis and Backer. *Pediatric Cardiac Surgery*, 3rd ed. New York: Mosby; 2003. Used with permission.)

upper descending thoracic aorta. Additional imaging should focus on determining whether a right-sided ductus arteriosus is present.

Right Aortic Arch With Aberrant Left Subclavian Artery

Involution of the embryonic left fourth arch results in formation of a right aortic arch. Mirror-image branching is present in 35% of patients with a right aortic arch and occurs when there is persistence of the right fourth arch and disappearance of the left arch between the left subclavian artery and the dorsal descending aorta. A vascular ring is formed when the ligamentum arteriosum originates from the descending aorta.

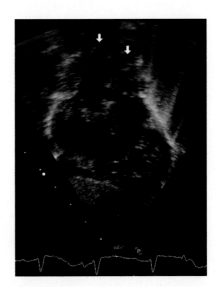

FIGURE 20.7. Vascular ring. Subcostal imaging plane demonstrating left aortic arch with right sided ductus arteriosus forming a vascular ring.

Echocardiographic identification of the first brachiocephalic vessel coursing leftward and superiorly in the suprasternal short-axis view, confirms the presence of a right aortic arch. Absence of the bifurcation of the left innominate artery with a right aortic arch suggests the presence of an aberrant left subclavian artery. Additional imaging modalities may be needed to confirm the presence of a left ligamentum arteriosum.

Right Aortic Arch With Retroesophageal Segment and Left Descending Aorta

Persistence of the embryonic right fourth arch with deletion of the left arch between the left carotid and left subclavian arteries results in a right aortic arch with a retroesophageal course of the left subclavian artery (Fig. 20.6). In 65% of patients with a right aortic arch, the left subclavian artery arises from the descending aorta and courses to the left behind the esophagus. In this case, a vascular ring may be formed when there is a ligmentum arteriosum extending from the descending aorta to the left pulmonary artery.

In the suprasternal long-axis view, echocardiographic identification of this arch anomaly may be difficult because the descending aorta descends to the left despite the arch being rightward. Often associated with a cervical arch, the arch can have a hairpin appearance. The transducer may need to be moved onto the neck to accurately demonstrate branching. The diagnosis of a right aortic arch is confirmed when the first brachiocephalic vessel courses leftward and superiorly.

Double Aortic Arch

A double aortic arch occurs when there is persistence of both the right and left aortic arches. A ring is formed around the trachea and esophagus by the two arches, as they arise from the ascending aorta. The posterior arch is rightward and typically the dominant arch in 75% of cases, giving rise to the right carotid and subclavian arteries. The anterior, leftward arch is usually smaller and gives rise to the left carotid and subclavian arteries. In 20% of cases, the left arch may be the dominant arch, while in 5% of cases the arches may be equal in size. Approximately 20% of patients with double aortic arch have associated congenital heart disease, including tetralogy of Fallot, ventricular septal defect, coarctation, patent ductus arteriosus, transposition of the great arteries, and truncus arteriosus.

Subcostal imaging of left ventricular outflow may show bifurcation into two separate arches and is often the first clue that a double aortic arch is present. From the suprasternal long-axis view, counterclockwise rotation of the transducer will bring both arches into view. Color Doppler is helpful in confirming these findings and in identifying the origins of the arch vessels.

Pulmonary Artery Sling

In this rare vascular malformation, the left pulmonary artery originates from the right pulmonary artery and passes between the esophagus and trachea as it courses toward the left hilum (Fig. 20.8). Symptoms are typically related to tracheal compression and include respiratory distress, stridor, cyanosis, wheezing, and retractions. Additional cardiac defects are often present and can include patent ductus arteriosus, atrial septal defect, ventricular septal defect, pulmonary atresia, left superior vena cava, and single ventricle. Tracheal stenosis, complete tracheal rings, and tracheoesophageal fistula are also common extracardiac associations.

Although there may be a suggestion of an abnormal origin of the left pulmonary artery in the subcostal and parasternal short-axis views, the suprasternal long-axis view provides the best acoustic window for imaging of a pulmonary artery sling. In this view, the left pulmonary artery is seen arising from the right pulmonary artery and coursing leftward, behind the trachea to the left lung (Fig. 20.9). Color and spectral Doppler are helpful for differentiating the left pulmonary artery from other structures that may be mistaken for the left pulmonary artery, such as a patent ductus arteriosus or left atrial appendage.

Additional Imaging Modalities

The diagnosis of aortic arch anomalies such as vascular rings can often be made echocardiographically. However, because of limited acoustic windows, it may not be the dominant imaging modality used. Initial evaluation of a patient with suspected vascular ring typically includes a chest radiograph for determination of arch sidedness and its relation to the trachea. When arch sidedness is not clearly evident, the presence of a double aortic arch should be suspected. Narrowing of the trachea in the lateral images may be seen with a right aortic arch or double aortic arch (Fig. 20.10). Unilateral hyperinflation of the right lung suggests the presence of a pulmonary artery sling.

The barium esophagogram has traditionally been used for the diagnosis of vascular rings. Indentation of the barium-filled esophagus by the anomalous arch vessel produces characteristic patterns

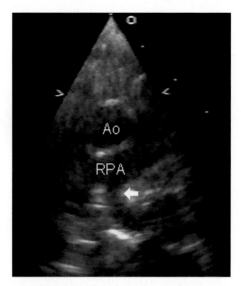

FIGURE 20.9. Pulmonary artery sling. Parasternal image demonstrating origin of the left pulmonary artery (arrow) from the right pulmonary artery. Ao, aorta.

for each specific lesion. For example, a right aortic arch with left ligamentum or double aortic arch produces an indentation of the posterior aspect of the esophagus (Fig. 20.11A). A double aortic arch results in bilateral compression of the esophagus in the anteroposterior view (Fig. 20.11B). A right aortic arch with a retroesophageal left subclavian artery creates an oblique indentation in the esophagus angled toward the left shoulder, whereas an aberrant right subclavian artery generates a high posterior oblique indentation of the esophagus directed from left to right. An anterior esophageal indentation is seen with pulmonary artery sling (Fig. 20.12).

Bronchoscopy may be helpful for establishing the diagnosis in children who present with respiratory distress in whom a vascular ring is suspected. Compression of the trachea can be seen with a double aortic arch or right aortic arch with a left ligamentum. Bronchoscopy can be used to exclude other causes of respiratory compromise, such as the presence of tracheal rings with a pulmonary artery sling.

Additional imaging modalities that provide accurate diagnosis of aortic arch anomalies, such as vascular rings, include computed tomography (CT) scanning and magnetic resonance imaging (MRI). Because not all vascular rings are completed by a patent vascular structure (i.e., some are completed by a ligamentum arteriosum or atretic lesser arch), recognition of the arterial branching pattern,

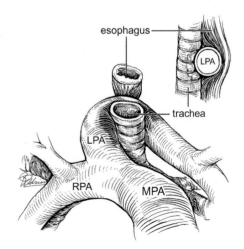

FIGURE 20.8. Diagram demonstrating a pulmonary artery sling. The left pulmonary artery (LPA) originates from the right pulmonary artery (RPA) rather than the from the normal bifurcation from the main pulmonary artery (MPA). (From Mavroudis and Backer. *Pediatric Cardiac Surgery*, 3rd ed. New York: Mosby; 2003. Used with permission.)

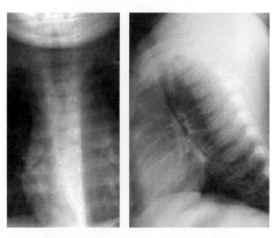

FIGURE 20.10. A. Frontal radiograph with tracheal narrowing consistent with a double aortic arch. **B.** Lateral radiograph demonstrating tracheal narrowing consistent with either a right or double aortic arch. (Courtesy of Cynthia Rigsby, MD.)

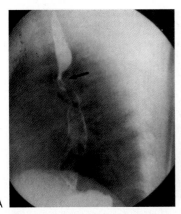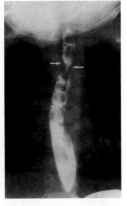

A   B

FIGURE 20.11. A. Barium esophagram from the lateral projection demonstrating an indentation (arrow) consistent with a vascular ring. **B.** Barium esophagram demonstrating bilateral compression (arrows) consistent with a double aortic arch. (Courtesy of Cynthia Rigsby, MD.)

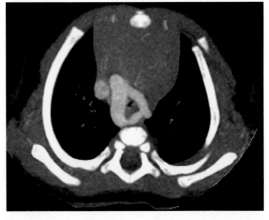

FIGURE 20.13. Chest CT scan demonstrating tracheal compression from a vascular ring. (Courtesy of Cynthia Rigsby, MD.)

arch sidedness, and narrowing of the airway remain important clues in establishing a correct diagnosis. CT scanning is often preferred because it can be performed quickly and does not necessarily require sedation. CT and MRI have essentially obviated the need for tracheograms and cardiac catheterization in the diagnosis of vascular rings (Figs. 20.13 through 20.16).

 ## COARCTATION OF THE AORTA

Coarctation of the aorta represents a congenital narrowing of the aorta, most often occurring just distal to the left subclavian artery and adjacent to the site of insertion of the ductus arteriosus. Coarctation occurs in 5% to 8% in patients with congenital heart disease and is slightly more predominant in males. Common associated anomalies include patent ductus arteriosus, bicuspid aortic valve, ventricular septal defect, and mitral valve abnormalities. More complex defects that may be seen in conjunction with coarctation include Shone syndrome, hypoplastic left heart syndrome, tricuspid atresia with transposed great arteries, and other forms of transposition, in which coexisting subaortic stenosis may lead to development of arch obstruction. Additional arterial abnormalities, such as steno-

sis of the origin of the left subclavian artery and anomalous origin of the right subclavian artery distal to the site of coarctation, have also been reported.

The clinical presentation of coarctation may be variable and depends on patient age, lesion severity, and location of the narrowing, as well as the presence and severity of additional cardiac defects. As the name implies, ductal-dependent, or critical, coarctation typically presents with cardiovascular collapse early in the newborn period once the ductus closes. The clinical presentation of severe coarctation may be delayed to later in infancy and includes symptoms of congestive heart failure, such as respiratory distress, pallor, and poor feeding. Children with less severe narrowing of the aorta may not have any significant symptoms until later in life, in which case they may present with systemic hypertension and their femoral pulses may be absent or weak and delayed in comparison with their brachial pulses.

Two-dimensional Imaging of Coarctation

Although coarctation of the aorta is best imaged from the suprasternal notch view, there are several intracardiac findings demonstrated in a combination of views that should suggest the possibility of arch obstruction. These include the presence of left ventricular obstruction, right or left ventricular hypertrophy and/or dysfunction without an obvious etiology, and reduced or absent pulsatility of the abdominal aorta.

The subcostal view is useful for demonstrating the position of the aorta as it traverses the diaphragm. The transducer is positioned just below the xiphoid process with the plane of sound oriented in a coronal section for the short-axis view. From here, 90-degree rotation of the transducer with leftward or rightward angulation (depending on position of the aorta in the abdomen) in the sagittal

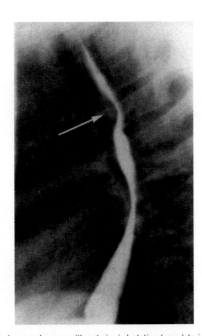

FIGURE 20.12. Barium esophagram with anterior indentation (arrow) typical of a pulmonary artery sling. (Courtesy of Cynthia Rigsby, MD.)

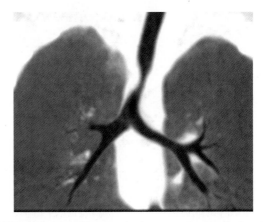

FIGURE 20.14. Tracheogram with compression from a vascular ring. (Courtesy of Cynthia Rigsby, MD.)

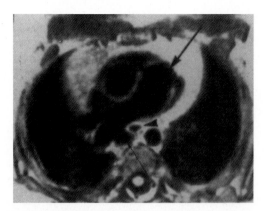

FIGURE 20.15. MRI scan demonstrating a pulmonary artery sling. The trachea (short arrow) is compressed by the left pulmonary artery (thin arrow). Main pulmonary artery (thick arrow). (Courtesy of Cynthia Rigsby, MD.)

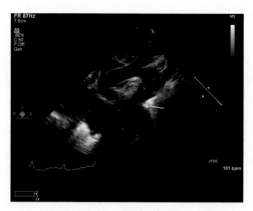

FIGURE 20.17. Coarctation of the aorta. Suprasternal long-axis view demonstrating a posterior shelf (arrow).

plane demonstrates a long segment of the descending, abdominal aorta. In small infants, it may be possible to visualize the entire aorta by scanning in a cranial direction in this plane. Left atrial enlargement, right ventricular enlargement, and dilation of the pulmonary artery may be evident. The presence of ventricular dysfunction should lead to careful assessment of both outflow tracts for potential obstruction.

Parasternal long-axis imaging shows right ventricular dilation and hypertrophy in coarctation. The left ventricle may also be dilated with poor systolic function. Anterior angulation of the transducer allows visualization of the dilated pulmonary artery and ductus arteriosus, if one is present. A high left or right parasternal view with angulation of the transducer toward the left shoulder may also reveal the site of coarctation. The parasternal short-axis view may demonstrate ventricular dilation. M-mode is used to quantify left ventricular wall thickness, chamber dimensions, left ventricular mass, and systolic function.

The apical view may reveal chamber enlargement and hypertrophy and allows additional assessment of the outflow tracts. Ventricular function can be further quantified by calculation of left ventricular ejection fraction.

The suprasternal arch view is considered the best window for imaging the aortic arch (Fig. 20.17). From the long-axis orientation, the aortic arch can usually be imaged in its entirety. The area of coarctation is typically found in the region of the left subclavian artery and is most often characterized by an echo-dense shelf of tissue arising from the posterior aspect of the aorta. It is important not to confuse an anterior shelf, which may be present in the location of the ductal ampulla, as coarctation. On occasion, a long segment narrowing may be present or the narrowed segment may be

located more distally in the aorta. For this reason, the entire aorta must be imaged so as not to miss this important diagnosis. The transverse aortic arch may be hypoplastic in neonates with coarctation and can contribute to residual obstruction following repair. Additional features of coarctation include an increased distance between the left common carotid artery and left subclavian artery and an isthmus diameter of less than two-thirds the diameter of the descending aorta. Determination of arch sidedness and branching, which can be obtained from the suprasternal short-axis view, is also important in the presurgical evaluation of patients with coarctation. If imaging of the aorta and arch is inadequate or in the presence of a large ductus arteriosus, other imaging modalities such as CT and MRI may be necessary to better define arch anatomy before surgical repair.

Doppler Features of Coarctation

Color Doppler demonstrates an area of flow acceleration proximal to the narrowed aortic segment, thus confirming the diagnosis of coarctation (Fig. 20.18). In severe coarctation, there is often aliasing of the color flow jet above the Nyquist limit, with continuation of flow in both systole and diastole. The width of the color jet has been shown to correlate well with the diameter of the coarctation measured angiographically.

In the presence of a significant coarctation, the pulsed Doppler examination of the abdominal aorta in the subcostal view will show a dampened, low-velocity signal with continuation of flow throughout diastole and absence of early diastolic flow reversal (Fig. 20.19). Time to peak velocity is delayed, and the mean acceleration rate is decreased (Fig. 20.20).

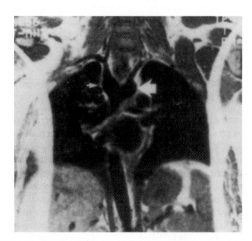

FIGURE 20.16. MRI scan demonstrating a double aortic arch (arrows). (Courtesy of Cynthia Rigsby, MD.)

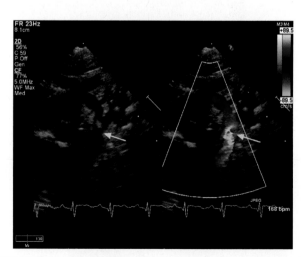

FIGURE 20.18. Coarctation of aorta. 2-dimensional imaging (left) demonstrates a discrete coarctation (arrow). Color Doppler (right) demonstrates aliased flow in the area of obstruction.

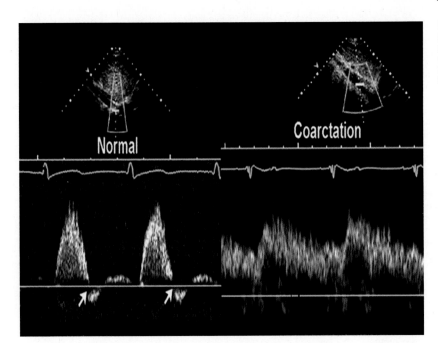

FIGURE 20.19. Abdominal aorta Doppler flow patterns. Left (normal): pulsed-wave Doppler evaluation of the abdominal aorta at the diaphragm demonstrates a brisk upstroke and downstroke with presence of an early diastolic flow reversal (EDR) signal (arrow). The EDR signal excludes proximal obstruction in the thoracic aorta. **Right** (coarctation): Upstroke and downstroke are delayed and the EDR is absent.

In the suprasternal notch view, placement of the pulsed Doppler sample volume parallel to, and just proximal to the site of coarctation, reveals increased flow velocity, usually exceeding the Nyquist limit. For this reason, use of guided and nonguided continuous-wave Doppler is necessary. The characteristic Doppler flow pattern is described as "sawtooth" in appearance, with antegrade flow extending into diastole. Two populations of flow are typically present and superimposed on one another: a high-velocity, outer envelope reflects flow across the site of coarctation (V_2), and a lower-velocity, dense inner envelope represents flow proximal to the coarctation (V_1) (Fig. 20.21). Because additional left heart obstructive lesions may be present in patients with coarctation, the velocity proximal to the site of coarctation may be increased. If the proximal velocity is greater than 1 m/s, then the modified Bernoulli equation ($\Delta P = 4[V_2^2 - V_1^2]$) should be used to calculate the maximum instantaneous gradient across the area of coarctation. Because the systolic velocities may overestimate the true blood pressure gradient, the mean gradient may be more reflective of the actual blood pressure gradient.

Certain limitations exist with Doppler evaluation of the coarctation gradient. It is important to note that in the presence of a large ductus arteriosus or significant collateral flow, the descending aortic Doppler pattern may be normal. If the Doppler beam is not aligned parallel to flow, the coarctation gradient may be underestimated. The severity of obstruction may also be masked by low cardiac output.

The presence of significant arch obstruction predisposes the left ventricle to increased afterload and the development of left ventricular hypertrophy. Diastolic dysfunction may be present and is manifested by abnormal mitral Doppler filling patterns consistent with impaired left ventricular relaxation that often persist after repair.

Imaging Following Coarctation Repair

Following successful coarctation repair without residual arch obstruction, it is not uncommon to detect an increase in the systolic

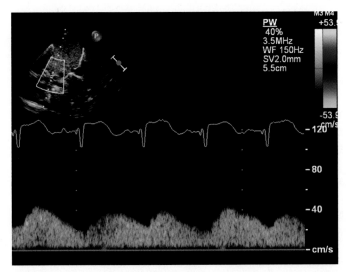

FIGURE 20.20. Abdominal aortic pulsed wave Doppler flow in a patient with severe coarctation of aorta.

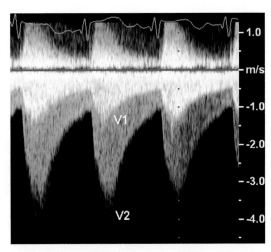

FIGURE 20.21. Continuous wave Doppler (CW) assessment of coarctation. This CW signal was obtained with a non-imaging probe from the suprasternal notch. Two populations of flow are demonstrated: flow proximal to the coarctation (V1) and high velocity flow across the coarctation site (V2).

peak velocity across the site of surgical repair. The Doppler profile is otherwise normal, with absence of continuation of flow in diastole. When a residual coarctation is present, the Doppler pattern is similar to that seen before repair with a delayed upstroke and continuation of flow into diastole. Abdominal aortic pulsatility may also be diminished. Color Doppler is helpful for identifying the site of residual obstruction.

Abnormalities of left ventricular systolic and diastolic function have been shown to persist, even after successful coarctation repair. These include decreased early diastolic filling with compensatory increased late diastolic filling during mitral inflow. Increased fractional shortening, greater left ventricular mass index, and lower left ventricular wall stress have also been reported at long-term follow-up, despite the absence of residual arch obstruction.

Associated defects that are commonly seen with coarctation include ventricular septal defects and multiple left-sided obstructive lesions. Following surgical repair of coarctation, the hemodynamic severity of these lesions may progress or become more apparent. Therefore, careful echocardiographic evaluation of the intracardiac anatomy and function should be included in the postoperative examination.

Interrupted Aortic Arch

IAA represents the most severe form of coarctation. This rare anomaly accounts for 1.5% of all congenital heart defects. It is often associated with other cardiac abnormalities, including a patent ductus arteriosus, ventricular septal defect, subaortic stenosis caused by posterior malalignment of the conal septum, bicuspid aortic valve with hypoplasia of the aortic annulus, and atrial septal defect. Less commonly associated cardiac anomalies include truncus arteriosus and aortopulmonary window. A complete echocardiographic evaluation of the intracardiac anatomy is warranted to identify additional abnormalities.

Interruption of the aortic arch may occur at three sites (Fig. 20.22). In IAA type A, the interruption occurs between the left subclavian artery and descending aorta at the level of the isthmus. IAA type B interruption is the most common form and occurs between the left common carotid artery and the left subclavian artery. A ventricular septal defect is present in up to 80% of cases, and aberrant origin of the right subclavian artery is also commonly associated with this type of interruption. IAA type C is the least frequent form of arch interruption and occurs between the innominate artery and left carotid artery.

Infants with IAA typically present with symptoms of cardiovascular collapse and pronounced acidosis on ductal closure. Injury to the heart muscle is reflected as poor cardiac output. Poor perfusion to the lower body causes ischemic injury to the liver, intestines, and kidneys. Severe systemic acidosis ultimately results in damage to the brain.

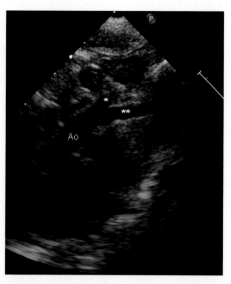

FIGURE 20.23. Interrupted aortic arch type B. Suprasternal long-axis image demonstrates the innominate artery (*) and left common carotid artery (**) arising from the aortic arch. The left subclavian artery arises distal to the interruption from the descending aorta.

Two-dimensional Imaging of Interrupted Aortic Arch – As with coarctation, IAA is best imaged from the suprasternal short-axis view. From this view, the ascending portion of the aorta appears smaller than the descending aorta. Inability to demonstrate continuity between the ascending and descending portions of the aortic arch confirms the diagnosis of arch interruption. From a surgical perspective, it is important to note whether the distance between the proximal and distal segments is long or short and to accurately determine which vessels arise from the proximal and distal aorta.

The type of IAA is determined by the position of the arch vessels in relation to the site of interruption. Origin of the subclavian artery from the distal descending aorta occurs with type B interruption (interruption between the left carotid and left subclavian arteries). This is best shown in the suprasternal long-axis view with the plane of the sound tilted toward the left (Fig. 20.23). In type A interruption (interruption between the left subclavian artery and the descending aorta), all of the head and neck vessels arise from the proximal aorta. Type C interruption is rare and occurs between the innominate and left subclavian artery.

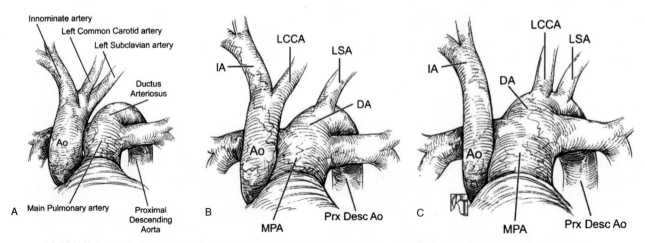

FIGURE 20.22. Three sites of aortic arch interruption are demonstrated. Type A: Interruption between the left subclavian artery (LSA) and descending aorta (Desc Ao). **Type B:** Interruption between the left common carotid artery (LCCA) and LSA. **Type C:** Interruption between innominate artery (IA) and LCCA. DA, ductus arteriosus; MPA, main pulmonary artery. (From Mavroudis and Backer. *Pediatric Cardiac Surgery*, 3rd ed. New York: Mosby; 2003. Used with permission.)

Doppler Features of Interrupted Aortic Arch – In the presence of a widely patent ductus arteriosus, the color flow Doppler pattern in the descending aorta may be normal, and the spectral Doppler pattern may show normal pulsatility. As the ductus closes, the color flow pattern will demonstrate a high-velocity jet in the descending aorta, similar to that seen with coarctation.

Imaging Following Interrupted Aortic Arch Repair – The echocardiographic examination following repair of IAA should focus on evaluating for residual obstruction at the site of the anastomosis. The severity of residual obstruction can be determined by employing the Doppler techniques described earlier, as well as assessing for abdominal aortic pulsatility, and the peak and mean Doppler gradients through the site of residual narrowing. In the presence of residual obstruction, the Doppler pattern will demonstrate a delay in upstroke and continuous flow in diastole, similar to that seen with residual coarctation.

Acknowledgment

The authors would like to acknowledge Dr. Constantine Mavroudis and Dr. Cynthia Rigsby for their contributions.

SUGGESTED READING

Abbott ME. *Atlas of congenital cardiac disease.* New York: American Heart Association; 1936.

Backer CL, Ilbawi MN, Idriss FS, et al. Vascular anomalies causing tracheo-esophageal compression. Review of experience in children. *J Thorac Cardiovasc Surg.* 1989;97:725.

Backer CB, Mavroudis C. Vascular rings and pulmonary artery sling. In: Mavroudis C, Backer CL, eds. *Pediatric cardiac surgery.* 3rd ed. Philadelphia: Mosby; 2003:234–250.

Bayford D. Account of singular case of obstructed deglutition. *Mem Med Soc Lond.* 1794;2:275.

Beabout JW, Steward JR, Kincaid OW. Aberrant right subclavian artery, dispute of commonly accepted concepts. *AJR Am J Roentgenol.* 1964;92:855.

Bonnard A, Auber F, Fourcade L, et al. Vascular ring abnormalities: a retrospective study of 62 cases. *J Pediatr Surg.* 2003;38:539.

Celano V, Pieroni DR, Gingell RL, et al. Two-dimensional echocardiographic recognition of the right aortic arch. *Am J Cardiol.* 1983;51:1507–1512.

Collins-Nakai RI, Dick M, Parisi-Buckley L, et al. Interrupted aortic arch in infancy. I 1976;88:959.

Edwards JE. Congenital cardiovascular causes of tracheobronchial and/or esophageal obstruction. In: Tucker BL, Lindesmith GC, eds. *First Clinical Conference on Congenital Heart Disease.* New York: Grune & Stratton; 1979:66–69.

Felson B, Palayew MJ. The two types of right aortic arch. *Radiology.* 1963;81:745.

Hollinger LD. Diagnostic endoscopy of the pediatric airway. *Laryngoscope.* 1989;99:346.

Huhta JC, Gutgesell HP, Latson LA, et al. Two-dimensional echocardiographic assessment of the aorta in infants and children with congenital heart disease. *Circulation.* 1984;70:417–4244.

Jonas RA. Vascular rings and pulmonary artery sling. In: Mavroudis C, Backer CL, eds. *Pediatric cardiac surgery.* 3rd ed. Philadelphia: Mosby; 2003:273–282.

Kersting-Sommerhoff BA, Sechtem UP, Fisher MR, et al. MR imaging of congenital anomalies of the aortic arch. *AJR Am J Roentgenol.* 1987;149:9.

Kveselis DA, Snider AR, Dick M II, et al. Echocardiographic diagnosis of right aortic arch with a retroesophageal sement and left descending aorta. *Am J Cardiol.* 1986;57:1198–1199.

Lu CW, et al. Noninvasive diagnosis of aortic coarctation in neonates with patent ductus arteriosus. *J Pediatr.* 2006;148:217–221.

Marx GR, Allen HD. Accuracy and pitfalls of Doppler evaluation of the pressure gradient in aortic coarctation. *J Am Coll Cardiol.* 1986;7:1379.

McLoughlin MJ, Weisbrod G, Wise DJ, et al. Computed tomography in congenital anomalies of the aortic arch and great vessels. *Radiology.* 1981;138:399.

Meliones JN, Snider AR, Serwer GA, et al. Pulsed Doppler assessment of left ventricular diastolic filling in children with left ventricular outflow obstruction before and after balloon angioplasty. *Am J Cardiol.* 1989;63:231.

Moes CAF. Vascular rings and related conditions. In: Freedom RM, Mawson JB, Yoo SJ, et al (eds). *Congenital heart disease: textbook of angiography.* Armonk, NY: Futura; 1997:947–983.

Morriss MJ, McNamara DG. Coarctation of the aorta and interrupted aortic arch. In: Garson Jr A, Bricker JT, Fisher DJ, et al. (eds). *The science and practice of pediatric cardiology.* 2nd ed. Baltimore: Williams & Wilkins; 1998.

Moskowitz WB, Schieken RM, Mosteller M, et al. Altered systolic and diastolic function in children after "successful" repair of coarctation of the aorta. *Am Heart J.* 1990;120:103.

Parikh SR, et al. Rings, slings and such things: diagnosis and management with special emphasis on the role of echocardiography. *J Am Soc Echocardiogr.* 1993;6:1.

Pickhardt PJ, Siegel MJ, Gutierrez FR. Vascular rings in symptomatic children: frequency of chest radiographic findings. *Radiology.* 1997;203:423.

Powell AJ, Mandell VS. Vascular rings and slings. In: Keane JF, Lock JE, Fyler DC, eds. *Nadas' pediatric cardiology.* 2nd ed. Philadelphia: Saunders Elesevier; 2006:811–823.

Riggs TW, et al. Two-dimensional echocardiographic features of interruption of the aortic arch. *Am J Cardiol.* 1982;50:1285.

Sell JE, Jonas RA, Mayer JE, et al. The results of a surgical program for interrupted aortic arch. *J Thorac Cardiovasc Surg.* 1988;96:864.

Shaddy RE, Snider AR, Silverman NH, et al. Pulsed Doppler findings in patients with coarctation of the aorta. *Circulation.* 1986;73:82–88.

Shrivastava S, Berry JM, Einzig S, et al. Parasternal cross-sectional echocardiographic determination of aortic arch situs: a new approach. *Am J Cardiol.* 1985;55:1236–1238.

Silverman NH. *Pediatric echocardiography.* Baltimore: Williams & Wilkins; 1993.

Simpson IA, et al. Color Doppler flow mapping in patients with coarctation of the aorta: new observations and improved evaluation with color flow diameter and proximal acceleration as predictors of severity. *Circulation.* 1988;77:736.

Smallhorn JT, Huhta JC, Adams PA, et al. Cross-sectional echocardiographic assessment of coarctation in the sick neonate and infant. *Br Heart J.* 1983;50:349–361.

Snider AR, Serwer GA, Ritter SB, eds. *Echocardiography in pediatric heart disease.* 2nd ed. St. Louis: Mosby–Year Book; 1997.

Snider AR, Silverman NH. Suprasternal notch echocardiography: a two-dimensional technique for evaluating congenital heart disease. *Circulation.* 1981;64:165–173.

Stark J, Roesler M, Chrispin A, et al. The diagnosis of airway obstruction in children. *J Pediatr.* 1985;20:113.

Tawes, RL Jr, Aberdeen E, Waterston DJ, et al: Coarctation of the aorta in infants and children. A review of 333 operative cases, including 179 infants. *Circulation.* 1969;39(5):1173.

Van Son JAM, Julsrud PR, Hagler DJ, et al. Imaging strategies for vascular rings. *Ann Thorac Surg.* 1994;57:604.

Yeager SB, Chin AJ, Sanders SP. Two-dimensional echocardiographic diagnosis of pulmonary artery sling in infancy. *J Am Coll Cardiol.* 1986;7:625–629.

Zapata H, Edwards JE, Titus JL. Aberrant right subclavian artery with left aortic arch: associated cardiac anomalies. *Pediatr Cardiol.* 1993;150–161.

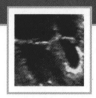

Chapter 21
Marfan Syndrome: Aortic Aneurysm and Dissection

Heidi M. Connolly

The primary cause of morbidity and mortality in patients with Marfan syndrome (MFS) is related to the abnormalities of the cardiovascular system, specifically the propensity to aortic aneurysm formation and associated dissection. Noninvasive cardiovascular imaging has contributed to the improved survival noted among patients with MFS in the current era. Ascending aortic dilatation is usually readily detected with transthoracic echocardiography (TTE) and transesophageal echocardiography (TEE). Echocardiography is a very important imaging tool in the management of patients with MFS.

MFS, an autosomal dominant multisystem disorder, is the most common systemic connective tissue disease, occurring in 2 to 3 per 10,000 individuals. Cardiovascular complications occur in the majority of patients. Classically MFS is caused by a mutation of the fibrillin-1 gene (FBN1), which maps to 15q21. FBN1 mutations increase the susceptibility of fibrillin-1 to proteolysis in vitro leading to fragmentation of microfibrils. Fragmentation of the elastic fibers in the aortic media is a histological marker of MFS, so-called medial degeneration. Transforming growth factor-beta (TGFβ) has been shown to bind to fibrillin, and it is hypothesized that these changes in fibrillin result in alterations in TGFβ signaling and ultimately to abnormal elastic properties that make the aorta stiffer and less distensible than normal.

More than 500 different mutations involving the fibrillin-1 gene have been identified to date, and the penetrance of the fibrillin mutation is high. However, no correlation has been recognized between the specific type of fibrillin-1 mutation and the clinical phenotype. In approximately 75% of cases, an individual with MFS inherits the disorder from an affected parent, the remaining 25% result from de novo mutation. Genetic counseling should be provided at the time of initial evaluation or diagnosis, as well as to potential parents.

There are important limitations to genetic testing in patients with MFS; thus, the diagnosis continues to depend primarily on clinical features that have been codified into the Ghent diagnostic nosology (Table 21.1). Confirmation of the diagnosis of MFS requires a complete personal and family history and a comprehensive multidisciplinary approach involving genetic, cardiac, ophthalmologic, and, in select cases, orthopedic consultations and various diagnostic tests.

ANATOMY AND PHYSIOLOGY OF THE CARDIAC LESION

The cardiovascular features of MFS were initially reported by McKusick et al. Dilatation of the ascending aorta at the level of the aortic sinuses is the most common and characteristic cardiovascular manifestation of MFS (Fig. 21.1). Progressive aortic sinus enlargement is present in approximately 50% of adults and children with MFS.

Ascending aortic aneurysm in MFS can be readily detected by TTE in most patients, and serial TTE studies of the ascending aorta can usually be performed to monitor the size of the aorta. Alternate imaging windows of the aorta such as TEE (Fig. 21.2), computed tomography (CT) scanning (Fig. 21.3), or magnetic resonance imaging (MRI) (Fig. 21.4) are used to assess the thoracic and abdominal aorta, and the ascending aorta in select patients with limited imaging opportunities. Aortic dissection (Fig. 21.5) or rupture accounts for most of the premature mortality in patients with MFS. Marked improvement in life expectancy in patients with MFS has been noted over the past 30 years. This change in prognosis is largely to the result of the early diagnosis of MFS, initiation of medical therapy, and aortic imaging with recognition of aortic aneurysmal disease and prophylactic aortic root replacement. Thus, it is critically important to consider the diagnosis and to perform serial

cardiovascular imaging studies in all patients with confirmed or suspected MFS.

Aortic dissection data suggest that MFS is present in 50% of patients presenting with aortic dissection who are younger than 40 years. Risk factors for aortic dissection in MFS include (a) aortic sinus diameter greater than 50 mm, (b) aortic dilatation extending beyond the sinuses of Valsalva, (c) more than 5% per year increase in aortic size in children, or an increase of more than 2 mm per year in adults, and (d) family history of aortic dissection. Aortic diameter should be measured at multiple levels by TTE and compared with normal values based on age and body surface area (Fig. 21.6). Serial measurements are indicated. When adequate assessment of the aorta is not possible by TTE, alternate imaging modalities are used such as CT, MRI, or TEE.

Patients with MFS are predisposed to dilatation or dissection of the descending thoracic aorta, although this is less common than involvement of the ascending aorta. (Fig. 21.7) Dilatation or dissection of the descending thoracic aorta is a recognized cardiovascular feature and complication of MFS when it occurs in patients younger than age 50. Nevertheless, imaging of the entire aorta is essential for the optimal management of patients with MFS.

Important cardiovascular manifestations in MFS other than aortic dilatation have been recognized. Mitral valve prolapse (Fig. 21.8) occurs in approximately 60% of patients with MFS. The mitral valve leaflets are longer and thinner, with less posterior leaflet prolapse and more anterior or bileaflet prolapse compared with mitral valve prolapse in non-patients with MFS. In addition, patients with MFS develop severe degrees of mitral valve regurgitation and present for surgery at a younger age than non-MFS patients. The pulmonary artery diameter is often significantly larger in patients with MFS at all ages than in non MFS patients, without associated pulmonary valve disease. Less common cardiovascular complications of MFS include mitral annular calcification (Fig. 21.9) occurring at less than 40 years and tricuspid valve prolapse (Fig. 21.10). Central aortic valve regurgitation caused by annular enlargement occurs as the aorta enlarges (Fig. 21.11). There are reports of left ventricular dilatation and systolic dysfunction, regardless of valvular regurgitation in patients with MFS, and other reports suggesting that ventricular dysfunction is uncommon in the absence of valve disease.

CLINICAL PRESENTATION

Despite the progress in management of patients with MFS and sophistication of the health care system, patients with MFS still die of aortic dissection before consideration and diagnosis of the disorder. In retrospect, many of these patients have physical features or a family history of MFS that should have prompted cardiovascular screening before the aortic catastrophe.

The majority of patients with MFS have a family history of the disorder and are identified during routine family screening. Skeletal, ocular, and occasionally pulmonary features may prompt cardiovascular screening of the patient and family. When a patient is initially diagnosed with MFS, screening of all first-degree relatives is recommended. When MFS is suspected, screening with TTE is recommended to identify the cardiovascular disease—most importantly, aortic aneurysmal disease.

Marfan Syndrome in Children

The diagnosis of MFS in children may be difficult to confirm if they do not meet the Ghent diagnostic criteria. The Ghent diagnostic features may be subtle initially and develop with age. Children with suspected MFS should have comprehensive evaluation in preschool, before puberty, and at age 18, because some of the clinical

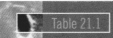 **Table 21.1**   SUMMARY OF THE MAJOR AND MINOR SUGGESTED GHENT CRITERIA USED TO ESTABLISH THE DIAGNOSIS OF MARFAN SYNDROME

Skeletal

Major (at least four of the following constitutes a major criterion)

Pectus carinatum

Pectus excavatum requiring surgery

Reduced upper–to–lower segment ratio OR arm span–to–height ratio >1.05

Wrist and thumb signs

Scoliosis of >20 degrees or spondylolisthesis

Reduced extension at the elbows (<170 degrees)

Medial displacement of the medial malleolus causing pes planus

Protrusio acetabuli of any degree

Minor

Pectus excavatum

Joint hypermobility

Highly arched palate with crowding of teeth

Facial appearance: dolichocephaly (long narrow skull)

Malar hypoplasia (flattening)

Enophthalmos (sunken eyes)

Retrognathia (recessed lower mandible)

Down-slanting palpebral fissures

For involvement of the skeletal system, at least two features contributing to major criteria, or one major and two minor criteria must be present.

Ocular

Major

Ectopia lentis

Minor

Flat cornea

Increased axial length of globe (<23.5 mm)

Hypoplastic iris OR hypoplastic ciliary muscle causing decreased miosis

For involvement of the ocular system, at least two of the minor criteria must be present.

Cardiovascular

Major (either of the following constitutes a major criterion)

Dilatation of the ascending aorta with or without aortic regurgitation and involving at least the sinuses of Valsalva

Dissection of the ascending aorta

Minor

Mitral valve prolapse with or without mitral valve regurgitation

Dilatation of the main pulmonary artery, in the absence of valvular or peripheral pulmonic stenosis, below the age of 40 years

Calcification of the mitral annulus below the age of 40 years

Dilatation or dissection of the descending thoracic or abdominal aorta below the age of 50 years

For involvement of the cardiovascular system, only one of the minor criteria must be present.

Pulmonary System

Major

None

Minor

Spontaneous pneumothorax

Apical blebs

For involvement of the pulmonary system, only one of the minor criteria must be present.

Skin and Integument

Major

None

Minor

Striae atrophicae (stretch marks) not related to marked weight gain, pregnancy, or repetitive stress

Recurrent or incisional herniae

For involvement of the skin and integument, only one of the minor criteria must be present.

Dura

Major

Lumbosacral dural ectasia by CT or MRI

Minor

None

Family/Genetic History

Major (one of the following constitutes a major criterion)

First-degree relative who independently meets the diagnostic criterion

Presence of mutation in FBN1

Presence of a haplotype around FBN1 inherited by descent and unequivocally associated with diagnosed Marfan syndrome in the family

Minor

None

manifestations of MFS become evident with time. Serial aortic imaging follow-up is recommended for children with MFS or when the aorta is enlarged regardless of diagnostic criteria.

The majority of patients with MFS demonstrate aortic root dilatation, mitral valve prolapse, or both before age 18 years. It is important to make the diagnosis and to initiate appropriate medical therapy and serial screening in an effort to prevent or slow aortic enlargement and thus delay aortic operative intervention. Beta-blockers have been demonstrated to significantly decrease the rate of aortic dilatation at the level of sinus of Valsalva in children and therefore should be prescribed either at the time of diagnosis or on documentation of aortic enlargement.

Neonatal MFS is a severe form of MFS apparent at birth that carries a poor prognosis. Aortic enlargement with associated severe aortic valve regurgitation is often present. In addition, progressive mitral and/or tricuspid valve prolapse with regurgitation leading to congestive heart failure is common and affects management and patient survival. Characteristic noncardiac features include infantile pulmonary emphysema, ectopia lentis, arachnodactyly, joint contractures, and loose skin.

 ## COMPLICATIONS OF CARDIAC LESION IN MARFAN SYNDROME

The most important, and life-threatening, complication of cardiovascular involvement in MFS is aortic dissection or rupture. This most commonly involves the ascending aorta but can also affect the descending thoracic aorta. Additional cardiovascular complications include progressive valvular regurgitation, such as aortic regurgitation caused by annular enlargement or mitral or tricuspid valve regurgitation caused by leaflet prolapse.

Prophylactic beta-blockade has been demonstrated to be effective in slowing the rate of aortic dilatation and reducing the development of aortic complications. These medications are generally recommended in patients with MFS. The angiotensin receptor blocker losartan has been demonstrated to have an important impact on vascular development in the mouse model of MFS. These data have not been confirmed in humans with MFS or other aortic disorders but are currently undergoing evaluation. These agents should be

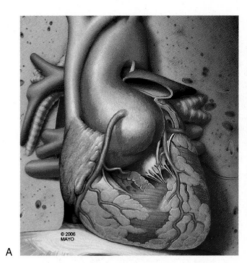
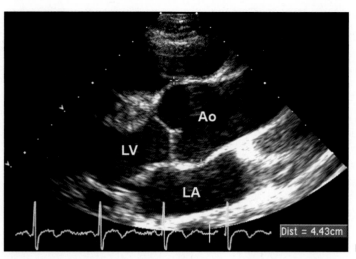

FIGURE 21.1. Aortic Enlargement in Marfan Syndrome. A: Schematic of the typical aortic enlargement in Marfan syndrome. This schematic demonstrates enlargement of the proximal aorta at the level of the aortic sinuses. **B:** Two-dimensional echocardiogram in the parasternal long-axis image orientation demonstrates dilatation of the ascending aorta at the level of the aortic sinuses. The electronic calipers demonstrate the leading edge–to–leading edge method for ascending aortic measurement. Ao, aorta; LA, left atrium; LV, left ventricle.

considered as an alternative medication option for patients with MFS intolerant of beta-blockers.

Genetic counseling is recommended for all patients with MFS. Because of the autosomal dominant nature of the disorder, with each offspring of an affected Marfan parent having a 50% chance of inheriting the genetic mutation, the risk of transmission to the fetus should also be discussed before pregnancy.

Cardiac Surgical Intervention

Aortic root replacement in patients with MFS is recommended when the ascending aorta reaches a diameter of 5 cm or more because of the increased risk of aortic rupture. Select patients are referred for aortic root replacement with an aortic dimension less than 5 cm; these include patients with a family history of aortic dissection, patients with a rapid rate of aortic dilatation (greater than 5% per year, or more than 2 mm per year in adults), those interested in future pregnancy with an aortic dimension greater than 40 to 45 mm, and those interested in the valve sparing aortic root replacement. Patients with aneurysms measuring less than 5 cm and no high-risk characteristics require serial follow-up studies to measure the aortic dimensions and decide the appropriate timing of intervention.

Cardiovascular surgery can be safely performed in children with MFS. Indications for surgical intervention in the pediatric population include (a) rapid rate of growth of the ascending aorta (greater than 5 mm/y), (b) progressive aortic valve regurgitation, or (c) the need for mitral valve surgery in patients with substantial aortic enlargement. The composite graft repair (Fig. 21.12) and the valve-sparing procedure (Fig. 21.13) have shown excellent results for prophylactic replacement of an enlarged aortic root in older children.

Pregnancy in Patients With MFS

The risk of aortic dissection during pregnancy is increased in patients with MFS. This is the result of a combination of the preexisting medial aortic disease with superimposed hormonal inhibition

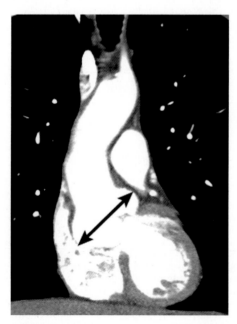

FIGURE 21.2. Transesophageal echocardiogram in the longitudinal image plane at 150 degrees. Dilatation of the ascending aorta at the level of the aortic sinuses *(arrow)*. Ao, aorta; LA, left atrium.

FIGURE 21.3. Computed tomography (CT) examination of the chest using a dual-source CT scanner with intravenous contrast material. Reformatted in the coronal plane, shows marked dilatation of the ascending aorta at the level of the aortic sinuses *(arrow)* in a patient with Marfan syndrome. Note that the rest of the aorta is near normal caliber.

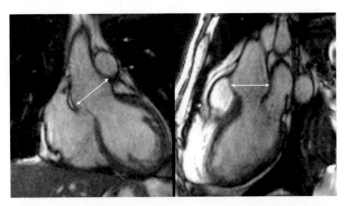

FIGURE 21.4. Electrocardiographic gated, steady state free precession magnetic resonance imaging. Performed in the coronal plane (**left**) and a plane corresponding to the echocardiographic parasternal long-axis plane (**right**) and showing dilatation of the ascending aorta at the level of the aortic sinuses (*arrows*).

of aortic collagen and elastin deposition, and the hyperdynamic, hypervolemic circulatory state of pregnancy. There is a reported 11% complication rate associated with pregnancy in patients with MFS, mostly related to aortic rupture and endocarditis. The overall risk of death during pregnancy is around 1%.

Women with MFS are counseled against proceeding with pregnancy when the ascending aorta exceeds 40 to 45 mm. The risk of aortic complication is increased during pregnancy in patients with MFS when the aortic root diameter exceeds 40 to 45 mm at the start of pregnancy, and the risk is further increased when the aorta dilates during pregnancy. The risk of dilatation of the aorta during pregnancy in the MFS patient has been reported to be lowest in the first trimester and greatest in the third trimester, as well as during labor and the early post partum period. Beta-blocker therapy should be continued throughout pregnancy, and patients should have serial follow-up echocardiograms to assess the change in the size of the aorta during pregnancy. The frequency of monitoring should be individualized. Aortic root replacement should be considered during pregnancy in patients with MFS with progressive aortic dilatation or for documented aortic dissection.

Assisted vaginal delivery can be considered in patients with MFS when the aortic root diameter is less than 40 mm, the aorta has not demonstrated change during pregnancy, and there is no associated severe cardiovascular disease. For patients with MFS with other characteristics, planned cesarean delivery is generally the preferred mode of delivery. Antibiotic prophylaxis administered around the

time of delivery is appropriate for those patients with prior root and valve replacement surgery or a past history of endocarditis. Postpartum uterine hemorrhage is a common complication of MFS, occurring in nearly 40% of women.

BASICS OF ECHOCARDIOGRAPHIC ANATOMY AND IMAGING

Classic Two-dimensional Echocardiographic Anatomy and Hemodynamics

A comprehensive TTE examination will often demonstrate the cardiovascular features of MFS in the involved patient but may be normal or near normal despite a confirmed diagnosis of MFS.

Echocardiographic imaging of the aorta includes the parasternal long-axis view to measure the dimensions of the aortic sinuses, sinotubular junction, and ascending aorta. The leading edge–to–leading edge technique is used to measure the ascending aorta (Fig. 21.1). An off-axis parasternal image also demonstrates the descending thoracic aorta in many patients (Fig. 21.14). The aortic arch and descending thoracic aorta are imaged using the suprasternal window (Fig. 21.15), and the abdominal aorta is imaged from the subcostal format (Fig. 21.16). Aortic dimensions should be compared to normal for patient age and body surface area (Fig. 21.6).

Aortic distensibility has been reported to be an independent predictor of progressive aortic dilatation, and therefore risk assessment and monitoring in patients with MFS may include not only serial assessment of aortic diameter but also assessment of aortic stiffness. M-mode echocardiography and Doppler tissue imaging assessment of aortic wall mechanics and stiffness have been reported. Systolic blood pressure, aortic stiffness index, maximum wall expansion velocity, and strain have been demonstrated to be predictors of aortic dilatation. Decreased aortic strain, maximum wall expansion velocity, and increased stiffness index have also been found to be predictive of aortic dissection. The clinical utility of these measurements has yet to be determined.

Aortic valve regurgitation is identified in the parasternal long-axis (Fig. 21.11), short-axis, and apical images by color-flow imaging and Doppler assessment. The severity is assessed according to American Society of Echocardiography recommendations. Similarly, mitral, tricuspid, and pulmonary valve prolapse and regurgitation are identified and the degree of regurgitation is similarly assessed.

Mitral annular calcification is readily identified on the parasternal long- and short-axis images as an echo-bright region in the posterior atrioventricular groove (Fig. 21.9). This is a common feature

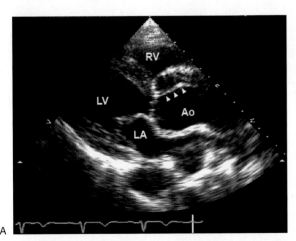

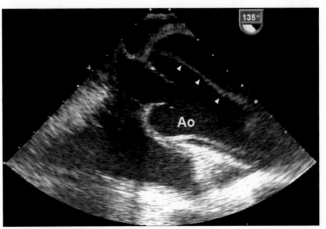

FIGURE 21.5. Aortic Dissection. A: Two-dimensional transthoracic echocardiogram in the parasternal long-axis image orientation showing dilatation of the ascending aorta and proximal aortic dissection (*arrowheads*). **B:** Transesophageal echocardiogram in a longitudinal image orientation showing dilatation of the ascending aorta and proximal aortic dissection (*arrowheads*). The transesophageal echocardiogram was performed in the operating room before surgical repair. Ao, aorta; LA, left atrium; LV, left ventricle; RV, right ventricle.

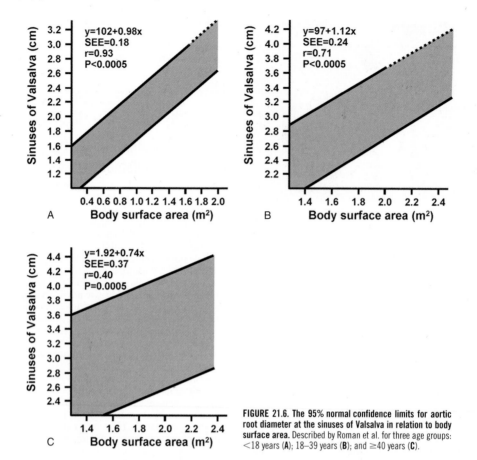

FIGURE 21.6. The 95% normal confidence limits for aortic root diameter at the sinuses of Valsalva in relation to body surface area. Described by Roman et al. for three age groups: <18 years (A); 18–39 years (B); and ≥40 years (C).

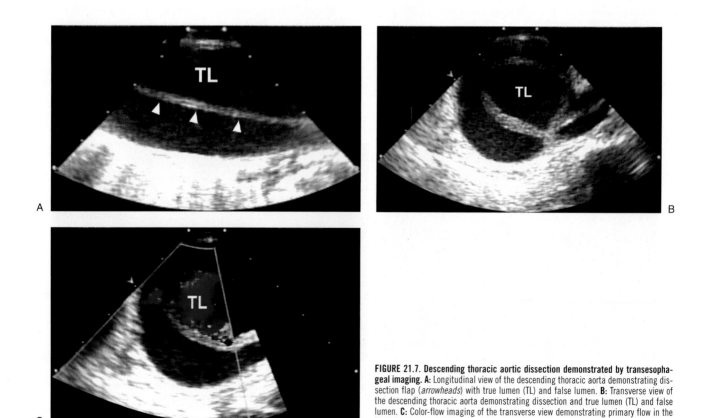

FIGURE 21.7. Descending thoracic aortic dissection demonstrated by transesophageal imaging. A: Longitudinal view of the descending thoracic aorta demonstrating dissection flap (*arrowheads*) with true lumen (TL) and false lumen. B: Transverse view of the descending thoracic aorta demonstrating dissection and true lumen (TL) and false lumen. C: Color-flow imaging of the transverse view demonstrating primary flow in the TL of the dissected descending thoracic aorta.

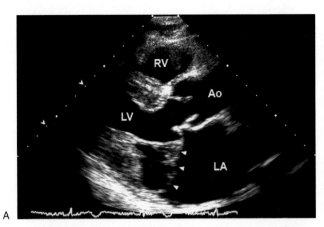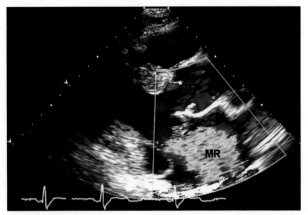

FIGURE 21.8. Mitral Valve Prolapse in Marfan Syndrome. A: Bileaflet mitral valve prolapse (*arrowheads*) noted by two-dimensional echocardiographic parasternal long-axis imaging in a patient with Marfan syndrome. **B:** Associated with severe mitral regurgitation by color flow imaging. Note enlargement of the left atrium and aortic sinuses. Ao, aorta; LA, left atrium; LV, left ventricle; MR, mitral regurgitation; RV, right ventricle.

in MFS and is a minor cardiovascular diagnostic criterion when present in a patient under age 40.

Left ventricular systolic and diastolic function is assessed using standard TTE imaging techniques, with parasternal long- and short-axis and apical imaging.

Echocardiographic Assessment of Aortic Dissection

TTE is a reasonable initial imaging modality for proximal aortic dissection because of its availability. The positive predictive value is high, but aortic dissection cannot be excluded in patients with negative findings. A dilated aorta is noted in most patients with aortic dissection by TTE; however, an intimal flap is seen in less than 80% (Fig. 21.5). False-positive diagnoses of aortic dissection occur in less than 10% of patients using TTE. Another concern regarding TTE in aortic imaging is that the descending thoracic aorta is not well visualized in many patients. Therefore, TTE is a rapid screening tool for aortic dissection, but negative findings or a suboptimal examination requires further diagnostic evaluation.

The anatomic relationship between the esophagus and the thoracic aorta usually allows visualization of the entire thoracic aorta using omniplane TEE. The distal portion of the ascending aorta and the proximal aortic arch may be difficult to visualize because of the interposed trachea using a horizontal TEE view. However, this blind area can usually be adequately visualized with the longitudinal view. Omniplane imaging provides a more complete view of the entire aorta; thus, the role of echocardiography has changed in the diagnosis and management of aortic dissection (Fig. 21.5).

The International Registry of Acute Aortic Dissection (IRAD) was established in 1996 to assess the presentation, management, and outcomes of acute aortic dissection. Acute aortic dissection was reviewed in 628 patients from 13 international medical centers. Imaging modalities used for diagnosis were assessed. TEE and computed tomography (CT) are now the most common initial imaging tests for the diagnosis of aortic dissection. Two thirds of the patients in IRAD had two or more imaging studies to confirm the diagnosis.

The European multicenter cooperative study was the first to demonstrate that TEE was at least equal to CT and aortography in the diagnosis of aortic dissection (99% sensitivity). Subsequent studies reinforced the diagnostic accuracy of TEE in aortic dissection. Increased clinical availability of TEE has decreased its diagnostic sensitivity (88%) in the IRAD, compared with CT (93%). Currently, the initial diagnostic procedure of choice for suspected aortic dissection is TEE or CT with contrast agent. Although the diagnostic accuracy of cardiac MRI is superb in aortic dissection, its clinical role is limited by the longer examination time, difficulties in monitoring patients during the procedure, and the location of the imaging facility from the emergency department.

ILLUSTRATIVE IMAGING EXAMPLES

Case 1: Aortic Root Enlargement in a Patient With MFS

This 25-year-old male patient with a family history of MFS has a TTE that demonstrates enlargement of the ascending aorta at the level of the aortic sinuses (Fig. 21.1). The presence of aortic root

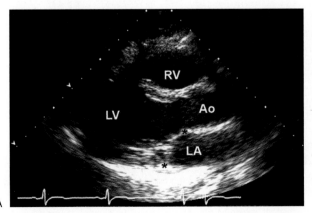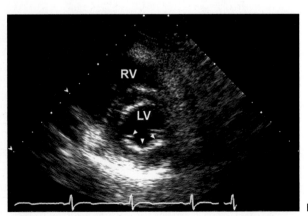

FIGURE 21.9. Mitral annular calcification in a 35-year-old woman with Marfan syndrome. A: Parasternal long-axis view (*asterisk*, mitral annular calcification). **B:** Parasternal short axis view (*arrowheads*, mitral annular calcification). Ao, aorta; LV, left ventricle; LA, left atrium; RV, right ventricle.

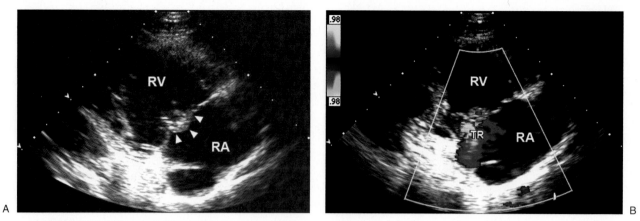

FIGURE 21.10. Tricuspid valve prolapse (*arrowheads*) in a patient with Marfan syndrome. A: Two-dimensional echocardiographic imaging with associated (**B**) moderate tricuspid regurgitation demonstrated by color-flow imaging. RA, right atrium; RV, right ventricle; TR, tricuspid regurgitation.

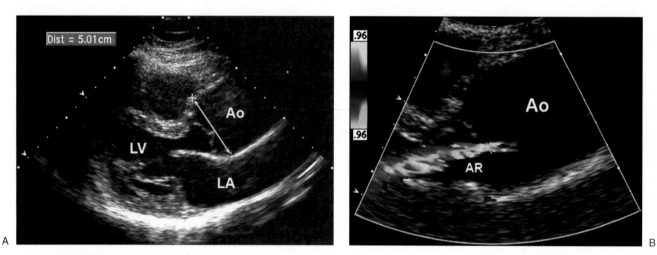

FIGURE 21.11. Aortic annular dilation and regurgitation. A: Parasternal long-axis image demonstrating aneurysmal enlargement of the ascending aorta (*arrow*). **B:** Color flow imaging demonstrating aortic valve regurgitation caused by annular dilatation. Ao, aorta; AR, aortic valve regurgitation; LA, left atrium; LV, left ventricle.

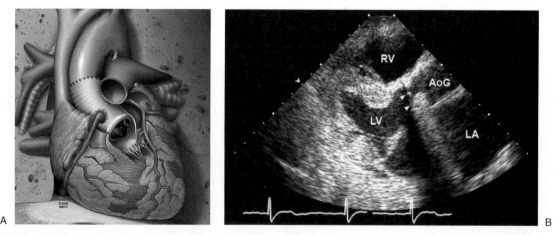

FIGURE 21.12. Bentall operation. A: Schematic of the Bentall operation. In this operative procedure, the proximal aorta is replaced with a valved conduit, and the coronary arteries are reimplanted. This schematic demonstrates a mechanical valve prosthesis. Biological prostheses can also be used. **B:** Transthoracic echocardiographic image of a patient with Marfan syndrome after a Bentall operation. The aortic valve and proximal ascending aorta are replaced with a mechanical valve prosthesis (*arrowheads*) and aortic graft, respectively. AoG, aortic graft; LA, left atrium; LV, left ventricle; RV, right ventricle.

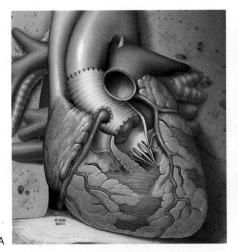
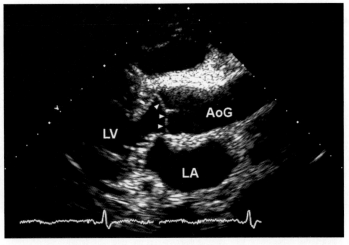

FIGURE 21.13. Valve-sparing aortic root replacement. A: Schematic of the valve-sparing aortic root replacement. The ascending aorta is replaced with a graft material, the native aortic valve is preserved, and the coronary arteries are reimplanted. **B:** Transthoracic echocardiographic image after a valve-sparing aortic root replacement operation. The native aortic valve remains (*arrowheads,* spared native aortic valve), and proximal ascending aorta is replaced with an aortic graft. AoG, aortic graft; LA, left atrium; LV, left ventricle.

enlargement, a family history of MFS, and skeletal involvement confirm the diagnosis of MFS in this patient. MRI confirmed the aortic sinus measurement noted by TTE and excluded aneurysmal disease involving the rest of the aorta. Beta-blocker therapy and regular clinical and TTE surveillance were recommended. This case emphasizes the clinical importance of echocardiographic imaging in the diagnosis and management of patients with MFS.

Case 2: Mitral Valve Prolapse and Mitral Regurgitation in a Patient With MFS

This 27-year-old male patient with a diagnosis of MFS presents with exertional dyspnea. His TTE demonstrates dilatation of the ascending aorta (47 mm) and bileaflet mitral valve prolapse with severe mitral valve regurgitation (Fig. 21.8). Operative intervention with mitral valve repair caused by severe symptomatic mitral valve regurgitation was recommended. Aortic valve sparing root replacement was also recommended given the degree of aortic enlargement and the propensity for progressive aortic dilatation. Individualized medical and surgical management is recommended for all patients with MFS. This patient wanted to avoid warfarin anticoagulation. Mitral valve repair and valve sparing root replacement provided that option for this patient.

Case 3: Imaging After Aortic Root and Valve Replacement in a Patient With MFS

This 85-year-old woman has a personal and family history of MFS. She underwent a Bentall procedure (Fig. 21.12; aortic valve and ascending aorta replaced) approximately 20 years before this echocardiogram. She has bileaflet mitral valve prolapse with moderate mitral valve regurgitation, chronic atrial fibrillation, and associated biatrial enlargement. She has two sons with MFS; both have had valve-sparing aortic root replacement (Fig. 21.13) for ascending aortic aneurysms. This case highlights some of the postoperative cardiovascular features in MFS, the need for continued surveillance, and the potential longevity of patients with MFS.

How to Obtain Proper Echocardiographic and Doppler Images

Standard TTE imaging windows are usually adequate for assessment of the ascending aorta and the cardiac valves in patients with MFS. Occasionally, nonstandard imaging windows are used to measure the ascending and descending thoracic aorta such as high left

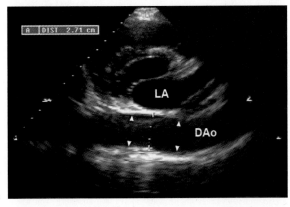
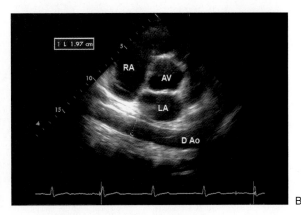

FIGURE 21.14. Two-dimensional echocardiographic images of the descending thoracic aorta visualized using off-axis imaging. A: Modified parasternal long-axis window. **B:** Modified parasternal short-axis window. AV, aortic valve; DAo, descending aorta; LA, left atrium; RA, right atrium.

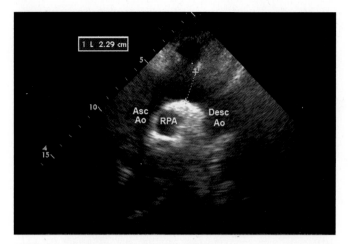

FIGURE 21.15. Suprasternal echocardiographic imaging demonstrates the ascending aorta (AscAo), aortic arch, and proximal descending thoracic aorta. DescAo, descending aorta; RPA, right pulmonary artery.

FIGURE 21.16. Subcostal two-dimensional echocardiographic imaging demonstrates the abdominal aorta in a longitudinal view where measurements can be performed. Note the dissection flap (*arrowheads*) in the abdominal aorta.

parasternal or right parasternal windows. In addition, patients with skeletal abnormalities such as pectus deformity or scoliosis related to MFS may require special imaging windows. TEE is used to complement the TTE evaluation of patients with MFS.

Differential Diagnoses

The differential diagnosis of MFS includes disorders that involve cardiac, skeletal, or ophthalmologic manifestations. Confirming the

clinical diagnosis of MFS is often challenging, especially in the child or adolescent without a family history. Clinical and imaging follow-up may be the only way to differentiate MFS from some of the other disorders.

1. *Congenital bicuspid aortic valve disease with associated aortopathy.* In patients with bicuspid aortic valve disease with associated aortopathy, the dilatation of the ascending aorta is most often seen at the mid-ascending aortic level (Fig. 21.17A)

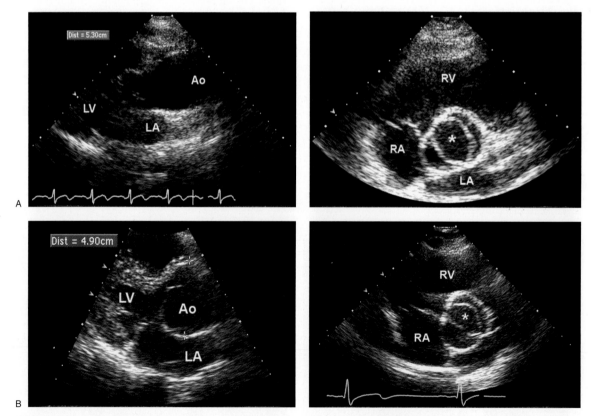

FIGURE 21.17. Bicuspid aortic valve. A: Two-dimensional echocardiogram in a parasternal long-axis image plane (*left*) demonstrates dilatation of the mid-ascending aorta in a patient with bicuspid aortic valve. The leading edge–to–leading edge method is used for ascending aortic measurement. The short-axis image (**right**) confirms the bicuspid aortic valve (*asterisk*). There was no aortic valve stenosis or regurgitation. **B:** Two-dimensional echocardiogram in a parasternal long-axis image plane (*left*) demonstrates dilation of the ascending aorta at the level of the aortic sinuses in a patient with bicuspid aortic valve. The leading edge–to–leading edge method is used for ascending aortic measurement. The bicuspid aortic valve (*asterisk*) functions normally (**right**). Ao, aorta; LA, left atrium; LV, left ventricle; RA, right atrium; RV, right ventricle.

rather than at the aortic sinuses (Fig. 21.17B) despite histologic similarities between the bicuspid aortic valve–related aortopathy and MFS. The presence of a bicuspid aortic valve is an independent risk factor for progressive aortic dilatation, aneurysm formation, and dissection. Bicuspid aortic valve is associated with accelerated degeneration of the aortic media, indicating that bicuspid aortic valve disease is an ongoing pathologic process. Focal abnormalities within the aortic media such as matrix disruption and smooth muscle cell loss have been identified, suggesting that a degenerative process causes the structural weakness of the aortic wall. The vascular complications in patients with bicuspid aortic valves are not thought to be secondary to valvular dysfunction and can manifest in young adults without significant aortic valve disease or in patients in whom the native bicuspid aortic valve was replaced with a prosthetic valve. Aortic root enlargement occurs in more than 50% of young patients with normally functioning bicuspid aortic valves. This disorder is also inherited in an autosomal dominant manner with reduced penetrance and variable age of aortic dilatation. Family members of the affected individual may demonstrate aortic dilatation without an abnormal valve. Echocardiographic screening is recommended for the first degree relatives of patients with bicuspid aortic valve with or without associated aortopathy.

2. *Coarctation of the aorta* may be associated with ascending or descending aortic aneurysm formation and increased risk of aortic dissection. More than 50% of patients with aortic coarctation also have bicuspid aortic valves. The propensity to aneurysm formation in patients with coarctation of the aorta is incompletely understood but may be related to a generalized structural abnormality of the arterial system caused by maldevelopment of the neural crest, which gives rise to the muscular arteries.

3. *Loeys-Dietz syndrome* is a disorder recently described that is characterized by arterial tortuosity and aneurysms with an increased risk of dissection throughout the arterial tree, often at small arterial sizes. Additional features include hypertelorism without ectopia lentis and a broad or bifid uvula (Fig. 21.18) Because of the high risk of lethal aortic complications, an aggressive surgical approach has been recommended in these patients.

4. *Ehlers-Danlos syndrome type IV* includes skin laxity, scars, easy bruising, and a propensity toward arterial dilatation and dissection.

5. *Familial thoracic aortic aneurysm* or *aortopathy* is a disorder characterized by a familial tendency to arterial dilatation and dissection in the thoracic aorta, abdominal aorta, and cerebral circulation. Individuals with this disorder do not show any other systemic manifestation of MFS. It may be inherited in an autosomal dominant manner with reduced penetrance and varying age of aortic dilatation. Familial thoracic aortic aneurysms may grow at a faster rate than other aortic disorders, exemplifying an aggressive course.

6. *MASS phenotype* is a familial disorder that includes features similar to MFS with mitral valve prolapse, aortic enlargement, and nonspecific skin and skeletal features. The aortic enlargement is usually mild and nonprogressive.

7. *Homocystinuria* shares several skeletal and ocular features of MFS, in addition to mitral valve prolapse. Aortic enlargement is not typically seen in this disorder. Homocystinuria is an autosomal recessive disorder that is characterized by an elevated urinary homocysteine excretion and can be diagnosed by measuring total plasma homocysteine. Affected individuals often have subnormal intelligence, a predisposition to thromboembolism, and coronary artery disease.

8. *Stickler syndrome* is characterized by retinal detachment rather than ectopia lentis; additional features include cleft palate and hearing loss.

9. *Congenital contractural arachnodactyly* or *Beals syndrome* is an autosomal dominant disorder manifest by joint contractures, scoliosis, and crumpled ear malformation in addition to a marfanoid appearance.

10. *Aneurysm of the sinus of Valsalva* is caused by localized absence of the media in the aortic wall that results in aneurysmal dilatation of one of the sinuses of Valsalva. Although commonly an incidental finding, it can cause compression of adjacent structures or rupture into the adjacent cardiac chambers, most commonly the right atrium or right ventricle, or into the ventricular septum. These aneurysms can be distinguished confidently from aneurysms of the aorta at the level of the aortic sinuses with comprehensive TTE and TEE examinations.

11. *Aortitis* refers to an inflammation of the aortic wall caused by infection such as syphilitic or mycotic involvement, giant cell arteritis, Takayasu disease, ankylosing spondylitis, rheumatoid arthritis, or relapsing polychondritis. The aortic involvement is usually an expression of the systemic nature of the underlying vasculitis or disease.

Potential Imaging Pitfalls

Aortic dissection can be missed by TTE and TEE. When there is clinical suspicion of aortic dissection with enlargement or abnormal TTE images of the ascending aorta, further imaging should be performed promptly. In the majority of patients, the descending thoracic aorta is not adequately visualized to exclude aneurysmal dilatation or dissection by TTE. Thus, when descending aortic aneurysm or dissection is suspected, an alternative imaging modality is recommended.

The ascending aorta can be visualized and reliably measured by TTE in the majority of patients. At the time of initial evaluation, it is reasonable to confirm the size of the aortic enlargement and exclude additional aneurysmal aortic disease using an alternative imaging modality. Importantly, aortic dilatation may be incompletely visualized

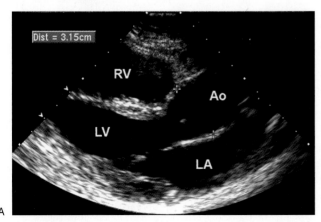
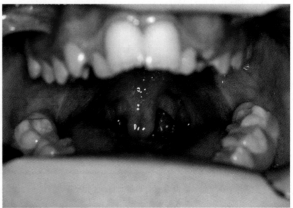

FIGURE 21.18. A 12-year-old patient with Loeys-Dietz syndrome. A: Two-dimensional echocardiogram in a parasternal long-axis image orientation demonstrates dilatation of the ascending aorta at the level of the aortic sinuses (electronic calipers). Ao, aorta; LA, left atrium; LV, left ventricle; RV, right ventricle. **B:** Photograph of the uvula. Note that the uvula is broad and bipartite.

because of imaging difficulties in select patients; thus, periodic aortic imaging using TEE, CT, or MRI is suggested in all patients with MFS.

Aortic imaging is limited in patients with MFS who have had prior aortic root replacement. Although routine TTE is used to assess ventricular and valve function in patients with MFS, regular aortic imaging using CT or MRI is recommended.

Variations on Classic Anatomy

Patients with confirmed MFS may have a normal echocardiogram; alternatively, patients with echocardiographic features suspicious for MFS may not meet Ghent diagnostic criteria. There is a range of normal aortic dimensions, which are related to age and body surface area (Fig. 21.6).

Ascending aortic enlargement at the sinus level is classic for patients with MFS; however, aortic enlargement and dissection can affect other parts of the aorta.

Common Associated Lesions and Findings

The Ghent diagnostic criteria for MFS represent the diagnostic features and should be sought when clinical features are suspicious, or TTE images demonstrate ascending sinus dilatation, with mitral and or tricuspid valve prolapse, or other cardiovascular features of MFS (Table 21.1).

Key Findings That Alter Clinical Management

1. Marked ascending aortic dilatation (Fig. 21.1)
2. Ascending aortic dissection (Fig. 21.5)
3. Mitral or tricuspid valve prolapse with regurgitation (Figs. 21.8 and 21.10)
4. Aortic valve regurgitation (Fig. 21.11)
5. Descending aortic aneurysm or dissection (Fig. 21.7)

Interventional and Postinterventional Imaging

Intraoperative TEE is routinely performed during operative intervention in patients with MFS and is particularly important for the patient undergoing valve-sparing aortic root replacement (Fig. 21.13). Immediate postbypass assessment of the spared aortic valve function affects patient management. When more than mild aortic valve regurgitation is present following the valve sparing operation, revision or valve replacement is commonly performed. Postbypass assessment of the replaced aortic valve function is also routinely performed to determine the prosthetic valve gradient. The aortic valve composite graft used in patients with MFS does not allow perivalvular regurgitation; thus, the postbypass imaging focuses on prosthetic valve function, gradient, and ventricular and native valve function.

Following the valve-sparing aortic root replacement (Fig. 21.13), patients with MFS require regular reevaluation of the aorta as well as assessment of aortic valve function. There is a recognized increased risk of requiring reoperation for aortic valve regurgitation following the valve sparing aortic root replacement. A multicenter study funded by the National Marfan Foundation is currently under way to determine the durability of the valve-sparing versus valve-replacement operation in patients with MFS undergoing aortic root replacement.

After the Bentall procedure (Fig. 21.12), a comprehensive TTE evaluation of the aortic valve prosthesis and graft is recommended early after surgery to provide a fingerprint for future assessment of the prosthetic valve and aorta performance. Although the ascending aorta has been replaced, the remaining aortic segments remain vulnerable to aortic dissection or rupture and regular reevaluation and aortic imaging are indicated.

Pseudoaneurysm of the aorta results from a tear or perforation in the aortic wall and subsequent leakage of blood from the aorta into a contained aneurysmal cavity. It is usually caused by prior operation, infection, or trauma and has been reported late after the Bentall operation. Because pseudoaneurysms tend to rupture, repair is usually recommended. A pseudoaneurysm has a different appearance from a true aneurysm, having a sharply demarcated rupture site where communication occurs between the aorta and the pseudoaneurysm (Fig. 21.19). Depending on the location and orientation, TTE or TEE may be able to identify the pseudoaneurysm. CT or MRI is an excellent imaging modality for further delineation. Another uncommon late complication of both composite and valve-sparing operation is the development of *coronary ostial aneurysms* (Fig. 21.20). These aneurysms develop at the site of coronary artery reimplantation as a result of the perioperative stretch of the weakened wall of the coronary ostium and can be visualized by TTE, TEE, CT angiography, MR angiography, and standard aortography. Operative intervention is usually recommended.

Potential Roles of Alternative Imaging Modalities

MRI and CT allow visualization and assessment of the entire thoracic and abdominal aorta and therefore provide critical complementary information to TTE and TEE in the assessment of patients with MFS and related disorders. MRI or CT should be performed at the time of initial assessment to confirm the size and extent of enlargement of the thoracic aorta and identify additional pathology, and periodically thereafter in the unoperated patient. Both

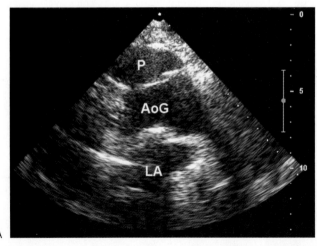
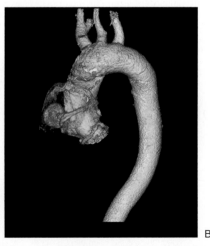

FIGURE 21.19. Patient with Marfan syndrome and prior Bentall procedure. A: Right parasternal imaging. The ascending aorta has been replaced with a graft, but there is a localized area of dilatation in the region of the proximal aorta adjacent to the right coronary artery anastomosis caused by a pseudoaneurysm. AoG, aortic graft; LA, left atrium; P, pseudoaneurysm. **B:** Gated computerized tomographic angiogram (CTA) with three-dimensional reconstruction from the same patient demonstrates composite graft replacement of the ascending aorta (Bentall procedure). There is a pseudoaneurysm involving the ascending thoracic aorta. A communication was noted adjacent to the implanted right coronary artery.

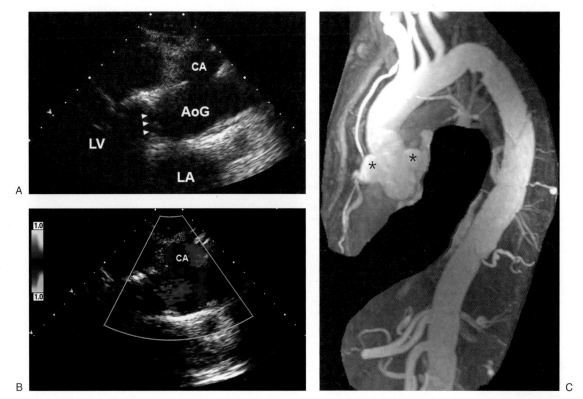

FIGURE 21.20. A: 43-year-old patient with Marfan syndrome had a Bentall procedure 15 years before this imaging study. The patient had subsequent descending thoracic aortic replacement for an aneurysm. Routine transthoracic echocardiogram demonstrates a composite graft replacement of the ascending aorta (Bentall procedure) with normally functioning aortic mechanical prosthesis (*arrowheads*) and aneurysmal dilatation of the anastomosis of the right coronary artery with the aortic graft (CA) noted by two-dimensional (**A**) and color flow imaging (**B**). AoG, ascending aortic graft; CA, coronary artery; LA, left atrium; LV, left ventricle. **C:** Magnetic resonance imaging confirmed that both proximal coronary arteries demonstrate aneurysmal dilatation (*asterisk*).

radiologic imaging modalities and TEE have high sensitivity and specificity in the diagnosis of aortic dissection. However, MRI is less often performed in the acute situation because of safety concerns in critically ill patients, longer imaging duration, and less availability.

Although TEE can be used to image the descending thoracic aorta serially, because of the importance of regular reevaluation of the aortic size at multiple levels and comparison with prior imaging studies, CT or MRI is preferred for following patients with descending thoracic aortic dissection or aneurysm because of the ability to make multiple serial aortic measurements at specific levels over time in most circumstances.

Patients with MFS with prior aortic surgery require regular surveillance of the descending thoracic and abdominal aortas. This is best performed by MRI or CT. Due to the life-long need for aortic surveillance, MRI is preferred by many physicians and patients in an effort to avoid repeated radiation exposure related to CT. However, an individualized imaging strategy is recommended.

 SUMMARY

MFS is a multisystem inherited disorder of connective tissue. The life expectancy of untreated patients with MFS is markedly decreased compared to the general population, with an early study reporting the average life span to be about 32 years. However, advances in the understanding of the cause of MFS, as well as timely and accurate diagnosis and implementation of appropriate prophylactic therapy, have dramatically reduced the mortality and morbidity associated with this disorder. In the current era, the median cumulative probability of survival has increased to over 72 years.

Echocardiography is the recommended screening tool for patients with suspected cardiovascular features of MFS, and the diagnosis of MFS may be confirmed based on the cardiovascular features identified by TTE. Echocardiographic imaging in patients with MFS also has had a major impact on serial follow-up and identification of

the appropriate timing for aortic intervention. Intraoperative TEE plays a pivotal role in identifying surgical success and potential need for revision. Finally, TTE is used for comprehensive life-long post-intervention monitoring of the cardiovascular system.

SUGGESTED READING

Abhayaratna W, Seward J, Appleton C, et al. Left atrial size: physiologic determinants and clinical applications. *J Am Coll Cardiol.* 2006;47: 2357–2363.

Albornoz G, Coady M, Roberts M, et al. Familial thoracic aortic aneurysms and dissections—incidence, modes of inheritance, and phenotypic patterns. *Ann Thorac Surg.* 2006;82:1400–1405.

Angiolillo D, Moreno R, Macaya C. Isolated distal coronary dissection in Marfan syndrome. *Ital Heart J.* 2004;5:305–306.

Anton E. Cerebral infarction in a young adult with Marfan syndrome. *Int J Cardiol.* 2006;112:378–379.

Armstrong W, Zoghbi W. Stress echocardiography: current methodology and clinical applications. *J Am Coll Cardiol.* 2005;45:1739–1747.

Banerjee S, Jagasia D. Unruptured sinus of Valsalva aneurysm in an asymptomatic patient. *J Am Soc Echocardiogr.* 2002;15:668–670.

Baumgartner C, Matyas G, Steinmann B, et al. A bioinformatics framework for genotype-phenotype correlation in humans with Marfan's syndrome caused by FBN1 gene mutations. *J Biomed Inform.* 2006;39:171–183.

Beroukhim R, Roosevelt G, Yetman A. Comparison of the pattern of aortic dilation in children with the Marfan's syndrome versus children with a bicuspid aortic valve. *Am J Cardiol.* 2006;98:1094–1095.

Cameron D, Vricella L. Valve-sparing aortic root replacement in Marfan syndrome. Seminars in Thoracic & Cardiovascular Surgery. *Pediatr Card Surg Annu.* 2005:103–111.

Cerqueira M, Weissman N, Dilsizian V, et al. Standardized myocardial segmentation and nomenclature for tomographic imaging of the heart. A statement for healthcare professionals from the Cardiac Imaging Committee of the Council on Clinical Cardiology of the American Heart Association. *Circulation.* 2002;105:539–542.

Chatrath R, Beauchesne L, Connolly H, et al. Left ventricular function in the Marfan syndrome without significant valvular regurgitation. *Am J Cardiol.* 2003;91:914–916.

De Backer J, Devos D, Segers P, et al. Primary impairment of left ventricular function in Marfan syndrome. *Int J Cardiol.* 2006;112:353–358.

De Backer J, Loeys B, Devos D, et al. A critical analysis of minor cardiovascular criteria in the diagnostic evaluation of patients with Marfan syndrome. *Genet Med.* 2006;8:401–408.

De Paepe A, Devereux R, Dietz H, et al. Revised diagnostic criteria for the Marfan syndrome. *Am J Med Genet.* 1996;62:417–426.

Dietz H, Cutting G, Pyeritz R, et al. Marfan syndrome caused by a recurrent do novo missense mutation in the fibrillin gene. *Lett Nat.* 1991;352:337–339.

Dokainish H, Zoghbi W, Lakkis N, et al. Optimal noninvasive assessment of left ventricular filling pressures: a comparison of tissue Doppler echocardiography and B-type natriuretic peptide in patients with pulmonary artery catheters. *Circulation.* 2004;109:2432–2439.

Elefteriades J. Natural history of thoracic aortic aneurysms: indications for surgery and surgical versus nonsurgical risks. *Ann Thorac Surg.* 2002;74:S1877–S1880.

Engelfriet P, Boersma E, Tijssen J, et al. Beyond the root: dilatation of the distal aorta in Marfan's syndrome. *Heart.* 2006;92:1238–1243.

Espinola-Zavaleta N, Casanova-Garces J, Munoz Castellanos L, et al. Echocardiometric evaluation of cardiovascular abnormalities in Marfan syndrome. *Arch Cardiol Mex.* 2005;75:133–140.

Gott V, Greene P, Alejo D, et al. Replacement of the aortic root in patients with Marfan's syndrome. *N Engl J Med.* 1999;340:1307–1313.

Habashi J, Judge D, Holm T, et al. Losartan, an AT1 antagonist, prevents aortic aneurysm in a mouse model of Marfan syndrome. *Science.* 2006;312:36–37.

Harrer J, Sasse A, Klotzsch C. Intimal flap in a common carotid artery in a patient with Marfan's syndrome. *Ultraschall Med.* 2006;27:487–488.

Januzzi J, Isselbacher E, Fattori R, et al. Characterizing the young patient with aortic dissection: results from the International Registry of Aortic Dissection (IRAD). *J Am Coll Cardiol.* 2004;43:665–669.

Januzzi J, Marayati F, Mehta R, et al. Comparison of aortic dissection in patient with and without Marfan's syndrome (results from the International Registry of Aortic Dissection). *Am J Cardiol.* 2004;94:400–402.

Judge D, Biery N, Dietz H. Characterization of microsatellite markers flanking FBN1: utility in the diagnostic evaluation for Marfan syndrome. *Am J Med Genet.* 2001;99:39–47.

Judge D, Dietz H. Marfan's syndrome. *Lancet.* 2005;366:1965–1976.

Loeys B, Chen J, Neptune E, et al. A syndrome of altered cardiovascular, craniofacial, neurocognitive and skeletal development caused by mutations in TGFBR1 or TGFBR2. *Nat Genet.* 2005;37:275–6281.

Marwick T. Measurement of strain and strain rate by echocardiography: ready for prime time? *J Am Coll Cardiol.* 2006;47:1313–1327.

McKusick V. The cardiovascular aspects of Marfan's syndrome: a heritable disorder of connective tissue. *Circulation.* 1955;(suppl XI):321–342.

Meijboom L, Drenthen W, Pieper P, et al. Obstetric complications in Marfan syndrome. *Int J Cardiol.* 2006;110:53–59.

Meijboom L, Vos F, Timmermans J, et al. Pregnancy and aortic root growth in the Marfan syndrome: a prospective study. *Eur Heart J.* 2005;26:914–920.

Milewicz D, Dietz H, Miller D. Treatment of aortic disease in patients with Marfan syndrome. *Circulation.* 2005;111:e150–e157.

Moore A, Eagle K, Bruckman D, et al. Choice of computed tomography, transesophageal echocardiography, magnetic resonance imaging, and aortography in acute aortic dissection: International Registry of Acute Aortic Dissection (IRAD). *Am J Cardiol.* 2002;89:1235–1238.

Neptune E, Frischmeyer P, Arking D, et al. Dysregulation of TGF-beta activation contributes to pathogenesis in Marfan syndrome. *Nat Genet.* 2003;33:407–411.

Nollen G, Groenink M, Tijssen J, et al. Aortic stiffness and diameter predict progressive aortic dilatation in patients with Marfan syndrome. *Eur Heart J.* 2004;25:1146–1152.

Robinson P, Arteaga-Solis E, Baldock C, et al. The molecular genetics of Marfan syndrome and related disorders. *J Med Genet.* 2006;43:769–787.

Roman M, Devereux R, Kramer-Fox R, et al. Two-dimensional echocardiographic aortic root dimensions in normal children and adults. *Am J Cardiol.* 1989;64:507–512.

Rossiter J, Repke J, Morales A, et al. A prospective longitudinal evaluation of pregnancy in the Marfan syndrome. *Am J Obstet Gynecol.* 1995;173:1599–1606.

Senior R, Monaghan M, Becher H, et al. Stress echocardiography for the diagnosis and risk stratification of patients with suspected or known coronary artery disease: a critical appraisal. *Heart.* 2005;91:427–436.

Shores J, Berger K, Murphy E, et al. Progression of aortic dilatation and the benefit of long-term β-adrenergic blockade in Marfan's syndrome. *N Engl J Med.* 1994;330:1335–1341.

Silverman D, Burton K, Gray J, et al. Life expectancy in the Marfan syndrome. *Am J Cardiol.* 1995;75:157–160.

Smiseth O, Stoylen A, Ihlen H. Tissue Doppler imaging for the diagnosis of coronary artery disease. *Curr Opin Cardiol.* 2004;19:421–429.

Vignon P. Hemodynamic assessment of critically ill patients using echocardiography Doppler. *Curr Opin Crit Care.* 2005;11:227–234.

Voigt J, Lindenmeier G, Exner B, et al. Incidence and characteristics of segmental postsystolic longitudinal shortening in normal, acutely ischemic, and scarred myocardium. *J Am Soc Echocardiogr.* 2003;16:415–423.

Webb G, David T, eds. *Marfan syndrome: a cardiovascular perspective.* Philadelphia: Churchill Livingstone; 2003.

Williams J, Loeys B, Nwakanma L, et al. Early surgical experience with Loeys-Dietz: a new syndrome of aggressive thoracic aortic aneurysm disease. *Ann Thorac Surg.* 2007;83:S757–S763.

Zoghbi W, Enriquez-Sarano M, Foster E, et al. Recommendations for evaluation of the severity of native valvular regurgitation with two-dimensional and Doppler echocardiography. *J Am Soc Echocardiogr.* 2003;16:777–802.

Chapter 22
Hypertrophic Cardiomyopathy

Patrick W. O'Leary

It has become clear that hypertrophic cardiomyopathy is a genetic disease. In fact, it is the most common inherited cardiovascular disorder, afflicting 1 of every 500 individuals. From a molecular perspective, hypertrophic cardiomyopathy is caused by mutations in at least one of the 10 proteins of the cardiac sarcomere. Despite our ever increasing understanding of the molecular etiologies of this complex disorder, the clinical diagnosis of hypertrophic cardiomyopathy remains within the realm of the echocardiographer. The most common clinical manifestation of hypertrophic cardiomyopathy is left ventricular outflow obstruction. However, diastolic heart failure and mitral regurgitation are also prominent features of this disease that can be evaluated with echocardiographic techniques in patients of all ages.

This chapter reviews the common echocardiographic features displayed by patients with hypertrophic cardiomyopathy. We will also outline a classification and examination strategy that will not only detect the presence of the disease, but also assist with planning both medical and surgical therapies. Finally, a review of both the intraoperative and postoperative echocardiographic challenges associated with hypertrophic cardiomyopathy will be presented.

 ## DIAGNOSIS OF AND CLASSIFICATION SYSTEMS FOR HYPERTROPHIC CARDIOMYOPATHY

The diagnosis of hypertrophic cardiomyopathy is made when one detects increased myocardial wall thickness that is not caused by another abnormality, such as hypertension or aortic valve stenosis. The most common manifestation of hypertrophic cardiomyopathy is an asymmetrically thickened ventricular septum (Fig. 22.1). This basal septal thickening narrows the left ventricular outflow tract. Accelerated blood flow within the narrowed left ventricular outflow tract creates a Venturi effect, drawing the mitral valve leaflets and chordal support forward into the subaortic area. This systolic anterior mitral valve motion has become known as "SAM." This combination of abnormalities leads to one of the hallmarks of this disorder—dynamic left ventricular outflow tract obstruction (Figs. 22.2 and 22.3). The systolic distortion of the mitral valve

leaflets can cause significant mitral regurgitation (Figs. 22.2 and 22.3), increasing the degree of symptoms experienced by the patient.

Echocardiography plays a major role not only in diagnosing this disorder but also in excluding secondary causes of hypertrophy. Diagnoses such as coarctation of the aorta and congenital aortic/subaortic stenosis are readily apparent during routine echocardiographic examinations. In older patients, after years of intense athletic training, two-dimensional echocardiographic findings similar to hypertrophic cardiomyopathy may develop. Features that distinguish the athletic heart from hypertrophic cardiomyopathy are summarized in Table 22.1. Clinical tests other than echocardiography are needed to identify patients with systemic hypertension, pheochromocytoma, renal artery stenosis, and/or other forms of renal disease. Diagnoses that are more difficult to exclude on echocardiographic criteria alone include metabolic and storage diseases (Fig. 22.4). The increases in wall thickness associated with these disorders are not caused by true myocyte hypertrophy but rather are caused by storage of abnormal molecules within the myocardial cell. These disorders require clinical correlation and appropriate metabolic screening for accurate identification.

In the normal heart, the ventricular septum and posterior left ventricular wall have similar thicknesses. The normal ventricular septum has a concave curvature, relative to the left ventricular cavity. This curvature is altered in the presence of hypertrophic cardiomyopathy. Patients with hypertrophic cardiomyopathy have been classified based on either this curvature (Fig. 22.5) or the distribution of left ventricular hypertrophy (Fig. 22.6). Both systems are valid. The type of curvature present seems to be related to the presence of an identifiable genetic mutation. Knowing the pattern of hypertrophy present identifies patients who are likely to have or develop obstruction and the surgical approach that may be most beneficial. Classic asymmetric septal hypertrophy (both basal and diffuse), and mid-ventricular hypertrophy usually show reversed septal curvatures and dynamic outflow obstruction, which can be relieved by transaortic myectomy and myotomy. Some patients with sigmoid curves also have typical dynamic outflow obstruction and are effectively treated by surgical interventions. The most severe subset of patients with reversed septal curvatures develops biventricular outflow obstruction. Those with significant biventricular

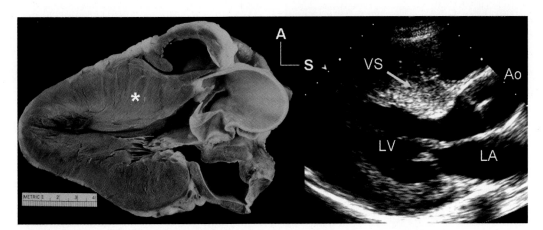

FIGURE 22.1. Long-axis anatomy typical of hypertrophic cardiomyopathy. Left: Anatomic specimen shows a tremendous increase in left ventricular wall thickness, but the increase in myocardial mass is most prominently displayed in the ventricular septum (*asterisk*). **Right:** Echocardiographic image displays similar anatomy. The increase in myocardial thickness is less prominent than in the anatomic example, but the basal septum (*yellow*) is still asymmetrically thickened relative to the posterior left ventricular wall. A, anterior; Ao, aorta; LA, left atrium; LV, left ventricle; S, superior; VS, ventricular septum.

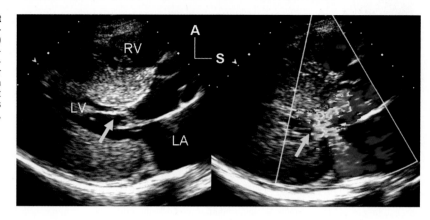

FIGURE 22.2. Systolic, parasternal long-axis frames demonstrating the left ventricular inflow and outflow tracts of a patient with hypertrophic cardiomyopathy. Left: Two-dimensional image shows systolic anterior motion (SAM) of the mitral valve chordal supports (*yellow arrow*). There was prolonged contact between the chords and the septum beginning in mid-systole and extending through the remainder of ventricular ejection. **Right:** Color-flow Doppler image shows not only turbulent flow in the left ventricular outflow tract (as a result of dynamic obstruction), but also an eccentric, posteriorly directed jet of mitral regurgitation (*yellow arrow*). The dysfunction of the mitral valve is related to the distortion of the leaflets caused by the SAM seen on the left. A, anterior; LA, left atrium; LV, left ventricle; RV, right ventricle; S, superior.

outflow gradients face the greatest risk for sudden, unexpected mortality.

Cases with diffuse, concentric hypertrophy, or hypertrophy that is isolated to the ventricular free wall, usually have a neutral curve and do not manifest obstruction. These morphologies tend to present with diastolic dysfunction and symptoms suggestive of pulmonary venous congestion. As a result, surgical therapy offers little

benefit, and medical therapy is the mainstay of treatment for these patients.

Patients with apical hypertrophy have a variable septal curvature, manifest intracavitary gradients, but not develop true outflow tract obstruction. Diastolic dysfunction is often their primary clinical problem. When the severity of hypertrophy compromises the size of the "functional" left ventricular cavity, apical myectomy designed to increase cavity size (and therefore diastolic filling) can reduce symptoms in this group.

ECHOCARDIOGRAPHIC IMAGING IN HYPERTROPHIC CARDIOMYOPATHY

A complete surface echocardiographic evaluation of the patient with hypertrophic cardiomyopathy should include a description of (a) the pattern and severity of myocardial thickening present, (b) the presence and nature of left and/or right ventricular outflow obstruction, (c) the nature of the mitral valve distortion and severity of the resulting regurgitation, (d) the size of the left atrium (shown to be associated with the clinical disease burden), (e) left ventricular diastolic filling, and (f) the pulmonary arterial pressure.

The typical anatomy of obstructive hypertrophic cardiomyopathy is often most easily recognized in the parasternal long-axis views. There is often a prominent basal septal bulge present and the distortion of the mitral support structures can be easily appreciated (Figs. 22.1 and 22.2). Apical four-chamber and long-axis views can reveal the same findings (Fig. 22.3) and are better suited for some Doppler echocardiographic interrogations. The magnitude of septal thickening has been associated with the incidence of sudden death. Patients with diastolic septal thicknesses greater than 30 mm have an increased risk of sudden death events, while sudden death

FIGURE 22.3. Images from the cardiac apex. Left: Images are oriented in a four-chamber format, but the plane of sound has been angled anteriorly, allowing visualization of the left ventricular outflow tract. **Right:** Images are displayed in an apical, long-axis format, also demonstrating the left ventricular inflow and outflow tracts. **Top left:** Diastolic frame, which demonstrates the asymmetric, basal ventricular septal thickening that is common with hypertrophic cardiomyopathy. **Top right:** Systolic frame, which demonstrates the systolic anterior motion of the mitral apparatus, as well as septal contact indicating significant obstruction. **Bottom:** Two color-flow Doppler images demonstrate the primary physiologic consequences of this disorder. The early systolic frame (**bottom left**) shows narrowing of the left ventricular outflow tract between the hypertrophied septum and the deviated mitral apparatus (*yellow arrow*). The color flow signal displays turbulence and aliasing at this level, indicating that the outflow tract obstruction extending at least to this level. The image on the **bottom right** was taken later in systole. The distortion of the mitral valve associated with systolic anterior motion results in inadequate coaptation and late systolic regurgitation. This series of events has been referred to as the "eject, obstruct, leak" phenomenon and can be seen in virtually all patients with the obstructive form of hypertrophic cardiomyopathy. L, left; LA, left atrium; LV, left ventricle; P, posterior; RV, right ventricle; S, superior.

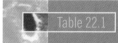

Table 22.1 ECHOCARDIOGRAPHIC FEATURES DISTINGUISHING HYPERTROPHIC CARDIOMYOPATHY FROM THE ATHLETIC HEART

Hypertrophic Cardiomyopathy	The Athletic Heart
• Asymmetrical hypertrophy	• Symmetrical increases in wall thickness
• Severely thickened ventricular walls (>17 mm)	• Milder hypertrophy (<17 mm)
• Reduced left ventricular diameter and diastolic volume	• Increased left ventricular diameter, diastolic volume, and stroke volumes
• Abnormal myocardial relaxation	
• Abnormal diastolic Doppler patterns	• Normal diastolic ventricular function and filling patterns
• Abnormal tissue Doppler and strain rate patterns	• Normal tissue Doppler and strain rate profiles
• Normal resting heart rates	• Decreased resting heart rates (sinus bradycardia)

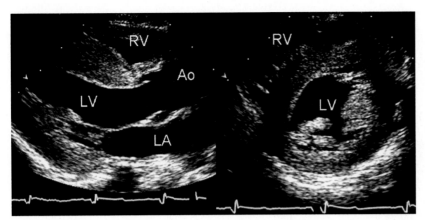

FIGURE 22.4. Parasternal long- and short-axis images of the left ventricle demonstrate diffuse thickening of the myocardium. The examination was performed in a neonate with no family history of cardiomyopathy. The appearance of these images is similar to the diffuse, nonobstructive form of hypertrophic cardiomyopathy. However, the increased thickness of the myocardium is not caused by hypertrophy in this case, but rather it is secondary to accumulation of glycogen within the myocardial cells. This child was found to have type II glycogen storage disease (Pompe disease). This type of case serves to remind one that echocardiography detects increased wall thickness rather than true hypertrophy and that a diagnosis of hypertrophic cardiomyopathy can only be made after other causes of increased myocardial wall thickness have been excluded. Ao, aorta; LA, left atrium; LV, left ventricle; RV, right ventricle.

events rarely occur if the septal diameter is less than 19 mm. This thickness is best assessed using parasternal two-dimensional scans (Fig. 22.1). These scans allow the examiner to determine the point of maximal diastolic thickness and to avoid inclusion of the right ventricular papillary muscles in the measurement. Systolic ventricular contraction is usually normal or hyperdynamic in this disorder. Systolic ventricular dysfunction is only seen in the most advanced stages of this disease, after years of obstruction and progressive myocardial fibrosis. In contrast, diastolic dysfunction is present in nearly all patients with hypertrophic cardiomyopathy. The associated elevations in left atrial and ventricular diastolic pressures contribute significantly to patient's symptoms.

Parasternal long-axis views also provide a unique insight into surgical planning. When obstruction is present, the examiner should define the distance between the anatomic aortic valve annulus and the point of contact between the mitral apparatus and the ventricular septum that is farthest from the aortic valve. This distance represents the minimum extent to which a septal myectomy should be performed (Fig. 22.7). Early surgical therapy, first proposed by Morrow, created a single trough in the hypertrophied ventricular septum, allowing an unobstructed channel for ejection (Fig. 22.8). In many patients, the obstructive zone involves the papillary muscles themselves. In these cases, an extended septal myectomy is required (Fig. 22.9) to provide adequate enlargement of the outflow tract. In patients with a small aortic annulus or obstructions extending deep into the ventricle (beyond the mid-papillary muscle level), a combination of transaortic and apical myectomies may be necessary (Fig. 22.10).

The diffuse, nonobstructive, and apical form of hypertrophic cardiomyopathy requires multiple planes of imaging for confident recognition. The ventricular walls are concentrically thickened. No accelerated color flow Doppler signals will be seen during systole, and the mitral apparatus will move normally. The prominent

diastolic dysfunction associated with this type of myopathy will usually cause significant left atrial enlargement.

The thickened segments of myocardium in patients with apical hypertrophic cardiomyopathy are often not visible from the parasternal window (Fig. 22.11). Apical four-chamber and long-axis scans will demonstrate obliteration of the apical portion of the left ventricular cavity by hypertrophied muscle (Fig. 22.12). High-velocity flow signals can be found in the left ventricular apex. These systolic flow accelerations are directed toward the mid-ventricular cavity, but the true outflow tract is usually widely patent. The potential left ventricular diastolic volume is often reduced in these patients, further compounding the diastolic dysfunction associated with this form of cardiomyopathy. In select cases, transapical resection of the inner myocardial segments may be helpful, increasing the potential diastolic ventricular stroke volume in these patients.

Left atrial size has become increasingly recognized as an accurate barometer of disease burden in many forms of adult cardiac disease. It has recently been shown that left atrial volume has a similar association to disease severity in children and adolescents with hypertrophic cardiomyopathy. This is not surprising given the fact that the obstruction and diastolic dysfunction associated with hypertrophic cardiomyopathy lead to elevations in diastolic filling pressures, and mitral regurgitation, both potent stimuli for left atrial distention.

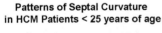
Patterns of Septal Curvature in HCM Patients < 25 years of age

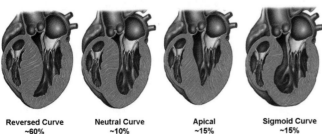

| Reversed Curve ~60% | Neutral Curve ~10% | Apical ~15% | Sigmoid Curve ~15% |

FIGURE 22.5. Variety of septal curvatures that can exist in patients with hypertrophic cardiomyopathy. By far the most common morphology seen in childhood is the reversed septal curve. Any of these patterns can be associated with outflow obstruction. Diastolic dysfunction also occurs in all of these groups but tends to be most severe in those with neutral septal curves or the apical variant of hypertrophic cardiomyopathy (HCM).

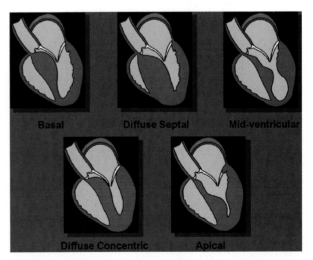

FIGURE 22.6. Shape of the ventricular septum in patients with hypertrophic cardiomyopathy. Top: Patients with these septal geometries often develop significant, dynamic outflow obstruction. The obstruction seen in these three morphologies will usually be effectively treated with transaortic, extended septal myectomy. **Bottom:** Combined transaortic and transapical approaches may be necessary when the hypertrophy is more diffuse. In the rare patient in whom apical hypertrophy limits ventricular diastolic filling, transapical myectomy may increase the diastolic filling potential.

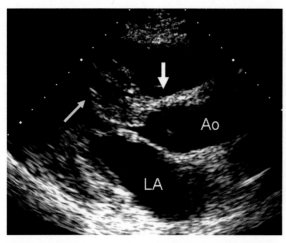

FIGURE 22.7. Impact of echocardiography on surgical planning. This parasternal long-axis image shows the relationship between the hypertrophied segment of basal ventricular septum and the aortic valve. The aortic valve annulus is indicated by the *white arrow*. The *yellow arrow* shows the point at which ventricular septal thickness decreases. This point is beyond the septal contact lesion and is approximately at the same level as the heads of the papillary muscles. This morphology and spatial relationship should be defined on the preoperative echocardiogram. The distance between the aortic annulus and the *yellow arrow* was approximately 4 cm. This information assists the surgeon in planning the septal myectomy and can be obtained both during the preoperative examination and with transesophageal echocardiography in the operating theater. Ao, aorta; LA, left atrium.

 DOPPLER ECHOCARDIOGRAPHY

Doppler echocardiography plays a major role in the evaluation of patients with hypertrophic cardiomyopathy. Color flow Doppler demonstrates and localizes the turbulence associated with dynamic outflow obstruction (Figs. 22.2 and 22.3). Mitral regurgitation can be detected and quantified as previously described. Continuous-wave Doppler allows quantitation of obstructive flow velocities and determination of ventricular-to-atrial pressure gradients. Pulsed-wave and tissue Doppler techniques enhance the assessment of left ventricular filling abnormalities.

Dynamic left ventricular outflow tract obstruction is the physiologic hallmark of the "obstructive" forms of hypertrophic cardio-

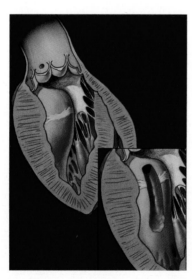

FIGURE 22.8. Anatomic relationships of the left ventricular outflow tract in typical hypertrophic cardiomyopathy with prominent basal hypertrophy and dynamic obstruction. The *white horizontal line* on the ventricular septum represents the fibrotic contact lesion associated with systolic anterior motion of the mitral valve. **Bottom right inset:** An example of an early septal myectomy. In essence, a long trough was created in the outflow of ventricular septal myocardium. This trough allowed left ventricular ejection, even though significant portions of the left ventricular outflow tract were still compromised.

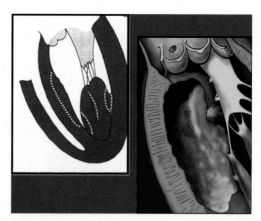

FIGURE 22.9. Areas targeted by an extended septal myectomy for hypertrophic cardiomyopathy. Top left (*dotted lines*): Areas in which myocardium is resected to increase the area available for left ventricular outflow. **Right:** The ventricular septum after such a myectomy. In comparison to the technique originally used (Fig. 22.8), this approach is much more likely to completely relieve left ventricular hypertension and has a much lower incidence of late recurrence of obstruction.

myopathy. The reduction in left ventricular outflow tract diameter associated with septal hypertrophy and systolic anterior mitral valve motion results in a late peaking left ventricular–to–aortic gradient and Doppler flow signal. Continuous-wave Doppler velocities provide convenient quantitation of these gradients. The Doppler signals associated with this obstruction are usually recorded from the apical transducer position. However, right parasternal and suprasternal positions may also provide good acoustic windows.

The Doppler signal of dynamic left ventricular outflow obstruction shows a characteristic "dagger-shape" profile (Fig. 22.13). The curved upstroke is a consequence of the gradually increasing severity of obstruction caused by progressive thickening of the outflow septum and mitral systolic anterior motion during systole. The late peaking nature of this obstruction causes left ventricular and aortic pressures to be maximal at nearly the same time. As a result, the maximum instantaneous Doppler gradient is usually closely correlated with the peak-to-peak gradient measured at cardiac catheterization. This situation is distinctly different from what is seen in more fixed obstructions, like aortic valve stenosis, in which the mean Doppler gradient best reflects the pressure drop across the stenotic valve.

In some patients, the left ventricular outflow tract Doppler signal is difficult to separate from the mitral regurgitation flow profile. In these cases, the left ventricular outflow gradient can be estimated by using the maximum mitral regurgitant velocity to determine the peak left ventricular pressure (Fig. 22.14). The regurgitant velocity is converted to a left ventricular–to–left atrial pressure difference with the simplified Bernoulli equation ($4V^2$). The patient's systolic blood pressure can then be subtracted from that gradient, providing a value for the left ventricular to aortic gradient (Fig. 22.15). Accuracy of this type of gradient determination is increased if one adds an estimate of left atrial pressure to the Doppler predicted ventricular to atrial gradient. Alternatively, the left ventricular outflow signal can be obtained from an alternative acoustic window, such as the suprasternal notch or high right parasternal areas (Fig. 22.15).

Evaluation of the mitral valve assists in defining the clinical burden of the disease. Even the patient with severe outflow obstruction often has no symptoms, if the mitral valve remains relatively competent. However, when the mitral valve is significantly distorted, mitral regurgitation will occur. As the volume of regurgitation increases, so does the size of the left atrium. The mitral regurgitation increases the left atrial and pulmonary venous pressures. These changes are associated with reduced exercise tolerance and exertional dyspnea.

The mitral leaflet distortion caused by systolic anterior motion creates a posteriorly directed regurgitant jet in patients with typical dynamic left ventricular outflow obstruction. Unlike many other diseases associated with mitral regurgitation, the parasternal long-axis

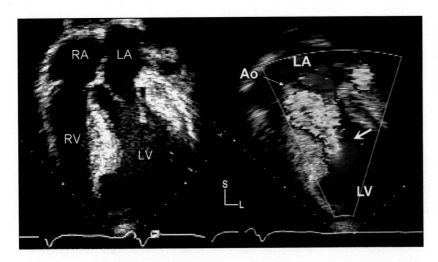

FIGURE 22.10. Apical echocardiographic images of a patient with prominent basal and mid-ventricular hypertrophy caused by hypertrophic cardiomyopathy. The area of thickened septum (**left**) extends beyond the true midpoint of the papillary muscles and the obstruction originates deep in the ventricular cavity (**right**, *white arrow*). When this is the case, a combined transaortic and transapical approach may be required to adequately relieve the obstruction. L, left; LA, left atrium; LV, left ventricle; RA, right atrium; RV, right ventricle; S, superior.

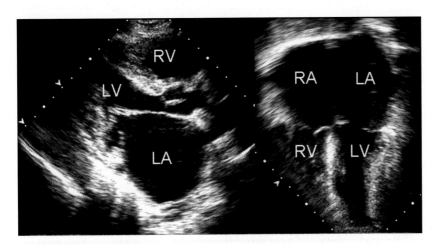

FIGURE 22.11. A 15-year-old patient with apical hypertrophic cardiomyopathy. Both ventricles showed evidence of diastolic dysfunction, as evidenced by the severe biatrial enlargement seen in these images. **Left:** The parasternal long-axis image on the left does not reveal significantly increased wall thicknesses. **Right:** The typical four-chamber view suggests prominent apical walls, primarily because of the tapering shape of the ventricular cavity. These images highlight the difficulties in making this diagnosis. When images are particularly challenging, contrast imaging can improve image definition at the apex. LA, left atrium; LV, left ventricle; RA, right atrium; RV, right ventricle.

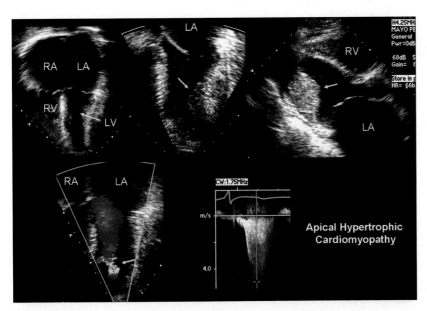

FIGURE 22.12. Same patient shown in Figure 22.11. Top left: The apical four-chamber view depicts the reduction in apical cavity size associated with this disorder. **Top middle:** Focused imaging, in the apical long-axis projection, revealed prominent apical hypertrophy, especially involving the posterior wall (*yellow arrow*). **Top right:** Oblique, parasternal long-axis view oriented more toward the cardiac apex than normal. Unlike the standard long-axis image shown in Figure 22.11, this view reveals the tremendously hypertrophied apical myocardium that is characteristic of this disorder. The color flow image and continuous-wave Doppler signal (**bottom**) document the intracavitary gradients that are common in this morphology. The obstruction in abnormal systolic flow is limited to the cardiac apex (**bottom left**, *yellow arrow*). Although the apical velocities reach nearly 5 m/s, most of the left ventricular cavity is not obstructed during systole, because the outflow septum is of normal thickness and there is no systolic anterior motion present. LA, left atrium; LV, left ventricle; RA, right atrium; RV, right ventricle.

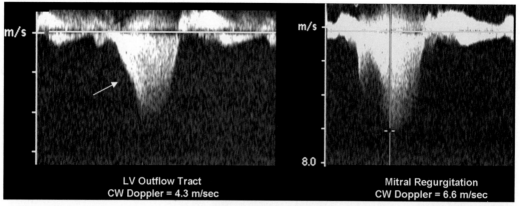

FIGURE 22.13. Continuous-wave Doppler signals from a patient with classic, dynamic left ventricular outflow obstruction caused by hypertrophic cardiomyopathy. Left: Late-peaking, "dagger"-shaped signal (*arrow*). The systolic upstroke is concave to the left. This is a manifestation of progressive narrowing in left ventricular outflow area caused by hyperdynamic contraction. **Right:** Mitral regurgitation signal reached a maximum velocity of 6.6 m/s. Occasionally, these two signals are difficult to separate in space. This is not surprising because the obstruction and regurgitation both originate from the point of contact between the septum and mitral valve tissue. When completely separated signals cannot be recorded, the left ventricular outflow gradient can be estimated by measurement of the maximal mitral regurgitation velocity. This velocity can be converted to a value representing the maximum left ventricular–to–left atrial pressure difference by Bernoulli's equation ($4V^2$). The example shown in Figure 22.13 would suggest a left ventricular–to–left atrial gradient of 172 mm Hg. The left atrium was enlarged and diastolic function was abnormal. As a result, we assumed the left atrial pressure to be 15 mm Hg, predicting a left ventricular maximal systolic pressure of 187 mm Hg. The patient's blood pressure was 105 mm Hg as measured by an arm cuff. These two values would suggest a left ventricular outflow gradient of 82 mm Hg. This correlates relatively well with the velocity of the outflow Doppler signal, which could be separated from the regurgitant flow in this case. This signal reached 4.3 m/s, suggesting a maximum instantaneous gradient of 74 mm Hg between the left ventricle and the aorta. CW, continuous wave; LV, left ventricular.

image frequently provides parallel alignment for Doppler interrogation of the mitral regurgitation (Fig. 22.2). Therefore, this view often provides an excellent acoustic window for Doppler interrogation of the mitral regurgitation, both for PISA analysis or for obtaining the maximum continuous-wave Doppler velocity profile.

ASSESSMENT OF DIASTOLIC DYSFUNCTION

Hearts with hypertrophic cardiomyopathy display markedly impaired myocardial relaxation. Left ventricular pressures fall more slowly after aortic valve closure as shown by prolongation of the isovolumic relaxation time and reduction in transmitral early filling velocity. While left ventricular compliance is still relatively normal, atrial contraction will produce significant augmentation of diastolic filling (Fig. 22.16, left). As myocardial fibrosis progresses, left atrial pressures rise and the transmitral Doppler diastolic filling profile shifts to a more restrictive pattern (Fig. 22.16, top right). These changes are also reflected in the pulmonary venous flow signal (Fig. 22.16, bottom right). The amount and duration of flow reversal within the pulmonary vein after atrial contraction are very sensitive markers for elevated diastolic filling pressure, even in children.

Early diastolic mitral annular tissue Doppler velocities are reduced in most patients with hypertrophic cardiomyopathy. Comparison of the pulsed-wave Doppler early transmitral diastolic filling velocity with the annular early tissue Doppler velocity (E/E' ratio) has provided noninvasive insight into pulmonary capillary wedge pressure and exercise tolerance. Larger values of this ratio are associated with more advanced disease.

Analysis of myocardial deformation is likely to provide additional insights into both systolic and diastolic ventricular performance. However, the clinical impact of these techniques, while promising, remains limited in children.

ROLE OF ECHOCARDIOGRAPHY DURING AND AFTER SURGICAL INTERVENTIONS

Medical and device therapies are important components of the treatment strategies used for patients with hypertrophic cardiomyopathy. However, in young patients with severe obstruction, surgical septal myectomy and myotomy provide significant therapeutic benefits. Adequate relief of the outflow gradient reduces the risk of sudden death, can eliminate mitral regurgitation (often without valve repair or replacement), and can significantly reduce clinical symptoms.

FIGURE 22.14. Patient in whom the obstructive zone extended for 3.7 cm below the aortic annulus (left). The color Doppler signals (**right**) depict a situation in which the left ventricular outflow and the mitral regurgitant Doppler signals could not be separated using Doppler examinations from the cardiac apex. The approach described in Figure 22.13 was used to determine the left ventricular outflow gradient (Fig. 22.15). Ao, aorta; LA, left atrium; LV, left ventricle; RV, right ventricle.

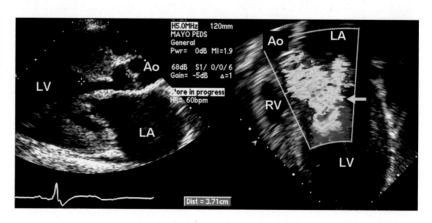

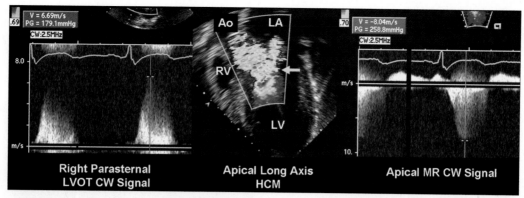

FIGURE 22.15. Same patient shown in Figure 22.14. Middle: Apical long-axis view, with overlapping color flow jets of outflow obstruction and mitral regurgitation. From the apex, separate obstructive and regurgitant signals could not be obtained. Therefore, the examiner concentrated on the mitral regurgitant signal, obtaining the maximum velocity of 8 m/s. The Bernoulli equation predicted that left ventricular systolic pressure was 260 mm Hg greater than the left atrial pressure. The systolic blood pressure was 90 mm Hg, suggesting a gradient of approximately 170 mm Hg between the ventricle and the aorta. Later in the examination, right parasternal imaging revealed the plane in which the outflow jet could be separately evaluated (**left**). A 6.7-m/s velocity was obtained, suggesting a maximum instantaneous gradient of 180 mm Hg and confirming the extremely severe nature of this obstruction. Ao, aorta; CW, continuous wave; HCM, hypertrophic cardiomyopathy; LA, left atrium; LV, left ventricle; LVOT, left ventricular outflow tract; MR, mitral regurgitation; RV, right ventricle.

Echocardiography should be a routine part of both the intraoperative and postoperative evaluation of these patients. Whether the examination is performed in the operating room or late after surgery, the postoperative evaluation of a patient with hypertrophic cardiomyopathy needs to include assessment of left ventricular outflow obstruction, diastolic ventricular filling, mitral regurgitation, and the unintended consequences of septal myectomy (if any). These unintended consequences may include aortic regurgitation, iatrogenic ventricular septal defect, or mitral valve perforation. Unusual color flows are often seen in the area of a ventricular septal myectomy. These flows are usually secondary to small septal coronary arteries that have been incised during the subaortic resection. These coronary–to–left ventricular communications are benign and can be distinguished from ventricular septal defects by their flow pattern. Ventricular septal defects will have a high-velocity, predominantly systolic flow pattern.

The small coronary artery–to–left ventricle communications will usually have exclusively diastolic flow.

Demonstrating absence of systolic anterior motion of the mitral support apparatus is one of the most important components of the postbypass intraoperative echocardiogram. If systolic anterior motion is present, then the dynamic component of the left ventricular outflow tract obstruction has not been relieved. The gradient may be low, but when systolic anterior motion persists, additional interventions are usually required to ensure a good outcome.

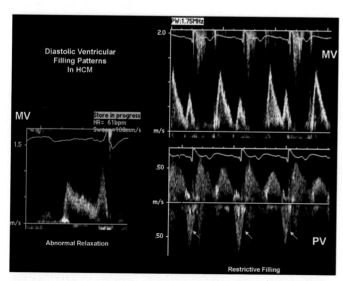

FIGURE 22.16. Pulsed-wave Doppler tracings demonstrate the spectrum of diastolic filling patterns seen in patients with hypertrophic cardiomyopathy. Left: Mitral inflow signal depicts a classic pattern of abnormal relaxation with a ratio between early and atrial diastolic filling velocity that is less than 1. Mid-diastolic deceleration time is prolonged (260 ms), as is isovolumic relaxation time (not shown). **Right:** Recording represents mitral inflow (**top**) and pulmonary venous Doppler flow patterns in a patient with restrictive ventricular filling, suggesting significant elevation of diastolic ventricular pressure. The early mitral diastolic filling wave is dominant; deceleration time and atrial filling waves are short; and pulmonary venous atrial reversal velocity and duration are severely increased (*yellow arrows*). HCM, hypertrophic cardiomyopathy; MV, mitral valve; PV, pulmonary vein.

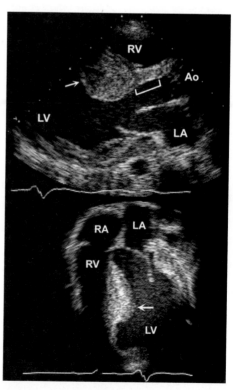

FIGURE 22.17. "Recurrent" left ventricular outflow obstruction in a 10-year-old with hypertrophic cardiomyopathy and a prior history of subaortic resection. The parasternal long-axis image (**top**) shows the area of the prior myectomy outlined by the *white bracket.* Unfortunately, the hypertrophy extends much farther into the ventricular cavity and the septal contact point was at the point indicated by the *white arrow.* This patient had an initial reduction in gradient after her first operation; however, the hypertrophy was far more extensive than could be addressed by the small myectomy that had been performed. Ao, aorta; LA, left atrium; LV, left ventricle; RA, right atrium; RV, right ventricle.

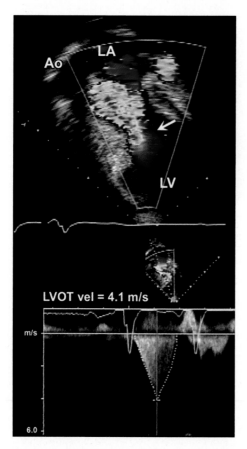

FIGURE 22.18. Color-flow and continuous-wave Doppler findings consistent with severe dynamic obstruction. The color-flow Doppler aliases deep within the ventricle, at the mid to papillary muscle level—well beyond the previous myectomy. The continuous-wave Doppler signal has the typical late-peaking morphology and predicts a 66 mm Hg maximum instantaneous outflow gradient. LA, left atrium; LV, left ventricle; LVOT, left ventricular outflow tract; vel, velocity.

Unfortunately, recurrent, symptomatic left ventricular outflow tract obstruction does occur in this disorder. Often this is secondary to the aggressive nature of the underlying disease. However, an incomplete or cautious initial myectomy can also contribute to redeveloping obstruction. Clear definition of the extent of and

FIGURE 22.19. Comparison of the preoperative (left) and postoperative (right) anatomic findings in the patient described Figures 22.17 and 22.18. An extensive resection has been performed, allowing an unobstructed passageway between the ventricular cavity and the aorta (*asterisk*). Despite the large amount of muscle that was removed, the ventricular septum remains quite thick. Ao, aorta; LA, left atrium; LV, left ventricle; RA, right atrium; RV, right ventricle.

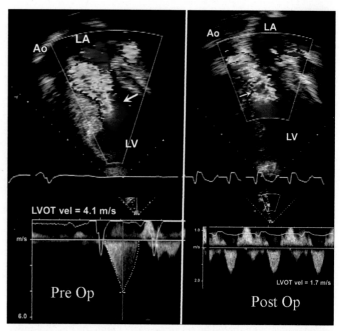

FIGURE 22.20. Comparison of the preoperative (left) and postoperative (right) physiology of the patient described Figures 22.17 and 22.18. The color-flow "wavefront" in the left ventricular outflow tract is still aliased (*top right*). However, systolic velocities only reach the upper limit of normal (1.7 m/s), likely because of the patient's hyperdynamic postoperative state rather than any residual obstruction. Note that the outflow signal is no longer late peaking, and does not have the concave upstroke that was seen preoperatively. Ao, aorta; LA, left atrium; LV, left ventricle; LVOT, left ventricular outflow tract; vel, velocity.

mechanism causing the obstruction is critical to planning and executing successful reintervention.

The 10-year-old girl illustrated in Figures 22.17, 22.18, and 22.19 provides a good example of this type of integrated case management. She clearly had extensive septal hypertrophy (Fig. 22.17). Unfortunately, the first attempt at surgical therapy removed only a small segment of basal myocardium (Fig. 22.17). The tremendously thickened segments of ventricular septum extended nearly 6.5 cm below the aortic annulus. Fig. 22.18 shows a typical, late-peaking left ventricular outflow Doppler signal consistent with severe dynamic obstruction. The color flow Doppler aliases deep within the ventricle, well beyond the previous myectomy. The surface images revealed that geometry and extent of the septal hypertrophy would not be successfully approached through

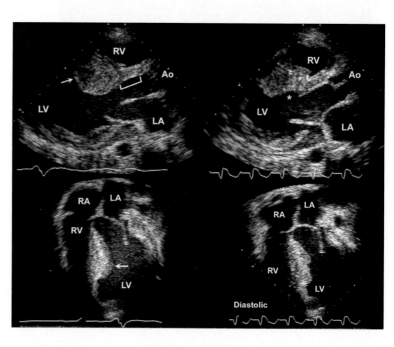

the patient's relatively small, but normal, aortic valve annulus (14 mm). These findings predicted that a combined transaortic and transapical approach was required to adequately relieve the obstruction present in this child. The results of this approach are demonstrated in Fig. 22.19 and 22.20.

SUGGESTED READING

Ackerman MJ, Van Driest SL, Ommen SR, et al. Prevalence and age dependence of malignant mutations in the beta-myosin heavy chain and troponin T genes in hypertrophic cardiomyopathy: a comprehensive outpatient perspective. *J Am Coll Cardiol.* 2002;39:2042–2048.

Arad M, Maron BJ, Gorham JM, et al. Glcogen storage diseases presenting as hypertrophic cardiomyopathy. *N Engl J Med.* 2005;352:362–372.

Binder J, Ommen SR, Gersh BJ, et al. Echocardiography-guided genetic testing in hypertrophic cardiomyopathy: septal morphological features predict the presence of myofilament mutations. *Mayo Clin Proc.* 2006;81:459–467.

Comparato C, Pipitone S, Sperandeo V, et al. Clinical profile and prognosis of hypertrophic cardiomyopathy when first diagnosed in infancy as opposed to childhood. *Cardiol Young.* 1997;7:410–416.

Dearani JA, Ommen SR, Gersh BJ, et al. Surgery insight: septal myectomy for obstructive hypertrophic cardiomyopathy—the Mayo Clinic experience. *Nat Clin Pract Cardiovasc Med.* 2007;4:503–512.

Klues HG, Roberts WC, Maron BJ. Morphologic determinants of echocardiographic patterns of mitral valve systolic anterior motion in obstructive hypertrophic cardiomyopathy. *Circulation.* 1993;87:1570–1579.

Klues HG, Schiffers A, Maron EJ. Phenotypic spectrum and patterns of left ventricular hypertrophy in hypertrophic cardiomyopathy: morphologic observations and significance as assessed by two-dimensional echocardiography in 600 patients. *J Am Coll Cardiol.* 1995;26:1699–1708.

Maron BJ. Hypertrophic cardiomyopathy in childhood. *Pediatr Clin North Am.* 2004;51:1305–1346.

Maron BJ, Henry WL, Clark CE, et al. Asymmetric septal hypertrophy in childhood. *Circulation.* 1976;53:9–19.

Maron BJ, McIntosh CL, Klues HG, et al. Morphologic basis for obstruction to right ventricular outflow in hypertrophic cardiomyopathy. *Am J Cardiol.* 1993;71:1089–1094.

Maron BJ, Pelliccia A. Athlete's heart, sudden death and related cardiovascular issues. *Circulation.* 2006;114:1633–1644.

Maron BJ, Pelliccia A, Spirito P. Cardiac disease in young trained athletes: Insights into methods for distinguishing athlete's heart from structural heart disease with particular emphasis on hypertrophic cardiomyopathy. *Circulation.* 1995;91:1596–1601.

McCully RB, Nishimura RA, Bailey KR, et al. Hypertrophic obstructive cardiomyopathy: preoperative echocardiographic predictors of outcome after septal myectomy. *J Am Coll Cardiol.* 1996;27:1491–1496.

McKenna W, Deanfield J, Faruqui A, et al. Prognosis in hypertrophic cardiomyopathy: role of age and clinical, electrocardiographic and hemodynamic features, *Am J Cardiol.* 1981;47:532–538.

McMahon CJ, Nagueh SF, Pignatelli RH, et al. Characterization of left ventricular diastolic function by tissue Doppler imaging and clinical status in children with hypertrophic cardiomyopathy, *Circulation.* 2004;109:1756–1762.

Menon SC, Ackerman MJ, Ommen SR, et al. Impact of septal myectomy on left atrial volume and left ventricular diastolic filling patterns: an echocardiographic study of young patients with obstructive hypertrophic cardiomyopathy. *J Am Soc Echocardiogr.* 2008;21:684–688.

Minakata K, Dearani JA, Nishimura RA, et al. Extended septal myectomy for hypertrophic obstructive cardiomyopathy with anomalous mitral papillary muscles or chordae. *J Thorac Cardiovasc Surg.* 2004;127:481–489.

Minakata K, Dearani JA, O'Leary PW, et al. Septal myectomy for obstructive hypertrophic cardiomyopathy in pediatric patients: early and late results. *Ann Thorac Surg.* 2005;80:1424–1430.

Minakata K, Dearani JA, Schaff HV, et al. Mechanisms for recurrent left ventricular outflow tract obstruction after septal myectomy for obstructive hypertrophic cardiomyopathy. *Ann Thorac Surg.* 2005;80:851–856.

Mohr R, Schaff HV, Danielson GK, et al. The outcome of surgical treatment of hypertrophic obstructive cardiomyopathy. Experience over 15 years, *J Thorac Cardiovasc Surg.* 1989;97:666–674.

Mohr R, Schaff HV, Puga FJ, et al. Results of operation for hypertrophic obstructive cardiomyopathy in children and adults less than 40 years of age. *Circulation.* 1989;80:1191–1196.

Nishimura RA, Appleton CP, Redfield MM, et al. Noninvasive Doppler echocardiographic evaluation of left ventricular filling pressures in patients with cardiomyopathies: a simultaneous Doppler echocardiographic and cardiac catheterization study, *J Am Coll Cardiol.* 1996;28.

Nishimura RA, Tajik AJ, Reeder GS, et al. Evaluation of hypertrophic cardiomyopathy by Doppler color flow imaging: initial observations. *Mayo Clin Proc.* 1986;61:631–639.

Ommen SR, Maron BJ, Olivotto I, et al. Long-term effects of surgical septal myectomy on survival in patients with obstructive hypertrophic cardiomyopathy. *J Am Coll Cardiol.* 2005;46:470–476.

Sasson Z, Yock PG, Hatle LK, et al. Doppler echocardiographic determination of the pressure gradient in hypertrophic cardiomyopathy. *J Am Coll Cardiol.* 1988;11:752–756.

Sorajja P, Nishimura RA, Ommen SR, et al. Use of echocardiography in patients with hypertrophic cardiomyopathy: clinical implications of massive hypertrophy. *J Am Soc Echocardiogr.* 2006;19:788–795.

Suda K, Kohl T, Kovalchin JP, et al. Echocardiographic predictors of poor outcome in infants with hypertrophic cardiomyopathy. *Am J Cardiol.* 1997;80:595–600.

Theodoro DA, Danielson GK, Feldt RH, et al. Hypertrophic obstructive cardiomyopathy in pediatric patients: results of surgical treatment. *J Thorac Cardiovasc Surg.* 1996;112:1589–1599.

Wigle ED, Rakowski H, Kimbal BP, et al. Hypertrophic cardiomyopathy. Clinical spectrum and treatment. *Circulation.* 1995;92:1680–1692.

Woo A, Williams WG, Choi R, et al. Clinical and echocardiographic determinants of long-term survival following surgical myectomy in obstructive hypertrophic cardiomyopathy. *Circulation.* 2005;111:2033–2041.

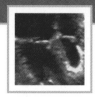

Chapter 23
Additional Cardiomyopathies

Colin J. McMahon • Ricardo H. Pignatelli

Cardiomyopathy is defined as an intrinsic abnormality in systolic and/or diastolic function of the myocardium and represents a significant morbidity and mortality to both pediatric and adult populations. In recent years, our understanding of the molecular and genetic mechanisms responsible for cardiomyopathy has increased exponentially. Although the disease process may appear similar in adults and children, children represent a unique population. Data regarding predictors of adverse clinical outcomes in this group are lacking. Echocardiographic assessment of children with cardiomyopathy often represents the first line of investigation. Proper assessment is critical in establishing the diagnosis, allowing a strategy of appropriate management and additionally providing prognostic information for the patient. This chapter aims to discuss the echocardiographic evaluation of all forms of cardiomyopathy excluding hypertrophic cardiomyopathy (HCM), which will be discussed in a separate chapter.

 ## CLASSIFICATION OF CARDIOMYOPATHY

There are several classification systems for cardiomyopathy and some groups have even advocated a molecular classification. The National Australian Childhood Cardiomyopathy Study, which studied all cases between 1987 and 1996 reported an annual incidence of 1.24 per 100,000 children younger than 10 years of age. The most common forms of cardiomyopathy in this cohort included dilated cardiomyopathy (DCM) (59%), HCM (26%), restrictive cardiomyopathy (RCM) (2.5%), and left ventricular noncompaction cardiomyopathy (LVNC) (9%). Among the study population, lymphocytic myocarditis was present in 25 of 62 cases (40%) of DCM. Sudden cardiac death (SCD) occurred in 11 cases (4%). The North American Cardiomyopathy study, which looked at the northeastern and southern United States, reported findings similar to those reported in the Australian study.

 ## GENETICS OF CARDIOMYOPATHY AMONG CHILDREN

There are characteristic racial and genetic factors that predispose to various forms of cardiomyopathy. For each form of cardiomyopathy, specific mutations have been determined that are responsible for encoding proteins that compose the cytoskeletal structure. A breakdown in cytoskeletal structure consequently translates to a defective phenotype in these children. Certain populations may also have a predisposition to cardiomyopathy. Arrhythmogenic right ventricular dysplasia (ARVD) has a dramatically increased prevalence among the Italian population, and there have been reports of increased risk of HCM among North American, western European, and Japanese populations.

 ## CHARACTERIZATION OF CARDIOMYOPATHIES

Cardiomyopathies can be classified as follows:

1. DCM
2. HCM
3. RCM
4. LVNC
5. ARVD
6. Neuromuscular disorders and storage disorder–induced cardiomyopathy
7. Others, including arrhythmia-induced and anthracycline-induced cardiomyopathy

Dilated Cardiomyopathy

DCM is the most common form of cardiomyopathy and is defined as a dilated and poorly contracting left ventricle, with a left ventricular ejection fraction (LVEF) of less than 40% and a left ventricular end-diastolic dimension (LVEDD) greater than 2 Z-scores. These patients develop congestive heart failure as a consequence of LV or RV systolic dysfunction, or both. The etiology underlying this disease comprises multiple genetic and metabolic disorders. Some of these diagnoses are provided in Table 23.1. Differentiation of DCM from myocarditis is important because myocarditis may have significant improvement in LV contractility following a quiescence of the viral process.

Causes and Prevalence of Dilated Cardiomyopathy–Approximately 50% of cases are idiopathic with an overall prevalence of 36.5 per 100,000 patients. The majority of cases of DCM become manifest in the fourth decade of life, but the disease will often declare itself in childhood.

The Cardiac Cytoskeleton – The myocardium acts as a mechanical syncytium, coupling individual myocytes to provide a concerted myocardial contraction. Force is generated by the actin–myosin

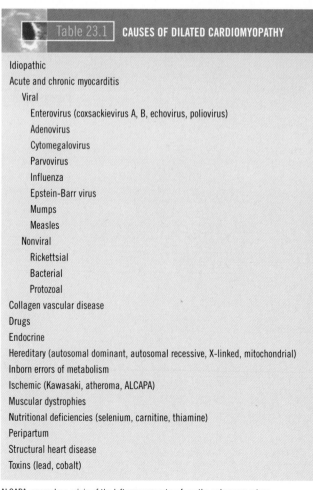

Table 23.1	CAUSES OF DILATED CARDIOMYOPATHY
Idiopathic	
Acute and chronic myocarditis	
Viral	
Enterovirus (coxsackievirus A, B, echovirus, poliovirus)	
Adenovirus	
Cytomegalovirus	
Parvovirus	
Influenza	
Epstein-Barr virus	
Mumps	
Measles	
Nonviral	
Rickettsial	
Bacterial	
Protozoal	
Collagen vascular disease	
Drugs	
Endocrine	
Hereditary (autosomal dominant, autosomal recessive, X-linked, mitochondrial)	
Inborn errors of metabolism	
Ischemic (Kawasaki, atheroma, ALCAPA)	
Muscular dystrophies	
Nutritional deficiencies (selenium, carnitine, thiamine)	
Peripartum	
Structural heart disease	
Toxins (lead, cobalt)	

ALCAPA, anomalous origin of the left coronary artery from the pulmonary artery.

Extracellular

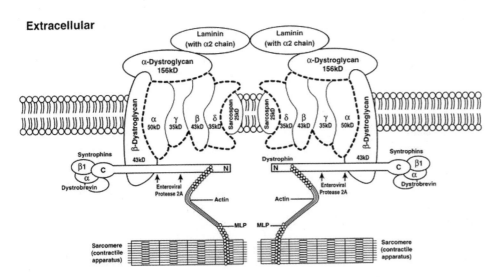

FIGURE 23.1. The cardiac cytoskeleton demonstrating dystrophin-associated glycoprotein complex linking actin and myosin. (Reproduced with permission from Bowles NE, Bowles K, Towbin JA. Prospects for gene therapy for inherited cardiomyopathies. *Progr Pediatr Cardiol.* 2000;12:133–145.)

Intracellular

interaction, and this energy is transmitted to adjacent sarcomeres at Z discs and between myocytes at the intercalated discs. There is an extensive network of proteins that link these sites. Dystrophin and actin represent two essential proteins in this process (Fig. 23.1) and mutations within these components often lead to defective force transmission, which is accompanied by progressive LV dilatation and failure (Frank-Starling curve exceeded). The progressive dilatation of the LV results in increased wall stress (LaPlace law) and increased mismatch of myocardial oxygen supply and demand. With continued ventricular remodeling with ongoing heart failure, cardiac fibroblasts proliferate and mechanically stable collagen is degraded by metalloproteinases resulting in an excess of poorly cross-linked collagen within the interstitium. This results in increased muscle mass, ventricular dilatation, and wall thinning. Eventually, cardiac apoptosis occurs with noninflammatory programmed cell death.

Genetics of Dilated Cardiomyopathy – Several genetic loci have been identified to be responsible for DCM. X-linked cardiomyopathy was one of the earliest detected genetic causes of DCM, highlighting the crucial role of dystrophin in maintaining integrity of the cytoskeleton. Other loci include *1p1-1q1, 1q32, 2q31, 3p22-p25, 9q13-q22, 10q21-23,* and *15q14.*

Clinical Features of Dilated Cardiomyopathy – The most common symptoms are dyspnea, failure to thrive, and orthopnea in older children. Physical examination will reveal tachycardia, elevated jugular venous pressure, and a displaced apex beat with a gallop rhythm. There may be a mitral or tricuspid regurgitation murmur if there is significant atrioventricular valvar dilatation or elevated LV end-diastolic pressure. Hepatomegaly is common, although peripheral edema is rarely seen in children compared with adults. The chest radiograph demonstrates cardiomegaly with increased pulmonary venous congestion.

Two-dimensional Echocardiographic Evaluation of Dilated Cardiomyopathy – Echocardiography is diagnostic in DCM, demonstrating a dilated left ventricle with depressed LV systolic function. DCM is defined as an LVEDD greater than 2 Z-scores and an LVEF of less than 40% (Fig. 23.2). The left ventricle assumes a more globular shape in DCM rather than the normal ellipsoid pattern. In the normal heart, the LV long axis–to–short axis ratio exceeds 1.6. In patients with DCM, this "sphericity index" ratio decreases to less than 1.5 and approaches 1.0. The LVEDD progressively increases, resulting in mitral annular dilatation. This results in noncoaptation of the anterior and posterior mitral valve leaflets, which results in mitral regurgitation (Fig. 23.3). The presence of elevated LV end-diastolic pressure exacerbates mitral regurgitation. With progressive mitral regurgitation, there is left atrial enlargement and retrograde flow into the pulmonary veins, eventually resulting in the development of pulmonary venous and arterial hypertension.

M-mode echocardiography allows for excellent spatial resolution and calculation of LV end-diastolic and end-systolic dimensions and hence derivation of LV shortening fraction (Fig. 23.4). Using Simpson's method, serial LV volumes in systole and diastole are measured and an LVEF is determined (Fig. 23.5). One limitation of calculating LVEF in DCM using Simpson's method results from LV dilatation, which may make it difficult to image the LV apex from the four-chamber and two-chamber views. Myocardial dropout in the region of the LV apex may be improved using contrast echocardiography. The presence of pulmonary arterial hypertension should be assessed from the TR jet velocity [Bernoulli equation: RV systolic pressure = $(TR\ velocity)^2$ + right atrial pressure]. In adult patients, a characteristic M-mode finding in DCM is an increased E-point–to–septal separation (EPSS), which is indicative of a reduced LVEF. EPSS is the distance in millimeters from the anterior septal myocardium to the maximal early opening point of the mitral valve (Fig. 23.6). As the LV internal dimension is proportional to LV diastolic volume and maximal diastolic mitral valve excursion relates to mitral stoke volume, a reduced LVEF correlates with a reduction in the mitral valve opening and hence an increased distance between E-point and septum. In normal adult patients, the EPSS measures approximately 6 mm.

Doppler evaluation of the patient with DCM yields much data regarding systolic and diastolic parameters. The stroke volume and hence cardiac output can be calculated from the time-velocity integral (TVI) in the LV outflow tract (LVOT). Cardiac output is the multiple of stroke volume and heart rate. The stroke volume is calculated by the product of the TVI and the cross-sectional area of the LVOT (measured as πr^2, where r = radius of LVOT) (Fig. 23.7). Errors in the measurement of the LVOT radius will exponentially

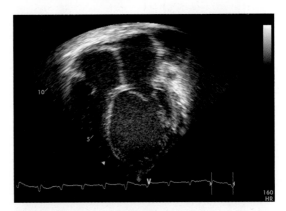

FIGURE 23.2. Apical four-chamber view demonstrating dilated left ventricle with depressed left ventricular systolic function.

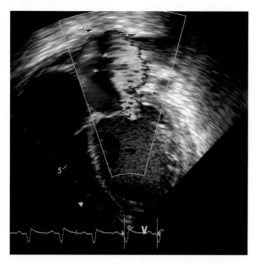

FIGURE 23.3. Moderate mitral regurgitation in a patient with dilated cardiomyopathy.

increase the error as this measure is squared in calculation of the cross-sectional area.

The transmitral inflow and pulmonary venous Doppler patterns are important in the evaluation of LV diastolic relaxation. The patterns of inflow include normal mitral inflow, abnormal relaxation, and decreased LV compliance (Fig. 23.8). With abnormal relaxation, there is a decrease in early inflow (E-wave) velocity, increase in A-wave velocity, and prolongation of E-wave deceleration time. The pulmonary venous inflow normally demonstrates a predominant systolic flow, but diastolic flow predominates in impaired relaxation states. The reverse Ar wave duration and velocity are typically normal. There are various states of decreased compliance with an initial phase of pseudo-normalization where E-and A-wave patterns are normal but there is predominant diastolic pulmonary venous flow, increased Ar-wave velocity/duration, and a reduction in the transmitral Ea velocity at the lateral mitral annulus. With further reductions in LV compliance, the E/A wave ratio increases, diastolic pulmonary venous filling predominates, and Ea and Aa tissue Doppler velocities are reduced further. End-stage (grade 4) diastolic dysfunction characterized by high E/A wave ratio, primary diastolic pulmonary venous filling, and severely reduced Ea and Aa lateral mitral tissue Doppler velocities is typically irreversible regardless of medical therapies.

Tissue Doppler Imaging Velocities in Patients With Dilated Cardiomyopathy – Descent of the base of the heart to the ventricular apex provides a nonvolumetric assessment of LV systolic function.

Tissue Doppler imaging velocities at the lateral and septal mitral annuli measure the velocity of relaxation (Ea and Aa velocities) and contractility (Sa velocity) (Fig. 23.9). These are relatively load-independent indices of systolic and diastolic relaxation. Combining the transmitral E-wave velocity and the lateral mitral Ea velocity as a ratio (E/Ea ratio) allows an indirect measurement of left heart filling pressures (Fig. 23.10). In adult patients, this has shown good correlation with LVEDP [$r = 0.86$, PCWP $= 1.55 + 1.47$(E/Ea)] (Fig. 23.11). Nagueh et al. demonstrated an E/Ea ratio greater than 10 predicted LVEDP higher than 15mm Hg with a sensitivity of 85% and specificity of 93% in adult patients in normal sinus rhythm or sinus tachycardia. Accurate acquisition of tissue Doppler velocities requires consistent perpendicular interrogation of the area of myocardium being examined. Changes in angle of interrogation will result in widely varying values. Color tissue Doppler imaging may be used to assess differential myocardial velocities throughout the LV wall, which is then analyzed using offline analysis.

Myocardial Performance Index (Tei Index) – In the 1990s, a novel combined index of systolic and diastolic relaxation, the myocardial performance index, was analyzed in several cohorts of patients with abnormal LV systolic and diastolic function. This ratio was measured as the summation of isovolumetric relaxation and contraction times divided by the LV ejection time (Fig. 23.12). Although this has shown some clinical utility in adult studies, its utility in providing prognostic information in children with DCM remains contentious.

dP/dt Measurement and Flow Propagation – Other indices of LV systolic function in patients with mitral regurgitation include measurement of dP/dt derived from continuous-wave Doppler analysis of the mitral regurgitant jet (Fig. 23.13). A high-quality Doppler signal is required with a high sweep speed. The time change in milliseconds is determined from the point at which the velocity is 1 m/s and 3 m/s. This represents the time required for a 32 mm Hg pressure change in the LV cavity. The dP/dt is then calculated = 32 ÷ time in milliseconds. A significantly reduced positive or negative dP/dt is associated with poor prognosis.

Color flow propagation (Vp) is measured using a combination of color Doppler and M-mode echocardiography. Mitral inflow propagation velocity is measured from the LV apex (Fig. 23.14). Reduced LV filling velocity is associated with delayed LV filling and a reduced slope of the color M-mode signal (Fig. 23.15). With progressive LV dysfunction, the propagation velocity decreases indicating a reduction in LV velocity with propagation to the apex and correlates with LV diastolic dysfunction. Although flow propagation has shown correlation with LV dysfunction in adults, its role in pediatric patients appears more limited, presumably due to the limited size of the distance of propagation (LV cavity) in this younger population.

Strain Rate Imaging in Dilated Cardiomyopathy – Strain rate imaging allows high-resolution interrogation of regional LV function. *Strain rate* is defined as the instantaneous rate of change in

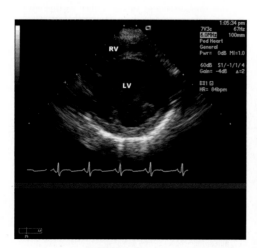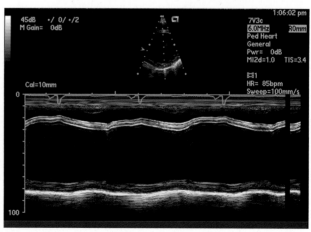

FIGURE 23.4. M-mode tracing demonstrating reduced left ventricular shortening fraction in dilated cardiomyopathy.

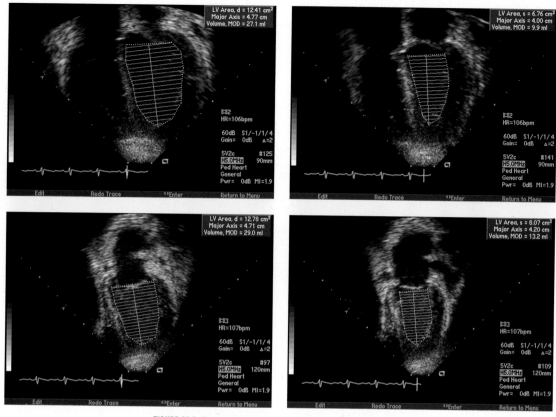

FIGURE 23.5. Simpson's calculation of left ventricular ejection fraction.

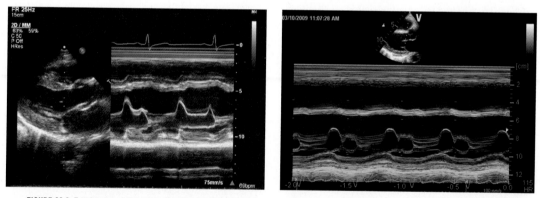

FIGURE 23.6. E-point–to–septal separation derived from M-mode echocardiography in normal (left) versus dilated cardiomyopathy (right).

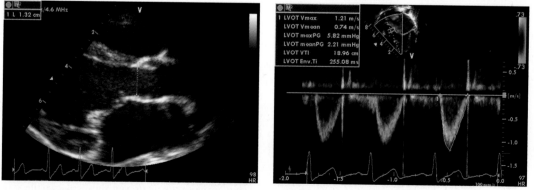

FIGURE 23.7. Cardiac output derived from time-velocity integral and cross-sectional area of left ventricular outflow tract.

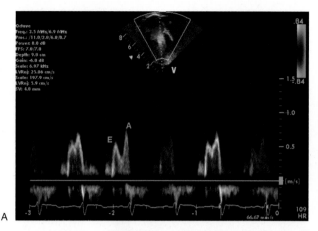
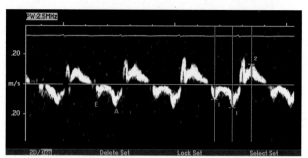

FIGURE 23.8. Transmitral inflow (A) and tissue Doppler (B) patterns in patients with impaired left ventricular relaxation.

two myocardial velocities divided by the instantaneous distance between the two points (Fig. 23.16). Negative values denote active myocardial contraction for longitudinal or circumferential myocardial fibers. Meanwhile, active radial tickening fibers are depicted as positive values. Strain rate has proved to be more robust than several other methodologies as an early and sensitive indicator of regional LV wall dysfunction. Subtle alterations in systolic and diastolic regional function are detectable using this technique because of its excellent spatial and temporal resolution.

Treatment of Dilated Cardiomyopathy – The mainstay of medical therapy includes diuretics, cardiac glycosides, and angiotensin-converting enzyme inhibitors (afterload reduction) if tolerated. Beta-blockers (carvedilol, metoprolol) are increasingly used to support the failing myocardium because they reduce myocardial wall stress and myocardial oxygen consumption. Carvedilol is a particularly attractive agent as it has beta-blocker and vasodilating actions. Patients in cardiogenic shock may require inotropic support. Dobutamine and milrinone (phosphodiesterase inhibitor) are the most appropriate inotropic agents. Epinephrine is associated with poorer outcomes in adult patients with congestive heart failure and probably results in further trauma to the cytoskeleton. Optimizing preload and minimizing afterload appear to be the optimal means of supporting the myocardium. Occasionally, patients on high inotropic support who continue to demonstrate end-organ failure require support of the myocardium using extracorporeal membrane oxygenation or ventricular assist devices.

Echocardiographic evaluation of patients with DCM who have undergone mechanical support using ventricular assist devices has demonstrated improvement in LV indices and systolic function. This is corroborated by regeneration of dystrophin in patients who have undergone mechanical assistance.

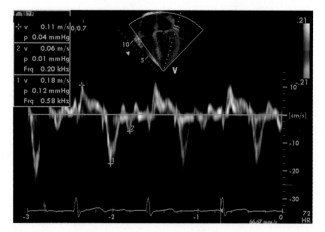

FIGURE 23.9. Tissue Doppler imaging velocities in a normal patient. Note: Ea, Aa, and Sa velocities.

In a subgroup of patients with severe mitral regurgitation, surgical repair of the atrioventricular valve is associated with an improvement in New York Heart Association functional class and a reduction in left heart dimensions. Vatta et al. have provided convincing evidence that resting the myocardium results in dystrophin remodeling in patients with DCM (Fig. 23.17). The mean survival for children with DCM is 63% to 90% at 1 year to 20% to 80% at 5 years.

Echocardiographic Predictors of Outcomes in Children With Dilated Cardiomyopathy – Several studies have evaluated echocardiographic parameters associated with a poor prognosis. These include older age at presentation (older than 2 years), elevated LVEDP greater than 20 mm Hg, presence of mural thrombus, coexistent atrial or ventricular arrhythmias, histologic evidence of endocardial fibroelastosis, right ventricular (RV) failure (in addition to LV dysfunction), and reduced heart rate variability. Echocardiographic predictors included lower LVEF, moderate-severe mitral regurgitation, decreased lateral mitral Ea velocities, and LV wall thinning.

Myocarditis – In 40% of patients presenting with acute DCM, a viral etiology of myocarditis will be responsible. It is crucial to differentiate genetic DCM from viral mediated cytoskeletal disruption because this has major implications for medical therapies and prognosis. There is the potential for cytoskeletal remodeling in cases of viral myocarditis and resting the myocardium may result in full recovery of myocyte function. One would defer cardiac transplantation if at all possible in this subset of patients. At this time, it is not possible echocardiographically to differentiate myocarditis from genetic etiologies of DCM. The echocardiographic findings are comparable to those in DCM, although early presentation may not be associated with severe LV dilatation. Regional wall motion abnormalities are common, but generalized hypocontractility is the most common presentation. Pericardial effusions are often present in the setting of myocarditis.

In the future, tissue Doppler imaging and strain rate imaging may provide some role in differentiating these diseases. Currently, cardiac magnetic resonance imaging (MRI) with delayed contrast hyperenhancement has been used to identify hot spots of viral myocyte infiltration. This can then be used for targeted endomyocardial biopsy to confirm the presence of virus using polymerase chain reaction (PCR). Viral agents causing myocarditis are outlined in Table 23.1.

Restrictive Cardiomyopathy

RCM is characterized by impaired diastolic relaxation, abnormal ventricular compliance, and elevated LV and RV end-diastolic pressures. Although these latter indices can only be quantified at cardiac catheterization, echocardiography can demonstrate particular transmitral inflow characteristics such as an elevation in the E:A wave ratio and increased E-wave deceleration time (DT). Later findings include severe biatrial enlargement. In some cases, the atrial volumes may actually exceed ventricular volumes (Fig. 23.18).

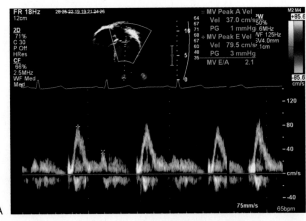 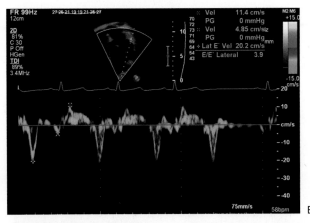

FIGURE 23.10. Transmitral E/Ea as a predictor of left ventricular end-diastolic pressure.

The findings in RCM are similar to those of constrictive pericarditis. The ventricular volumes are decreased, and in association with impaired relaxation, progressive enlargement of both atria occurs. RCM is relatively rare in children. Recent evidence has demonstrated a particularly poor prognosis once children become symptomatic. Certain institutions advocate early transplantation especially in the setting of acute abdominal or thoracic pain, which is associated with sudden cardiac death. Mutations within desmin have been implicated in the development of RCM.

Left Ventricular Noncompaction Cardiomyopathy

Noncompaction of the ventricular myocardium, also known as LV noncompaction (LVNC), represents an arrest in the normal process of myocardial compaction, resulting in persistence of multiple prominent ventricular trabeculations and deep intertrabecular recesses. The disorder has only recently been recognized as a distinct form of cardiomyopathy. It was previously termed "spongy myocardium," although this term has been abandoned as it underscores the hypothesis that the basic morphogenetic abnormality may be arrest of normal compaction of the loose interwoven mesh of myocardial fibers in the embryo. It typically involves the left ventricle, although involvement of the right ventricle has been reported. Clinical presentations include depressed systolic and diastolic function, systemic embolism, and the development of ventricular tachyarrhythmias in both adult and pediatric populations. Children with LVNC may manifest an undulating phenotype with initial DCM that progresses to HCM. The medical management of LVNC depends on the clinical phenotype. To date, a small number of patients have been identified with mutations in *G4.5* (taffazin gene) and in *CYPHER/ZASP,* but in the majority of cases there is no identified genetic locus. A small number of patients may also manifest Barth's syndrome, characterized by a dilated phenotype, neutropenia, and elevated 3,5-methylgluconic aciduria.

Echocardiographic Features of Left Ventricular Noncompaction Cardiomyopathy – Characteristic features include multiple apical trabeculations (more than three), deep recesses between the trabeculations, and a noncompact-to-compact myocardial ratio exceeding 2:1 (Fig. 23.19). The location of the trabeculations may vary from apical, to LV free wall, septal wall, and LV posterior wall. The transmitral inflow Doppler pattern demonstrates a restrictive pattern with increased E-wave velocity, decreased A-wave velocity, increased E/A ratio, and a shortened E-wave deceleration time. The transmitral E/Ea ratio is often increased, reflecting elevated LV end-diastolic pressure. Color Doppler imaging is useful, focusing on blood flow into the recesses between the trabeculations. Tissue Doppler imaging velocities are decreased in children with LVNC compared with age- and gender-matched controls (Fig. 23.20). One study of children with LVNC demonstrated decreased ejection fraction and lateral mitral Ea velocity to be useful in predicting risk of death, transplantation, and need for hospital admission.

FIGURE 23.11. Correlation of pulmonary capillary wedge pressure and E/Ea. (Reproduced with permission from Nagueh SF, Mikati I, Kopelen HA, et al. Doppler estimation of left ventricular filling pressure in sinus tachycardia. A new application of tissue Doppler imaging. *Circulation.* 1998;98:1644–1650.)

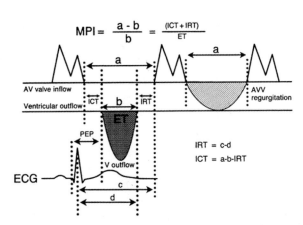

FIGURE 23.12. Derivation of myocardial performance index (Tei index). (Used with permission: Eidem BW, Tei C, O'Leary PW, et al. Right and Left Ventricular Function: Myocardial Performance Index in Normal Children and Patients with Ebstein Anomaly. *J Am Soc Echocardiogr* 1998;11: 849-56.)

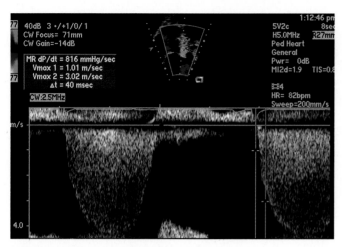

FIGURE 23.13. Measurement of dP/dT. (Used with permission: Eidem BW, Tei C, O'Leary PW, et al. Right and Left Ventricular Function: Myocardial Performance Index in Normal Children and Patients with Ebstein Anomaly. *J Am Soc Echocardiogr* 1998;11:849-56.)

Arrhythmogenic Right Ventricular Dysplasia

ARVD is a highly lethal disease and well-recognized cause of sudden cardiac death. There is a high prevalence of this disease in the Italian population. It is characterized by RV regional wall motion abnormalities, replacement of the RV outflow tract by fibrofatty infiltration, and dilatation of the right ventricle and atrium. These findings are best delineated using cardiac MRI with fat saturation sequences. Familial occurrence is well recognized with an autosomal dominant inheritance pattern. Genetic heterogeneity has been established with linkage analysis identifying four specific loci on chromosomes 14q23-q24 (*ARVD1*), 1q42-q43 (*ARVD2*), 14q12-q22 (*ARVD3*), and 2q32.1-q32.3 (*ARVD4*). The ventricular tachycardia associated with this disorder has a left bundle-branch block morphology, indicating its origin from the right ventricle.

Echocardiographic evaluation of children with ARVD is challenging. Cardiac MRI is more sensitive in detecting RV dilatation, regional RV systolic/diastolic abnormalities, and fibrofatty infiltration of the RV outflow tract. Right atrial and ventricular dilatation may, however, be recognized on routine two-dimensional echocardiography. Complete evaluation for this condition, though, warrants cardiac MRI.

Neuromuscular Disorders and Storage Disorder–Induced Cardiomyopathy

Dilated Cardiomyopathy Associated With Duchenne Muscular Dystrophy– Duchenne's muscular dystrophy arises secondary to a mutation in the dystrophin gene located at Xp21. This results in cytoskeletal

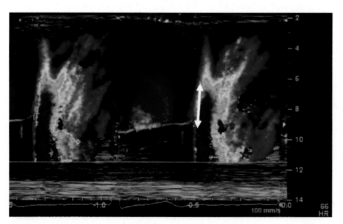

FIGURE 23.14. Flow propagation velocity with color Doppler M-mode.

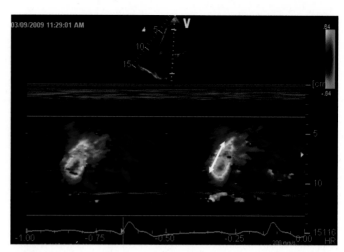

FIGURE 23.15. Reduced Vp curve in patient with depressed left ventricular systolic and diastolic function.

disruption and impaired force transmission that results in progressive LV dilatation and LV systolic dysfunction. The echocardiographic findings are consistent with DCM. Earlier detection of DCM has resulted in earlier treatment in these patients. Some investigators maintain that earlier medical intervention in this disease may delay the progression of LV systolic dysfunction, although this remains contentious.

Storage Disorders Associated With Cardiomyopathy – Several storage disorders may result in cardiomyopathy, with the majority associated with HCM. Pompe disease (acid maltase deficiency), Danon disease (lysosomal associated protein-2 mutation), and Fabry disease (alpha-galactosidase A deficiency) are among the most common metabolic disorders associated with hypertrophic phenotypes. Mitochondrial disorders are also commonly associated with cardiomyopathy, manifesting as either dilated or hypertrophic phenotypes.

Chagas Disease – This condition mimics myocarditis following infection with *Trypanosoma cruzi*. This disease demonstrates a propensity to involve the apical segment of the left ventricle and may even give rise to aneurysm formation. Although the condition is endemic to South America, it is rarely encountered in the United States or Europe.

Pospartum Cardiomyopathy – The etiology of this condition remains poorly understood, with some women developing cardiomyopathy late in the third trimester or early following childbirth. The findings are similar to DCM with progressive LV dilatation,

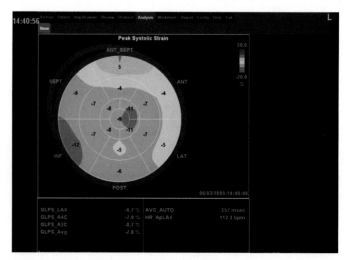

FIGURE 23.16. Strain imaging bullseye in a patient with dilated cardiomyopathy. Note the significantly decreased strain in all myocardial segments.

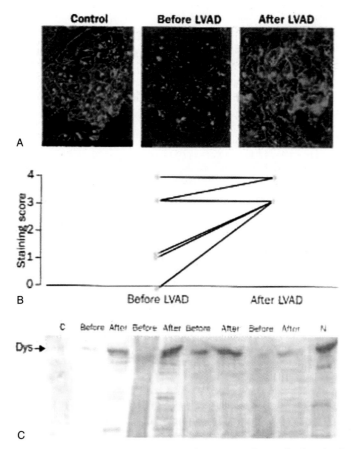

FIGURE 23.17. Dystrophin remodeling in patients with dilated cardiomyopathy. (Reproduced from Vatta M, Stetson SJ, Perez-Verdia A, et al. Molecular remodeling of dystrophin in patients with end-stage cardiomyopathies and reversal in patients on assistance-device therapy. *Lancet* 2002;359:936–941, with permission.)

depressed LV systolic function, and mitral regurgitation. Potential causes may be related to preeclampsia, viral etiology, or idiopathic. The prognosis is variable, some women experiencing a full recovery and others with long-standing LV dysfunction.

Other Cardiomyopathies

Arrhythmia-Induced Cardiomyopathy – Intractable atrial or ventricular tachyarrhythmias may induce LV and/or RV dysfunction.

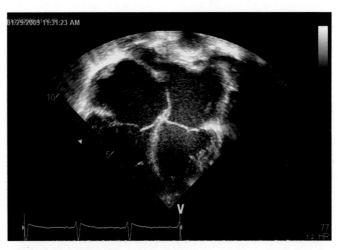

FIGURE 23.18. Apical four-chamber view demonstrating severe biatrial enlargement in restrictive cardiomyopathy.

The most common tachycardia in this setting is atrial ectopic tachycardia. It may be difficult to prove whether the tachycardia or cardiomyopathy is the initial insult. Echocardiographic parameters are similar to those presenting with DCM. Termination of the arrhythmia and medical therapy with beta-blockage, afterload reduction, and cardiac glycosides often result in normalization of the ventricular function.

Anthracycline-Induced Cardiomyopathy – Anthracyclines (doxorubicin and epirubicin) are well-established chemotherapy agents that have cardiac toxicity as a side effect. This is mediated via oxygen free radicals. With higher cumulative doses, there is a substantial risk of cardiac dysfunction, which may occur many years after the cessation of treatment. Administration of oxygen free radical scavengers (doxrezoxane) may reduce the risk of cardiomyopathy and is undergoing clinical trials. Echocardiographic findings in anthracycline cardiomyopathy are similar to those found in DCM. Interestingly, a recent study has demonstrated strain rate abnormalities in patients after a single dose of anthracycline therapy.

Takotsubo Cardiomyopathy – In recent years, a new form of cardiomyopathy has been recognized in association with chest pain, ST-segment changes, and transient LV apical ballooning in the absence of coronary arterial disease. Rarely, LVOT obstruction

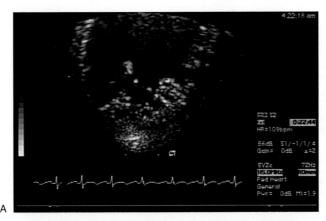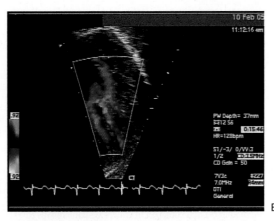

FIGURE 23.19. Apical four-chamber view demonstrating characteristic findings of left ventricular noncompaction cardiomyopathy. A. Multiple apical trabeculations with deep recesses and a noncompacted: compacted ratio of 2:1. **B.** Color Doppler within deep trabeculations in LUNC. (Reproduced with permission from Ganame J, et al. Left ventricular noncompaction, a recently recognized form of cardiomyopathy. *Insuficiencia Cardiaca.* 1[3], 2006.)

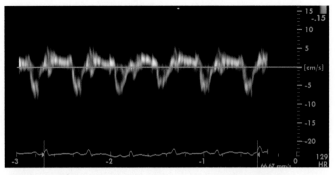

FIGURE 23.20. Decreased lateral mitral Ea velocity in a patient with left ventricular noncompaction cardiomyopathy requiring hospitalization for management of heart failure.

may occur in association with systolic anterior motion (SAM) of the mitral valve. This is typically a benign and reversible process. Differentiation from acute coronary syndrome is essential because inotropic support may exacerbate the condition. Echocardiographic findings may include apical distention of the left ventricle and LVOT obstruction secondary to SAM.

FETAL ECHOCARDIOGRAPHIC DIAGNOSIS OF CARDIOMYOPATHY

Several forms of cardiomyopathy may be diagnosed antenatally. This is often the case in DCM secondary to parvovirus, which may be associated with pericardial effusion, pleural effusion, and hydrops fetalis.

CONCLUSIONS

Echocardiography, including two-dimensional imaging, M-mode echocardiography, color Doppler, tissue Doppler imaging, and strain and strain rate imaging, is crucial in the complete evaluation of children with cardiomyopathy. Further studies are required to clarify prognostic factors that will allow stratification of patients into high-risk group of patients who require closer evaluation and potentially more aggressive intervention.

SUGGESTED READING

Abbara S, Migrino RQ, Sosnovik DE, et al. Value of fat suppression in the MRI evaluation of suspected arrhythmogenic right ventricular dysplasia. *AJR Am J Roentgenol.* 2004;182:587–591.

Abramson SV, Burke JF, Kelly JJ Jr, et al. Pulmonary hypertension predicts mortality and morbidity in patients with dilated cardiomyopathy. *Ann Intern Med.* 1992;116:888–895.

Akagi T, Benson LN, Lightfoot NE, et al. Natural history of dilated cardiomyopathy. *Am Heart J.* 1991;121:1502–1506.

Anselme F, Boyle N, Josephson M. Incessant fascicular tachycardia: a cause of arrhythmia induced cardiomyopathy. *Pacing Clin Electrophysiol.* 1998;21: 760–763.

Arbustini E, Morbini P, Grasso M, et al. Restrictive cardiomyopathy, atrioventricular block and mild to subclinical myopathy in patients with desmin-immunoreactive material deposits. *J Am Coll Cardiol.* 1998;31:645–653.

Arola A, Tuominen J, Ruuskanen O, et al. Idiopathic dilated cardiomyopathy in children: prognostic indicators and outcome. *Pediatrics.* 1998;101:369–376.

Azeka E, Ramires JA, Ebaid M, et al. Clinical outcome after starting carvedilol in infants and children with severe dilated cardiomyopathy: candidates for heart transplantation. *J Heart Lung Transplant.* 2001;20:222.

Bestetti RB, Muccillo G. Clinical course of Chagas' heart disease: a comparison with dilated cardiomyopathy. *Int J Cardiol.* 1997;60:187–193.

Biagini E, Ragni L, Ferlito M, et al. Different types of cardiomyopathy associated with isolated ventricular noncompaction. *Am J Cardiol.* 2006;98: 821–824.

Border WL, Michelfelder EC, Glascock BJ, et al. Color M-mode and Doppler tissue evaluation of diastolic function in children: simultaneous correlation with invasive indices. *J Am Soc Echocardiogr.* 2003;16:988–994.

Bowles KR, Gajarski R, Porter R, et al. Gene mapping of familial autosomal dominant dilated cardiomyopathy to chromosome 10q21-23. *J Clin Invest.* 1996;98:1355–1360.

Brecker SJ, Xiao HB, Mbaissouroum M, et al. Effects of intravenous milrinone on left ventricular function in ischemic and idiopathic dilated cardiomyopathy. *Am J Cardiol.* 1993;71:203–209.

Breinholt JP, Fraser CD, Dreyer WJ, et al. The efficacy of mitral valve surgery in children with dilated cardiomyopathy and severe mitral regurgitation. *Pediatr Cardiol.* 2007. Epub.

Brunetti ND, Ieva R, Rossi G, et al. Ventricular outflow tract obstruction, systolic anterior motion and acute mitral regurgitation in Tako-Tsubo syndrome. *Int J Cardiol.* 2007. Epub.

Burch M, Siddiqi SA, Celermajer DS, et al. Dilated cardiomyopathy in children: determinants of outcome. *Br Heart J.* 1994;72:246–250.

Carvalho JS, Silva CM, Shinebourne EA, et al. Prognostic value of posterior wall thickness in childhood dilated cardiomyopathy and myocarditis. *Eur Heart J.* 1996;17:1233–1238.

Chin TK, Perloff JK, Williams RG, et al. Isolated noncompaction of the left ventricular myocardium. A study of eight cases. *Circulation.* 1990;82:507–513.

Ciszewski A, Bilinska ZT, Lubiszewska B, et al. Dilated cardiomyopathy in children: clinical course and prognosis. *Pediatr Cardiol.* 1994;15:121–126.

Corya BC, Rasmussen S, Knoebel SB, et al. M-mode echocardiography in evaluating left ventricular function and surgical risk in patients with coronary artery disease. *Chest.* 1977;72:181–185.

DeGroff CG, Shandas R, Kwon J, et al. Accuracy of the Bernoulli equation for estimation of pressure gradient across stenotic Blalock-Taussig shunts: an in vitro and numerical study. *Pediatr Cardiol.* 2000;21:439–447.

Doppler echocardiography. In: Allen HD, Driscoll DJ, Feltes TF, Shaddy RE, eds. *Moss and Adams' Heart disease in infants, children and adolescents.* Philadelphia, PA: Lippincott Williams & Wilkins; 2008:257–259.

Dujardin KS, Tei C, Yeo TC, et al. Doppler index combining systolic and diastolic performance in idiopathic dilated cardiomyopathy. *Am J Cardiol.* 1998;82:1071–1076.

Durand J-B, Bachinski LL, Bieling LC, et al. Localization of a gene responsible for familial dilated cardiomyopathy to chromosome 1q32. *Circulation.* 1995;92:3387–3389.

Eidem BW, McMahon CJ, Cohen RR, et al. Impact of cardiac growth on Doppler tissue imaging velocity: a study in healthy children. *J Am Soc Echocardiogr.* 2004;17:212–221.

Eidem BW, Tei C, O'Leary PW, et al. Nongeometric quantitative assessment of right and left ventricular function: myocardial performance index in normal children and patients with Ebstein anomaly. *J Am Soc Echocardiogr.* 1998;11:849–856.

Fontaine G, Fontaliran F, Frank R. Arrhythmogenic right ventricular cardiomyopathies. Clinical forms and main differential diagnoses. *Circulation.* 1998;97:1532–1535.

Friedrich MG, Strohm O, Schulz-Menger J, et al. Contrast media-enhanced magnetic resonance imaging visualizes myocardial changes in the course of viral myocarditis. *Circulation.* 1998;97:1802–1809.

Ganame J, Claus P, Uyttebroeck A, et al. Myocardial dysfunction late after low dose anthracycline treatment in asymptomatic patients. *J Am Soc Echocardiogr.* 2007. Epub.

Garcia-Rubira JC, Cobos MA, Fernandez-Ortiz AI. Calculation of left ventricular flow velocity propagation from M-mode echocardiography. *Eur J Echocardiogr.* 2004;5:405–406.

Gianni M, Dentali F, Grandi AM, et al. Apical ballooning syndrome or Takotsubo cardiomyopathy: a systematic review. *Eur Heart J.* 2006;27:1523–1529.

Gunja-Smith Z, Morales AR, Romanelli R, et al. Remodeling of human myocardial collagen in idiopathic dilated cardiomyopathy. Role of metalloproteinases and pyridinoline cross-links. *Am J Pathol.* 1996;148:1639–1648.

Gussenhoven WJ, Busch HF, Kleijer WJ, et al. Echocardiographic features in the cardiac type of glycogen storage disease II. *Eur Heart J.* 1983;4:41–43.

Hale JP, Lewis JJ. Anthracyclines: cardiotoxicity and its prevention. *Arch Dis Child.* 1994;71:457–462.

Harada K, Tamura M, Toyono M, et al. Comparison of the right ventricular Tei index by tissue Doppler imaging to that obtained by pulsed Doppler in children without heart disease. *Am J Cardiol.* 2002;90:566–569.

Hellmann K. Preventing the cardiotoxicity of anthracyclines by dexrazoxane. *BMJ.* 1999;319:1085–1086.

Ichida F, Tsubata S, Bowles KR, et al. Novel gene mutations in patients with left ventricular noncompaction or Barth syndrome. *Circulation.* 2001;103: 1256–1263.

Jefferies JL, Eidem BW, Belmont JW, et al. Genetic predictors and remodeling of dilated cardiomyopathy in muscular dystrophy. *Circulation.* 2005;112:2799–2804.

Jin SM, Noh CI, Bae EJ, et al. Decreased left ventricular torsion and untwisting in children with dilated cardiomyopathy. *J Korean Med Sci.* 2007;22: 633–640.

Karakurt C, Aytemir K, Karademir S, et al. Prognostic value of heart rate turbulence and heart rate variability in children with dilated cardiomyopathy. *Acta Cardiol.* 2007;62:31–37.

Kass S, MacRae AC, Graber HL, et al. A gene defect that causes conduction system disease and dilated cardiomyopathy maps to chromosome 1p1-1q1. *Nat Genet.* 1994;7:546–551.

Kimberling MT, Balzer DT, Hirsch R, et al. Cardiac transplantation for pediatric restrictive cardiomyopathy: presentation, evaluation, and short-term outcome. *J Heart Lung Transplant.* 2002;21:455–459.

Lewis AB. Late recovery of ventricular function in children with idiopathic dilated cardiomyopathy. *Am Heart J.* 1999;138:334–338.

Lipschultz SE, Sleeper LA, Towbin JA, et al. The incidence of pediatric cardiomyopathy in two regions of the United States. *N Engl J Med.* 2003;348:1647–1655.

Manolio TA, Baughman KL, Rodeheffer R, et al. Prevalence and etiology of idiopathic dilated cardiomyopathy (summary of a National Heart, Lung and Blood Institute workshop). *Am J Cardiol.* 1992;69:1458–1466.

Marcus FI, Fontaine G. Arrhythmogenic right ventricular dysplasia/cardiomyopathy: a review. *Pacing Clin Electrophysiol.* 1995;18:1298–1314.

Marin Huerta E, Erice A, Fernandez Espino R, et al. Postpartum cardiomyopathy and acute myocarditis. *Am Heart J.* 1985;110:1079–1081.

Maron BJ. Hypertrophic cardiomyopathy. In: Allen HD, Driscoll DJ, Feltes TF, Shaddy RE, eds. *Moss and Adams' Heart disease in infants, children and adolescents.* Philadelphia, PA: Lippincott Williams & Wilkins; 2008:1167.

Marton T, Martin WL, Whittle MJ. Hydrops fetalis and neonatal death from human parvovirus B19: an unusual complication. *Prenat Diagn.* 2005;25:543–545.

McMahon CJ, Nagueh SF, Eapen RS, et al. Echocardiographic predictors of adverse clinical events in children with dilated cardiomyopathy: a prospective clinical study. *Heart.* 2004;90:908–915.

McMahon CJ, Pignatelli RH, Nagueh SF, et al. Left ventricular noncompaction cardiomyopathy in children: characterization of clinical status using tissue Doppler derived indices of left ventricular diastolic relaxation. *Heart.* 2007;93:676–681.

Muntoni F, Cau M, Ganau A, et al. Brief report: deletion of the dystrophin muscle-promoter region associated with x-linked dilated cardiomyopathy. *N Engl J Med.* 1993;329:921–925.

Naccarella F, Naccarelli G, Fattori R, et al. Arrhythmogenic right ventricular dysplasia cardiomyopathy: current opinions on diagnostic and therapeautic aspects. *Curr Opin Cardiol.* 2001;16:8–16.

Nagueh SF, Mikati I, Kopelen HA, et al. Doppler estimation of left ventricular filling pressure in sinus tachycardia. A new application of tissue Doppler imaging. *Circulation.* 1998;98:1644–1650.

Narula J, Haider N, Virmani R, et al. Apoptosis in myocytes in end-stage heart failure. *N Engl J Med.* 1996;335:1182–1189.

Nugent AW, Daubeney PE, Chondros P, et al. National Australian Childhood Cardiomyopathy Study. *N Engl J Med.* 2003;348:1639–1646.

Nugent AW, Davis AM, Kleinert S, et al. Clinical, electrocardiographic, and histological correlations in children with dilated cardiomyopathy. *J Heart Lung Transplant.* 2001;20:1152–1157.

Oechslin EN, Attenhofer JCH, Rojas JR, et al. Long-term follow-up of 34 adults with isolated left ventricular noncompaction: a distinct cardiomyopathy with poor prognosis. *J Am Coll Cardiol.* 2000;36:493–500.

Ogata H, Nakatani S, Ishikawa Y, et al. Myocardial strain changes in Duchenne muscular dystrophy without overt cardiomyopathy. *Int J Cardiol.* 2007;115:190–195.

Ogunyankin KO. Color and spectral modes of tissue Doppler imaging have similar diagnostic utility but different numerical values. *J Am Soc Echocardiogr.* 2006;19:1411.

Palecek T, Linhart A, Bultas J, et al. Comparison of early diastolic mitral annular velocity and flow propagation velocity in detection of mild to moderate left ventricular diastolic dysfunction. *Eur J Echocardiogr.* 2004;5:196–204.

Parthenakis FI, Patrianakos AP, Tzerakis PG, et al. Late left ventricular diastolic flow propagation velocity determined by color M-mode Doppler in the assessment of diastolic dysfunction. *J Am Soc Echocardiogr.* 2004;17:139–145.

Pauschinger M, Chandrasekharan K, Schultheiss HP. Myocardial remodeling in viral heart disease: possible interactions between inflammatory mediators and MMP-TIMP system. *Heart Fail Rev.* 2004;9:21–31.

Pignatelli RH, McMahon CJ, Dreyer WJ, et al. Clinical characterization of left ventricular noncompaction in children: a relatively common form of cardiomyopathy. *Circulation.* 2003;108:2672–2678.

Rivenes SM, Kearney DL, Smith EO, et al. Sudden death and cardiovascular collapse in children with restrictive cardiomyopathy. *Circulation.* 2000;102:876–882.

Russo LM, Webber SA. Idiopathic restrictive cardiomyopathy in children. *Heart.* 2005;91:1199–1202.

Sachdev B, Takenaka T, Teraguchi H, et al. Prevalence of Anderson-Fabry disease in male patients with late onset hypertrophic cardiomyopathy. *Circulation.* 2002;105:1407–1411.

Scaglia F, Towbin JA, Craigen WJ, et al. Clinical spectrum, morbidity, and mortality in 113 patients with mitochondrial disease. *Pediatrics.* 2004;114:925–931.

Schwartz ML, Cox GF, Lin AE, et al. Clinical approach to genetic cardiomyopathy in children. *Circulation.* 1996;94:2021–2038.

Silverstein JR, Laffely NH, Rifkin RD. Quantitative estimation of left ventricular ejection fraction from mitral valve E-point to septal separation and comparison to magnetic resonance imaging. *Am J Cardiol.* 2006;97:137–140.

Siu BL, Nimura H, Osborne JA, et al. Familial dilated cardiomyopathy locus maps to chromosome 2q31. *Circulation.* 1999;99:1022–1026.

Tani LY, Minich LL, Williams RV, et al. Ventricular remodeling in children with left ventricular dysfunction secondary to various cardiomyopathies. *Am J Cardiol.* 2005;96:1157–1161.

Thiene G, Corrado D, Basso C. Cardiomyopathies: is it time for a molecular classification? *Eur Heart J.* 2004;25:1772–1775.

Towbin JA. Pediatric myocardial disease. *Pediatr Clin North Am.* 1999;46:289–312.

Towbin JA, Hejtmancik JF, Brink P, et al. X-linked dilated cardiomyopathy: molecular genetic evidence of linkage to the Duchenne muscular dystrophy (dystrophin) gene at the Xp21 locus. *Circulation.* 1993;87:1854–1865.

Towbin JA, Lowe AM, Colan SD, et al. Incidence, causes and outcomes of dilated cardiomyopathy in children. *JAMA.* 2006;296:1867–1876.

Towbin JA, Vatta M, Li H. Genetics of Brugada, long QT, and arrhythmogenic right ventricular dysplasia. *J Electrocardiol.* 2000;33:11–22.

Van Doorn C, Karimova A, Burch M, et al. Sequential use of extracorporeal membrane oxygenation and the Berlin Heart Left Ventricular Assist Device for 106-day bridge to transplant in a two-year-old child. *ASAIO J.* 2005;51:668–669.

Vatta M, Mohapatra B, Jimenez S, et al. Mutations in Cypher/ZASP in patients with dilated cardiomyopathy and left ventricular non-compaction. *J Am Coll Cardiol* 2003;42:2014–2027.

Vatta M, Stetson SJ, Perez-Verdia A, et al. Molecular remodeling of dystrophin in patients with end-stage cardiomyopathies and reversal in patients on assistance-device therapy. *Lancet.* 2002;359:936–941.

Vicario ML, Caso P, Martiniello AR, et al. Effects of volume loading on strain rate and tissue Doppler velocity imaging in patients with idiopathic dilated cardiomyopathy. *J Cardiovasc Med.* 2006;7:852–858.

Wahr DW, Wang YS, Schiller NB. Left ventricular volumes determined by two-dimensional echocardiography in a normal adult population. *J Am Coll Cardiol.* 1983;1:863–868.

Weidemann F, Eyskens B, Jamal F, et al. Quantification of regional left and right ventricular radial and longitudinal function in healthy children using ultrasound based strain rate and strain imaging. *J Am Soc Echocardiogr.* 2002;15:20–28.

Weller RJ, Weintraub R, Addonizio LJ, et al. Outcome of idiopathic restrictive cardiomyopathy. *Am J Cardiol.* 2002;90:501–506.

Wierzbowska-Drabik K, Drozdz J, Plewka M, et al. Assessment of mitral inflow during standardized Valsalva maneuver in stratification of diastolic dysfunction. *Echocardiography.* 2007;24:464–471.

Williams RV, Ritter S, Tani LY, et al. Quantitative assessment of ventricular function in children with single ventricles using the Doppler myocardial performance index. *Am J Cardiol.* 2000;86:1106–1110.

Yang Z, McMahon CJ, Smith LR, et al. Danon disease as an underrecognized cuase of hypertrophic cardioymopathy. *Circulation.* 2005;112:1612–1617.

Yildirim A, Soylu O, Dagdeviren B, et al. Correlation between Doppler derived dP/dT and left ventricular asynchrony in patients with dilated cardiomyopathy: a combined study using strain rate imaging and conventional Doppler echocardiography. *Echocardiography.* 2007;24:508–514.

Yinon Y, Yagel S, Hegesh J, et al. Fetal cardiomyopathy: in utero evaluation and clinical significance. *Prenat Diagn.* 2007;27:23–28.

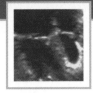

Chapter 24
Pericardial Disorders

Martha Grogan • Jae K. Oh

*Note: This Chapter is adapted from Oh JK, Seward JB, Tajik AJ. The echo manual. 3rd ed.
Philadelphia, PA: Lippincott Williams & Wilkins; 2006, with permission.*

The evaluation of pericardial disorders is of increasing importance in the management of patients with congenital heart disease. Previous cardiac surgery now accounts for over 25% of cases of constrictive pericarditis and diagnosis can be challenging, especially in patients with congenital heart disease and co-existing myocardial dysfunction. This chapter will outline the echocardiographic evaluation of pericardial disorders, including the distinction between constrictive pericarditis and restrictive myocardial disease.

Normal pericardium consists of an outer sac, the fibrous pericardium, and an inner double-layered sac, the serous pericardium. The visceral layer of the serous pericardium, or epicardium, covers the heart and proximal great vessels. It is reflected to form the parietal pericardium, which lines the fibrous pericardium (Fig. 24.1). The pericardium provides mechanical protection for the heart and lubrication to reduce friction between the heart and surrounding structures. The pericardium also has a significant hemodynamic impact on the atria and ventricles. The nondistendible pericardium limits acute distention of the heart. Ventricular volume is greater at any given ventricular filling pressure with the pericardium removed than with the pericardium intact. The pericardium also contributes to diastolic coupling between two ventricles: the distention of one ventricle alters the filling of the other, an effect that is important in the pathophysiology of cardiac tamponade and constrictive pericarditis. Ventricular interdependence becomes more marked at high ventricular filling pressures. Abnormalities of the pericardium can range from the pleuritic chest pain of pericarditis to marked heart failure and even death from tamponade or constriction.

Echocardiography is the most important clinical tool in the diagnosis and management of various pericardial diseases. Pericardial effusion, tamponade, pericardial cyst, and absent pericardium are readily recognized on two-dimensional (2D) echocardiography. The detection of pericardial effusion was clinically very difficult before the advent of echocardiography and was one of the most exciting initial clinical applications of cardiac ultrasonography 40 years ago. When a pericardial effusion needs to be drained, pericardiocentesis can be performed most safely under the guidance of 2D echocardiography. Although it usually is difficult to establish the diagnosis of constrictive pericarditis with 2D echocardiography alone, the characteristic respiratory variation in mitral inflow and hepatic vein Doppler velocities and tissue Doppler recording of mitral annulus velocity have added reliability and confidence to the noninvasive diagnosis of constrictive pericarditis. Transesophageal echocardiography (TEE) is helpful in measuring pericardial thickness, in evaluating diastolic function (for tamponade or constrictive physiology) from the pulmonary vein, and in detecting loculated pericardial effusion or other structural abnormalities of the pericardium. The various applications of echocardiography in the evaluation of pericardial diseases are illustrated in this chapter.

 ## CONGENITALLY ABSENT PERICARDIUM

The congenital absence of the pericardium usually involves the left side of the pericardium. Complete absence of the pericardium on the right side is uncommon. The defect is more frequent in males, and it rarely creates symptoms such as chest pain, dyspnea, or syncope. Because of the pericardial defect, cardiac motion is exaggerated, especially the posterior wall of the left ventricle. The entire cardiac structure is shifted to the left; hence, the right ventricular (RV) cavity appears enlarged from the standard parasternal windows, mimicking the RV volume overload pattern on echocardiography. The absence of pericardium should be considered when the right ventricle appears enlarged from the parasternal window and is at the center of the usual apical image (Fig. 24.2A). This condition is also associated with a high incidence of atrial septal defect, bicuspid aortic valve, and bronchogenic cysts. It is readily recognized because of its typical 2D echocardiographic features, and the diagnosis can be confirmed with computed tomography (CT) or magnetic resonance imaging (MRI) (Fig. 24.2B).

Pericardial Cyst

A pericardial cyst typically is a benign structural abnormality of the pericardium that usually is detected as an incidental mass lesion on a chest radiograph or as a cystic mass on echocardiography (Fig. 24.3A). Most frequently, pericardial cysts are located in the right costophrenic angle, but they also are found in the left costophrenic angle, hilum, and superior mediastinum. Pericardial cysts need to be differentiated from malignant tumors, cardiac chamber enlargement, and diaphragmatic hernia. Two-dimensional echocardiography is useful in differentiating a pericardial cyst from other solid structures, because a cyst is filled with clear fluid and appears as an echo-free structure. It also has a characteristic appearance on CT or MRI (Fig. 24.3B).

Pericardial Effusion/Tamponade

When the potential pericardial space is filled with fluid or blood, it is detected as an echo-free space. When the amount of effusion is greater than 25 mL, an echo-free space persists throughout the cardiac cycle. A smaller amount of pericardial effusion may be detected as a posterior echo-free space that is present only during the systolic phase. As pericardial effusion increases, movement of the parietal pericardium decreases. When the amount of pericardial effusion is massive, the heart may have a "swinging" motion in the pericardial cavity (Fig. 24.4A), which is responsible for the electrocardiographic manifestation of cardiac tamponade, "electrical alternans" (Fig. 24.4B). The swinging motion is not always present in cardiac tamponade, however. Cardiac tamponade can occur with a small amount of pericardial effusion, if the accumulation of pericardial effusion happens rapidly. A clinical example is myocardial perforation after acute myocardial infarction or during implantation of a pacemaker. Various M-mode and 2D echocardiographic signs have been reported in this life-threatening condition: early diastolic collapse of the right ventricle, late diastolic right atrial (RA) inversion,

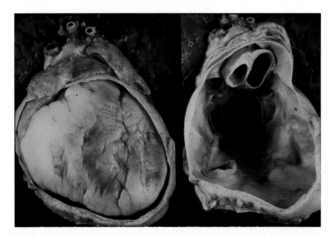

FIGURE 24.1. Pathology specimens demonstrating the double-layered pericardium with and without the heart in the fibrous pericardial cavity. (Courtesy of William Edwards, MD.)

x

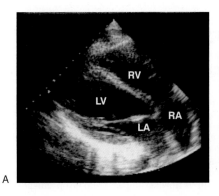
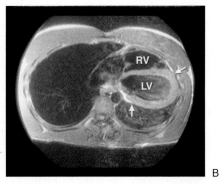

FIGURE 24.2. Patient with a congenitally absent pericardium. A: Two-dimensional still-frame obtained from the normal apical position (left fifth intercostal space at the midclavicular line). Because of the leftward shift of the heart, the right ventricle (RV) is at the center of the apical image rather than the left ventricular (LV) apex; this is often confused with RV volume overload. Cardiac catheterization was performed elsewhere to evaluate an atrial septal defect and showed no shunt before this evaluation. **B:** Magnetic resonance image of the chest showing a marked shift of the heart to the left side of the chest because of the partial absence of the pericardium on the left side. *Arrows* indicate area of absent pericardium.

abnormal ventricular septal motion, respiratory variation in ventricle chamber size (Fig. 24.5), and plethora of the inferior vena cava with blunted respiratory changes. These findings are caused by the characteristic hemodynamics of tamponade. Diastolic collapse of the right atrium and right ventricle is related to intrapericardial pressure rising above the intracardiac pressures, and abnormal ventricular septal motion is related to respiratory variation in ventricular filling. Diastolic collapse of the right heart may not occur if right heart pressure is elevated. In case of acute myocardial rupture or proximal aortic dissection, clotted blood may be seen in the pericardial sac; this finding is highly suggestive of hemopericardium (Fig. 24.6). When there is air in the pericardial sac (pneumopericardium) as a result of esophageal perforation, cardiac imaging (both transthoracic echocardiography (TTE) and TEE) is difficult because ultrasound does not penetrate air well.

Doppler echocardiographic features of pericardial effusion/tamponade are more sensitive than the 2D echocardiographic features mentioned earlier. The Doppler findings of cardiac tamponade are based on the following characteristic respiratory variations in intrathoracic and intracardiac hemodynamics (Fig. 24.7). Normally, intrapericardial pressure (hence, left atrial [LA] and left ventricular [LV] diastolic pressures) and intrathoracic pressure (hence, pulmonary capillary wedge pressure) fall the same degree during inspiration, but in cardiac tamponade intrapericardial (and intracardiac) pressure falls substantially less than intrathoracic pressure. Therefore, the LV filling pressure gradient (from pulmonary wedge pressure to LV diastolic pressure [the shaded area in Fig. 24.7]) decreases with inspiration. Consequently, mitral valve opening is delayed, which lengthens the isovolumic relaxation time (IVRT) and decreases mitral E velocity. In cardiac tamponade, the degree of ventricular filling depends on the other ventricle because of the relatively fixed combined cardiac volume (ventricular interdependence); thus, reciprocal changes occur in the right heart chambers (Fig. 24.8). Increased venous return to the right heart chambers with inspiration also contributes to the increased ventricular interdependence.

The respiratory flow velocity changes across the mitral and tricuspid valves are also reflected in the pulmonary and hepatic venous flow velocities, respectively: inspiratory decrease and expiratory increase in pulmonary vein diastolic forward flow and expiratory decrease in hepatic vein forward flow and increase in expiratory reversal flow (Fig. 24.9).

Echocardiographically Guided Pericardiocentesis

The most effective treatment for cardiac tamponade is removal of the pericardial fluid. Although pericardiocentesis is lifesaving, a blind percutaneous attempt has a high rate of complications, including pneumothorax, puncture of the cardiac wall, or death. Two-dimensional echocardiography can guide pericardiocentesis by locating the optimal site of puncture (Fig. 24.10) by determining the depth of the pericardial effusion and the distance from the puncture site to the effusion and by monitoring the results of the pericardiocentesis, usually from the subcostal view. The position of the pericardiocentesis needle can be checked by imaging with administration of agitated saline. Fig. 24.11 demonstrates contrast (arrows) in the pericardial space, not in the right ventricle. Under most circumstances, a pig-tail (6 or 7 French) catheter is introduced and left in the pericardial sac for several days with intermittent drainage (every 4 to 6 hours), which has markedly curtailed the rate of recurrent effusion and use of a sclerosing agent. At the Mayo Clinic, most pericardiocentesis procedures are performed by an echocardiographer with the guidance of 2D echocardiography. The most common location of needle entry is in the parasternal area, but this depends on 2D echocardiographic findings. In our consecutive 1127 echo-guided pericardiocenteses, malignant effusion was most common (34%), followed by postoperative (25%), complication of catheter-bases procedure (10%), and other (Fig. 24.12). The procedure was successful in 97%, and complications occurred in 4.4%, mostly minor. Major complications were death (1 patient), cardiac laceration (5), vessel laceration (1), pneumothorax (5), infection (1), and sustained ventricular tachycardia (1).

PERICARDIAL EFFUSION VERSUS PLEURAL EFFUSION

A pericardial effusion usually is located circumferentially. If there is an echo-free space anteriorly only, it more likely is an epicardial fat pad than pericardial effusion. Posteriorly, a pericardial effusion is located anterior to the descending thoracic aorta, whereas a pleural effusion is present posterior to the aorta (Fig. 24.13). Two-dimensional ultrasonographic imaging of pleural effusion is

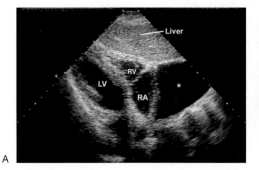
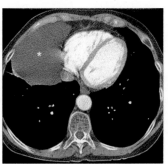

FIGURE 24.3. Pericardial cyst. A: Subcostal view showing a large pericardial cyst (*asterisk*) adjacent to the right atrium (RA). It has a typical echo-free appearance with a smooth boundary. LV, left ventricle. RV, right ventricle. **B:** MRI of the same patient as in **A** with a large pericardial cyst (*asterisk*).

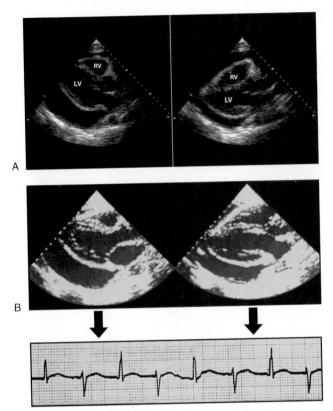

FIGURE 24.4. Pericardial effusion. A: Parasternal long-axis views showing a large pericardial effusion with a swinging motion of the heart. LV, left ventricle. **B:** With a large amount of pericardial effusion, the heart has a swinging motion, which is an ominous sign of cardiac tamponade. When the left ventricular cavity is close to the surface (**left**), the QRS voltage increases on the electrocardiogram, but it decreases when the LV swings away from the surface (**right**), producing electrical alternans.

also helpful in planning for a thoracentesis to locate the optimal puncture site. Pleural effusion on the left side allows cardiac imaging from the back (Fig.24.14).

Constrictive Pericarditis

Constrictive pericarditis is caused by thickened, inflamed, adherent, or calcific pericardium limiting the diastolic filling of the heart (Fig. 24.15). Constrictive pericarditis is not an uncommon condition but frequently escapes clinical detection because it is not clinically considered in many cases and no one diagnostic test alone can ensure the diagnosis of constrictive pericarditis with high confidence. Since this is a curable entity causing severe heart failure, constrictive pericarditis should be considered in all patients with heart failure, especially when systolic function is normal and/or there is a predisposing factor. Currently, previous cardiac surgery is the most common cause for constriction, followed by pericarditis, episode of pericardial effusion, and radiation therapy. Fig. 24.16 demonstrates the multiple underlying etiologies of constriction in more than 400 patients who underwent pericardiectomy since 1985 at Mayo Clinic. Patients with constrictive pericarditis present with dyspnea, peripheral edema, ascites, pleural effusion, fatigue, or anasarca. Jugular venous pressure is almost always elevated with typical rapid "y" descent (Fig. 24.17). Kussmaul sign and pericardial knock are other typical physical findings. Because of their abdominal symptoms and elevation of liver enzymes because of hepatic venous congestion, many patients are labeled as having a liver or gastrointestinal disease and undergo noncardiac procedures such as liver biopsy, endoscopy, or even abdominal exploration before the diagnosis of constrictive pericarditis. The diagnosis of pericardial constriction can be particularly challenging in patients with operated or unoperated congenital heart disease as a result of coexisting lesions and myocardial dysfunction, making the correct diagnosis more elusive. In many patients with congenital heart disease and pericardial constriction, restrictive myocardial disease and residual hemodynamic lesions may contribute to the clinical presentation and findings.

Pericardial calcification on chest radiography is helpful but is present in only 23% of cases (Fig. 24.18). Thickened pericardium is

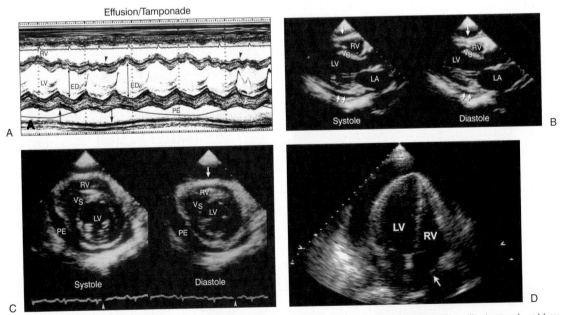

FIGURE 24.5. Pericardial effusion with tamponade. A: M-mode echocardiogram from the parasternal window in a patient with cardiac tamponade and large circumferential pericardial effusion (PE). The M-mode was recorded simultaneously with the respirometer tracing at the bottom (*upward arrow* indicates onset of inspiration and *downward arrow* indicates onset of expiration). The left ventricular (LV) dimension during inspiration (EDi) becomes smaller than with expiration (EDe). The opposite changes occur in the right ventricle (RV). The ventricular septum (*arrowheads*) moves toward the LV with inspiration and toward the RV with expiration, accounting for the abnormal ventricular septum in patients with cardiac tamponade. Parasternal long-axis (**B**) and short-axis (**C**) views of a patient with tamponade during systole and diastole. The pericardial effusion (*double arrows* in **B**; PE in **C**) appears small in the long axis and moderate in the short axis during systole, but during early diastole, the RV free wall collapses (*arrow at top*). VS, ventricular septum. **D:** Apical four-chamber view demonstrating late diastolic (*arrowhead* on electrocardiograph) collapse of right atrium (RA) wall (*arrow*). This sign is sensitive but not specific for tamponade. When RA inversion lasts longer than a third of the RR interval, it is specific for hemodynamically significant pericardial effusion.

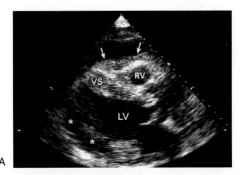
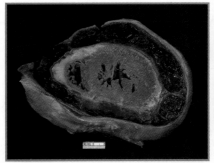
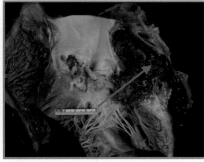

FIGURE 24.6. Hemopericardium. A: This echocardiogram was obtained from a 73-year-old man who is septic with Streptococcus mitis and is hypotensive. There was a moderate amount of circumferential pericardial effusion with soft-tissue density (*arrows*) over the right ventricle (RV), characteristic for coagulae tamponade or hemopericardium. **B:** Soon after this echocardiogram, the patient died. Pathology showed hemopericardium (**left**) because of a perforation of the proximal aorta (*arrow*) with aortic valve endocarditis (**right**).

a usual finding in this condition, but pericardial thickness may be normal in up to 20% of cases. Pericardial thickness can be evaluated by echocardiography (most accurately by transesophageal study) and by CT and MRI). In patients with congenital heart disease and univentricular physiology, the evaluation of pericardial thickness is of increased importance in suspected constrictive pericarditis, given the inability to evaluate interventricular hemodynamics. Traditional invasive hemodynamic features do have a large overlap with those found in restrictive cardiomyopathy or other myocardial diseases. New insights into the mechanism of constrictive pericarditis have allowed development of more reliable and specific diagnostic criteria for constriction using comprehensive echocardiography including 2D, Doppler and tissue Doppler imaging. Subsequent to this observation, new diagnostic criteria of invasive hemodynamic features of constriction have been proposed.

The M-mode (Fig. 24.19) and 2D echocardiographic features of constrictive pericarditis include thickened pericardium, abnormal ventricular septal motion, flattening of the LV posterior wall during diastole, respiratory variation in ventricular size, and a dilated inferior vena cava, but these findings are not sensitive or specific. Hatle et al. described the Doppler features typical of constriction, which are distinct from those of restrictive hemodynamics. Although the underlying pathologic mechanism is different from that of cardiac tamponade, the hemodynamic events of constriction in regard to respiratory variation in LV and RV filling are similar to those of tamponade.

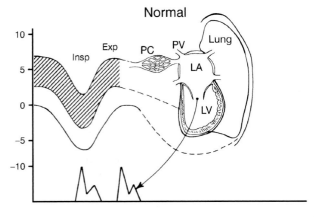

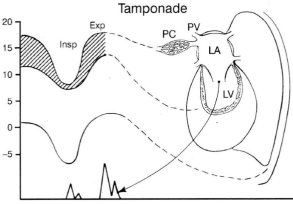

FIGURE 24.7. Diagram of intrathoracic and intracardiac pressure changes with respiration in normal and tamponade physiology. The shaded area indicates left ventricle (*LV*) filling pressure gradients (difference between pulmonary capillary wedge pressure and LV diastolic pressure). At the bottom of each drawing is a schematic mitral inflow Doppler velocity profile reflecting LV diastolic filling. In tamponade, there is a decrease in LV filling after inspiration (Insp) because the pressure decrease in the pericardium and LV cavity is smaller than the pressure fall in the pulmonary capillaries (PC). LV filling is restored after expiration (Exp). PV, pulmonary vein. (Modified from Sharp JT, Bunnell IL, Holland JF, et al. Hemodynamics during induced cardiac tamponade in man. *Am J Med.* 1960;29:640–646, with permission.)

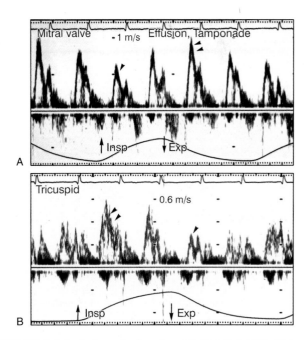

FIGURE 24.8. Typical pulsed-wave Doppler pattern of tamponade recorded with a nasal respirometer. A: Mitral inflow velocity decreases (*single arrowhead*) after inspiration (Insp) and increases (*double arrowheads*) after expiration (Exp). **B:** Tricuspid inflow velocity has the opposite changes. E velocity increases (*double arrowheads*) after inspiration and decreases (*single arrowhead*) after expiration. (From Oh JK, Hatle LK, Mulvagh SL, Tajik AJ. Transient constrictive pericarditis: diagnosis by two-dimensional Doppler echocardiography. *Mayo Clin Proc.* 1993;68:1158–1164, with permission.)

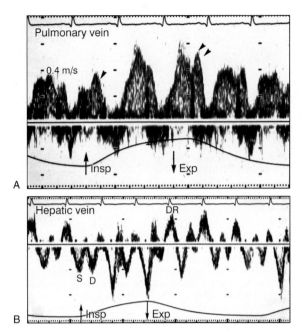

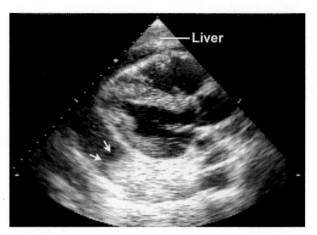

FIGURE 24.11. Appearance of agitated saline in the pericardial sac (*arrows*). If agitated saline is seen in any of cardiac chambers, surgical consultation should be obtained immediately before any attempt to remove pericardiocentesis needle or catheter.

FIGURE 24.9. Pulmonary vein and hepatic vein Doppler patterns of tamponade. **A:** Diastolic forward pulmonary venous flow decreases (*single arrowhead*) after inspiration (Insp) and increases (*double arrowheads*) after expiration (Esp). **B:** The hepatic vein has a significant reduction in diastolic forward flow and an increase in diastolic reversals (DR) after expiration. D, diastolic flow; S, systolic flow. (From Oh JK, Hatle LK, Mulvagh SL, Tajik AJ. Transient constrictive pericarditis: diagnosis by two-dimensional Doppler echocardiography. *Mayo Clin Proc.* 1993;68:1158–1164, with permission.)

To establish the diagnosis of constrictive pericarditis, the following two hemodynamic characteristics need to be demonstrated either by 2D/Doppler echocardiography or by cardiac catheterization.

1. Disassociation between intrathoracic and intracardiac pressures
2. Exaggerated ventricular interdependence

A thickened or inflamed pericardium prevents full transmission of the intrathoracic pressure changes that occur with respiration to the pericardial and intracardiac cavities, creating respiratory variations in the left-side filling pressure gradient (the pressure difference between the pulmonary vein and the left atrium). With inspiration, intrathoracic pressure falls (3 to 5 mm Hg normally) and the pressure in other intrathoracic structures (pulmonary vein, pulmonary capillaries) falls to a similar degree. This inspiratory pressure change is not fully transmitted to the intrapericardial and intracardiac cavities. As a result, the driving pressure gradient for LV filling decreases immediately after inspiration and increases with expiration. This characteristic hemodynamic pattern is best illustrated by simultaneous pressure recordings from the left ventricle and the pulmonary capillary wedge together with mitral inflow velocities (Fig. 24.20).

Diastolic filling (or distensibility) of the left and right ventricles rely on each other because the overall cardiac volume is relatively fixed within the thickened or noncompliant (adherent) pericardium. Hence, reciprocal respiratory changes occur in the filling of the left and right ventricles. With inspiration, decreased LV filling allows increased filling in the right ventricle. As a result, the ventricular septum shifts to the left, and tricuspid inflow E velocity and hepatic vein diastolic forward flow velocity increase (Fig. 24.21). With expiration, LV filling increases, causing the ventricular septum to shift

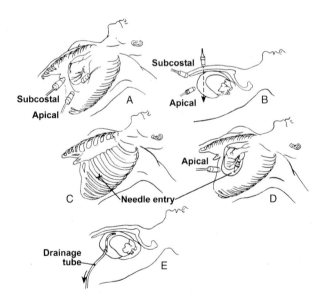

FIGURE 24.10. Echocardiographically guided pericardiocentesis.
STEP 1. Locate an area on the chest or subcostal region from which the largest amount of pericardial effusion can be visualized, and mark it (**A–C**).
STEP 2. Determine the depth of effusion from the marked position and the optimal angulation.
STEP 3. After sterile preparation and local anesthesia, perform pericardiocentesis (**D**).
STEP 4. When in doubt about the location of the needle, inject saline solution through the needle and image it from a remote site to locate the bubbles.
STEP 5. Monitor the completeness of the pericardiocentesis by repeat echocardiography.
STEP 6. Place a 6F or 7F pigtail catheter in the pericardial space to minimize reaccumulation of fluid (**E**).
STEP 7. Drain any residual fluid or fluid that has reaccumulated via the pigtail catheter every 4 to 6 hours. If after 2 to 3 days pericardial fluid has not reaccumulated, as demonstrated echocardiographically, the pigtail catheter may be removed. Always have the pericardial fluid analyzed: cell counts, glucose and protein measurements, culture, and cytology. (Modified from Callahan JA, Seward JB, Tajik AJ, et al. Pericardiocentesis assisted by two-dimensional echocardiography. *J Thorac Cardiovasc Surg.* 1983;85:877–879, with permission.)

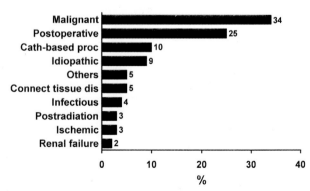

FIGURE 24.12. Distribution of underlying etiologies for pericardial effusion requiring pericardiocentesis.

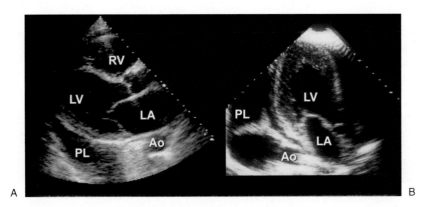

A B

FIGURE 24.13. Two-dimensional imaging of pleural effusion (PL) from the parasternal long-axis (A) and apical long-axis (B) views. Pericardial effusion is present between the descending thoracic aorta (Ao) and the posterior cardiac walls, whereas pleural effusion is present behind the descending thoracic aorta.

to the right, which limits RV filling. Tricuspid inflow decreases and hepatic vein diastolic forward flow decreases, with significant flow reversals during diastole. Usually, diastolic forward flow velocity is higher than systolic forward flow velocity in the hepatic vein, which corresponds to the Y and X waves of systemic venous pressure, respectively. It needs to be emphasized that the respiratory variation in ventricular filling is initiated from the left side, which is also evident from careful inspection of simultaneous pressure tracings from the left and right ventricles.

Ideally, demonstration of a respiratory variation of 25% or greater in the mitral inflow E velocity and increased diastolic flow reversal with expiration in the hepatic vein establish the diagnosis of constrictive pericarditis (Fig. 24.22). Further clinical observations, however, indicate that up to 50% of patients with constrictive pericarditis demonstrate less than 25% of respiratory variation in mitral E velocity. This may be related to (a) mixed constriction and restriction, (b) marked increase of atrial pressures, or (c) more clinical experience of using 2D/Doppler echocardiography in the diagnosis of constrictive pericarditis. If LA pressure is markedly increased, mitral valve opening occurs at the steep portion of the LV pressure curve, when the respiratory change has little effect on the transmitral pressure gradient. In this case, a Doppler echocardiographic examination may be repeated after an attempt to reduce preload (i.e., head-up tilt or sitting position). In any event, the lack of respiratory variation in mitral inflow velocities does not, and should not, exclude the diagnosis of constrictive pericarditis. Other features of constriction should be looked for such as hepatic vein velocity changes or mitral septal annular velocity of greater than 7 cm/s, especially when mitral inflow velocity indicates restrictive filling or high filling pressures (i.e., E/A ratio of 1.5 with deceleration time of less than 160 ms). Mitral annular velocity recorded by TDI has become a valuable Doppler parameter in establishing the diagnosis of constriction and in differentiating it from a myocardial

disease or restrictive cardiomyopathy (Fig. 24.23). In myocardial disease, mitral septal annular velocity is reduced (less than 7 cm/s) since myocardial relaxation is abnormal, but in constrictive pericarditis, the mitral annular velocity, especially the septal annular velocity, is relatively normal or even increased (Fig. 24.23A). This is because of the limitation of ventricular filling by lateral expansion of the heart caused by the constrictive pericardium with most of ventricular filling accomplished by exaggerated longitudinal motion of the heart. Myocardial relaxation is relatively well preserved in constriction unless the myocardium is also involved, as is seen in radiation heart injury. The longitudinal motion, hence mitral septal annular velocity, becomes more increased as the constriction worsens with resultant higher filling pressure, paradoxical to its change in myocardial disease. The phenomenon has been termed *annulus paradoxus*. E/E' is, therefore, inversely proportional to pulmonary capillary wedge pressure in constriction, whereas E/E' is positively related to pulmonary capillary wedge pressure in myocardial disease. More recently, Sohn and his colleagues reported that E' also varies with respiration, but usually in the opposite direction compared to mitral inflow.

Pitfalls and Caveats

Several other clinical entities can produce a similar respiratory variation in mitral inflow velocities: acute dilatation of the heart, pulmonary embolism, RV infarct, pleural effusion, and chronic obstructive lung disease. Most of these conditions do not present a significant diagnostic problem in the interpretation of Doppler findings because their clinical and 2D echocardiographic features are different from those of constrictive pericarditis. Patients with chronic lung disease, however, may have symptoms of right-sided heart failure similar to those of constrictive pericarditis.

Several Doppler echocardiographic features can be used to distinguish between chronic obstructive lung disease and constrictive pericarditis:

1. In chronic obstructive lung disease, individual mitral inflow velocities usually are not restrictive because the LV filling pressure is not increased.
2. In chronic obstructive lung disease, the highest mitral E velocity occurs toward the end of expiration, but it occurs immediately after the onset of expiration in constrictive pericarditis. This difference, however, may not be that helpful especially when patient is tachypneic.
3. The Doppler finding that most reliably distinguishes between these two entities is superior vena caval flow velocities. In chronic obstructive lung disease, superior vena cava flow is markedly increased with inspiration (Fig. 24.24), because the underlying mechanism for respiratory variation in chronic obstructive lung disease is a greater decrease in intrathoracic pressure with inspiration, which generates greater negative pressure changes in the thorax. This enhances flow to the right atrium from the superior vena cava with inspiration. In constrictive pericarditis, superior vena caval systolic flow velocities do not change significantly with respiration (Fig. 24.25); the difference in systolic forward flow velocity between inspiration and expiration is rarely 20 cm/s in constrictive pericarditis. It needs to be emphasized

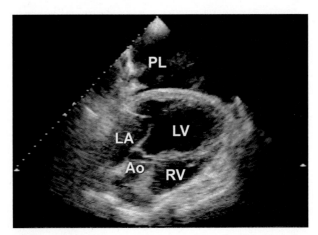

FIGURE 24.14. Two-dimensional echocardiographic examination from the back through a pleural effusion (PL). This unique view may be the only available ultrasound window to the heart in some patients. Ao, aorta.

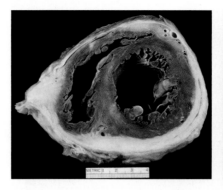
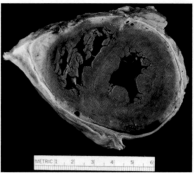

FIGURE 24.15. Cardiac specimens from two patients who died with constrictive pericarditis. Left: The pericardium is thickened and calcified. **Right:** The pericardial thickness is relatively normal, but adhered to the epicardium. In both situations, diastolic filling to right and left cardiac chambers was markedly reduced.

that it is important to compare systolic, not diastolic, flow velocities in the superior vena cava with respiration.

4. Hepatic vein Doppler may not be helpful if there is superimposed severe tricuspid regurgitation.

5. In patients after mitral valve replacement, mitral inflow Doppler will still demonstrate respiratory variation with a deceleration time shorter than expected for a mitral prosthesis (Fig. 24.26). Mitral annular velocity may not be increased because of the mitral prosthesis sewn to the annulus. However, hepatic vein should demonstrate characteristic Doppler changes.

6. Mitral annular velocity is reduced when the adjacent myocardium is abnormal, such as after previous cardiac surgery or myocardial infarction. In a patient with an inferior wall myocardial infarction, the septal mitral annular velocity is reduced even when the patient has constrictive pericarditis. Hepatic vein Doppler velocity still should have characteristic diastolic flow reversal with expiration.

7. Hepatic vein Doppler velocities are mostly lower than 60 cm/s and reversal flow velocities are even lower. To augment the display of characteristic hepatic vein Doppler velocities in constriction, the pulsed-wave Doppler filter and velocity scale should be set low.

Atrial fibrillation makes the interpretation of respiratory variation in Doppler velocities difficult. Patients with constrictive pericarditis and atrial fibrillation will still have the typical 2D echocardiographic features but will require longer observation of Doppler velocities to detect velocity variation with respiration, regardless of the underlying cardiac cycle length. Hepatic vein diastolic flow reversal with expiration is an important Doppler finding to suggest constrictive pericarditis, even when mitral inflow velocity pattern is not diagnostic. Occasionally, it may be necessary to achieve a regular rhythm, even with a temporary pacemaker, to evaluate the respiratory variation of Doppler velocities. Respirometer recording may have a phase delay up to 1000 ms, which may make the timing of velocity variation erroneous. A good rule is to remember that the lowest mitral inflow velocity usually occurs during inspiration. It

also is important to instruct the patient to breathe smoothly during Doppler recording. An erratic breathing pattern distorts the timing of Doppler flow velocities.

Complex congenital heart disease, including univentricular physiology, presents a particular challenge in the diagnosis of pericardial constriction, despite an increased risk of this diagnosis in those who have undergone previous cardiac surgery. Patients with previous surgical intervention for congenital heart disease are also at increased risk of coexisting myocardial disease, further confounding the diagnosis of pericardial constriction. Tissue Doppler imaging may be helpful in such patients, particularly if higher than expected E' velocity is present. In addition, the lack of variation in superior vena cava Doppler flow velocity also suggests pericardial constriction.

 RESTRICTION VERSUS CONSTRICTION

The clinical and hemodynamic profiles of restriction (myocardial diastolic heart failure) and constriction (pericardial diastolic heart failure) are similar, although their pathophysiologic mechanisms are distinctly different. Both are caused by limited or restricted diastolic filling, with relatively preserved global systolic function. Diastolic dysfunction in restrictive cardiomyopathy or myocardial disease is the result of stiff and noncompliant ventricular myocardium, but in constrictive pericarditis, it is related to a thickened and/or noncompliant pericardium. Both disease processes limit diastolic filling and result in diastolic heart failure. Restrictive cardiomyopathy resulting from infiltrative cardiomyopathy is the abnormality easiest to diagnose because it has typical 2D echocardiographic and biochemical features. A noninfiltrative type of restrictive cardiomyopathy is more difficult to diagnose. The myocardium becomes noncompliant because of fibrosis and scarring, and systolic function (or at least ejection fraction) is usually maintained. Because of limited diastolic filling and increased diastolic pressure, the atria become enlarged. In contrast, myocardial

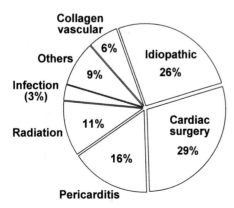

FIGURE 24.16. Distribution of underlying etiologies for constrictive pericarditis. There was only one patient with tuberculosis since 1985 at Mayo Clinic, Rochester.

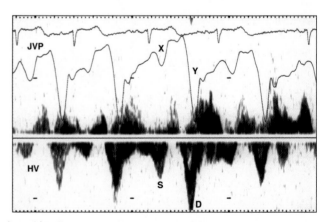

FIGURE 24.17. Simultaneous jugular venous pressure (JVP) tracing and pulsed-wave Doppler recording of hepatic vein (HV) velocities. There is the characteristic Y descent. D, diastolic flow; S, systolic flow; X and Y, jugular venous pressure waveforms.

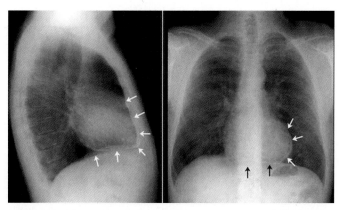
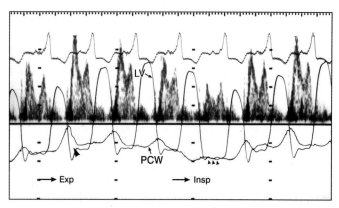

FIGURE 24.18. Lateral and posteroanterior (PA) chest radiographs showing pericardial calcification (arrows). This calcification is most common in the diaphragmatic portion of the pericardium.

FIGURE 24.20. Simultaneous pressure recordings from the left ventricle (LV) and pulmonary capillary wedge together with mitral inflow velocity on a Doppler echocardiogram. The onset of the respiratory phase is indicated at the bottom. Exp, expiration; Insp, inspiration. With the onset of expiration, pulmonary capillary wedge pressure (PCW) increases much more than LV diastolic pressure, creating a large driving pressure gradient (large arrowhead). With inspiration, however, PCW decreases much more than LV diastolic pressure, with a very small driving pressure gradient (three small arrowheads). These respiratory changes in the LV filling gradient are well reflected by the changes in the mitral inflow velocities recorded on Doppler echocardiography.

compliance usually is not decreased in constrictive pericarditis. The thickened and/or adherent pericardium limits diastolic filling, resulting in hemodynamic features that are similar but distinctly different from those of restrictive cardiomyopathy. Atrial enlargement is less prominent in constriction than in restrictive cardiomyopathy, but it can be as large. When restrictive cardiomyopathy affects both ventricles, clinical signs because of abnormalities of right-sided heart failure are apparent, with increased jugular venous pressure and peripheral edema. An early diastolic gallop (S_3) is a rule in restriction, but it often is difficult to differentiate this sound from a pericardial knock which occurs at the nadir of the rapid "y" descent. Similar physical findings are present in patients with constrictive pericarditis although ascites is more common in patients with constrictive pericarditis.

Electrocardiographic and chest radiographic findings are nonspecific. A calcified pericardium (which is present in 23% of patients with constriction) should point to constrictive pericarditis. Low QRS voltage on the electrocardiogram suggests cardiac amyloidosis, but may also be seen in constriction. Echocardiographically, it is difficult to distinguish between restriction and constriction only on the basis of M-mode and 2D findings, although diagnostic abnormalities may be detected with careful observation. In constrictive pericarditis, the most striking finding is ventricular septal motion abnormalities, which can be explained on the basis of respiratory variation in ventricular filling. The pericardium usually is thickened, but this may not be obvious on TTE. TEE measurements of pericardial thickness correlate well with those of electron-beam CT; however, other 2D, Doppler, and TDI findings should be able to differentiate a myopathic restrictive process from a pericardial constriction process as described above. In restrictive cardiomyopathy, mitral inflow Doppler velocity rarely shows respiratory variation (unless the patient also has chronic obstructive lung disease). However, each Doppler velocity pattern appears similar to that of constriction, with increased E velocity, an E/A ratio usually

greater than 2.0 and a short deceleration time (DT) usually less than 160 ms. Hepatic vein flow reversals are more prominent with inspiration in restrictive cardiomyopathy, although it is not unusual to see significant diastolic flow reversals in the hepatic vein during both inspiration and expiration in patients with advanced constriction or with combined constriction and restriction. The Doppler features of constriction and restriction are summarized in Fig. 24.27. Mitral inflow propagation velocity (PFV) measured by color M-mode is also helpful in distinguishing restriction (PFV < 45 cm/s) from constriction (PFV > 45 cm/s). However, this is more difficult to perform than TDI.

Despite the significant difference in the pathophysiologic mechanisms of restriction and constriction, there is significant overlap in hemodynamic parameters between these two entities. Increased atrial pressures, equalization of end-diastolic pressures, and a dip-and-plateau or square root sign of the ventricular diastolic pressure recording have been advocated as hemodynamic features typical of constrictive pericarditis (Table 24.1). Hemodynamic pressure tracings can also be almost identical in constriction versus restrictive cardiomyopathy. Therefore, in addition to these hemodynamic features, respiratory variation in ventricular filling should be demonstrated to diagnose constriction, either invasively or noninvasively. The dissociation between intrathoracic and intracardiac pressure changes with inspiration are well demonstrated in simultaneous recordings of LV and pulmonary capillary wedge pressures. In constrictive pericarditis, the fluctuation in the pulmonary capillary wedge pressure is more marked in parallel with intrathoracic pressure changes than with changes in LA and LV diastolic pressure. Ventricular interdependence also is observed in simultaneous recordings of LV and RV pressures.

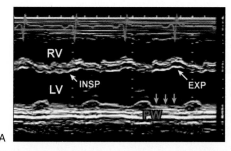
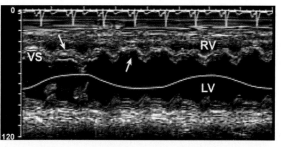

FIGURE 24.19. Typical M-mode echocardiograms of constrictive pericarditis. A: There is a typical respiratory shift of the ventricular septal motion, which comes toward the left ventricle (LV) with inspiration (INSP) and toward the right ventricle (RV) with expiration (EXP). This is a result of increased interventricular dependence. Posterior wall (PW) is flattened soon after early diastole (arrows). B. With tachycardia, flattening of the posterior wall could not be well demonstrated, but there is a typical ventricular septal shift with respiration (downward arrow indicates inspiration and upward arrow indicates expiration).

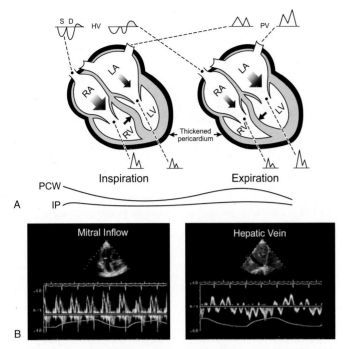

FIGURE 24.21 Hemodynamic filling patterns in constriction. A: Diagram of a heart with a thickened pericardium to illustrate the respiratory variation in ventricular filling and the corresponding Doppler features of the mitral valve, tricuspid valve, pulmonary vein (PV), and hepatic vein (HV). These changes are related to discordant pressure changes in the vessels in the thorax, such as pulmonary capillary wedge pressure (PCW) and intrapericardial (IP) and intracardiac pressures. *Hatched area under* curve indicates the reversal of flow. *Thicker arrows* indicate greater filling. D, diastolic flow; S, systolic flow. **B:** Typical mitral inflow and hepatic vein pulsed wave Doppler recordings in constrictive pericarditis along with simultaneous recording of respiration at the bottom (onset of inspiration at upward deflection and onset at expiration at downward deflection). **Left:** The first mitral inflow is at the onset of inspiration and the fourth mitral inflow is soon after the onset of expiration. Mitral inflow E velocity is decreased with inspiration (first and sixth beats). **Right:** There is a marked diastolic flow reversal (*arrow*) with expiration in the hepatic vein (sixth beat soon after the downward deflection of respirometer recording). Insp, inspiration; Exp, expiration.

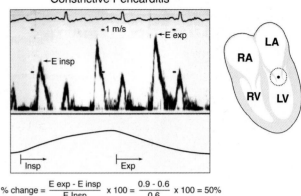

$$\% \text{ change} = \frac{E\ exp - E\ insp}{E\ Insp} \times 100 = \frac{0.9 - 0.6}{0.6} \times 100 = 50\%$$

FIGURE 24.22. Calculation of the extent of respiratory variation in mitral inflow E velocity is shown in the diagram and Doppler recording. Percent respiratory changes calculated as the difference between peak E velocity at expiration (E exp) and peak E velocity at inspiration (E insp) divided by E insp. In this example, E exp is 0.9 m/s and E insp is 0.6 m/s. Therefore, the difference in E velocity is 0.3 m/s, or 50% of E insp.

With inspiration, which induces less filling of the left ventricle, LV peak systolic pressure decreases; the opposite changes occur in the right ventricle so that RV peak systolic pressure increases with inspiration. Ejection time also varies with respiration in opposite directions in the left and right ventricles. This discordant pressure change between the left and right ventricles in constrictive pericarditis does not occur in restrictive cardiomyopathy (Fig. 24.28).

EFFUSIVE-CONSTRICTIVE PERICARDITIS

Effusive-constrictive pericarditis is an interesting condition that represents a unique clinical situation of combined pericardial effusion and constrictive pericarditis. Usually, a patient presents initially with pericardial effusion and clinical/hemodynamic evidence of increased filling pressures or tamponade/constriction. These constrictive hemodynamics persist even after removal or disappearance of the pericardial effusion. In some patients, the underlying constrictive pericarditis requires pericardiectomy, while in other patients, constrictive pericarditis is caused by a reversible inflammation of the pericardium (related to the same cause for pericardial effusion) and may resolve spontaneously or after treatment with anti-inflammatory agent(s). The later condition has been termed transient constrictive pericarditis.

TRANSIENT CONSTRICTIVE PERICARDITIS

About 7% to 10% of patients with acute pericarditis have a transient constrictive phase. These patients usually have a moderate amount of pericardial effusion, and as the pericardial effusion disappears, the pericardium remains inflamed, thickened, and

noncompliant, resulting in constrictive hemodynamics. The typical patient presents with dyspnea, peripheral edema, increased jugular venous pressure, and, sometimes, ascites, as in patients with chronic constrictive pericarditis. This transient constrictive phase may last 2 to 3 months before it gradually resolves either spontaneously or with treatment with anti-inflammatory agents (Fig. 24.29). When hemodynamics and findings typical of constriction develop in patients with acute pericarditis, initial treatment is indomethacin (Indocin) for 2 to 3 weeks and, if there is no response, the use of steroids for an additional 1 to 2 months (60 mg daily for 1 week, then tapered over 6 to 8 weeks). A bacterial etiology of the pericarditis should be ruled out before steroid therapy. Increased pericardial thickness usually returns to normal thickness with concomitant resolution of constrictive hemodynamics.

PERICARDIAL EFFUSION, ASSOCIATED WITH MALIGNANCY

One of the more common primary tumors of the heart associated with pericardial effusion (PE) is angiosarcoma. A characteristic example is shown in Fig. 24.30 in which a mass in the right atrium infiltrates the RA wall. The prognosis is very poor. Other malignant tumors associated with pericardial effusion include lymphoma, breast cancer, and lung cancer.

TRANSESOPHAGEAL ECHOCARDIOGRAPHY

When TTE is not adequate for obtaining satisfactory imaging of the pericardium and hemodynamic assessment of ventricular filling, TEE should be considered. A hemodynamically compromising loculated pericardial effusion may be difficult to detect on TTE.

Table 24.1	TRADITIONAL HEMODYNAMIC CRITERIA FOR CONSTRICTION VERSUS RESTRICTION	
Criterion	Constriction	Restriction
LVEDP – RVEDP (mm Hg)	≤5	>5
RV systolic pressure (mm Hg)	≤50	>50
RVEDP/RVSP	≥0.33	<0.3

LVEDP, left ventricular end-diastolic pressure; RVEDP, right ventricular end-diastolic pressure; RVSP, right ventricular systolic pressure.

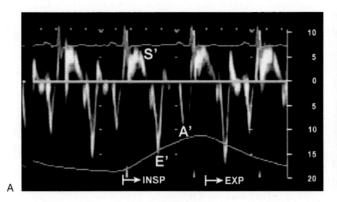

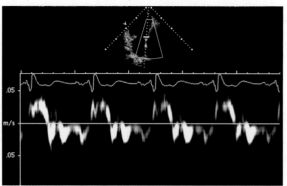

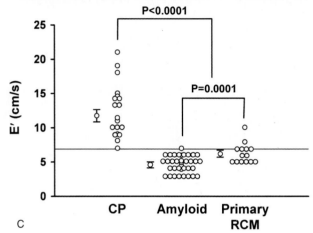

FIGURE 24.23. Tissue Doppler imaging of the septal mitral annulus in constriction (A) and restriction (B). A: Early diastolic septal mitral annulus velocity (E') is 15 cm/s, which indicates relatively normal or even greater than normal longitudinal motion of the mitral annulus. In patients with heart failure and elevated jugular venous pressure, E' velocity ≥8 cm/s should be equated with constrictive pericarditis (CP) until proved otherwise. **B:** E' is markedly reduced (3 cm/s) in this patient with myocardial disease and heart failure. Reduced E' correlates with abnormality in myocardial relaxation, which is reduced in almost all forms of cardiomyopathies. **C:** There is a very little overlap of E' between constriction (CP) and myocardial disease. Distribution of septal mitral annulus E' velocity in CP, cardiac amyloid, and primary restrictive cardiomyopathy (RCM). From Ha J, Ommen S, Tajik A, et al. Differentiation of constrictive pericarditis from restrictive cardiomyopathy using mitral annular velocity by tissue Doppler echocardiography. *Am J Cardiol* 2004; 94:316–319, with permission.

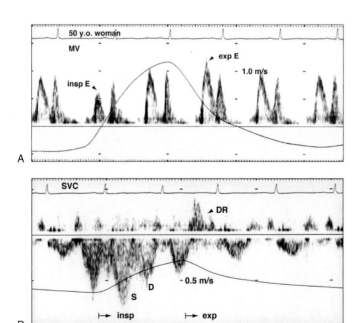

FIGURE 24.24. Doppler echocardiography in chronic obstructive lung disease. A: Pulsed-wave Doppler recording of mitral inflow velocity (MV) showing respiratory variation in a 50-year-old woman with chronic obstructive lung disease. There is 100% change in E velocity (from 0.6 m/s with inspiration to 1.2 m/s with expiration. insp, inspiration; exp, expiration. **B:** Pulsed-wave Doppler recording from the superior vena cava (SVC) showing a marked increase in SVC flow velocity with inspiration and a marked diminution with expiration. D, diastolic flow; DR, diastolic flow reversal; S, systolic flow.

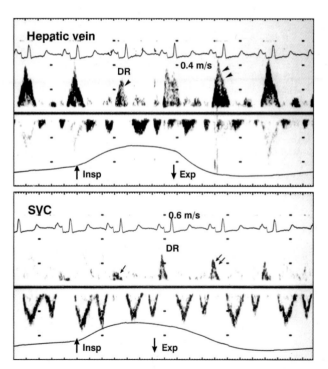

FIGURE 24.25. Pulsed-wave Doppler recording from the hepatic vein and superior vena cava (SVC) in a patient with constrictive pericarditis. Diastolic flow reversal (DR) increases (*double arrowheads*) in the hepatic vein with expiration (Exp) compared with DR with inspiration (Insp) (*single arrowhead*). However, there is a smaller diastolic flow reversal (*double arrows*) in the SVC during expiration compared with that in the hepatic vein. Diastolic flow reversal during inspiration is minimal (*single arrow*). Also, there was no significant change in the SVC forward flow velocity during inspiration and expiration, compared with SVC flow in chronic obstructive lung disease.

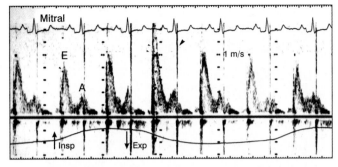

FIGURE 24.26. Mitral inflow velocity in a patient who developed constriction after mitral valve replacement. There is the typical respiratory variation in mitral E (early diastolic) velocity. Deceleration time is shortened despite the presence of mechanical mitral prosthesis because of increased left atrial pressure. *Arrowhead*, Closing of mitral prosthesis. Exp, expiration; Insp, inspiration.

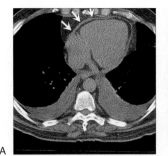
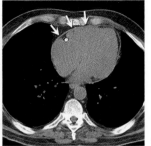

FIGURE 24.29. Computed tomography of the chest demonstrating increased pericardial thickness and pleural effusion (A), which disappeared after a course of steroid treatment (B). The patient has been free of constrictive symptoms since.

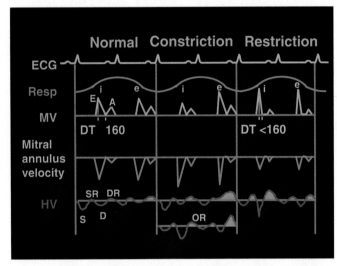

FIGURE 24.27. Diagram of Doppler velocities from mitral inflow (MV), mitral annulus velocity, and hepatic vein (HV) and the electrocardiographic (ECG) and respirometer recordings (Resp) indicating inspiration (i) and expiration (e). D, diastolic flow; DR, diastolic flow reversal; DT, deceleration time; S, systolic flow; SR, systolic flow reversal; *Blackened areas under curve*, flow reversal. Typically, mitral inflow has respiratory variation, but not always.

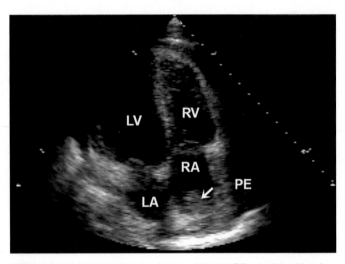

FIGURE 24.30. Apical four-chamber view showing a right atrial (RA) mass along with pericardial effusion. This is an example of malignant angiosarcoma.

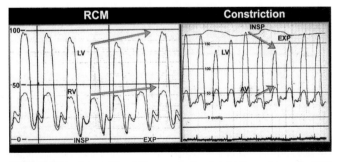

FIGURE 24.28. Simultaneous LV and RV pressure tracings in restrictive cardiomyopathy (RCM) and constriction. See text for details. Again, the changes in LV and RV are opposite between RCM and constriction.

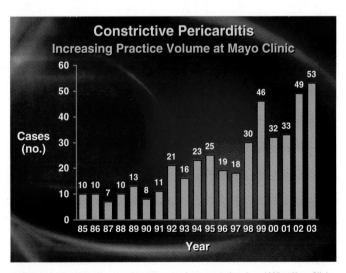

FIGURE 24.31. Number of pericardiectomy cases for constriction since 1985 at Mayo Clinic.

TEE has been especially helpful in postoperative patients with tamponade because of loculated hemopericardium. TEE also is useful to obtain pulmonary venous pulsed-wave Doppler velocities with a simultaneous respirometer recording to more optimally evaluate constrictive pericarditis. Furthermore, TEE is helpful in measuring the thickness of the pericardium and in evaluating abnormal structures near the pericardium (e.g., pericardial cyst, metastatic tumor).

 ## CLINICAL IMPACT

Echocardiography is typically one of the first diagnostic procedures used in patients in whom a pericardial abnormality is suspected. This noninvasive modality is capable of providing a complete assessment of the pericardial effusion (how much and how significant), identifying the best site for pericardiocentesis, and helping to establish or suggest the diagnosis of constrictive pericarditis. In some patients, constrictive pericarditis is transient, usually after acute pericarditis. The development and resolution of transient constrictive hemodynamics are readily assessed with serial 2D Doppler echocardiography. Detection of respiratory variation in mitral flow and central venous flow velocities may be the initial diagnostic clue to constrictive pericarditis, even in patients without any clinical suspicion of a pericardial abnormality. Comprehensive 2D and Doppler echocardiography with simultaneous recording of respiration should be able to distinguish constriction from restriction in nearly all patients. Detection of the patients with constrictive pericarditis has improved greatly using echocardiography over the past 20 years at the Mayo Clinic as evident in the increasing volume of pericardiectomy for constrictive pericarditis (Fig. 24.31).

SUGGESTED READING

Appleton C, Hatle L, Popp R. Cardiac tamponade and pericardial effusion: respiratory variation in transvalvular flow velocities studied by Doppler echocardiography. *J Am Coll Cardiol.* 1988;11:1020–1030.

Armstrong W, Schilt B, Helper D, et al. Diastolic collapse of the right ventricle with cardiac tamponade: an echocardiographic study. *Circulation.* 1982;65:1491–1496.

Bertog S, Thambidorai S, Parakh K, et al. Constrictive pericarditis: etiology and cause-specific survival after pericardiectomy. *J Am Coll Cardiol.* 2004;43:1445–1452.

Bloomfield R, Lauson H, Cournand A, et al. Recording of right heart pressures in normal subjects and in patients with chronic pulmonary disease and various types of cardio-circulatory disease. *J Clin Invest.* 1946;25:639–664.

Boonyaratavej S, Oh J, Appleton C. Superior vena cava Doppler can distinguish chronic obstructive lung disease from constrictive pericarditis despite similar respiratory variation in mitral flow velocity. *J Am Soc Echocardiogr.* 1996;9:370(8A).

Burstow D, Oh J, Bailey K, et al. Cardiac tamponade: characteristic Doppler observations. *Mayo Clin Proc.* 1989;64:312–324.

Callahan J, Seward J, Tajik A. Cardiac tamponade: pericardicentesis directed by two-dimensional echocardiography. *Mayo Clin Proc.* 1985;60:344–347.

Candell-Riera J, Garcia del Castillo H, Permanyer-Miralda G, et al. Echocardiographic features of the interventricular septum in chronic constrictive pericarditis. *Circulation.* 1978;57:1154–1158.

Connolly H, Click R, Schattenberg T, et al. Congenital absence of the pericardium: echocardiography as a diagnostic tool. *J Am Soc Echocardiogr.* 1995;8:87–92.

Engel P, Fowler N, Tei C, et al. M-mode echocardiography in constrictive pericarditis. *J Am Coll Cardiol.* 1985;6:471–474.

Feigenbaum H, Waldhausen J, Hyde L. Ultrasound diagnosis of pericardial effusion. *JAMA.* 1965;191:711–714.

Feigenbaum H, Zaky A, Waldhausen J. Use of ultrasound in the diagnosis of pericardial effusion. *Ann Intern Med.* 1966;65:443–452.

Garcia M, Rodriguez L, Ares M, et al. Differentiation of constrictive pericarditis from restrictive cardiomyopathy: assessment of left ventricular diastolic velocities in longitudinal axis by Doppler tissue imaging. *J Am Coll Cardiol.* 1996;27:108–114.

Gibson T, Grossman W, McLaurin L, et al. An echocardiographic study of the interventricular septum in constrictive pericarditis. *Br Heart J.* 1976;38:738–743.

Gillam L, Guyer D, Gibson T, et al. Hydrodynamic compression of the right atrium: a new echocardiographic sign of cardiac tamponade. *Circulation.* 1983;68:294–301.

Ha J, Oh J, Ling L, et al. Annulus Paradoxus. Transmitral flow velocity to mitral annular velocity ratio is inversely proportional to pulmonary capillary wedge pressure in patients with constrictive pericarditis. *Circulation.* 2001;104:976–978.

Ha J, Oh J, Ommen S, et al. Diagnostic value of mitral annular velocity for constrictive pericarditis in the absence of respiratory variation in mitral inflow velocity. *J Am Soc Echocardiogr.* 2002;15:1468–1471.

Ha J, Ommen S, Tajik A, et al. Differentiation of constrictive pericarditis from restrictive cardiomyopathy using mitral annular velocity by tissue Doppler echocardiography. *Am J Cardiol.* 2004;94:316–9.

Haley J, Tajik A, Danielson G, et al. Transient constrictive pericarditis: causes and natural history. *J Am Coll Cardiol.* 2004;43:271–275.

Hatle L, Appleton C, Popp R. Differentiation of constrictive pericarditis and restrictive cardiomyopathy by Doppler echocardiography. *Circulation.* 1989;79:357–370.

Hurrell D, Nishimura R, Higano S, et al. Value of dynamic respiratory changes in left and right ventricular pressures for the diagnosis of constrictive pericarditis. *Circulation.* 1996;93:2007–2013.

Ling L, Oh J, Breen J, et al. Calcific constrictive pericarditis: is it still with us? *Ann Intern Med.* 2000;132:444–450.

Ling L, Oh J, Schaff H, et al. Constrictive pericarditis in the modern era. Evolving clinical spectrum and impact on outcome after pericardiectomy. *Circulation.* 1999;100:1380–1386.

Ling L, Oh J, Tei C, et al. Pericardial thickness measured with transesophageal echocardiography: feasibility and potential clinical usefulness. *J Am Coll Cardiol.* 1997;29:1317–1323.

Nasser W, Helmen C, Tavel M, et al. Congenital absence of the left pericardium: clinical, electrocardiographic, radiographic, hemodynamic, and angiographic findings in six cases. *Circulation.* 1970;41:469–478.

Oh J, Hatle L, Seward J, et al. Diagnostic role of Doppler echocardiography in constrictive pericarditis. *J Am Coll Cardiol.* 1994;23:154–162.

Oh J, Tajik A, Appleton C, et al. Preload reduction to unmask the characteristic Doppler features of constrictive pericarditis: a new observation. *Circulation.* 1997;95:796–799.

Rajagopalan N, Garcia M, Rodriquez L, et al. Comparison of new Doppler echocardiographic methods to differentiate constrictive pericardial heart disease and restrictive cardiomyopathy. *Am J Cardiol.* 2001;87:86–94.

Sagrista-Sauleda J, Angel J, Sanchez A, et al. Effusive-constrictive pericarditis. *N Engl J Med.* 2004;350:469–475.

Sohn D, Kim Y, Kim H, et al. Unique features of early diastolic mitral annulus velocity in constrictive pericarditis. *J Am Soc Echocardiogr.* 2004;17:222–226.

Spodick D. Current concepts: acute cardiac tamponade. *N Engl J Med.* 2003;349:684–690.

Tajik A. Echocardiography in pericardial effusion. *Am J Med.* 1977;63:29–40.

Tsang T, Sarano M, Freeman W, et al. Consecutive 1127 therapeutic echocardiographically guided pericardiocenteses: clinical profile, practice patterns, and outcomes spanning 21 years. *Mayo Clin Proc.* 2002;77:429–436.

Vaitkus P, Kussmaul W. Constrictive pericarditis versus restrictive cardiomyopathy: a reappraisal and update of diagnostic criteria. *Am Heart J.* 1991;122:1431–1441.

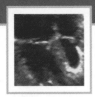

Chapter 25
Vascular Abnormalities

Michele A. Frommelt • Peter C. Frommelt

 ## ARTERIOVENOUS MALFORMATIONS

Systemic Arteriovenous Malformations

Systemic arteriovenous malformations in children result from errors in the formation and development of the normal arterial–capillary–venous connections that occur very early in gestation. They can arise anywhere in the body but are most commonly seen in the brain. Most arteriovenous malformations are clinically silent, with symptoms developing in adulthood. There are rare examples of arteriovenous malformations presenting at birth with life-threatening high output heart failure. A large arteriovenous malformation should be included in the differential diagnosis of an infant presenting with severe congestive heart failure.

Vein of Galen malformations are the most common form of symptomatic cerebrovascular malformation in neonates and infants. The clinical manifestations demonstrated early in life reflect both the large size and low resistance of the vascular malformation. There typically is torrential blood flow into the malformation, leading to increased cardiac output, increased cardiac chamber volumes, and congestive heart failure. Blood flow to the body is reduced and may result in ischemic multisystem organ failure, lactic acidosis, and death. Along with signs of severe congestive heart failure, unique physical findings include the presence of a cranial bruit, often heard over the posterior cranium, as well as bounding carotid pulses. The neonate who presents with a vein of Galen malformation may also be cyanotic, related to patency of the ductus arteriosus and elevated pulmonary vascular resistance.

The clinical signs and symptoms of a neonate or infant with a vein of Galen malformation mimic those of a patient with critical congenital heart disease, leading to the request for echocardiography. Although structural anatomy is typically normal, there are distinct anatomic and hemodynamic echocardiographic features that should lead the echocardiographer to suspect the diagnosis.

Echocardiography – Cardiac output can be over twice normal in these patients, resulting in enlargement of all cardiac chambers. Increased blood flow into the vein of Galen malformation may lead to dilatation of the ascending aorta and carotid arteries (Fig. 25.1A). The left subclavian artery and descending aorta are typically of normal caliber but may appear relatively small, suggestive of aortic coarctation. Because coarctation of the aorta has been described with increased frequency in patients with vein of Galen malformations, careful two-dimensional imaging of the aortic arch is critical. Color Doppler interrogation of the descending thoracic aorta reveals marked holodiastolic retrograde flow into the cerebral circulation (Fig. 25.1B); this is confirmed with pulsed Doppler examination of the descending aorta, which also reveals very limited antegrade systolic flow to the body (Fig. 25.1C). Increased systemic venous return

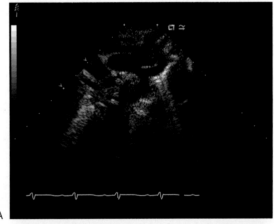

A

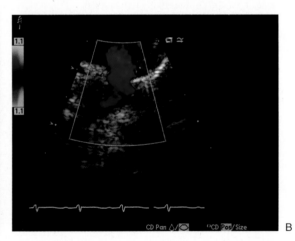

B

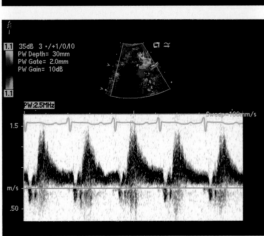

C

FIGURE 25.1. Suprasternal notch imaging in a newborn with a large vein of Galen malformation. A: Long-axis image reveals dilatation of the ascending aorta and brachiocephalic vessels, with mild distal transverse arch hypoplasia. There is no posterior shelf seen in the descending thoracic aorta. B: Color Doppler interrogation of the descending thoracic aorta demonstrates marked retrograde diastolic flow (*red signal*) into the cerebral circulation. C: Pulsed Doppler with the sample volume positioned in the descending aorta confirms dramatic retrograde flow from the aorta into the cerebral circulation, with little antegrade systolic flow to the body.

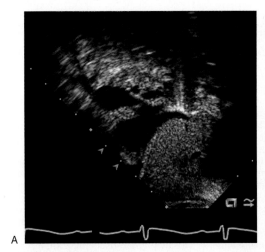 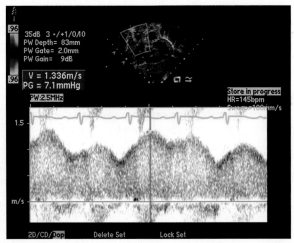

FIGURE 25.2. Subcostal sagittal view in a newborn with a large vein of Galen malformation. A: Aneurysmal dilatation of the superior vena cava is seen as it enters the right atrium. **B:** Pulsed Doppler with the sample volume positioned in the superior vena cava reveals abnormally high velocities with a continuous flow pattern.

from the malformation leads to dilatation of the superior vena cava (Fig. 25.2A), with abnormal high-velocity continuous flow identified by pulsed and color Doppler (Fig. 25.2B). Increased frequency of sinus venosus atrial septal defects has also been reported, with some postulating the increased superior caval return in utero may interfere with absorption of the right horn of the sinus venosus into the right atrium.

The newborn with a vein of Galen malformation demonstrates unique hemodynamics secondary to elevation in pulmonary vascular resistance and the presence of a patent ductus arteriosus and patent foramen ovale. The elevated pulmonary resistance in combination with the low systemic resistance from the malformation promotes right-to-left ductal shunting. Decreased flow into the pulmonary arteries and left atrium combined with increased flow in the superior vena cava and right atrium promotes right-to-left atrial level shunting as well. The right heart structures are often markedly enlarged, with right ventricular dysfunction, tricuspid insufficiency, and Doppler evidence of systemic pulmonary artery hypertension.

Although much less common, the infant with a large hepatic arteriovenous malformation may present in a similar fashion. The echocardiographic findings are a bit different, as the site of the malformation in the lower body alters the distribution of blood flow. Increased blood flow into the liver may lead to dilatation of the descending aorta prior to the origin of the celiac axis. Doppler in the descending thoracic aorta will reveal augmented systolic antegrade flow, with persistence of antegrade flow throughout diastole. Increased systemic venous return from the malformation will lead to dilatation of the inferior vena cava. Again, because cardiac output is often twice normal, all of the cardiac chambers may appear dilated.

Treatment – Before the advent of sophisticated imaging techniques and endovascular therapies, the mortality associated with large systemic arteriovenous malformation in the newborn was extremely high, with some series quoting only 50% survival at 1 month of age. As interventional therapy has progressed with catheter-based occlusion of the malformation, survival has improved. Initial medical management of the congestive heart failure often helps alleviate symptoms, so that direct therapy of the malformation can be delayed until an older age.

Pulmonary Arteriovenous Malformations

Pulmonary arteriovenous malformations are caused by abnormal communications between pulmonary arteries and pulmonary veins. They are commonly congenital in nature, are often multiple, and have a tendency to involve the lower lobes. It is estimated that about

70% of pulmonary arteriovenous malformations occur in patients with hereditary hemorrhagic telangiectasia, also known as Rendu-Osler-Weber disease. Hereditary hemorrhagic telangiectasia is an autosomal dominant disorder characterized by arteriovenous malformations in the skin, mucous membranes and visceral organs. Pulmonary arteriovenous malformations are rarely identified in infancy or childhood, with a peak incidence in the fourth and fifth decades.

Pulmonary arteriovenous malformations create a right-to-left shunt from the pulmonary arteries to the pulmonary veins, leading to systemic arterial desaturation. Because pulmonary vascular resistance is also low, flow into the malformation is not torrential; therefore cardiac output is typically normal or only mildly elevated. Most patients develop symptoms of dyspnea and cyanosis later in life, although life-threatening presentations including severe hemoptysis have been described. The intrapulmonary right-to-left shunt also may facilitate passage of emboli into the cerebral circulation, placing patients at risk for stroke and brain abscess. Presentation early in life is rare, but the classic triad of cyanosis, tachypnea, and an audible bruit over the lung fields in an infant should raise the question of a pulmonary arteriovenous malformation.

Pulmonary arteriovenous malformations can also be acquired. In the pediatric age group, acquired pulmonary arteriovenous malformations have been well described in the patient with single-ventricle physiology palliated with a cavopulmonary anastomosis. The development of pulmonary malformations appears to be related to exclusion of hepatic venous blood from the pulmonary circulation, supported by evidence that these malformations regress after completion of the Fontan when hepatic venous blood is again directed into the pulmonary circulation. Acquired pulmonary arteriovenous malformations also occur in the setting of mitral stenosis, chronic liver disease, schistosomiasis, trauma, and metastatic thyroid carcinoma.

Echocardiography – Although the diagnosis of pulmonary arteriovenous malformations can be made with use of many different imaging modalities, contrast echocardiography has become the preferred tool for screening and diagnosis, as it is readily available and noninvasive. The technique involves injection of 5 to 10 mL of agitated saline into a peripheral vein, while simultaneously imaging the heart with two-dimensional echocardiography. The agitated saline contains microbubbles, which are easily visualized by echocardiography because of their echo-reflectivity. In the patient with normal intracardiac anatomy, no intracardiac or intrapulmonary shunt, and normal systemic venous drainage, the microbubbles quickly appear in the right heart, with gradual dissipation as the bubbles are cleared by the pulmonary capillary circulation, never appearing in the left heart. In the patient with a patent foramen ovale or atrial level shunt, contrast can be visualized in the left atrium within one cardiac cycle of its appearance in the right atrium; the sensitivity of this procedure can be enhanced with the patient performing a Valsalva maneuver, which raises right atrial pressure to facilitate right-to-left atrial shunting. In the patient with a pulmonary arteriovenous malformation, contrast is also visualized in the left atrium, as the microbubbles bypass the pulmonary capillaries through the abnormal arteriovenous channels. However, as opposed to the atrial level shunt, there is a delay of about three to eight cardiac cycles before the contrast appears in the left atrium, because it takes time for the microbubbles to traverse the pulmonary vascular bed.

Contrast echocardiography in the patient with a cavopulmonary anastomosis is also helpful in the diagnosis of pulmonary arteriovenous malformations but is not diagnostic. In this patient group, the superior vena cava is excluded from the atria and is directly connected to the pulmonary arteries. Therefore, injection of agitated saline into an upper extremity peripheral vein should not produce contrast echoes within the right or left atria, as they should be cleared by the pulmonary capillary bed. If contrast echoes are visualized within the heart, pulmonary arteriovenous malformations need to be considered; however, venovenous collaterals will also bypass the pulmonary vasculature, leading to return of microbubbles to the atria via the abnormal venous channels. It is critical to differentiate pulmonary arteriovenous malformations from venovenous collaterals in these patients, because both can result in marked cyanosis, yet treatment is completely different. Angiography is a better way to evaluate the venous collaterals and, if demonstrated, permits catheter-based interventional closure of the collaterals.

Treatment – Pulmonary arteriovenous malformations can be treated with catheter embolization or surgical resection. Close observation may be reasonable in the asymptomatic patient with only mild desaturation. In the patient with acquired pulmonary arteriovenous malfomations, treatment of the underlying disease process will often cause regression of the lesions. Incorporation of the hepatic circulation into the pulmonary vascular bed is the treatment of choice in the patient with pulmonary arteriovenous malformations after cavopulmonary anastomosis.

 ## CORONARY ARTERY ABNORMALITIES

Isolated coronary artery anomalies have been described in approximately 1% to 5% of patients undergoing coronary angiography and approximately 0.3% of patients at autopsy. Many patients are asymptomatic, but signs of myocardial ischemia may present in childhood. Although visualization of coronary artery anatomy has traditionally been obtained using invasive procedures such as coronary angiography, transthoracic echocardiography has become the most important screening procedure for detection of these abnormalities in the pediatric population.

It is worthwhile considering coronary anomalies in children under three classifications: (a) anomalies involving *obligatory ischemia*, such as anomalous origin of the left coronary artery from the pulmonary artery, where clinical symptoms are frequent and presentation during childhood with evidence of myocardial dysfunction and injury is common; (b) anomalies involving *exceptional ischemia,* such as anomalous origin of a coronary artery from the opposite sinus of Valsalva, where ischemia can occur under severe clinical stress but there is no evidence of myocardial dysfunction at rest; and (c) anomalies involving *absent ischemia*, such as coronary artery fistulas, with minimal risk of myocardial dysfunction in childhood.

Echocardiography

Transthoracic echocardiographic imaging of coronary artery origins is critical and should be a part of the routine complete examination in every child. This is usually best accomplished from parasternal short-axis imaging, where both origins can be visualized by scanning superior to the aortic valve with careful interrogation of the aortic sinuses. The left coronary generally rises at approximately 4 o'clock if you consider the aortic root as a clock face, and the right coronary artery arises at approximately 12 o'clock (Fig. 25.3). Rotation of the transducer clockwise from the standard short-axis position frequently improves imaging of the length of the main coronary

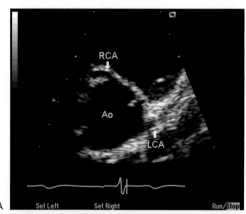

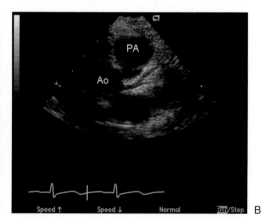

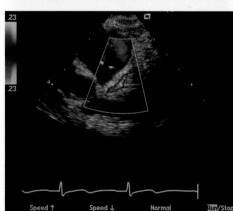

FIGURE 25.3. Short-axis images of the normal coronary origins from the aortic root (Ao). A: Normal origins of the left main coronary artery (LCA) from the left sinus of Valsalva and right coronary artery (RCA) from the right sinus of Valsalva are well visualized. With clockwise rotation of the probe from this position in **B**, a longer length of the left main coronary and its bifurcation into the left anterior descending and circumflex branches are visualized. Finally, color Doppler assessment of flow direction in the coronaries can obtained **(C)** by lowering the color Nyquist limit (in this case to 23 cm/s) to visualize the low-velocity diastolic antegrade flow in the left main coronary seen as a red flow signal coursing appropriately toward the transducer and away from the Ao.

artery and its early branches, the left anterior descending coronary artery and the left circumflex coronary artery. In contrast, counterclockwise rotation from the standard short axis view can facilitate imaging of the origin of the right coronary artery. Color Doppler flow interrogation of the left and right main coronaries is also important, as documentation of direction of and timing of flow is also helpful in diagnosing anomalies (as described later). Normal coronary artery flow is predominantly diastolic, because that is the time that aortic pressure (and thus coronary pressure) exceeds ventricular pressure. To see these coronary flow signals, which are usually low velocity, the Nyquist limit of the color Doppler map must be decreased to 20 to 40 cm/s. Many machines allow presets for coronary imaging to facilitate altering the setup to better identify coronary flow signals. Using the highest frequency transducer that allows adequate penetration is also important in coronary imaging, because fine-detail resolution is required to optimally image these small structures.

Anomalous Origin of a Coronary Artery from the Pulmonary Artery

Anomalous origin of the left coronary artery from the pulmonary artery (ALCAPA) is a rare congenital abnormality, occurring in approximately 1 in 300,000 children. The anomalous left coronary usually arises from the main pulmonary artery, although anomalous origin from the right pulmonary artery has also been described. The timing of presentation during childhood is quite variable and is related to adequacy of collateralization from the right coronary artery. In fetal life, the pressure in the pulmonary artery is high, allowing antegrade perfusion of the left coronary artery. However, shortly after birth, when pulmonary artery pressures fall, the left coronary artery system becomes dependent on the development of right coronary artery collaterals to supply the left ventricular myocardium. When few collaterals to supply left coronary flow are present, there is significant myocardial ischemia in infancy, leading to symptoms such as irritability, tachypnea, diaphoresis, and congestive heart failure. The clinical picture mimics the presentation of a patient with idiopathic dilated cardiomyopathy. In the patient with adequate right coronary collaterals, presentation is often delayed until adolescence or young adulthood, because myocardial function can be well preserved. Sudden cardiac death can occur in this age group, particularly with exercise, and is likely related to limited coronary reserve with development of pathologic ventricular arrhythmias during times of increased myocardial demands.

Echocardiography – Prospective identification of ALCAPA using echocardiography has been well described, and this technique should be diagnostic in most patients. Two-dimensional imaging may provide direct visualization of the anomalous coronary insertion into the pulmonary artery from parasternal long- and short-axis imaging, with the coronary usually inserting into the posterior and leftward aspect of the main pulmonary artery (Fig. 25.4). The anomalous left coronary artery frequently courses close to its normal site of origin near the left sinus of Valsalva, however, and so recognition of associated echo findings is often critical to the diagnosis (Table 25.1). The right coronary artery is dilated because of the obligate collateral circulation needed to perfuse the left ventricular myocardium, but this may not be striking in the infant with limited collateralization who presents early with a severe dilated cardiomyopathy. Dramatic right coronary dilatation and tortuosity are characteristic of the older asymptomatic child (Fig. 25.5). In addition, the older patient is likely to have prominent coronary collaterals that can be identified using color Doppler flow mapping as abnormal diastolic flow signals within the myocardium of the ventricular septum (Fig. 25.6).

Because the anomalous left coronary artery is perfused retrograde from the right coronary artery collaterals, identification of retrograde filling of the left coronary is critical for diagnosis (Fig. 25.7). This can be accomplished by documenting direction of flow in the left main coronary artery using color or spectral Doppler, with the expectation that appropriate flow will progress away from the aortic root (usually seen as a red Doppler signal in the normal patient because the left coronary arises from the more posteriorly positioned left sinus and courses anteriorly toward the transducer from parasternal windows). Careful screening for diastolic flow signals in the main pulmonary artery

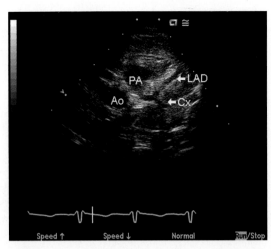

FIGURE 25.4. Two-dimensional image of anomalous insertion of the left main coronary artery into the posterior aspect of the proximal main PA from a parasternal short-axis view in a 4-month-old infant with anomalous left coronary artery from the pulmonary artery (PA). The left anterior descending (LAD) and circumflex (Cx) arteries are both seen entering the PA through a short left main coronary segment, clearly a long distance from the normal entrance into the aortic root (Ao).

by color Doppler is also important. Mitral valve abnormalities are variable, but fibrotic changes of the chordae and papillary muscles secondary to chronic ischemia are common and can lead to the development of mitral valve prolapse and mitral insufficiency (Fig. 25.8). Left ventricular dysfunction should always increase suspicion of ALCAPA, especially when endocardial fibrotic changes are also seen, but left ventricular function can be well preserved, particularly in older children with well-developed collaterals.

Surgical Therapy – Surgery to reconnect the left coronary artery with the aortic root is indicated in all patients when this lesion is identified, even in the patient with good left ventricular function, to normalize perfusion to the left coronary bed. Initial surgical techniques involved ligation of the anomalous coronary to prevent continued "steal" of left coronary flow into the pulmonary artery, but this did not alter left ventricular dependence on right coronary collateral circulation for left coronary artery perfusion and resulted in significant surgical and late mortality. More recently, direct coronary reimplantation into the aorta or creation of an intrapulmonary tunnel that connected the aorta with the anomalous coronary have been used to provide antegrade flow from the aorta into the left coronary system. Imaging of the left main coronary origin and course after reimplantation should be obtained by postoperative echocardiography with documentation of laminar antegrade flow from the

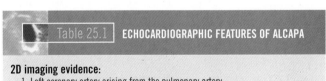

Table 25.1	ECHOCARDIOGRAPHIC FEATURES OF ALCAPA

2D imaging evidence:
1. Left coronary artery arising from the pulmonary artery
2. Dilated right coronary artery
3. Left ventricular chamber dilatation and systolic dysfunction/dilated cardiomyopathy
4. Mitral papillary and chordal fibrotic changes ± mitral valve prolapse

Color Doppler evidence:
1. Retrograde flow in the left coronary artery
2. Diastolic flow signals in the main pulmonary artery
3. Diastolic flow signals in the ventricular septum and left ventricular free wall
4. Mitral insufficiency related to mitral apparatus ischemia

ALCAPA, anomalous origin of the left coronary artery from the pulmonary artery.

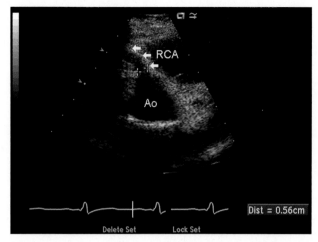

FIGURE 25.5. Short-axis image of the origin of the right coronary artery (RCA) in a 10-year-old child with anomalous origin of the left coronary from the pulmonary artery. The right coronary arises appropriately from the anterior aspect of the aorta (Ao) and is markedly dilated (*arrows*) because of the increased flow into that coronary, which measured 5.6 mm in diameter proximally.

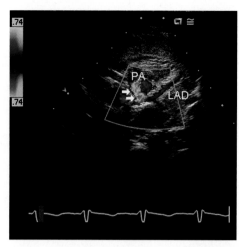

FIGURE 25.7. Short-axis image using color Doppler to identify retrograde flow in the left anterior descending coronary artery (LAD) in the same 4-month-old infant with anomalous left coronary artery from the pulmonary artery shown in Figure 25.4. Flow in the LAD is blue as it moves away the transducer toward the pulmonary artery (PA), which is abnormal because it should be flowing away from the aortic root (red Doppler signal) rather than toward it. A turbulent flow signal (*arrows*) is also seen in the pulmonary artery as the anomalous left coronary artery empties into the low-pressure pulmonary artery.

aortic root into the coronary bed by color Doppler. Serial evaluation of left ventricular function is important after surgery, because revascularization frequently results in dramatic remodeling of the left ventricle, with progressive normalization of function. Because mitral papillary muscle ischemia is common with ALCAPA, recovery of mitral function is variable after surgery and frequently does not correlate with recovery of left ventricular function. Late reoperation for mitral valve repair or replacement is required in a minority of patients with chronic severe insufficiency.

Anomalous Origin of a Coronary Artery from the Opposite Sinus of Valsalva

Anomalous origin of a coronary artery (AOCA) from the opposite sinus of Valsalva has been associated with myocardial ischemia, ventricular arrhythmias, and sudden death, particularly when the anomalous coronary (left coronary from the right sinus or right

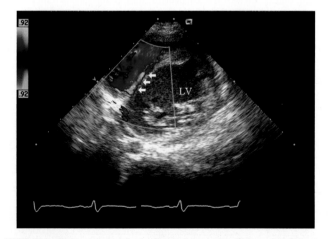

FIGURE 25.6. Short-axis image of color Doppler interrogation of the ventricular septum shows septal coronary collateral flow in the same 10-year-old child as Figure 25.5. The child was initially referred for evaluation of a heart murmur and was found to have anomalous origin of the left coronary from the pulmonary artery. A low-velocity linear diastolic flow signal is seen in the ventricular septum (*arrows*). The color Doppler and spectral Doppler timing of flow in diastole help differentiate this septal collateral from a ventricular septal defect, which is generally characterized by a high-velocity *systolic* flow signal. The identification of this septal flow signal was the initial echo finding that led to the diagnosis of ALCAPA in this boy.

coronary from the left sinus) courses in between the great arteries (Fig. 25.9). The anomalous coronary can arise from the opposite sinus and course anterior or posterior to the great arteries rather than between them, but the risk of coronary complications appears to be much lower. Although AOCA from the noncoronary or posterior sinus of Valsalva has also been described, it is quite rare and not generally associated with myocardial ischemia or sudden death. When the anomalous coronary is interarterial, it can course within the myocardial sulcus between the great arteries (intramyocardial) or within the anterior wall of the aorta between the great arteries (intramural).

Anomalous origin of the left coronary artery from the right sinus of Valsalva with the anomalous coronary coursing in between the great arteries is quite rare (with an estimated incidence of 0.03% to 0.05%) but is clearly associated with sudden cardiac death. The majority of patients who died suddenly with this anomaly had the sudden death episode during or shortly after vigorous exertion. More important, the highest-risk groups for exercise-induced sudden cardiac death are children and adolescents, and the majority are asymptomatic without previous complaints of chest pain, palpitations, syncope, or an identified arrhythmia. Sudden death in older patients was much less common, and cardiac death in the older group is generally associated with atherosclerotic disease. The lower risk of sudden death in older patients with this anomaly is likely related to the fact that they rarely participate in high-intensity competitive sports. Anomalous origin of the right coronary artery from the left sinus of Valsalva is more common (estimated incidence of 0.1%) and has also been associated with exercise-induced sudden cardiac death in children and young adults. Although anomalous origin of either coronary artery from the opposite sinus with an interarterial course carries a risk of sudden cardiac death, particularly for the young athlete, assessment of that risk in an individual patient remains difficult and controversial, because symptoms are rare and provocative stress testing is typically normal. Finally, a subset of patients present with sudden death in infancy, related to severe coronary ostial stenosis at the origin of the anomalous coronary.

The mechanisms that lead to myocardial ischemia in the patient with AOCA from the opposite sinus with an interarterial course between the pulmonary and aortic roots are unclear, but several theories have been proposed. The ostium of the anomalously arising coronary artery is frequently slitlike, likely compromising flow reserve. In addition, the anomalous coronary artery usually arises at an acute angle from the aorta, rather than perpendicularly, and this may alter flow patterns into that coronary artery bed. Finally, it has been hypothesized that the interarterial course places the anomalous coronary at risk of compression between the great arteries. This seems unlikely given the low pressure in the pulmonary

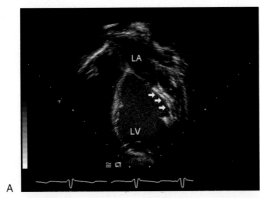 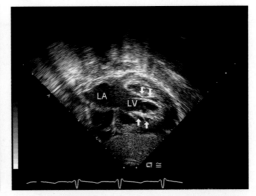

FIGURE 25.8. Apical four-chamber (A) and subcostal four-chamber (figure B) images of an infant with dilated cardiomyopathy and anomalous origin of left coronary artery from the pulmonary artery. These images demonstrate marked left atrial (LA) and left ventricular (LV) chamber dilatation with echo bright fibrotic changes of the mitral papillary muscles (arrows), consistent with chronic endocardial ischemia.

artery in normal individuals, even during exercise. The ischemia is more likely due to deformation of the anomalous coronary within the aortic wall during periods of arterial hypertension with exercise, particularly in patients with an intramural course. Because wall tension is determined by the radius of a vessel, the aorta will have greater wall tension than the intramural coronary with its wall, resulting in deformation of the coronary and diminished cross-sectional area. As aortic wall tension increases with increasing aortic pressure during exercise, the anomalous coronary becomes flattened and coronary reserve is reduced to a point where myocardial oxygen requirements are not met.

Echocardiography – Transthoracic echocardiography has become an important noninvasive tool for prospectively identifying anomalous origin of the left coronary from the right sinus of Valsalva and anomalous origin of the right coronary from the left sinus of Valsalva. Identification of either anomaly requires focused two-dimensional and color Doppler imaging of the coronary arteries. Intramyocardial anomalous coronary arteries from the opposite sinus can be seen running within the muscle immediately behind the right ventricular outflow tract between the great arteries, and they frequently stand out prominently within the muscle (Fig. 25.10). This form is very rare and appears to occur almost exclusively with anomalous origin of the left coronary from the right sinus. It is usually characterized by a single coronary ostia from the right sinus with early bifurcation into the left and right coronary branches

(Fig. 25.11). It appears to carry less risk for coronary complications than the intramural form of anomalous left coronary from the right sinus.

The intramural course of an anomalous coronary from the opposite sinus is much more common but can be more difficult to detect, particularly because the coronary exits the aortic wall from the usual or appropriate sinus of Valsalva (Fig. 25.12). Interestingly, the intramural segment in patients with anomalous origin of the left coronary from the right sinus is longer and usually traverses at least half of the right sinus before exiting the aortic wall from the left sinus (Fig. 25.13). In contrast, the intramural form of anomalous right coronary from the left sinus is usually characterized by a shorter (2 to 3 mm) intramural segment from the left sinus with the anomalous coronary ostia arising adjacent to the commissure between the right and left cusps (Fig. 25.14). Color Doppler imaging is critical in making this diagnosis, as it can help identify that intramural segment. In many cases, the intramural segment of the anomalous coronary is often only suspected after color Doppler interrogation of the aortic root identifies an abnormal color signal within the anterior aortic wall (Figs. 25.15 and 25.16). Color Doppler is also useful in diagnosing AOCA from the opposite sinus with an intramural course, because the technique can give the additional information of direction of flow in the intramural segment. This helps in differentiating whether the anomalous coronary arises from the right or left sinus. When the left coronary arises anomalously from the right sinus, a blue Doppler signal will be seen in the intramural segment as flow moves away

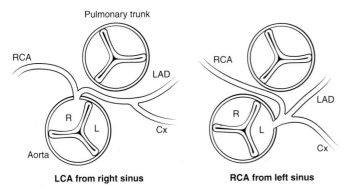

FIGURE 25.9. Schematic diagram of the two forms of anomalous origin of a coronary from the wrong sinus associated with myocardial ischemia—anomalous origin of the left coronary artery (LCA) from the right sinus of Valsalva (left) and anomalous origin of the right coronary artery (RCA) from the left sinus of Valsalva (right). In each case, the anomalous coronary can be seen coursing between the aorta and pulmonary artery (PA). With anomalous origin of the left coronary, the left main coronary artery (LMCA) arises from the right aortic sinus (R) and passes between the great arteries before dividing into its two usual branches—the left anterior descending (LAD) and left circumflex (LCx) coronary arteries. With anomalous origin of the right coronary, the right coronary artery (RCA) arises from the left aortic sinus (L) and passes between the great arteries before coursing in its usual distribution. P, posterior or noncoronary sinus.

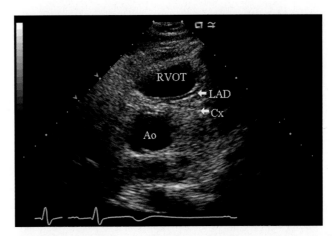

FIGURE 25.10. Short-axis image through the aortic root in a patient with anomalous origin of the left coronary artery from the right sinus of Valsalva and an intramyocardial course of the anomalous coronary. The anomalous left coronary artery can be seen coursing between the aorta (Ao) and right ventricular outflow tract (RVOT) within the myocardial wall before bifurcating into the left anterior descending (LAD) and circumflex (Cx) branches. No coronary artery is seen arising from the left coronary sinus.

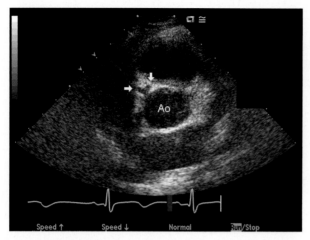

FIGURE 25.11. Short-axis image in a patient with anomalous origin of the left coronary artery from the right sinus of Valsalva and an intramyocardial course of the anomalous coronary. There is a single coronary origin from aorta (Ao) arising from the right sinus of Valsalva and immediately bifurcating into the right and left main coronary arteries (*arrows*). Again, no coronary artery is seen arising from the left aortic sinus.

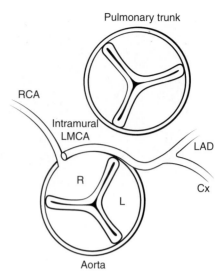

FIGURE 25.13. Schematic diagram of anomalous origin of the left coronary artery (LCA) from the right sinus of Valsalva with an intramural course between the great arteries. The left main coronary artery (LMCA) arises from the right aortic sinus (R) and passes between the great arteries through a long intramural segment before exiting the aortic wall from the left sinus. The exit site from the aortic wall in the left sinus is usually more anterior (nearer the commissure between the left and right cusps) than the normal or usual origin. It then divides into its two usual branches—the left anterior descending (LAD) and left circumflex (LCx) coronary arteries.

from the right sinus toward the more posteriorly positioned left sinus (Fig. 25.15). This is the opposite of anomalous origin of the right coronary from the left sinus, where a red Doppler signal will be seen in the intramural segment as flow moves toward the right sinus from its origin in the left sinus (Fig. 25.16).

Other transthoracic windows can also provide imaging evidence that a coronary has an anomalous origin from the aortic root. From the parasternal long-axis view, the anomalous coronary running between the great arteries can be seen as a discrete circle anterior to the aortic root as an initial clue (Fig. 25.17). In addition, in children who undergo high-quality subcostal imaging, scanning from the aortic root more anteriorly to the pulmonary root can identify a length of the anomalous coronary running between the great arteries (Fig. 25.18).

Transesophageal echocardiography has also been very useful in identifying or confirming anomalous origin of a coronary from the opposite sinus with an interarterial course, again particularly when that course is intramural. Imaging of the aortic root with

the multiplane sector at 25 to 40 degrees in the standard transesophageal position frequently provides excellent imaging of the coronary anatomy, and the intramural segment is usually well delineated by both imaging and color Doppler interrogation (Fig. 25.19). Intravascular ultrasound has documented both coronary hypoplasia and localized systolic lateral compression of the intramural segment of anomalous coronaries that run within the aortic wall. Not surprisingly, this degree of compression appears to have individual variations that likely explain the individual and

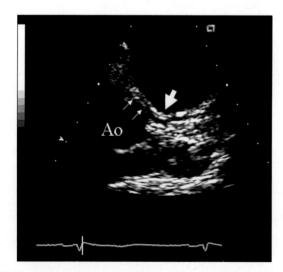

FIGURE 25.12. Short-axis image in a patient with anomalous origin of the left coronary artery from the right sinus of Valsalva and an intramural course of the anomalous coronary. The left coronary artery appears to be exiting the aorta (Ao) appropriately from the left sinus of Valsalva (*large arrow*); however, on closer inspection, the anomalous intramural segment of the proximal left coronary can be appreciated coursing within the anterior aortic wall (*small arrows*).

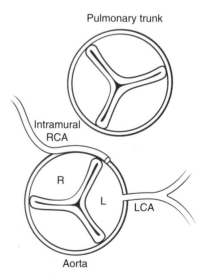

FIGURE 25.14. Schematic diagram of anomalous origin of the right coronary artery (RCA) from the left sinus of Valsalva with an intramural course between the great arteries. The RCA arises from the left aortic sinus (R) and passes between the great arteries through an intramural segment before exiting the aortic wall from the right sinus. In contrast to anomalous origin of the left coronary from the right sinus with an intramural course, the origin of the anomalous right coronary is usually near the commissure between the left and right cusps (within 2 to 3 mm) with a clearly separate origin and short intramural course, and so it can sometimes be difficult to determine if the coronary is actually arising from the left or right sinus. It then courses through the anterior aortic wall to exit the aorta near its usual site of origin in the right sinus. N, noncoronary sinus.

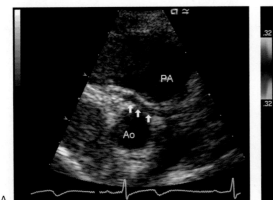
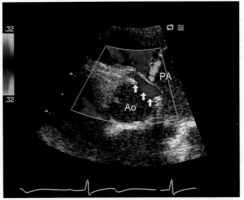

FIGURE 25.15. Short-axis imaging in a patient with anomalous origin of the left coronary artery from the right sinus of Valsalva and an intramural course of the anomalous coronary. A: Two-dimensional image shows the anomalous left main coronary artery running intramural within the anterior aortic wall (*arrows*) between the aorta (Ao) and pulmonary artery before exiting the wall in the left sinus of Valsalva. Note the long length of the left coronary within the anterior wall as courses along the right sinus. **B:** Color Doppler imaging shows the linear diastolic flow of the anomalous coronary within the anterior aortic wall (*arrows*); the blue signal confirms anomalous coronary flow away from the transducer, consistent with the coronary originating from the right sinus and coursing toward the more posteriorly positioned left sinus. Note the low velocity Nyquist limit (32 cm/s) needed to visualize the low-velocity coronary flow signal.

unpredictable responses to exercise in this patient group. The coronary narrowing is exacerbated by pharmacologic challenge that likely mimics exercise conditions. In addition, the length of the intramural segment may play a role in development of ischemia, as longer segments may accentuate the degree of stenosis caused by luminal distortion during exercise (which may explain

the perceived higher risk of anomalous origin of the left coronary from the right sinus). Finally, risk is almost certainly influenced by the precipitating conditions (usually vigorous exercise) at the time of the ischemic insult as well as the location/amount of myocardium supplied by the anomalous coronary. Again, there is currently no effective technique for quantifying these risks.

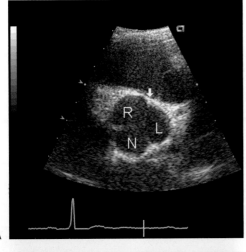
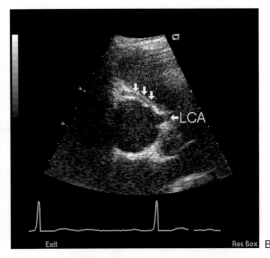
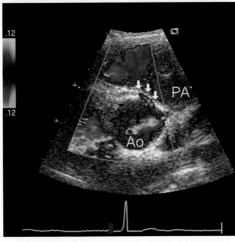

FIGURE 25.16. Short-axis imaging in a patient with anomalous origin of the right coronary artery from the left sinus of Valsalva and an intramural course of the anomalous coronary. A: position of the aortic sinuses at the level of the aortic valve; the commissure between the right (R) and left (L) cusps is well visualized (*arrow*). The noncoronary sinus (N) is seen posteriorly. **B:** Angling the transducer more superiorly above the valve leaflets, the anomalous right coronary artery can be seen arising from the left sinus of Valsalva near the origin of the left main coronary artery (LCA) and coursing intramural within the anterior aortic wall (*arrows*) between the aorta and the right ventricular outflow tract toward the right sinus of Valsalva. Comparing **A** and **B**, it is easy to appreciate that the anomalous coronary originates close to the commissure but clearly from the left sinus. **C:** Color Doppler imaging shows the linear diastolic flow of the anomalous coronary within the anterior aortic wall (*arrows*) between the aorta (Ao) and pulmonary artery (PA); the red signal confirms anomalous coronary flow toward the transducer, consistent with the coronary originating from the left sinus and coursing toward the more anteriorly positioned right sinus. Again, note the low-velocity Nyquist limit (12 cm/s) needed to visualize the low-velocity coronary flow signal.

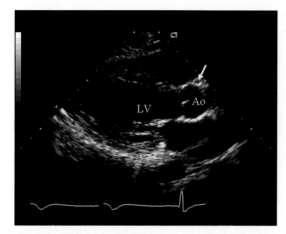

FIGURE 25.17. Parasternal long-axis image through the left ventricle (LV) in a patient with anomalous origin of a coronary from the opposite sinus with an intra-arterial course. The anomalous coronary is seen coursing anterior to the aorta (Ao) between the great arteries as a discreet circle (*arrow*); this may be the first clue that there is an anomalous coronary, as visualization of a coronary anterior to the aorta from this view is never seen with normal coronary origins.

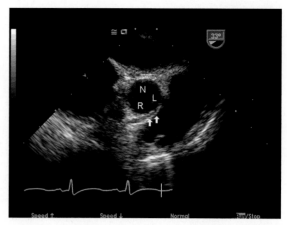

FIGURE 25.19. Transesophageal echocardiographic image from a mid-esophageal short-axis window through the aortic root in a patient with anomalous origin of the right coronary artery from the left sinus of Valsalva and an intramural course of the anomalous coronary. The anomalous right coronary artery can be seen arising from the left sinus of Valsalva (L) and coursing intramural within the anterior aortic wall (*arrows*) between the aorta and the right ventricular outflow tract toward the right sinus of Valsalva (R). The noncoronary cusp (N) is seen posteriorly.

Treatment – Surgical repair of AOCA has generally been reserved for patients with known symptoms of myocardial ischemia. Multiple surgical techniques have been used, including coronary bypass graft placement, patch enlargement of the anomalous coronary origin, reimplantation of the anomalous coronary to the appropriate sinus, and unroofing of the intramural segment of the anomalous coronary. The unroofing procedure has several advantages over other coronary repair techniques and is ideally suited for the patient with an intramural course of the anomalous coronary. The management of asymptomatic patients with AOCA remains controversial.

Coronary Artery Fistulas

Congenital coronary artery fistulas (CAFs) involve a abnormal communication between a coronary artery and a chamber of the heart or any segment of the systemic or pulmonary circulation. The origin of the coronary is normal; it is the termination or emptying segment of the coronary that is pathologic. The majority of fistulas arise from the right coronary artery (60%) and empty into the right

side of the heart (90%). The most frequent sites of termination of a CAF are the right ventricle, right atrium, coronary sinus, and pulmonary vascular bed. Coronary fistulous communications can be seen in the context of other congenital cardiac anomalies, most frequently pulmonary atresia with intact ventricular septum. The pathophysiology of CAF is the steal of coronary blood flow related to runoff from the coronary fistula into a low-pressure receiving cavity; this puts the myocardium beyond the site of the fistula at risk for ischemia because blood will preferentially empty into the low-pressure chamber. Most patients with CAF are asymptomatic in childhood and present because of a continuous murmur appreciated along the precordium. This murmur can sound similar to a patent ductus arteriosus, although its parasternal location frequently suggests a different etiology. Late complications have been described in older adults and include bacterial endocarditis, congestive heart failure, and angina.

Echocardiography – Two-dimensional echocardiographic findings are most striking for enlargement of the coronary that supplies the fistula; this coronary can be quite dilated and tortuous (Fig. 25.20). Flow into the involved coronary is easily identified by color Doppler and is associated with high-volume shunts through

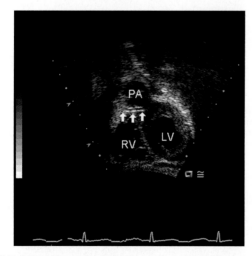

FIGURE 25.18. Subcostal image of a child with anomalous origin of left coronary from the right sinus of Valsalva and an interarterial course. This image demonstrates the anomalous coronary (*arrows*) immediately behind the pulmonary artery as the transducer is angled anteriorly from the left ventricle (LV) toward the right ventricular (RV) outflow. A coronary artery should never be imaged in this plane when there are normal origins.

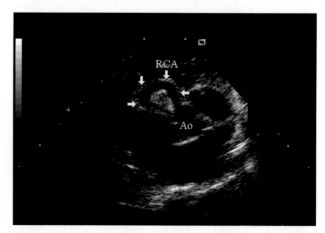

FIGURE 25.20. Parasternal short-axis image of the dilated origin of the right coronary artery (RCA) in a child with a right coronary–to–right ventricular fistula. The coronary is markedly dilated, measuring 5 mm in diameter, and tortuous (*arrows*) as it arises from the aorta (Ao) because of the increased flow through the fistula.

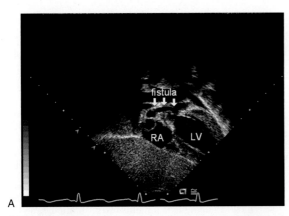 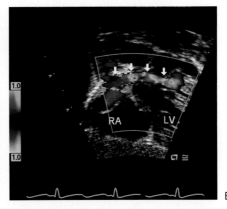

FIGURE 25.21. Subcostal images of a coronary fistula entering the right atrium in a child with a left coronary–to–right atrial fistula. **A:** Fistula courses posterior to the aorta (*arrows*) above the left ventricle (LV) with the terminal segment of the fistula emptying into the right atrium (RA). **B:** With color Doppler, the turbulent flow throughout the length of the fistula as it courses toward the right atrium is well visualized (*arrows*).

the fistula. The entire course of the coronary fistula can sometimes be tracked using imaging and color Doppler (Fig. 25.21), and the site of drainage is best identified by color Doppler because a high-velocity continuous color signal is evident where the coronary empties into the lower-pressure receiving chamber (Fig. 25.22). Cardiac chamber dilatation is unusual but may be present in the patient with a large left-to-right shunt. Large-volume fistulas can demonstrate retrograde steal from the aorta during diastole by color and spectral Doppler (Fig. 25.23).

Treatment – Closure of the fistula is indicated in any child with symptoms, and this can be accomplished either surgically or with interventional devices that obstruct the fistulous opening placed in the cardiac catheterization laboratory. Most children are asymptomatic, and so timing and need for fistula closure depend on the size and location of the shunt. Because the natural history of larger fistulas is to continue to dilate over time with a progressively increasing risk of thrombosis, endocarditis, and/or rupture, all except small fistulas are generally recommended for closure. Transesophageal echo guidance during surgical or device intervention can be useful in confirming successful closure.

Coronary Artery Aneurysms

Coronary artery aneurysms are uncommon and usually acquired, with an incidence that varies from 1.5% to 5% in postmortem series

(likely reflecting varying criteria in defining a coronary aneurysm). They are usually defined as an area of dilatation that is 1.5 times the size of the adjacent normal coronary segment and can be classified as saccular (ball-like with nearly equal axial and lateral diameters) or fusiform (gradual tapering of a symmetrically dilated segment on either end of the aneurysm). Diffuse dilatation of a coronary without localized enlargement is described as "ectasia." The possible causes of coronary aneurysms are summarized in Table 25.2, but the vast majority of aneurysms seen in pediatric patients are related to Kawasaki disease.

Kawasaki Disease

Kawasaki disease is an acute febrile vasculitis of unknown etiology with potential for serious morbidity and mortality attributable to the development of coronary artery aneurysms. Although the widespread use of intravenous immunoglobulin has improved outcome, Kawasaki disease remains the leading cause of acquired heart disease among children in the United States and Japan, surpassing acute rheumatic fever.

Because there is no specific diagnostic assay for Kawasaki disease, the diagnosis is based on clinical criteria that include fever for at least 5 days and four or more of the five major clinical features (conjunctival injection, cervical lymphadenopathy, oral mucosal changes, rash, and swelling/erythema of the extremities). Cardiovascular manifestations are prominent in the acute phase of

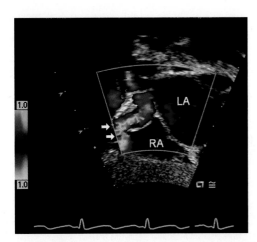 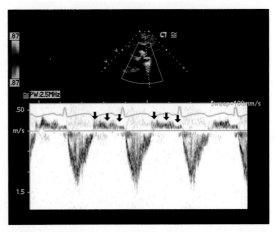

FIGURE 25.22. Subcostal image of the coronary fistula drainage site in a child with a left coronary–to–right atrial fistula. Color Doppler of the fistula shows a turbulent jet of flow where the fistula empties into the right atrium (RA), with the jet of flow striking the atrial wall (*arrows*).

FIGURE 25.23. Pulsed Doppler tracing in the descending thoracic aorta in a child with a large left coronary–to–right atrial fistula. Because of significant diastolic steal of flow into the coronary as it empties into the low resistance right atrium, holodiastolic retrograde aortic flow (*arrows*) is appreciated from the Doppler signal; this would suggest a significant volume shunt through the fistula.

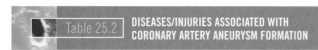

Table 25.2   DISEASES/INJURIES ASSOCIATED WITH CORONARY ARTERY ANEURYSM FORMATION

- Kawasaki disease
- Arteritis (polyarteritis nodosa, systemic lupus erythematosus, Takayasu, syphilis)
- Connective tissue disorders (Marfan and Ehlers-Danlos syndromes)
- Mycotic
- Dissection
- Atherosclerosis
- Complications of coronary angioplasty
- Trauma

the disease, and chronic changes in the coronary arteries continue to be the leading cause of morbidity and mortality. Two-dimensional and Doppler echocardiography remains the gold standard in the cardiac assessment of children with Kawasaki disease, because it is noninvasive and has a high sensitivity and specificity for detection of proximal coronary artery abnormalities.

Echocardiography – Complete two-dimensional and Doppler echocardiography should be performed as soon as the diagnosis of Kawasaki disease is suspected. Although the echocardiographic examination of patients with Kawasaki disease is focused on the coronary arteries, histologic evidence suggests that myocarditis

is universal in the acute phase of the disease. Measurement of left ventricular dimensions and ejection fraction should be a standard part of the initial examination and should be followed serially. Pericardial effusions can also be seen but typically are not hemodynamically important. Valvular insufficiency has also been reported, so all valves should be interrogated using color Doppler. The initial echocardiographic study will serve as a baseline for longitudinal follow-up of left ventricular function and coronary artery dimensions/morphology. Although the parasternal short-axis view provides ideal images of the proximal left and right coronary arteries (Fig. 25.24), multiple imaging planes and unique transducer positions are required when trying to image all major coronary artery segments. The apical four-chamber (Fig. 25.25) and subcostal (Fig. 25.26) views will often provide additional information, especially when trying to visualize the mid and distal right coronary artery. Transesophageal echocardiography may optimize coronary imaging in patients with limited transthoracic windows, and especially evaluation of the proximal right and left coronary arteries.

Coronary artery aneurysm formation rarely occurs before day 10 of the illness, but subtle changes in the coronary arteries can be seen at presentation. Coronary artery dilatation often occurs in the acute phase and may be a very early marker of coronary arteritis. Criteria for diagnosis of coronary artery ectasia have been characterized and vary with patient size; aneurysms have also been classified by size, with the largest ones clearly associated with late development of coronary insufficiency and myocardial ischemia. Individual measurements of the left main coronary artery, left anterior descending coronary artery, and proximal right coronary artery should be made. Measurements should be made from inner edge to

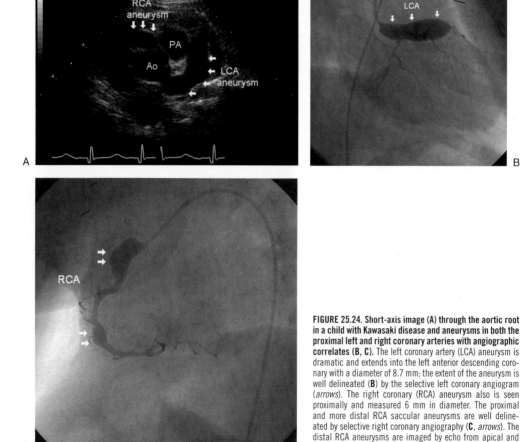

FIGURE 25.24. Short-axis image (A) through the aortic root in a child with Kawasaki disease and aneurysms in both the proximal left and right coronary arteries with angiographic correlates (B, C). The left coronary artery (LCA) aneurysm is dramatic and extends into the left anterior descending coronary with a diameter of 8.7 mm; the extent of the aneurysm is well delineated (**B**) by the selective left coronary angiogram (*arrows*). The right coronary (RCA) aneurysm also is seen proximally and measured 6 mm in diameter. The proximal and more distal RCA saccular aneurysms are well delineated by selective right coronary angiography (**C**, *arrows*). The distal RCA aneurysms are imaged by echo from apical and subcostal imaging (Figs. 25.25 and 25.26).

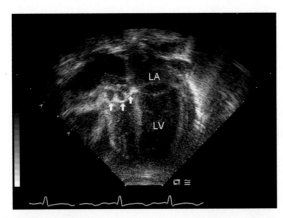

FIGURE 25.25. Apical image in the same child with Kawasaki disease as shown in Figure 25.24, identifying multiple aneurysms in the posterior descending branch of the right coronary artery (*arrows*). The scanning plane has been angled posteriorly through the right heart to visualize the atrioventricular groove behind the tricuspid valve to image this distal coronary branch, which was important in characterizing the extent of the disease. The left atrium (LA) and left ventricle (LV) are also imaged, with a pericardial effusion posteriorly as well.

inner edge and should exclude points of branching. In the setting of incomplete Kawasaki disease, it is suggested that the echocardiogram be considered "positive" if the z-score of the left anterior descending coronary artery or right coronary artery is equal to or exceeds 2.5. Other features suggestive of Kawasaki disease include perivascular brightness and lack of tapering of the coronary arteries (Fig. 25.27).

In the patient with detected coronary artery aneurysms, it is important to recognize the limitations of echocardiography. The detection of coronary artery stenosis and thrombosis is much more difficult using transthoracic echocardiography; other imaging modalities may be required if ischemic disease is suspected. Evaluation of the cardiovascular manifestations of Kawasaki disease requires serial echocardiography and should be performed using equipment with appropriate transducers. In the uncomplicated case of Kawasaki disease, echocardiographic assessment should be performed at the time of diagnosis, at 2 weeks, and at 6 to 8 weeks after disease onset. If the echocardiographic findings are normal at the 8-week evaluation, further studies are unlikely to reveal any coronary artery changes.

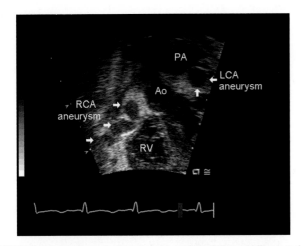

FIGURE 25.26. Subcostal transverse image in the same child with Kawasaki disease as shown in Figures 25.24 and 25.25. Image identifies aneurysmal dilation (*arrows*) of the proximal right coronary artery (RCA) as it courses down the anterior right ventricle (RV) adjacent to the aorta (Ao). A cross section of the proximal left coronary aneurysm is also seen (LCA).

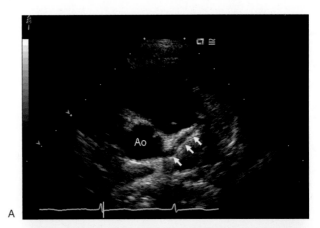

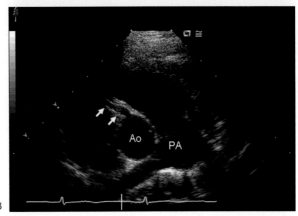

FIGURE 25.27. Short-axis image through the aortic root (Ao) to visualize the proximal left coronary (A) and right coronary (B) arteries in a child with Kawasaki disease. Diffuse coronary dilatation (ectasia) of both proximal branches is appreciated with a lack of the normal tapering (*arrows*). Although subjective, there also appears to be perivascular brightness of the tissue around the vessels, and the walls of the coronaries appear prominent. No aneurysms are seen. PA, pulmonary artery.

SUGGESTED READING

Barzilai B, Waggoner AD, Spessert C, et al. Two-dimensional contrast echocardiography in the detection and follow-up of congenital pulmonary arteriovenous malformations. *Am J Cardiol.* 1991;68:1507–1510.

Bhattacharya JJ, Thammaroj J. Vein of Galen malformations. *J Neurol Neurosurg Psychiatry.* 2003;74(suppl 1):i42–i44.

Cerebral arteriovenous malformations in children. *Can J Anaesth.* 1994;41:321–331.

Frommelt MA, Frommelt PC, Pelech AN, et al. Detection of septal coronary collaterals by Doppler color flow mapping is a marker for anomalous origin of the coronary artery from the pulmonary artery. *J Am Soc Echocardiogr.* 1996;9:388.

Frommelt PC, Frommelt MA, Tweddell JS, et al. Prospective echocardiographic diagnosis and surgical repair of anomalous origin of a coronary artery from the opposite sinus with an interarterial course. *J Am Coll Cardiol.* 2003;42:148–154.

Higuera S, Gordley K, Metry DW, et al. Management of hemangiomas and pediatric vascular malformations. *J Craniofac Surg.* 2006;12:738–739.

Hsieh KS, Huang TC, Lee CL. Coronary artery fistulas in neonates, infants, and children: clinical findings and outcome. *Pediatr Cardiol.* 2002;23:415–419.

Imoto Y, Sese A, Joh K. Redirection of the hepatic venous flow for the treatment of pulmonary arteriovenous malformations after Fontan operation. *Pediatr Cardiol.* 2006;27:490–492.

Liechty KW, Flake AW. Pulmonary vascular malformations. *Semin Pediatr Surg.* 2008;17:9–16.

McElhinney DB, Halbach VV, Silverman NH, et al. Congenital cardiac anomalies with vein of Galen malformations in infants. *Arch Dis Child.* 1998;78:548–551.

Newburger JW, Takahashi M, Gerber MA, et al. Diagnosis, treatment, and long-term management of Kawasaki disease: a statement for health professionals from the Committee on Rheumatic Fever, Endocarditis and Kawasaki Disease, Council on Cardiovascular Disease in the Young, American Heart Association. *Circulation.* 2004;110:2747–2771.

Patel N, Millis JF, Cheung MMH, et al. Systemic haemodynamics in infants with vein of Galen malformation: assessment and basis for therapy. *J Perinatol.* 2007;27:460–463.

Roberts WC. Major anomalies of coronary arterial origin seen in adulthood. *Am Heart J.* 1986;111:941–963.

Ruey-Kang R, Chang J, Alejos C, et al. Bubble contrast echocardiography in detecting pulmonary arteriovenous shunting in children with univentricular heart after cavopulmonary anastomosis. *J Am Coll Cardiol.* 1999;33; 2052–2058.

Sadick H, Sadick M, Gotte K, et al. Hereditary hemorrhagic telangiectasia: an update on clinical manifestations and diagnostic measures. *Wien Klin Wochenschr.* 2006;118:72–80.

Sanders SP, Parness IA, Colan SD. Recognition of abnormal connections of coronary arteries with the use of Doppler color flow mapping. *J Am Coll Cardiol.* 1989;13:922–926.

Shah MJU, Rychik J, Fogel MA, et al. Pulmonary AV malformations after superior cavopulmonary connection: resolution after inclusion of hepatic veins in the pulmonary circulation. *Ann Thorac Surg.* 1997;63:960–963.

Snider AR, Serwer GA, Ritter SB: Abnormal vascular connections and structures. In: DeYoung L, ed. *Echocardiography in pediatric heart disease.* St. Louis: CV Mosby; 1997:452–496.

Srivastave D, Preminger T, Lock JE, et al. Hepatic venous blood and the development of pulmonary arteriovenous malformations in congenital heart disease. *Circulation.* 1995;92:1217–1222.

Chapter 26
Cardiac Tumors

David J. Driscoll • Frank Cetta • Benjamin W. Eidem

Before the advent of echocardiography, the true incidence of primary cardiac tumors in children was elusive. With echocardiography, the incidence per echocardiogram performed approximates 0.08%. In children, the vast majority of primary cardiac tumors are histologically benign; fewer than 10% are malignant. Secondary or metastatic tumors of the heart are relatively rare in children. In children, rhabdomyomas are the most common primary cardiac tumor, whereas in adults, myxomas are the most common (Table 26.1, Fig. 26.1). Echocardiography is the primary imaging modality to diagnose cardiac tumors, whereas magnetic resonance imaging (MRI) and computed tomography can be useful adjunctive imaging modalities. Although most cardiac tumors in children are histologically benign, if their location in the heart jeopardizes cardiac, valvar, or conduction system function, then they can be associated with serious hemodynamic compromise and death.

SYMPTOMS AND PHYSICAL FINDINGS

In general, the physical findings of cardiac tumors depend on the location and size of the mass. If the mass is causing restriction to flow through a valve, there may be a murmur suggestive of stenosis, or if the obstruction is severe, there may be evidence of reduced cardiac output and even shock. Obstruction of the tricuspid valve, especially in a neonate, can be associated with cyanosis. Mitral valve obstruction or pulmonary venous obstruction can cause pulmonary edema and evidence of pulmonary hypertension. If the mass is preventing normal closure of a valve, there may be a murmur of valvar insufficiency.

Myxomas and papillary fibroelastomas have the potential for embolism and physical findings associated with pulmonary, or systemic embolic phenomenon can be apparent. Because these tumors can be sessile, sudden occlusion of a cardiac valve or a coronary artery can produce sudden death.

Pericardial teratomas may cause a pericardial effusion. Hence, the heart sounds may be muffled, and pulsus paradoxicus can occur along with hepatomegaly. Teratomas can cause distortion of the heart, which can be associated with superior or inferior vena cava obstruction and the physical findings attendant to the obstruction.

RHABDOMYOMA

Rhabdomyomas are the most common primary tumor in infants and children. They consist of well-circumscribed, nonencapsulated white or white gray masses that contain vacuolated cells filled with glycogen. They are classified as hamartomas and do not undergo mitotic division. They can exist entirely intramurally or extend into the atrial or ventricular cavities. Most frequently, they involve the ventricular walls and cavities. There are multiple rhabdomyomas in 90% of cases.

Most patients with rhabdomyomas are asymptomatic. However, sudden death has occurred with these tumors. Protrusion of the mass underneath the pulmonary or aortic valve can produce significant left or right ventricular outflow tract obstruction. As noted, arrhythmias can be associated with rhabdomyomas as well.

Rhabdomyomas are quite echogenic and usually are multiple, homogeneous, and well circumscribed. They frequently have a speckled pattern. Usually they are intramural but they can be intracavitary (Fig. 26.2). Although they can occur anywhere in the heart, usually they are present within the ventricular walls and often have a variable amount of extension into the ventricular cavity. Occasionally they can be pedunculated. In contrast to thrombi, myxomas, and vascular tumors, rhabdomyomas do not have echolucent areas indicative of hemorrhage or areas of calcification. These tumors can cause either right or left ventricular outflow tract obstruction but characteristically do not embolize to the pulmonary or systemic circulation. Serial echocardiography often reveals decreasing rhabdomyoma size, and, if present, right or left ventricular outflow tract obstruction may decrease over time.

There is a strong association of rhabdomyomas with tuberous sclerosis. Tuberous sclerosis is an autosomal dominant condition manifest by subungual fibromas, café au lait pigmentation, and subcutaneous nodules. From 30% to 50% of patients with tuberous sclerosis have rhabdomyomas, and 50% to 80% of fetuses with rhabdomyomas have tuberous sclerosis. Two disease genes have been described for tuberous sclerosis; *TSC-1* gene encodes a protein called hamartin, and *TSC-2* gene encodes a protein called tuberin.

Because rhabdomyomas frequently regress, if they are causing no hemodynamic compromise and there appears to be no potential for them to embolize, they should be observed. Operation is indicated to remove them only if they are causing hemodynamic compromise or there is high risk of embolization.

MYXOMA

Considering patients of all ages, myxomas are the most common cardiac tumor generally coming to medical attention in the third to sixth decades of life. In children, however, they are second in frequency to rhabdomyomas. Three-quarters of myxomas are located in the left atrium (Fig. 26.3), and 25% are in the right atrium (Fig. 26.4A) They can be readily demonstrated by echocardiography in the subcostal and apical views. They occur rarely in the ventricles (Fig. 26.4B). They are friable pedunculated red lobular tumors (Fig. 26.5). They consist of a paucicellular myxoid background and contain multiple small blood vessels, lymphocytes, and histiocytes. In the atrium, the stalk typically is attached to the region of the fossa ovalis (Fig. 26.6). They can be multiple. Myxomas are rarely malignant.

In infants, a myxoma can mimic a variety of congenital heart defects. In children, they frequently cause relative obstruction of the tricuspid or mitral valve. Doppler echocardiography is very helpful to evaluate the hemodynamic impact of these tumors to atrioventricular valve inflow. Large myxomas can entirely obstruct the valve and be lethal. Partial obstruction of the mitral valve can cause pulmonary hypertension. The symptoms of valvar obstruction can be positional as the mass moves in and out of the valve orifice with changing from the standing to supine positions. The patient may experience positional dyspnea, dizziness, and/or syncope. Myxomas can be associated with the triad of (a) valvar obstruction, (b) embolic events, and (c) systemic illness. Constitutional symptoms include

Table 26.1	RELATIVE FREQUENCY OF CARDIAC TUMORS			
	Pediatric	Fetal	Neonatal	Adult
Rhabdomyoma	40–61%	64%	47%	3–4%
Myxoma	5–14%	0%	4%	77–96%
Fibroma	8%	7%	16%	3–4%
Pericardial teratoma	1.6%	22%	15%	2%
"Hemangioma"	<5%	7%	5%	1%
Papillary fibroelastoma	<10%	...	...	8%
Malignant tumors	4%	...	...	10%
Lipoma	...	...	...	1–4%
Purkinje cell hamartoma	...	0%	11%	...

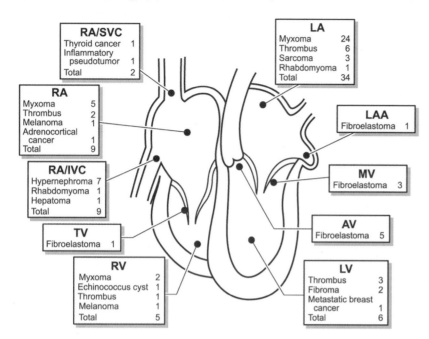

fever, malaise, weight loss, arthralgias, and myalgias. The patient also may exhibit anemia, thrombocytopenia, elevated sedimentation rate, and elevated gamma-globulin levels. The constitutional symptoms may be related to secretion of interleukin 6 by the tumor. The manifestations of a myxoma can be protean and be confused with rheumatic fever, endocarditis, septicemia, myocarditis, and collagen vascular diseases.

Carney syndrome is a familial form of myxoma that also includes lentigines (Fig. 26.7) and noncardiac as well as cardiac myxomas and endocrine abnormalities. If Carney syndrome is suspected, family members should be screened for the presence of myxomas.

The treatment of myxomas is surgical removal. It is important to remove the stalk of the tumor; with incomplete removal, the tumor can recur.

FIBROMA

Fibromas are the second or third most common cardiac tumor in children. They occur in infancy and rarely are identified in older children, adolescents, or adults. Fibromas consist of firm, white,

nonencapsulated tumors most characteristically in the left ventricular free wall or septum and frequently at the left ventricular apex (Figs. 26.8 and 26.9). They can be broad based or pedunculated. Fibromas can affect the right atrium and ventricle and the atrial free wall and septum. These tumors may also compromise atrioventricular valve architecture and function, resulting in significant valvar regurgitation. Echocardiographically, fibromas appear as a single, bright, intramural echogenic mass that may invade the ventricular cavity resulting in impaired filling or significant outflow tract obstruction (Figs. 26.10 and 26.11). They are distinguished from rhabdomyomas by having multiple areas of calcification and cystic degeneration. Using strain imaging, fibromas are not compressed during the cardiac cycle. MRI may be useful in distinguishing them from rhabdomyomas. The clinical features of fibroma are similar to those of rhabdomyomas.

Gorlin syndrome consists of cardiac fibromas, multiple basal cell carcinomas, jaw cysts, and skeletal abnormalities. Due to the risk of sudden death from refractory ventricular arrhythmia, our center has favored surgical removal of large fibromas. If the fibroma is located within the atrioventricular groove and is intimate with a coronary artery, then surgical removal may be hazardous and these patients may be observed.

TERATOMA (GERM CELL TUMORS)

Intrapericardial teratomas usually are single encapsulated tumors containing multiple cysts within a mucoid stroma and are attached to the aorta or pulmonary artery at the base of the heart. Rarely are they malignant. Typically they are diagnosed in the neonate or newborn. Intrapericardial teratomas can be associated with pericardial effusion and can compress cardiac structures such as the right atrium and ventricle. If they cause rotational displacement of the heart, superior vena cava obstruction can occur. Intracardiac teratomas are less frequent than intra-pericardial teratomas and usually occur on the right side of the heart.

Infants with a teratoma typically present with respiratory distress, pericardial effusion, signs of cardiac compression, cardiac tamponade, and/or nonimmune hydrops fetalis. Death can occur from rupture of cysts within the teratoma, causing cardiac tamponade. These tumors should be removed surgically.

Echocardiographically, they are usually a single nonhomogeneous, lobular, intrapericardial mass and almost always are associated with pericardial effusion. They can be confused with a bronchogenic cyst, but the two can be distinguished by using MRI.

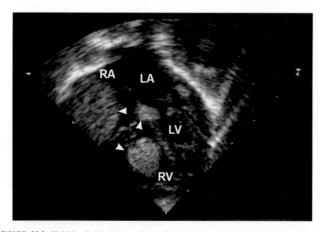

FIGURE 26.2. Multiple rhabdomyomas (arrows) demonstrated as homogeneous echogenic masses in the ventricular septum, right atrium (RA), and right ventricle (RV).

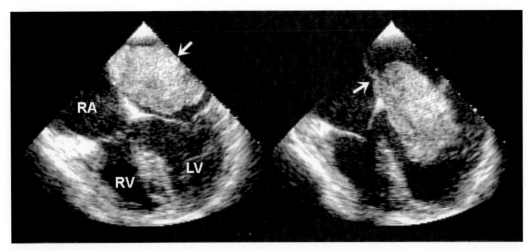

FIGURE 26.3. Large myxoma in the left atrium attached to the atrial septum. Movement with the cardiac cycle can be appreciated in these systolic (*left*) and diastolic (*right*) images. (From Oh JK, Seward JB, Tajik AJ. *The Echo Manual,* 3rd ed, Lippincott Williams & Wilkins. © 2006 Mayo Foundation for Medical Education and Research, with permission.)

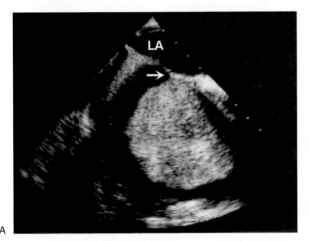

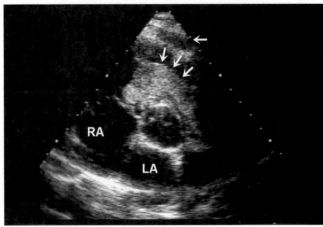

A   B

FIGURE 26.4. Myxoma A: Large myxoma in the right atrium. **B:** Parasternal short-axis view demonstrating a large myxoma in the right ventricular outflow tract. In young patients, a myxoma in an unusual location is probably related to familial myxoma syndrome. (From Oh JK, Seward JB, Tajik AJ. *The Echo Manual,* 3rd ed, Lippincott Williams & Wilkins. © 2006 Mayo Foundation for Medical Education and Research, with permission.)

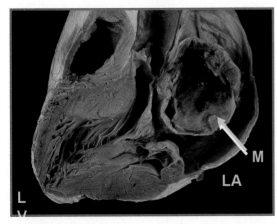

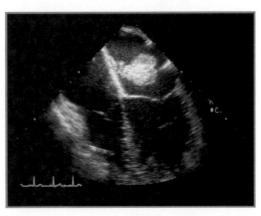

FIGURE 26.5. Pathologic specimen demonstrating a large myxoma (M) in the left atrium.

FIGURE 26.6. Transesophageal four-chamber image demonstrating an atrial myxoma with attachment of the stalk to the region of the fossa ovalis.

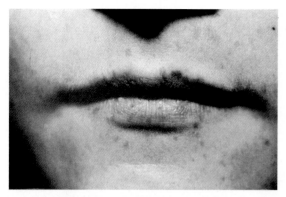

FIGURE 26.7. Typical facies of a patient with Carney syndrome. Note numerous lentigines. (Courtesy of Dr. James Seward.)

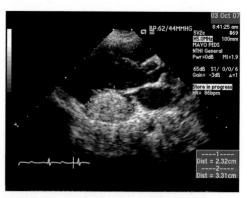

FIGURE 26.10. Parasternal long-axis image of the large cardiac excised fibroma shown in Figure 26-9. Note the homogeneous echogenic appearance.

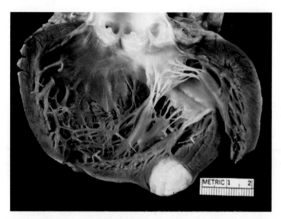

FIGURE 26.8. Pathologic specimen demonstrating a bright white fibroma at the left ventricular apex.

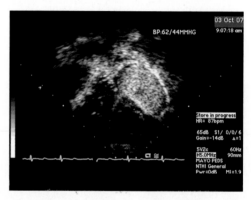

FIGURE 26.11. Para-apical four-chamber image demonstrating the lateral and apical extent of the excised fibroma shown in Figure 26-9.

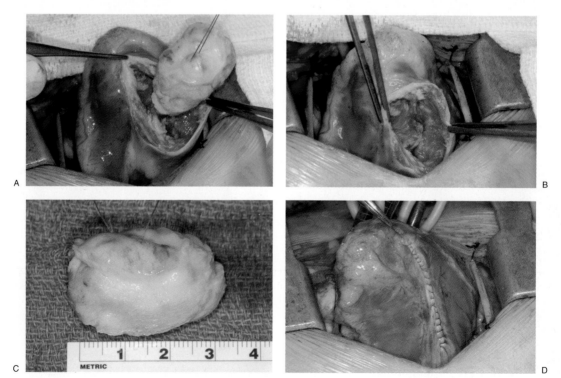

FIGURE 26.9. A–D: Sequential intraoperative photographs during excision of a large fibroma from the left ventricular apex in a 3-year-old child. (Courtesy Dr. Joseph Dearani.)

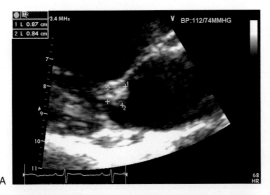

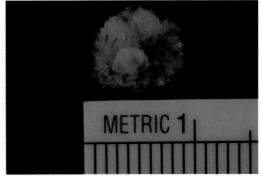

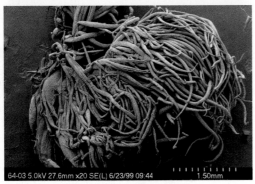

FIGURE 26.12. A papillary fibroelastoma on the atrial surface of the anterior mitral leaflet. A: Parasternal long-axis image. Surgical excision is recommended due to the risk of embolization. **B:** Pathologic specimen of a papillary fibroelastoma that had been removed from the anterior leaflet of the mitral valve in an adult patient. **C:** Electron micrograph of a papillary fibromoelastoma with multiple fronds resembling a sea anemone.

VASCULAR MALFORMATION ("HEMANGIOMA")

Vascular malformations of the heart (incorrectly referred to as "hemangiomas") usually are single and can occur on the epicardium or within the myocardium or can be intracavitary in location. Often they are polypoid or sessile and have central areas of necrosis or calcification. They may be associated with a nonbloody pericardial effusion.

PAPILLARY FIBROELASTOMA

In adults, papillary fibroelastoma is the third most common cardiac tumor. They usually are single, small (less than 1.5 cm) and echocardiographically have a dense central core with a shimmering appearance (Fig. 26.12A). Pathologic specimens demonstrate fronds and have been likened to sea anemones (Figs. 26.12B, C). They occur most frequently on the aortic (Fig. 26.13) and mitral valves. Most patients are asymptomatic but papillary fibroelastomas can be associated with embolization and resultant stroke, angina, and sudden death. Therefore, surgical excision is recommended.

PHEOCHROMOCYTOMA

Primary cardiac pheochromocytomas are very rare. These tumors have been reported primarily in women, and they have a unique and characteristic location along the atrioventricular groove. They are typically well circumscribed and are intimate with the coronary arteries and receive a coronary blood supply (Fig. 26.14).

MALIGNANT CARDIAC TUMORS

Primary malignant cardiac tumors comprise fewer than 10% of cardiac tumors in children. The most common is angiosarcoma, which

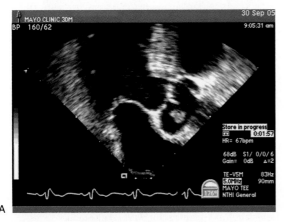

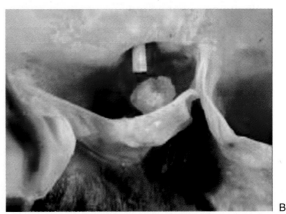

FIGURE 26.13. A large papillary fibroelastoma on the aortic surface of the valve. A: Transesophageal echocardiographic image of the aortic valve in longitudinal projection. **B:** Pathologic specimen demonstrating a papillary fibroelastoma attached to an aortic valve cusp.

FIGURE 26.14. Large pheochromocytoma in the right atrioventricular groove. Left: Subcostal frontal scan. **Right:** Right coronary artery angiogram demonstrating the vascular tumor (T) adjacent to the proximal coronary artery (RCA) CS, coronary sinus.

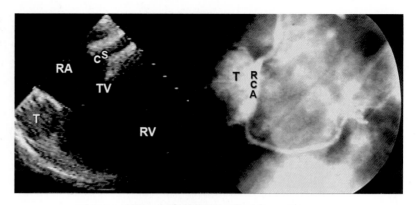

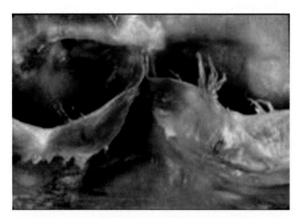

FIGURE 26.15. Pathologic specimen of an aortic valve with Lambl excrescences. These strands of fibrous tissue are typically present on the ventricular side of the semilunar valve cusps and rarely are of any clinical significance. They should not be confused with thrombi or papillary fibroelastomas.

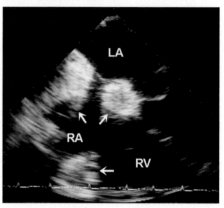

FIGURE 26.16. Lipomatous atrial septum. Transesophageal longitudinal view of the atrial septum demonstrating lipomatous thickening of the superior and inferior limbus (*arrows*) and the lateral tricuspid annulus.

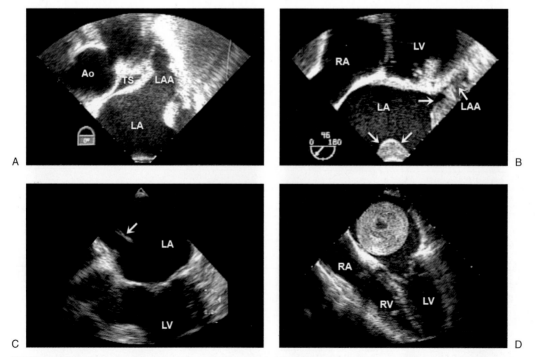

FIGURE 26.17. Masses in the heart that are not tumors. A: Transesophageal echocardiogram at the base of the heart in the short axis projection demonstrating the transverse sinus (TS) between the great arteries and the left atrial appendage (LAA). **B:** Large thrombus layered along the posterior surface of the left atrium (LA) into the LAA. **C:** Transesophageal four-chamber view demonstrating a retained left atrial infusion catheter. **D:** Large circular LA thrombus in a patient with mitral valve stenosis.

can be associated with hemorrhagic pericardial effusion, cardiac tamponade, and obstruction to cardiac venous inflow channels. Other primary malignant cardiac tumors include fibrosarcomas, lymphosarcomas, giant cell sarcomas, fibromyxosarcoma, sarcomas, rhabdomyosarcomas, undifferentiated sarcomas, leiomyosarcomas, and neurogenic sarcoma. The most common types of secondary (metastatic) cardiac tumors in children include non-Hodgkin lymphoma, leukemia, and neuroblastoma.

 INTRACARDIAC "NONTUMORS"

As two-dimensional imaging has advanced over the years and with the introduction of transesophageal echocardiography and intracardiac echocardiography, other unusual structures have been identified in the heart that may be mistaken for tumors. These include Lambl excrescences (Fig. 26.15), usually observed on the ventricular surface of the aortic valve. Lipomatous atrial septum (Fig. 26.16), thrombi, retained foreign bodies, and normal structures such as the transverse sinus may also be mistaken for a cardiac tumor (Fig. 26.17). Before labeling any of these structures as a "tumor," the echocardiographer should communicate with the referring physician regarding the clinical context of such observations.

SUGGESTED READING

Burke A, Jeudy J Jr, Virmani R. Cardiac tumours: an update. *Heart.* 2008; 94:117–123.
Burke A, Virmani R. Pediatric heart tumors. *Cardiovasc Pathol.* 2008;17: 193–198.
Carney JA. Differences between nonfamilial and familial cardiac myxoma. *Am J Surg Pathol.* 1985;9:53–55.

Cho JM, Danielson GK, Puga FJ, et al. Surgical resection of ventricular cardiac fibromas: early and late results. *Ann Thorac Surg.* 2003;76:1929–1934.
Dujardin KS, Click RL, Oh JK. The role of intraoperative transesophageal echocardiography in patients undergoing cardiac mass removal. *J Am Soc Echocardiogr* 2000;13:1080–1083.
Ekmektzoglou KA, Samelis GF, Xanthos T. Heart and tumors: location, metastasis, clinical manifestations, diagnostic approaches and therapeutic considerations. *J Cardiovasc Med.* 2008;9:769–777.
Filho JDF, Lucchese FA, Leaes P, et al. Primary cardiac angiosarcoma. A therapeutic dilemma. *Arq Bras Cardiol.* 2002;78:589–591.
Freedom RM, Lee KJ, Madonald C, et al. Selected aspects of cardiac tumors in infancy and childhood. *Pediat Cardiol.* 2000;21:299–316.
Gowda RM, Khan IA, Nair CK, et al. Cardiac papillary fibroelastoma: a comprehensive analysis of 725 cases. *Am Heart J.* 2003;146:404–410.
Grebenc ML, Rosado-de-Christenson ML, Green CE, et al. Cardiac myxoma: imaging features in 83 patients. *RadioGraphics* 2002;22:673–689.
Klarich KW, Enriquez-Sarano M, Gura G, et al. Papillary fibroelastoma: echocardiographic characteristics for diagnosis and pathologic correlation. *J Am Coll Cardiol.* 1997;30:784–790.
Lam KY, Dickens P, Chan AC. Tumors of the heart. A 20-year experience with a review of 12 485 consecutive autopsies. *Arch Pathol Lab Med.* 1993;117:1207–1031.
Marx G, Moran A. Cardiac tumors, In: Allen HD, Driscoll DJ, Feltes TF, Shaddy RE, eds. *Moss and Adams' Heart disease in infants, children and adolescents.* Philadelphia, PA: Lippincott Williams & Wilkins; 2008:1479–1495.
McCarthy PM, Piehler JM, Schaff HV, et al. The significance of multiple, recurrent, and "complex" cardiac myxomas. *J Thorac Cardiovasc Surg.* 1986;91:389–396.
Pinede L, Duhaut P, Loire R. Clinical presentation of left atrial cardiac myxoma. A series of 112 consecutive cases. *Medicine* 2001;80:150–172.
Reynen K. Frequency of primary tumors of the heart. *Am J Cardiol.* 1996;77:107.
Sallee D, Spector ML, van Heeckeren DW, et al. Primary pediatric cardiac tumors: a 17 year experience. *Cardiol Young.* 1999;9:155–162.
Silverman NA. Primary cardiac tumors. *Ann Surg.* 1980;191:127–138.
Vaughan CJ, Veugelers M, Basson CT. Tumors and the heart: molecular genetic advances. *Curr Opin Cardiol.* 2001;16:195–200.

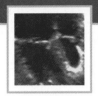

Chapter 27
Evaluation of the Transplanted Heart

William T. Mahle

Heart transplantation is an effective mode of treatment for children with end-stage heart failure. Each year in the United States more than 300 children undergo heart transplantation, of whom 20% are less than 1 year of age. Congenital heart disease is the most common reason for transplantation in infants, whereas cardiomyopathy represents the predominant indication in the school-age child and adolescent. In some young children, heart transplantation is used as the primary treatment for the congenital heart defect. Hypoplastic left heart syndrome (HLHS) and pulmonary atresia with intact ventricular septum are the most common congenital heart lesions treated primarily with heart transplantation. The number of infants with HLHS who are managed with heart transplantation has decreased dramatically in the past 15 years because of improved results with palliative surgery—the Norwood procedure—and a scarcity of donors for infants.

The outcome following pediatric heart transplantation has steadily improved over the past 25 years. The survival rate at 1 year, 5 years, and 10 years after transplantation is 85%, 73%, and 58%, respectively. The major causes of graft failure are coronary allograft vasculopathy, nonspecific graft failure, acute rejection, and malignancy. When the transplanted heart fails, retransplantation may be considered. Retransplantation now accounts for over 7% of heart transplant procedures in children, and this number is increasing annually.

The mainstay of therapy post cardiac transplantation is chronic immunosuppressive therapy. Most centers use calcineurin inhibitors (cyclosporine or tacrolimus) and antimetabolites (azathioprine or mycophenolate mofetil), while corticosteroids may be used either initially or on a chronic basis. More recently, rapamycin inhibitors, such as sirolimus or everolimus, have been incorporated into routine immunosuppression as these agents may be more efficacious in inhibiting the development or progression of coronary allograft vasculopathy (CAV).

ECHOCARDIOGRAPHY IN EVALUATION OF POTENTIAL HEART TRANSPLANT RECIPIENTS

In addition to the physical examination and history, echocardiography plays a fundamental role in the assessment of the child with advanced heart failure. Echocardiography not only quantifies ventricular systolic function but also provides critical hemodynamic information regarding left atrial pressures, right heart function, and valve performance (Table 27.1). Numerous studies have shown that left ventricular (LV) ejection fraction, as assessed by echocardiography, is a predictor of death or need for transplantation in both children and adults. Nonetheless, the correlation of LV ejection fraction is not as strong as a number of other echocardiographic measures. In fact, right heart systolic function appears to be a more important predictor of outcome than left heart function. Right ventricular ejection fraction determined by planimetry has been shown to be valuable in identifying cardiomyopathy patients at greatest risk of adverse outcome. Tissue Doppler imaging, which is less cumbersome than planimetry, has also been found to be valuable in predicting outcome in children with dilated cardiomyopathy. In one study of children with cardiomyopathy, tricuspid annular Ea velocity had the greatest specificity for determining children at greatest risk of adverse events. Left atrial size has been reported to provide additional prognostic value in adults with cardiomyopathy.

It is important to realize that current recommendations regarding the evaluation of the potential transplant recipient do not include echocardiographic measures. Rather advanced symptoms of heart failure, maximal oxygen consumption measured by exercise testing,

nutritional status, and the presence of malignant arrhythmias represent the most common indications for cardiac transplantation. Currently, children with cardiomyopathy or heart failure are not listed for heart transplantation based on echocardiographic measures alone.

For those patients with significant ventricular dysfunction, one should consider the potential role of cardiac resynchronization therapy (CRT). While the exact role of CRT is not fully understood, a number of publications have suggested that a subset of children with ventricular dyssynchrony may benefit from CRT. Current echocardiographic criteria that identify subjects who might benefit from CRT remain a matter of debate. M-mode measures such a delay of the septal to posterior wall systolic motion (greater than 130 ms) or various tissue Doppler indices (TDIs) have been proposed.

When evaluating children with suspected restrictive cardiomyopathy, it is important to exclude constrictive pericardial disease. TDIs have proved to be extremely valuable in distinguishing between these two entities. Importantly, constrictive pericardial disease can be present even in subjects who do not have significant pericardial thickening on other imaging modalities such as CT or MRI.

EVALUATING POTENTIAL DONORS

An important component of achieving a successful heart transplant is the identification of appropriate donors. Refusal to accept a donor heart for transplantation is multifactorial, with LV dysfunction being the most common cause in approximately 25% of cases. Brainstem death is associated with intensive sympathetic nervous system activity with the release of pathophysiologic amounts of catecholamines into the circulation. This sympathetic storm can produce both myocardial ischemia and an intense inflammatory reaction. Altered vascular resistance, a variable volume status, and abnormalities of myocardial wall motion characterize this sympathetic activation.

The best method to assess the donor heart remains controversial. Currently, selection involves a review of the present and past medical history, invasive monitoring of donor heart function with central venous and pulmonary arterial catheters, and direct surgical inspection. Direct surgical inspection may offer the best clinical assessment; however, logistical challenges of organ harvesting limit this options as the primary evaluation of organ suitability. Rather, echocardiography, because of its extensive availability and ability to comprehensively evaluate donor heart performance, should serve as the primary modality to determine the adequacy of the potential donor heart.

LV dysfunction is a common finding in patients with neurologic injury and brainstem death. Global or regional LV dysfunction is identified in approximately 20% of patients with subarachnoid hemorrhage. Regional wall motion abnormalities often occur in the absence of coronary artery disease. Apical LV function is often preserved despite the presence of other regional abnormalities. LV dysfunction documented on echocardiography in donors with brainstem death does not appear to correlate with any demonstrable pathologic abnormality at postmortem evaluation. In addition, it has been shown that donor hearts with mild abnormalities in LV function can be successfully transplanted. Even donor hearts with more significant regional wall abnormalities may improve immediately post-transplantation.

There are less data regarding evaluation of donor hearts in children. In one study of urgent cardiac transplantation in critically ill pediatric recipients, the use of donor hearts despite the presence of mild LV dysfunction and mitral regurgitation did not result in increased mortality or the need for additional inotropic support compared to donor organs with normal function. In this

Table 27.1	ECHOCARDIOGRAPHIC ASSESSMENT OF POTENTIAL HEART TRANSPLANT CANDIDATES	
	Area of Interest	**Key Point**
Congenital heart surgery (repair or palliation)	Residual lesions	Additional surgery or transcatheter intervention may improve hemo-dynamics and avoid need for transplantation.
Valve function	Valve regurgitation	Mitral regurgitation may be secondary to ventricular remodeling; outcomes for surgical repair of mitral regurgitation in primary myopathy are poor.
Chamber dimensions	LV dimensions, left atrial size	Higher LVEDD Z-score is associated with poorer outcome.
Ventricular systolic function	LV ejection fraction or shortening fraction (M-mode, 2D)	Correlated with risk of death while awaiting transplant.
Ventricular dyssynchrony	Various measures from M-mode, tissue Doppler	Cardiac resynchronization therapy may benefit subset of children with advanced heart failure.
Right heart function	RV fractional area change, TDI of tricuspid annulus	Strong predictor of clinical deterioration.
Right heart pressure	Tricuspid regurgitation or pulmonary regurgitation velocity	Assessment of pulmonary artery pressure is important in transplant evaluation (risk and timing of listing).
Restrictive cardiomyopathy versus constrictive pericardial disease	Tissue Doppler Imaging	Children with constrictive pericardial disease can be treated without transplantation.

2D, two-dimensional; LV, left ventricular; LVEDD, left ventricular end-diastolic dimension; RV, right ventricular; TDI, tissue Doppler imaging.

study LV function was normal on echocardiography at 30 days post-transplantation. Clearly, the presence of regional wall abnormalities in a young donor is likely to be of less significance than those found in an older donor in whom the likelihood of ischemic heart disease is greater.

Tissue Doppler imaging (TDI) has also been proposed as a valuable adjunct in the assessment of potential donors. In particular isovolumic acceleration, which is thought to be load independent, has been proposed as a method to discriminate suitability of a marginal donor heart.

Transthoracic echocardiography is often limited. In the evaluation of the potential adolescent or adult donor. In such cases, transesophageal echocardiography (TEE) may be useful. While it should be recognized that TEE is seldom needed in the evaluation of younger children, it may be required in adolescents. Moreover, adolescents may receive organs from adult donors.

EVALUATION OF THE HEART IMMEDIATELY FOLLOWING HEART TRANSPLANTATION

The surgical technique of orthotopic heart transplantation is well established, and complications related to the surgical procedure are uncommon in experienced centers. Potential complications can occur at the anastomotic site of the great vessels resulting in either supravalvar pulmonary stenosis or supravalvar aortic stenosis. There are two techniques to anastomose the donor heart. The traditional biatrial surgical approach involves anastomosis to retained cuffs of the recipient's left and right atria. This technique seldom results in obstruction to venous inflow. However, on echocardiography one appreciates the enlarged atria because of redundant atrial tissue. More recent investigators have advocated a bicaval technique. The latter approach involves anastomosis of the donor heart to the superior and inferior venae cavae and to a small left atrial cuff corresponding to the orifices of the pulmonary veins (Fig. 27.1). When a bicaval anastomosis is performed, stenosis of the superior vena cava may occur—although this is relatively rare. Lastly, on rare occasions, the native heart may be left in situ and the donor heart is placed in the thorax next to the native heart. This is termed a "heterotopic" heart transplant. The heterotopic approach can be used in patients with elevated pulmonary vascular resistance. While the surgical anastomosis is technically more challenging, this approach could allow cardiac transplantation in the child with moderately elevated pulmonary vascular resistance who might otherwise not be an acceptable candidate for orthotopic heart transplantation.

Postsurgical complications occur more commonly in patients with prior congenital heart disease, which represents more than 40% of all pediatric heart transplants. Some patients have not undergone prior surgery, but they may have significant vascular abnormalities, including aortic arch hypoplasia, pulmonary artery anomalies, or venous anomalies. These congenital defects may require additional surgical procedures or significant modifications to the surgical technique that require careful evaluation on postoperative echocardiographic studies. Up to 20% of those who undergo infant heart transplantation develop significant recoarctation. A growing number of heart transplant recipients have congenital heart disease and have undergone prior cardiac surgeries. In some cases, these prior procedures may include complex venous baffles as in the Senning or Fontan procedures. In such cases, the surgeon may undertake a more complex reconstruction at the time of cardiac transplantation with particular attention paid to the systemic venous connections and pulmonary arteries.

The primary role for echocardiography in the immediate post-transplantation period is to provide a comprehensive assessment of graft function and hemodynamics. In this timeframe, transient graft dysfunction is common. The reasons for graft dysfunction are many and include prolonged ischemic time. In addition, it is

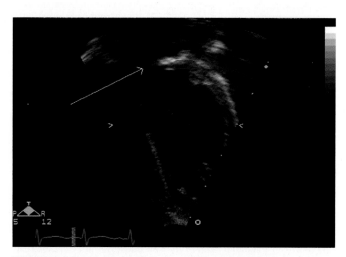

FIGURE 27.1. Apical four-chamber image demonstrating left atrial suture line in bicaval anastomosis.

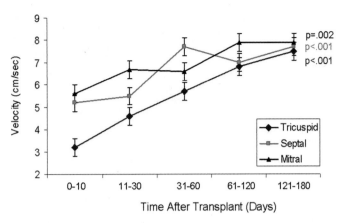

FIGURE 27.2. Changes in tricuspid annular tissue Doppler imaging velocities following heart transplantation. Note gradual improvement of these velocities on serial evaluation.

not uncommon for heart transplant recipients to have elevations in pulmonary vascular resistance because of longstanding heart failure or as a consequence of congenital heart disease. The right ventricle of the donor heart may be unable to adapt to this elevation of pulmonary vascular resistance in this setting. Therefore, assessment of right heart function is vital in the immediate post-transplant period. This comprehensive noninvasive assessment should include an estimate of right heart pressure from spectral Doppler tracings. Semiquantitative evaluation of right ventricular ejection fraction can also be derived via other methods, including planimetry. More recently, tissue Doppler imaging has been used to evaluate right heart function. It is important to realize that tissue Doppler velocities are decreased in children following cardiac transplantation. A recent study reported a gradual increase in tricuspid annular TDI velocities from the time of initial transplantation to 6-month follow-up (Fig. 27.2). However, even at inter-mediate-term follow-up, these velocities were less than those for age-matched controls.

Early graft failure occurs in less than 5% of heart transplants. Early graft failure can be the result of poor protection of the donor organ, a marginal donor heart, early humoral or cellular rejection, or, rarely, hyperacute rejection. Assessment of graft function using a variety of techniques such as M-mode, two-dimensional imaging, and tissue Doppler can provide important prognostic information.

An increase in LV mass also occurs soon after transplantation. In adults the mean LV mass is 35% greater than that in age-matched controls. There are several potential factors that lead to an increase in LV mass, including transient myocardial injury, denervation, and hypertension. One study suggested that hypertension was the factor most strongly associated with LV hypertrophy. Interestingly, significant LV hypertrophy has been identified in other solid-organ recipients. There are reports that this hypertrophy resolves when the immunosuppressant regimens are modified. In infants, it is not uncommon to see ventricular hypertrophy that may mimics hyper-trophic cardiomyopathy. Hypertrophy is often most prominent in the ventricular septum and may predispose to an outflow gradient. This phenomenon occurs in most cases after a child receives a heart from a relatively large donor. The ratio of weight of the donor to that of the recipient can be as high as 3:1. As such, the end-diastolic volume and relative wall thicknesses are increased. In such cases, the wall thickness–to–cavity ratio normalizes over the course of several months.

 ## ASSESSMENT FOR REJECTION

One of the greatest concerns following heart transplantation is the development of rejection. Rejection may be T-cell mediated (cellu-lar) or B-cell mediated (humoral). The diagnosis of rejection rests on pathologic examination of myocardial tissue that is typically obtained from right heart endomyocardial biopsy. This technique

is expensive and invasive and has the risk of complications such as myocardial perforation and arrhythmias.

There has been a longstanding interest in developing noninva-sive techniques to identify rejection. Beginning with the introduc-tion of M-mode technology, investigators have proposed that various echocardiographic techniques could reduce or eliminate the need for invasive surveillance biopsies following cardiac transplantation. To date, most of these studies have suggested that echocardiography is not sufficiently sensitive and/or does not identify cardiac rejec-tion. One of the clear limitations of these studies relates to the lack of precision of the gold standard pathologic grading. The current International Society for Heart and Lung Transplantation (ISHLT) grading system consists of four grades: 0, 1R, 2R, and 3R with only the latter two grades being clinically significant. One recent study suggested significant discrepancies exist when comparing biopsy grading between local hospital pathologists and those pathologists at a study core center (interobserver correlation = 0.77). Therefore, it should not come as a surprise that echocardiographic measures have relatively poor agreement with pathologic interpretation of endomyocardial biopsies. Nonetheless, it is important to understand how various echocardiographic techniques compare to the ISHLT grading system and to consider what role echocardiography has in routine surveillance.

Endomyocardial biopsy is commonly performed under fluoros-copy guidance in the cardiac catheterization laboratory. However, this procedure exposes the patient to radiation and may involve trans-porting a critically ill patient from the intensive care unit. Therefore, echocardiography has increasingly been used to guide both bedside and outpatient endomyocardial biopsies. Reported biopsy success rates of greater than 95% without the need for fluoroscopic guidance have been reported using a transthoracic two-dimensional approach. Real-time three-dimensional echocardiography may offer improved guidance compared to two-dimensional imaging (Fig. 27.3). To date, most published studies evaluating three-dimensional echocardiogra-phy have used this technique as an adjunct to fluoroscopy. No ran-domized trials using the two approaches to compare incidence of tricuspid valve injury and sufficiency of myocardial specimens have been performed to date.

While acute adverse events are uncommon following endo-myocardial biopsy, significant tricuspid regurgitation occurs in up to 30% of patients. Tricuspid valve surgery, either annuloplasty or valve replacement, is the most common indication for heart surgery among heart transplant recipients. The bioptome may compromise tricuspid valve function in several ways, including leaflet perfora-tion, disruption of the chordae tendinae, or injury to the papillary muscles. Identification of the mechanism of injury by echocardio-graphy can aid in planning potential surgical intervention. The deci-sion to surgically intervene is determined by right atrial and right ventricular size, right heart pressures, and associated symptoms.

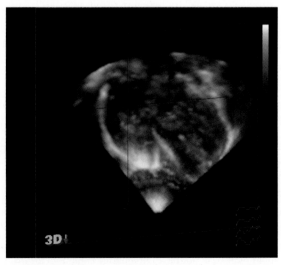

FIGURE 27.3. Still image of bioptome in right ventricle.

It is important to recognize that tricuspid regurgitation may occur less commonly as a result of myocardial ischemia secondary to CAV. This possibility needs to be evaluated before proceeding with surgical intervention.

ACUTE REJECTION

Acute cellular rejection is characterized by lymphocyte infiltration, myocardial inflammation, and eventually myocardial necrosis in severe cases. Acute rejection results in myocardial edema and impairment in myocyte function, which are manifest by myocardial thickening, pericardial effusion, and compromised systolic and diastolic ventricular function. Diastolic dysfunction with restrictive physiology may precede overt systolic compromise. M-mode measurements of ventricular thickness and ventricular contractility provide important insights into the rejection process. However, there are limitations of using M-mode–derived LVEF to identify rejection, including its load-dependent nature. A number of investigators have attempted to enhance the capabilities of M-mode by offline analysis of digitized tracings to evaluate a number of additional variables, including wall motion in systole and diastole. This offline technique combines these various measures into a single score that can be used to predict the likelihood of cellular rejection. However, the proprietary software and the need for postprocessing have limited its widespread use. Boucek and colleagues, who developed the methodology, subsequently proposed a modified scoring system termed "Echo B" to improve specificity. However, this strategy has not been widely accepted to date.

One of the important considerations in using M-mode, or any other echocardiographic technique, is to define a reference range. Numerous investigators have suggested cutoffs to distinguish those children at increased risk of rejection from the rest of the pediatric heart transplant population. However, many studies have suggested that to detect heart transplant rejection, it may be better to use the patient as his or her own control. Therefore, a child would be considered at risk for rejection not when the LV mass reached a population-defined threshold but rather when LV mass increased significantly compared to previous studies. Recent studies have demonstrated that population variability among all echo parameters is substantial. Intrapatient variability of measures such as TDI values, velocity of circumferential fiber shortening (VCFc), and mitral inflow velocities are comparatively small, suggesting that serial comparison is of greater clinical value than adherence to population norms.

More than 20 separate echocardiographic variables have been proposed to assay for cardiac rejection. Those measures that have been studied in children are reported in Table 27.2. While it is not practical for any single echocardiography laboratory to use all of these techniques, it is important to devise an echo-based surveillance strategy that measures both systolic and diastolic function and that can be performed and interpreted in a reproducible manner. Among these methodologies, automatic border detection (ABD) theoretically provides some particular advantages over conventional M-mode techniques. ABD provides real-time assessment of ventricular area. Moreover, proprietary software programs provide measures of peak filling rate. One study from Kimball and colleagues identified several ABD-derived variables that correlated to biopsy-proved rejection in children. The percentage of total ventricular filling during diastasis increased significantly during rejection (10% ± 6% versus 15% ± 8%, $p = .02$), and the percentage of filling during the rapid filling phase decreased during rejection (82% ± 8% versus 77% ± 11%, $p = .08$). Analyzing adult heart transplant recipients, Moidl et al. reported that a decline in peak filling rate of 18% or greater from baseline had high sensitivity and specificity in detecting rejection.

Spectral Doppler techniques have been applied to the transplant population as well. Based on the belief that abnormalities in ventricular relaxation precede the development of systolic dysfunction, a number of investigators have proposed that Doppler-derived measures of relaxation are best suited to identify cardiac rejection. LV isovolumic relaxation time and mitral valve pressure half-time can be determined by using the mitral inflow and LV outflow spectral tracings. Several studies have suggested that isovolumic relaxation time and mitral valve pressure half-time are statistically associated with biopsy-proved rejection. However, the additive value of these measurements is limited and sensitivity is not sufficient to replace surveillance biopsy. A more recent methodology has been to use a global measure of ventricular function based on spectral Doppler measurement. The myocardial performance index has been proposed a simple measure that can identify rejection in a significant proportion of those with rejection. However, other investigators have suggested that this measure has marginal sensitivity.

TDI has become integrated into the routine echocardiographic examination of children and adults. TDI derives measurements of contraction and relaxation velocities directly from the myocardium and has been proposed as a more robust method to detect transplant rejection of adults undergoing endomyocardial biopsy for suspected rejection. Dandel and colleagues reported that TDI-derived early relaxation velocities had sufficient sensitivity and negative predictive values, 90% and 96%, respectively, to limit the need for surveillance biopsies. Similarly, these investigators suggested that relaxation time derived by TDI also showed a strong sensitivity for identifying biopsy-proved rejection. Systolic TDI velocities had poor sensitivity and specificity for identifying rejection. In this study, a positive finding was defined as a change of greater than 10% from baseline in myocardial velocities or time intervals. This was proposed as a more valuable measure than specific myocardial velocity cutoff values that might be applied to the entire transplant population. In fact, other investigators who have attempted to identify myocardial velocity thresholds for detecting rejection have found a relatively low sensitivity. Mankad and colleagues, however, did report that mitral annular velocity of greater than 135 mm/s had a high sensitivity and negative-predictive value for detecting rejection (93% and 98%, respectively).

Less is known about the utility of TDI to identify rejection in children following transplantation. One study suggested that because wall motion abnormalities are common in transplant recipients, TDI may have a limited role to identify rejection (Fig. 27.4). Pauliks and colleagues reported that transplanted hearts have decreased myocardial longitudinal velocities relative to radial velocities but that this myocardial pattern varied significantly from patient to patient and may be related to a unique process of "untwisting" of LV fibers in diastole in the transplanted heart. Many of these factors have led investigators to suggest that TDI velocities cannot be used to supplant surveillance biopsies. While it is true that depressed TDI velocities are commonly seen in both systole and diastole in rejection episodes, there are a number of other processes that can also produce this pattern including coronary artery disease and cardiac infection. Isovolumic acceleration (IVA) does appear to be a more robust method to identify rejection. IVA is the peak isovolumic contraction wave velocity divided by the acceleration time. Accurate calculation of IVA requires a clear TDI tracing and offline calculation, but the process is not so cumbersome as to preclude clinical usefulness.

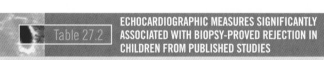

ECHOCARDIOGRAPHIC MEASURES SIGNIFICANTLY ASSOCIATED WITH BIOPSY-PROVED REJECTION IN CHILDREN FROM PUBLISHED STUDIES
Measure
LV contractility (fractional shortening)
Velocity of circumferential fiber contractility
LV posterior wall diastolic thinning
LV mass
Mitral valve pressure half-time
Mitral valve spectral E velocity
Isovolumic relaxation time
Automatic border detection (% ventricular filling during diastasis)
Myocardial performance index
Mitral valve propagation velocity
Tissue Doppler S velocity
Tissue Doppler E velocity

LV, left ventricular.

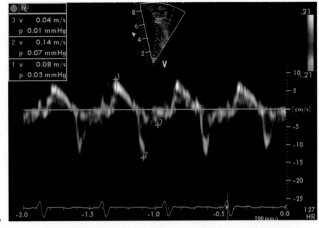
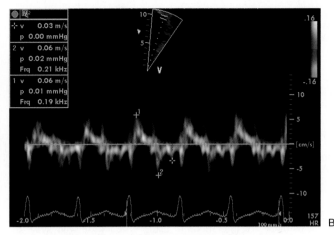

FIGURE 27.4. Tissue Doppler imaging velocities at lateral mitral valve annulus in transplant patient when clinically well (A) and with evidence of rejection (B). Note depression in both systolic and diastolic velocities.

Identification of rejection by echocardiography remains a major challenge. There is considerable overlap in echocardiographic measures of systolic and diastolic dysfunction in subjects with and without rejection. The published literature supports serial comparison of echocardiographic measurements as more valuable than comparisons of data from the entire transplant population. Moreover, given the advances in digital archiving and review, it is now quite feasible to compare current and prior studies in a side-by-side fashion to assess for qualitative and quantitative changes in myocardial function.

IDENTIFICATION OF CORONARY ALLOGRAFT VASCULOPATHY

The most common cause of graft failure and patient death following pediatric heart transplantation is CAV. CAV is characterized by diffuse intimal thickening and narrowing of the vessel lumen and has traditionally been diagnosed with annual coronary angiography. CAV is often considered severe when the lumen of a major coronary artery has greater than 50% occlusion. While coronary angiography is well suited to identify advanced CAV, it has limited sensitivity to detect the early process of CAV. Detecting CAV in the early phase is of significant clinical importance because it allows changes in the immunosuppression regimen once it has been identified. In this setting, rapamycin, a novel immunosuppressant, may be introduced because of its reported ability to halt or reverse CAV in some series. In addition, it is important to realize that the outcome of patients identified with CAV varies considerably. Noninvasive methods to both identify and predict the outcome of CAV can contribute to improved outcome in children who have undergone heart transplantation.

Intravascular ultrasound (IVUS) is now widely used in adults with coronary artery disease as well as adults who have undergone heart transplantation. IVUS provides circumferential cross-sectional tomographic images of coronary vessel (Fig. 27.5), enabling detection of early CAV, including intimal thickening and lipid deposition within the media. However, IVUS is expensive and highly operator dependent and requires advanced experience. To date, a number of published series have reported that IVUS can be safely performed in young children and can identify CAV not evident on coronary angiography. Nonetheless, IVUS is currently used in a minority of pediatric transplant centers.

Stress echocardiography has been found to have a strong correlation with angiographic CAV. More importantly, there are data to suggest that even in the absence of angiographic CAV, stress echocardiography can identify heart transplant patients at greatest risk of death or graft failure. It is likely that many "false-positive" stress echocardiography studies may actively identify early CAV because of its diffuse and microvascular nature, which may not be detected by angiography.

A number of pediatric centers have explored the potential role of stress echocardiography in the evaluation of CAV. Di Filippo examined 18 pediatric heart transplant patients and found that subjects with a normal dobutamine stress echocardiogram (DSE) were free of CAV on coronary angiography. Larsen and colleagues found that DSE could identify subjects at increased risk of coronary-related events. This study reported a sensitivity and specificity of 72% and 80%, respectively, for the identification of CAV at angiography. However, stress echocardiography has not gained widespread use in pediatric centers because of limited experience with this modality.

Doppler echocardiography has also been helpful to identify decreased myocardial function associated with CAV. The majority of patients with CAV have elevated LV filling pressure. This restrictive process usually precedes impairment in systolic function. Therefore, noninvasive methods that evaluate for the presence of CAV must include a measure of both diastolic and systolic function. TDI has been proposed as an important method to assess ventricular performance in patients with suspected CAV. Fyfe and colleagues reported that decreased TDI velocities were predictive of death or need for retransplantation within 6 months (Fig. 27.6). Importantly, decreased TDI velocities, both systolic and early diastolic, at the lateral tricuspid annulus appeared to precede similar changes in mitral annular velocities. This TDI pattern is important and may facilitate identification of the high-risk patient and allow sufficient time to plan cardiac retransplantation.

SUMMARY

Heart transplantation is the definitive therapy for advanced heart failure in children. Echocardiography plays a major role in the

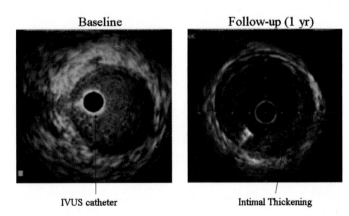

FIGURE 27.5. Intravascular ultrasound (IVUS) of the left main coronary artery at baseline and at follow-up. Intimal thickening, the hallmark of CAV, is shown.

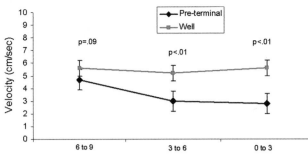

A

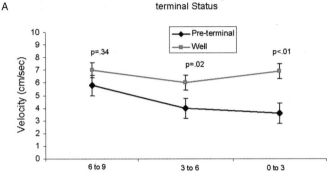

B

FIGURE 27.6. Tissue Doppler imaging (TDI) velocities. A: TDI systolic velocities in children who have undergone heart transplantation. The majority (n = 45) were clinically "well"; 8 children developed progressive heart failure as a result of coronary allograft vasculopathy leading to death or retransplantation "preterminal." **B:** TDI early diastolic velocities (Em) in children who have undergone heart transplantation, comparing clinically "well" to "preterminal." (Adapted from Fyfe DA, Ketchum D, Lewis R, et al. Tissue Doppler imaging detects severely abnormal myocardial velocities that identify children with pre-terminal cardiac graft failure after heart transplantation. *J Heart Lung Transplant.* 2006;5:510–517.)

selection of potential recipients and donors and is also vital to the management of the child following heart transplantation. The major role of echocardiography is in surveillance for cardiac rejection and assessment of potential graft dysfunction secondary to CAV. Novel methods such as tissue Doppler imaging are likely to favorably affect patient outcome following heart transplantation.

SUGGESTED READING

Aggarwal M, Drachenberg C, Douglass L, et al. The efficacy of real-time 3-dimensional echocardiography for right ventricular biopsy. *J Am Soc Echocardiogr.* 2005;18:1208–1212.

Asante-Korang A, Fickey M, Boucek MM, et al. Diastolic performance assessed by tissue Doppler after pediatric heart transplantation. *J Heart Lung Transplant.* 2004;23:865–872.

Boucek MM, Mathis CM, Kanakriyeh MS, et al. Donor shortage: use of the dysfunctional donor heart. *J Heart Lung Transplant.* 1993;12(6 Pt 2):S186–S190.

Boucek MM, Mathis CM, Kanakriyeh MS, et al. Serial echocardiographic evaluation of cardiac graft rejection after infant heart transplantation. *J Heart Lung Transplant.* 1993;12:824–831.

Canter CE, Shaddy RE, Bernstein D, et al. Indications for heart transplantation in pediatric heart disease: a scientific statement from the American Heart Association Council on Cardiovascular Disease in the Young; the Councils on Clinical Cardiology, Cardiovascular Nursing, and Cardiovascular Surgery and Anesthesia; and the Quality of Care and Outcomes Research Interdisciplinary Working Group. *Circulation.* 2007;115:658–676.

Cheung MM, Redington AN. Assessment of myocardial ventricular function in donor hearts: is isovolumic acceleration measured by tissue Doppler the Holy Grail? *J Heart Lung Transplant.* 2004;23(9 Suppl):S253–S256.

Costello JM, Wax DF, Binns HJ, et al. A comparison of intravascular ultrasound with coronary angiography for evaluation of transplant coronary disease in pediatric heart transplant recipients. *J Heart Lung Transplant.* 2003;22:44–49.

Dandel M, Hummel M, Muller J, et al. Reliability of tissue Doppler wall motion monitoring after heart transplantation for replacement of invasive routine screenings by optimally timed cardiac biopsies and catheterizations. *Circulation.* 2001;104(12 Suppl 1):I184–I191.

Di Filippo S, Semiond B, Roriz R, et al. Non-invasive detection of coronary artery disease by dobutamine-stress echocardiography in children after heart transplantation. *J Heart Lung Transplant.* 2003;22:876–882.

Fyfe DA, Ketchum D, Lewis R, et al. Tissue Doppler imaging detects severely abnormal myocardial velocities that identify children with pre-terminal cardiac graft failure after heart transplantation. *J Heart Lung Transplant.* 2006;5:510–517.

Kuhn MA, Jutzy KR, Deming DD, et al. The medium-term findings in coronary arteries by intravascular ultrasound in infants and children after heart transplantation. *J Am Coll Cardiol.* 2000;36:250–254.

Larsen RL, Applegate PM, Dyar DA, et al. Dobutamine stress echocardiography for assessing coronary artery disease after transplantation in children. *J Am Coll Cardiol.* 1998;2:515–520.

Mahle WT, Cardis BM, Ketchum D, et al. Reduction in initial ventricular systolic and diastolic velocities after heart transplantation in children: improvement over time identified by tissue Doppler imaging. *J Heart Lung Transplant.* 2006;25:1290–1296.

Mankad S, Murali S, Kormos RL, et al. Evaluation of the potential role of color-coded tissue Doppler echocardiography in the detection of allograft rejection in heart transplant recipients. *Am Heart J.* 1999;138(4 Pt 1):721–730.

McMahon CJ, Nagueh SF, Eapen RS, et al. Echocardiographic predictors of adverse clinical events in children with dilated cardiomyopathy: a prospective-clinical study. *Heart.* 2004;90:908–915.

Mouly-Bandini A, Vion-Dury J, Viout P, et al. Value of Doppler echocardiography in the detection of low-grade rejections after cardiac transplantation. *Transpl Int.* 1996;9:131–136.

Palka P, Lange A, Galbraith A, et al. The role of left and right ventricular early diastolic Doppler tissue echocardiographic indices in the evaluation of acute rejection in orthotopic heart transplant. *J Am Soc Echocardiogr.* 2005;18:107–115.

Pauliks LB, Pietra BA, DeGroff CG, et al. Non-invasive detection of acute allograft rejection in children by tissue Doppler imaging: myocardial velocities and myocardial acceleration during isovolumic contraction. *J Heart Lung Transplant.* 2005;24(7 suppl):S239–S248.

Pauliks LB, Pietra BA, Kirby S, et al. Altered ventricular mechanics in cardiac allografts: a tissue Doppler study in 30 children without prior rejection events. *J Heart Lung Transplant.* 2005;24:1804–1813.

Prakash A, Printz BF, Lamour JM, et al. Myocardial performance index in pediatric patients after cardiac transplantation. *J Am Soc Echocardiogr.* 2004;17:439–442.

Shirali GS, Cephus CE, Kuhn MA, et al. Posttransplant recoarctation of the aorta: a twelve year experience. *J Am Coll Cardiol.* 1998;32:509–514.

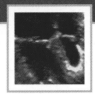

Chapter 28
Pulmonary Hypertension

Peter Bartz • Stuart Berger

PULMONARY HYPERTENSION DEFINITION

Pulmonary hypertension is defined as an elevation in pulmonary artery pressure, with pulmonary artery mean pressure greater than 25 mm Hg at rest and/or greater than 30 mm Hg with exercise. This classic definition applies to both adults and children. There are multiple etiologies of pulmonary hypertension. Many of these causes are much more common in the adult population. Table 28.1 presents the WHO classification scheme for pulmonary hypertension.

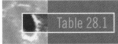

Table 28.1	WHO CLASSIFICATION SCHEME FOR PULMONARY HYPERTENSION

Class 1: Pulmonary artery hypertension

1.1   Idiopathic pulmonary hypertension

1.2   Familial pulmonary hypertension

1.3   Pulmonary hypertension associated with

    a. Collagen vascular disease

    b. Congenital heart disease with left-to-right shunt

    c. Portal hypertension

    d. HIV disease

    e. Drugs: anorexigens or other toxins

    f. Thyroid disorders

    g. Other entities: Gaucher disease, hereditary hemorrhagic telangectasia, hemoglobinopathies

1.4   Persistent pulmonary hypertension of the newborn

1.5   Pulmonary venoocclusive disease

Class 2: Pulmonary hypertension with left heart disease

2.1   Left atrial or left ventricular disease

2.2   Left-sided valvular disease

Class 3: Pulmonary hypertension associated with respiratory disorders or hypoxemia

3.1   Chronic obstructive lung disease

3.2   Interstitial lung disease

3.3   Sleep-disordered breathing

3.4   Alveolar hypoventilation

3.5   Chronic exposure to high altitude

3.6   Neonatal lung disease

3.7   Alveolar-capillary dysplasia

3.8   Other

Class 4: Pulmonary hypertension caused by chronic thrombotic/ embolic disease

4.1   Thrombotic obstruction of proximal pulmonary arteries

4.2   Obstruction of distal pulmonary arteries

    Pulmonary embolism (thrombus, tumor, parasites)

    In situ thrombosis

Class 5: Miscellaneous (e.g., sarcoid)

CLINICAL PRESENTATION

The symptoms associated with pulmonary hypertension in children are variable with symptomatology depending on the etiology and severity of disease as well as the age of the patient. At critical levels of pulmonary artery hypertension, symptoms may be attributed to low cardiac output. Although these symptoms may be nonspecific, they are likely to be significant and may include poor appetite and poor growth in infants, while older children may present with nausea, vomiting, activity intolerance, lethargy, or overt syncope.

INCIDENCE

The true incidence of pulmonary hypertension is not entirely clear. In recent years, the diagnosis has become more common—most likely because of a greater awareness of the disease. This is likely associated with a better understanding of the classification and underlying pathophysiology, as well as better diagnostic modalities such as echocardiography. It does appear that the frequency of disease may vary by gender, perhaps more so in adults than in children. The gender ratio in adult women is 1.7:1 compared to men, but some have suggested an equal ratio in females and males before adolescence. The relatively newly recognized entity of familial pulmonary hypertension comprises anywhere from 6% to 12% of cases of "idiopathic" pulmonary hypertension. It has been suggested that the mode of inheritance is autosomal dominant with incomplete penetrance. In addition, a gene for familial idiopathic pulmonary hypertension has been identified on chromosome 2q33. This gene is also believed to cause defects in bone morphogenetic protein receptor 2 (*BMPR-2*) and may lead to abnormalities in vascular smooth muscle, including uncontrolled proliferation. Genetic screening for *BMPR-2* is available and is recommended for first-degree relatives of patients with idiopathic pulmonary hypertension.

CLINICAL EVALUATION

The clinical evaluation of pulmonary hypertension should be directed at determining the etiology of the disease, as well as the severity of disease, and should establish a baseline for clinical follow-up. Table 28.2 lists studies that are important in the evaluations of the patient with newly diagnosed or suspected pulmonary hypertension. Echocardiography and its clinical utility will be discussed in great detail.

Noninvasive assessment of pulmonary arterial pressure is a routine component of a comprehensive echocardiographic evaluation. The two-dimensional scan can suggest an elevation in right-sided pressures. Doppler is used both to confirm the presence of pulmonary hypertension and quantify its severity. As a result, the echocardiogram plays a pivotal role in the diagnosis, identification, and treatment of pulmonary hypertension.

TWO-DIMENSIONAL ECHOCARDIOGRAPHY

Severe pulmonary hypertension can often be recognizable by routine two-dimensional echocardiography. In the normal heart, parasternal short-axis imaging demonstrates a circular left ventricle. Because normal left ventricular pressure is greater than right ventricular pressure, the septal curvature is convex toward the right ventricle and concave toward the left ventricle. During ventricular systole, the septum moves toward the center of the left ventricle. The septum retains its convex curvature toward the right ventricle

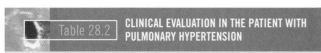

Table 28.2 CLINICAL EVALUATION IN THE PATIENT WITH PULMONARY HYPERTENSION

Chest radiograph

Electrocardiogram

Echocardiogram

Cardiac catheterization with acute vasodilator testing

Complete blood count

Urinalysis

Liver studies

- Liver function studies
- Hepatitis profile
- Abdominal ultrasound

Collagen vascular studies

- Antinuclear antibody
- Rheumatoid factor
- Erythrocyte sedimentation rate
- C-reactive protein
- Complement studies

Lung studies

- Pulmonary function studies with appropriate parameters to rule out COPD
- Sleep study with pulse oximetry
- Ventilation perfusion scan
- Lung biopsy
- CT scan to rule out pulmonary embolic disease

HIV studies

Thyroid function studies

Coagulation workup

Stress test and/or 6-minute walk distance

Toxicology studies for stimulants such as cocaine and methamphetamine

Brain natriuretic peptide

and diastolic function may be impaired. Right ventricular systolic dysfunction can be suggested by visual estimates or quantitatively estimated as discussed elsewhere in this text. With all the above, clinical clues and findings may be subtle, particularly with mild or moderate elevation in pulmonary arterial pressures. Therefore, the echocardiographer must maintain a high level of suspicion during image acquisition and interpretation.

Once pulmonary hypertension has been suggested by clinical examination or initial echocardiographic imaging, a comprehensive, detailed examination should be undertaken to evaluate for congenital heart disease that may lead to pulmonary hypertension. The segmental approach using a complete two-dimensional assessment should be carried out with the goal of identifying potential sources of pulmonary hypertension including left-to-right shunts and obstructive lesions. Since many of the two-dimensional echocardiographic features as well as Doppler gradients actually predict right ventricular systolic pressure and not pulmonary artery pressure, one must take particular care to exclude obstructive lesions such as pulmonary stenosis and branch pulmonary artery stenosis (Fig. 28.3). Once right ventricular outflow tract obstruction has been excluded, right ventricular pressure can be considered as a surrogate of pulmonary artery pressure.

Mean pulmonary artery pressure is derived by the product of pulmonary vascular resistance and pulmonary blood flow, which both can be greatly affected by left-to-right intracardiac shunts. Early in the disease course, significant left-to-right shunt lesions result in increased flow to the pulmonary vascular bed. This intracardiac shunt can be found at any level (atrial, ventricular, or great arteries). The increased flow results in increased mean arterial pulmonary pressure. Over time, increased pulmonary flow results in a progressive increase in pulmonary resistance with a concomitant increase in pulmonary artery pressure. As the pulmonary pressure approaches systemic pressure, as a result of either increased flow or resistance, care must be taken to not rely on color Doppler to identify these intracardiac shunts since low velocity shunting is often present because of equalization of systemic and pulmonary arterial pressure.

 DOPPLER ECHOCARDIOGRAPHY

Although qualitative data can be obtained by two-dimensional echocardiography, actual hemodynamic data should be estimated by Doppler echocardiography.

Tricuspid Regurgitation

Tricuspid regurgitation is common in patients with and without pulmonary hypertension. Doppler measurement of tricuspid regurgitation velocity accurately predicts right ventricular systolic pressure in patients with a wide spectrum of both acquired and congenital heart disease. The maximal right ventricular to right atrial systolic velocity via continuous-wave Doppler interrogation of the tricuspid regurgitation jet is used. Typically, the apical

and concave curvature toward the left ventricle throughout the cardiac cycle. Pulmonary hypertension results in right ventricular pressure that may equal or exceed left ventricular pressure, causing septal flattening or a reverse septal curvature during systole. This may result in left ventricular compression, best seen in both parasternal long- and short-axis imaging (Fig. 28.1). The majority of patients with pulmonary hypertension will have significant right ventricular and right atrial dilatation. Right ventricular hypertrophy is also common (Fig. 28.2). Additionally, right ventricular systolic

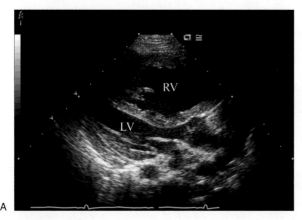
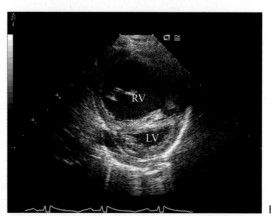

FIGURE 28.1. Severe right ventricular (RV) hypertension resulting in septal flattening and reverse septal curvature bowing toward the left ventricle (LV). Also note the RV dilation and RV hypertrophy. **A:** Parasternal long-axis imaging of severe RV hypertension resulting in compression of the LV. **B:** Parasternal short-axis imaging demonstrating the D-shaped LV.

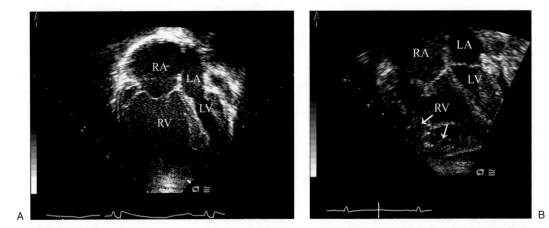

FIGURE 28.2. RV dilation and hypertrophy in pulmonary hypertension. A: Apical four-chamber imaging will typically demonstrate right ventricular (RV) dilation with significant pulmonary hypertension. This may often be the first echocardiographic sign of elevated pulmonary pressures. **B:** Also, with longstanding hypertension, there will be significant RV hypertrophy (*arrows*). RA, right atrium; LV, left ventricle; LA, left atrium.

four-chamber view or parasternal short- and long-axis planes allow for optimal alignment of continuous-wave Doppler using either an imaging or a nonimaging transducer. However, nonstandard "off-axis" views may be needed to achieve optimal alignment with the tricuspid regurgitant jet.

With careful adjustment of the transducer orientation with color Doppler guidance to ensure an optimal incident angle, Doppler echocardiography offers an accurate, noninvasive approach to determining right ventricular systolic pressure (RVSP). Currie et al. confirmed this with simultaneous continuous-wave Doppler echocardiography

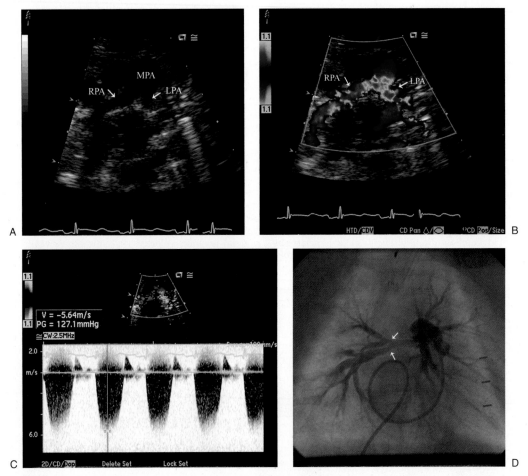

FIGURE 28.3. The presence of severe right ventricular hypertension was suggested by right-to-left shunting through a ventricular septal defect. A: Suprasternal notch imaging revealed bilateral branch pulmonary artery hypoplasia. LPA, left pulmonary artery; MPA, main pulmonary artery; RPA, right pulmonary artery. **B:** Color Doppler imaging demonstrates marked flow acceleration. **C:** confirmed by continuous-wave Doppler interrogation calculating a gradient of 127 mm Hg. The patient was found to have Williams Syndrome. **D:** Angiography demonstrated severe branch pulmonary artery hypoplasia with multiple areas of segmental stenosis (*arrows*).

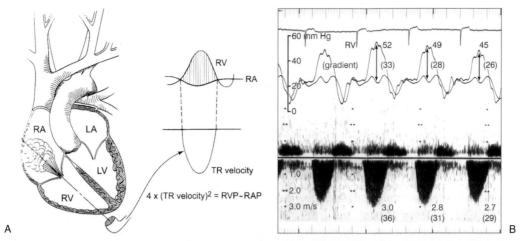

FIGURE 28.4. Quantitation of RV systolic pressure. A: Diagram demonstrating how to measure systolic right ventricular (RV) pressure from the tricuspid regurgitation (TR) continuous-wave Doppler velocity. The peak systolic tricuspid pressure gradient from the RV to the right atrium (RA) is represented by 4(peak TR velocity)^2. Therefore, systolic RV pressure is estimated by adding estimated or measured RA pressure to the pressure derived from the TR velocity. LA, left atrium; LV, left ventricle; RAP, right atrial pressure; RVP, right ventricle pressure. **B:** Simultaneous RV and RA pressure tracings and TR velocity recording by continuous-wave Doppler echocardiography. Pressure gradients (36, 31, and 29 mm Hg, respectively) derived from the peak Doppler velocities of the second, third, and fourth beats (3.0, 2.8, and 2.7 m/s, respectively) are similar to the catheter-derived RV-to-RA gradients (*arrows*, 33, 28, and 26 mm Hg). (From Oh JK, Seward JB, Tajik AJ, eds. *The echo manual.* 3rd ed. Philadelphia: Lippincott Williams & Wilkins. (c) 2006 Mayo Foundation for Medical Education and Research, with permission.)

and invasive right-sided cardiac pressure measurements (Fig. 28.4). The tricuspid regurgitant velocity (TRV) reflects the peak right ventricular–to–right atrial pressure (RA) difference, as stated by the modified Bernoulli equation:

$$RVSP - RA = 4 (TR)^2$$

and

$$RVSP = 4 (TR)^2 + RA$$

Right atrial pressure can be estimated via several techniques. If a central venous catheter is present, direct right atrial pressure measurements can be obtained. The right atrial pressure can be estimated clinically by evaluating the jugular venous distention; however, this is difficult in children and impractical in a busy echocardiography laboratory. Kirchner et al. demonstrated that two-dimensional echocardiographic estimates of right atrial pressure can be obtained by evaluating the inferior vena cava. Subcostal imaging of inferior vena caval collapse within 2 cm of the right atrium correlates with right atrial pressure. Patients with an inspiratory collapse of the inferior vena cava greater than 50% tend to have a right atrial pressure less than 10 mm Hg, while those having less than 50% collapse tend to have right atrial pressure greater than 10 mm Hg. Ommen et al. suggested that a combination of hepatic venous Doppler evaluation in addition to inferior vena cava diameter changes with respiration can further predict right atrial pressure. In adults, if the inferior vena caval diameter is less than 15 mm Hg and the systolic forward flow Doppler velocity is greater than the velocity of atrial reversal in the hepatic vein, an estimated right atrial pressure of 5 mm Hg can be used. Alternately, if the inferior vena cava diameter is greater than 20 mm Hg and systolic forward flow is less than the velocity at atrial reversal, an estimated right atrial pressure of 25 mm Hg can be used. All other patients can be assumed to have a right atrial pressure of 14 mm Hg.

Practically, the importance of accurate right atrial pressure is greatest at intermediate tricuspid regurgitant Doppler velocities. For example, a tricuspid regurgitation velocity of 2.5 m/s with a right atrial pressure of 5 mm Hg results in a calculated systolic pulmonary pressure of 30 mm Hg. However, if the right atrial pressure is 20 mm Hg, the same 2.5 m/s Doppler velocity would estimate a pulmonary pressure of 45 mm Hg. In contrast, if the tricuspid regurgitant velocity is 5 m/s, the error associated with accurate right atrial pressure estimation is of little clinical importance (105 mm Hg versus 120 mm Hg) since both values suggest severe pulmonary hypertension.

Pulmonary Regurgitation

Pulmonary regurgitation is present in many normal individuals as well as in a large percentage of patients with congenital heart disease and nearly all patients with pulmonary hypertension. Pulmonary artery diastolic pressure can be estimated from the end-diastolic velocity of pulmonary regurgitation Doppler signal (Fig. 28.5). At end-diastole, the pulmonary regurgitation end-diastolic velocity (PREDV) jet represents the pressure difference between the pulmonary artery end diastolic pressure and the right ventricular end-diastolic pressure. In the absence of tricuspid stenosis, the right ventricular end-diastolic pressure can be assumed to be equal to right atrial pressure (RAP). Therefore, pulmonary artery end-diastolic pressure (PAEDP) can be estimated using the modified Bernoulli equation:

$$PAEDP = 4 (PREDV)^2 + RAP$$

Underestimation of the pressure gradient by the Doppler method may be caused in part by the inability to align the Doppler angle of interrogation parallel to the direction of the pulmonary regurgitant jet. Therefore, color Doppler should be used to guide the incident angle since the direction of the regurgitant jet is not predictable from the anatomy of the surrounding anatomic structures.

Ventricular Septal Defect

The presence of a ventricular septal defect affords an additional opportunity to noninvasively estimate right ventricular pressure. Continuous-wave Doppler can accurately measure the instantaneous pressure gradient across the ventricular septal defect and thereby can be used to estimate right ventricular systolic pressure. In the absence of LV outflow tract obstruction, the left ventricular systolic pressure (LVSP) is essentially equal to the systemic systolic blood pressure (SBP). By once again applying the modified Bernoulli equation, the right ventricular systolic pressure (RVSP) can be estimated by using the ventricular septal defect Doppler velocity (VSDV):

$$RVSP = SBP - 4 (VSDV)^2$$

In general, when appropriately aligning the Doppler beam, the jet through a perimembranous ventricular septal defect is directed anteriorly and rightward. Often, adequate alignment can be obtained from the left parasternal view. However, alternative views, such as a subcostal view or a peri-apical view, where the transducer is positioned toward the right ventricle, may be needed (Fig. 28.6).

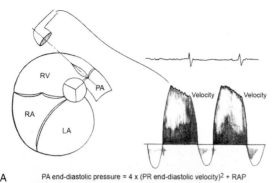

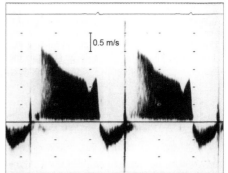

A   PA end-diastolic pressure = 4 x (PR end-diastolic velocity)^2 + RAP

B

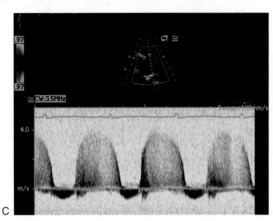

C

FIGURE 28.5. Quantitation of PA end diastolic pressure. A: Diagram of continuous-wave Doppler interrogation of pulmonary regurgitation (PR) for the left parasternal window. If end-diastolic pulmonary velocity is 3 m/s, end-diastolic pulmonary artery (PA) pressure = $4(3)^2 + 14 = 50$ mm Hg, assuming a right atrial (RA) pressure of 14 mm Hg. LA, left atrium; RV, right ventricle. **B:** Continuous-wave Doppler of PR velocity in a patient with normal PA pressure. Because the pressure difference between the PA and right ventricle is small during diastole, contraction of the right atrium decreases the PA–right ventricular pressure gradient, resulting in a dip in pulmonary regurgitation velocity. **C:** When pulmonary pressure is high, RA contraction typically does not make a notable change in the PA–right ventricular pressure gradient—hence, no dip in the continuous-wave Doppler signal of pulmonary regurgitation. (From Oh JK, Seward JB, Tajik AJ, eds. *The echo manual.* 3rd ed. Philadelphia: Lippincott Williams & Wilkins. (c) 2006 Mayo Foundation for Medical Education and Research, with permission.)

Doppler gradients across a ventricular septal defect predict peak instantaneous pressure gradients between the left and right ventricles. The majority of ventricular septal defect Doppler signals will have a plateau appearance, allowing for accurate estimation of the peak-to-peak gradient between the left and right ventricles. However, when interpreting these gradients when asynchronous peaking of left ventricle and right ventricle pressures is present, care must be taken not to underestimate the right ventricular pressure in this setting. In these patients, the ventricular septal defect Doppler signal will peak early in systole, creating a sloped appearance. The right ventricular peak pressure occurs later than the left ventricular peak pressure. The clinical consequence of using the instantaneous peak Doppler gradients is the underestimation of the right ventricular pressure by overestimating the true peak-to-peak gradient. In the presence of a sloped Doppler signal, using the end-systolic or the mean gradient across the ventricular septal defect may better predict the right ventricular systolic pressure.

Patent Ductus Arteriosus

The Doppler flow pattern and derived pressure gradient across a patent ductus arteriosus can also be used to predict pulmonary artery pressure. Optimal alignment is usually best achieved with the high left parasternal short-axis view. Continuous left-to-right ductal shunting is interrogated with continuous-wave or pulsed-wave Doppler. The peak systolic ductus arteriosus velocity (PDAV) can be used to estimate the pressure gradient between the aorta (Ao) and pulmonary artery. Therefore, with the modified

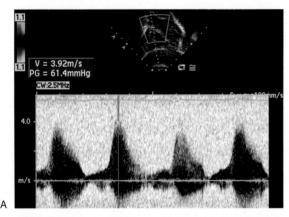

A

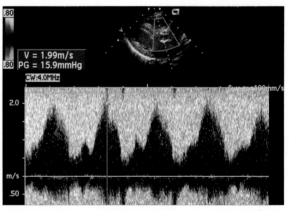

B

FIGURE 28.6. Utilization of VSD velocity to estimate RV systolic pressure. A: Continuous-wave Doppler image obtained from a subcostal imaging plane predicting normal right ventricular pressure in an infant with a small perimembranous ventricular septal defect. **B:** Alternatively, continuous-wave Doppler image obtained from a left parasternal position in a patient with a large ventricular septal defect demonstrating low-velocity (2 m/s) left-to-right shunting consistent with elevated right ventricular pressure. Both Doppler signals have a more typical plateau appearance.

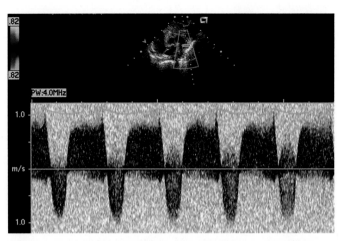

FIGURE 28.7. Pulmonary artery hypertension is confirmed with pulsed-wave Doppler from high left parasternal imaging of a patent ductus arteriosus. There is diastolic left-to-right shunting (above baseline) and systolic right-to-left shunting predicting near systemic pulmonary artery pressure.

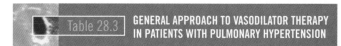

	GENERAL APPROACH TO VASODILATOR THERAPY IN PATIENTS WITH PULMONARY HYPERTENSION

Table 28.3

1. Acute response to vasodilator testing with inhaled nitric oxide or prostacyclin in the catheterization laboratory
   - Reasonable to use a trial of oral calcium channel blockade, typically nifedipine
2. Absence of an acute response to vasodilator therapy but in the **absence** of symptoms of right heart failure and/or syncope
   - Reasonable to use oral agents including endothelin receptor antagonists (bosentan, sitaxsentan) and/or phosphodiesterase-5 inhibitors (sidenafil)
   - May consider prostacyclin-based agents (epoprostenol, treprostenil, or iloprost) depending on the degree of symptomatology and practitioner preference
3. Absence of an acute response to vasodilator therapy in the **presence** of symptoms of right heart failure and/or syncope
   - A prostacyclin derivative is preferred
4. Failure of therapy or progression of symptoms in any of the above groups
   - Additional medications may be added from one of the therapeutic groups of medications that the patient may not be on, including the addition of any of the forms of prostacyclin agents

Bernoulli equation, the pulmonary artery pressure (PAP) can be estimated as:

$$PAP = Ao - 4(PDAV)^2$$

Aortic pressure is assumed to be equal to systolic pressure obtained by cuff or arterial line measurements.

Early systolic right-to-left shunting is associated with systemic or near systemic pulmonary pressures (Fig. 28.7). In patients with suprasystemic pulmonary pressure, a prolonged duration of right-to-left ductal flow may be observed. Severe pulmonary hypertension with a concomitant patent ductus arteriosus may result in reversal of transverse aortic arch flow because of the decrease in left ventricular cardiac output.

Pulmonary Artery Velocity Curve

The pulmonary artery Doppler velocity curve can be used to estimate pulmonary artery pressures in the absence of adequate tricuspid or pulmonary insufficiency, ventricular septal defect, or patent ductus arteriosus. With normal pulmonary pressure, the right ventricular ejection curve tends to have a longer time from onset of flow to peak flow, giving a "rounded" appearance. As pulmonary pressure increases, the curve more closely resembles the left ventricular ejection curve with very rapid acceleration and a short time period from flow onset to maximum velocity. Clearly, these patterns can be subtle and should be reserved for instances when all other methodologies just described are not available.

 ## MANAGEMENT

Management of pulmonary hypertension varies based on the specific etiology of the disease. For discussion purposes, management can be divided into general measures, as well as measures directed specifically at the pulmonary vascular bed. In any case, efficacy of therapy can be determined by a combination of symptoms, chemical measures such as BNP, noninvasive measures (echocardiography), and more invasive measures such as cardiac catheterization.

General therapeutic measures have included anticoagulation with warfarin. This has been based on adult studies prior to the historical advent of vasodilator therapy. These studies suggested a survival benefit in patients who received warfarin therapy. The rationale for this therapy is supported by the observed presence of microthrombi in the pulmonary vasculature of patients with pulmonary hypertension discovered at either lung biopsy or autopsy. It

is unclear if this is a primary or a secondary finding. There are no data to suggest that the use of warfarin is an effective therapy for children with pulmonary hypertension.

Digoxin has also been traditionally used for the treatment of pulmonary hypertension, especially in the face of right ventricular dysfunction. Similarly, no data exist to demonstrate the efficacy of this therapy.

Pulmonary vasodilator therapy has been a major advancement in patients with pulmonary hypertension. Table 28.3 represents a vasodilator treatment protocol for patients with pulmonary hypertension. Many believe that patients with newly diagnosed pulmonary hypertension should undergo acute drug testing in the cardiac catheterization laboratory to determine reactivity and allow for a rational approach to therapy. Pulmonary vascular reactivity is defined as a 20% or greater decrease in pulmonary vascular resistance and/or increase cardiac output with acute drug testing in the catheterization laboratory. This evaluation is typically performed with a combination of inhaled nitric oxide, intravenous prostacyclin, and oxygen. It is recommended that the patient with proved pulmonary vascular reactivity have therapy with an oral calcium channel blocker, such as nifedipine. In the absence of reactivity, and in the presence of systemic–to–suprasystemic pulmonary artery pressure, symptoms of low cardiac output, or right ventricular dysfunction as demonstrated by echocardiography, therapy with continuous intravenous prostacyclin is recommended. This implies the need for long-term central venous access. As depicted in Table 28.3, therapy with oral agents such as endothelin inhibitors and/or sildenafil may be used as an adjunctive therapy to prostacyclin or an initial therapy in the patient with subsystemic pulmonary artery pressure and good right ventricular function. Studies assessing oral prostacyclin derivatives are ongoing; their use has yet to be approved in the United States.

An exhaustive review of the efficacies of therapies and multiple agents available for the treatment of pulmonary hypertension is beyond the scope of this chapter. By way of a very brief summary, it should be noted that therapy with intravenous prostacyclin has resulted in significant improvement in outcomes for patients with pulmonary hypertension, with most studies suggesting a 5-year survival of nearly 95% in children treated with continuous intravenous prostacyclin therapy. Additional forms of prostacyclin (subcutaneous and oral), as well as other agents, such as the endothelin receptor blockers (bosentan, sitaxsentan, etc.) and phosphodiesterase-5 inhibitors (sildenafil, etc.), are currently being widely used, with evidence suggesting very good efficacy. Further studies are on the horizon detailing the efficacy of the above drugs as well as combination drug therapy targeted at forms of pulmonary hypertension in specific etiologic groups.

Finally, much work continues with regard to the use of additional heretofore-untapped medical therapies for pulmonary hypertension. The genomic approach, including further identification of candidate genes, may allow for manipulation of selected genes as well as allow for a further understanding of the pathobiology and genetics of pulmonary hypertension. Perhaps this approach will someday allow for the prevention of this potentially devastating disease.

SUGGESTED READING

Berger M, Haimowitz A, Van Tosh A, et al. Quantitative assessment of pulmonary hypertension in patients with tricuspid regurgitation using continuous wave Doppler ultrasound. *J Am Coll Cardiol.* 1985;6:359–365.

Chan KL, Currie PJ, Seward JB, et al. Comparison of three Doppler ultrasound methods in the prediction of pulmonary artery pressure. *J Am Coll Cardiol.* 1987;9:549–554.

Currie PJ, Hagler DJ, Seward JB, et al. Instantaneous pressure gradient: a simultaneous Doppler and dual catheter correlative study. *J Am Coll Cardiol.* 1986;7:800–806.

Currie PJ, Seward JB, Chan KL, et al. Continuous wave Doppler determination of right ventricular pressure: a simultaneous Doppler-catheterization study in 127 patients. *J Am Coll Cardiol.* 1985;6:750–756.

Hatle L, Angelsen BA, Tromsdal A. Non-invasive estimation of pulmonary artery systolic pressure with Doppler ultrasound. *Br Heart J.* 1981;45:157–165.

Hiraishi S, Horiguchi Y, Misawa H, et al. Noninvasive Doppler echocardiographic evaluation of shunt flow dynamics of the ductus arteriosus. *Circulation.* 1987;75:1146–1153.

Kircher BJ, Himelman RB, Schiller NB. Noninvasive estimation of right atrial pressure from the inspiratory collapse of the inferior vena cava. *Am J Cardiol.* 1990;66:493–496.

Lane J, Acherman RJ, Khongphattanayothin A, et al. Reverse aortic arch flow secondary to severe pulmonary hypertension in the neonate. *Am J Perinatol.* 1999;16:143–149.

Lindblade CL, Schamberger MS, Darragh RK, et al. Use of peak Doppler gradient across ventricular septal defect leads to underestimation of right-sided pressures in a patient with M-shaped Doppler signal: a case report. *J Am Soc Echocardiogr.* 2004;17:1207–1209.

Marx GR, Allen HD, Goldberg SJ. Doppler echocardiographic estimation of systolic pulmonary artery pressure in pediatric patients with interventricular communications. *J Am Coll Cardiol.* 1985;6:1132–1137.

Masuyama T, Kodama K, Kitabatake A, et al. Continuous-wave Doppler echocardiographic detection of pulmonary regurgitation and its application to noninvasive estimation of pulmonary artery pressure. *Circulation.* 1986;74:484–492.

Murphy DJ Jr, Ludomirsky A, Huhta JC. Continuous-wave Doppler in children with ventricular septal defect: noninvasive estimation of interventricular pressure gradient. *Am J Cardiol.* 1986;57:428–432.

Musewe NN, Poppe D, Smallhorn JF, et al. Doppler echocardiographic measurement of pulmonary artery pressure from ductal Doppler velocities in the newborn. *J Am Coll Cardiol.* 1990;15:446–456.

Musewe NN, Smallhorn JF, Benson LN, et al. Validation of Doppler-derived pulmonary arterial pressure in patients with ductus arteriosus under different hemodynamic states. *Circulation.* 1987;76:1081–1091.

Nanda NC, Gramiak R, Robinson TI, et al. Echocardiographic evaluation of pulmonary hypertension. *Circulation.* 1974;50:575–581.

Oh JK, Seward JB, Tajik AJ, eds. *The echo manual.* 3rd ed. Philadelphia: JB Lippincott; 2006.

Ommen SR, Nishimura RA, Hurrell DG, et al. Assessment of right atrial pressure with 2-dimensional and Doppler echocardiography: a simultaneous catheterization and echocardiographic study. *Mayo Clin Proc.* 2000;75:24–29.

Schamberger MS, Farrell AG, Darragh RK, et al. Use of peak Doppler gradient across ventricular septal defects leads to underestimation of right-sided pressures in patients with "sloped" Doppler signals. *J Am Soc Echocardiogr.* 2001;14:1197–1202.

Silbert DR, Brunson SC, Schiff R, et al. Determination of right ventricular pressure in the presence of a ventricular septal defect using continuous wave Doppler ultrasound. *J Am Coll Cardiol.* 1986;8:379–384.

Waggoner AD, Quinones MA, Young JB, et al. Pulsed Doppler echocardiographic detection of right-sided valve regurgitation. Experimental results and clinical significance. *Am J Cardiol.* 1981;47:279–286.

Yock PG, Popp RL. Noninvasive estimation of right ventricular systolic pressure by Doppler ultrasound in patients with tricuspid regurgitation. *Circulation.* 1984;70:657–662.

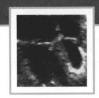

Chapter 29
Echocardiography in the Diagnosis and Management of Endocarditis

L. LuAnn Minich • Lloyd Y. Tani

BACKGROUND

The clinical picture of infective endocarditis continues to evolve with changes in the populations at risk, development of new diagnostic tools, improvements in surgical management, and evolution of antibiotic susceptibilities of organisms. The frequency of endocarditis in children appears to be increasing with the current incidence estimated at 0.8 to 3.3 per 1000 pediatric hospitalizations. This increase is often attributed to three major sources: (a) the growing population of individuals with repaired or palliated congenital heart disease, (b) the explosion in the use of indwelling intravenous lines in both neonatal and pediatric intensive care units, and (c) an increase in the use of intracardiac devices and prostheses. Although mortality has decreased from 100% in the preantibiotic era to the current rate of 6% to 30% at most pediatric institutions, endocarditis remains a severe disease often accompanied by a high morbidity. At best, endocarditis in children requires prolonged hospitalization and usually 4 to 6 weeks of intravenous antibiotics.

RISK FACTORS

Endocarditis may occur in anyone. However, populations at risk have been defined (Table 29.1), and the index of suspicion should be high in these cases. This is particularly true in the child who has multiple risk factors such as the premature infant with underlying congenital heart disease, an immature immune system, and an indwelling intravenous line for parenteral nutrition. Rheumatic fever, now rare except in specific areas of the United States, has been replaced by indwelling lines and congenital heart disease as the highest risk factors for endocarditis.

PATHOGENESIS

Bacteria that commonly lead to endocarditis include viridans streptococci, *Staphylococcus aureus* and *S. epidermidis*, beta-hemolytic streptococci, and some gram-negative organisms. Polymicrobial endocarditis is uncommon in children, but when it does occur, it is largely limited to intravenous drug users. The most common fungal etiologies of endocarditis are *Candida* and *Aspergillus*. Regardless of the organism involved, the pathogenesis is similar. Bacteremia frequently occurs in all individuals in many settings, including postoperatively, with intravenous drug use, or with daily activities such as chewing, tooth brushing, or flossing. Although bacteremia

occurs frequently, it rarely leads to endocarditis. Endocarditis only occurs when virulence factors and a unique cytokine milieu allow bacteria to adhere to exposed fibronectin. For example, turbulent blood flow from congenital or acquired heart disease, especially in lesions with high pressure gradients, may traumatize and disrupt endothelium, exposing fibronectin and initiating the clotting cascade and fibrin deposition that leads to clot formation (nonbacterial thrombotic endocarditis). In the setting of bacteremia, bacteria can invade the clot and vegetation growth encases the original nidas of infection. As the infection progresses, it destroys surrounding tissue. The location and amount of tissue destroyed determine the degree of valve regurgitation as well as the presence and size of an abscess cavity.

CLINICAL PRESENTATION

The clinical presentation of the child with endocarditis depends on age, general state of health, and causative organism. Presentations vary widely within age groups and with the causative organism, so the terms "acute" and "subacute" are no longer widely used. Premature or sick neonates requiring central indwelling lines for parenteral nutrition (Fig. 29.1) are at risk regardless of the presence or absence of a cardiac anomaly. Coagulase-negative staphylococci and enterococci are important pathogens in this age group. The sick neonate may or may not have fever, and other systemic signs may be nonspecific, making the diagnosis of endocarditis difficult. Therefore, the standard of care at many institutions includes a complete echocardiogram in all neonates with indwelling lines who have recurrent or persistent bacteremia to look for vegetations and determine the need for line removal.

The clinical presentation in older children is also variable. Although Osler's triad of pneumonia, endocarditis, and meningitis is considered the classic finding in adults, it rarely occurs in children. In children, the disease is often indolent and characterized by fever, weight loss, fatigue, and night sweats. Myalgia, arthralgia, headache, and general malaise are common. Nearly all children with endocarditis have a murmur. Some investigators report an average of 35 to 90 days between the first symptom and diagnosis and suggest that the nonspecific and insidious development of symptoms may delay the diagnosis. Viridans group streptococci remain

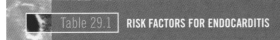

Table 29.1 **RISK FACTORS FOR ENDOCARDITIS**

- Congenital heart disease
- Acquired heart disease (including rheumatic fever)
- Indwelling vascular catheters
- Intracardiac devices and prostheses
- Immunodeficiency
- Intravenous drug use
- Staphylococcal septicemia
- Fungal septicemia

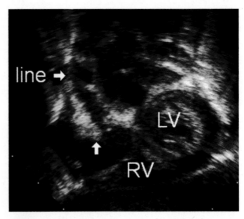

FIGURE 29.1. Modified subcostal view of a central venous line in the right atrium. The use of B color allows easy identification of the dense vegetation (*arrow*), giving a thickened, irregular appearance to the catheter. LV, left ventricle; RV, right ventricle.

the most frequent cause of endocarditis in children. It commonly presents with an indolent course and rarely leads to complications, especially if diagnosed early and treated with proper antibiotic therapy. Because endocarditis can result in generalized, nonspecific symptoms in children with normal hearts or those with minor unrecognized congenital heart disease, it should be considered in the differential for all children with prolonged, unexplained fever with persistent bacteremia.

Severe infection with valve destruction and significant regurgitation leads to symptoms of congestive heart failure and a severely ill child. In this scenario, a skilled clinician with a high index of suspicion readily makes the diagnosis. The challenge in evaluating a febrile child with less involvement, however, lies in differentiating the innocent murmur associated with the high-output state often associated with fever from the murmur of valve regurgitation. When in doubt, echocardiography should readily resolve the question. However, it should be noted that the yield for a positive study indicative of endocarditis is low in the absence of positive blood cultures and appropriate clinical setting.

As stated above, bacteremia is common with daily activities but rarely results in endocarditis. The exception to this rule is when *S. aureus* is a causative organism. *S. aureus* causes many pyogenic infections in children and may lead to sepsis. Endocarditis develops in about 20% of cases of staphylococcal sepsis, even in the absence of underlying heart disease. Because the classic findings of endocarditis are seldom present and the clinical picture is often nonspecific, many experts recommend the routine use of echocardiography with all cases of *S. aureus* sepsis.

Circulating immune complexes and rheumatoid factor occur in 84% to 100% of cases of endocarditis and are deposited in the skin, spleen, synovium of joints, and glomeular basement membrane. These cause the classic noncardiac manifestations associated with endocarditis including splenomegaly, polyarthritis, glomerulonephritis, splinter hemorrhages, Osler nodes (painful bluish nodules at the fingertips), Janeway lesions (painless hemorrhagic lesions on the palms and soles), and Roth spots (retinal hemorrhages).

Complications of endocarditis may occur early and alter the presentation as described in the next section.

 ## COMPLICATIONS

Complications (Table 29.2) from endocarditis are common and contribute to the morbidity and mortality. Risk factors for complications include prosthetic valves, *S. aureus* or fungal causative agents, prior episodes of endocarditis, cyanotic heart disease, left-sided involvement, and clinical symptoms for longer than 3 months.

Congestive heart failure is one of the most common complications of endocarditis. Heart failure may occur acutely and abruptly as a result of valvular regurgitation occurring when native valve leaflets or support structures are disrupted (Fig. 29.2) or from dehiscence of a valve prosthesis resulting in a significant perivalvar leak. In other

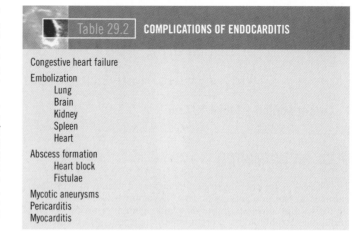

| Table 29.2 | COMPLICATIONS OF ENDOCARDITIS |

Congestive heart failure

Embolization
  Lung
  Brain
  Kidney
  Spleen
  Heart

Abscess formation
  Heart block
  Fistulae

Mycotic aneurysms
Pericarditis
Myocarditis

cases, heart failure symptoms may develop more slowly or insidiously. In either case (acute or insidious), heart failure is secondary to valve regurgitation with or without accompanying ventricular dysfunction. Surgical intervention should be considered in patients with endocarditis and heart failure.

Embolization of vegetation fragments complicates endocarditis in 20% to 40% of cases. The risk is highest during the first days after antibiotic therapy is initiated and drops to 9% to 21% after 2 weeks of treatment. The lungs, brain, kidney, and spleen are the most common organs affected. Coronary artery embolism is a less common but potentially lethal complication.

Embolism occurs frequently in gram-negative, pneumococcal, or fungal endocarditis. In children, gram-negative endocarditis is most commonly caused by one of the HACEK organisms (*Haemophilus, Actinobacillus, Cardiobacterium, Eikenella,* and *Kingella* spp.) and is associated with embolism in 31% of cases. About one third of cases of HACEK endocarditis occur in the absence of underlying heart disease. Because these organisms are fastidious and slow growing and require special growth factors and carbon dioxide for isolation, diagnosis and appropriate treatment are typically delayed, allowing the vegetations to become large and friable, increasing the risk of embolization.

There has been a resurgence of pneumococcal endocarditis in parallel with the increase in its antibiotic resistance. Pneumococcal endocarditis is associated with meningitis, pneumonia, otitis media, or mastoiditis in 50% of pediatric cases. The mitral valve is involved (either alone or in association with aortic or tricuspid valve) in 68% of cases, and 80% have large vegetations, predisposed to embolization.

Fungal organisms account for approximately 1.1% of cases of endocarditis in children, occurring most commonly in developing countries where it is often fatal. *Candida* causes about 63%, and *Aspergillus,* 26%, of cases. Approximately two thirds of cases involve

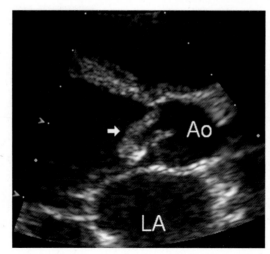 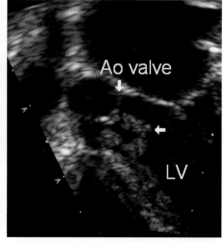

FIGURE 29.2. Aortic valve vegetation. Left: Parasternal long-axis view shows a vegetation on the aortic valve (*arrow*) that prolapses into the left ventricle during diastole. The valve cusps are partially destroyed and prolapse, resulting in severe aortic regurgitation. Ao, aorta; LA, left atrial. **Right:** Apical four-chamber view demonstrates the extensive involvement of the vegetation (*horizontal arrow*) on the aortic valve (*vertical arrow*) that extends along the interventricular septum. Ao, aortic; LV, left ventricle.

children younger than 1 year. In developed nations, premature neonates undergoing medical instrumentation and children who have had congenital heart surgery using prosthetic material are at highest risk of developing fungal endocarditis. Diagnosis is often delayed until large, friable vegetations are formed or after embolization has occurred. The major obstacle to diagnosis is the difficulty in reliably growing fungi in automated blood culture systems. Polymerase chain reaction (PCR) has been useful for the detection and identification of fungal organisms.

One of the most severe complications of endocarditis is an abscess. A perivalvar abscess may be seen when the infection extends beyond the valve annulus. Although this is a rare complication, it is strongly associated with a poor outcome. In both children and adults, *S. aureus* is the most common cause and nearly all abscesses involve the aortic valve. In adults, the incidence of perivalvar abscess is approximately 20% to 40% with native aortic valve endocarditis and 60% in the setting of a prosthetic aortic valve. Similar data are not available for children as only small series or case reports comprise the literature. The literature suggests that the underlying native valve anatomy is normal in 66% of cases of endocarditis complicated by abscess formation in children. Although a perivalvar abscess may have an indolent presentation, the more typical picture is that of acute, severe illness. The child has a new pathologic murmur and may also have a rub indicating pericarditis. The abscess disrupts the aortic annulus, creating severe regurgitation that results in intractable congestive heart failure (Fig. 29.3). The infection may extend into the mitral-aortic fibrosa and involve the anterior mitral leaflet so that the mitral valve becomes regurgitant as well. When the structural integrity of the aortic wall is further weakened, a sinus of Valsalva aneurysm may form and ultimately rupture into the right ventricular outflow tract or either atria, creating a shunt that is poorly tolerated. Fever and bacteremia usually persist despite appropriate antibiotic therapy and recurrent emboli are common. The new development of bundle branch block or complete heart block is highly specific for a perivalvar abscess. Most experts recommend serial echocardiographic evaluations looking for development of perivalvar abscess in the following settings: (a) *S. aureus* endocarditis regardless of whether a native or prosthetic valve is involved, (b) persistent fever or bacteremia despite appropriate antibiotic therapy, and (c) a persistent bundle branch block or complete heart block, especially when there has been a prolonged period of symptoms before diagnosis and treatment.

 DIAGNOSIS

Endocarditis is largely diagnosed by positive blood cultures for a typical organism and the presence of vegetations and/or abscess formation on echocardiography. Systemic, vascular, and/or immunologic findings support the diagnosis. Typical laboratory findings include anemia and elevated white blood count, erythrocyte sedimentation rate, and C-reactive protein. Blood cultures are positive in over 90% of cases but may be negative with prior use of antibiotics, with right-sided endocarditis, or when the pathogen is intracellular or fastidious. Serology may prove useful in these circumstances. Serology is the only method that allows diagnosis of *Coxiella burnetii* (Q fever), *Brucella*, *Bartonella*, and chlamydial endocarditis.

Early diagnosis and aggressive treatment are warranted to avoid the serious complications associated with endocarditis. At the same time, overdiagnosis must be avoided as treatment involves weeks or months of intravenous antimicrobial therapy. When the classic noncardiac findings and/or new-onset regurgitant murmurs are present in the febrile child with bacteremia and an echocardiogram shows vegetations and/or abscess, the diagnosis of endocarditis can readily be made. The picture is seldom so clear, however. Fever may be absent if the child is debilitated, immunocompromised, or pretreated with antibiotics. Innocent murmurs are common in children during illness and may be difficult to differentiate from those of valvar regurgitation. Noncardiac manifestations may not be present. In a series of 76 episodes of endocarditis in children, splenomegaly occurred in 5%, splinter hemorrhages in 4%, Roth spots in 4%, and Osler nodes in 3%.

A team of pediatricians, infectious disease specialists, cardiologists, and cardiovascular surgeons may be needed for optimal evaluation and management. The modified Duke criteria (Table 29.3) have been validated in children and should be used when the clinical picture is unclear. The Duke criteria function similar to the Jones criteria for rheumatic fever by dividing clinical, microbiological, and echocardiographic findings into major and minor categories. The two major criteria typically include (a) microbiologic evidence and (b) evidence of endocardial involvement (positive echocardiogram or new valvular regurgitation). It is worth noting that three echocardiographic findings qualify as major criteria: (a) discrete, echogenic, oscillating intracardiac mass at site of endocardial injury, (b) perivalvar abscess, or (c) new dehiscence of a prosthetic valve. The 15 minor criteria include the presence of specific known risk factors, evidence of emboli, classic findings resulting from immunologic phenomenon, and laboratory findings. Endocarditis is definitively diagnosed if (a) there is pathologic evidence of an intracardiac or embolized vegetation or intracardiac abscess or (b) fulfillment of clinical criteria, requiring the presence of (i) two major or (ii) one major and three minor or (iii) five minor criteria. Endocarditis is considered possible if one major and one minor or three minor criteria are present. A firm alternative diagnosis, resolution of symptoms within 4 days of antimicrobial therapy, and absence of surgical or autopsy evidence of endocarditis within 4 days of antimicrobial therapy points away from a diagnosis of endocarditis.

Blood cultures are central to the diagnosis and effective treatment of endocarditis. Contrary to earlier teaching, it is not necessary to obtain blood sampling at the time of fever, as the bacteremia of endocarditis is continuous. The volume of blood drawn is important, however, and experts recommend 1 to 3 mL in infants and 5 to 7 mL in older children. Three cultures over a minimum time of 1 hour should be drawn before administering empiric antibiotics. Despite numerous cultures with adequate volumes, prolonged culture periods, and examination of surgically excised tissue, about 5% of cases of

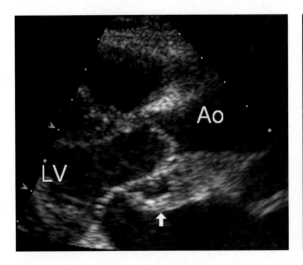
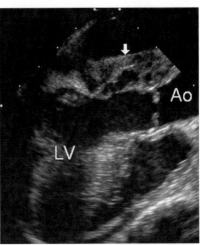

FIGURE 29.3. Perivalve abscess. Left: Parasternal long-axis view of the left ventricular outflow tract shows the shaggy appearance of a hypoechoic space posterior to the aortic outflow tract representing a perivalvar abscess (*arrow*). Ao, aorta; LV, left ventricle. **Right:** Transesophageal echocardiogram using a longitudinal view of the left ventricular outflow tract in the same patient demonstrates the abscess cavity (*arrow*). The aortic valve leaflets are thickened and distorted and fail to coapt with significant aortic regurgitation. Ao, aorta; LV, left ventricle.

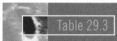

Table 29.3	MODIFIED MAJOR AND MINOR (DUKE) CRITERIA FOR THE DIAGNOSIS OF ENDOCARDITIS

Major

1. Microbiologic evidence (Positive blood cultures)
   a. Typical organism from 2 separate cultures
   b. Persistently positive cultures with a typical organism drawn >12 hours apart
   c. All 3 or a majority of ≥4 cultures with the first and last drawn at least 1 hour apart
   d. Positive serology for Q fever
2. Evidence of endocardial involvement
   a. Two-dimensional echocardiographic evidence
      I. Oscillating intracardiac mass on valve apparatus, implanted materials, or in the path of regurgitant jets without a satisfactory alternative explanation
      II. Perivalvar Abscess
      III. New partial dehiscence of a prosthetic valve
   b. Doppler evidence of new valvular regurgitation

Minor

Predisposing heart disease or intravenous drug use

Fever (38°C)

Vascular phenomena

Major arterial emboli

Septic pulmonary artifacts

Mycotic aneurysm

Intracranial hemorrhage

Conjunctival hemorrhages

Janeway lesions

Immunologic phenomena

　Osler's nodes

　Roth spots

　Glomerulonephritis

　Rheumatoid factor

Microbiologic evidence

　Positive blood culture not meeting major criteria

　Positive serology for active infection with a typical organism

Modified from Milazzo AS, Jr., Li JS. Bacterial endocarditis in infants and children. Pediatr Infect Dis J 2001;20(8):799-801. Mylonakis E, Calderwood SB. Infective endocarditis in adults. *N Engl J Med* 2001;345(18):1318-1330.

endocarditis are culture negative. Attempts to obtain an organism through antibody titers and polymerase chain reaction techniques may also fail. Several reasons for "culture-negative" endocarditis include inability to grow a fastidious organism, antibiotic use prior to culturing, pulmonary filtering of bacteria for right-sided lesions, and sequestration of the organism within the vegetation.

 ## MANAGEMENT

It is important to note that the Duke criteria provide guidelines for the diagnosis but not the management of endocarditis. Prolonged use of intravenous antibiotics is clearly indicated for those with definite endocarditis, but their use for possible or rejected cases must be considered on an individual basis. The team of experts must weigh the risk factors, evaluate the reliability of the blood cultures, and determine the likelihood that endocarditis best explains the clinical picture.

Once diagnosed, the patient's condition and causative organism dictates the course and length of treatment. All patients require medical therapy and some will require surgery. If antibiotics are started before culture results become available, treatment is usually directed toward the most common bacteria—streptococci and staphylococci. Once the organism is isolated, susceptibilities are determined and antibiotics adjusted accordingly. Antibiotics may

be combined to provide synergy and must be given intravenously to achieve concentrations sufficiently high to treat infection in the poorly vascularized valve leaflets as well as penetrate infected vegetations. Treatment is typically for 4 to 6 weeks but may be longer in those patients with prosthetic valves or those who are immunocompromised or have other extenuating circumstance. Anticoagulation is not indicated (unless given for a reason other than endocarditis) and is actually contraindicated with severe cerebral complications or mycotic aneurysms. Afterload reduction in the setting of significant acute aortic or mitral regurgitation is limited to stabilization of the patient before surgical intervention.

Surgery is indicated in cases of abscess formation, severe valvar regurgitation with intractable congestive heart failure, recurrent arterial emboli, or persistent bacteremia after 2 weeks of appropriate antibiotic therapy. Typically, patients with infected pacing systems (Fig. 29.4), intracardiac devices (Fig. 29.5), and prosthetic valves are managed surgically. Some experts recommend surgery for vegetations greater than 1 cm in size, increasing vegetation size while on appropriate antibiotics, marked mobility of the vegetation, and fungal etiology, but data are conflicting and these indications remain controversial. Closure of a hemodynamically insignificant ventricular septal defect is warranted after successful treatment of endocarditis to decrease the risk of recurrence.

 ## PROGNOSIS

Prognosis depends on several factors. Patients with a more severe course leading to hospitalization within 1 week of onset of the first symptom also have higher mortality rates. The prognosis is worse for younger children (younger than 3 years) compared with older children, even when the time to diagnosis is similar. In terms of bacterial etiology, *S. aureus* infection carries the highest mortality rates in most published series. In contrast to adults, left-sided and right-sided vegetations appear to carry a similar mortality in children. The primary causes of death include congestive heart failure, renal failure, rupture of a mycotic aneurysm, or consequences of emboli.

 ## PROPHYLAXIS

The American Heart Association guidelines regarding antibiotic prophylaxis for endocarditis have evolved over the past 50 years. The latest revision, published in 2007, substantially revised the indications for antibiotics in at-risk groups. Prophylaxis is no longer recommended for genitourinary or gastrointestinal tract procedures. Prophylaxis for dental procedures is recommended only

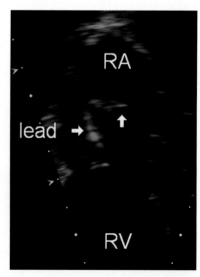

FIGURE 29.4. The apical four-chamber view shows a pacemaker lead (horizontal arrow) as it passes through the tricuspid valve in this patient with endocarditis. A vegetation is well defined with B color (*vertical arrow*). RA, right atrium; RV, right ventricle.

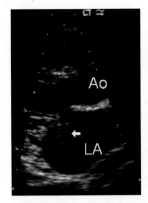 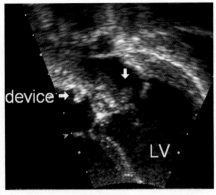 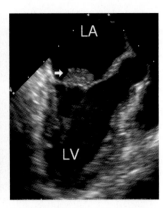

FIGURE 29.5. ASD device endocarditis. Left: Parasternal long-axis view of a patient after device closure of an atrial septal defect shows an arm of the device into the mitral valve funnel. A vegetation (*arrow*) is seen attached to this arm. Ao, aorta; LA, left atrium. **Middle:** Off-axis apical four-chamber view demonstrating the device (*horizontal arrow*) and the thickened irregular vegetation (*vertical arrow*) attached to it. LV, left ventricle. **Right:** Transesophageal echocardiogram at the level of the mitral valve and left ventricular outflow tract level demonstrates an additional vegetation (*arrow*) on the posterior leaflet of the mitral valve. LA, left atrium; LV, left ventricle.

in the following circumstances: (a) prosthetic valve, (b) history of endocarditis, (c) unrepaired cyanotic congenital heart disease (including after palliation with shunts and conduits), (d) for 6 months after completely repaired heart defects using prosthetic materials, (e) repaired defects with residual lesions at, or adjacent to, the site of prosthetic material or device, and (f) cardiac transplant patients with valvulopathy. In contrast to previous guidelines, antibiotic prophylaxis is not recommended for any other congenital heart defect. Good oral hygiene to decrease the incidence of bacteremia is probably the best way of reducing the risk of endocarditis.

 IMPORTANT ECHOCARDIOGRAPHIC CONSIDERATIONS

Echocardiography should be performed in any child suspected of having endocarditis to allow earlier diagnosis and prevent complications. That being said, not all masses seen on an echocardiogram are vegetations (Fig. 29.6). The echocardiographic appearance of vegetations, noninfectious thrombi, and other intracardiac masses may be indistinguishable. In the absence of microbiological, serologic, or physical evidence to support the diagnosis, the positive predictive value of echocardiography is poor. Therefore, the incidental echocardiographic finding of a mass in a child who has no associated clinical suspicion of endocarditis likely warrants further investigation and follow-up but should not be considered a vegetation without supporting clinical features (see modified Duke criteria, Table 29.3).

Vegetations

Echocardiographic findings typical of endocarditis are present in more than 90% of cases. False negative examinations may occur when preexisting pathology obscures the vegetations or when the vegetations are too small to be seen with the ultrasound equipment or imaging approach used (including when imaging is suboptimal). Detection rates may improve with the transesophageal approach, especially in older children and adolescents, allowing visualization of vegetations as small as 1 mm. Vegetations large enough to be visualized by current ultrasound machines appear as echogenic masses attached to a cardiac valve, papillary muscle, chordae, endocardium, prosthetic patch, or indwelling line or device. The typical vegetation forms downstream from the turbulent flow—on the right ventricular side of a ventricular septal defect, the ventricular side of the regurgitant aortic valve, or the left atrial side of the regurgitant mitral valve. When vegetations are seen on one valve, care should be taken to determine if other cardiac valves are also involved or if abscesses are present. This is particularly true with intravenous drug abuse, where multivalvar involvement is common. In some cases, the vegetations themselves may disrupt valve function and cause varying degrees of regurgitation. More frequently, however, infection destroys the leaflets or supporting apparatus resulting in significant regurgitation. Chordae may rupture resulting in a flail leaflet and significant regurgitation, but this must also be considered in the clinical setting where it occurs. The flail leaflet as a result of infection may appear identical to the flail leaflet resulting from trauma or bioprosthesis degeneration. Color Doppler echocardiography is useful for differentiating transvalvular and paravalvular jets when a prosthesis is involved.

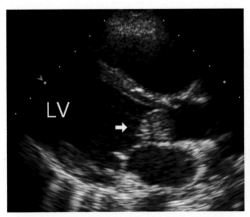 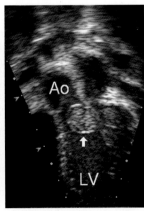

FIGURE 29.6. Example of a cardiac mass not related to endocarditis. Left: This patient presented with the new onset of a cardiac murmur. He had no associated fever, bacteremia, or other systemic or laboratory findings. A large mass (*arrow*) is demonstrated attached to the ventricular side of the mitral valve that moves into and partially obstructs the left ventricular outflow tract during systole. Although endocarditis was considered, neither the clinical picture nor the location of the mass supported the diagnosis. **Right:** Apical four-chamber view demonstrates the attachments of the mass (*arrow*) to the ventricular side of the anterior mitral valve leaflet. The mass was excised and pathology demonstrated a ventricular myxoma. Ao, aorta; LV, left ventricle.

Attempts have been made to determine echocardiographic predictors of complications. Patients with larger vegetations have a higher incidence of embolization, abscess formation, heart failure, failure of medical therapy, and death. The echogenicity of the vegetation appears to have no relationship to the risk of embolization. Spontaneous echocardiographic contrast is thought to imply increased platelet aggregation involved in the formation and growth of vegetations. In one series, the dynamic clouds of slowly curling or spiraling echoes characteristic of spontaneous contrast were seen within the left ventricular cavity in 26% of patients with endocarditis. These investigators found spontaneous contrast had a specificity and sensitivity for predicting an embolic event of 83% and 38%, respectively. The presence of spontaneous contrast was also associated with an increased risk for valve replacement, prolonged healing, and death. Although controversial, size and mobility of vegetations are frequently considered risk factors. Vegetation size greater than 1 cm and marked mobility predict embolization with odds ratios of 9 and 2.4, respectively. Vegetations greater than 1.5 cm have the worst prognosis.

Valve regurgitation is an important finding in endocarditis, and while its presence does not prove endocarditis, its absence makes the diagnosis extremely unlikely. Echocardiography may allow determination of the mechanism of regurgitation, such as visualization of leaflet perforation, loss of leaflet coaptation, chordal rupture, or disruption of the annular support.

Abscesses and Fistulae

With careful attention to imaging detail, echocardiography allows detection of more than 90% of perivalvar abscesses; other imaging modalities are rarely needed. Vegetations involving the right coronary cusp of the aortic valve have the highest association with abscess formation. The abscess cavity appears as marked thickening or enlargement of the aortic wall or sinuses of Valsalva (anteriorly or posteriorly), frequently associated with a hypoechoic space or a spontaneous contrast appearance (Fig. 29.7). Similar densities may extend to the interventricular septum or the ventricular wall adjacent to the native or prosthetic valve annulus. Significant regurgitation and the formation of fistulae into the pulmonary artery or cardiac chambers are common. In the setting of a prosthetic valve, there is a rocking or asynchronous movement of the valve between the annulus and the sewing ring. If the transthoracic examination is equivocal and the index of suspicion for endocarditis is high, the transesophageal approach should be used. The long- and short-axis views with the transducer at the level of the aortic valve allow visualization of the abscess cavity as a circumscribed pocket with reduced echo density. The total extent of involvement can usually be defined but often requires nonstandard, off-axis views. Color Doppler aids in detecting fistulae draining to other vessels and/or cardiac chambers.

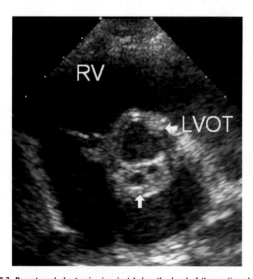

FIGURE 29.7. Parasternal short-axis view just below the level of the aortic valve demon-strates the left ventricular outflow tract (LVOT) in cross section. An abscess cavity is imaged posterior to it (*vertical arrow*), creating a double-circle appearance. RV, right ventricle.

Embolism, Ventricular Dysfunction, and Pericarditis

Embolism is a relatively common complication of endocarditis and should be considered when symptoms develop or when there is a sudden decrease in the size of the vegetation. Embolism may occur to any organ system most commonly, the lungs, brain, kidney, or spleen. Left ventricular dysfunction is unusual but may occur in the setting of acute volume overload secondary to valvar regurgitation or a sizeable fistulous connection, after coronary embolism, or when myocarditis complicates the clinical picture. Coronary embolism will be accompanied by typical electrocardiographic changes as well as new regional wall motion abnormalities or global impairment of ventricular function on echocardiography.

A pericardial effusion may result from inflammation or direct extension of the infection into the adjacent pericardium, mycotic aneurysm of the proximal aorta, septic coronary embolus, or myocardial abscess (Fig. 29.8). Although reported in only 6% of patients with endocarditis without abscess, 52% of patients with a perivalvar abscess have a pericardial effusion. Purulent pericarditis is associated with an extremely high mortality.

Prosthetic Valves and Conduits

Prosthetic valves are associated with a significantly increased risk of endocarditis in children and adults. Because the prosthesis produces reverberation artifact and acoustic shadowing, it may be difficult to differentiate postoperative from inflammatory changes. It may be useful to note that isolated mild perivalvar regurgitation does not predict endocarditis and should not be considered as an echocardiographic finding suggestive of endocarditis. In contrast, vegetations, perivalvar abscesses, valve dehiscence, pseudoaneurysms, fistulae, or moderate or greater regurgitation is useful for making the diagnosis with a positive and negative predictive value of 94% and 96%, respectively, for any of these findings.

Even stentless aortic tissue valves present diagnostic challenges. The postoperative echocardiographic appearance varies with the implantation technique. Most surgical implantation methods retain part of the native aortic root, resulting in a double-lumen appearance that may be mistaken for a perivalvar abscess in the postoperative patient with a fever. The development of paravalvular thickening, diffuse leaflet thickening, or new valvar regurgitation or the presence of vegetation or fistula is indicative of endocarditis. In addition, because the typical postoperative double-lumen densities resolve within the first few months after surgery, an interval increase in the size of the densities on serial examinations suggests endocarditis.

Valved conduits are often used to establish continuity between the ventricles and the pulmonary arteries in many types of congenital heart disease. In such cases, echocardiographic evaluation should focus not only on the valve within the conduit but also on the proximal or distal anastamoses.

Role of Transesophageal Echocardiography

It is clear that the transesophageal approach is superior to the transthoracic approach in adults, but such evidence is lacking in children. Transesophageal echocardiography is not as widely used because of the need for sedation or general anesthesia and intubation in children, who often have favorable transthoracic acoustic windows. When the two approaches were systematically studied in a pediatric population (ages 0.3 to 17.5 years), the transesophageal approach added little when a vegetation was imaged transthoracically. Therefore, most pediatric cardiologists reserve transesophageal echocardiography for special circumstances: (a) poor transthoracic acoustic windows, (b) prosthetic valves that may obscure vegetations by acoustic shadowing, (c) persistent clinical and microbial evidence of endocarditis but a normal transthoracic study, or (d) older children and adolescents who are closer to adult size. Similar to the adult practice, most pediatric cardiologists adhere to the principle that transesophageal echocardiography should be performed if the transthoracic examination is negative when there is strong clinical evidence of endocarditis.

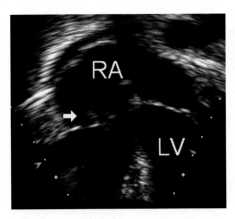
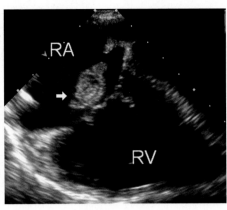

FIGURE 29.8. Tricuspid valve vegetation. Left: Apical four-chamber view shows a vegetation on the tricuspid valve (*arrow*). Note the small pericardial effusion adjacent to the right atrial wall. RA, right atrium; LV, left ventricle. **Right:** Transesophageal imaging and B-color allow better visualization of this large vegetation (*arrow*) associated with the tricuspid valve. RA, right atrium; RV, right ventricle.

Important Echocardiographic Suggestions

Careful attention to both machine and examination settings is important (Table 29.4). The highest-frequency transducer that allows adequate penetration to image cardiac structures should be used to both optimize detection as well as to resolve the edges of a vegetation and/or delineate abscess cavities. Gains must be set high enough to detect small, subtle vegetations and clearly visualize the blood–endocardium interface but not so high that low attenuation creates artifacts. All acoustic windows (both standard and nonstandard) should be used to image cardiac structures, detect vegetations, and abscesses and to differentiate subtle positive findings from artifacts. In contrast to artifacts that cannot consistently be seen in multiple planes, true abnormalities can be confirmed by imaging them from orthogonal and off-axis views. Color-encoded tissue processing (B-color), where real-time images are displayed with a dynamic compression of varying colors, should routinely be used. Compared with gray-scale imaging, B-color allows better differentiation of the extent of the mass and increases the user's ability to detect small vegetations.

The etiology of an intracardiac mass can seldom be determined by echocardiography alone. Both the sonographer performing the examination and the physician interpreting the study require extensive knowledge of normal and congenitally abnormal structures of the heart including the Eustachian valve, dilated coronary sinus, Chiari's network, and atrial or ventricular septal aneurysms that may appear as masses or abscesses. All abnormalities seen by echocardiography must be considered in the setting in which they occur. Vegetations cannot be distinguished from other intracardiac masses solely by echocardiography. The positive predictive value of echocardiography for endocarditis is low in the absence of microbiologic, serologic, and/or clinical evidence for systemic infection.

Serial echocardiograms are important during the course of the illness. Vegetations too small to be resolved on the initial study may subsequently be seen as they grow in size. Large vegetations may show a sudden decrease in size or disappear completely if embolization occurs. Valvar regurgitation may progress and volume overload may ultimately impair ventricular function. Complications such as abscesses or fistulae may not be present until later in the course of the disease. With appropriate therapy, the vegetations slowly decrease in size as the mass organizes, but serial exams have shown that they may persist for months or even years after the acute episode. These "healed vegetations" have no distinguishing echocardiographic features from the masses that present during the acute phase of the disease. Therefore, it is important to obtain an echocardiogram at the end of medical therapy when blood cultures are negative after completion of antibiotics. This end-of-therapy "baseline study" can then serve as a comparison should the patient develop clinical findings suggesting persistent or recurrent infection.

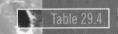 Table 29.4	ECHOCARDIOGRAPHIC CAVEATS IN THE CONSIDERATION OF ENDOCARDITIS

Machine and settings must be optimized
- Highest transducer frequency that allows adequate penetration
- Gain settings
- Color encoded tissue processing (B-color)

Optimal examination settings
- All acoustic windows (both standard and off-axis views)
- Imaging of masses in at least 2 planes
- Awareness of normal structures and common congenital abnormalities

Echo findings must be considered within the clinical setting
- History
- Risk factors
- Physical examination findings
- Laboratory findings

Serial echocardiograms are indicated
- Development of vegetations
- Change in vegetation size
- Development of abscesses
- Development of fistulae
- Progression of valve regurgitation
- Progressive impairment of ventricular function

SUGGESTED READING

Ali AS, Alam M, Singireddy S, et al. The clinical implications (or lack thereof) of vegetations detected by echocardiography in patients not thought to have endocarditis. *Clin Cardiol.* 1998;21:191–193.

Bonow RO, Carabello BA, Kanu C, et al. ACC/AHA 2006 guidelines for the management of patients with valvular heart disease: a report of the American College of Cardiology/American Heart Association Task Force on Practice Guidelines (Writing Committee to Revise the 1998 Guidelines for the Management of Patients With Valvular Heart Disease): developed in collaboration with the Society of Cardiovascular Anesthesiologists: endorsed by the Society for Cardiovascular Angiography and Interventions and the Society of Thoracic Surgeons. *Circulation.* 2006;114:e84–e231.

Caksen H, Uzum K, Yuksel S, et al. Cardiac findings in childhood staphylococcal sepsis. *Jpn Heart J.* 2002;43:9–11.

Choi M, Mailman TL. Pneumococcal endocarditis in infants and children. *Pediatr Infect Dis J.* 2004;23:166–171.

Davis JA, Weisman MH, Dail DH. Vascular disease in infective endocarditis. Report of immune-mediated events in skin and brain. *Arch Intern Med.* 1978;138:480–483.

De Castro S, Magni G, Beni S, et al. Role of transthoracic and transesophageal echocardiography in predicting embolic events in patients with active infective endocarditis involving native cardiac valves. *Am J Cardiol.* 1997;80:1030–1034.

Erbel R, Liu F, Ge J, et al. Identification of high-risk subgroups in infective endocarditis and the role of echocardiography. *Eur Heart J.* 1995;16:588–602.

Feder HM Jr, Roberts JC, Salazar JC, et al. HACEK endocarditis in infants and children: two cases and a literature review. *Pediatr Infect Dis J.* 2003;22: 557–562.

Ferrieri P, Gewitz MH, Gerber MA, et al. Unique features of infective endocarditis in childhood. *Pediatrics.* 2002;109:931–943.

Habib G. Management of infective endocarditis. *Heart.* 2006;92:124–130.

Hansen D, Schmiegelow K, Jacobsen JR. Bacterial endocarditis in children: trends in its diagnosis, course, and prognosis. *Pediatr Cardiol.* 1992;13: 198–203.

Hoyer A, Silberbach M. Infective endocarditis. *Pediatr Rev.* 2005;26:394–400.

Humpl T, McCrindle BW, Smallhorn JF. The relative roles of transthoracic compared with transesophageal echocardiography in children with suspected infective endocarditis. *J Am Coll Cardiol.* 2003;41:2068–2071.

Martin-Davila P, Navas E, Fortun J, et al. Analysis of mortality and risk factors associated with native valve endocarditis in drug users: the importance of vegetation size. *Am Heart J.* 2005;150:1099–1106.

Martin JM, Neches WH, Wald ER. Infective endocarditis: 35 years of experience at a children's hospital. *Clin Infect Dis.* 1997;24:669–675.

Milazzo AS Jr, Li JS. Bacterial endocarditis in infants and children. *Pediatr Infect Dis J.* 2001;20:799–801.

Millar BC, Jugo J, Moore JE. Fungal endocarditis in neonates and children. *Pediatr Cardiol.* 2005;26:517–536.

Mugge A, Daniel WG. Echocardiographic assessment of vegetations in patients with infective endocarditis: prognostic implications. *Echocardiography.* 1995;12:651–661.

Mylonakis E, Calderwood SB. Infective endocarditis in adults. *N Engl J Med.* 2001;345:1318–1330.

Nast CC, Colodro IH, Cohen AH. Splenic immune deposits in bacterial endocarditis. *Clin Immunol Immunopathol.* 1986;40:209–213.

Otto C. Infective endocarditis. In: Otto C, ed. *Valvular heart disease.* 2nd ed. Philadelphia: Elsevier; 2004:482–522.

Rastogi A, Luken JA, Pildes RS, et al. Endocarditis in neonatal intensive care unit. *Pediatr Cardiol.* 1993;14:183–186.

Rohmann S, Erbel R, Darius H, et al. Spontaneous echo contrast imaging in infective endocarditis: a predictor of complications? *Int J Card Imaging.* 1992;8:197–207.

Rohmann S, Erbel R, Mohr-Kahaly S, et al. Use of transoesophageal echocardiography in the diagnosis of abscess in infective endocarditis. *Eur Heart J.* 1995;16(suppl B):54–62.

Ronderos RE, Portis M, Stoermann W, et al. Are all echocardiographic findings equally predictive for diagnosis in prosthetic endocarditis? *J Am Soc Echocardiogr.* 2004;17:664–669.

Runge MS. The role of transesophageal echocardiography in the diagnosis and management of patients with aortic perivalvar abscesses. *Am J Med Sci.* 2001;321:152–155.

Shah FS, Fennelly G, Weingarten-Arams J, et al. Endocardial abscesses in children: case report and review of the literature. *Clin Infect Dis.* 1999;29: 1478–1482.

Strelich K, Deeb GM, Bach DS. Echocardiographic correlates of Freestyle stentless tissue aortic valve endocarditis. *Semin Thorac Cardiovasc Surg.* 2001;13(suppl 1):113–119.

Sutton MS, Lee RT. Diagnosis and medical management of infective endocarditis: transthoracic and transesophageal echocardiography. *J Card Surg.* 1990;5:39–43.

Tingleff J, Egeblad H, Gotzsche CO, et al. Perivalvular cavities in endocarditis: abscesses versus pseudoaneurysms? A transesophageal Doppler echocardiographic study in 118 patients with endocarditis. *Am Heart J.* 1995;130: 93–100.

Wilson W, Taubert KA, Gewitz M, et al. Prevention of infective endocarditis: guidelines from the American Heart Association: a guideline from the American Heart Association Rheumatic Fever, Endocarditis, and Kawasaki Disease Committee, Council on Cardiovascular Disease in the Young, and the Council on Clinical Cardiology, Council on Cardiovascular Surgery and Anesthesia, and the Quality of Care and Outcomes Research Interdisciplinary Working Group. *Circulation.* 2007;116:1736–1754.

Zuberbuhler JR NW, Park SC. Infectious endocarditis: an experience spanning three decades. *Cardiol Young.* 1994;244–251.

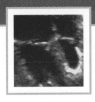

Chapter 30
Evaluation of Prosthetic Valves

Sabrina Phillips • Fletcher Miller

Replacement of dysfunctional native cardiac valves is very common in the practice of congenital heart disease. A subset of patients with congenital heart disease will require multiple "re-replacements" of valvular prostheses secondary to growth or prosthesis degeneration. Therefore, appropriate longitudinal evaluation of prosthetic valves is critical to clinical practice. Transthoracic echocardiography is the most useful tool in the routine evaluation of valve prostheses, but transesophageal echocardiography, cardiac catheterization, and fluoroscopy are all important adjuncts to the clinical evaluation of a dysfunctional prosthesis. As a reference for longitudinal follow-up, a transthoracic echocardiogram should be obtained early after valve implantation in all patients.

Prosthetic valves can be divided into two large categories: tissue and mechanical. The tissue prostheses include porcine or bovine heterografts and human allografts/homografts (Fig. 30.1). The mechanical prostheses include tilting disc prosthetics (e.g., the St. Jude bileaflet and the Medtronic-Hall single disc) and the ball-cage prosthesis (e.g., the Starr-Edwards) (Fig. 30.1). To accurately interpret echocardiographic findings, the exact type and size of the prosthesis should be known, as the various valve types demonstrate different hemodynamic profiles (Tables 30.1 through Table 30.4) and regurgitation characteristics. Prosthetic valve dysfunction may be caused by valve thrombosis, pannus formation, senescent changes (bioprostheses), and infection (Fig. 30.2).

EVALUATION OF THE MITRAL PROSTHESIS

Doppler interrogation of a mitral prosthesis is crucial in determining the functional status of the valve. However, the transthoracic echocardiographic evaluation of a mitral prosthesis should begin with a two-dimensional evaluation of valve stability and surrounding structures. Large vegetation, thrombus, and valve dehiscence can be identified. The leaflets of a bioprosthetic valve can be evaluated for symmetric excursion and evidence of calcification. The mechanical mitral prosthesis produces reverberation artifact, which limits the two-dimensional interrogation of the prosthesis itself and the surrounding structures, especially the left atrium (Fig. 30.3). Flow velocity through the prosthetic valve and determination of the maximal and mean pressure gradients should be obtained using continuous-wave Doppler interrogation. The pressure gradient can be elevated secondary to valve stenosis, regurgitation, or increased cardiac output. The pressure half-time measurement and the left ventricular outflow tract (LVOT) velocity can help distinguish between these two scenarios. The pressure half-time should be prolonged if the valve is obstructed, but normal or shortened if the increased pressure gradient across the valve is secondary to regurgitation. The LVOT velocity will be decreased if the increased velocity across the mitral prosthesis is secondary to severe regurgitation, as the

forward flow across the LVOT will be decreased (Table 30.5). It is important to recall that the pressure half-time method used to determine the area of a native mitral valve will overestimate the area of a mitral prosthesis. If there is no significant aortic or mitral regurgitation, the continuity equation is a valid and more optimal method for determining the area of a mitral prosthesis. The continuity equation for this calculation is as follows:

$$\text{MP area} = \text{LVOT area} \times ([\text{LVOT TVI}]/[\text{MP TVI}])$$
$$= \text{LVOT diameter}^2 \times 0.785 \times ([\text{LVOT TVI}]/[\text{MP TVI}])$$

where MP is mitral prosthesis, LVOT TVI is the LVOT time-velocity integral, and MP TVI is the time-velocity integral of the mitral prosthesis inflow velocity obtained by continuous-wave Doppler.

Regurgitation should be evaluated with color-flow imaging, spectral Doppler interrogation, and two-dimensional evaluation of the valve. If there is regurgitation, it is important to distinguish periprosthetic regurgitation from prosthetic regurgitation (Fig. 30.4), as the mechanism for each is different. The degree of regurgitation should then be assessed. The degree of prosthetic regurgitation can be assessed both by semiquantitative methods and quantitative methods (proximal isovelocity surface area [PISA]) if the jet is well seen. Severe regurgitation is indicated by the following:

1. Increased mitral inflow peak velocity 2.5 m/s or greater with normal mitral inflow pressure half-time (≤150 m/s)
2. Dense mitral regurgitant continuous-wave Doppler signals
3. Regurgitant fraction 55% or greater
4. Systolic Doppler flow reversals in the pulmonary vein

While prosthetic regurgitation can be detected by color flow imaging, the mechanical mitral prosthesis poses special challenges. The artifact produced in the left atrium may limit the ability to detect even significant degrees of prosthetic and periprosthetic regurgitation. In this situation, indirect indicators of significant regurgitation should be used. These include two-dimensional evidence of valve instability or periprosthetic tissue changes, increased left ventricular dimension, increased inflow gradient with a normal or reduced pressure half-time, and decreased LVOT velocity. Transesophageal echocardiography is very useful in defining the presence and degree of mechanical mitral prosthesis regurgitation (Fig. 30.5), as the posterior-to-anterior direction of the ultrasound beam allows visualization of the left atrium without imaging artifact.

When evaluating a prosthesis for regurgitation, it must be remembered that a small degree of prosthetic regurgitation is inherent for most mechanical prosthesis. The Doppler fingerprint of this regurgitation varies by prosthesis type. A Medtronic-Hall prosthesis

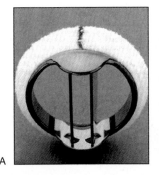

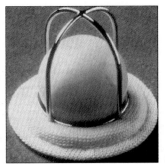

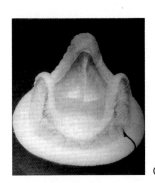

FIGURE 30.1. Prosthetic valves. (A) St. Jude bileaflet mechanical prosthesis. **(B)** Starr-Edwards prosthesis. **(C)** Porcine bioprosthesis.

Table 30.1	DOPPLER HEMODYNAMIC PROFILES OF 609 NORMAL AORTIC VALVE PROSTHESES			
Type of Prosthesis	No. of Prostheses	Peak Velocity (m/s)	Mean Gradient (mm Hg)	[LVOT TVI]/ [AV TVI]
Heterograft	214	2.4 ± 0.5	13.3 ± 6.1	0.44 ± 0.21
Ball-cage	160	3.2 ± 0.6	23.0 ± 8.8	0.32 ± 0.09
Björk-Shiley	141	2.5 ± 0.6	13.9 ± 7.0	0.40 ± 0.10
St. Jude Medical	44	2.5 ± 0.6	14.4 ± 7.7	0.41 ± 0.12
Homograft	30	1.9 ± 0.4	7.7 ± 2.7	0.56 ± 0.10
Medtronic-Hall	20	2.4 ± 0.2	13.6 ± 3.3	0.39 ± 0.09
Total	609	2.6 ± 0.7	15.8 ± 8.3	0.40 ± 0.16

AV, aortic valve; LVOT, left ventricular outflow tract; TVI, time-velocity integral. From Miller F, et al. Normal aortic valve prosthesis hemodynamics: 609 prospective Doppler examinations [abstract]. Circulation. 1989;80(suppl 2):II-169, with permission.

has one central jet of regurgitation, the St. Jude Medical mechanical prosthesis has two side and one central jet, the Starr-Edwards prosthesis has two curved side jets, and the Björk-Shiley prosthesis has two unequal side jets (Fig. 30.6). These normal regurgitant jets should be small, with a jet area less than 2 cm² and a jet length of less than 2.5 cm. Periprosthetic regurgitation is always abnormal. It may be a small amount of regurgitation related to a gap in the sutures placed at the anastomosis, or it may be secondary to an infectious process with perivalvular extension. Periprosthetic regurgitation that is significant may require treatment. Surgical intervention has traditionally been required, but transcatheter placement of devices to eliminate periprosthetic leakage is now possible in selected patients without evidence of active infection who are not surgical candidates.

EVALUATION OF THE AORTIC PROSTHESIS

An aortic valve prosthesis should be evaluated with an approach similar to the evaluation of the mitral prosthesis, with a few caveats. The spectral Doppler assessment of the left ventricular outflow tract and the aortic valve are usually best obtained with transthoracic imaging. Transesophageal imaging often does not allow optimal alignment of the Doppler beam to obtain the most accurate velocities through the valve and outflow tract. Left ventricular size, wall thickness, and function are also often most reliably measured during transthoracic imaging. Regurgitation can be demonstrated by both transthoracic and transesophageal imaging, but anterior periprosthetic jets are best seen on transthoracic images and posterior jets are best demonstrated by transesophageal images secondary to the location of the transducer and the artifact produced by the valve. Transesophageal images in general are better for the detection of vegetation.

Obstruction of an aortic prosthesis results in increased flow velocity across the prosthesis and is best quantitated by Doppler

Table 30.3	DOPPLER HEMODYNAMIC PROFILES OF 82 NORMAL TRICUSPID VALVE PROSTHESES			
Type of Prosthesis	No. of Prostheses	Peak Velocity (m/s)	Mean Gradient (mm Hg)	Pressure Half-time (ms)
Heterograft	41	1.3 ± 0.2	13.3 ± 1.1	146 ± 39
Ball-cage	33	1.3 ± 0.2	3.1 ± 0.8	144 ± 46
St. Jude Medical	7	1.2 ± 0.3	2.7 ± 1.1	108 ± 32
Björk-Shiley	1	1.3	2.2	144
Total	82	1.3 ± 0.2	3.1 ± 1.0	142 ± 42

From Connolly HM, et al. Doppler hemodynamic profiles of 82 clinically and echocardiographically normal tricuspid valve prostheses. Circulation. 1993;88:2722–2727, with permission.

echocardiography. Doppler interrogation should be performed in multiple imaging windows to obtain the maximal velocity across the prosthesis. To completely evaluate the prosthesis, continuous-wave Doppler should be obtained. From the highest velocity signal, a maximum instantaneous pressure gradient and a mean pressure gradient should be calculated. Pulsed-wave Doppler interrogation of the LVOT and measurement of the LVOT TVI is critical in determining the etiology of the increased blood flow velocity across the aortic prosthesis. Care should be taken to place the Doppler sample volume for this measurement below the area of flow acceleration. If the valve is truly obstructed, the LVOT velocity should not be increased. If the increased velocity across the valve is secondary to aortic regurgitation or a high output state, the LVOT velocity will be increased. The ratio of LVOT velocity or TVI versus AV velocity or TVI is helpful. If the prosthesis is obstructed, the ratio decreases (LVOT TVI/AV TVI ≤0.2 with normal ≥0.3) (Table 30.2).

The area of the aortic prosthesis can be estimated by the continuity equation as follows:

$$AP\ area = LVOT\ area \times ([LVOT\ TVI]/[AP\ TVI])$$
$$= SROD^2 \times 0.785 \times ([LVOT\ TVI]/[AP\ TVI])$$

where AP is aortic prosthesis and SROD is sewing ring diameter.

Evaluation of aortic prosthetic regurgitation should include two-dimensional evaluation of the valve and surrounding structures, color-flow imaging to determine the jet characteristics and location

Table 30.2	DOPPLER HEMODYNAMIC PROFILES OF 456 NORMAL MITRAL VALVE PROSTHESES			
Type of Prosthesis	No. of Prostheses	Peak Velocity m/s	Mean Gradient (mm Hg)	Effective Area (cm2)
Heterograft	150	1.6 ± 0.3	4.1 ± 1.5	2.3 ± 0.7
Ball-cage	161	1.8 ± 0.3	4.9 ± 1.8	2.4 ± 0.7
Björk-Shiley	79	1.7 ± 0.3	4.1 ± 1.6	2.6 ± 0.6
St. Jude Medical	66	1.6 ± 0.4	4.0 ± 1.8	3.0 ± 0.8

From Lengyel M, et al. Doppler hemodynamic profiles in 456 clinically and echo-normal mitral valve prostheses [abstract]. Circulation. 1990;82(suppl 3):III-43, with permission.

Table 30.4	DOPPLER ECHOCARDIOGRAPHIC DATA FOR PULMONARY VALVE PROSTHESES				
Type of Prosthesis	No.	Size (mm)	Peak Velocity (m/s)	Mean Gradient (mm Hg)	Trivial/Mild Prosthetic Regurgitation (No.)
Carpentier-Edwards	24	26.5 ± 1.8	2.4 ± 0.5	12.1 ± 5.3	7
Pulmonary homograft	17	24.2 ± 1.8	1.8 ± 0.6[a]	8.4 ± 4.8	15
Aortic homograft	3	22.3 ± 1.2	2.5 ± 0.4	14.4 ± 3.4	3
Hancock	3	26.0 ± 3.0	2.4 ± 0.5	14.0 ± 5.7	1
Ionescu-Shiley	2	25.0 ± 0.0	2.4 ± 0.4	12.5 ± 3.5	2
St. Jude Medical	1	25	2.6	12.0	1
Björk-Shiley	1	25	2.0	7.0	1

[a]Compared with all heterografts combined, P = .002.
From Novaro GM, et al. Doppler hemodynamic of 51 clinically and echocardiographically normal pulmonary valve prostheses. Mayo Clin Proc. 2001;76:155–160, with permission of Mayo Foundation for Medical Education and Research.

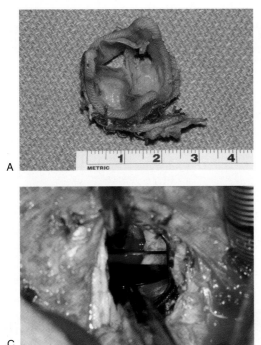
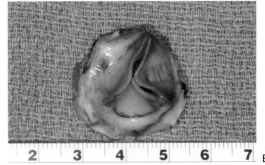

FIGURE 30.2. Prosthetic valve dysfunction. (A) Bioprosthetic valve with cusp perforation secondary to senescent changes. **(B)** Bioprosthetic valve with severe cusp thickening. **(C)** Mechanical valve compromised by pannus formation.

(prosthetic versus periprosthetic), pressure half-time of the regurgitant jet, mitral inflow pattern, diastolic reversal flow in the descending thoracic aorta, and regurgitation fraction (if the jet is suitable for quantification). The normal regurgitation patterns of mechanical prosthetic valves should be kept in mind so as not to be confused with pathologic regurgitation. Severe aortic valve regurgitation is indicated by:

1. Pressure half-time of regurgitant jet of 250 ms or less
2. Restrictive mitral inflow pattern (if the aortic regurgitation is acute)
3. Holodiastolic reversal in the descending thoracic aorta Doppler
4. Regurgitant fraction of 55% or greater

EVALUATION OF TRICUSPID AND PULMONARY PROSTHESES

Tricuspid and pulmonary valve replacements are much more common in patients with congenital heart disease. The evaluation of these prostheses is analogous to the evaluation of the aortic and mitral prosthetic valves with a few exceptions. The tricuspid and pulmonary valves are usually anterior structures. Therefore, imaging of these valves is often best with transthoracic imaging. The posterior location of the echo transducer in transesophageal imaging can diminish the ability to evaluate these anterior structures. If transesophageal imaging is used, transgastric images are usually best for evaluation.

Several forms of congenital heart disease require placement of an extraanatomic conduit and valve to establish continuity between the subpulmonary ventricle and the pulmonary arteries. These conduits are best evaluated with transthoracic images. Unique imaging windows must be obtained to completely determine the functional status of these prostheses. Imaging windows can often be found by palpation of the chest wall. Since the valve prosthesis is very close to the chest wall in these situations, flow through the valve is often felt as a vibratory sensation or "thrill." Placing the transducer at the site of the thrill may provide the best visualization of the valve. Often, the valve prosthesis itself is not seen and one must rely on Doppler interrogation and other indirect findings to determine the status of the prosthesis. Indirect findings include calculation of the right ventricular systolic pressure from the tricuspid valve regurgitation velocity using the modified Bernoulli equation: $\Delta P = 4V^2$. The velocity (and hence the calculated pressure gradient) across the pulmonary conduit cannot exceed the velocity through the tricuspid valve. Other indirect findings include right ventricular size, wall thickness, and function. The interventricular septal motion may also provide clues to right ventricular pressure or volume overload. If the septum flattens only in diastole, volume overload should be suspected. Septal flattening in both systole and diastole is indicative of right ventricular pressure overload.

Pulmonary valve prosthetic regurgitation may be brief in duration. The spectral Doppler pattern may be helpful in determining the degree of regurgitation. Rapid equalization of pulmonary artery and right ventricular diastolic pressure will occur if the degree of regurgitation is severe. This will result in a Doppler pattern of regurgitation that returns to the baseline before the end of diastole (Fig. 30.7). This pattern does not always signify significant regurgitation, however. If the right ventricle has poor compliance, smaller volumes of regurgitation cause greater changes in the diastolic pressure and can lead to a similar Doppler pattern. Significant noncompliance may result in diastolic forward flow with atrial contraction (Fig. 30.8).

Tricuspid prosthetic valves are often large and have lower flow velocity across them. Therefore, a lower calculated pressure

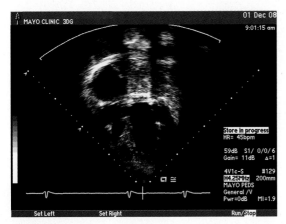

FIGURE 30.3. Apical four-chamber view showing reverberation artifact obscuring the left atrium in a patient with a mechanical mitral prosthesis.

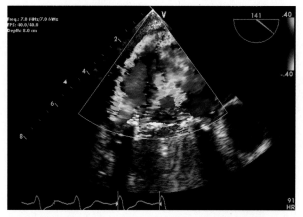

FIGURE 30.4. Transesophageal echocardiogram showing mechanical mitral prosthesis with both periprosthetic (*white arrow*) and prosthetic regurgitation (*yellow arrow*).

Table 30.5	INTERPRETATION OF INCREASED PROSTHESIS FLOW VELOCITY		
Mitral Prosthesis	**PHT**	**LVOT Velocity**	
Obstruction	↑	↔, ↓	
Regurgitation	↔, ↓	↓	
High output	↔	↑	
Aortic Prosthesis	**Mitral Inflow**	**LVOT Velocity**	**LVOT/AV TVI Ratio**
Obstruction	↔	↔, ↓	↓
Regurgitation	↔, ↓	↑	↔
High output	↑	↑	↔

AV, aortic valve; LVOT, left ventricular outflow tract; PHT, pressure half-time; TVI, time-velocity integral. ↑, increased; ↓, decreased; ↔, no change.

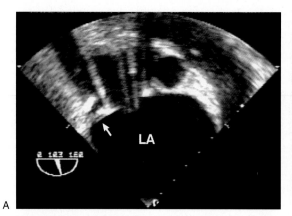
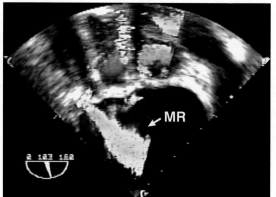

FIGURE 30.5. Mechanical mitral prosthesis visualized by transesophageal echocardiography. Note that there is no artifact obscuring the left atrium (**A**), allowing better visualization of the periprosthetic regurgitation jet (**B**).

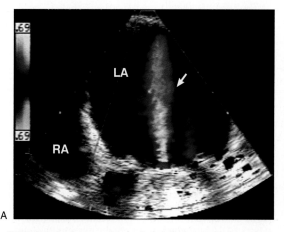
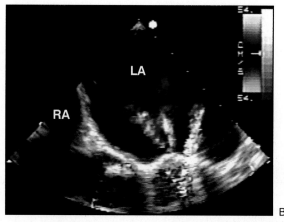

FIGURE 30.6. Appearance of normally functioning mechanical mitral prosthesis. (**A**) Medtronic-Hall prosthesis with a single central jet of normal regurgitation. (**B**) St. Jude prosthesis with three jets of normal regurgitation.

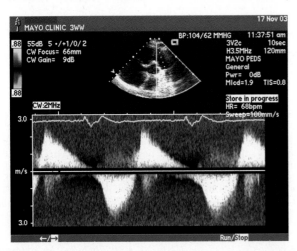

FIGURE 30.7. Spectral Doppler pattern consistent with severe pulmonary prosthetic regurgitation. Note the diastolic signal returns to the baseline prior to the start of systole.

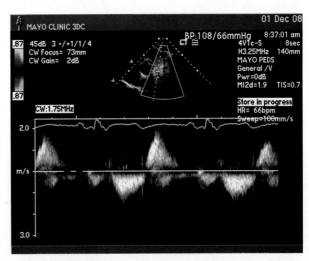

FIGURE 30.8. Spectral Doppler pattern through the pulmonary valve consistent with right ventricular noncompliance. Note the diastolic forward flow through the pulmonary valve with atrial contraction.

gradient is expected compared with the mitral valve prosthesis. Respiratory variation in transtricuspid flow is greater than that in transmitral flow. Flow is increased across the tricuspid prosthesis during inspiration and decreased during expiration. Measurement of the prosthetic gradient either should be obtained over several cardiac cycles and averaged or should be obtained during held expiration.

Tricuspid valve prosthetic regurgitation, when severe, may be laminar. Systolic flow reversals in the hepatic veins are a marker of severe tricuspid prosthetic regurgitation but are not always present. If the right atrium is very large, the systolic flow reversals in the hepatic veins are diminished or absent.

 ## PATIENT–PROSTHESIS MISMATCH

Prosthetic valves are manufactured in multiple different diameters. At surgery, the largest possible prosthesis should be implanted to provide the largest effective orifice area. If a prosthesis has an effective orifice area that is too small in relation to the patient's body surface area, an increased gradient will be present without inherent stenosis of the valve. This is known as patient–prosthesis mismatch. Patient–prosthesis mismatch is determined by calculating the effective orifice area of the prosthesis and dividing that area by the body surface area of the patient to obtain an indexed effective orifice area. If the indexed effective orifice area is greater than 0.85 cm^2/m^2, the

degree of mismatch is mild. Severe patient–prosthesis mismatch is defined as an indexed effective orifice area of 0.6 cm^2/m^2 or less. Patient–prosthesis mismatch has been shown in several studies to correlate with poor patient outcomes.

SUGGESTED READING

Connolly HM, et al. Doppler hemodynamic profiles of 82 clinically and echocardiographically normal tricuspid valve prostheses. *Circulation.* 1993;88:2722–2727.

Lengyel M, et al. Doppler hemodynamic profiles in 456 clinically and echo-normal mitral valve prostheses [abstract]. *Circulation.* 1990;82(suppl 3):III-43.

Miller F, et al. Normal aortic valve prosthesis hemodynamics: 609 prospective Doppler examinations [abstract]. *Circulation.* 1989;80(suppl 2):II-169.

Mohr-Kahaly S, et al. Regurgitant flow in apparently normal valve prostheses: improved detection and semiquantitative analysis by transesophageal two-dimensional color-coded Doppler echocardiography. *J Am Soc Echocardiogr.* 1990;3:187–195.

Novaro GM, et al. Doppler hemodynamic of 51 clinically and echocardiographically normal pulmonary valve prostheses. *Mayo Clin Proc.* 2001;76:155–160.

Rahimtoola SH. The problem of valve prosthesis-patient mismatch. *Circulation.* 1978;58:20–24.

Sorajja P, et al. Successful percutaneous repair of perivalvular prosthetic regurgitation. *Cathet Cardiovasc Interv.* 2007;70:815–823.

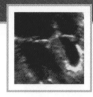

Chapter 31
Three-dimensional Echocardiography in Congenital Heart Diseases

Girish S. Shirali • Ivan Salgo

Complex intracardiac anatomy and spatial relationships are inherent to congenital heart defects. Beginning over 30 years ago and until recently, the clinician's ability to image the heart by echocardiography has been limited to two-dimensional techniques. In the interim, there have been important advances in 2D echocardiography (2DE). Improved transducer technology, beam-forming, and miniaturization have led to significant improvements in spatial and temporal resolution using 2DE. However, 2DE has fundamental limitations. The very nature of a 2DE slice, which has no thickness, necessitates the use of multiple orthogonal "sweeps." The echocardiographer then mentally reconstructs the anatomy and uses the structure of the report to express this mentally reconstructed vision. This means that the only three-dimensional image of the heart is the "virtual image" that exists in the echocardiographer's mind and is then translated into words. It is not easy for an untrained—albeit interested—observer to understand the images obtained in the course of a sweep: expert interpretation is required. Since myocardial motion occurs in three dimensions, 2DE techniques inherently do not lend themselves to accurate quantitation.

Recognition of these limitations of 2DE led to burgeoning research and clinical interest in the modality of three-dimensional echocardiography (3DE). Early reconstructive approaches were based on 2DE image acquisitions that were subsequently stacked and aligned based on phases of the cardiac cycle, to recreate a 3DE dataset. While these approaches proved to be accurate, the need for time and offline processing equipment imposed fundamental limitations on their clinical applicability. In 1990, von Ramm and Smith published their early results with a matrix array transducer that provided real-time images of the heart in three dimensions. While this was an important breakthrough, this transducer was unable to be steered in the third (elevation) dimension. Over the past 5 years, dramatic technological advances have facilitated the ability to perform live 3DE scanning, including the ability to steer the beam in three dimensions and to render the image in real-time.

THREE-DIMENSIONAL ECHOCARDIOGRAPHIC TECHNOLOGY

Technologic advances that have facilitated the maturation of 3DE techniques include the following:

- Matrix transducers
- Beam forming and steering in three spatial dimensions
- Display of three-dimensional information
- Software for quantification

Matrix Transducers

Two important advances in transducer technology—the organization of elements and the use of novel piezoelectric materials—have been the structural basis for improvements in 3DE matrix transducers. The organization of elements within the transducer is best understood by starting with a brief review of 2DE transducers.

Elements: Two-dimensional Transducers – Current 2DE transducers transmit and receive acoustic beams in a flat 2DE scanning plane. As opposed to M-mode, which provides one spatial and one temporal dimension, 2DE scanning systems sweep a scan line to and fro within this 2DE imaging plane. The angular position of the beam is said to vary in the azimuthal dimension. Even though traditional, flat 2DE scanning comprises two spatial dimensions plus one temporal dimension, this is not three-dimensional imaging. The 2DE transducer itself consists of elements that work in concert to create a scan line. Typically, a conventional transducer consists of 64 to 128 elements arranged along a single row (technically referred to

as a one-dimensional array of elements). These elements are spaced according to the ultimate frequency (and hence wavelength) of the acoustic vibrations; these propagate radially along the direction of the scan line. The two spatial dimensions in the image come from sweeping the beam by firing along this row at different times. This array of elements steers the outward ultrasound beam or scan line by using interference patterns generated by varying the spatiotemporal phase of each element's transmit event.

Elements: Primitive Matrix Array Transducers – An innovation applied in the past decade was to increase the number of rows of elements from one (in the 2DE transducer described earlier) to five to seven rows of elements. This "sparse-element" model generated a primitive matrix array transducer with 5 × 64 = 320 elements. While this represented a dramatic increase in the number of elements, not all elements were electrically active, and the individual elements were not electrically independent from each other. As a result, this transducer did not steer in the third (elevation) dimension. Poor image quality, a large footprint, and the lack of portability limited the mainstream acceptability of this approach.

Elements: Contemporary Matrix Array Transducers – Contemporary matrix-array transducers comprise as many elements in the elevational dimension as they do in the azimuthal dimension, with more than 60 elements in each of these dimensions. While the elements are arranged in a two-dimensional grid, this array generates 3DE images. To be able to steer in the elevational plane, each element must be electrically independent from all other elements, and each element must be electrically active. The technology and electrical circuitry to electrically insulate and connect each element became commercially available in 2002. As a result, the contemporary matrix array transducer consists of thousands of electrically active elements that independently steer a scan line left and right, as well as up and down.

Transducers: Piezoelectric Materials – The piezoelectric material in an ultrasound transducer is a fundamental determinant of system image quality. Piezoelectric transducer elements are responsible for delivery of ultrasound energy into the scanned tissue and for converting returning ultrasound echoes into electric signals. Their coupling efficiency in converting electrical energy to mechanical energy, or vice versa, is a key determinant of image quality, Doppler sensitivity, and penetration. To create an overall piezoelectric effect, these elements must be subject to the application of an external electric field to align dipoles within polycrystalline materials. For almost 40 years, a ceramic polycrystalline material, PZT (lead-zirconate-titanate) or PZT composites, has been the standard piezoelectric material used in medical imaging. This material is a uniform powder that is mixed with an organic binder; the resulting compound is baked into a dense polycrystalline structure. At its best, it achieves about 70% alignment of dipoles because of imperfect alignment of the individual dipoles. This leads to a corresponding constraint in the electromechanical coupling efficiency of the material.

One example of new piezoelectric material involves growing crystals from a molten ceramic material, resulting in a homogeneous crystal with fewer defects, lower losses, and no grain boundaries. When these crystals are poled at the preferred orientation(s), near-perfect alignment of dipoles (≈100%) is achievable resulting in dramatically enhanced electromechanical properties (Fig. 31.1). The efficiency of conversion of electrical to mechanical energy improves by as much as 68% to 85% compared with PZT ceramics currently used in ultrasound transducers. The new piezoelectric materials provide increased bandwidth and sensitivity, resulting in both improved penetration and high resolution. The improved arrangement of atoms in these new piezoelectric materials, and their superior strain energy density, translates into advances in transducer miniaturization. The recent implementation of these advances has

Traditional PZT Ceramics

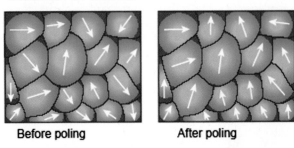

Before poling   After poling

New Technology: Ceramics

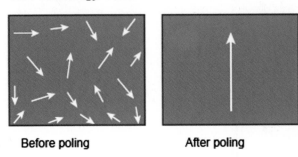

Before poling   After poling

FIGURE 31.1. Comparison of piezoelectric ceramics. Top: Imperfect alignment of dipoles in traditional piezoelectric (PZT) crystals after poling (application of an external electrical field). **Bottom:** Almost perfect alignment of dipoles in new piezoelectric material.

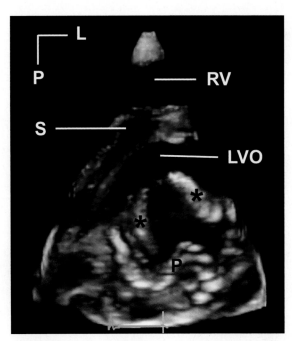

FIGURE 31.2. Parasternal short-axis image of a cleft in the anterior mitral leaflet. *Asterisks* mark the edges of the cleft. A tissue colorization map has been applied to the image. This has the effect of coloring tissues in the near field (near to either the transducer or the front of the three-dimensional image) in an orange color. Tissues in the far field are colored blue. This is a dynamic aftereffect, which means that as the operator rotates, tilts, or otherwise manipulates the image, the color effect correspondingly changes in real-time. L, left; LVO, left ventricular outflow tract; P, posterior; RV, right ventricle; S, septum.

led to the availability of a high frequency matrix 3DE transthoracic transducer that has dramatically enhanced the applicability of 3DE to pediatric populations.

Three-dimensional Beam Forming and Steering

Beam forming constitutes the steering and focusing of transmitted and received scan lines. For 3DE, this means that the beam former must be steered toward both the azimuthal and elevational planes. This is achieved both in the ultrasound system and within the transducer itself, using highly specialized integrated circuits to create a 3D trapezoid of acoustic information that is processed. These 3DE data are summed, processed, and finally placed into rectangular space using a 3D scan converter.

Display of Three-dimensional Echocardiographic Images

Two-dimensional computer displays consist of rows and blocks of picture elements, termed *pixels*, that comprise a 2D image. In contrast, a 3DE dataset consists of bricks of pixels, termed *volume elements* or *voxels*. However, even for a 3DE dataset, the two-dimensional nature of the display imposes restrictions on the ability to appreciate depth. As shown initially by the ancient Greeks and subsequently rediscovered during the Renaissance, perspective is used to simulate the appearance of 3D depth, providing objects the appearance of being close to or deeper/farther from the screen. The process of adding perspective is done by casting a light beam through the collection of voxels. The light beam either hits enough tissue so as to render it opaque, or it keeps shining through transparent voxels so as to render it transparent. More recent algorithms apply different hues to the front of the dataset (nearest to the screen) as opposed to voxels that are far from the screen (Fig. 31.2). The user has the ability to rotate and tilt the dataset on the computer screen. Tools are available to "cut away" interfering structures, thus performing "virtual dissection."

Software for Quantification

Quantification requires segmentation of structures of interest from the acquired data. Since myocardial motion occurs in three spatial dimensions, 2DE planes are inherently incapable of capturing

the entire motion. Two-dimensional techniques for quantitation are based on geometric formulas that rely on assumptions regarding the shapes of cardiac structures. However, these assumptions are frequently incorrect. In contrast, 3DE acquisitions include the entire extent of the structure, thus minimizing the possibility of foreshortening of the apex or any geometric assumptions regarding shape. Three-dimensional quantitative software tools have the potential to quantify cardiac structures accurately regardless of their shape. Advances in the software tools for processing 3DE datasets have mirrored the rapid advances in transducer technology that have occurred over the past 5 years.

The 3DE volumetric techniques rely on definition of chamber cavities, that is, the blood–endocardium interface. The software constructs this interface by using a process known as *surface rendering* and represents it as a mesh of points and lines. This software-generated mesh is calculated for every frame of acquisition, thus providing a moving cast of the cavity of the ventricle during the cardiac cycle. Because this is digital data, it provides for ease of computation of global and regional volumes, synchrony, as well as parametric displays of endocardial excursion and timing of contraction (Fig. 31.3).

The 3DE quantification tools for the left ventricle are more technologically advanced than those for other cardiac structures. Until recently, 3DE left ventricular (LV) quantification tools used the method of disk summation. With improvements in computing speeds and programming, newer tools have been developed to provide instantaneous tracking of the blood pool–endocardium interface at each frame of acquisition. This provides a surface-rendered model that is displayed as a mesh of lines and points. However, these approaches are still based on some basic 3D geometric assumptions regarding LV shape, and therefore their application cannot be extended to the right ventricle or to univentricular hearts. Given the complex shape and architecture of the right ventricle, it is not surprising that tools for quantifying RV volume have been slower to mature. Until very recently, these tools used the method of disks for volumetrics. Novel software now provides instantaneous tracking of the blood pool–endocardium interface at each frame of acquisition (Fig. 31.4). This yields a surface-rendered model that is displayed as a mesh of lines and points.

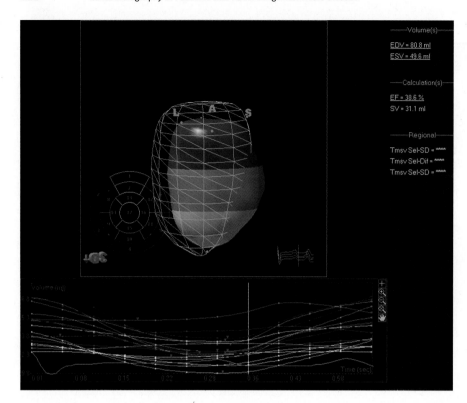

FIGURE 31.3. Software for processing three-dimensional echocardiography enables quantitation of left ventricular volumes throughout the cardiac cycle, providing end-diastolic and end-systolic volumes as well as ejection fraction. The mesh represents left ventricular volume at end-diastole. The cast of the left ventricular cavity consists of segments of varying colors, each of which represents a subvolume of the ventricular cavity based on the American Society of Echocardiography 16-segment model. The change in volume of each subvolume is represented graphically, with time on the *x*-axis and volume on the *y*-axis.

Quantitative software for the mitral valve provides the ability to perform sophisticated analyses of the nonplanar shape of the mitral annulus and to measure 3D structures including annular diameters, commissural lengths, and leaflet surface areas. Quantitative techniques have also been developed to provide volumetric measurements of 3D color flow using nonaliased color flow data.

MODES OF THREE-DIMENSIONAL ECHOCARDIOGRAPHY

Electronically steered 3DE systems have two major modes of scanning: live and electrocardiographically (ECG) gated. The live mode is the only modality where the system scans in 3D real-time. A defining characteristic of this mode is if the transducer comes off the chest, the image disappears. The live 3D mode can also be operated within a three-dimensionally shaped zoom box. Live 3DE modes provide narrow (20 to 30 degrees in the elevation plane) datasets that have high voxel density. This modality can be obtained on patients with arrhythmias or with an active precordium with no potential for motion or stitch artifacts.

ECG-gated modes are required to provide wider volumes while maintaining adequate frame rates (Fig. 31.5). Gating allows for four to eight smaller volumes to be stitched together to generate volumes that are greater than 90 degrees wide in the elevation plane, at frame rates exceeding 30 Hz. Gated modes have comparatively lower voxel density and are subject to both motion and stitch artifacts. Recent enhancements have improved the ability to acquire gated full-volume data among patients with arrhythmias. Gated modes are available using grayscale or color flow Doppler.

Contemporary 3DE systems provide the user with tools to vary frame rate, 3D volume size, and image resolution. Increasing the requirement in one of these causes a drop in the other two, all things being equal.

Given the potential for motion and stitch artifacts with gated modes and the need for high spatial and temporal resolution, it has been our practice to use live 3DE to delineate anatomy. We reserve the use of gated modes for the following:

- Targets that do not fit within a live 3DE window
- Quantitation of chamber volumes
- The 3DE color flow demonstrations of regurgitant jets or shunt flows.

Live 3DE imaging has been commercially available for transthoracic and fetal applications since 2002. Live 3DE transesophageal echocardiographic imaging became commercially available in 2007. This has yielded images never before seen on the beating heart (Fig. 31.6). We anticipate that continuing improvements in transducer technology and the wider applicability of advances in piezoelectrics will enable the application of 3DE technology to an ever-increasing range of patient sizes, windows, and applications.

CLINICAL APPLICATIONS IN CONGENITAL HEART DISEASE

The 3DE imaging has three broad areas of clinical application among patients with congenital heart disease: visualization of morphology, volumetric quantitation of chamber sizes and flows, and image-guided interventions.

Visualization of Morphology

Dating from an early stage in the development of 3DE technology, the structural complexity that is inherent to congenital heart disease has been identified as fertile substrate for exploration using 3DE.

Atrioventricular Valves – Use of 3DE is valuable in delineating the morphology of the atrioventricular valves. Espinola-Zavaleta et al. described the role of 3DE in delineating congenital abnormalities of the mitral valve. Lu et al. demonstrated that 3DE allowed comprehensive assessment of the anatomy of double-orifice mitral valve. Rawlins et al. demonstrated the additive value of 3DE and improved image quality using intraoperative epicardial 3DE to delineate the anatomy of atrioventricular valves. Seliem et al. studied 41 patients with atrioventricular valve abnormalities and found that 3DE imaging was helpful in delineating the morphology of the valve leaflets and their chordal attachments, the subchordal apparatus, the mech-

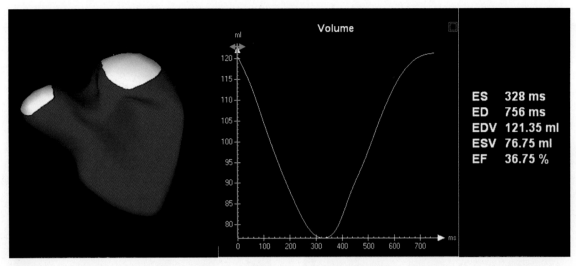

FIGURE 31.4. Novel software provides the ability to measure right ventricular volume throughout the cardiac cycle. This yields a surface-rendered model that is displayed as a mesh of lines and points. The change in volume of each subvolume is represented graphically, with time on the *x*-axis and volume on the *y*-axis.

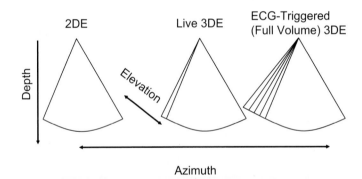

FIGURE 31.5. Differences between two-dimensional, live three-dimensional, and full-volume (electrocardiographically triggered) three-dimensional echocardiography (3DE). Left: Conventional 2DE. **Middle:** Live 3DE imaging adds the elevation plane. The shape of the image is therefore trapezoidal rather than pie-shaped. **Right:** Electocardiographically triggered (full volume) 3DE imaging, which provides a wider trapezoid.

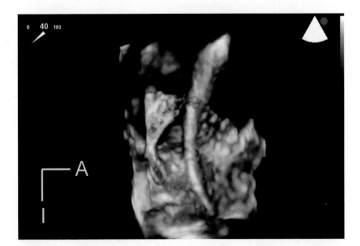

FIGURE 31.6. Live three-dimensional transesophageal echocardiography demonstrates a catheter passing through a large atrial septal defect. The viewing perspective is unique: the observer is virtually located within the left atrium, looking rightward. A, anterior; I, inferior.

anism and origin of regurgitation, and the geometry of the regurgitant volume. Vettukatil et al. examined the role of 3DE in patients with Ebstein's anomaly of the tricuspid valve. They demonstrated that 3DE provided clear visualization of the morphology of the valve leaflets, including the extent of their formation, the level of their attachment, and their degree of coaptation. They were also able to visualize the mechanism of regurgitation or stenosis. We have found that 3DE provides unparalleled surgeon's views of the tricuspid valve en face.

Atrioventricular Septal Defect – Hlavacek et al. studied 52 datasets on 51 patients with atrioventricular septal defects (AVSDs) and showed that gated 3DE views could be cropped to obtain en face views of the atrial and ventricular septa. These views provide a clear understanding of the relationships of the bridging leaflets to the septal structures (Figs. 31.7 and 31.8). These views have been useful to determine the precise location of the interventricular communication relative to the bridging leaflets and to demonstrate how these relationships determine the level of shunting (atrial, ventricular, or both atrial and ventricular). They found that 3DE on unrepaired balanced AVSDs and repaired AVSDs with residual lesions was more often additive/useful (33 of 36 [92%]) than on repaired AVSDs without residual lesions or unbalanced AVSDs (9 of 16 [56%]; *P* = .009). Use of 3DE was additive or useful in all three patients with unbalanced AVSDs being considered for biventricular repair. Useful information obtained by 3DE included precise characterization of mitral regurgitation and leaflet anatomy, unique viewing perspectives such as the surgeon's view of a cleft mitral valve, substrate for subaortic stenosis, valve anatomy, and presence and location of additional septal defects.

Atrial and Ventricular Septa – Tantengco et al. showed that 3DE reconstructions provided unique en face views of atrial and ventricular septal defects. Cheng et al. studied 38 patients with atrial and/or ventricular septal defects using 3DE and compared their results to 2DE and surgical findings. They demonstrated novel 3DE views of both atrial and ventricular septal defects and improved accuracy of quantification of the size of the defect by 3DE compared with 2DE (*r* = 0.92 versus *r* = 0.69). This approach has also been used to demonstrate the morphology of muscular ventricular septal defects. We have found live 3DE to be of great value in evaluating the ventricular septum en face and to assess malformations of the outflow tract that involve malalignment of the outlet septum.

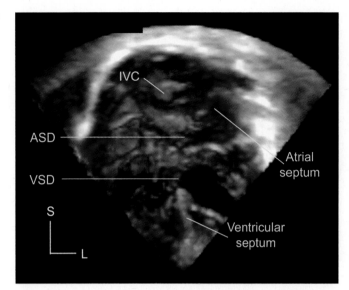

FIGURE 31.7. Apical four-chamber three-dimensional echocardiogram in a patient with an atrioventricular septal defect. The bridging leaflets divide the defect into an interatrial (ASD) and interventricular (VSD) component. Note the posterior location of the inferior vena caval orifice (IVC) relative to the septal structures. L, left; S, superior.

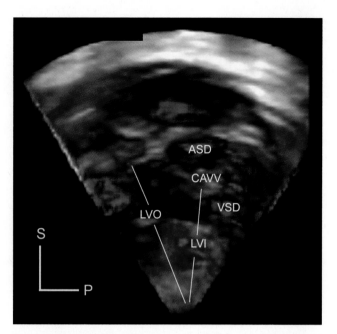

FIGURE 31.8. En face view of the left ventricular aspect of the ventricular septum in a patient with atrioventricular (AV) septal defect. The free walls of the left atrium and left ventricle have been cropped. The viewer is looking from left to right. This view demonstrates the left ventricular inflow-outflow disproportion that characterizes an AV septal defect. Note the crescentic inferior margin of the atrial septum and the scooped-out edge of the interventricular septum. This view provides excellent anatomic detail regarding the relationships between the bridging leaflets of the common AV valve (CAVV) and the septal structures. P, posterior; S, superior.

Aortic Arch, Pulmonary Arteries, and Aortopulmonary Shunts – The 3DE color flow Doppler has been used to provide echocardiographic "angiograms" of flow patterns in the aortic arch (coarctation of the aorta), the branch pulmonary arteries (the Lecompte maneuver), and across Blalock-Taussig shunts. Hlavacek et al examined echocardiographic "angiograms" in 26 patients (Fig. 31.9). The 3DE provided additional diagnostic information in 10 of 26 patients (38%). In 17 of 26 patients (65%), validation of the 3DE diagnosis was available with surgery, cardiac catheterization, magnetic resonance imaging (MRI), or computed tomography (CT) angiography.

Aortic Valve and Outflow Tract – Sadagopan et al. examined the role of 3DE in eight children who subsequently underwent surgery for congenital aortic valvar stenosis. They showed that 3DE was accurate in providing measurements of the aortic valve annulus and the number of valve leaflets, in identifying the sites of fusion of the leaflets, and in characterizing nodules and excrescences in dysplastic valves. Bharucha et al. studied 16 patients with subaortic stenosis. Using a form of 3DE reconstruction known as multiplanar reconstruction, which provides access to an unlimited number of 2DE planes, they demonstrated abnormalities of mitral valve leaflet or chordal apparatus attachments (14 patients), abnormal ventricular muscle band (11 patients), and abnormal increased aortomitral separation (2 patients).

Characterization of Left Ventricular Noncompaction – Baker et al. evaluated four patients with LV noncompaction using 3DE. They found that 3DE enabled diagnosis and provided detailed characterization of the affected myocardium, including easy visualization of entire trabecular projections, intertrabecular recesses, endocardial borders, and wall motion abnormalities of the affected myocardium. 3DE enabled easy differentiation between compacted and noncompacted portions of the myocardium.

Quantitation of Chamber Dimensions, Valve Apparatus, Function, and Flows

Left Ventricular Volumetrics – The 3DE quantitation provides both proven and potential value for pediatric echocardiography. Bu et al. compared 3DE measurements of LV volumetrics to those obtained using MRI. Their study showed that 3DE measurements of LV end-systolic volume, end-diastolic volume, mass, stroke vol-

ume, and ejection fraction in children using a rapid full-volume acquisition strategy are feasible, reproducible, and comparable with MRI measurements. They found good correlations between the two methods but a tendency toward mild underestimation of volumes by 3DE. Interestingly, estimates of ejection fraction were

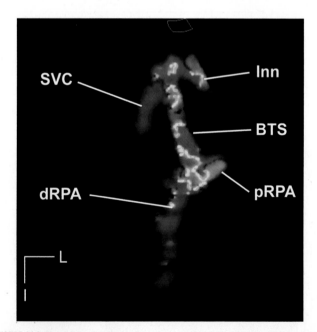

FIGURE 31.9. Three-dimensional color flow, electrocardiographically triggered (full-volume) echocardiographic acquisition demonstrating a right-sided Blalock-Taussig shunt (BTS). The grayscale image has been suppressed, thus providing an echocardiographic angiogram. The shunt is seen in its entirety from its origin from the innominate artery (Inn) to its insertion. The proximal and distal right pulmonary artery (pRPA and dRPA, respectively) are well seen. Note the proximity of the superior vena cava (SVC) to the cranial end of the shunt. This dataset can be rotated, tilted, and examined in an infinite number of planes to delineate the location of stenosis. I, inferior; L, left.

in closer agreement. Baker et al. evaluated the feasibility of 3DE LV volumetrics, as well as the resource utilization, learning curve, and interobserver and intraobserver reproducibility of this technique. The study design involved 15 datasets and four observers who had varying degrees of (self-rated) experience with 3DE quantitation. They found that in 59 of 60 instances, observers were able to obtain 3D LV ejection fraction in less than 3 minutes (median time, 1 minute 27 seconds). They demonstrated a learning curve for the observer with the lowest level of self-rated experience. Their study also showed excellent interobserver and intraobserver reproducibilities for 3DE LV volumetrics.

Left Ventricular Mass – Studies in adults have validated 3DE as an accurate method for measuring LV mass. While studies in children have been limited in number and scope, Riehle et al. recently demonstrated excellent correlations between 3DE and MRI for LV mass.

Left Ventricular Dyssynchrony – The 3DE approach to measuring intra-LV dyssynchrony uses the American Society of Echocardiography's 16-segment model of the left ventricle. It measures the time of each subvolume from maximal (end-diastolic) volume to minimal volume and the standard deviation of these time intervals. The higher the value of the standard deviation, the higher is the implied degree of intra-LV dyssynchrony. Baker et al. examined the association between LV dysfunction and intra-LV dyssynchrony in children using 3DE. They studied nine children with dilated cardiomyopathy and an equal number of age- and body size–matched normal volunteers. They found that normal patients had 3DE dyssynchrony indices that were below 3%. Among children with dilated cardiomyopathy, there was a clear threshold value of LV ejection fraction (LVEF): at an LVEF below 35% to 40%, intra-LV dyssynchrony was the rule. In contrast, patients whose LVEF was higher than 40% exhibited no significant dyssynchrony.

Right Ventricular Volumetrics – Until recently, the accuracy of 3DE measurement of right ventricular (RV) volume and ejection fraction had not been evaluated. This is not surprising given the complex architecture of the right ventricle and the technical difficulty of imaging it adequately. Recently, Gopal et al. reported a large series of adults who underwent RV volumetric measurements with MRI and 3DE using the disk summation method. In 16 children with congenital heart disease, Niemann et al. studied RV volumes by 3DE using a new and robust protocol that uses multiplanar reconstruction and tracing with semiautomated border detection. They found excellent correlations between MRI and 3DE for measurement of RV volumes and ejection fraction. As these tools become more widely available, user-friendly, and accurate, we may well see the emergence of a new paradigm in the use of echocardiographic parameters as surrogate outcome measures in clinical trials of medications and pacing strategies. The Pediatric Heart Disease Clinical Research Network is examining RV volumetrics as a secondary outcome measure in the Single Ventricle Reconstruction Study, which examines differences between initial shunt type on survival following the Norwood procedure for neonates with hypoplastic left heart syndrome (unpublished data, http://www.pediatricheartnetwork.org/svrforhealthcareproviders.asp).

Visualization and Quantitation of Three-dimensional Echocardiography Color Flow – Multiplanar reconstruction tools provide the ability to not only visualize but also to trace and measure the area of valvar regurgitant orifices at the level of the *vena contracta*. While this technique is new and has not been validated, it has been shown to be feasible and has already yielded new insights into the shape of regurgitant jets, and it holds promise as a tool to enhance the echocardiographer's ability to serially quantify valve regurgitation.

Pemberton et al. developed a technique for quantifying nonaliased 3DE color flow jets in vitro. They validated this technique on open-chest pigs; compared with measurements obtained from flow probes positioned on the ascending aorta, they obtained excellent correlations between the two methods. They compared 143 individual measurements of cardiac output and found excellent correlation between the two techniques ($r^2 = 0.93$). The 3DE quantification of color flow has recently been validated in adults

by comparison to cardiac outputs obtained by thermodilution. Application of this technique to pathologic states could lead to potentially more accurate measurements of regurgitant volumes and fractions.

Image-Guided Interventions

The high temporal and spatial resolution of transthoracic and particularly transesophageal echocardiography has ignited interest in the potential uses of live 3DE to guide interventions. Scheurer et al. demonstrated the use of live 3DE to guide the performance of endomyocardial biopsy in children. In their experience, the use of live 3DE guidance was associated with no complications, including no new tricuspid valve leaflet flail or pericardial effusion. The 3DE proved to be a reliable noninvasive modality to accurately direct the bioptome to the desired site of biopsy within the right ventricle. As familiarity with this technique increased, the need for fluoroscopic guidance of bioptome manipulation in the right ventricle was minimized. Del Nido et al. extended the concept of image-guided intervention to the very novel approach of epicardial live 3DE-guided, open-chest, closed-heart, off-bypass cardiac surgery. They began with in vitro validation of the ability of live 3DE to guide the performance of common surgical tasks. More recently, they have undertaken closure of small atrial septal defects in the porcine model using live 3DE guidance. With the recent introduction of live 3D TEE, we have been able to obtain spectacular images of cardiac chambers, septal structures, and valves. Live 3D TEE is being used to guide catheter manipulations, transseptal procedures, and closure of septal defects (Figs. 31.10 and 31.11).

 LEARNING CURVE

The learning curve with 3DE is steep but negotiable. Our experience suggests that the success of 3DE in a program requires advocacy and an investment of time by both echocardiographers and sonographers. The acceptance of 3DE is improving on a global level, albeit at an early stage of the technology cycle. We have developed and implemented an interactive teaching course that uses simulations with 3DE datasets with rehearsal and direct mentoring; this has been shown to be useful in overcoming the steep part of the learning curve.

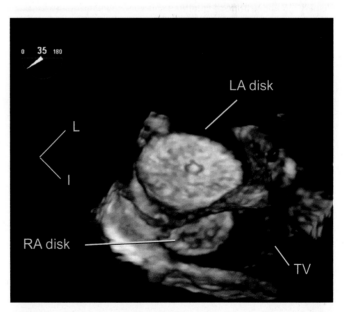

FIGURE 31.10. Live three-dimensional transesophageal echocardiogram immediately following device closure of a fenestrated atrial septum with a cribriform Amplatzer septal occluder. The viewer is "virtually" placed inside the left atrium, looking rightward and posteriorly. The entire left atrial disk of the device is seen, with its central umbilication and the meshwork of metal that constitutes its frame. Part of the inferior portion of the right atrial disk (RA disk) and the tricuspid valve apparatus (TV) are also seen. I, inferior; L, left.

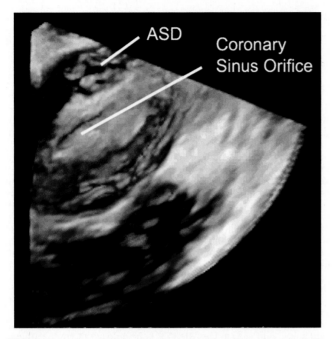

FIGURE 31.11. Live three-dimensional transesophageal echocardiogram in a patient with a low secundum atrial septal defect. Two-dimensional echocardiography imaging demonstrated that the defect was in proximity to the coronary sinus, raising doubts about candidacy for device closure. In this three-dimensional echocardiography image, the free walls and appendage of the right atrium have been removed. The viewer is looking posteriorly and leftward. Note the high resolution of anatomic detail. The atrial septal defect is separated from the coronary sinus orifice by a reasonable distance. Based on the shape and size of the defect, this patient was thought, on the basis of three-dimensional echocardiography, to be a reasonable candidate for device closure, which was successfully accomplished. A, anterior; S, superior.

 ## FUTURE DIRECTIONS

Over the next decade, advances in the 3DE arena will involve technical enhancements such as improved image resolution, holographic displays, a wide range of validated software tools for quantification, and enhancements to work flow. New, multimodality applications will increasingly bring 3DE into the mainstream. Refinements in transducer technology will make high-resolution 3DE available across the spectrum of patient sizes. We anticipate a 3DE TEE probe miniaturized for pediatric use. With the growing interest in multimodality imaging, 3DE volumetric data will eventually be integrated with the pressure data that are available during cardiac catheterization, yielding pressure-volume loops that can be obtained as a matter of routine clinical practice.

SUGGESTED READING

Acar P, Abadir S, Paranon S, et al. Live 3D echocardiography with the pediatric matrix probe. *Echocardiography.* Aug 2007;24:750–755.

Ariet M, Geiser EA, Lupkiewicz SM, et al. Evaluation of a three-dimensional reconstruction to compute left ventricular volume and mass. *Am J Cardiol.* 1984;54:415–420.

Baker GH, Flack EC, Hlavacek AM, et al. Variability and resource utilization of bedside three-dimensional echocardiographic quantitative measurements of left ventricular volume in congenital heart disease. *Congenital Heart Dis.* 2006;1:318–323.

Baker GH, Hlavacek AM, Chessa KS, et al. Left ventricular dysfunction is associated with intraventricular dyssynchrony by 3-dimensional echocardiography in children. *J Am Soc Echocardiogr.* 2008;21:230–233.

Baker GH, Pereira NL, Hlavacek AM, et al. Transthoracic real-time three-dimensional echocardiography in the diagnosis and description of noncompaction of ventricular myocardium. *Echocardiography.* 2006;23:490:494.

Baker GH, Shirali GS, Bandisode V. Transseptal left heart catheterization for a patient with a prosthetic mitral valve using live three-dimensional transesophageal echocardiography. *Pediatr Cardiol.* 2008:29:690–691.

Bharucha T, Ho SY, Vettukattil JJ. Multiplanar review analysis of three-dimensional echocardiographic datasets gives new insights into the morphology of subaortic stenosis. *Eur J Echocardiogr.* 2008.

Bu L, Munns S, Zhang H, et al. Rapid full volume data acquisition by real-time 3-dimensional echocardiography for assessment of left ventricular indexes in children: a validation study compared with magnetic resonance imaging. *J Am Soc Echocardiogr.* 2005;18:299–305.

Caiani EG, Corsi C, Zamorano J, et al. Improved semiautomated quantification of left ventricular volumes and ejection fraction using 3-dimensional echocardiography with a full matrix-array transducer: comparison with magnetic resonance imaging. *J Am Soc Echocardiogr.* 2005;18:779–788.

Cheng TO, Xie MX, Wang XF, et al. Real-time 3-dimensional echocardiography in assessing atrial and ventricular septal defects: an echocardiographic-surgical correlative study. *Am Heart J.* 2004;148:1091–1095.

Dekker DL, Piziali RL, Dong E Jr. A system for ultrasonically imaging the human heart in three dimensions. *Comput Biomed Res.* 1974;7:544–553.

Espinola-Zavaleta N, Vargas-Barron J, Keirns C, et al. Three-dimensional echocardiography in congenital malformations of the mitral valve. *J Am Soc Echocardiogr.* 2002;15:468–472.

Gopal AS, Chukwu EO, Iwuchukwu CJ, et al. Normal values of right ventricular size and function by real-time 3-dimensional echocardiography: comparison with cardiac magnetic resonance imaging. *J Am Soc Echocardiogr.* 2007;20:445–455.

Gururaja TR, Panda RK, Chen J, et al. Single crystal transducers for medical imaging applications. Ultrasonics Symposium, 1999. Proceedings. 1999 IEEE. 1999;2:969–972.

Hlavacek A, Lucas J, Baker H, et al. Feasibility and utility of three-dimensional color flow echocardiography of the aortic arch: The "echocardiographic angiogram". *Echocardiography.* 2006;23(10):860–864.

Hlavacek AM, Chessa K, Crawford FA, et al. Real-time three-dimensional echocardiography is useful in the evaluation of patients with atrioventricular septal defects. *Echocardiography.* 2006;23:225–231.

Jenkins C, Monaghan M, Shirali G, et al. An intensive interactive course for 3D echocardiography: Is "Crop Till You Drop" an effective learning strategy? *Eur J Echocardiogr.* 2008:9:373–380.

Kapetanakis S, Kearney MT, Siva A, et al. Real-time three-dimensional echocardiography: a novel technique to quantify global left ventricular mechanical dyssynchrony. *Circulation.* 2005;112:992–1000.

Kuwata J, Uchino K, Nomura S. Dielectric and piezoelectric properties of 0.91Pb(Zn1/3Nb2/3)O3–0.09PbTiO3 single crystals. *Jpn J Appl Phys.* 1982; 21:1298–1302.

Linker DT, Moritz WE, Pearlman AS. A new three-dimensional echocardiographic method of right ventricular volume measurement: in vitro validation. *J Am Coll Cardiol.* 1986;8:101–106.

Lodato JA, Weinert L, Baumann R, et al. Use of 3-dimensional color Doppler echocardiography to measure stroke volume in human beings: comparison with thermodilution. *J Am Soc Echocardiogr.* 2007;20:103–112.

Lu Q, Lu X, Xie M, et al. Real-time three-dimensional echocardiography in assessment of congenital double orifice mitral valve. J Huazhong Univ Sci Technolog Med Sci. 2006;26:625–628.

Matsumoto M, Matsuo H, Kitabatake A, et al. Three-dimensional echocardiograms and two-dimensional echocardiographic images at desired planes by a computerized system. *Ultrasound Med Biol.* 1977;3:163–178.

Matsumura Y, Fukuda S, Tran H, et al. Geometry of the proximal isovelocity surface area in mitral regurgitation by 3-dimensional color Doppler echocardiography: difference between functional mitral regurgitation and prolapse regurgitation. *Am Heart J.* 2008;155:231–238.

Mercer-Rosa L, Seliem MA, Fedec A, et al. Illustration of the additional value of real-time 3-dimensional echocardiography to conventional transthoracic and transesophageal 2-dimensional echocardiography in imaging muscular ventricular septal defects: does this have any impact on individual patient treatment? *J Am Soc Echocardiogr.* 2006;19(12):1511–1519.

Mor-Avi V, Sugeng L, Weinert L, et al. Fast measurement of left ventricular mass with real-time three-dimensional echocardiography: comparison with magnetic resonance imaging. *Circulation.* 2004;110(13):1814–1818.

Niemann PS, Pinho L, Balbach T, et al. Anatomically oriented right ventricular volume measurements with dynamic three-dimensional echocardiography validated by 3-Tesla magnetic resonance imaging. *J Am Coll Cardiol.* 2007;50:1668–1676.

Park SE, Shrout TR. Characteristics of relaxor-based piezoelectric single crystals for ultrasonic transducers. *IEEE Trans Ultrason Ferroelectr Freq Control.* 1997;44.

Pemberton J, Ge S, Thiele K, et al. Real-time three-dimensional color Doppler echocardiography overcomes the inaccuracies of spectral Doppler for stroke volume calculation. *J Am Soc Echocardiogr.* 2006;19:1403–1410.

Pemberton J, Hui L, Young M, et al. Accuracy of 3-dimensional color Doppler-derived flow volumes with increasing image depth. *J Ultrasound Med.* 2005;24:1109–1115.

Pemberton J, Li X, Karamlou T, et al. The use of live three-dimensional Doppler echocardiography in the measurement of cardiac output: an in vivo animal study. *J Am Coll Cardiol.* 2005;45:433–438.

Pouleur AC, le Polain de Waroux JB, Pasquet A, et al. Assessment of left ventricular mass and volumes by three-dimensional echocardiography in patients with or without wall motion abnormalities: comparison against cine magnetic resonance imaging. *Heart.* 2007:94:1050–1057.

Rawlins DB, Austin C, Simpson JM. Live three-dimensional paediatric intra-operative epicardial echocardiography as a guide to surgical repair of atrioventricular valves. *Cardiol Young.* 2006;16:34–39.

Riehle TJ, Mahle WT, Parks WJ, et al. Real-time three-dimensional echo-cardiographic acquisition and quantification of left ventricular indices in children and young adults with congenital heart disease: comparison with magnetic resonance imaging. *J Am Soc Echocardiogr.* 2008;21:78–83.

Sadagopan SN, Veldtman GR, Sivaprakasam MC, et al. Correlations with oper-ative anatomy of real-time three-dimensional echocardiographic imaging of congenital aortic valvar stenosis. *Cardiol Young.* 2006;16:490–494.

Salgo IS, Gorman JH 3rd, Gorman RC, et al. Effect of annular shape on leaflet curvature in reducing mitral leaflet stress. *Circulation.* 2002;106:711–717.

Salgo IS. Three-dimensional echocardiographic technology. *Cardiol Clin.* 2007;25:231–239.

Scheurer M, Bandisode V, Ruff P, et al. Early experience with real-time three-dimensional echocardiographic guidance of right ventricular biopsy in chil-dren. *Echocardiography.* 2006;23:45–49.

Seliem MA, Fedec A, Szwast A, et al. Atrioventricular valve morphology and dynamics in congenital heart disease as imaged with real-time 3-dimen-sional matrix-array echocardiography: comparison with 2-dimensional imaging and surgical findings. *J Am Soc Echocardiogr.* 2007;20:869–876.

Simpson JM. Real-time three-dimensional echocardiography of congenital heart disease using a high frequency paediatric matrix transducer. *Eur J Echocardiogr.* 2008:9:222–224.

Suematsu Y, Martinez JF, Wolf BK, et al. Three-dimensional echo-guided beating heart surgery without cardiopulmonary bypass: atrial septal defect closure in a swine model. *J Thorac Cardiovasc Surg.* 2005;130:1348–1357.

Suematsu Y, Marx GR, Stoll JA, et al. Three-dimensional echocardiography-guided beating-heart surgery without cardiopulmonary bypass: a feasibility study. *J Thorac Cardiovasc Surg.* 2004;128:579–587.

Suematsu Y, Marx GR, Triedman JK, et al. Three-dimensional echocardiogra-phy-guided atrial septectomy: an experimental study. *J Thorac Cardiovasc Surg.* 2004;128:53–59.

Sugeng L, Spencer KT, Mor-Avi V, et al. Dynamic three-dimensional color flow Doppler: an improved technique for the assessment of mitral regurgitation. *Echocardiography.* 2003;20:265–273.

Sugeng L, Weinert L, Lang RM. Real-time 3-dimensional color Doppler flow of mitral and tricuspid regurgitation: feasibility and initial quantita-tive comparison with 2-dimensional methods. *J Am Soc Echocardiogr.* 2007;20:1050–1057.

Tajik AJ, Seward JB, Hagler DJ, et al. Two-dimensional real-time ultrasonic imaging of the heart and great vessels. Technique, image orientation, struc-ture identification, and validation. *Mayo Clin Proc.* 1978;53:271–303.

Tantengco MV, Bates JR, Ryan T, et al. Dynamic three-dimensional echocar-diographic reconstruction of congenital cardiac septation defects. *Pediatr Cardiol.* 1997;18:184–190.

Vasilyev NV, Martinez JF, Freudenthal FP, et al. Three-dimensional echo and videocardioscopy-guided atrial septal defect closure. *Ann Thorac Surg.* 2006;82:1322–1326.

Vettukattil JJ, Bharucha T, Anderson RH. Defining Ebstein's malformation using three-dimensional echocardiography. *Interact Cardiovasc Thorac Surg.* 2007;6:685–690.

Vogel M, Ho SY, Anderson RH. Comparison of three dimensional echocardio-graphic findings with anatomical specimens of various congenitally mal-formed hearts. *Br Heart J.* 1995;73:566–570.

Vogel M, Ho SY, Buhlmeyer K, et al. Assessment of congenital heart defects by dynamic three-dimensional echocardiography: methods of data acquisition and clinical potential. *Acta Paediatr Suppl.* 1995;410:34–39.

Vogel M, Losch S. Dynamic three-dimensional echocardiography with a com-puted tomography imaging probe: initial clinical experience with transtho-racic application in infants and children with congenital heart defects. *Br Heart J.* 1994;71:462–467.

Von Ramm OT, Smith SW. Real-time volumetric ultrasound imaging system. *J Digital Imaging.* 1990;3:261–266.

Watanabe N, Ogasawara Y, Yamaura Y, et al. Mitral annulus flattens in isch-emic mitral regurgitation: geometric differences between inferior and ante-rior myocardial infarction: a real-time 3-dimensional echocardiographic study. *Circulation.* 2005;112(suppl):I458–1462.

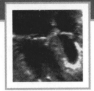

Chapter 32
Stress Echocardiography

Thomas R. Kimball

Robert A. Bruce, the father of exercise cardiology, once quipped, "You would never buy a used car without taking it out for a drive and seeing how the engine performed while it was running, and the same is true for evaluating the function of the heart." This eloquent statement succinctly explains both the past motivation of early cardiologists to develop exercise protocols and the current need to modernize our evaluation of pediatric cardiovascular disease.

With the creation of, first, the Master's Two-Step test and, second, the Bruce standardized treadmill test, cardiologists were provided, for the first time a standardized means to examine their patients outside of the resting condition. The ensuing introduction of the Bruce exercise protocol into the patient evaluation of congenital heart disease allowed cardiologists not only to predict the success of cardiac surgery but also to detect occult cardiovascular problems in otherwise asymptomatic individuals. The continued use of not only exercise but also other forms of stress in evaluating cardiac patients represents an extension of the resting physical examination. As Bruce stated in 1956, "an exercise test represents physical examination of the patient in relation to a reproducible amount of work."

Despite the advances in and documented usefulness of stress testing, most cardiovascular assessment today unfortunately continues to be performed almost exclusively while the patient is comfortably resting (sometimes even sleeping) in a clinic or echocardiographic examination room. These appraisals, while yielding valuable information about resting conditions, afford little clue as to the behavior of the cardiovascular system when the patient becomes active, which is the typical state during most of the patient's waking moments. Applying stress assessment in the clinical setting provides the means to observe the patient under conditions that closely mimic these more typically active states.

Further, in the relatively few cases when they are used, stress assessments rely heavily on electrocardiographic responses. Interestingly, when he conceived of the exercise evaluation, Bruce focused attention on and found predictive ability with the hemodynamic responses, not the electrocardiographic changes, occurring with exercise. For instance, he not only discovered that the mechanism of exercise-induced hypotension is a consequence of fixed stroke volume but also that these hemodynamic changes were predictive of adverse long-term outcome. These conclusions acquired both during and after the exercise test were founded on physical examination alone. Since then, echocardiography has revolutionized cardiovascular diagnostics. The coupling of echocardiography with exercise or other forms of stress is a natural progression of exercise science because it provides the window for more direct, accurate, and robust observations of the important and predictive hemodynamic responses discovered by Bruce more than 50 years ago.

EVOLUTION OF STRESS ECHOCARDIOGRAPHY SCIENCE

Stress echocardiography is the culmination of the parallel evolutions of *exercise science* and cardiac *ultrasound imaging* driven, primarily, by coronary artery disease as a major public health problem. Exercise science had its beginnings in 1918 when the first objective measure of cardiac dysfunction during stress was made by Bousfield, who observed ST-segment depression occurring with angina. Systematic electrocardiographic exercise testing began 10 years later in patients with angina. In 1935, Master became the first to standardize the exercise test by developing an exercise protocol using a 9-inch two-step. However, this test was too strenuous for most patients and did not allow continuous data acquisition, prompting Bruce to develop first, the one-stage treadmill exercise

test in 1949 and then, the multistage test (the Bruce protocol) in 1963.

The origins of *stress imaging* began in 1935, when Tennant and Wiggers noted by direct observation that interruption of coronary blood flow resulted in abnormal myocardial wall motion. However, it was not until 1970 that this phenomenon was visualized by ultrasound when Kraunz and Kennedy detected abnormal wall motion in patients with coronary artery disease immediately following exercise. The introduction of dobutamine stress echocardiography in 1986 improved image resolution because hyperpnea and patient motion associated with exercise were eliminated. In addition, dobutamine stress echocardiography provided a means to evaluate nonambulatory patients.

Pediatric stress echocardiography use began in 1980 when Alpert et al. performed simultaneous high-fidelity catheter pressure measurements and M-mode echocardiography during supine cycle ergometry in children with left-sided congenital heart disease to assess functional reserve. Exercise echocardiography was used throughout the 1980s in children for detection of subclinical left ventricular dysfunction in aortic insufficiency, insulin-dependent diabetes mellitus, and coarctation of the aorta. In addition, normal pediatric exercise physiology could now be more thoroughly evaluated. Pharmacologic stress echocardiography in children began in 1992, first using dipyridamole in patients after repair of anomalous left coronary artery from the pulmonary artery and, later, using dobutamine in children with a variety of cardiac pathology. Stress echocardiography has now become part of the standard offerings of clinical stress testing in pediatrics.

THEORY BEHIND STRESS ECHOCARDIOGRAPHY

Stress echocardiography is a specific diagnostic modality categorized within a broader scheme of stress imaging protocols. However, all stress imaging protocols, including stress echocardiography, are unified by the concept that all use one of many stressors designed to stimulate patient hemodynamics and thereafter evaluate the cardiovascular effects elicited by the specific stressor with one of many sensors.

Stress echocardiography is applied for two basic diagnostic issues: (a) suspected impairment in myocardial perfusion or (b) hemodynamic behavior during stress of noncoronary cardiac pathology. In evaluating the first pathologic type, impaired myocardial perfusion, the theory underlying the utility of stress echocardiography, simply relates to supply and demand. Myocardial oxygen demand is increased by applying the stressor. If the coronary arteries are normal, perfusion and myocardial oxygen supply also increase to meet the increased demands. However, if the coronary arteries are diseased, perfusion may not increase, creating a demand/supply mismatch, resulting in myocardial ischemia. The sensor is used to detect the resulting abnormality caused by this mismatch. For example, in the case of electrocardiography, demand/supply mismatch is manifest by ST-segment elevation. In the case of echocardiography, ischemia is manifest by a new or worsened myocardial wall motion abnormality. The manifestation of these abnormalities, and, therefore, the sensitivity of the sensors, is dependent on the degree of induced ischemic load (Fig. 32.1). Some sensors (e.g., positron emission tomography) are highly sensitive, and abnormalities (e.g., metabolic derangements) become evident with a brief and light ischemic load. Other sensors (e.g., ECG) are less sensitive, and the abnormalities sensed by them (e.g., ST-segment changes) become evident only with a long and heavy ischemic burden. The ischemia-induced wall motion abnormalities detected by echocardiography require an intermediate level of ischemic

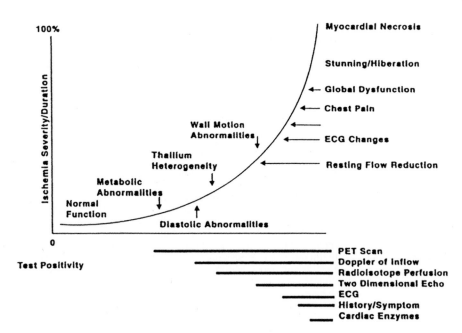

FIGURE 32.1. The ischemic cascade portrays the physiologic derangements (and the diagnostic sensors required to detect these derangements) occurring with a progressive ischemic burden. A low ischemic burden produces metabolic abnormalities that are detected by only highly sensitive sensors (e.g., positron emission tomography). A larger ischemic burden results in progressively deleterious derangements including diastolic dysfunction, wall motion abnormalities, myocardial stunning, and eventually myocardial necrosis. Angina develops with only a marked ischemic burden, making it a relatively insensitive indicator of coronary perfusion abnormalities. Wall motion abnormalities develop with an intermediate ischemic burden so that stress echocardiography has an intermediate sensitivity. (Reprinted with kind permission of Springer Science and Business Media.)

burden to become manifest and, therefore, echocardiography has an intermediate sensitivity.

In evaluating the second pathologic type, *hemodynamic behavior of noncoronary heart disease*, the theory underlying the utility of stress echocardiography, is founded on the premise that stress data are more reflective of a patient's typical diurnal activity state than are traditional data acquired in the resting state. In fact, data acquired during the resting state may be so dissimilar from data acquired during activity that the resting data may lead clinicians to a false sense of security regarding patient health. This premise has been similarly invoked for other cardiovascular tests that currently extend the patient evaluation beyond the office examination room such as ambulatory blood pressure and Holter monitoring. When using these two modalities, the clinician realizes that because symptomatology may

not be present in the office milieu, additional data acquired during an active state are needed to capture symptoms and explore etiologies. Likewise, stress echocardiography, as a simulation of the patient's active state, is used by clinicians to elicit and understand symptoms.

 INDICATIONS

Bayes Theorem

Bayes theorem is a result in probability theory that demonstrates the accuracy of a test with imperfect sensitivity and specificity is related to the prevalence of that disease in the population undergoing testing (Fig. 32.2, Table 32.1). Specifically, the positive and

A) Disease with High Prevalence (90%)
Sensitivity of test=90%, Specificity=80%, n=1000

		With + test	With - test
With Disease	900	810(0.9x900)	90
Without Disease	100	20	80(0.8x100)
TOTAL	**1000**	**830**	**170**

Positive predictive value = 810/830 = 98%
Negative predictive value = 80/170 = 47%

B) Disease with Low Prevalence (3%)
Sensitivity of test=90%, Specificity=80%, n=1000

		With + test	With - test
With Disease	30	27(0.9x30)	3
Without Disease	970	194	776(0.8x970)
TOTAL	**1000**	**221**	**779**

Positive predictive value = 27/221 = 12%
Negative predictive value = 776/779 = 99%

FIGURE 32.2. In general, diagnostic tests are evaluated by their sensitivity (the proportion of patients with disease who have a positive test) and specificity (the proportion of patients without the disease who have a negative test). However, Bayes theorem demonstrates that even with good sensitivity and specificity, a test may have limited clinical usefulness. Positive predictive value (the probability that a person with a positive result actually has the disease) and negative predictive value (the probability that person with a negative result does not have the disease) are better measures of overall clinical usefulness of a test, because they incorporate information on both the test (i.e., sensitivity and specificity) and the population being tested (i.e., prevalence). With high prevalence of disease in the population being tested (90% in Example A here), of 1000 patients, 900 will have the disease and 100 will not. A test with 90% sensitivity and 80% specificity will correctly identify 810 of the 900 patients with disease (90% of 900) and 80 of the 100 patients without disease (80% of 100). Bayes theorem demonstrates that the test has excellent positive predictive value; the likelihood of disease in a patient with a positive test is very high. On the other hand, a negative test would not rule out the disease; the patient would still have more than a 50% chance of having the disease. With low prevalence of disease (3% in Example B here), the test with the same sensitivity and specificity has poor positive predictive value. In other words, it is likely that a patient with a positive test does not have the disease. The test, therefore, would not be useful as a screening test because it would not be able to identify diseased individuals. On the other hand, a patient with a negative test result would be virtually ensured of not having the disease.

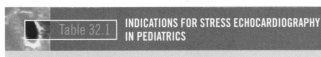

Table 32.1 INDICATIONS FOR STRESS ECHOCARDIOGRAPHY IN PEDIATRICS

- **Coronary artery disease**
  Adult coronary heart disease
  Post cardiac transplant graft vasculopathy
  Kawasaki disease
  Post arterial switch operation
  Supravalvar aortic stenosis and other conditions with suspected coronary ostial stenosis
  Anomalous origin of coronary arteries
  Coronary artery fistulas
  Obstructive left heart lesions
  Coronary pathology in pulmonary atresia with intact ventricular septum
- **Ventricular contractile reserve**
  Postoperative tetralogy of Fallot
  Postoperative coarctation of the aorta
  Anthracycline treatment
  Fontan circulation
  Obstructive sleep apnea
  Diabetes mellitus
  Dilated cardiomyopathy
  Aortic and mitral insufficiency
- **Pressure dynamics**
  Valvar stenosis
  Postoperative coarctation of the aorta
  Hypertrophic cardiomyopathy
  Pulmonary artery pressure

negative predictive values of a test are dependent on the prevalence of the disease so that low disease prevalence is associated with a high false-positive rate but a low false-negative rate. For example, in the evaluation of chest pain in an elderly, hypertensive adult patient, the positive predictive value of stress echocardiography would be appropriate and useful because the prevalence of coronary artery disease is high in elderly, hypertensive adults. A positive test result would be highly likely to reflect advanced coronary artery disease. However, performing stress echocardiography in a healthy, thin adolescent complaining of chest pain would be of little help in detecting coronary artery disease because its prevalence is so low in healthy, thin adolescents. In this instance, Bayes theorem would predict that the test would have a high false-positive rate so that a physician receiving a positive test result would still be left wondering if the patient truly has coronary artery pathology or, worse, establishing a false diagnosis of coronary artery disease. On the other hand, because Bayes theorem also predicts a low false-negative rate in this setting, the test is not totally without value. If the test were negative, a physician could conclude with very high certainty that the patient does not have coronary artery disease because Bayes theorem predicts a low false-negative rate in this setting. Proper application and interpretation of stress echocardiography are, therefore, essential in the pediatric population.

Coronary Artery Disease – Like most pathology, coronary artery disease consists of an anatomic substrate with physiologic consequences. It is important to assess both aspects of coronary pathology because even an impressive coronary artery narrowing may have minor or no physiologic consequences as a result of the development of collateral circulation. Intervention in such a case may be unwarranted because it will not improve physiology any more than has already occurred with the natural development of these collateral vessels. Before the advent of stress echocardiography, clinicians were only able to assess the anatomic severity of coronary artery disease. Diagnostic modalities such as coronary arteriography yield detailed images of coronary anatomy but reveal little information regarding actual myocardial perfusion. The application of stress echocardiography provides assessment of physiologic severity of coronary artery disease because it evaluates the degree of compromise in myocardial perfusion for any given anatomic abnormality. A main indication for performing stress echocardiography, therefore,

is determining physiologic significance of anatomically abnormal coronary arteries.

THE CHILD WITH ADULT CORONARY HEART DISEASE Much emphasis has appropriately been placed on the adult with congenital heart disease. Because congenital heart surgery survival rates have markedly improved, this heretofore uncommon population is growing.

A parallel situation is occurring in the pediatric population. It is known that the atherosclerotic process begins in childhood. For most children, vascular involvement has been minor so that treatment has been preventive. However, in some disease states, such as familial hypercholesterolemia, diabetes mellitus, chronic kidney disease, Kawasaki disease, and rheumatologic diseases, the childhood atherosclerotic process is hastened, leading to coronary events in childhood. An even more disturbing problem is that society is in the midst of a childhood obesity epidemic, which is accelerating this process even in children without other disease. Not only has childhood obesity resulted in more adults with cardiovascular disease, but it has also caused adverse cardiovascular risk factor changes during childhood. The presence of coronary artery disease and risk factors in children has resulted in a burgeoning of a heretofore uncommon pediatric population—the child with adult coronary artery disease, which similarly finds itself in the pediatric-adult netherworld previously reserved only for the adult patients with congenital heart disease. These patients are also falling between the cracks and receiving imperfect care. A concerted collaborative effort such as is occurring for the latter population needs to begin for these children. Recent reports demonstrate that myocardial infarction may occur in adolescents. In children with coronary risk factors such as insulin-dependent diabetes mellitus, left ventricular wall motion is compromised at an age as young as 10 years. The etiology of this remains unclear but may be related to damaged endothelial function. Stress echocardiography will be an important diagnostic tool in evaluating this population.

POST CARDIAC TRANSPLANT CORONARY ARTERY DISEASE Coronary artery pathology in children is most prevalent in the post cardiac transplant population. Transplant graft vasculopathy remains a major cause of late transplant mortality because it can result in chronic graft failure and arrhythmogenic sudden death. The disease is insidious and rapidly progressive. Because the coronary arteries are affected in a diffuse manner, the sensitivity of coronary angiography, which relies on having normal coronary segments adjacent to diseased segments for diagnosis of arterial disease, is imperfect and more accurate surveillance methods have been required. Intracoronary ultrasound is likely the most sensitive method but it is invasive and may also produce false-negative results. Dobutamine stress echocardiography has proved to be the most sensitive noninvasive test in detecting its presence and has been recommended by the American Heart Association as a means to follow these patients.

KAWASAKI DISEASE Myocardial perfusion may be impaired in patients who have had Kawasaki disease because of thrombosed aneurysms and/or strictures at aneurysm sites. In addition, there is evidence that patients without any echocardiographic coronary artery involvement have abnormal endothelial function, putting them at risk for early atherosclerotic heart disease. Even so, attention must be given to Bayes theorem when using stress echocardiography in the Kawasaki population. Nevertheless, stress echocardiography using both exercise and dobutamine has proved effective in following these patients for myocardial perfusion abnormalities. In addition, dobutamine stress echocardiography has been useful in the risk stratification of patients with coronary artery aneurysms and stenoses. Specifically, using dobutamine stress echocardiography, it has been shown that patients in the lowest four American Heart Association risk levels are unlikely to have coronary perfusion abnormalities. Patients in the highest risk level (Category 5) may or may not have perfusion abnormalities depending on the presence/absence of collateral circulation. Kawasaki disease is another example of how coronary artery physiology may be different in children versus adults. Children and adolescents may have very impressive coronary artery obstruction but have normal stress tests because of the development of collateral vessels. In most of these instances, bypass grafting would not be indicated. Stress echocardiography is an important tool in differentiating those patients who need revascularization from those who may safely undergo observation alone.

ARTERIAL SWITCH OPERATION FOR TRANSPOSITION OF THE GREAT VESSELS   The arterial switch operation involves reimplanting the coronary arteries from the native aorta to the main pulmonary artery stump (the neoaorta). Following the arterial switch operation, coronary artery lesions are common and progressive, necessitating routine serial evaluation of perfusion with stress echocardiography and sometimes resulting in the need for revascularization. In addition, stress echocardiography has been able to detect perfusion abnormalities in the absence of symptoms or arteriographic stenoses. The significance of such findings has yet to be determined; a constant finding in these patients is right coronary artery dominance with a hypoplastic distal left anterior descending coronary artery, which may result in the perfusion abnormality. Interestingly, these abnormalities are usually not present after the Ross operation, a procedure that also involves coronary reimplantation.

CORONARY OSTIAL STENOSIS   Ischemia can occur in patients with supravalvar aortic stenosis, particularly those with Williams syndrome, because of coronary ostial stenosis, fusion of an aortic valve leaflet to the supravalvar ridge, or diffuse left main coronary artery narrowing. Coronary ostial stenosis may also be seen with an anomalous origin of the left coronary artery from the right sinus of Valsalva or in patients with transposition of the great vessels, This pathology may be very difficult to diagnose angiographically because the catheter is usually engaged in the coronary artery downstream from the narrowing. Stress echocardiography may therefore be particularly helpful in these individuals.

OTHER CONGENITAL HEART DISEASE   Dobutamine and dipyridamole stress echocardiography has been useful in delineating the need for surgical management of anomalous origin of the left coronary artery from the pulmonary artery and in documentation of ischemia in coronary artery fistula. Other anomalies of the coronary artery origins such as the left main coronary artery from the right sinus of Valsalva or the circumflex coronary artery from the right main coronary artery have a higher incidence of atherosclerosis. Obstruction of left heart structures (valvar aortic stenosis, coarctation of the aorta, hypertrophic cardiomyopathy) is also associated with premature atherosclerosis. Finally, infants with pulmonary atresia and intact ventricular septum may have right ventricular–dependent coronary circulation and focal areas of coronary narrowing or frank coronary arterial interruption or aortocoronary atresia. Stress echocardiography could help to risk stratify these patients.

Ventricular Contractile Reserve

A second indication for stress echocardiography is in the evaluation of ventricular reserve. Patients with compromised ventricular function have elevated circulating catecholamines, decreased myocardial beta-receptor density, and downregulation of myocardial receptors. The contractile response to exogenous catecholamines has prognostic value. Patients with poor cardiac performance will have downregulation of beta receptors and have minimal response to exogenous catecholamines. Patients with better ventricular performance will have better beta-receptor responsiveness and better response to catecholamine administration. The magnitude of augmentation of cardiac performance during cardiovascular stress is the contractile reserve.

Measurement of left ventricular contractile reserve by stress echocardiography has been helpful in the detection and management of subclinical compromise of ventricular function in pediatric patients at risk for cardiomyopathy. For instance, stress echocardiography has shown that right and left ventricular reserve is depressed in children following repair of tetralogy of Fallot and enhanced after coarctation of the aorta repair (Fig. 32.3). Other investigators have shown that stress echo can detect subclinical left ventricular dysfunction in childhood cancer survivors who have received cardiotoxic chemotherapeutic agents. Some investigators have combined echocardiography with catheter-derived intracardiac pressure measurements during exercise to provide sophisticated contractility data helpful in differentiating mechanisms of ventricular reserve in

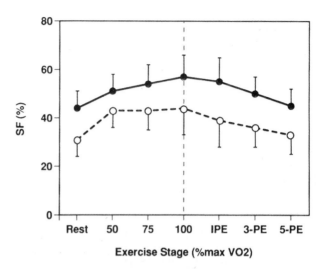

FIGURE 32.3 Contractile reserve in postoperative coarctation of the aorta patients (*filled circles*) is enhanced relative to that in control children (*open circles*) as assessed by measurement of left ventricular shortening fraction (SF) during exercise. Data are expressed as mean +/− standard deviation. IPE, 3-PE, and 5-PE indicate immediately and 3 and 5 minutes after exercise, respectively; Max VO2, maximal oxygen consumption; 50, 75, and 100, 50%, 75%, and 100% of maximal oxygen consumption, respectively. (Reprinted by permission of Elsevier Publishing Company.)

congenital left-sided lesions. In patients after Fontan operation as the result of single-ventricle physiology, exercise echocardiography demonstrates normal increases in stroke and cardiac index during exercise until late submaximal levels at which point these indices decrease.

Many of the other studies documenting the utility of contractile reserve have been performed in adult patients only. For example, the technique has also proved valuable in evaluating contractile reserve in adult patients with obstructive sleep apnea and diabetes mellitus. In addition, left ventricular contractile reserve assessed by dobutamine stress echocardiography predicts 5-year mortality in patients with dilated cardiomyopathy. Evaluation of contractile reserve has also proved valuable in the evaluation of aortic and mitral insufficiency. In adult patients with aortic and mitral insufficiency, contractile reserve by exercise echocardiography is a better predictor of myocardial function after medical or surgical therapy than resting ejection fraction. These results in adult patients are encouraging and, as with most other echocardiographic indices, have found their utility first in the adult population. Similar studies need to be performed in children as pediatric cardiologists are currently perplexed as to timing and efficacy of interventions in these patients. Stress echocardiography would be a robust tool to help answer these dilemmas.

Pressure Dynamics

The final indication for stress echocardiography is to evaluate pressure dynamics during a simulated active state. As discussed previously, traditional evaluation of hemodynamics is performed during the resting state and, therefore, affords little information regarding how these parameters change during a child's normally active life. Such data might prove helpful in conditions such as hypertrophic cardiomyopathy, valve stenosis, and pulmonary hypertension. In patients with rheumatic mitral stenosis, a mean mitral valve gradient of greater than 18 mm Hg at peak dobutamine is predictive of future clinical events (hospitalization, acute pulmonary edema, or supraventricular tachyarrhythmias). In asymptomatic patients with aortic stenosis, the degree of increase in aortic valve gradient during exercise provides incremental predictive value over resting echocardiographic and exercise electrocardiographic indices. In children after the Ross procedure, stress echocardiography has demonstrated that the aortic autograft hemodynamics during exercise are no different than those of normal aortic valves but that transpulmonary gradients are significantly different during exercise compared with normal control patients.

Exercise echocardiography has been used in children after repair of coarctation of the aorta to show that, despite a normal resting gradient, significant hypertension and arch gradients can develop during exercise. In keeping with the theme espoused by early exercise pioneers, these authors emphasize that "clinical assessment and definition of an 'acceptable' surgical repair of aortic coarctation should be viewed in the context of the patient's functional exercise response as well as resting studies."

In patients with hypertrophic cardiomyopathy, application of stress echocardiography has facilitated our understanding of the disease pathology that is now believed to be a disease predominantly of left ventricular outflow tract obstruction. Traditionally, nonobstructive hypertrophic cardiomyopathy has been regarded as the predominant form of the disease, but the application of stress demonstrates that even these patients develop marked left ventricular outflow tract gradients. Others have used dobutamine stress echocardiography to assess the effectiveness of surgical myomectomy in relieving the left ventricular outflow gradient. Clinicians now suggest that such patients may also be candidates for septal reduction therapy and advocate that stress echocardiography should be a routine component of the evaluation of hypertrophic cardiomyopathy patients without resting gradients.

Stress echocardiography has also been used to assess changes in pulmonary artery pressure. For instance, the technique has been helpful in understanding the elevation of pulmonary artery pressure during exercise in a subgroup of symptomatic patients with mitral stenosis with a relatively large mitral valve area. Exercise echocardiography demonstrates that this is because of poor left atrial compliance. Others have used exercise echocardiography to understand the mechanism of pulmonary hypertension in a variety of chronic lung diseases.

 ## PREPARATION

Training

Administration of almost all stressors requires performing the echocardiogram in unique and sometimes challenging settings. For example, the hyperpnea and tachypnea caused by exercise are significant impediments to diagnostic images. Administration of a pharmacologic agent for the distinct purpose of eliciting myocardial ischemia is by definition a potentially dangerous act. Therefore, training in performance and interpretation of stress echoes is essential. General guidelines for the knowledge and training required to perform and interpret stress echocardiography have been established, but the clinical practice of stress echocardiography in pediatric laboratories varies considerably. Whereas administration of stress tests and evaluation of regional wall motion are staples of adult cardiology training, these topics are not broached in pediatric cardiology training. Pediatric cardiologists with an interest in performing stress echocardiography should obtain training from experienced adult cardiologists before beginning such an endeavor. Further, they should establish an ongoing relationship with adult cardiologists for the purpose of consultation in difficult cases or interpretation of questionable images. Pediatric nurses and cardiac sonographers could also benefit from obtaining training from their adult counterparts.

Stressor

Exercise is just one of many different stressors and may consist of either dynamic exercise (upright or supine cycle and treadmill) or isometric exercise (handgrip). Other stressors include pharmacologic agents (dobutamine, adenosine, dipyridamole, and isoproterenol), electrophysiologic pacing, mental (e.g., time-pressured computer-based tasks), and cold pressor (Table 32.2).

The specific stressor that is to be used is a clinical decision tailored to the patient's age, exercise ability, cardiac pathology, and type of information desired. Each stressor has its unique advantages and disadvantages. For example, exercise has the advantage of most closely mimicking an athlete's activity outside the office but carries the disadvantages of (a) negatively affecting the image quality of most sensors because of body motion and heavy breathing

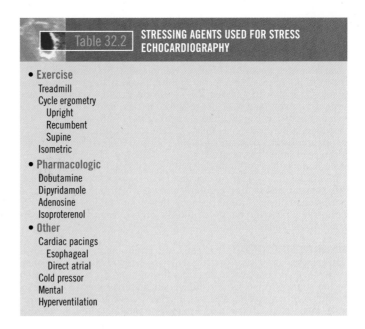

| Table 32.2 | STRESSING AGENTS USED FOR STRESS ECHOCARDIOGRAPHY |

- **Exercise**
  Treadmill
  Cycle ergometry
    Upright
    Recumbent
    Supine
  Isometric
- **Pharmacologic**
  Dobutamine
  Dipyridamole
  Adenosine
  Isoproterenol
- **Other**
  Cardiac pacings
    Esophageal
    Direct atrial
  Cold pressor
  Mental
  Hyperventilation

and (c) inability to use in younger patients (generally, younger than 7 years). Intravenous dobutamine administration is a stressor that has no age limitations, but the hemodynamic changes with dobutamine may be different than those occurring with physical exercise. In general, with exercise a maximal "stress dose" is administered, immediately after which the sensor (e.g., echocardiography) is used, whereas with pharmacologic stressors, submaximal "stress doses" are given while echocardiography is used continuously. This is advantageous for the patient as the test can be terminated at lesser (i.e., submaximal) stress doses if pathology or a serious adverse reaction is elicited.

Exercise Echocardiography – Exercise testing is a mainstay of pediatric cardiovascular evaluation, yet it is almost always obtained with electrocardiography as the sole diagnostic modality. With the simple addition of echocardiography, which adds no further annoyance to the patient, the test becomes much more robust. Dynamic exercise is the physiologic reference standard. In performing a treadmill test, the patient is exercised until exhaustion at which point he or she is immediately and quickly moved to a supine, left lateral decubitus position on an examination table. Echocardiographic data must be obtained within 60 to 90 seconds of test termination to ensure that the stress effects are still operative. Cycle ergometry can be performed in upright or semirecumbent postures and affords the opportunity of not only obtaining immediate postexercise test as is done with the treadmill test but also acquiring echocardiographic data during the test itself. While the patient is exercising in an upright position, the sonographer places his or her "nonimaging" hand on the back of the patient to stabilize the chest, reduce patient thorax movement, and enhance imaging. With the patient in a semirecumbent position, the examination table serves this purpose. Using these techniques, it is possible to obtain submaximal and, more important, peak exercise data. These modalities are therefore useful in detecting the hemodynamic differences that sometimes occur between peak exercise and immediate postexercise. In addition, the inclusion of images during the intermediate stages of exercise improves the sensitivity of detecting ischemia.

Sometimes the clinical question does not focus on issues of dynamic exercise. For example, the issue of interest may be the hemodynamic changes occurring in an adolescent wishing to participate in an isometric activity such as high school weight training or wrestling. In these instances, an isometric exercise echocardiogram would be appropriate. Investigators have used isometric exercise (e.g., 3 minutes of handgrip pressure at 33% of patient-specific maximum) echocardiography to demonstrate that children with aortic insufficiency and normal resting function have accentuated systolic blood pressure response and decreased left ventricular systolic performance compared with control subjects.

Pharmacologic Echocardiography – Dobutamine, disopyramide, adenosine, and isoproterenol are the agents used for pharmacologic echocardiography. Dobutamine stimulates beta$_1$-adrenergic receptors, causing increased contractility, heart rate, and myocardial oxygen demand, with little effect on beta$_2$- or alpha-receptors. It is administered intravenously beginning with a dose of 5 to 10 µg/kg per minute and is progressively increased every 4 minutes by 10 µg/kg per minute up to a maximal dose of 50 µg/kg per minute as necessary. Echocardiographic images are obtained at each stage. Atropine (0.01 mg/kg up to 0.25-mg aliquots given every 1 to 2 minutes to a maximum dose of 1 mg) should be given to augment heart rate as needed. In children, maximal dobutamine dose and atropine are usually needed to achieve a target heart rate. Esmolol (10 mg/mL dilution (not the 250 mg/mL dilution used for drips)) at a dose of 0.5 mg/kg should be available to rapidly reverse dobutamine in the event of ischemia or adverse events.

Isoproterenol stimulates beta$_1$- and beta$_2$-receptors, increasing heart rate and contractility and also causing systemic arterial vasodilation. It is administered intravenously at doses ranging from 0.05 to 2 µg/kg per minute. With each of these medications, the test termination points are achievement of target heart rate (85% of age-related maximal heart rate [220 – age in years]) or the presence of ischemia (either greater than 2-mm ST-segment depression or a new or worsened regional wall motion abnormality) or a serious adverse event. Adenosine and dipyridamole are lesser-used agents. Adenosine causes dilatation of normal coronary artery segments, resulting in a steal from diseased segments. Dipyridamole inhibits adenosine reuptake, resulting in the same action. Adenosine is infused at a maximum dose of 140 µg/kg per minute with simultaneous imaging over 4 minutes. Dipyridamole is administered in two stages with continuous imaging. The first stage consists of a dose of 0.56 mg/kg over 4 minutes. The second stage is performed if there are no adverse effects and consists of a dose of 0.28 mg/kg over 2 minutes. Atropine can be used to augment heart rate. Aminophylline should be available for an adverse dipyridamole reaction.

Although similar, the cardiac effects of the pharmacologic agents are not identical to those of exercise. Cnota et al. compared the hemodynamic effects of peak dobutamine to peak exercise. Dobutamine infusion resulted in lower cardiac output, heart rates, and systolic blood pressure. At peak dobutamine (versus exercise), there was smaller left ventricular end-diastolic dimension, higher fractional shortening, and higher contractility as measured by velocity of circumferential fiber shortening.

Other Stressors – Other stressing methods are either rarely used or used only for unique situations. Mental stress can be delivered by a variety of means but the easiest are time-pressured computer-based tasks such as arithmetic or word problems. Electrophysiologic pacing can also be used as a stressing method. Cold pressor is a cardiovascular challenge resulting from immersion of one hand in ice water for 2 or more minutes, which increases systemic blood pressure and ventricular afterload.

Sensors

Echocardiography is only one of many potential sensors that can be used to assess the effects of the above stressors. Although echocardiography is a valuable and robust sensing tool, it is important to remember that one of the other sensors may be more applicable (or combined with echocardiography) in a certain situation. These sensors include electrocardiography, magnetic resonance imaging, nuclear imaging, computed tomography imaging, and positron emission tomography.

Personnel

It is essential to have not only a qualified, trained physician but also an experienced sonographer administer the test as described earlier. In the case of pharmacologic stress, a nurse is needed for intravenous line placement, administration of medications, and monitoring of the patient.

Equipment

The ultrasound system should have the capability of storing motion clips digitally and a display that allows side-by-side comparison of clips from different stress stages. A system equipped with four-dimensional imaging capabilities makes acquisition and interpretation of wall motion particularly easy.

Monitoring equipment should include continuous electrocardiographic monitoring with a system that allows for easy detection of ST-segment changes—ideally, with the capability of comparing current ST segments to resting ST segments. An oxygen saturation probe and intermittent blood pressure monitors are also needed. Resuscitation equipment should be readily available.

Transpulmonary Contrast Agents

Transpulmonary contrast agents are protein microspheres filled with inert gases that pass through the pulmonary capillary bed to opacify the left ventricle. The use of transpulmonary contrast agents for left ventricular opacification during stress echocardiography has been helpful in adult patients. In these situations, particularly difficult-to-image wall segments, such as the left ventricular apex, can be imaged much more clearly with the addition of a transpulmonary contrast agent.

In general, stress images in children are of sufficient quality that contrast agents are not necessary. However, in certain patients, the images may be limited so that contrast can be helpful. These agents have been shown to be safe and efficacious in children.

Commercially marketed contrast agents to date have had a somewhat checkered history. Questions of sterility, potential paradoxical emboli across intracardiac shunts, and possible cardiopulmonary adverse reactions have tempered initial enthusiasm. Contrast agents should not be administered in patients with worsening or clinically unstable heart failure, acute myocardial infarction or acute coronary syndrome, serious ventricular arrhythmias, or respiratory failure. Until these issues become resolved, transpulmonary contrast agents should be limited in use to those patients in whom standard imaging modalities are not diagnostic and, even in those cases, should be administered with caution.

 ## CONTRAINDICATIONS AND POTENTIAL COMPLICATIONS

In adults with aortic valve stenosis, dobutamine stress echocardiography can precipitate atrial and ventricular tachyarrhythmias. Even so, this high risk population can undergo the test safely. There are no absolute documented contraindications to performing stress echocardiography in children. Nevertheless, careful thought should be given before administering the test to patients in very high risk populations such as patients with hypertrophic cardiomyopathy, significant aortic valve stenosis, and/or dysrhythmias.

It is known that individuals with structurally normal hearts, particularly if they have refrained from drinking or eating for any considerable time, may develop left ventricular outflow tract gradients during dobutamine stress echocardiography, which, in rare circumstances, could result in diminished cardiac output with syncope or angina. This has not been reported in children.

The most frequent potential complication in the pediatric population with dobutamine stress echocardiography is emesis. This occurs in approximately 10% to 20% of children undergoing the test. When it occurs, it does so most commonly at the peak dobutamine dose and usually after concomitant administration of atropine. In most studies, the peak heart rate images can be obtained and the dobutamine discontinued with prompt (within seconds) improvement in patient symptoms.

 ## OUTPUTS AND INTERPRETATION

Ischemia manifests itself on the echocardiogram as a new or worsened regional wall motion abnormality. Traditionally, four echocardiographic views (parasternal long and short axes, apical two and four chambers) are acquired. From these four views, 16 different wall segments can be evaluated (6 of these segments can be evaluated in two different views). A wall motion abnormality in a given segment corresponds to a perfusion abnormality of the coronary artery supplying the given segment (Fig. 32.4).

FIGURE 32.4. The 16 myocardial segments imaged during a stress echocardiogram. The parasternal long- and short-axis and the apical two- and four-chamber views are obtained. From these four views, 16 segments (6 segments can be visualized in two views) are obtained. Each myocardial segment is perfused by one of the three coronary arteries. A regional wall motion abnormality in a specific myocardial segment corresponds to a perfusion abnormality in the coronary artery serving that wall segment. (Reprinted with permission of Springer Science and Business Media.)

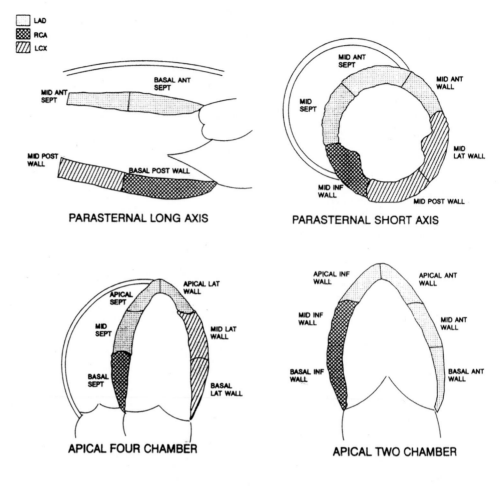

Identifying a wall motion abnormality may be difficult, particularly for a pediatric cardiologist. It is emphasized that pediatric cardiologists should receive training from adult cardiologists expert in stress echocardiography and maintain these relationships so that consultation advice remains readily available. In evaluating the left ventricle for wall motion abnormalities, it is helpful to first survey global left ventricular function. It would be unusual for a regional wall motion abnormality to be present in the face of normal global function. *Abnormal regional wall motion* is defined as both poorer endocardial excursion and lesser wall thickening. Each segment must be examined methodically for these two features.

Some ultrasound systems are equipped with quantitative or semiquantitative modalities that may assist in detecting regional wall motion abnormalities. These include regional assessment of strain and strain rate using Doppler tissue technology. With these modalities, a sample volume is placed directly on a wall segment of interest and the strain and strain rate is determined for that specific segment. Similar quantitative wall motion can be performed using standard two-dimensional imaging, using speckle tracking, which measures the velocity of the natural "speckles" or echo-densities in the myocardium.

For evaluations other than coronary perfusion, the output data will be specific to the question being asked. For example, this might include Doppler interrogation of antegrade valve flow to determine valve behavior during stress, Doppler interrogation of tricuspid insufficiency to estimate right ventricular/pulmonary artery pressure during stress, or assessment of ventricular function for an evaluation of contractile reserve. Evaluation often includes a combination of these assessments.

Prognostic Significance

The validity of using stress-elicited valve gradients, intracardiac pressure determinations and ventricular function values for prognostic purposes have been questioned because the natural history of such stress results is unknown. For example, it is unclear whether a mean Doppler aortic valve stenosis gradient of 100 mm Hg elicited during maximal exercise carries the same serious implications of a similar gradient obtained at rest. Admittedly, it probably does not; but, on the other hand, such data should not be dismissed, particularly in light of the fact that the maximal exercise mean semilunar gradient in patients without valvar disease never exceeds 10 to 20 mm Hg.

An interesting study investigating exercise hemodynamics and subsequent cardiac changes in children with hypertension sheds some light. In this study, Mahoney et al. investigated, in hypertensive children, determinants of not only systolic blood pressure but also left ventricular mass, a known cardiovascular risk factor. These investigators found that follow-up (mean duration of 3.4 years) systolic blood pressure was predicted by initial resting blood pressure and initial maximal exercise blood pressure. More important, subsequent left ventricular mass was predicted by initial maximal exercise blood pressure alone, *having no relation to initial resting blood pressure.* These data support previous reports in adults that show left ventricular mass has only a modest relationship to resting blood pressure but strong relationships to mean 24-hour systolic blood pressure, blood pressure at work, and home blood pressures on a workday. The authors emphasize that exercise measures, not resting measures, are more valuable because they are predictive of future adverse cardiac changes.

 ## RESEARCH

Stress echocardiography has been used to elucidate the mechanisms during exercise for maintenance of cardiac output, on the one hand, and exhaustion on the other. While exercising, children exhibit an initial rise in stroke volume that reaches a plateau at mild-moderate intensities. The initial rise in stroke volume is caused by (a) increased preload from skeletal muscle contraction, thereby mobilizing blood that is "pumped" into the heart and (b) decreased systemic vascular resistance caused by peripheral vasodilatation in the skeletal muscle. The plateau of stroke volume during moderate intensity relates to increased heart rate and shortening of diastole and systole. Although both systolic ejection and diastolic filling periods progressively decrease with exercise, the latter decreases more, so that at higher levels of exercise, the relative durations of diastole and systole are reversed compared with at rest. Decreased filling leads to decreased left ventricular volume, decreased preload, and decreased stroke volume. Rowland et al. performed exercise echocardiography in children with cardiomyopathic states (because of anthracycline toxicity primarily) to demonstrate that to sustain stroke volume at peak exercise (when diastolic filling and ejection times are short), there must be an increase in contractility.

Stress echocardiography in children has also been used to examine the adaptations occurring from training. During exercise, trained children increase cardiac output by increasing stroke volume (even at higher intensities), but in untrained children, higher cardiac output is achieved only by increasing heart rate.

 ## CONCLUSION

The stress echocardiography work that has been highlighted in this chapter has revealed many insights into stress physiology. However, one of the most important is that despite a significant prevalence and diversity of anatomic coronary artery pathology, actual physiologic derangement in the form of ischemia is remarkably uncommon in the pediatric population. Perhaps this is related to a lesser disease severity in children than in the adult population. However, this appears unlikely because there are children who have anatomically severe coronary disease without symptoms or perfusion abnormalities. More likely, this phenomenon is caused by an increased adaptive ability for development of collateral vessels and/or for ischemic tolerance of the myocardium. It is hoped that cardiologists will learn from pediatric stress echocardiography that, in some instances, diagnosis of coronary artery anatomic pathology does not necessarily translate into a need for intervention and that the heart of a child has a robust adaptive ability to treat itself.

Stress echocardiography has provided clinicians and researchers with a window to examine and investigate children outside of the traditional setting of a quiet, resting state. The pediatric responses to stress as evaluated by echocardiography enable clinicians, on the one hand, to diagnose disease earlier in the disease process or, on the other hand, to reassure themselves and their patients that untoward events are unlikely. These modalities have also enabled researchers to establish the mechanisms for cardiac output increase and exhaustion in both trained and untrained children. Stress echocardiography is a powerful, robust tool that extends resting evaluations, thereby improving diagnostic capability and enhancing medical care to children.

SUGGESTED READING

Aggeli C, Giannopoulos G, Misovoulos P, et al. Real-time three-dimensional dobutamine stress echocardiography for coronary artery disease diagnosis: validation with coronary angiography. *Heart.* 2007;93:672–675.

Alpert BS, Bloom KR, Olley PM. Assessment of left ventricular contractility during supine exercise in children with left-sided cardiac disease. Br *Heart J.* 1980;44:703–710.

Apostolopoulou SC, Laskari CV, Tsoutsinos A, et al. Doppler tissue imaging evaluation of right ventricular function at rest and during dobutamine infusion in patients after repair of tetralogy of Fallot. Int *J Cardiovasc Imaging.* 2007;23:25–31.

Armstrong WF, Pellikka PA, Ryan T, et al. Stress echocardiography: recommendations for performance and interpretation of stress echocardiography. Stress Echocardiography Task Force of the Nomenclature and Standards Committee of the American Society of Echocardiography. *J Am Soc Echocardiogr.* 1998;11:97–104.

Bach DS. Stress echocardiography for evaluation of hemodynamics: valvular heart disease, prosthetic valve function, and pulmonary hypertension. *Prog Cardiovasc Dis.* 1997;39:543–554.

Baspinar O, Alehan D. Dobutamine stress echocardiography in the evaluation of cardiac haemodynamics after repair of tetralogy of Fallot in children: negative effects of pulmonary regurgitation. *Acta Cardiol.* 2006;61:279–283.

Baum VC, Levitsky LL, Englander RM. Abnormal cardiac function after exercise in insulin-dependent diabetic children and adolescents. *Diabetes Care.* 1987;10:319–323.

Berthe C, Pierard LA, Hiernaux M, et al. Predicting the extent and location of coronary artery disease in acute myocardial infarction by echocardiography during dobutamine infusion. *Am J Cardiol.* 1986;58:1167–1172.

Bountioukos M, Kertai MD, Schinkel AF, et al. Safety of dobutamine stress echocardiography in patients with aortic stenosis. *J Heart Valve Dis.* 2003;12:441–446.

Bruce RA, Blackmon JR, Jones JW, Strait G. Exercising testing in adult normal subjects and cardiac patients. *Pediatrics.* 1963;32:742–756.

Bruce RA, Pearson R, et al. Variability of respiratory and circulatory performance during standardized exercise. *J Clin Invest.* 1949;28:1431–1438.

Carpenter MA, Dammann JF, Watson DD, et al. Left ventricular hyperkinesia at rest and during exercise in normotensive patients 2 to 27 years after coarctation repair. *J Am Coll Cardiol.* 1985;6:879–886.

Chang RK, Qi N, Larson J, et al. Comparison of upright and semi-recumbent postures for exercise echocardiography in healthy children. *Am J Cardiol.* 2005;95:918–921.

Cnota JF, Mays WA, Knecht SK, et al. Cardiovascular physiology during supine cycle ergometry and dobutamine stress. *Med Sci Sports Exerc.* 2003;35:1503–1510.

Cortes RG, Satomi G, Yoshigi M, et al. Maximal hemodynamic response after the Fontan procedure: Doppler evaluation during the treadmill test. *Pediatr Cardiol.* 1994;15:170–177.

Cyran SE, Grzeszczak M, Kaufman K, et al. Aortic "recoarctation" at rest versus at exercise in children as evaluated by stress Doppler echocardiography after a "good" operative result. *Am J Cardiol.* 1993;71:963–970.

Daniels SR, Witt SA, Glascock B, et al. Left atrial size in children with hypertension: the influence of obesity, blood pressure, and left ventricular mass. *J Pediatr.* 2002;141:186–190.

Dawn B, Paliwal VS, Raza ST, et al. Left ventricular outflow tract obstruction provoked during dobutamine stress echocardiography predicts future chest pain, syncope, and near syncope. *Am Heart J.* 2005;149:908–916.

De Wolf D, Suys B, Verhaaren H, et al. Low-dose dobutamine stress echocardiography in children and young adults. *Am J Cardiol.* 1998;81:895–901.

Deng YB, Li TL, Xiang HJ, et al. Impaired endothelial function in the brachial artery after Kawasaki disease and the effects of intravenous administration of vitamin C. *Pediatr Infect Dis J.* 2003;22:34–39.

Devereux RB, Pickering TG, Harshfield GA, et al. Left ventricular hypertrophy in patients with hypertension: importance of blood pressure response to regularly recurring stress. *Circulation.* 1983;68:470–476.

Dhillon R, Clarkson P, Donald AE, et al. Endothelial dysfunction late after Kawasaki disease. *Circulation.* 1996;94:2103–2106.

Di Filippo S, Semiond B, Roriz R, et al. Non-invasive detection of coronary artery disease by dobutamine-stress echocardiography in children after heart transplantation. *J Heart Lung Transplant.* 2003;22:876–882.

Dunning DW, Hussey ME, Riggs T, et al. Long-term follow-up with stress echocardiograms of patients with Kawasaki's disease. *Cardiology.* 2002; 97:43–48.

Elhendy A, Nierop PR, Roelandt JR, et al. Myocardial ischemia assessed by dobutamine stress echocardiography in a patient with bicoronary to pulmonary artery fistulas. *J Am Soc Echocardiogr.* 1997;10:189–191.

Ferrara LA, Mainenti G, Fasano ML, et al. Cardiovascular response to mental stress and to handgrip in children. The role of physical activity. *Jpn Heart J.* 1991;32:645–654.

Geny B, Mettauer B, Muan B, et al. Safety and efficacy of a new transpulmonary echo contrast agent in echocardiographic studies in patients. *J Am Coll Cardiol.* 1993;22:1193–1198.

Gidding SS. Dyslipidemia in the metabolic syndrome in children. *J Cardiometab Syndr.* 2006;1:282–285.

Glowinska B, Urban M, Koput A. Cardiovascular risk factors in children with obesity, hypertension and diabetes: lipoprotein(a) levels and body mass index correlate with family history of cardiovascular disease. *Eur J Pediatr.* 2002;161:511–518.

Gol MK, Emir M, Keles T, et al. Septal myectomy in hypertrophic obstructive cardiomyopathy: late results with stress echocardiography. *Ann Thorac Surg.* 1997;64:739–745.

Guleserian KJ, Armsby LB, Thiagarajan RR, et al. Natural history of pulmonary atresia with intact ventricular septum and right-ventricle-dependent coronary circulation managed by the single-ventricle approach. *Ann Thorac Surg.* 2006;81:2250–2258.

Gumbiner CH, Gutgesell HP. Response to isometric exercise in children and young adults with aortic regurgitation. *Am Heart J.* 1983;106:540–547.

Hanekom L, Cho GY, Leano R, et al. Comparison of two-dimensional speckle and tissue Doppler strain measurement during dobutamine stress echocardiography: an angiographic correlation. *Eur Heart J.* 2007;28:1765–1772.

Hanekom L, Jenkins C, Jeffries L, et al. Incremental value of strain rate analysis as an adjunct to wall-motion scoring for assessment of myocardial viability by dobutamine echocardiography: a follow-up study after revascularization. *Circulation.* 2005;112:3892–3900.

Harpaz D, Rozenman Y, Medalion B, et al. Anomalous origin of the left coronary artery from the pulmonary artery accompanied by mitral valve prolapse and regurgitation: Surgical implication of dobutamine stress echocardiography. *J Am Soc Echocardiogr.* 2004;17:73–77.

Hauser M, Bengel FM, Kuhn A, et al. Myocardial blood flow and flow reserve after coronary reimplantation in patients after arterial switch and Ross operation. *Circulation.* 2001;103:1875–1880.

Henein MY, Dinarevic S, O'Sullivan CA, et al. Exercise echocardiography in children with Kawasaki disease: ventricular long axis is selectively abnormal. *Am J Cardiol.* 1998;81:1356–1359.

Hui L, Chau AK, Leung MP, et al. Assessment of left ventricular function long term after arterial switch operation for transposition of the great arteries by dobutamine stress echocardiography. *Heart.* 2005;91:68–72.

Kass M, Allan R, Haddad H. Diagnosis of graft coronary artery disease. *Curr Opin Cardiol.* 2007;22:139–145.

Kavey RE, Allada V, Daniels SR, et al. Cardiovascular risk reduction in high-risk pediatric patients: a scientific statement from the American Heart Association Expert Panel on Population and Prevention Science; the Councils on Cardiovascular Disease in the Young, Epidemiology and Prevention, Nutrition, Physical Activity and Metabolism, High Blood Pressure Research, Cardiovascular Nursing, and the Kidney in Heart Disease; and the Interdisciplinary Working Group on Quality of Care and Outcomes Research: endorsed by the American Academy of Pediatrics. *Circulation.* 2006;114:2710–2738.

Kelishadi R. Childhood overweight, obesity, and the metabolic syndrome in developing countries. *Epidemiol Rev.* 2007;29:62–76.

Kimball TR, Mays WA, Khoury PR, et al. Echocardiographic determination of left ventricular preload, afterload, and contractility during and after exercise. *J Pediatr.* 1993;122:S89–S94.

Kimball TR, Reynolds JM, Mays WA, et al. Persistent hyperdynamic cardiovascular state at rest and during exercise in children after successful repair of coarctation of the aorta. *J Am Coll Cardiol.* 1994;24:194–200.

Kimball TR, Witt SA, Daniels SR. Dobutamine stress echocardiography in the assessment of suspected myocardial ischemia in children and young adults. *Am J Cardiol.* 1997;79:380–384.

Kimball TR. Pediatric stress echocardiography. *Pediatr Cardiol.* 2002;23:347–357.

Klewer SE, Goldberg SJ, Donnerstein RL, et al. Dobutamine stress echocardiography: a sensitive indicator of diminished myocardial function in asymptomatic doxorubicin-treated long-term survivors of childhood cancer. *J Am Coll Cardiol.* 1992;19:394–401.

Koenigsberg J, Boyd GS, Gidding SS, et al. Association of age and sex with cardiovascular risk factors and insulin sensitivity in overweight children and adolescents. *J Cardiometab Syndr.* 2006;1:253–258.

Kraunz RF, Kennedy JW. Ultrasonic determination of left ventricular wall motion in normal man. Studies at rest and after exercise. *Am Heart J.* 1970;79:36–43.

Lancellotti P, Lebois F, Simon M, et al. Prognostic importance of quantitative exercise Doppler echocardiography in asymptomatic valvular aortic stenosis. *Circulation.* 2005;112:I377–I382.

Lane JR, Ben-Shachar G. Myocardial infarction in healthy adolescents. *Pediatrics.* 2007;120:e938–e943.

Lang D, Hilger F, Binswanger J, et al. Late effects of anthracycline therapy in childhood in relation to the function of the heart at rest and under physical stress. *Eur J Pediatr.* 1995;154:340–345.

Lanzarini L, Bossi G, Laudisa ML, et al. Lack of clinically significant cardiac dysfunction during intermediate dobutamine doses in long-term childhood cancer survivors exposed to anthracyclines. *Am Heart J.* 2000;140:315–323.

L'Ecuyer TJ, Poulik JM, Vincent JA. Myocardial infarction due to coronary abnormalities in pulmonary atresia with intact ventricular septum. *Pediatr Cardiol.* 2001;22:68–70.

Lee R, Haluska B, Leung DY, et al. Functional and prognostic implications of left ventricular contractile reserve in patients with asymptomatic severe mitral regurgitation. *Heart.* 2005;91:1407–1412.

Legendre A, Losay J, Touchot-Kone A, et al. Coronary events after arterial switch operation for transposition of the great arteries. *Circulation.* 2003;108(suppl 1):II-186–II-190.

Leung DY, Griffin BP, Stewart WJ, et al. Left ventricular function after valve repair for chronic mitral regurgitation: predictive value of preoperative assessment of contractile reserve by exercise echocardiography. *J Am Coll Cardiol.* 1996;28:1198–1205.

Lewis JF, Selman SB, Murphy JD, et al. Dobutamine echocardiography for prediction of ischemic events in heart transplant recipients. *J Heart Lung Transplant.* 1997;16:390–393.

Lin SS, Roger VL, Pascoe R, et al. Dobutamine stress Doppler hemodynamics in patients with aortic stenosis: feasibility, safety, and surgical correlations. *Am Heart J.* 1998;136:1010–1016.

Mahoney LT, Schieken RM, Clarke WR, et al. Left ventricular mass and exercise responses predict future blood pressure. The Muscatine Study. *Hypertension.* 1988;12:206–213.

Maron MS, Olivotto I, Zenovich AG, et al. Hypertrophic cardiomyopathy is predominantly a disease of left ventricular outflow tract obstruction. *Circulation.* 2006;114:2232–2239.

Marwick TH. Application of stress echocardiography to the evaluation of noncoronary heart disease. *Eur J Echocardiogr.* 2000;1:171–179.

Master AM. The two-step exercise electrocardiogram: a test for coronary insufficiency. *Ann Intern Med.* 1950;32:842–863.

McGiffin DC, Savunen T, Kirklin JK, et al. Cardiac transplant coronary artery disease. A multivariable analysis of pretransplantation risk factors for disease development and morbid events. *J Thorac Cardiovasc Surg.* 1995;109:1081–1089.

Michelfelder EC, Witt SA, Khoury P, et al. Moderate-dose dobutamine maximizes left ventricular contractile response during dobutamine stress echocardiography in children. *J Am Soc Echocardiogr.* 2003;16:140–146.

Moir S, Hanekom L, Fang ZY, et al. Relationship between myocardial perfusion and dysfunction in diabetic cardiomyopathy: a study of quantitative contrast echocardiography and strain rate imaging. *Heart.* 2006;92:1414–1419.

Nicolas RT, Kort HW, Balzer DT, et al. Surveillance for transplant coronary artery disease in infant, child and adolescent heart transplant recipients: an intravascular ultrasound study. *J Heart Lung Transplant.* 2006;25:921–927.

Noto N, Ayusawa M, Karasawa K, et al. Dobutamine stress echocardiography for detection of coronary artery stenosis in children with Kawasaki disease. *J Am Coll Cardiol.* 1996;27:1251–1256.

Nottin S, Vinet A, Stecken F, et al. Central and peripheral cardiovascular adaptations during a maximal cycle exercise in boys and men. *Med Sci Sports Exerc.* 2002;34:456–463.

Ogawa S, Fukazawa R, Ohkubo T, et al. Silent myocardial ischemia in Kawasaki disease: evaluation of percutaneous transluminal coronary angioplasty by dobutamine stress testing. *Circulation.* 1997;96:3384–3389.

Okuda N, Ito T, Emura N, et al. Depressed myocardial contractile reserve in patients with obstructive sleep apnea assessed by tissue Doppler imaging with dobutamine stress echocardiography. *Chest.* 2007;131:1082–1089.

Otasevic P, Popovic ZB, Vasiljevic JD, et al. Head-to-head comparison of indices of left ventricular contractile reserve assessed by high-dose dobutamine stress echocardiography in idiopathic dilated cardiomyopathy: five-year follow up. *Heart.* 2006;92:1253–1258.

Otoiu ME. Non-invasive assessment of left ventricular performance at rest and during exercise by T-M mode echocardiography. *Ann Clin Res.* 1982;14(suppl 34):146–159.

Oyen EM, Ignatzy K, Ingerfeld G, et al. Echocardiographic evaluation of left ventricular reserve in normal children during supine bicycle exercise. *Int J Cardiol.* 1987;14:145–154.

Oyen EM, Ingerfeld G, Ignatzy K, et al. Dynamic exercise echocardiography in children with congenital heart disease affecting the left heart. *Int J Cardiol.* 1987;17:315–325.

Oyen EM, Schuster S, Brode PE. Dynamic exercise echocardiography of the left ventricle in physically trained children compared to untrained healthy children. *Int J Cardiol.* 1990;29:29–33.

Pahl E, Crawford SE, Swenson JM, et al. Dobutamine stress echocardiography: experience in pediatric heart transplant recipients. *J Heart Lung Transplant.* 1999;18:725–732.

Pahl E, Duffy CE, Chaudhry FA. The role of stress echocardiography in children. *Echocardiography.* 2000;17:507–512.

Pahl E, Sehgal R, Chrystof D, et al. Feasibility of exercise stress echocardiography for the follow-up of children with coronary involvement secondary to Kawasaki disease. *Circulation.* 1995;91:122–128.

Paridon SM, Alpert BS, Boas SR, et al. Clinical stress testing in the pediatric age group: a statement from the American Heart Association Council on Cardiovascular Disease in the Young, Committee on Atherosclerosis, Hypertension, and Obesity in Youth. *Circulation.* 2006;113:1905–1920.

Park TH, Tayan N, Takeda K, et al. Supine bicycle echocardiography improved diagnostic accuracy and physiologic assessment of coronary artery disease with the incorporation of intermediate stages of exercise. *J Am Coll Cardiol.* 2007;50:1857–1863.

Phillips JR, Daniels CJ, Orsinelli DA, et al. Valvular hemodynamics and arrhythmias with exercise following the Ross procedure. *Am J Cardiol.* 2001;87:577–583.

Picano E, Lattanzi F, Masini M, et al. Usefulness of the dipyridamole-exercise echocardiography test for diagnosis of coronary artery disease. *Am J Cardiol.* 1988;62:67–70.

Pierard LA, Lancellotti P. Stress testing in valve disease. *Heart.* 2007;93:766–772.

Quinones MA, Douglas PS, Foster E, et al. American College of Cardiology/American Heart Association clinical competence statement on echocardiography: a report of the American College of Cardiology/American Heart Association/American College of Physicians--American Society of Internal Medicine Task Force on Clinical Competence. *Circulation.* 2003;107:1068–1089.

Raisky O, Bergoend E, Agnoletti G, et al. Late coronary artery lesions after neonatal arterial switch operation: results of surgical coronary revascularization. *Eur J Cardiothorac Surg.* 2007;31:894–898.

Reis G, Motta MS, Barbosa MM, et al. Dobutamine stress echocardiography for noninvasive assessment and risk stratification of patients with rheumatic mitral stenosis. *J Am Coll Cardiol.* 2004;43:393–401.

Ren JF, Hakki AH, Kotler MN, et al. Exercise systolic blood pressure: a powerful determinant of increased left ventricular mass in patients with hypertension. *J Am Coll Cardiol.* 1985;5:1224–1231.

Roberts WC. Major anomalies of coronary arterial origin seen in adulthood. *Am Heart J.* 1986;111:941–963.

Rowland T, Goff D, Popowski B, et al. Cardiac responses to exercise in child distance runners. *Int J Sports Med.* 1998;19:385–390.

Rowland T, Potts J, Potts T, et al. Cardiac responses to progressive exercise in normal children: a synthesis. *Med Sci Sports Exerc.* 2000;32:253–259.

Rowland T, Potts J, Potts T, et al. Cardiovascular responses to exercise in children and adolescents with myocardial dysfunction. *Am Heart J.* 1999;137:126–133.

Rowland T, Wehnert M, Miller K. Cardiac responses to exercise in competitive child cyclists. *Med Sci Sports Exerc.* 2000;32:747–752.

Rowlands DB, Glover DR, Ireland MA, et al. Assessment of left-ventricular mass and its response to antihypertensive treatment. *Lancet.* 1982;1:467–470.

Sadaniantz A, Katz A, Wu WC. Miscellaneous use of exercise echocardiography in patients with chronic pulmonary disease or congenital heart defect. *Echocardiography.* 2004;21:477–484.

Savoye M, Shaw M, Dziura J, et al. Effects of a weight management program on body composition and metabolic parameters in overweight children: a randomized controlled trial. *JAMA.* 2007;297:2697–2704.

Schowengerdt KO. Advances in pediatric heart transplantation. *Curr Opin Pediatr.* 2006;18:512–517.

Schwammenthal E, Vered Z, Agranat O, et al. Impact of atrioventricular compliance on pulmonary artery pressure in mitral stenosis: an exercise echocardiographic study. *Circulation.* 2000;102:2378–2384.

Sharples LD, Jackson CH, Parameshwar J, et al. Diagnostic accuracy of coronary angiography and risk factors for post-heart-transplant cardiac allograft vasculopathy. *Transplantation.* 2003;76:679–682.

Sorof J, Daniels S. Obesity hypertension in children: a problem of epidemic proportions. *Hypertension.* 2002;40:441–447.

Sorrentino MJ, Marcus RH, Lang RM. Left ventricular outflow tract obstruction as a cause for hypotension and symptoms during dobutamine stress echocardiography. *Clin Cardiol.* 1996;19:225–230.

Steinberger J, Daniels SR. Obesity, insulin resistance, diabetes, and cardiovascular risk in children: an American Heart Association scientific statement from the Atherosclerosis, Hypertension, and Obesity in the Young Committee (Council on Cardiovascular Disease in the Young) and the Diabetes Committee (Council on Nutrition, Physical Activity, and Metabolism). *Circulation.* 2003;107:1448–1453.

Stern H, Sauer U, Locher D, et al. Left ventricular function assessed with echocardiography and myocardial perfusion assessed with scintigraphy under dipyridamole stress in pediatric patients after repair for anomalous origin of the left coronary artery from the pulmonary artery. *J Thorac Cardiovasc Surg.* 1993;106:723–732.

Thistlethwaite PA, Madani MM, Kriett JM, et al. Surgical management of congenital obstruction of the left main coronary artery with supravalvular aortic stenosis. *J Thorac Cardiovasc Surg.* 2000;120:1040–1046.

Wahi S, Haluska B, Pasquet A, et al. Exercise echocardiography predicts development of left ventricular dysfunction in medically and surgically treated patients with asymptomatic severe aortic regurgitation. *Heart.* 2000;84:606–614.

Weber HS, Cyran SE, Grzeszczak M, et al. Discrepancies in aortic growth explain aortic arch gradients during exercise. *J Am Coll Cardiol.* 1993; 21:1002–1007.

Weesner KM, Bledsoe M, Chauvenet A, et al. Exercise echocardiography in the detection of anthracycline cardiotoxicity. *Cancer.* 1991;68:435–438.

Welch GE, Bruce RA, Bridges WC, et al. Comparison of a new step test with a treadmill test for the evaluation of cardio-respiratory working capacity. *Am J Med Sci.* 1952;223:607–617.

Zilberman MV, Goya G, Witt SA, et al. Dobutamine stress echocardiography in the evaluation of young patients with Kawasaki disease. *Pediatr Cardiol.* 2003;24:338–343.

Zilberman MV, Witt SA, Kimball TR. Is there a role for intravenous transpulmonary contrast imaging in pediatric stress echocardiography? *J Am Soc Echocardiogr.* 2003;16:9–14.

Chapter 33
Intracardiac and Intraoperative Transesophageal Echocardiography

Donald J. Hagler

Transesophageal echocardiography (TEE) and intracardiac echocardiography (ICE) have revolutionized the ability to monitor and direct intraoperative surgical procedures and interventional cardiac catheterization procedures for patients with congenital heart disease. TEE has been the traditional imaging modality of choice for the past two decades in the operating suite and catheterization laboratory. More recently, the miniaturization of echocardiography technology has permitted ICE probes to be used in children and adults. Each imaging modality has advantages, disadvantages, and limitations but the availability of both modalities has improved patient care in the operating suite and cardiac catheterization laboratory. Important limitations of TEE include the need for general anesthesia and potential problems related to airway management during prolonged use in the supine patient. Imaging limitations of TEE include some views of the posterior and inferior atrial septum that may be inadequate to exclude significant defects or shunts. The close proximity of the TEE probe to that area of the atrial septum creates this imaging issue. During atrial septal defect (ASD) device placement, with TEE there may be struggles with artifact when attempting to image through the device. In addition, the apical ventricular septum may be relatively inaccessible with TEE in some patients. For these reasons, the availability of high quality intracardiac imaging has successfully merged the cardiac catheterization and echocardiography practices for patients with congenital heart disease.

 INTRACARDIAC ECHOCARDIOGRAPHY

Equipment

Mechanical ICE systems were introduced in the 1980s; the current ICE system using an 8 or a 10 French (Fr) phased-array system was developed from single-array TEE prototype probes. The initial ICE probe was a 10 Fr catheter (Acunav Diagnostic Ultrasound Catheter; Siemens Corporation, Mountain View, CA). This is a 64-element vector, phased-array transducer that is multifrequency (5.5 to 10 MHz) and mounted on a 3.3-mm (10 Fr) catheter with a maneuverable four-way tip (Fig. 33.1). The probe is capable of high-resolution two-dimensional and full Doppler imaging (pulsed wave, continuous wave, and tissue Doppler). The longitudinal plane

provides a 90-degree sector image with tissue penetration of 2 to 12 cm. Currently, the probe is also available as an 8 Fr catheter. This catheter has similar echo capabilities but is longer than the 10 Fr catheter. The added length of the 8 Fr probe makes it more difficult to manipulate. The ICE catheter is advanced to the right atrium under fluoroscopic guidance. Image quality is optimized by adjusting gain, depth, frequency, and focal length controls. Complete ICE evaluation of both sides of the heart is then performed, sometimes with assistance of fluoroscopy to guide orientation and position of the ICE catheter.

Examination

The movements described in this chapter relate to the manipulation of the control mechanisms on the handle of the ICE catheter. Movement of the control handle to the left of midline results in movement of the catheter tip to the left as visualized from the front of the probe handle. However, these movements may not result in movement of the catheter tip in the same direction as illustrated outside of the body because, during an examination, the imaging palette is also being rotated in various directions to achieve a particular image plane. The imaging palette of the probe can be identified by the black stripe on the outside of the catheter and the black side of the probe evident on fluoroscopy. Thus, if the probe has been rotated to visualize a posterior structure (palette-directed posterior), posterior or rightward movement of the probe handle controls results in a more medial position of the catheter tip toward the atrial septum. When the catheter is angulated into unusual positions, such as the position required to achieve a short-axis image plane (anterior and leftward control movement), simple rotation of the catheter does not result in the longitudinal scanning effect as in TEE, but, rather, the tip of the probe moves in a large 360-degree arch. In practice, either the echo images can be followed and the probe manipulated to obtain the desired images, or the position of the probe tip can be monitored by fluoroscopy to obtain a standard probe position.

Image Acquisition

By advancing the ICE catheter from the inferior vena cava with the control mechanism in a free or neutral position, the catheter is placed in the midright atrium, and a tricuspid valve inlet view is obtained by rotating the imaging palette of the catheter anteriorly and slightly leftward (Fig. 33.2). The catheter tip is then rotated clockwise to visualize the aorta and left ventricular outflow tract (Fig. 33.3). The lower atrial septum (cardiac crux) and mitral valve are then visualized by further clockwise catheter rotation (Fig. 33.4). In some cases, with some posterior control movement there is posterior deflection of the catheter tip, and a classic four-chamber view of the cardiac crux may be obtained as shown in Figure 33.4D. With continued clockwise rotation and cranial advancement of the catheter, a long-axis view of the atrial septum is obtained (Fig. 33.5).

In most cases, some leftward or anterior control movement with resultant lateral deflection of the catheter tip is needed to optimize this long-axis image by moving the transducer tip back and away from the atrial septum. With further cranial and caudal positioning of the catheter and slight counterclockwise and clockwise rotation, the entire atrial septum is evaluated with two-dimensional and color flow imaging. Usually, the lipomatous superior margin of the atrial septum (septum secundum) is clearly recognized, as is the membrane of the fossa ovalis (Fig. 33.6). From this same position, posterior, leftward imaging beyond the atrial septum allows visualization and evaluation of the left atrium and the left upper and lower pulmonary veins as they course in front of the descending thoracic aorta (Fig. 33.5). The pulmonary veins are evaluated further by color flow imaging and pulsed-wave Doppler interrogation. Continued clockwise rotation

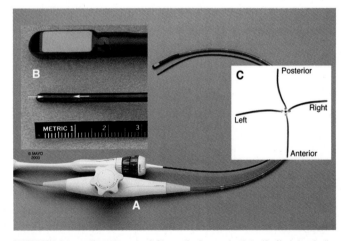

FIGURE 33.1. Intracardiac echo probe. A: Diagnostic ultrasound catheter (AcuNav) placed adjacent to a pediatric transesophageal echocardiography probe shows the relatively small size of the 10 Fr catheter. **B:** Close-up of the 3.3-mm-diameter catheter tip (*arrows*) shows the longitudinally oriented crystal array (palette). **C:** Overhead view of the four-way tip maneuverability of the diagnostic catheter.

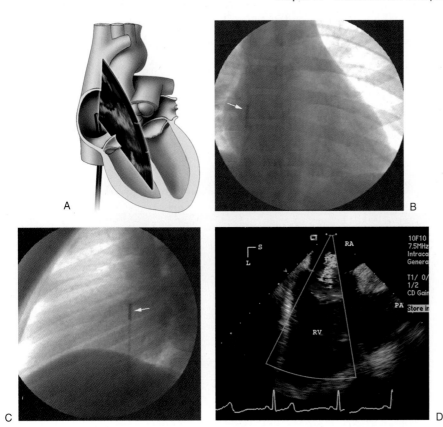

FIGURE 33.2. Tricuspid valve inflow view with ICE. A: Illustration of catheter course and probe position for right ventricular inflow view. **B:** Anteroposterior radiograph reveals the intracardiac echocardiography catheter tip in the right atrium (*arrow*) with the transducer palette pointed toward the tricuspid valve. **C:** Lateral radiograph shows the corresponding lateral image with the transducer tip (*arrow*) pointed anteriorly. **D:** Corresponding intracardiac echocardiography image of the tricuspid valve and right ventricle (RV) with mild tricuspid insufficiency shown with color flow imaging. L, left; PA, pulmonary artery; RA, right atrium; S, superior.

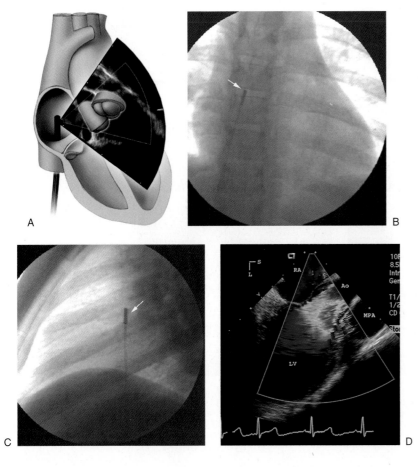

FIGURE 33.3. Evaluation of aorta and left ventricular outflow tract with ICE. A: Illustration of catheter course and probe position for view of the left ventricular outflow tract and aortic valve. **B:** Anteroposterior radiograph shows the intracardiac echocardiography catheter (*arrow*) now rotated slightly clockwise to point to the left ventricular (LV) outflow tract. **C:** Lateral image of the same catheter position (*arrow*). **D:** Corresponding intracardiac echocardiography image of the left ventricular outflow tract with color flow imaging. Ao, ascending aorta; L, left; MPA, main pulmonary artery; RA, right atrium; S, superior.

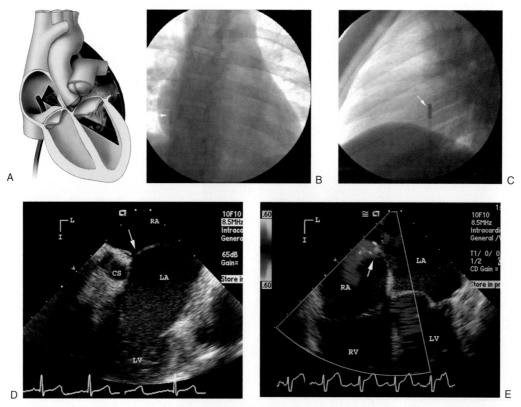

FIGURE 33.4. Evaluation of atrial septum and cardiac crux with ICE. A: Illustration of catheter course and probe position for view of the lower atrial septum and crux of the heart. **B:** Anteroposterior radiograph shows the intracardiac echocardiography catheter (*arrow*) further rotated clockwise to image the cardiac crux portion of the atrial septum above the mitral valve. **C:** Lateral image of this catheter position (*arrow*). **D:** Corresponding intracardiac echocardiography image of the cardiac crux (*arrow*) just above the mitral valve and coronary sinus (CS). **E:** Four-chamber view of the cardiac crux shows small right-to-left shunt across patent foramen ovale (*arrow*). I, inferior; L, left; LA, left atrium; LV, left ventricle; RA, right atrium; RV, right ventricle.

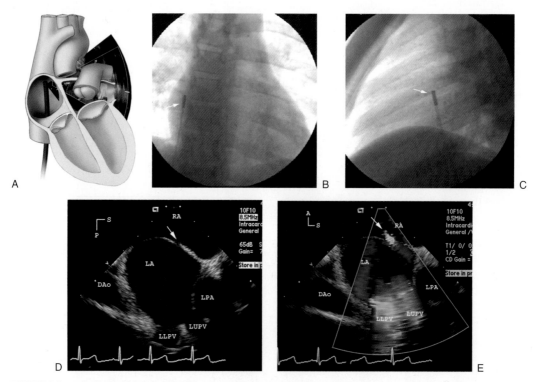

FIGURE 33.5. Long axis view of atrial septum with ICE. A: Illustration of the catheter course and probe position for the long-axis view of the atrial septum. **B:** Anteroposterior radiograph of the intracardiac echocardiography catheter (*arrow*) after further clockwise rotation and slight anterior and lateral retroflexion of the catheter reveals a long-axis intracardiac echocardiography image of the atrial septum. **C:** Lateral image of the catheter position (*arrow*) shows the slight anterior flexion of the catheter. **D:** Corresponding intracardiac echocardiography image of the long axis of the atrial septum (*arrow*) thus obtained. **E:** Color flow image of left pulmonary venous return and a small left-to-right atrial shunt (*arrow*). A, anterior; DAo, descending aorta; LA, left atrium; LLPV, left lower pulmonary vein; LPA, left pulmonary artery; LUPV, left upper pulmonary vein; P, posterior; RA, right atrium; S, superior.

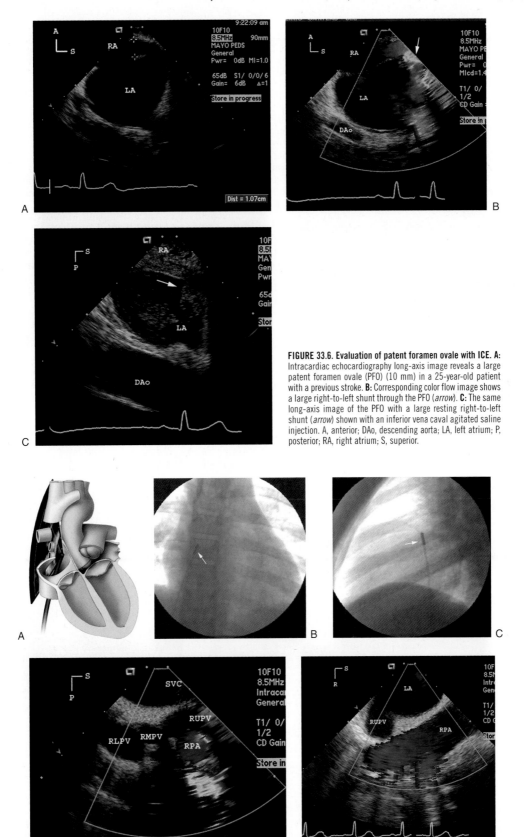

FIGURE 33.6. Evaluation of patent foramen ovale with ICE. A: Intracardiac echocardiography long-axis image reveals a large patent foramen ovale (PFO) (10 mm) in a 25-year-old patient with a previous stroke. **B:** Corresponding color flow image shows a large right-to-left shunt through the PFO (*arrow*). **C:** The same long-axis image of the PFO with a large resting right-to-left shunt (*arrow*) shown with an inferior vena caval agitated saline injection. A, anterior; DAo, descending aorta; LA, left atrium; P, posterior; RA, right atrium; S, superior.

FIGURE 33.7. Evaluation of right pulmonary veins with ICE. A: Illustration of the catheter course and probe position for viewing the right pulmonary veins. **B:** Anteroposterior radiograph reveals intracardiac echocardiography catheter tip position (*arrow*) after further clockwise catheter rotation to the right to image the right pulmonary veins. **C:** Lateral radiograph shows catheter position (*arrow*). **D:** Corresponding intracardiac echocardiography image shows all three right pulmonary veins. Note that the right upper pulmonary vein (RUPV) courses anterior and then inferior to the right pulmonary artery (RPA). **E:** With the catheter tip moved across the atrial defect, the image then reveals a long-axis view of the RPA with the RUPV just inferior to the RPA. LA, left atrium; P, posterior; R, right; RLPV, right lower pulmonary vein; RMPV, right middle pulmonary vein; S, superior; SVC, superior vena cava.

then allows subsequent evaluation of the right lower pulmonary vein and subsequently the right upper pulmonary vein (Fig. 33.7), which is anterior and inferior to the right pulmonary artery. In some patients, visualization of the right pulmonary veins requires not only clockwise rotation but also some cranial advancement of the probe. With anterior flexion of the catheter tip by anterior and leftward control movement, the superior vena cava (SVC) is then evaluated (Fig. 33.8). The crista terminalis is often visible near the SVC.

A short-axis image of the atrial septum and aortic root can be obtained with combined anterior and leftward control movement and with some clockwise rotation of the handle. This directs the tip anteriorly and medially toward and sometimes across the tricuspid valve annulus (Fig. 33.9). Short-axis images are important to access appropriate device positioning near the aortic root and provide a typical transverse image of the aortic valve and the atrial septum. The right lower pulmonary veins are visible near the back wall of the left atrium.

To cross the atrial septum, the catheter tip is repositioned in the midright atrium and, with the imaging palette facing posterior to the atrial septum, is manipulated with posterior or rightward control movement to move the catheter tip toward the atrial septum. With the catheter tip seated adjacent to the atrial septum or, in many cases, across the interatrial defect, the pulmonary veins are again evaluated. Once across the septal defect, with further posterior and rightward control movement (catheter flexion), an en face mitral inflow view is obtained (Fig. 33.10). With the catheter across the atrial septum, in a neutral position and rotated anteriorly (counterclockwise), a detailed short-axis view of the aortic valve is obtained, and with slight clockwise rotation of the catheter, the right ventricular outflow tract and pulmonary valve are observed (Fig. 33.11). With posterior and rightward movement of the controls similar to the mitral valve view, the probe can be advanced into the

left ventricle or near the lateral atrioventricular groove where scans of the ventricular septum, both atrioventricular (AV) valves, and the ventricles can be obtained similar in appearance to a four-chamber view (Fig. 33.12). This view provides excellent imaging of the inlet and membranous ventricular septum.

Returning to the right atrium, with combined anterior and leftward control movement similar to that to obtain a short-axis image, the curved probe can be manipulated across the tricuspid valve to visualize structures within the right ventricle. With advancement of the probe into the right ventricle, scans of the right ventricular outflow tract and pulmonary valve are easily obtained (Fig. 33.13). By releasing the curvature on the probe, it can then be rotated to scan inferiorly to obtain short-axis images of the left ventricle and the ventricular septum. These same views can be used to scan the membranous and muscular portions of the ventricular to visualized ventricular septal defects (VSDs) (Fig. 33.14).

Imaging Note: ALL ICE PROBE MANIPULATIONS WITHIN THE LEFT ATRIUM, LEFT VENTRICLE AND RIGHT VENTRICLE SHOULD BE GRADUAL, GENTLE, AND PERFORMED WITH FLUOROSCOPIC GUIDANCE BECAUSE THE STIFF ICE PROBE MAY CAUSE DAMAGE TO THE VALVULAR APPARATUS AND OTHER STRUCTURES.

Applications

The potential applications of ICE to interventional cardiac catheterization continue to expand, not only with respect to catheter-based treatment of congenital and acquired heart disease but also to the management of cardiac arrhythmias. ICE imaging results in improved patient comfort compared with TEE. ICE imaging bypasses potentially poor acoustic windows that are commonly encountered during transthoracic echocardiography. In addition, the use of ICE imaging allows a "single operator" concept, thereby alleviating the

FIGURE 33.8. Evaluation of superior vena cava with ICE. A: Illustration of the catheter course and probe position to view the superior vena cava. **B:** Anteroposterior radiograph reveals anterior and lateral flexion of the catheter (*arrow*) to scan superiorly into the superior vena cava (SVC). **C:** Lateral image of the same catheter position (*arrow*) scanning superiorly. **D:** Corresponding intracardiac echocardiography image shows flow from the SVC into the right atrium (RA). The right upper pulmonary vein (RUPV) is noted as it courses anterior (A) and inferior to the right pulmonary artery (RPA). S, superior.

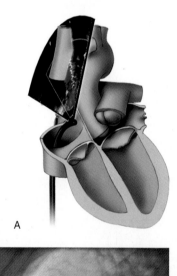
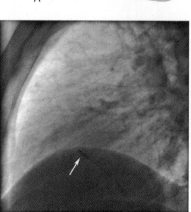
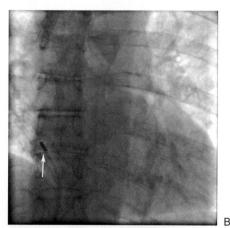
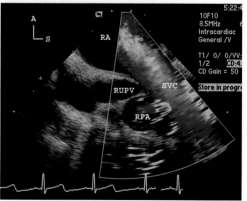

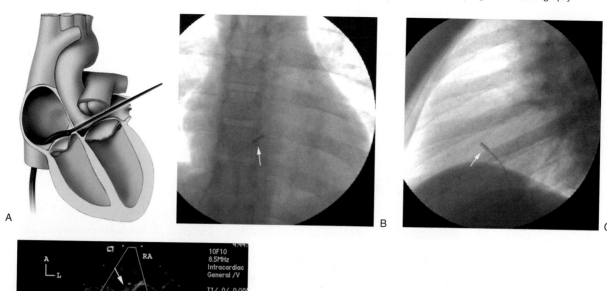

FIGURE 33.9. Short axis view of atrial septum and aorta with ICE. **A:** Illustration of the catheter course and probe position for the short-axis view of the atrial septum and aorta. **B:** Anteroposterior radiograph shows retroflexion of the catheter tip by anterior and leftward movement of the probe controls and subsequent rotation of the catheter tip clockwise to place the tip (*arrow*) near or through the tricuspid valve. **C:** Lateral image reveals the catheter position (*arrow*) near the tricuspid valve. **D:** Corresponding intracardiac echocardiography image reveals a typical short-axis image of the heart at the level of the aortic valve. A small left-to-right shunt (*arrow*) is observed through the superior margin of the atrial septal defect. The main pulmonary artery (MPA) is also noted posterior to the aorta. A, anterior; Ao, ascending aorta; L, left; LA, left atrium; RA, right atrium.

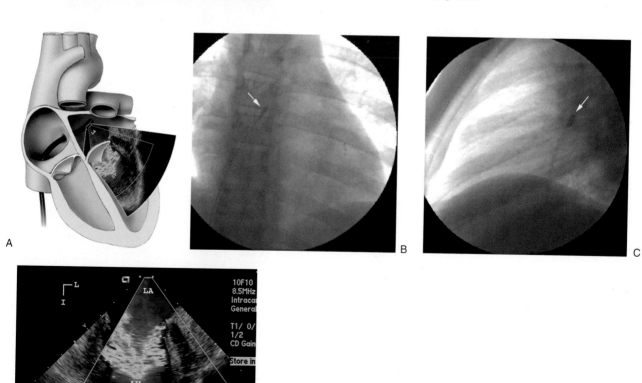

FIGURE 33.10. Evaluation of the mitral valve with ICE. **A:** Illustration of the catheter course and probe position for an en face view of the mitral valve from the left atrium. **B:** Anteroposterior radiograph shows the intracardiac echocardiography catheter (*arrow*) advanced across the atrial septal defect and flexed inferiorly to view the mitral valve orifice. **C:** Lateral radiograph reveals the same catheter position (*arrow*). Note the posterior location of the catheter in the left atrium. **D:** Corresponding intracardiac echocardiography image of the en face view of the mitral orifice. I, inferior; L, left; LA, left atrium; LV, left ventricle.

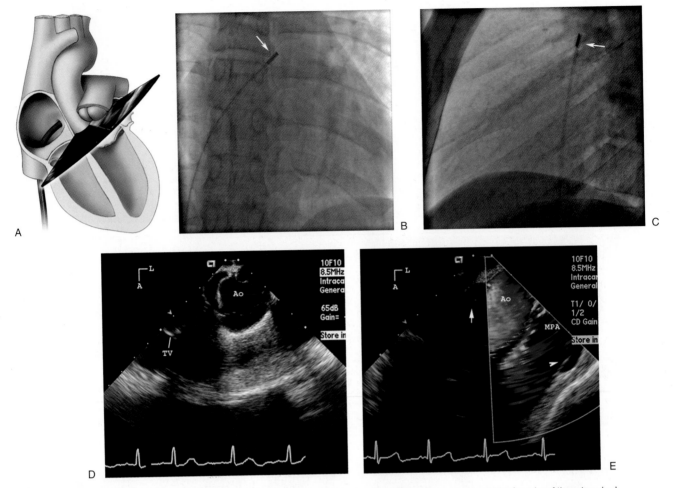

FIGURE 33.11. Evaluation of aorta, RVOT, and pulmonary artery with ICE. A: Illustration of the catheter course and probe position for a view of the aorta and pulmonary artery from the left atrium. **B:** Anteroposterior radiograph of the intracardiac echocardiography catheter tip (*arrow*) placed across the atrial septal defect into the left atrium but rotated counterclockwise to an anterior position immediately behind the aortic valve. **C:** Lateral image of the same catheter position (*arrow*). Note that the transducer is pointing anteriorly. **D:** Corresponding intracardiac echocardiography image shows in the short axis the fine detail of the aortic valve leaflets. **E:** With additional clockwise catheter rotation, a view of the right ventricular outflow tract and main pulmonary artery (MPA) is obtained. Arrow points to aortic valve and arrowhead points to pulmonary valve. A, anterior; Ao, ascending aorta; L, left; TV, tricuspid valve.

need for an additional echocardiographer in the catheterization laboratory, provided the primary operator is familiar with ICE imaging and interpretation. The interventionalist has control of the echocardiographic ICE images and must be able to provide the appropriate image planes for diagnosis and catheter intervention. The ability to provide this imaging rapidly and without the need for other echocardiographic support expedites the procedure and shortens interventional procedure time.

Superior image quality and visualization of intracardiac structures allow accurate guidance of interventional procedures, thereby reducing both fluoroscopic and procedure times. Procedures where ICE imaging has been reported to be of benefit include, but are not limited to, guidance of transseptal puncture to gain access to the left atrium, transcatheter closure device placement, radiofrequency ablation, cardiac biopsy, mitral valvuloplasty, and left atrial appendage occlusion.

Electrophysiology Procedures – The first reports of intracardiac ultrasound during electrophysiology procedures (EPS) were for use of a mechanical, single-element intracardiac echo probe. Anatomic definition was thought to be of great benefit for ablation procedures, as fluoroscopic guidance did not provide adequate tissue definition. Intracardiac imaging with the newer phased-array ICE catheter has been incorporated to guide electrophysiology procedures. Proper location of the transseptal puncture as guided by ICE has been useful in conjunction with EPS. Anatomic landmarks that are important for a successful ablation are best visualized by

ICE and are not easily seen fluoroscopically. One of the most common uses of ICE imaging during EPS has been during pulmonary vein isolation for atrial flutter ablation. ICE imaging provides exact determination of the pulmonary vein anatomy (number and position), including the presence or absence of an antrum that may receive the left upper and lower pulmonary veins before joining the left atrium. Visualization of pulmonary vein ostia by ICE facilitates catheter positioning to ensure adequate tip-tissue contact for delivery of radiofrequency energy, thereby improving the success of the ablation procedure and reducing fluoroscopic times. Additionally, anatomic definition reduces the risk of inadvertent ablation deeper within the vein itself, which should reduce the occurrence of subsequent pulmonary vein stenosis. ICE imaging during ablation of ventricular arrhythmias is of particular use for the evaluation of known anatomic landmarks for certain tachycardia circuits and to evaluate catheter proximity to valves and coronary arteries.

Device Closure Procedures – Another application of ICE imaging, rapidly adopted into clinical practice, has been for guidance during device closure of interatrial defects, such as secundum ASD or patent foramen ovale (PFO). ICE images provide superior imaging of the atrial septum. Assessment of the defect(s) and relationship to the surrounding cardiac structures is critical to a successful procedure and is facilitated by the proximity of the ICE catheter to the atrial walls, appendage, Eustachian valve, limbus of

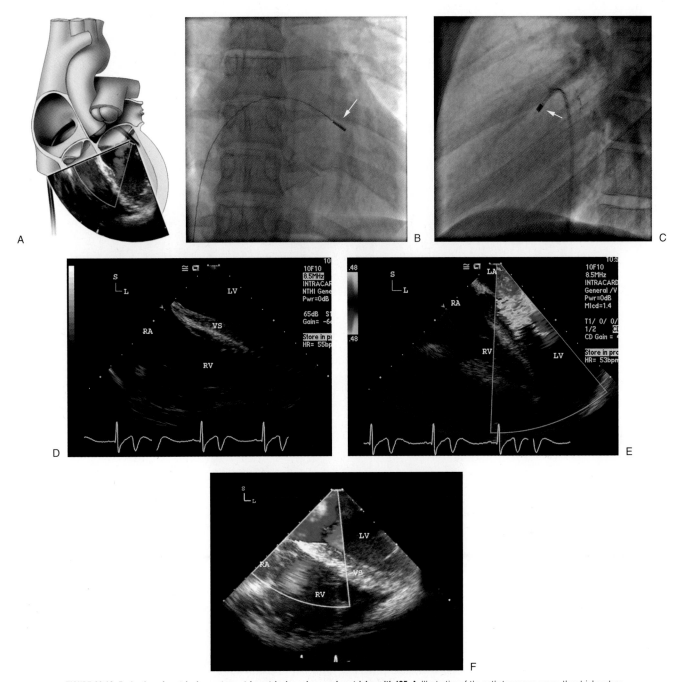

FIGURE 33.12. Evaluation of ventricular septum, atrioventricular valves, and ventricles with ICE. A: Illustration of the catheter course across the atrial septum and the probe position just inside the left ventricle near the left atrioventricular groove. Rightward and posterior control movement results in angulation of the probe to view the ventricular septum and both ventricles. **B:** Anteroposterior radiograph of the intracardiac echocardiography catheter tip(*arrow*)at the left atrioventricular groove. **C:** Lateral radiograph demonstrating this catheter position. **D:** Corresponding intracardiac echocardiography image showing a four-chamber–like view of both ventricles and the ventricular septum. The membranous to inlet portion of the ventricular septum is well visualized. **E:** Color flow image showing mitral inflow. **F:** Similar view in another patient demonstrating a systolic image.

the fossa ovalis, and pulmonary veins. Documentation of normal pulmonary venous return to the left atrium (Figs. 33.5 and 33.7) is an important aspect of ASD closure and is easily accomplished by ICE. Long-axis and short-axis views (Fig. 33.15) aid in dimensional analysis of the ASD and allow very accurate measurement of both static diameter and balloon-stretched diameter (used to select the appropriate device size) compared with fluoroscopy (Fig. 33.16). Spatial orientation of devices in relationship to surrounding cardiac structures are better visualized by ICE compared with TEE. During deployment and subsequent delivery of an occlusion device there is no shadowing of the right atrial disc of the device by the left atrial disc when ICE guidance is utilized. Therefore, ICE imaging provides

superior visualization of septal rims in relationship to device position before final deployment is accomplished, reducing the risk of device embolization. In contrast, when TEE is used for evaluation of device placement, significant acoustic shadowing from the left atrial disc may preclude adequate imaging of each disc and its relationship to the atrial septum, increasing the time needed for imaging before delivery of the device in an optimal position.

Transcatheter closure of muscular VSD (congenital or post myocardial infarction) is now possible. In a patient with post–myocardial infarction VSD, TEE imaging may not be tolerated by the more clinically compromised patient. ICE is an additional imaging modality that can be used to aid visualization of cardiac structures during

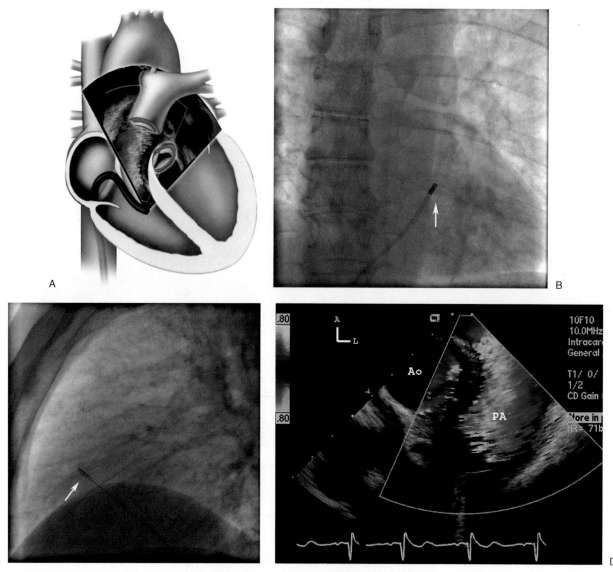

FIGURE 33.13. Evaluation of RVOT and pulmonary valve with ICE. A: Illustration of the catheter course and probe position across the tricuspid valve in the right ventricle. Because of the leftward and anterior control manipulation the probe is angulated to visualized the pulmonary outflow tract and valve superiorly. **B:** Anteroposterior radiograph of the intracardiac echocardiography catheter in the right ventricle. **C:** Lateral radiograph demonstrating the anterior catheter location. **D:** Corresponding intracardiac echocardiography image of the pulmonary outflow and color flow through the pulmonary valve.

defect sizing, delivery, and deployment of a septal closure device. Monitoring of tricuspid valve regurgitation is facilitated by ICE during such procedures. To visualize the VSD properly, manipulation of the ICE catheter through the tricuspid valve orifice into the right ventricle may be needed (as described earlier).

Periprosthesis Valvular Regurgitation – In patients with both acquired heart disease (e.g., rheumatic valvular disease) and congenital heart disease who have undergone mechanical valve replacement, perivalvular leak is a reported phenomenon. Often, acoustic shadowing by the mechanical valve precludes adequate echo imaging from one side of the valve. Depending on the intracardiac anatomy, both ICE and TEE may be needed to facilitate evaluation of such defects for location, proximity to the mechanical valve, and size of the defect. In addition, during deployment of closure devices, assurance of valve function during and after device placement is critical. Evaluation of leaflet mobility is important, and the device must not interfere with normal valve function. Continuous monitoring during device deployment, positioning, and delivery is easily accomplished with ICE (Fig. 33.17). Judicious use of TEE may be needed to fully evaluate some

patients during closure of perivalvular leak but can then be minimized to facilitate patient comfort during supine imaging with the additional use of ICE.

Additional Applications – Device closure of the left atrial appendage has been under investigation as a treatment to reduce embolic risk with chronic atrial fibrillation. ICE imaging of the appendage before device closure facilitates evaluation of thrombus in the appendage. Continuous monitoring during the interventional procedure is typically performed from the right atrium, with proximity to the left atrial structures allowing adequate visualization of the device during deployment and final delivery. Intracardiac thrombus related to the procedure can be evaluated by ICE. During mitral valvuloplasty, the use of ICE may aid in monitoring the location of the initial transseptal puncture, particularly in situations where the atrial septum is excessively thickened. Additionally, ICE may be used for assessment of valve morphology, annulus measurement, and monitoring of the results of the balloon valvuloplasty.

Instantaneous monitoring for catheter-related complications is also possible with the use of ICE. Detection of left-sided thrombus or

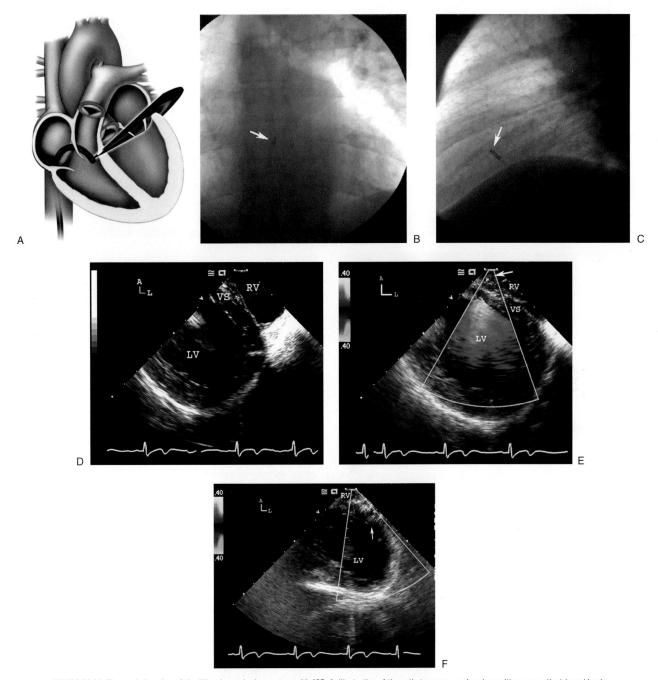

FIGURE 33.14. Short axis imaging of the LV and ventricular septum with ICE. A: Illustration of the catheter course and probe position across the tricuspid valve and with the probe directed posterior to the ventricular septum to visualize the left ventricle in short axis. **B:** Anteroposterior radiograph demonstrating this catheter position in the right ventricle. **C:** Lateral radiograph demonstrating the same catheter position. **D:** Corresponding echocardiographic images demonstrating the right ventricle (RV) anteriorly and the left ventricle (LV) in short axis. **E:** Color flow imaging demonstrating flow in the LV and the *arrow* points to a small jet near the ventricular septum (VS) which represents flow from a muscular ventricular septal defect (VSD). **F:** More apical view demonstrating the origin (*arrow*) of the VSD in the LV. A, anterior; L, left.

spontaneous contrast in a cardiac chamber as a precursor to thrombus is facilitated by the use of ICE. Pericardial effusion can easily be visualized by ICE and then promptly treated to prevent complications.

 # CONGENITAL INTRAOPERATIVE TRANSESOPHAGEAL ECHOCARDIOGRAPHY

Intraoperative transesophageal echocardiography (IOTEE) has been used in the care of patients with congenital heart defects since the late 1980s. Previous reports have suggested that IOTEE can provide important additional information during intracardiac repair of congenital heart defects. Recommendations for the use of IOTEE have been broad, in part because of the small sample size in prior studies. The preliminary experience with IOTEE during surgery for congenital heart defects at the Mayo Clinic confirmed the accuracy of IOTEE and identified select patients who would benefit from IOTEE based on a small study population of 104 patients. Bezold and colleagues at Texas Children's Hospital reported a larger experience with IOTEE in 341 patients. They concluded that biplane imaging was far superior to monoplane imaging. IOTEE

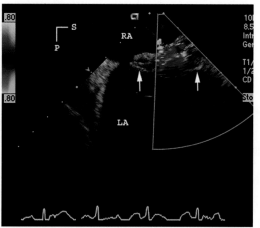

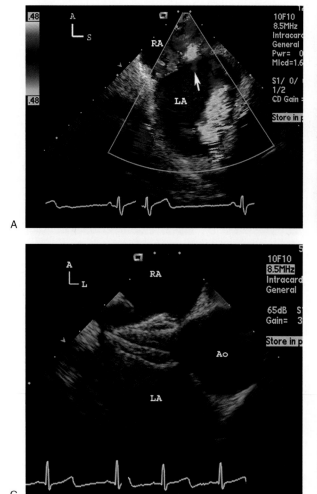

FIGURE 33.15. Evaluation of ASD device closure with ICE during interventional cardiac catheterization. A: Intracardiac echocardiography image demonstrating the long axis of the atrial septum with a moderate left-to-right shunt (*arrow*) through a secundum atrial septal defect. **B:** Similar image showing an occluder device in place (*arrows*) with a small residual central shunt. **C:** A short-axis image showing a device in place behind the aortic root (Ao). RA, right atrium; LA, left atrium; A, anterior; L, left; S, superior.

also seemed to be most beneficial in patients with select diagnoses and surgical procedures in this series. Stevenson concluded that IOTEE had a very low complication rate (about 3%). The largest experience specifically evaluating the utility of intraoperative echocardiography was published by Ungerleider and colleagues, involving over 1000 cases. Their study evaluated both epicardial and transesophageal echocardiography. Disadvantages of epicardial imaging include invasion of the surgical field, limited windows, possible induction of ventricular ectopic beats, and possible transient hypotension. Therefore, IOTEE has become the preferred modality of imaging during surgery for congenital heart defects. IOTEE is useful for recognition of intracardiac air before coming off cardiopulmonary bypass and to provide a routine assessment of postbypass ventricular function.

Equipment

The multiplane TEE transducer is now the standard probe preferred for all intraoperative TEE studies. The probe consists of a single array of crystals that can be rotated electronically or mechanically around the long axis of the ultrasound beam in an arc of 180 degrees. With rotation of the transducer array, multiplane TEE can obtain a continuum of transverse and longitudinal image planes. Newer adult-size TEE probes have 3- to 7-MHz ultrasound frequency ranges, and some are capable of harmonic imaging as well. Usually with a 64-crystal array, they range in size from 12- to 14-mm diameter tip (Fig. 33.18). Some IOTEE probes have increase shielding to protect them from the effects of intraoperative electrocautery. Recently developed systems will have software capability to obtain live three-dimensional reconstructed images. Unfortunately, pediatric TEE probes have not

achieved the degree of sophisticated development as the adult counterpart. The currently available multiplane pediatric TEE probe has a 48-crystal array with a tip diameter of 9 mm (Fig. 33.18). The frequency agility is from 5 to 7 MHz, and the mobility is limited to movement in one plane. No additional probe shielding from the electrocautery is yet available. As discussed later, we have also used the intracardiac Acunav probe for TEE imaging in small infants (weighing less than 3 kg). Table 33.1 lists the general weight guidelines we have used for probe selection in infants and children.

Image Acquisition

Four primary multiplane TEE views can be obtained by rotating the transducer array from 0 to 135 degrees (Fig. 33.19). At 0 degrees, a typical transverse image plane is obtained allowing the typical four-chamber view; at 30 to 45 degrees, transverse

Table 33.1	WEIGHT GUIDELINES FOR TRANSESOPHAGEAL ECHOCARDIOGRAPHY PROBE SELECTION IN INFANTS AND CHILDREN
Weight (kg)	**Probe Type**
1.5–3	Intracardiac echo longitudinal plane probe
3–15	Pediatric multiplane probe
15–20	Variable depending on other patient factors.
>20	Adult multiplane probe

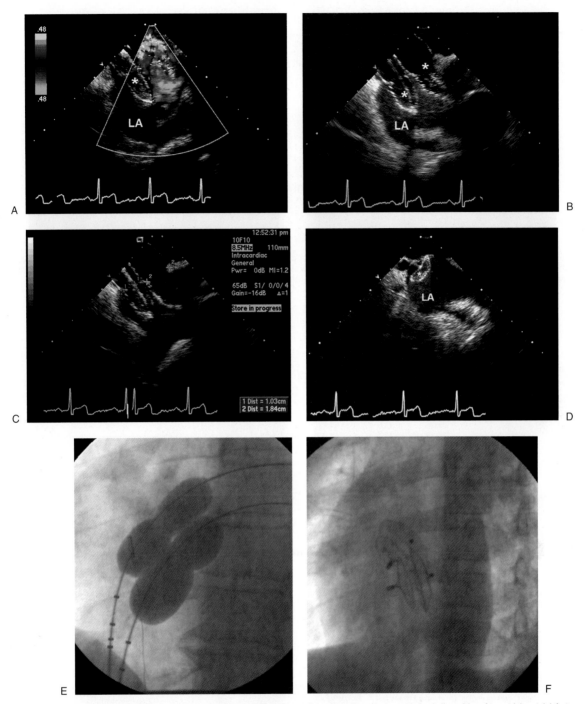

FIGURE 33.16. ICE imaging during interventional device closure of ASD. A: Intracardiac echocardiography image during balloon sizing of two atrial septal defects (ASDs). A balloon (*asterisk*) is inflated across the more inferior defect. Color Doppler imaging demonstrates a large left-to-right shunt across the more superior defect at this time. **B:** Two balloons (*asterisks*) now occlude the defects. **C:** Measurement of the respective balloon waists to size the ASDs. Inferior defect, 10 mm; superior defect, 18 mm. **D:** Device deployment. The left atrium (LA) side of the device (*arrow*) has been deployed across the more inferior defect. **E:** Anteroposterior fluoroscopic image while both balloons are inflated across the atrial septum. Note the plane of the atrial septum as identified by the balloon waists. **F:** Fluoroscopic image after deployment of two Amplatzer septal occluders. A, anterior; S, superior.

plane short-axis images are obtained similar to the TTE parasternal short-axis views of the aortic valve as well as short-axis transgastric images of the left ventricle; 90 degrees provides a typical longitudinal transducer orientation and produces images somewhat oblique to the long axis of the heart; and 120 to 135 degrees provides a true long-axis image of the left ventricular outflow tract analogous to the parasternal long-axis view. Additional images and modifications of typical transverse and longitudinal scan

images can also be obtained by typical TEE probe tip manipulation for flexion or right/left angulation (Fig. 33.20). Basic image orientation for TEE imaging has followed the standard image orientation used for transthoracic imaging (Fig. 33.21). The various transverse and longitudinal image planes obtained by probe position, rotation, tip angulation, and image plane angulation have been previously described by Seward et al. and are illustrated in Figs 33.22 through 33.28.

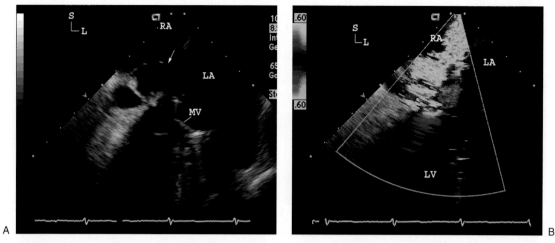

FIGURE 33.17. Evaluation of prosthetic perivalvar leak with ICE. A: Intracardiac echocardiography image obtained from the right atrium (RA) in a patient with a left ventricular (LV)-to- RA shunt following mitral valve (MV) replacement. This view of the crux of the heart shows the entrance (*arrow*) of the fistula in the RA. **B:** Color flow imaging demonstrating a moderate shunt from LV to RA. LA, left atrium; L, left; S, superior.

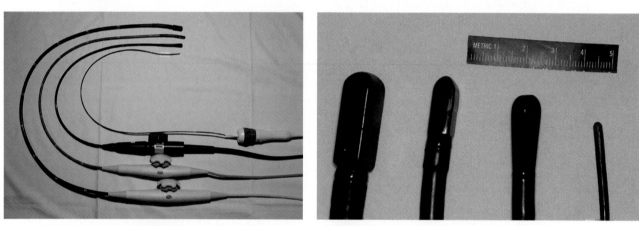

FIGURE 33.18. TEE imaging probes. A: Comparison view of pediatric transesophageal echocardiography probes ranging from the adult-sized multiplane probe, the pediatric biplane probe, the pediatric multiplane probe, and the intracardiac catheter. **B:** Comparison view of the same probe tips. From **left** to **right:** The adult multiplane is 13 mm with 64 elements; the pediatric biplane probe has a 9-mm tip with 64 elements; the pediatric multiplane probe has a 10-mm tip with 48 elements; and the intracardiac echocardiography catheter has a 64-element longitudinal array and is 3.3 mm in diameter.

FIGURE 33.19. Diagrammatic illustration of multiplane transesophageal echocardiography scan planes corresponding to standard transthoracic short- and long-axis views. The 0-degree transverse orientation corresponds to the standard horizontal plane of biplane transesophageal echocardiography systems, and the 90-degree longitudinal orientation corresponds to the standard vertical plane.

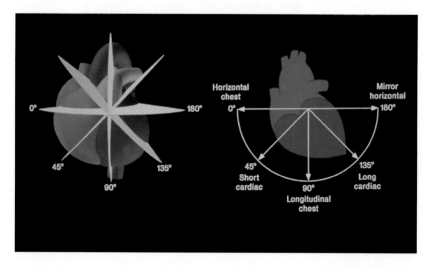

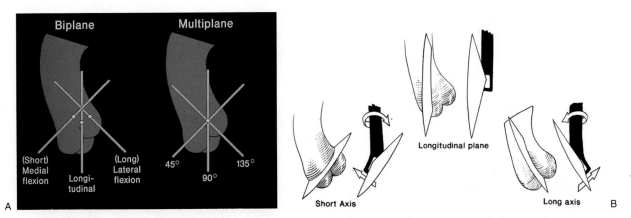

FIGURE 33.20. TEE imaging planes to evalvate aorta. A: Illustrates a similar comparison of biplane and multiplane transesophageal echocardiography images as they relate to the long axis of the aorta. **B:** Illustrates the typical transesophageal echocardiography tip deflection used for both biplane and multiplane images to obtain images similar to transthoracic image orientation.

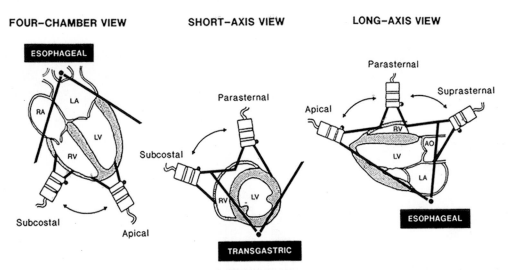

FIGURE 33-21. Diagrammatic illustration of comparable transthoracic and transesophageal echocardiography images and appropriate orientation as observed with four-chamber, short-axis, and long-axis images.

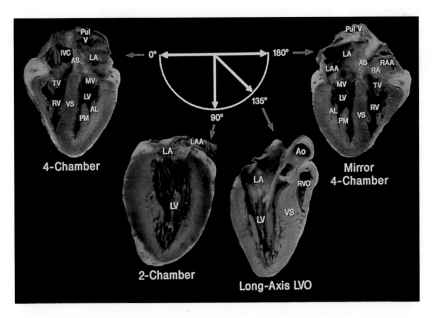

FIGURE 33.22. Pathologic correlation of images obtained with various multiplane images from 0 degrees to 135 degrees representing horizontal (four-chamber and longitudinal scan planes). AS, atrial septum; AW, anterior LV wall; AL, anterolateral papillary muscle; B, bronchus; CS, coronary sinus; E, esophagus; IVC, inferior vena cava; LAA, left atrial appendage; LVO, LV outflow; L, left coronary cusp; MPA, main pulmonary artery; N, noncoronary cusp; PM, posteromedial papillary muscle; PV, pulmonary valve; Pul V, pulmonary veins; R, right coronary cusp; RAA, right atrial appendage; RVO, RV outflow; SVC, superior vena cava; T, trachea; VS, ventricular septum.

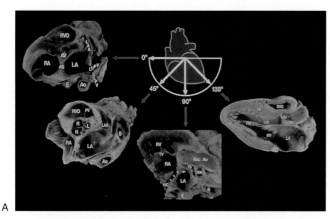
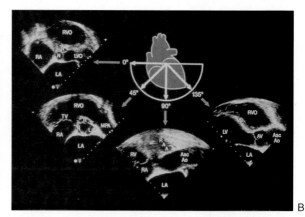

FIGURE 33.23. TEE imaging planes obtained from midesophagus. A: Tomographic anatomy of the heart at the midesophagus. Specimens are presented from the perspective of 0-degree rotation of imaging to 135-degree rotation. The 30- to 45-degree rotation results in short-axis images, while the 120- to 135-degree rotation obtain images similar to parasternal long-axis images. **B:** Composite transesophageal echocardiography images obtained at the various tomographic sections illustrated in **A.** The image orientation is similar to those obtained with standard transthoracic imaging. AS, atrial septum; AW, anterior LV wall; AL, anterolateral papillary muscle; B, bronchus; CS, coronary sinus; E, esophagus; IVC, inferior vena cava; LAA, left atrial appendage; LVO, LV outflow; L, left coronary cusp; MPA, main pulmonary artery; N, noncoronary cusp; PM, posteromedial papillary muscle; PV, pulmonary valve; Pul V, pulmonary veins; R, right coronary cusp; RAA, right atrial appendage; RVO, RV outflow; SVC, superior vena cava; T, trachea; VS, ventricular septum.

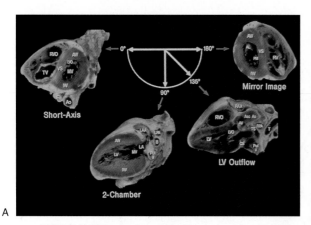
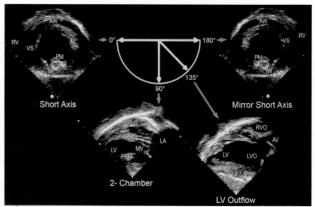

FIGURE 33.24. TEE imaging planes obtained from transgastric position. A: Tomographic short- and long-axis anatomic specimens corresponding to transesophageal echocardiography views obtained with transgastric imaging. True short- and long-axis images can be obtained at 45- and 135-degree rotation, respectively. **B:** Corresponding transesophageal echocardiography images obtained from the transgastric position illustrating short-axis images at 45 degrees and long-axis images obtained at 135-degree array rotation. AS, atrial septum; AW, anterior LV wall; AL, anterolateral papillary muscle; B, bronchus; CS, coronary sinus; E, esophagus; IVC, inferior vena cava; LAA, left atrial appendage; LVO, LV outflow; L, left coronary cusp; MPA, main pulmonary artery; N, noncoronary cusp; PM, posteromedial papillary muscle; PV, pulmonary valve; Pul V, pulmonary veins; R, right coronary cusp; RAA, right atrial appendage; RVO, RV outflow; SVC, superior vena cava; T, trachea; VS, ventricular septum.

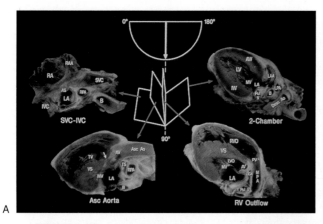
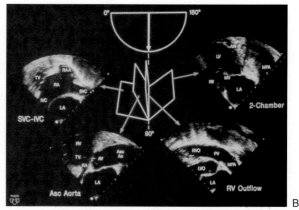

FIGURE 33.25. TEE imaging from the longitudal scan plane at the midesophagus. A: Midesophageal longitudinal tomographic anatomic sections cut to corresponding to longitudinal plane echocardiographic images obtained by rotating the transesophageal echocardiography probe from the patient's right to left. **B:** A series of longitudinal echocardiographic views obtained from the midesophagus by rotating the transesophageal echocardiography probe while maintaining the array at 90 degrees throughout the probe rotation to the patient's left. The first image is obtained on the patient's right side illustrating a long-axis bicaval view of the right atrium. With progressive probe rotation subsequent images of the proximal ascending aorta, the right ventricular outflow tract, and finally a two-chamber view of the left ventricle are obtained. AS, atrial septum; AW, anterior LV wall; AL, anterolateral papillary muscle; B, bronchus; CS, coronary sinus; E, esophagus; IVC, inferior vena cava; LAA, left atrial appendage; LVO, LV outflow; L, left coronary cusp; MPA, main pulmonary artery; N, noncoronary cusp; PM, posteromedial papillary muscle; PV, pulmonary valve; Pul V, pulmonary veins; R, right coronary cusp; RAA, right atrial appendage; SVC, superior vena cava; T, trachea; VS, ventricular septum.

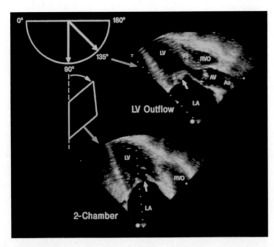

FIGURE 33.26. TEE imaging of LV long axis. Transesophageal echocardiography images obtained from the midesophagus illustrating the standard longitudinal images at 90 degrees and movement to typical LV long-axis images obtain by rotating the crystal array to 135 degrees. AS, atrial septum; AW, anterior LV wall; AL, anterolateral papillary muscle; B, bronchus; CS, coronary sinus; E, esophagus; IVC, inferior vena cava; LAA, left atrial appendage; LVO, LV outflow; L, left coronary cusp; MPA, main pulmonary artery; N, noncoronary cusp; PM, posteromedial papillary muscle; PV, pulmonary valve; Pul V, pulmonary veins; R, right coronary cusp; RAA, right atrial appendage; RVO, RV outflow; SVC, superior vena cava; T, trachea; VS, ventricular septum.

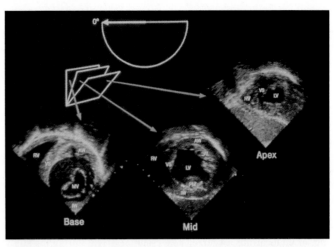

FIGURE 33.27. TEE imaging of LV short axis. Transesophageal echocardiography images obtained from the transgastric position demonstrating a series of short-axis images obtained with the crystal array at 0 degree and by retroflexing the probe to obtain short-axis images closer to the apex of the left ventricle. AS, atrial septum; AW, anterior LV wall; AL, anterolateral papillary muscle; B, bronchus; CS, coronary sinus; E, esophagus; IVC, inferior vena cava; LAA, left atrial appendage; LVO, LV outflow; L, left coronary cusp; MPA, main pulmonary artery; N, noncoronary cusp; PM, posteromedial papillary muscle; PV, pulmonary valve; Pul V, pulmonary veins; R, right coronary cusp; RAA, right atrial appendage; RVO, RV outflow; SVC, superior vena cava; T, trachea; VS, ventricular septum.

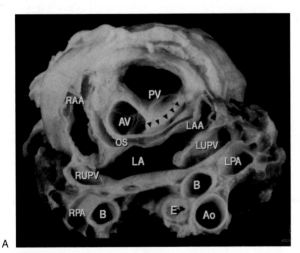

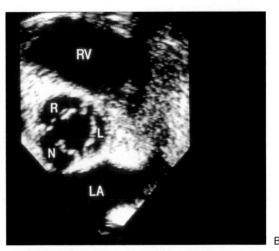

FIGURE 33.28. TEE imaging at the cardiac base. A: Anatomic cross section of the base of the heart just above the level of the aortic valve demonstrating the proximity of the esophagus to the left atrium and cardiac structures. The cross section illustrates the type of aortic valve image observed in the standard transesophageal echocardiography short-axis image. AS, atrial septum; AW, anterior LV wall; AL, anterolateral papillary muscle; B, bronchus; CS, coronary sinus; E, esophagus; IVC, inferior vena cava; LAA, left atrial appendage; LVO, LV outflow; L, left coronary cusp; MPA, main pulmonary artery; N, noncoronary cusp; PM, posteromedial papillary muscle; PV, pulmonary valve; Pul V, pulmonary veins; R, right coronary cusp; RAA, right atrial appendage; RVO, RV outflow; SVC, superior vena cava; T, trachea; VS, ventricular septum.

Mayo Clinic Congenital Intraoperative Transesophageal Echocardiography Experience

Randolph et al. reported the Mayo Clinic IOTEE experience with examinations performed in 1002 patients during congenital heart surgery. Impact of IOTEE was assigned prospectively by the surgeon and cardiologist who performed the IOTEE, while the patient was still in the operating suite. The combined major impact rate for the series was 14%. Separate rates of preoperative and postoperative major impact were 9% and 6%, respectively. Of the 22 primary diagnostic categories analyzed, complex right ventricular outflow tract obstruction, defined as lesions requiring more than a valvotomy or transannular patch, had the highest combined impact rate—48% (Table 33.2). Surgical procedures involving younger patients (Table 33.3) and those with VSD repair, valve repair, complex cyanotic disease, or great artery modifications were indications for IOTEE study with the greatest impact.

Table 33.2	MAJOR IMPACT OF INTRAOPERATIVE TRANSESOPHAGEAL ECHOCARDIOGRAPHY BASED ON PRIMARY DIAGNOSIS		
Primary Diagnosis	**No. of Patients**	**Impact (%)**	**Odds Ratio**
Complex RVOT obstruction	23	48	6.0
Double-outlet right ventricle	29	31	2.9
TGA ± VSD	44	27	2.4
Complex AV discordance	33	24	2.0
Subaortic stenosis	57	21	1.7
Partial AV septal defect	55	20	1.6

AV, atrioventricular; RVOT, right ventricular outflow tract; TGA, transposition of the great arteries; VSD, ventricular septal defect.

Table 33.3	MAJOR IMPACT OF INTRAOPERATIVE TRANSESOPHAGEAL ECHOCARDIOGRAPHY BASED ON AGE	
Age (y)	No. of Patients	Major Impact (%)
<6	377	16
6 to <18	289	15
>18	336	11*

*P value = .018 compared with those patients younger than 18 years at the time of the operation.

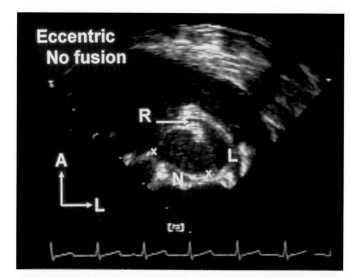

FIGURE 33.29. Transesophageal echocardiography short-axis image of bicuspid aortic valve showing a very eccentric valve orifice with a raphe (fused commissure) between the right and left aortic cusps. There is some nodular thickening at the raphe but no other evidence of commissural fusion. The orifice commissure is marked by the two x's. R, right cusp; L, left cusp; N, noncoronary cusp; A, anterior; L, left; AS, atrial septum; AW, anterior LV wall; AL, anterolateral papillary muscle; B, bronchus; CS, coronary sinus; E, esophagus; IVC, inferior vena cava; LAA, left atrial appendage; LVO, LV outflow; L, left coronary cusp; MPA, main pulmonary artery; N, noncoronary cusp; PM, posteromedial papillary muscle; PV, pulmonary valve; Pul V, pulmonary veins; R, right coronary cusp; RAA, right atrial appendage; RVO, RV outflow; SVC, superior vena cava; T, trachea; VS, ventricular septum.

No major complications, defined as death, esophageal or gastric perforations, accidental extubations, upper gastrointestinal bleeding, or endocarditis, occurred as a result of IOTEE during the study period. Minor complications, defined as transient airway compression, problems with ventilation, or compression of the descending aorta by the probe, were observed in 10 patients, or 1% of the study population. Minor complications were most common in patients weighing less than 4 kg. IOTEE was performed in 51 patients weighing less than 4 kg. Minor complications occurred in 6 of these infants, representing a minor complication rate of 12% in this subset of patients.

Some examples of valvular anomalies demonstrated by TEE are exemplified by short-axis TEE images of a bicuspid aortic valve. TEE imaging allows excellent valve imaging to identify the anatomic configuration and degree of commissural fusion as well as leaflet thickening. Figures 33.29 and 33.30 identify the fused leaflets in two examples of bicuspid aortic valve that were significantly stenotic but had little commissural fusion. The stenosis was secondary to eccentricity of the valve leaflets that resulted in a small effective valve orifice. Similarly, Figure 33.31 illustrates aortic valve prolapse and left-to-right shunt in an intraoperative study on a patient with a supracristal VSD. Atrioventricular septal defects (AVSDs) were frequently listed as being impacted by IOTEE. Figure 33.32 illustrates features often observed in AVSDs. Repair of complex congenital defects also ranked high with IOTEE impact. Based on these data and reports from other large institutions, our practice has been to routinely perform IOTEE during intracardiac surgery for all congenital heart defects.

Intraoperative Transesophageal Echocardiography Using the Intracardiac Echocardiography Probe

The ICE probe has also been used for transesophageal imaging in small infants during congenital cardiac surgery. The small size of this probe facilitates its placement in children weighing less than 3.0 kg. To date, our center has performed approximately 100 studies in children less than 3 kg with this probe. Initial reports of the TEE use of the ICE probe in animal models and small children have been encouraging. Bruce and colleagues demonstrated in 2002 that the probe could successfully be used in a group of 17 infants who weighed between 2.1 and 5.6 kg. No major complications were reported. In 13 of 22 studies performed in that study, the standard biplane pediatric TEE probe could not be advanced into the esophagus due to the patient's small size. Therefore, TEE imaging would not have been performed if the ICE probe was unavailable. High-quality two-dimensional and Doppler images of the descending thoracic aorta (Fig. 33.33), both ventricles (Fig. 33.34), and apical and outlet ventricular septa are obtained with the ICE probe. In addition, the systemic and pulmonary venous connections to the atria and the atrial septum are adequately visualized with this probe.

The major disadvantage of the ICE probe is that it is monoplane. Longitudinal imaging is effective, but the crux of the heart and the inlet ventricular septum are not adequately visualized. This probe has not been suitable during repair of AVSDs. However, these defects are rarely repaired in the newborn period. Transgastric

imaging is also suboptimal with this probe because the orientation of the phased-array pallet does not permit articulation near the probe tip. To avoid thermal injury, it is recommended that imaging time be succinct and that the probe be powered only when in use. While there are technical limitations to performing TEE with this probe, it provides reliable and adequate imaging in patients who otherwise would not be able to have TEE performed during cardiac surgery.

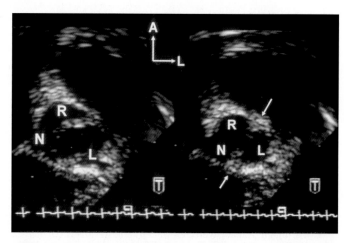

FIGURE 33.30. Transesophageal echocardiography short-axis images of bicuspid aortic valve. The aortic orifice is fairly symmetric and opens widely without commissural fusion. There is mild leaflet thickening. AS, atrial septum; AW, anterior LV wall; AL, anterolateral papillary muscle; B, bronchus; CS, coronary sinus; E, esophagus; IVC, inferior vena cava; LAA, left atrial appendage; LVO, LV outflow; L, left coronary cusp; MPA, main pulmonary artery; N, noncoronary cusp; PM, posteromedial papillary muscle; PV, pulmonary valve; Pul V, pulmonary veins; R, right coronary cusp; RAA, right atrial appendage; RVO, RV outflow; SVC, superior vena cava; T, trachea; VS, ventricular septum.

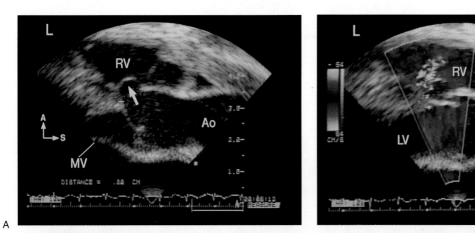

FIGURE 33.31. Aortic CUSP prolapse. A: Intraoperative transesophageal echocardiography long-axis image showing a subarterial ("supracristal") ventricular septal defect with a prolapsed aortic cusp. The defect margins are marked with +s. **B:** Color flow imaging during a systolic frame showing a left-to-right shunt through the defect. RV, right ventricle; LV, left ventricle; Ao, aorta; L, longitudinal plane; A, anterior; S, superior; MV, mitral valve.

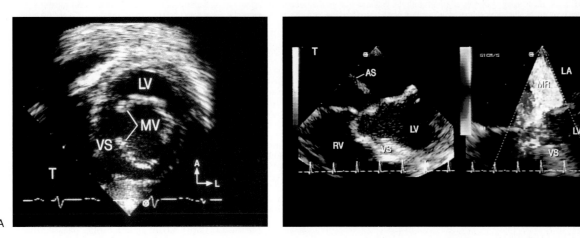

FIGURE 33.32. TEE imaging in AVSD. A: Transgastric intraoperative transesophageal echocardiography LV short-axis image showing a large cleft in the anterior mitral leaflet in a patient with an ostium primum atrial septal defect (ASD) (partial AV septal defect). **B:** Transverse (four-chamber) views of partial AV septal defect showing the ASD and both atrioventricular valves that are aligned on the same horizontal plane. The cleft in the anterior mitral leaflet results in significant regurgitation (MR) into the left atrium (LA). RV, right ventricle; LV, left ventricle; AS, atrial septum; VS, ventricular septum; s, superior; L, left.

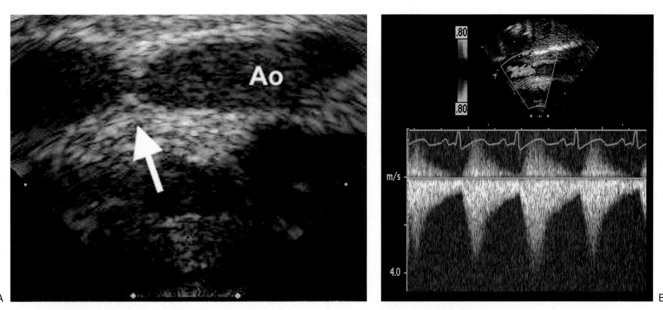

FIGURE 33.33. TEE imaging of descending aorta with ICE probe. A: Trans-esophageal echocardiography image with the intracardiac echocardiography catheter obtained in a small infant with critical discrete coarctation (*arrow*) of the aorta (Ao). **B:** Color flow imaging demonstrates aliased flow through the obstruction with a 4 m/s velocity recorded with continuous-wave Doppler.

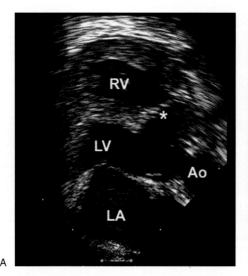
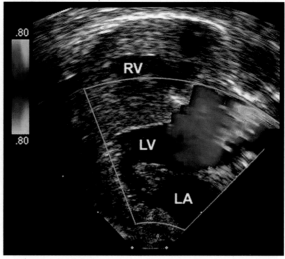

FIGURE 33.34. TEE imaging of truncus arteriosus with ICE probe. A: Transesophageal echocardiography image with the intracardiac echocardiography catheter obtained in an infant after repair of truncus arteriosus. A patch (*asterisk*) is observed closing the ventricular septal defect between the right ventricle (RV) and the left ventricle (LV). **B:** Color flow imaging demonstrated an intact patch. LA, left atrium; Ao, aorta.

SUGGESTED READING

Alboliras ET, Gotteiner NL, Berdusis K, et al. Transesophageal echocardiographic imaging for congenital lesions of the left ventricular outflow tract and the aorta. *Echocardiography.* 1996;13:439–446.

Bartel T, Konorza T, Arjumand J, et al. Intracardiac echocardiography is superior to conventional monitoring for guiding device closure of interatrial communications. *Circulation.* 2003;107:795–797.

Bezold LI, Pignatelli R, Altman CA, et al. Intraoperative transesophageal echocardiography in congenital heart surgery. The Texas Children's Hospital experience. *Tex Heart Inst J.* 1996;23:108–115.

Bruce CJ, O'Leary PW, Hagler DJ, et al. Miniaturized transesophageal echocardiography in newborn infants. *J Am Soc Echocardiogr.* 2002;15:791–797.

Bruce CJ, Nishimura RA, Rihal CS, et al. Intracardiac echocardiography in the interventional catheterization laboratory: preliminary experience with a novel, phased-array transducer. *Am J Cardiol.* 2002;89:635–640.

Bruce C, Packer D, O'Leary P, et al. Feasibility study: transesophageal echocardiography with a 10F (3.2 mm), multifrequency (5.5–10 MHz) ultrasound catheter in a small rabbit model. *J Am Soc Echocardiogr.* 1999;12:596–600.

Cabalka AK, Hagler DJ, Mookadam F, et al. Percutaneous closure of left ventricular-to-right atrial fistula after prosthetic mitral valve rereplacement using the Amplatzer duct occluder. *Catheter Cardiovasc Interv.* 2005;64:522–527.

Chu E, Fitzpatrick AP, Chin MC, et al. Radiofrequency catheter ablation guided by intracardiac echocardiography. *Circulation.* 1994;89:1301–1305.

Cyran SE, Kimball TR, Meyer RA, et al. Efficacy of intraoperative transesophageal echocardiography in children with congenital heart disease. *Am J Cardiol.* 1989;63:594.

Earing MG, Cabalka AK, Seward JB, et al. Intracardiac echocardiographic guidance during transcatheter device closure of atrial septal defect and patent foramen ovale. *Mayo Clin Proc.* 2004;79:24–34.

Fyfe DA, Kline CH. Transesophageal echocardiography for congenital heart disease. *Echocardiography.* 1991;8:573–586.

Gentles TL, Rosenfeld HM, Sanders SP, et al. Pediatric biplane transesophageal echocardiography: preliminary experience. *Am Heart J.* 1994;128:1225–1233.

Hijazi Z, Wang Z, Cao Q, et al. Transcatheter closure of atrial septal defects and patent foramen ovale under intracardiac echocardiographic guidance: feasibility and comparison with transesophageal echocardiography. *Catheter Cardiovasc Interv.* 2001;52:194–199.

Holzer R, Balzer D, Amin Z, et al. Transcatheter closure of postinfarction ventricular septal defects using the new Amplatzer muscular VSD occluder: results of a U.S. Registry. *Cathet Cardiovasc Interv.* 2004;61:196–201.

Jongbloed MRM, Schalij MJ, Zeppenfeld K, et al. Clinical applications of intracardiac echocardiography in interventional procedures. *Heart.* 2005;91:981–990.

Khositseth A, Cabalka AK, Sweeney JP, et al. Transcatheter Amplatzer device closure of atrial septal defect and patent foramen ovale in patients with presumed paradoxical embolism. *Mayo Clin Proc.* 2004;79:35–41.

Mullen MJ, Dias BF, Walker F, et al. Intracardiac echocardiography guided device closure of atrial septal defects. *J Am Coll Cardiol.* 2003;41:285–292.

O'Leary PW, Hagler DJ, Seward JB, et al. Biplane intraoperative transesophageal echocardiography in congenital heart disease. *Mayo Clin Proc.* 1995;70:317–326.

Packer DL, Stevens CL, Curley MG, et al. Intracardiac phased-array imaging: methods and initial clinical experience with high resolution, under blood visualization: initial experience with intracardiac phased-array ultrasound. *J Am Coll Cardiol.* 2002;39:509–516.

Rosenfeld HM, Gentles TL, Wernovsky G, et al. Utility of intraoperative transesophageal echocardiography in the assessment of residual cardiac defects. *Pediatr Cardiol.* 1998;19:346–351.

Sharma S, Stamper T, Dhar P, et al. The usefulness of transesophageal echocardiography in the surgical management of older children with subaortic stenosis. *Echocardiography.* 1996;13:653–661.

Stevenson JG. Incidence of complications in pediatric transesophageal echocardiography: experience in 1650 cases. *J Am Soc Echocardiogr.* 1999;12:527–532.

Stevenson JG, Sorensen GK, Gartman DM, et al. Transesophageal echocardiography during repair of congenital cardiac defects: identification of residual problems necessitating reoperation. *J Am Soc Echocardiogr.* 1993;6:356–365.

Stumper OF, Elzenga NJ, Hess J, et al. Transesophageal echocardiography in children with congenital heart disease: an initial experience. *J Am Coll Cardiol.* 1990;16:433–441.

Tardif JC. Cao QL. Schwartz SL, et al. Intracardiac echocardiography with a steerable low-frequency linear-array probe for left-sided heart imaging from the right side: experimental studies. *J Am Soc Echocardiogr.* 1995;8:132–138.

Chapter 34
Cardiac Magnetic Resonance in Congenital Heart Disease

Mark A. Fogel

To some, cardiac magnetic resonance (CMR) is a "new" and "novel" imaging technique, exotic in infants and children, with limited niche uses in congenital heart disease (CHD); this could not be further from the truth. Cardiac imaging using the principles of magnetic resonance began in earnest over 25 years ago and is now firmly established in the evaluation of anatomy, physiology, and function in patients with CHD. Its use in CHD has been limited by access to the magnetic resonance (MR) scanner, lack of appropriate training, and issues of control and personnel to operate the system. In many institutions throughout the country, these limitations are changing and CMR is growing in its popularity. The CMR volume at The Children's Hospital of Philadelphia has grown in double digits in 5 of the past 7 years; the rate of growth is currently 36%, which represents a nearly fivefold increase in the number of examinations performed over a 7-year period.

ADVANTAGES AND DISADVANTAGES OF CARDIAC MAGNETIC RESONANCE

Presently, CMR is used in conjunction with other imaging modalities; however, in a number of areas such as vascular rings, CMR has become the imaging modality of choice. For ventricular volumes and mass, it has become the gold standard even in the echocardiographic community. In addition, CMR offers several advantages over other imaging modalities, including (a) freely selectable imaging planes without limitations to "windows" (e.g., in echocardiography) or overlapping structures (e.g., in angiography), (b) lack of ionizing radiation (e.g., in computed tomography [CT]), (c) excellent soft tissue contrast, (d) a capacity for true three-dimensional imaging of both anatomy and physiology/function, (e) accurate flow quantification using phase contrast velocity mapping, (f) noninvasive labeling of the myocardium or blood (myocardial tagging), (g) assessment of myocardial viability, and (h) perfusion and coronary imaging.

Because patient size plays an important role in the ability of echocardiography to visualize structures, CMR has a distinct advantage in the older child, adolescent, and adult. In complex CHD, the overlapping of structures in angiography or the "sweeps" used in echocardiography may not be sufficient to conceptualize the entire anatomic picture. With CMR, because images can be obtained in contiguous, parallel slices, computers can stack these images one atop the other offline and slice the volumetric data set in any plane desired (called multiplanar reconstruction), yielding the salient points of the anatomy. This same ability allows a three-dimensional volume-rendered image to be created, which can itself be sectioned in any plane, viewed from any angle, and have individual structures removed to reveal the necessary information. With high-resolution three-dimensional time-resolved gadolinium angiography, temporal information is obtained and each time point can be reconstructed into a high-resolution three-dimensional image. Even "curved planes" are used clinically.

A difference between echocardiography and CMR is that for nearly all types of images, the data are obtained from multiple heartbeats, unlike echocardiography and angiography, where the imaging is instantaneous. A single CMR image can be created from two to many hundreds of heartbeats. While an echocardiographer may have to sit and view many heartbeats and average it to obtain a functional assessment of ventricular performance, the CMR image itself is an average of many heartbeats and, therefore, CMR functional analysis can give a better handle on long-term performance. However, if instantaneous imaging is needed, "real-time" as well as "interactive" CMR can be used.

There are a number of CMR capabilities that have been in use for years such as myocardial tissue tagging (Fig. 34.1), which allows calculation of regional wall strain and wall motion similar to the newer speckle tracking techniques of echocardiography. Other capabilities are unique to CMR such as viability and delayed enhancement (Fig. 34.2) which allows for identification of myocardial scar tissue as well as foreign bodies such as patches. Another unique CMR application is the T2* technique, which has the capability of quantifying the amount of myocardial iron present. This technique is useful in patients with thalassemia and sickle cell disease. More recently developed CMR capabilities include two- and three-dimensional coronary artery imaging and myocardial perfusion/stress imaging. Not surprisingly, CMR has been called the "one-stop-shop" for cardiac imaging.

These advantages are some of the many reasons for the increasing popularity of CMR for both clinical and research purposes in CHD. Continued advances in MR hardware, software, and imaging techniques are making CMR faster and even more robust. With the advent of relatively new techniques such as fast imaging with steady-state free precession (e.g., "true FISP"), "real-time" cine, and high-resolution three-dimensional time-resolved gadolinium angiography, CMR is poised to become a first-line imaging modality in a number of clinical areas in CHD.

There are limitations and challenges with CMR as with any imaging modality. Conscious sedation, similar to what may occur in echocardiography, and occasionally general anesthesia may be needed for young patients to remain motionless in the CMR scanner. In addition, cooperation by the preteen or teenager may be problematic (e.g., breath-holding). Some may also experience claustrophobia. Also, wires, stents, intravascular coils, and clips may all cause imaging artifacts if they are near the structure of interest. Although recent literature suggests that selected patients with pacemakers can safely undergo CMR, it is still not performed routinely in patients with pacemakers and implanted defibrillators. Because CMR is not portable, the critically ill infant who would need to be scanned would require transport to the CMR suite to be imaged. And, finally, patients with arrhythmias may cause difficulty for proper data acquisition including abnormalities of their electrocardiogram

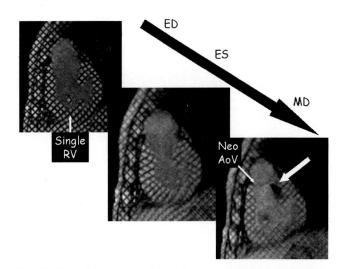

FIGURE 34.1. Myocardial tissue tagging. This technique uses spatial modulation of magnetization (SPAMM) to lay a series of black parallel lines onto the myocardium dividing the myocardium up into "cubes of magnetization." As the cardiac cycle progresses from end-diastole (ED), the deformation of the regional myocardium can be tracked and strain/wall motion can be quantified. This is an example of a patient with hypoplastic left heart syndrome after the Fontan procedure in a short-axis orientation at ED (top left), end-systole (ES) (middle), and mid-diastole (MD) (bottom right). This cine sequence can identify turbulent jets of blood by a loss of signal. In this example, the bottom right image demonstrates insufficiency from the neoaortic valve (NeoAoV). RV, right ventricle.

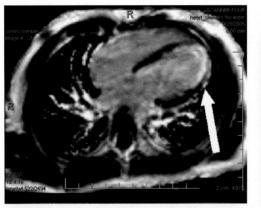
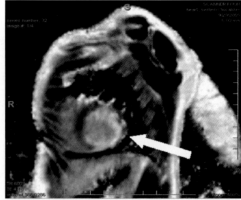
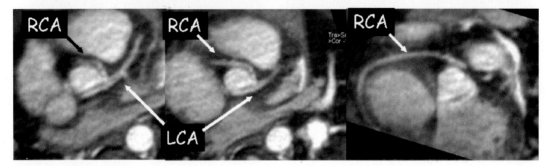

FIGURE 34.2. Viability/delayed enhancement and coronary imaging. Top: Four-chamber view (left) and ventricular short-axis view (right) in an infant post myocardial infarction. The infarcted sites are shown by a bright signal in the myocardium (*arrow*), whereas the darker areas are viable tissue. Gadolinium remains in the infarcted tissue, whereas it is washed out of viable tissue by normal coronary flow. **Bottom:** This patient has a single left coronary artery (LCA) with the right coronary artery (RCA) coursing between the aorta and the pulmonary artery. **Left and middle:** Slightly different angles of the single LCA. **Right:** Image lays out the RCA in its entire length.

(ECG) (e.g., bizarre T waves or bundle branch block), which may not allow for appropriate triggering. This is becoming less of an issue now that "real-time" CMR (images continually created without ECG triggering), "single-shot" CMR (entire image constructed in one heartbeat), "self-gating" CMR (scanner uses the motion of the heart to trigger similar to using M-mode in echocardiography), and sequences with "arrhythmia rejection" (data are ignored if extra heartbeats are detected) are realities.

CARDIAC MAGNETIC RESONANCE AS AN IMAGING MODALITY

The Physics of Cardiac Magnetic Resonance

Although the detailed physics of MR image generation is beyond the scope of this text, a simplistic, broad-based general concept is appropriate.

A powerful magnet is used to align the spins of a tiny percentage of the hydrogen atoms in the body. A radiofrequency pulse (electromagnetic energy) combined with a special magnetic field creates a magnetic "gradient" that is used to perturb a small percentage of these molecules in a specific part of the body into a higher energy state. The alignment of the protons is said to have "flipped" by a certain angle relative to their resting state of alignment in the magnetic field. This magnetic gradient relative to position in space enables the localization of specific pieces of tissue—that is, the amount of "flip" of the proton is proportional to the magnetic field strength along the gradient. When the radiofrequency pulse is turned off, the hydrogen atoms return to their normal state, releasing energy in the process. This energy is then collected by the scanner and is analyzed by a complex series of mathematical computations to yield at least one (sometimes multiple) line(s) of imaging data. An image is divided into a checkerboard (matrix), with each box called a pixel, and rows of pixels forming each line. Generally, between 64 and 512 lines of data make up an image. Depending on the type of CMR being performed, this process is repeated numerous times over the course of many heartbeats to create the image. The time from one repetition to the next repetition of this sequence of events is called the repetition time (TR), and the time from the initial radiofrequency pulse to the time the scanner "listens" for the release of energy as the protons return to their resting state is called the echo time (TE). At different line acquisitions of the image, the "phase" of the incoming signal is changed slightly—the phase is where a certain part of the signal is located at a given period of time. Changing the phase of each signal gives positional information to allow for a full two-dimensional image to be created. In broad terms, the magnetic gradient determines where the signal is coming from on the x-axis of the image and the altered phase of each signal determines where that signal is coming from on the y-axis of the image. To allow for "noise" in the system (false data) as well as to alleviate artifacts from breathing, each line can be obtained two or three times and averaged (with breath-holding techniques, this is typically not necessary). To image the heart, the scanner generally uses the ECG (or pulse recording) to determine at what part of the cardiac cycle to obtain the image. Generally, static images are obtained in mid or late diastole, whereas cine imaging occurs throughout the cardiac cycle.

CMR differentiates tissue by its magnetic properties based on the above imaging approach. The release of energy occurs when the protons relax to their resting state. The two essential ways that this relaxation occurs is T1 relaxation, also called longitudinal, vertical, or spin-lattice relaxation, and T2 relaxation, also called horizontal, transverse, or spin-spin relaxation. Different types of CMR imaging take advantage of one or both of these properties. In addition, the hydrogen/proton density and the motion/flow properties of the tissue (if any) are also important factors in differentiating tissue by CMR. Different types of images are generated by changing the magnetic gradients, timing the radiofrequency pulses differently, and altering their magnitude.

Cardiac Magnetic Resonance for Anatomy

There are many types of CMR in clinical use. To define anatomy, double inversion (DI) dark blood T1-weighted CMR yields high-resolution images of myocardial tissue and blood vessel walls where the

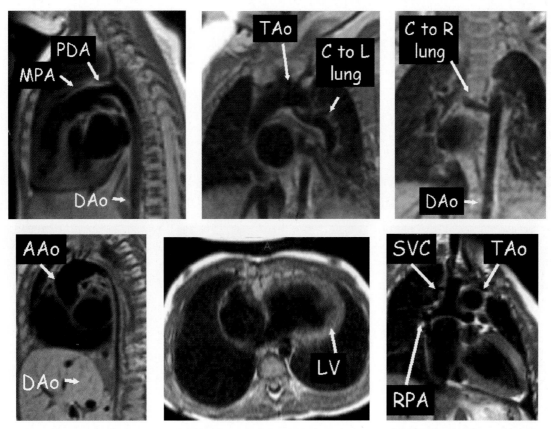

FIGURE 34.3. Examples of dark blood imaging. Top left: Patent ductus arteriosus (PDA) in a 3-week-old infant, **Top middle** and **right**: A 3-month-old with tetralogy of Fallot with pulmonary atresia. A collateral (C) off the underside of the transverse aortic arch (TAo) going to the left (L) lung (**top middle**) and an additional collateral coming off the descending aorta (DAo) going to the right (R) lung (**top right**) are clearly visualized. **Bottom left:** Diffuse DAo hypoplasia in a 2-year-old with William syndrome. **Bottom middle:** A 1-year-old with tricuspid atresia who has undergone a hemi-Fontan procedure. **Bottom right:** Ventricular long-axis view of the atretic tricuspid valve and the left ventricle (LV). Superior vena cava (SVC)–to–right pulmonary artery (RPA) anastomosis. AAo, ascending aorta; MPA, main pulmonary artery.

blood remains signal poor and dark (Fig. 34.3). Another technique called half-Fourier acquisition single-shot turbo spin echo (HASTE) can also be used to quickly acquire dark blood images, albeit at a lower resolution than the DI dark blood images; for many applications, however, this may be all that is needed. Steady state free precession (SSFP) imaging also yields high-resolution images of myocardial tissue and blood vessels; however, the blood is bright and imaging is dependent on the contrast between the high signal of the blood and the decreased signal from tissue. This type of imaging is currently the state of the art (Fig. 34.4). To delineate valve morphology, cine CMR (see later) and dark blood CMR can be used by obtaining a cross-sectional plane at the level of the valve annulus.

For anatomy, CMR also uses contrast enhanced imaging with a gadolinium-based agent. This agent is an element with seven unpaired electrons in its outer shell and is paramagnetic. It is toxic in its native form and must be bound to a chelator such as diethylenetriamine penta-acetic acid (DPTA) to be used. This chelation increases renal excretion of gadolinium by a factor of approximately 500 relative to prechelation. The half-life is approximately 1.5 hours. Gadolinium works by increasing the relaxation of the surrounding protons in a dose-dependent fashion. It decreases the T1 relaxation constant and therefore increases the signal of the surrounding tissue (i.e., it reduces the T1 relaxation rate of blood from 1200 ms to 100 ms). Once gadolinium is injected into the cardiovascular system, the target structure (e.g., aorta) takes up the agent, whereas the background tissue does not. One way to perform this type of CMR is to inject the gadolinium while using a "real-time" sequence to monitor the course of the circulating gadolinium (called bolus tracking). Once the agent arrives at the target structure, a T1-weighted, generally short TR and moderately short TE three-dimensional sequence is used to obtain a three-dimensional image of the cardiovascular system.

These images can then be formatted as multiple two-dimensional images, as a maximum intensity projection (MIP), or as a volume-rendered object (Fig. 34.5). This type of imaging may be used, for example, to localize collateral vessels off of the aorta in a patient with tetralogy of Fallot with pulmonary atresia. Another way to perform this type of imaging is to use advanced hardware and software to obtain a series of three-dimensional high-resolution images extremely quickly and follow the gadolinium as it traverses the cardiovascular system (similar to the bolus tracking technique). With this "time-resolved three-dimensional gadolinium" technique, each phase can be made into a high-resolution three-dimensional volume-rendered display with temporal information incorporated into the sequence as well (Fig. 34.6).

Coronary imaging by CMR has been attempted since the 1980s and has had wide clinical use since the mid-1990s (Fig. 34.2). Presently, coronary imaging is performed as a free breathing technique using a "navigator" that monitors diaphragmatic motion, similar to performing an M-mode across the diaphragm. For some patients, breath-hold imaging can be done and is often more time efficient. CMR imaging of the coronary arteries relies on minimizing the motion of these arteries (both cardiac and respiratory motion) by acquiring all of the CMR data for the image at the same point in the respiratory cycle (typically expiration) and cardiac cycle (typically mid to late-diastole). Imaging in mid-late diastole also is advantageous in that this is the part of the cardiac cycle in which the coronary arteries contain the most blood. To optimize the image, destroying the signal from fat (fat saturation) and using a T2 preparation to help destroy spins of the myocardium are also techniques that are used. Recently, "whole heart" T2 preparation coronary imaging has been developed, which allows the creation of a three-dimensional image of the heart and coronary arteries similar to CT scans.

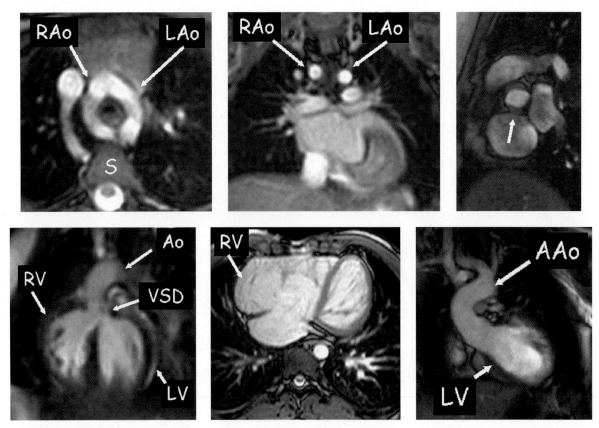

FIGURE 34.4. Steady state free precession (SSFP) bright blood imaging and gradient echo imaging. Top left and **top middle:** Bright blood static images from a 6-month-old infant with a double aortic arch in the axial (left) and coronal (middle) planes. The right (RAo) and left (LAo) aortic arches can clearly be seen. **Top right:** Spoiled gradient echo cine image from a 6-month-old with coarctation of the aorta and a bicuspid aortic valve (*arrow*). **Bottom left:** Bright blood cine image from a 4.6-kg 10-day-old neonate with tetralogy of Fallot, which highlights the ventricular septal defect (VSD) and the overriding aorta. **Bottom middle:** Static bright blood image from a 4-year-old with tetralogy of Fallot after transannular patch repair demonstrating significant right ventricular (RV) enlargement. **Bottom right:** Cine image of the left ventricular outflow tract of the patient with tricuspid atresia from Figure 34.2. Ao, aorta; AAo, ascending aorta; LV, left ventricle; S, spine.

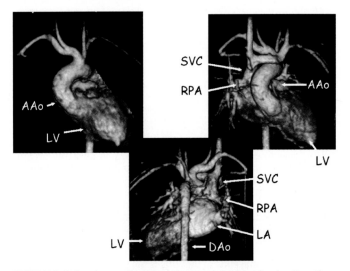

FIGURE 34.5. Static volume-rendered three-dimensional gadolinium imaging. These three-dimensional images are from a 1-year-old child with tricuspid atresia who has undergone a hemi-Fontan procedure. **Top left:** Left ventricular outflow tract from an anterior view without the venous phase. **Top right:** Venous phase from an anterior view where the superior vena cava (SVC)–to–right pulmonary artery (RPA) anastomosis can be clearly seen. **Bottom:** Resultant image if this scan is rotated to a posterior orientation, where the hemi-Fontan connection is clearly seen along with the left atrium (LA). AAo, ascending aorta; LV, left ventricle; DAo, descending aorta.

Cardiac Magnetic Resonance for Physiology and Function

Besides evaluating anatomy and morphology, one of the more powerful applications of CMR is in the assessment of cardiovascular physiology and function by the use of cine (Fig. 34.7). In this technique, the protons are flipped quickly but not to the same degree as when performing anatomic imaging. Multiple lines of imaging data are obtained at multiple phases of the cardiac cycle in a given plane, allowing the visualization of both cardiac motion and flowing blood. In this type of imaging, CMR produces a high signal from the blood and a lower-amplitude signal from the tissue. Calculation of cardiac index, ventricular volume and mass, regional wall motion, and blood flow is visualized in this manner. If turbulence is present, cine CMR will demonstrate a signal void in the region (Fig. 34.1). This is used to detect valvular regurgitation, stenosis, or blood vessel stenosis. Cine MR is generally of two types. The older form is termed spoiled gradient echo (SGE), where the signal of blood is high and that of tissue is lower. The more recent commonly used type is SSFP), where blood is exceptionally bright and there is a very high contrast between blood and tissue signals. SSFP is a much faster sequence and has elements of both T1- and T2-weighting. It is used when performing "real-time" cine or when using "interactive real-time" to allow "sweeps" to be performed interactively in real-time.

The MRI signal that is generated typically contains both amplitude and phase information. Phase-encoded velocity mapping (Fig. 34.8) encodes velocity data in a special sequence that can be used

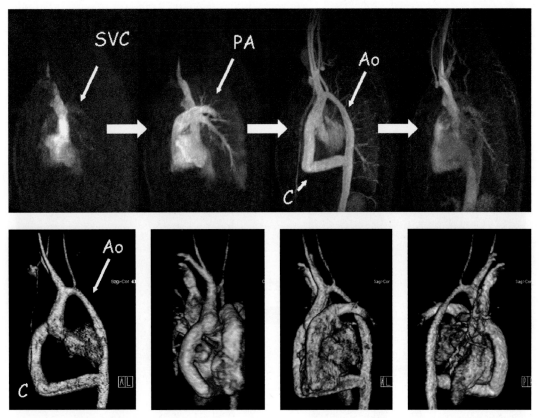

FIGURE 34.6. Time-resolved three-dimensional gadolinium imaging. Top: Four phases of flow after a gadolinium injection in this sagittal view of a patient with an ascending-to-descending aortic conduit (C) for coarctation of the aorta. As the panels progress (**left** to **right**), the flow of gadolinium is seen to flow from the right superior vena cava (SVC) and right atrium (**left**) to the pulmonary arteries (PA) (**second from left**) to the aorta (Ao) and conduit (**second from right**) and then back to the superior vena cava (**right**). **Bottom:** Volume-rendered images obtained from this series of images. **Left:** Aorta, coarctation, and conduit in a sagittal view. If the pulmonary phase and the arterial phase are combined, a volume-rendered image of the entire heart is created as in the **right three** panels (**third from right**, anterior view; **second from right**, sagittal view looking from the left; **right**, off-axis sagittal view looking from the right). The course of the conduit and its relationship to various structures are clearly seen. Ao, aorta; C, conduit.

to determine the velocity of blood (or tissue) as well as the flow to any organ (such as cardiac output or relative flow to each lung). A magnetic gradient is applied along with a radiofrequency pulse followed by a second radiofrequency of equal amplitude but in the opposite direction. Protons of the stationary tissue are flipped by the first radiofrequency pulse and then flipped back immediately to their resting state by the second opposite pulse because they have not changed position. However, protons of moving tissue, such as blood, are flipped a certain amount during the initial radiofrequency pulse but are flipped back a different amount during the second equal and opposite radiofrequency pulse; since they have moved and are not at the same part of the magnetic gradient, the amount of "flip" of the proton is proportional to the magnetic field strength along the gradient. In this way, moving tissue is labeled by the phase change of these protons along the magnetic gradient. By knowing how the magnetic gradient changes with the position and timing of the radiofrequency pulses, corresponding velocity can be measured.

Phase contrast velocity maps come in two forms: (a) *through plane* velocity mapping, where velocity is encoded into and out of the plane of the image, and (b) *in-plane* velocity mapping, where velocity is encoded in the plane of the image (similar to Doppler echocardiography). The advantage of through plane velocity mapping is that if a blood vessel is imaged in cross section, all of the pixels that encode for velocity in the blood vessel can be summed over the entire cross-sectional area of the vessel integrated over the entire cardiac cycle. This can therefore be used to obtain flow (as in liters per minute, not just velocity). Directionality of flow is coded as a positive signal in one direction (bright on the image) and a negative signal in the other direction (dark on the image). For example, cardiac index can be obtained by performing phase-encoded velocity mapping across the aortic valve. A pulmonary-to-systemic flow ratio (Qp/Qs) in a patient with an atrial septal defect

can be obtained by comparing this value with the phase-encoded velocity mapping of the pulmonary artery. The regurgitant fraction of the aortic valve is easily calculated by CMR by dividing the reverse flow by the forward flow and multiplying by 100 (Fig. 34.8). In addition, because the aortic valve is obtained in cross section to obtain flow across it, an added advantage of this technique is that valve morphology is easily seen (Fig. 34.8).

Because of the quantitative nature of CMR, internal consistencies of the data can be easily evaluated. For example, cardiac index is measured from both the aorta and pulmonary artery and, in the absence of any intracardiac shunt, these values should be similar (within 10% of each other). Flow in the right and left pulmonary arteries should equal flow in the main pulmonary artery. Similarly, in the absence of atrioventricular valve insufficiency, the stroke volume of the left ventricle by cine CMR should equal the forward flow in the aorta by phase-encoded velocity mapping. This approach ensures data integrity and is one of the unique features of CMR.

Myocardial tissue tagging (Fig. 34.1) is a CMR technique used to assess ventricular function. This methodology "magnetically labels" the walls of the myocardium and divides it into "cubes of magnetization." This can be tracked to demonstrate myocardial deformation. This technique is similar to speckle tracking in echocardiography and allows for the calculation of regional wall strain, wall motion, and torsion. A set of radiofrequency pulses are used to destroy the spins of the protons in parallel lines, resulting in dark bands on the image. This can be done in a "grid" pattern or as a series of one set of parallel lines using a CMR technique termed spatial modulation of magnetization (SPAMM). Finally, blood tagging is similar to tissue tagging except that blood is labeled, allowing for visualization of velocity profiles. This labeling can be by bolus tagging, where only a thin stripe is laid down on the blood vessel to label it, or this technique can use a large stripe that is laid down on the blood to detect shunt flow.

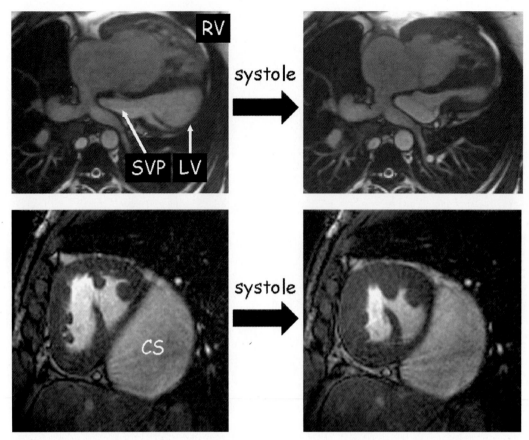

FIGURE 34.7. Cine cardiac magnetic resonance (CMR). Left: End-diastolic images. **Right:** Images in mid systole. **Top:** Patient with transposition of the great arteries who underwent a Senning procedure. **Bottom:** Single-ventricle patient who has a severely dilated coronary sinus (CS) that is connected to the systemic venous pathway (SVP). LV, left ventricle; RV, right ventricle.

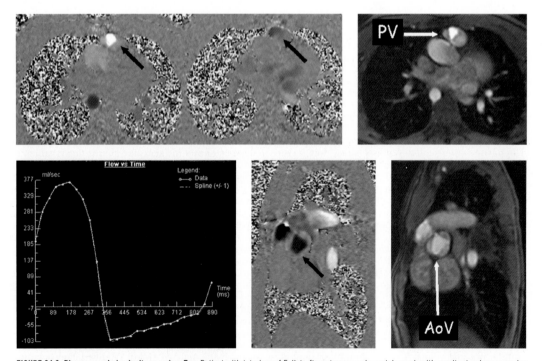

FIGURE 34.8. Phase-encoded velocity mapping. Top: Patient with tetralogy of Fallot after a transannular patch repair with resultant pulmonary valve (PV) insufficiency. **Right:** Anatomic image of the pulmonary valve in cross section. Through-plane phase-encoded velocity mapping is used to quantify flow (see text) and direction is encoded as dark or bright. **Left:** Phase map at mid-systole. The signal is bright (*arrow*) across the pulmonary valve, demonstrating antegrade flow. **Middle:** Captured in early diastole and black across the pulmonary valve, demonstrating retrograde flow (*arrow*). **Bottom left:** Flow-time curve generated from this PV velocity map. **Bottom middle** and **right:** Phase-encoded velocity map and anatomic image, respectively, demonstrate a cross section of the trileaflet aortic valve (AoV) of the same patient with tetralogy of Fallot (*arrow*).

Cardiac Magnetic Resonance for Tissue Characterization

Regional myocardial perfusion and viability (Fig. 34.2) have come into routine clinical use in CMR. By using gadolinium enhancement, CMR assesses regional wall perfusion via a "first-pass" technique. Typically, short-axis views of the ventricle are obtained and the CMR sequence is set up such that the heart is imaged relatively motionless. Gadolinium is injected intravenously while the CMR scanner continuously images the ventricle (up to four or five short-axis slices may be imaged at once). The gadolinium bolus is followed from right ventricular (RV) cavity to left ventricular cavity and eventually to the ventricular myocardium. Defects in perfusion show up as dark portions of the myocardium while the remainder of the ventricle is signal intense. Images are obtained prior to administration of a pharmacologic agent as well as in conjunction with a coronary vasodilator, such as adenosine, which is administered as an infusion of 140 µg/kg per minute over 4 to 6 minutes. Along with viability imaging, the CMR data can be accurately interpreted as being characteristic of ischemic tissue, infarcted tissue, or artifact. In addition, lung perfusion can also be assessed qualitatively using time-resolved gadolinium techniques.

Infarcted myocardium can be identified by a contrast-enhanced technique called viability or delayed enhancement (Fig. 34.2). Gadolinium is avidly taken up by scarred myocardium and remains in scarred tissue for an extended period of time, whereas it is "washed" out by coronary blood flow in normally perfused myocardium. In this way, the signal intensity-time curves of both infarcted myocardium and perfused myocardial tissue separate, with the infarcted myocardium's gadolinium curve remaining highly signal intense after 5 to 10 minutes, whereas normal myocardium becomes much less so. The contrast between normal and infarcted myocardium can be of the order of 500%. This technique has been demonstrated to accurately delineate the presence, extent, and location of both acute and chronic myocardial infarction. Foreign bodies such as ventricular septal defect patches or RV outflow tract (RVOT) patches after tetralogy of Fallot repair have also been shown to become signal intense with this technique. In addition, various cardiac tumors can take up gadolinium, whereas others will not, and CMR uses this tissue property, along with T1-weighted images, T2-weighted images, and fat saturation to predict the type of tumor that is present.

The measurement of T2* in the relaxation process of the protons can be used to assess the amount of myocardial iron present in the tissue. By obtaining multiple images at various TEs using a gradient echo sequence, the myocardium and liver can be seen to become increasingly dark with longer TEs. Because iron is ferromagnetic, it changes the magnetic properties of the myocardium. Increasing iron concentration decreases the measured T2* and makes the myocardium even darker. Values below 20 ms are at risk for poor ventricular function; therefore, chelation therapy in cases of thalassemia and sickle cell disease can be modified based on CMR data.

GENERALIZED PROTOCOL OF CARDIAC MAGNETIC RESONANCE FOR CONGENITAL HEART DISEASE

The following, in the author's opinion, is the most efficient and complete way to accomplish the CMR examination. As in echocardiography, the CMR protocol needs to be individualized to the patient and the disease process. It is important to initially delineate cardiac anatomy since physiologic and functional data must be interpreted in this context.

Anatomic Imaging

After localizers, anatomic data are acquired. The purpose of this sequence is not only to survey cardiovascular anatomy and enable an "anatomic diagnosis" but also to act as a localizer for subsequent physiologic and functional imaging. A full contiguous set of axial images from the diaphragm to the thoracic inlet is obtained (typically 40 to 50 images). The author prefers "static" SSFP images (e.g., true-FISP) (Fig. 34.4) in which the images are acquired in diastole. This must be extended outside the thorax for evaluation of congenital heart lesions such as infracardiac total anomalous pulmonary venous connections. Imaging that uses SSFP depends on contrast between the blood pool and the surrounding tissue. Therefore, the highest flip angle possible should be used. Generally, the axial images in this stack are "averaged," allowing breath-holding to be reserved for later imaging. These axial images form the anatomic basis of the cardiac anatomy.

One disadvantage to using "static" SSFP is that diastolic turbulence will be manifested as signal loss on the image and may be misinterpreted as the absence of a structure. In the case of a systemic–to–pulmonary artery shunt (e.g., Blalock-Taussing shunt) after a Norwood Stage I reconstruction, the pulmonary arteries are very difficult to visualize. This limitation can be compensated for by performing an axial stack of HASTE images, which yields a rapid set of dark blood images. This can be performed while multiplanar reconstruction (MPR) is being done (see later) so that no time is lost during the examination. Alternatively, a set of axial cine images can be used to visualize these structures in the hope that a phase of the cardiac cycle will demonstrate the "missing" structure. With the advent of "T2-prepared SSFP," institutions have begun using this technique instead to obtain "whole-heart" three-dimensional imaging. This can not only be used to survey the cardiac anatomy and be used as a localizer for subsequent imaging but can also be used to create a three-dimensional volume-rendered image without the use of contrast agents.

MPR is a reformatting technique whereby a set of contiguous images (e.g., axial) are stacked together, enabling any plane to be reconstructed by computer. Cardiac anatomy can then be inspected from multiple orientations from a single set of axial images. Not only can any double oblique imaging plane be reconstructed, but a "curved" imaging plane can be created to demonstrate salient anatomic features in one plane. MPR can be used with any type of imaging (e.g., SSFP or HASTE). By using MPR, if the scan is terminated prematurely because of patient instability or technical issues, the important points of the anatomy can still be reconstructed offline if a single set of axial images has already been obtained.

Next, a set of high-resolution double-inversion recovery dark blood images can be obtained to examine regions of interest (e.g., candy cane view of the aorta in the case of coarctation) after being delineated via MPR (Fig. 34.3). This type of imaging is used judiciously since it requires relatively long scanning times. If there are time constraints, this part of the CMR examination can be omitted with cine imaging performed instead to delineate the region of interest. However, if turbulence degrades the area of interest, then double-inversion dark blood imaging should be done. For evaluation of arrhythmogenic RV dysplasia (ARVD), visualization of the pericardium, or to perform tumor characterization, the additional time investment to obtain these dark blood images is an important component to the examination. It may be combined with "fat saturation" or contrast enhancement to evaluate, for example, what type of tumor is present (e.g., a lipoma is suggested if the structure is signal intense without a fat saturation but is signal poor with fat saturation).

Cine CMR (Fig. 34.7) and phase-contrast velocity mapping (PC-MR) (Fig. 34.8) are also included in anatomic imaging because both can be used to determine the morphology of cardiac valves. To determine whether an aortic valve is bicuspid or trileaflet, both SSF and gradient echo (GRE) cine may be used. The author prefers GRE with a high flip angle (e.g., 25 degrees) that allows blood flowing into the imaging plane to be highly signal intense and outlines the valve leaflets optimally (Fig. 34.8). This is also how PC-MR is used to determine valve morphology. For example, to visualize a bicuspid aortic valve, the most common CHD, an en face view of the valve, is performed by lining up the imaging plane perpendicular to the left ventricular outflow tract in two orthogonal views (obtained by MPR, double-inversion dark blood or cine) at the level of the aortic valve. This typically results in the equivalent of a "parasternal short-axis view" by echocardiography and the anatomy is delineated similarly (Fig. 34.8).

Physiologic and Functional Imaging

Cine Cardiac Magnetic Resonance – Cine CMR is one of the workhorses of physiologic and functional imaging in CHD (either SSFP or GRE sequences) and is tailored to the cardiac lesion (Fig. 34.7). These bright blood techniques visualize both the motion of the heart and the flow of blood and can be used to detect turbulence in vessels (e.g., coarctation of the aorta) or at the valve level (e.g., aortic stenosis or insufficiency).

Cine CMR is used in two basic ways:

1. *To image the physiologic consequences of abnormal cardiac anatomy.* If branch pulmonary artery stenosis is visualized on dark blood imaging or MPR of the contiguous axial images, turbulence should be noted on cine imaging. If there is prolapse of the mitral valve, a loss of signal should be seen originating from the valve. A stack of cines can be obtained to localize these jets, while off-axis images can be set up from this stack to optimally profile the jet. Similar to echocardiography, caution must be used when using this signal void to grade the degree of stenosis or insufficiency as it must be viewed in the context of CMR physics from which the image was created (e.g., frame rate, angle of incidence, etc.). The size of the signal void is a function of a number of factors such as the TE, where longer TEs increase the size of the signal void and shorter TEs decrease its size. In addition, the size of the signal void is also a function of the direction of the stenotic jet relative to the orientation of the image voxel. Finally, SSFP imaging may underestimate the signal void seen on gradient echo sequences.

2. *To directly assess function.* To determine left ventricular volume overload in a patient with ventricular septal defect, a stack of contiguous left ventricular short-axis images are acquired (typically 8 to 12 slices). This allows for measurement of left ventricular volumes, mass, ejection fraction, stroke volume, and cardiac index. CMR techniques are now in place to perform an entire volume set in one breath-hold. Even in children who cannot hold their breath, a full volume data set rarely takes longer than 5 minutes to acquire. This method does not rely on any geometric assumptions, which is advantageous because of the bizarre ventricular shapes found in CHD. Cines at all slice levels are obtained at the same temporal resolution (typically 20 to 35 phases in the cardiac cycle, depending on the heart rate), and the data are sorted by time. The results are multiple full-volume data sets at, for example, 20-ms time intervals. *Ventricular volume* at a given time (usually end-diastole and end-systole) is obtained by tracing the endocardial borders on all images at that specific time, planimeterizing the areas, multiplying by the slice thickness, and then summing. *Ventricular mass* is obtained by tracing the epicardial borders on all images, planimeterizing the areas, multiplying by the slice thickness, summing, and then subtracting the ventricular volume. *Stroke volume* is simply the ventricular volume at end-diastole minus the ventricular volume at end-systole. Once this is known, *ejection fraction* is calculated in the usual fashion. *Cardiac index* is simply the stroke volume multiplied by heart rate divided by body surface area. A Qp/Qs and *semilunar valve regurgitant fraction* may also be calculated by obtaining the differences in stroke volumes between right and left ventricles.

Phase Contrast Velocity Mapping

Phase Contrast Velocity Mapping – After cine imaging, blood flow data are obtained. Similar to cine CMR, PC-MRI is tailored to the cardiac lesion (Fig. 34.8). Directionality of blood flow is encoded as "bright" in one direction (signal intense) and "dark" in another direction (signal poor) although many vendors now offer color coding similar to echocardiographic color flow mapping. There are two different ways to use the ECG to obtain blood flow information:

1. The state of the art is "retrospectively" acquired images where the CMR scanner continuously acquires data along with recording the ECG and then "retrospectively" fits the imaging data into the proper points in the ECG. Retrospectively gated images allow for flow during the entire cardiac cycle to be measured.

2. "Prospectively" triggered images where the scanner uses the ECG to begin its acquisition of data for each heart beat and must leave some "dead space" prior to the next acquisition (e.g., the next R wave).

There are also two ways to obtain flow images relative to flow in the body:

1. *Through-plane PC-MRI* measures velocity and flow into and out of the imaging plane and is the most useful type of velocity mapping since "flow" can be measured. If the imaging plane is perpendicular to the direction of blood flow (e.g., obtaining a cross-sectional area of the vessel such as the branch pulmonary arteries), summing all velocities in each pixel in a given cross section of blood vessel, and multiplying by the area of each pixel will yield flow at that given period of time. Summing the flow in all phases of the cardiac cycle will yield the stroke volume across that cross-sectional area of the vessel. The product of this stroke volume with the heart rate will yield the cardiac output across this blood vessel. Most software on present day CMR scanners have a temporal resolution of approximately 20 ms, and if the examiner is willing to invest the time, this software can yield a temporal resolution well below that. For example, in the patient with pulmonary insufficiency, a velocity map across the pulmonary valve is used to measure the regurgitant fraction and can confirm the cardiac index measured by cine CMR. The regurgitant fraction is simply the area under the curve of the reverse flow minus the area under the curve of the forward flow in a flow-time curve multiplied by 100. Care should be taken to place the imaging plane as close to the valve as possible as erroneous results can be obtained otherwise. In a patient with an atrial septal defect, through-plane velocity mapping can measure the Qp/Qs by placing velocity maps across the aortic and pulmonary valves. Measurements of Qp/Qs by velocity mapping have been validated against oximetry.

2. *In-plane velocity mapping* (Fig. 34.9 and 34.10) encodes flow in the plane of the image similar to that done in echocardiography. Velocities can be encoded along either axis of the image and can be directed in any direction (e.g., superoinferior dimension in the case of a coarctation). This type of imaging is useful in visualizing flow across an atrial septal defect along with its direction. In addition, this type of imaging can be used to aid in determining maximum velocities across a stenotic region (e.g., aortic stenosis).

Velocity mapping can be used in conjunction with cine CMR to calculate additional important parameters of ventricular performance. For example, patients who have undergone repair of a complete atrioventricular canal defect can have significant left atrioventricular valve insufficiency as a sequelae. To assess this quantitatively, the stroke volume of the left ventricle minus the forward flow across the aortic valve would be equal to the absolute regurgitant flow across the left atrioventricular valve. If this regurgitant flow is divided by the stroke volume of the left ventricle and then multiplied by 100, the left atrioventricular valve regurgitant fraction can be obtained.

Gadolinium-Based Anatomic CMR

Gadolinium-Based Anatomic CMR – Contrast enhancement based on gadolinium can be used to determine detailed cardiac anatomy and physiology (Figs. 34.5, 34.6, and 34.11). Gadolinium is an extracellular paramagnetic chemical that changes the magnetic property of the tissue or vessel in which it is in. Specifically, it markedly decreases T1 relaxation and uses this property to distinguish the target structure (e.g., the aorta) from background (e.g., other mediastinal structures). It is considered a highly safe substance with adverse events occurring in 1 in 200,000 to 400,000 uses.

Generally, this component of the CMR examination is performed after cine-CMR imaging but before PC-MRI. Because 5 to 10 minutes need to elapse after gadolinium administration before delayed enhancement imaging can be performed, the time after gadolinium administration is used to perform PC-MRI. There are four types of gadolinium techniques commonly used:

1. *Static three-dimensional imaging* is used to create a three-dimensional image of the cardiovascular system, which can then be rotated and cut in any desired image plane (Figs. 34.5 and 34.11). This sequence can be viewed in its raw data format, as an MIP, or as a volume-rendered object. Multiple three-dimensional data sets can be acquired to separate out the systemic and pulmonary circulations or simply to enhance the probability of successful imaging. This imaging sequence can be used to visualize smaller vessels much better than other techniques (e.g., to "label" the collaterals from the aorta in pulmonary atresia/intact ventricular septum). This CMR technique is generally performed in either of two ways:

   • *Bolus tracking*: The target structure (e.g., the aorta in the case of a coarctation) is imaged in real-time and gadolinium is injected. Once the contrast agent arrives at the target structure, the three-dimensional image is obtained.

   • *Timing bolus*: A small amount of contrast agent is injected and timed to determine when it will arrive at the target

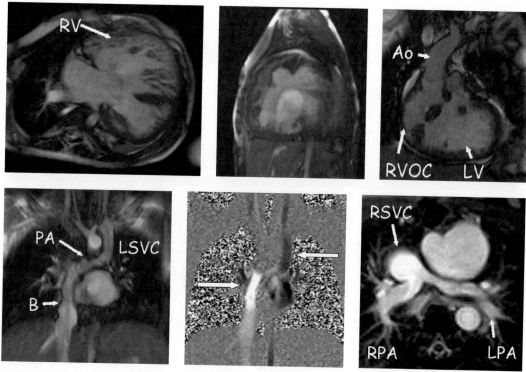

FIGURE 34.9. Cardiac magnetic resonance (CMR) of single ventricle. Top left and **middle:** Four-chamber and short-axis views, respectively, in a patient with a right ventricular (RV)-dominant unbalanced atrioventricular canal defect. **Middle:** Note that the common atrioventricular valve can be seen en face. **Top right:** Off-axis coronal image of a patient with congenitally corrected transposition of the great arteries with a right ventricular outflow chamber (RVOC) and aorta (Ao) arising from it. Note how the entire cardiac output must traverse two small ventricular septal defects connecting the RVOC and the left ventricle (LV). **Bottom left** and **middle:** Anatomic and "in-plane" phase-encoded velocity map of a patient post Fontan palliation with a left superior vena cava (LSVC) and an absent right superior vena cava. The Fontan baffle (B) connects the inferior vena cava to the right pulmonary artery (PA). The LSVC is connected to the left pulmonary artery. In the "in-plane" phase encoded velocity map, bright signal encodes the blood flow toward the head, while black encodes blood flow toward the feet (*arrows*). **Right bottom:** Off-axis axial SSFP image of the right superior vena cava–to–right pulmonary artery (RPA) connection. LPA, left pulmonary artery.

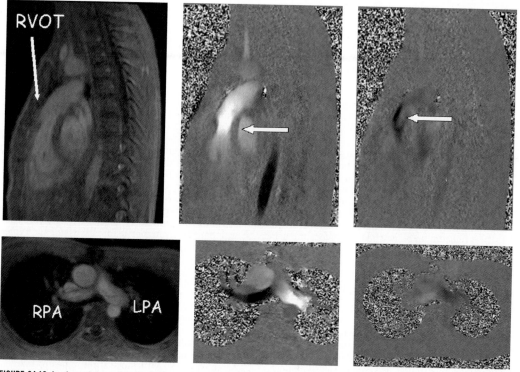

FIGURE 34.10. In-plane phase-encoded velocity mapping in a patient with tetralogy of Fallot after a transannular patch repair with pulmonary insufficiency. Top: Right ventricular outflow tract. **Bottom:** Pulmonary arteries in the bifurcation view. **Left:** Anatomic images. **Top middle** and **right:** Antegrade (bright signal encodes flow toward the head) flow in systole and retrograde (dark signal encodes flow toward the feet) flow in diastole through the pulmonary valve (*arrows*). **Bottom middle** (systole) and **right** (diastole) images demonstrate antegrade (bright signal encodes flow to the left) and retrograde (dark signal encodes flow to the right) in the branch pulmonary arteries.

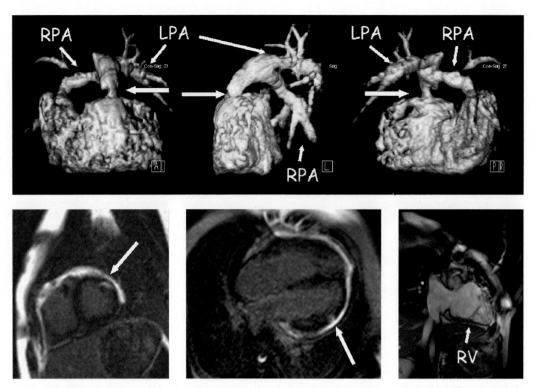

FIGURE 34.11. Cardiac magnetic resonance (CMR) imaging in tetralogy of Fallot: three-dimensional imaging, viability, and cine. Top: Volume-rendered three-dimensional gadolinium images of a patient after a transannular patch repair of tetralogy of Fallot with residual pulmonary valve obstruction (*arrows*). The right (RPA) and left pulmonary arteries (LPA) demonstrate varying degrees of hypoplasia. **Top left:** Anterior view. **Top middle:** Sagittal view. **Top right:** Posterior view. This patient was also found to have a left ventricular free wall myocardial scar (*arrow*) demonstrated by the bright signal in an otherwise dark myocardium in the four-chamber (**bottom left**) and short-axis views (**bottom middle**). Note the right ventricular (RV) volume overload. **Bottom right:** RV long-axis view by cine that also demonstrates RV volume overload

organ. The injection of the full dose of gadolinium is then performed followed by the three-dimensional sequence with a delay placed based on the small amount of contrast agent initially given.

2. *Time-resolved three-dimensional gadolinium imaging* is similar to the static version mentioned earlier; however, multiple three-dimensional data sets are obtained in an extremely short period of time (subsecond) and the bolus of gadolinium is followed through the cardiovascular system (Fig. 34.6). This sequence can be used to image cardiovascular physiology (to demonstrate shunt flow or small connections) as well as in determining lung perfusion (e.g., regions of lung with higher flows will be much brighter than regions of lung with low flow or no flow such as with a pulmonary embolism). In the past, time-resolved gadolinium had a low spatial resolution as a tradeoff to obtain improved temporal resolution. With the advent of newer and faster hardware and software, the spatial resolution of this technique can be on par with the static version. If both static and time-resolved imaging is performed in the same patient, they should be separated in time (approximately 15 to 20 minutes) to allow for the gadolinium of the first injection to be washed out before the second injection.

3. *Delayed enhancement (DE) imaging* (i.e., "viability") (Fig. 34.2). In simplistic terms, scar tissue preferentially accumulates gadolinium for a longer period of time than viable myocardium, where it is "washed out" quickly by coronary perfusion. DE takes advantage of the contrast between the gadolinium laden scar tissue and the gadolinium poor viable myocardium to "label" the scar tissue. In other words, the signal intensity-time curves separate, with the signal intensity curve of infarcted myocardium remaining highly signal intense after 5 to 10 minutes, whereas normal myocardium becomes much less so. Pulse sequences, first described in the mid-1980s, have taken advantage of this property, which is unique in noninvasive, nonionizing imaging. With the development of segmented inversion recovery fast gradient echo sequences and other techniques such as SSFP,

signal intensity differences between normal and infarcted myocardium of up to 500% have been achieved. The technique has been shown to accurately delineate the presence, extent, and location of acute and chronic myocardial infarction. DE is not just the province of adult heart disease, however. Hearts that have undergone surgical reconstruction can utilize DE to assess for myocardial scar tissue in both unoperated areas of myocardium and the areas that were surgically reconstructed such as the infundibulum and the pulmonary annulus in a patient after transannular patch repair of tetralogy of Fallot. In addition, surgically placed patches and valves can become bright with this technique.

4. *Perfusion.* Assessment of myocardial perfusion can be a very important component of the evaluation of the patient with CHD. Patients with congenital abnormalities of the coronary arteries (e.g., anomalous left coronary artery from the pulmonary artery), who have had surgical manipulation of the coronary arteries (e.g., transposition of the great arteries after arterial switch procedure or Ross procedure) as well as patients who have had specific inflammatory diseases (e.g., Kawasaki's disease) can all benefit from perfusion assessment. Typically, "adenosine" stress is performed initially at 140 µg/kg per minute for 4 to 6 minutes. This is followed by gadolinium administration using a time-resolved sequence that images the gadolinium as it courses through the body. A signal intense "blush" of the myocardium is seen uniformly in patients without coronary artery disease; however, in those with coronary compromise, a signal poor region of the myocardium will be observed. This is followed after 15 to 20 minutes with a similar injection and imaging sequence except that no adenosine is infused as a "resting" comparison. Finally, this sequence is followed approximately 10 minutes later by DE (see earlier). With these three types of images, it can be delineated if myocardial perfusion is normal, ischemic, or infarcted or has artifact. This type of imaging sequence can also be done with dobutamine stress or dipyridamole; however, in CHD, adenosine stress perfusion is more common.

There are special techniques that do not fall into this generalized protocol that may be inserted at different points, depending on the lesion:

- *Myocardial and blood tagging*: In patients where there is a question of regional wall motion abnormalities (e.g., cardiomyopathies or single ventricle) or whether a region of the myocardium is even contracting (e.g., tumor such as a rhabdomyoma), myocardial tagging can be used to assess this both qualitatively and quantitatively (Fig. 34.1). With myocardial tagging, the ventricle is noninvasively divided up into "cubes of magnetization" and local deformation of the myocardium can be visualized. This can be performed by laying down two sets of parallel black lines perpendicular to each other (two-dimensional tagging) or one series of lines (one-dimensional tagging) on bright blood cine imaging using a technique called spatial modulation of magnetization (SPAMM). This can quantify strain as well as regional wall motion.

  In addition, if there are questions regarding the presence of an atrial or a ventricular septal defect, a "saturation band" can be laid down on the blood to "tag" it as dark on a gradient echo image. This dark blood can be followed so that shunting can be visualized (Fig. 34.9, bottom left).
- *Real-time interactive cine imaging*: Small atrial and ventricular septal defects may be difficult to visualize using the standard imaging techniques of CMR. Real-time interactive cine imaging can be used to "sweep" the atrial or ventricular septum to identify these defects with the imager controlling the imaging plane in "real-time." In addition, these sweeps can be used to survey the cardiovascular anatomy in conjunction with static SSFP imaging.
- *Coronary artery imaging*: Using navigator sequences, and in some patients breath-hold imaging, this technique may be used to image patients with CHD who have had coronary manipulation (e.g., transposition of the great arteries after arterial switch) or who have native or acquired coronary disease such as anomalous left coronary artery from the pulmonary artery or in patients with Kawasaki's disease to assess for coronary aneurysms (Fig. 34.2). This technique relies on minimizing the motion of the coronary arteries (both cardiac and respiratory motion). A "navigator" pulse is used to monitor diaphragmatic motion, and the coronary arteries are imaged during inspiration. In addition, the images are triggered to the cardiac cycle and are acquired in diastole as this minimizes cardiac motion and is the time in the cardiac cycle when the coronary arteries are most filled with blood. Fat saturation and, in certain sequences, T2 preparation, are included in this type of imaging. Recently, "whole-heart" T2 prepared SSFP coronary imaging has been developed to create a three-dimensional image of the coronary arteries.

There are three special situations worth mentioning that require specific protocols that use many of the techniques mentioned here and some that were not detailed:

- *ARVD*: In this disease, replacement of RV myocardium by fatty or fibrofatty tissue results in (a) a dilated and poorly functioning right ventricle, (b) dyskinetic regional RV wall motion, (c) ECG abnormalities including RV conduction delay, inverted T waves, and (d) left bundle branch block tachycardia. Imaging is one of multiple criteria set forth in the 1994 Task Force guidelines. CMR has been successfully used in adults to identify this disease; however, considerable debate remains regarding its clinical value in children. The adult CMR criteria used to characterize ARVD vary from study to study but in general, there is (a) fatty substitution of the myocardium, (b) ectasia of the RVOT, (c) dyskinetic bulges or dyskinesia of RV wall motion, (d) a dilated RV, (e) a dilated RA, and (f) fixed RV wall thinning with decreased RV wall thickening. The CMR protocol includes T1-weighted imaging, cine MR imaging for ventricular function, one-dimensional RV myocardial tagging, if needed, to assess regional wall motion, phase-encoded velocity mapping, and finally DE.
- *Tumor/mass characterization*: Many cardiac tumors and masses can be differentiated from each other by their characteristics on CMR, the location where they occur in the heart, the clinical symptoms they cause, and at what age they occur. For example, lipomas are signal intense on T1-weighted images but become signal poor after fat saturation. Tumor characterization by CMR typically includes T1- and T2-weighted images, images with fat saturation, GRE imaging (e.g., for thrombus), perfusion (e.g., for hemangiomas), DE imaging,

T1-weighted images after gadolinium administration, and myocardial tagging. If time permits, functional imaging can also be used to assess for detrimental physiologic effects of the tumor such as obstruction to flow and decreased cardiac output.
- *Measurement of myocardial iron*: Because iron is a ferromagnetic element, tissues containing iron can have different magnetic properties than those without it. The "T2 star" technique takes advantage of this property and can quantify the amount of iron in the myocardium as well as liver. This is important in patients with thalessemia where heart failure caused by increased iron deposition within the myocardium is the leading cause of death. Similarly, patients with sickle cell disease also have myocardial iron deposition. CMR can be used to adjust chelation therapy in these patients. Increasing amounts of iron drive down the value of the CMR parameter T2 star (related to proton relaxation). A gradient echo sequence is used with multiple echo times (TE) to measure T2 star in the heart. Values under 20 ms have been correlated with increasingly poor ventricular function. A typical CMR protocol includes not only the measurement of T2 star but also cine CMR for ventricular function and PC-MRI.

CARDIAC MAGNETIC RESONANCE IN CONGENITAL HEART DISEASE

Functional Single Ventricles

The approach to the repair of single ventricle lesions is staged surgical reconstruction (two or three stages, depending on the anatomy and physiology) eventually culminating in the Fontan procedure (Fig. 34.1, 34.3, 34.4, 34.5, 34.7, and 34.9). Understanding the various forms of functional single ventricles, their associated anomalies and physiologic/functional sequelae, as well as the various surgical reconstructive techniques is important for optimal medical and surgical management of these very complex patients.

As the single-ventricle patient progresses through staged surgical reconstruction, the CMR examination changes, but the overall goal of assessing cardiac anatomy, physiology, and function remains the same. The CMR study, however, needs to be tailored to the individual needs of each patient. In all stages of surgical reconstruction, it is important to assess the following:

- Pulmonary arterial anatomy including pulmonary artery stenosis, hypoplasia, and discontinuity (Figs. 34.3, 34.5, and 34.9)
- Aortic arch anatomy, especially in patients with an aortic-to-pulmonary anastomosis to rule out aortic arch obstruction (Fig. 34.5)
- Systemic and pulmonary venous pathways (Fig. 34.9)
- Ventricular outflow tract obstruction, especially in patients with a bulboventricular foramen (Fig. 34.9)
- Anomalous systemic and pulmonary venous structures
- Aortic-pulmonary collaterals (typically by three-dimensional gadolinium sequences)
- Sites of intracardiac and extracardiac shunting
- Ventricular function, including regional wall motion abnormalities, ejection fraction, end-diastolic volume and mass, stroke volume, cardiac index, and atrioventricular valve regurgitant fraction
- Velocity mapping to assess cardiac index, Q_p/Q_s, relative flows to both lungs and regurgitant fraction of the semilunar (and indirectly) atrioventricular valve, and assess ventricular outflow tract obstruction

After the Stage I palliation procedure (e.g., hypoplastic left heart syndrome), focused CMR imaging of the aortic arch to rule out obstruction as well as evaluation of the RV-to–pulmonary artery shunt need to be areas of focused attention. Because of turbulence in these shunts, double-inversion dark blood imaging (or gadolinium) is used because cine generally causes signal loss. After the bidirectional Glenn or hemi-Fontan stage (Fig. 34.3), visualizing the superior vena cava–to–pulmonary artery anastomosis is a major focus of CMR imaging. After the Fontan procedure, it is important to image the entire systemic venous pathway (Fontan baffle) for the presence of obstruction or thrombus (Fig. 34.9). Quantitative evaluation of ventricular function after the Fontan, including delayed enhancement to assess for myocardial scar tissue, is also important.

Tetralogy of Fallot

Tetralogy of Fallot (TOF) is one of the more common congenital heart lesions referred to CMR (Figs. 34.4, 34.8, 34.10, and 34.11). TOF consists of four major cardiac abnormalities: (a) malalignment ventricular septal defect, (b) RVOT obstruction, (c) RV hypertrophy, and (d) overriding aorta. There may be any number of associated abnormalities including right aortic arch, pulmonary atresia, and absent pulmonary valve syndrome. Surgical repair consists of patch closure of the ventricular septal defect and relief of RVOT obstruction. Historically, a transannular patch was used to relieve RVOT obstruction leading to chronic severe pulmonary regurgitation. Recently, the surgical approach has been to limit this RVOT incision with valve-sparing techniques. Insertion of a competent pulmonary valve years after surgery has been advocated for patients with clinical symptomatology and those with significant RV dilation or dysfunction.

CMR can provide exquisite detail of the anatomy and physiology needed for diagnosis, treatment, and serial follow-up after surgical repair. Preoperatively, echocardiography remains the first-line imaging modality. However, CMR can be used not only to confirm the diagnosis but also to identify associated abnormalities, especially those of the great vessels (e.g., vascular ring) and systemic or pulmonary venous anomalies. Postoperatively, CMR is used routinely for the assessment of pulmonary regurgitation (Figs. 34.8 and 34.10) as well as right ventricular volumes and function. Because of the quantitative nature of CMR and its high accuracy and reproducibility, cine for ventricular volumes, mass, ejection, and cardiac output along with velocity mapping for pulmonary regurgitant fraction, cardiac index, and quantitation of pulmonary flow is considered the standard of care. Delayed enhancement imaging can be used to search for myocardial scar tissue (Fig. 34.11), especially as a correlate for regional ventricular wall motion abnormalities. In addition, CMR is used for assessment of residual RVOT obstruction, residual ventricular septal defect, and the status of the pulmonary arteries (Fig. 34.11).

FUTURE TRENDS IN CARDIAC MAGNETIC RESONANCE

With the many fast-paced advances in CMR over the last several years, the future holds great promise for continued applications of this modality in congenital heart disease. Interventional CMR is currently evolving and is being used for balloon valvuloplasty, stent placement, and occluder device insertion. Molecular imaging can now identify targets for therapy. T2* techniques can be used to evaluate myocardial oxygen content, and advances in hardware and software have enabled "real-time" flow assessment. These advances are readily seen in the ongoing research in the field of functional fetal CMR. Work recently published using "real-time" imaging demonstrated the feasibility of this approach in patients with an in utero diagnosis of hypoplastic left heart syndrome to quantify ventricular volumes and cardiac output. An increase in spatial and temporal resolution along with unique ways of "gating" may allow for phase contrast flow assessments and the routine use of functional fetal CMR in the near future.

CONCLUSION

The use of CMR in infants, children, adolescents, and adults with CHD is a rapidly evolving field with multiple clinical applications. CMR is used in conjunction with other imaging modalities to provide state-of-the-art care of patients both preoperatively and postoperatively. Continued advances in the field will lead to even more indications and applications to varying disciplines within pediatric cardiology. If past progress in the field is any indication of the future, we are in for a wild ride.

SUGGESTED READING

Adams R, Fellows KE, Fogel MA, et al. Anatomic delineation of congenital heart disease with 3D magnetic resonance imaging. *Proc SPIE Med Imaging.* 1994; 2168:184–194.

Anderson LJ, Holden S, Davis B, et al. Cardiovascular T2-star (T2*) magnetic resonance for the early diagnosis of myocardial iron overload. *Eur Heart J.* 2001;22:2171–2179.

Arai AE, Epstein FH, Bove KE, et al. Visualization of aortic valve leaflets using black blood MRI. *J Magn Reson Imaging.* 199;10:771–777.

Ashford MW, Liu W, Lin SJ, et al. Occult cardiac contractile dysfunction in dystrophin-deficient children revealed by cardiac magnetic resonance strain imaging. *Circulation.* 2005;112:2462–2467.

Bank ER. Magnetic resonance of congenital cardiovascular disease. An update. *Radiol Clin North Am.* 1993; 31:553–572.

Basso C, Thiene G, Corrado D, et al. Arrhythmogenic right ventricular cardiomyopathy: dysplasia, dystrophy or myocarditis. *Circulation.* 1996;94:983–991.

Beekman R, Hazekamp M, Sobotka M, et al. A new diagnostic approach to vascular rings and pulmonary slings: the role of MRI. *Magn Reson Imaging.* 1998;16:137–145.

Beerbaum P, Korperich H, Barth P, et al. Non-invasive quantification of left-to-right shunt in pediatric patients. Phase-contrast cine magnetic resonance imaging compared with invasive oxymetry. *Circulation.* 2001;10:2476–2482.

Bornemeier RA, Weinberg PM, Fogel MA. Angiographic, echocardiographic and three-dimensional magnetic resonance imaging of extracardiac conduits in congenital heart disease *Am J Cardiol.* 1996;78:713–717.

Bu L, Munns S, Zhang H, et al. Rapid full volume data acquisition by real-time three-dimensional echocardiography for assessment of LV indexes in children: a validation study compared with MRI. *J Am Soc Echocardiogr.* 2005;18:299–305.

Didier D, Higgins CB, Fisher M, et al. Congenital heart disease: gated magnetic resonance imaging in 72 patients. *Radiology.* 1986;158:227–235.

Didier D, Ratib O, Beghetti M, et al. Morphologic and functional evaluation of congenital heart disease by magnetic resonance imaging. *J Magn Reson Imaging.* 1999;10:639–655.

Donofrio MT, Clark BJ, Ramaciotti C, et al. Regional wall motion and strain of transplanted hearts in pediatric patients using magnetic resonance tagging. *Am J Physiol* 1999;277:R1481–R1487.

Edelman RR, Chien D, Kim D. Fast selective black blood MR imaging. *Radiology* 1991;181:655–660.

Eyskens B, Reybrouck T, Bagaert J, et al.. Homograft insertion for pulmonary regurgitation after repair of tetralogy of Fallot improves cardiorespiratory exercise performance. *Am J Cardiol.* 2000;85:221–225.

Finn JP, Baskaran V, Carr JC, et al. Low-dose contrast-enhanced three-dimensional MR angiography with subsecond temporal resolution: initial results. *Radiology.* 2002;224:896–904.

Fleenor JT, Weinberg PM, Kramer SS, et al. Vascular rings and their effect on tracheal geometry. *Pediatr Cardiol.* 2003;24:430–435.

Fletcher BD, Jacobsteink MD, Nelson AD, et al. Gated magnetic resonance imaging of congenital cardiac malformations. *Radiology.* 1984;150:137–140.

Fogel MA. Cardiac magnetic resonance of single ventricles. *J Cardiovasc Magn Reson.* 2006;8:661–670.

Fogel MA. Considerations in the single ventricle. In: Fogel MA, ed. *Ventricular Function and Blood Flow in Congenital Heart Disease,* Malden, MA: Blackwell Futura; 2005:286–308.

Fogel MA, Gupta KB, Weinberg PW, et al. Regional wall motion and strain analysis across stages of Fontan reconstruction by magnetic resonance tagging. *Am J Physiol.* 1995;269:H1132–H1152.

Fogel MA, Hubbard A, Weinberg PM. A simplified approach for assessment of intracardiac baffles and extracardiac conduits in congenital heart surgery with two- and three-dimensional magnetic resonance imaging. *Am Heart J.* 2001;142:1028–1036.

Fogel MA, Ramaciotti C, Hubbard AM, et al. Magnetic resonance and echocardiographic imaging of pulmonary artery size throughout stages of Fontan reconstruction *Circulation.* 1994;90:2927–2936.

Fogel MA, Rychik J, Chin A, et al. Evaluation and follow-up of patients with left ventricular apical to aortic conduits using two and three-dimensional magnetic resonance imaging and Doppler echocardiography: a new look at an old operation. *Am Heart J.* 2001;141:630–636.

Fogel MA, Rychik J. Right ventricular function in congenital heart disease: volume and pressure overload lesions. *Prog Cardiovasc Dis.* 1998;40:343–356.

Fogel MA, Weinberg PM, Chin AJ, et al. Late ventricular geometry and performance changes of functional single ventricle throughout staged Fontan reconstruction assessed by magnetic resonance imaging. *J Am Coll Cardiol.* 1996;28:212–221.

Fogel MA, Weinberg PM, Fellows KE, et al. A study in ventricular-ventricular interaction: single right ventricles compared with systemic right ventricles in a dual chambered circulation. *Circulation.* 1995;92:219–230.

Fogel MA, Weinberg PM, Gupta KB, et al. Mechanics of the single left ventricle: a study in ventricular-ventricular interaction, II. *Circulation.* 1998;98:330–338.

Fogel MA, Weinberg PM, Hoydu A, et al. The nature of flow in the systemic venous pathway in Fontan patients utilizing magnetic resonance blood tagging. *J Thorac Cardiovasc Surg.* 1997;114:1032–1041.

Fogel MA, Weinberg PM, Hubbard A, et al. Diastolic biomechanics in normal infants utilizing MRI tissue tagging. *Circulation.* 2000;102:218–224.

Fogel MA, Weinberg PM, Rhodes L. Usefulness of magnetic resonance imaging for the diagnosis of right ventricular dysplasia in children. 2006;97:1232–1237.

Fogel MA, Weinberg PM, Rychik J, et al. Caval contribution to flow in the branch pulmonary arteries of Fontan patients using a novel application of magnetic resonance presaturation pulse. *Circulation.* 1999;99:1215–1221.

Fogel MA, Wilson DR, Flake A, et al. A new method of functional assessment of the fetal heart using a novel application of "real time" cardiac magnetic resonance imaging. *Fetal Diagn Ther.* 2005;20:475–480.

Fontan F, Baudet E. Surgical repair of tricuspid atresia. *Thorax.* 1971;26:240–248.

Frahm J, Merboldt KD, Bruhn H, et al. 0.3 Second FLASH MRI of the human heart. *Magn Reson Med.* 1990;13:150–157.

Gutberlet M, Boeckel T, Hosten N, et al. Arterial switch procedure for d-transposition of the great arteries: quantitative midterm evaluation of hemodynamic changes with cine MR imaging and phase-shift velocity mapping. Initial experience. *Radiology.* 2000;214;467–475.

Harris M. Johnson T, Weinberg P, et al.. Delayed enhancement cardiovascular magnetic resonance identifies fibrous tissue in children after congenital heart surgery. *J Thorac Cardiovasc Surg.* 2007;133:676–681.

Harris MA, Weinberg PM, Fogel MA. Cardiac magnetic resonance atrial level shunt detection utilizing presaturation tagging. Presented at the 4th World Congress of Pediatric Cardiology and Cardiac Surgery, Buenos Aires, Argentina, 2005.

Higgins CB, Byrd BF, Farmer DW, et al. Magnetic resonance imaging in patients with congenital heart disease. *Circulation.* 1984;70:851–860.

Ho V, Prince M. Thoracic MR aortography: imaging techniques and strategies. *Radiographics.* 1998;18:287–309.

Kiaffas MG, Powell AJ, Geva T. Magnetic resonance imaging evaluation of cardiac tumor characteristics in infants and children. *Am J Cardiol.* 2002;89:1229–1233.

Kim WY, Danias PG, Stuber M, et al. Coronary magnetic resonance angiography for the detection of coronary stenosis. *N Engl J Med.* 2001;345:1863–1869.

Kuhl HP, et al. High-resolution transthoracic real-time three-dimensional echocardiography: quantitation of cardiac volumes and function using semi-automatic border detection and comparison with cardiac MRI. *J Am Coll Cardiol.* 2004;43:2083–2090.

Lee VS, Resnick D, Bundy JM, et al. MR evaluation in one breath hold with real-time true FAST imaging with steady-state precision. *Radiology.* 2002;222:835–842.

Martin ET, Coman JA, Shellock FG, et al. Magnetic resonance imaging and cardiac pacemaker safety at 1.5-Tesla. *J Am Coll Cardiol.* 2004;43:1315–1324.

McConnell MV, Ganz P, Selwyn AP, et al. Identification of anomalous coronary arteries and their anatomic course by magnetic resonance coronary angiography. *Circulation.* 1995;92:3158–3162.

McKenna WJ, Thiene G, Nava A, et al. Diagnosis of arrhythmogenic right ventricular dysplasia/cardiomyopathy. Task Force of the Working Group Myocardial and Pericardial Disease of the European Society of Cardiology and of the Scientific Council on Cardiomyopathies of the International Society and Federation of Cardiology. *Br Heart J.* 1994;71:215–218.

Midiri M, Finazzo M, Brancato M, et al. Arrhythmogenic right ventricular dysplasia: MR features. *Eur Radiol.* 1997;7:307–312.

Mor-Avi V, Sugeng L, Weinert L, et al. Fast measurement of LV mass with real-time three-dimensional echocardiography: comparison with MRI. *Circulation.* 2004;110:1814–1818.

Niezen RA, Helgbing WA, van der Wall EE, et al. Biventricular systolic function and mass studied with MRI imaging in children with pulmonary regurgitation after repair for tetralogy of Fallot. *Radiology.* 1996; 201:135–140.

Prakash A, Powell AJ, Krishnamurthy R, et al. Magnetic resonance imaging evaluation of myocardial perfusion and viability in congenital and acquired pediatric heart disease. *Am J Cardiol.* 2004;93:657–661.

Rebergen SA, Chin JGJ, Ottenkamp J, et al. Pulmonary regurgitaion in the late postoperative follow-up of tetralogy of Fallot. Volumetric quantification by MR velocity mapping. *Circulation.* 1993;88:2257–2266.

Rebergen SA, Ottenkamp J, van der Wall EE, et al. Postoperative pulmonary flow dynamics after Fontan surgery: Assessment with nuclear magnetic resonance velocity mapping. *J Am Coll Cardiol* 1993; 21:123–131.

Taylor AM, Dymarkowski S, Hamaekers P, et al. MR coronary angiography and late-enhancement myocardial MR in children who underwent arterial switch surgery for transposition of great arteries. *Radiology.* 2005;234:542–547.

van Son J, Julsrud P, Hagler D, et al. Imaging strategies for vascular rings. *Ann Thorac Surg.* 1994;57:604–610.

Weinberg PM, Hubbard AM, Fogel MA. Aortic arch and pulmonary artery anomalies in children. *Semin Roentgenol.* 1998;33:262–280.

Chapter 35
Aging and Congenital Heart Disease

James B. Seward

PREVALENCE OF ADULT CONGENITAL HEART DISEASE

Adult Congenital Heart Disease

More than 85% of children born with congenital heart disease (CHD) now survive to adulthood, and the number of adults with CHD is growing at 5% per year. In 2001, the number of adults with CHD living in the United States was estimated to be more than 800,000, a number that has grown steadily as more survivors of childhood surgery reach maturity. Of these, about 45% have mild forms of CHD (e.g., atrial septal defect, pulmonary valve stenosis), 40% have moderate disease (e.g., tetralogy of Fallot, Ebstein anomaly), and 15% have complex disease (e.g., transposition complexes, truncus arteriosus, single ventricle). There are significantly more females than males in both the adult and the pediatric CHD populations. From 1985 to 2000, the prevalence of CHD in adults in the United States increased to 49%, an 85% increase, and the median age of CHD patients increased from 11 years to 17 years. This finding is in part attributed to the detection of less severe CHD by more extensive use of echocardiography. However, better surgical outcomes also appeared to account for increased numbers of adults with more severe forms of CHD.

Severe Adult Congenital Heart Disease

The prevalence of severe CHD in adults in 2000 was estimated to be greater than 1 per 245 adults (9% of adults with CHD in the United States, or approximately 80,000 persons, have severe CHD). In 2000, there were nearly equal numbers of adults and children with severe CHD. The trends suggest that adults with severe CHD will ultimately have higher mortality rates than children with severe CHD.

CONGENITAL HEART DISEASE IS A LIFELONG DISEASE

Aging

In general, CHD—whether operated or unoperated—is associated with accelerated deterioration (aging) of the cardiovascular system. As CHD patients mature from adolescence to adulthood, the rate of hospitalizations nearly doubles (from about 20% to about 45%) and stays high thereafter. A large percentage of children and adults with CHD are lost to follow-up. However, all indicators confirm that adults with CHD increasingly receive general medical attention.

CHD patients typically receive no cardiology follow-up care through childhood and adolescence; only about 39% receive care from a cardiologist as young adults. Absolute numbers and mortality rates among CHD patients have increased, and the age distribution for CHD deaths has shifted from younger to older patients (Fig. 35.1). The survival of CHD patients is lower than that of the general population (relative 45-year survival, 89%) (Fig. 35.2). Most CHD patients die as a direct consequence of CHD; however, adult CHD patients have a higher mortality rate from respiratory deaths (because of pneumonia or heart failure).

Accelerated Mortality

Even if they have operative correction or palliation of CHD, patients continue to have variable risk related to either the evolution of the congenital abnormality or the physiologic abnormalities, which are a consequence of structural factors (abnormal cardiac or great vessel

morphology) or of the emergence of age-associated cardiovascular risk factors (heart failure, atrial fibrillation, secondary pulmonary hypertension, ischemic heart disease, etc.) (Fig. 35.2).

In the current era of sophisticated imaging modalities, such as x-ray computed tomography (CT), there are long-term concerns for young adults, females, and children who receive large amounts of poorly monitored diagnostic radiation. Because CHD is a lifelong condition, there is a greater impetus to reduce radiation exposure in young adults with CHD (mean age, older than 17 years). For example, the radiation exposure from multislice CT is comparable to about 400 chest radiographs and is associated with a measurable

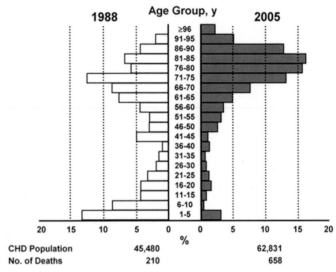

FIGURE 35.1. Distribution of age at death from congenital heart disease (CHD) for 1988 and 2005. The distribution has shifted away from the young and toward the adult. (From Khairy P, Mackie AS, Ionescu-Ittu R, et al. Changing age distribution of death in congenital heart disease from 1988 to 2005: a population based study [abstract]. *J Am Coll Cardiol.* 2007;49[suppl. 1]:268A. Used with permission.)

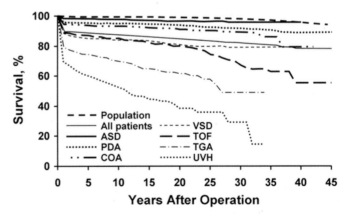

FIGURE 35.2. Survival rates for patients with various types of congenital heart disease in relation to the general population. ASD, atrial septal defect; COA, coarctation of aorta; PDA, patent ductus arteriosus; TGA, transposition of the great arteries; TOF, tetralogy of Fallot; UVH, univentricular heart; VSD, ventricular septal defect. (From Nieminen HP, Jokinen EV, Sairanen HI. Causes of late deaths after pediatric cardiac surgery: a population-based study. *J Am Coll Cardiol.* 2007;50:1263–1271. Used with permission.)

lifetime risk of cancer. Repeated radiographic studies should be kept to a minimum. Doppler echocardiography and magnetic resonance imaging are preferred imaging techniques. Doppler echocardiography, with its superior temporal resolution, mobile configurability, and ability to quantify pathophysiologic features, is the preferred means of determining cardiovascular function.

Pregnancy

CHD in the mother is associated with a much higher complication rate during pregnancy. Arrhythmias, heart failure, and cardiovascular events have been reported in 11% of women with CHD and completed pregnancies, but these complications rarely occur in healthy women in the general population. Compared with the general population in the industrialized world, women with CHD have a higher premature birth rate (16% versus 10% to 12%) and higher offspring mortality (4% versus <1%), especially among women with CHD who have premature delivery or complicated CHD. Mortality is particularly high for patients with Eisenmenger syndrome, and in general, pregnancy is discouraged in these patients.

Coronary Artery Disease

Coronary artery disease in adults with CHD appears to have a natural history similar to that of coronary artery disease in adults in the general population. Most CHD patients with coronary artery disease have one or more cardiovascular risk factors. Patients with cyanotic CHD and low cholesterol levels have a very low propensity for the development of coronary atherosclerosis.

Most sudden death in older adults with CHD is caused by coronary thrombosis or severe coronary artery disease (or both). Sudden cardiac death, especially with congenital coronary artery anomalies, occurs almost exclusively in adults younger than 35 years. Anomalous coronary arteries are associated with a high incidence of CHD but do not appear to be associated with an increased risk of coronary atherosclerosis.

Surgery for Adult Congenital Heart Disease

In adult patients with CHD, preoperative arrhythmia and systolic dysfunction are common, and postoperative adverse events are frequently encountered. Risk factors predictive of postoperative adverse events include older age, atrial fibrillation, New York Heart Association functional Class III or greater, and functional single ventricle. Age-associated risk factors (atrial fibrillation, stroke, heart failure, etc.) are similar to those in the general population.

Associated Disease in the Adult

Many problems that are unfamiliar to pediatric specialists (e.g., coronary artery disease, age-associated risk, stroke, adult-onset atrial fibrillation, chronic congestive heart failure) are best handled by clinicians with both pediatric and adult training in CHD and with expertise in adult cardiac and noncardiac diseases. In many respects, the adult patient with CHD appears to be affected equally by age-associated cardiovascular disease and emergent cardiovascular risk.

 # HEART FAILURE ASSOCIATED WITH AGING AND CONGENITAL HEART DISEASE

Background

Because of the inherent cardiac and extracardiac structural abnormalities associated with CHD, lifelong deterioration in cardiovascular function is nearly uniformly observed. The long-term effects of diagnostic and therapeutic procedures are not well understood. Premature occurrence of restrictive physiologic changes and secondary pulmonary hypertension after two to three decades is common.

Normal Cardiac Function

For the left ventricle to function as an effective pump, it must be able to empty and fill without requiring abnormal elevation of left atrial pressure. The stroke volume must increase in response to stress, such as exercise, without an appreciable increase in left atrial pressure. Elevation of atrial pressure is directly related to the inability of the left atrium to efficiently empty its contents into the ventricle. In turn, heart failure symptoms (breathlessness, exercise intolerance, fluid retention, etc.) are related to increased pressure reflected backward into the left atrium and pulmonary veins during atrial emptying (diastole). Abnormal cardiovascular anatomy and physiology typical of CHD contribute to an accelerated deterioration of cardiovascular function with advancing age. Age-associated cardiovascular risk appears much earlier in patients with either operated or unoperated CHD.

Age-Associated Congenital Heart Disease Events

Cardiovascular dysfunction leading to elevation of filling pressure can be broadly grouped as a consequence of (a) altered cardiomyocyte function, which is most strongly associated with abnormal ventricular geometry as encountered in CHD, or (b) abnormal cardiac loading, which most commonly begins as a consequence of extracardiac stiffening of the conduit arterial system (dilated great arteries, coarctation, etc.), or (c) both. With either of these sentinel features, compensatory mechanisms are propagated throughout the contiguous cardiovascular system and portend the emergence of increased cardiovascular risk (heart failure, atrial fibrillation, stroke, etc.). Cyclical and self-perpetuating mechanisms account for the clustering of common adverse events. Emergent risk factors (atrial fibrillation, heart failure, etc.), which appear to have a common physiologic basis, are best viewed as *consequences* and not as *causes*.

Conduit Arterial Stiffening

Normally, the great arteries are compliant, expanding outward during systole and recoiling during diastole. The cardiovascular system is best viewed as a contiguous system (pump, arteries, and reservoir). The heart is a pump delivering pulsatile flow to the conduit arterial and capillary system, which acts as an extensive hydraulic filter that converts pulsatile flow to continuous flow at the end organ. Blood returns to the atria and veins, which act as a distensible reservoir storing blood during ventricular contraction and filling the ventricle during diastole. The conversion of continuous flow back to pulsatile flow is initiated in the atrial and venous reservoir.

Elastin, which runs in the longitudinal dimension of the aorta and pulmonary trunk, has the tensile characteristics of compliant rubber and accounts for the normal expansion and recoil of the great arteries (normal arterial elastance). Conversely, collagen, which runs in the circumferential dimension of the great arteries, has the tensile characteristics of steel. With aging or structural change in the arterial wall, a conduit artery becomes less compliant and more dependent on the characteristics of collagen. For example, aortic valve stenosis associated with bicuspid valve has a clinical progression that is similar to the natural history of age-associated degenerative cardiovascular disease (Fig. 35.3). The great arteries and ventricle are connected to one another and undergo simultaneous stiffening, altering how the heart and arterial system interact at rest and particularly under stress and exertional demands. Delayed active and passive relaxation of the stiff ventricle during early diastole disturbs the normal suction gradient between ventricle and atrium. The concept of "continuity disease and ventriculoarterial coupling" has been proposed to describe the shared physiology between the aorta and the contiguous cardiovascular system (arteries, heart pump, and atrial reservoir).

CHD, which is associated with lifelong and often progressive arterial outflow obstruction, dilated aortic root (e.g., tetralogy of Fallot, Marfan syndrome, bicuspid aortic valve), or reduced arterial elastance, results in a variable yet chronic increase in ventricular afterload. Stiffening of arterial and ventricular components is referred to as "coupling disease" and is considered to be the principal contributor to age-associated cardiovascular adverse events such as heart failure, atrial fibrillation, stroke, and cognitive dysfunction. CHD of the great arteries is accompanied by premature deterioration of the normal relationship of the contiguous pump (ventricles) and atrial and venous reservoir.

Abnormal Ventricular Geometry

Abnormal suction of blood into the left ventricle has been replicated with various heart failure models of abnormal ventricular geometry

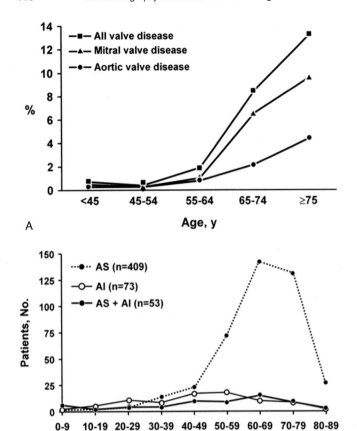

A

B

FIGURE 35.3. Similarities between age-associated degenerative valve disease and aortic stenosis associated with bicuspid aortic valve. A: The increased prevalence of degenerative valve disease in the general population begins to occur after the age of 45 and continues to escalate thereafter (prevalence in males and females is similar). **B:** Note the similarly increased frequency of aortic valve stenosis associated with bicuspid aortic valve, which occurs after the age of 40 and increases thereafter. AI, aortic insufficiency; AS, aortic stenosis. [**A,** From Nkomo VT, Gardin JM, Skelton TN, et al. Burden of valvular heart diseases: a population-based study. Lancet. 2006;368:1005–1011. Used with permission. **B,** From Sabet HY, Edwards WD, Tazelaar HD, et al. Congenitally bicuspid aortic valves: a surgical pathology study of 542 cases (1991 through 1996) and a literature review of 2,715 additional cases. *Mayo Clin Proc* 1999;74:14–26. Used with permission.]

algorithms. Prevention of emergent consequences relies on accurate prediction and quantification of subclinical risk and cardiovascular function and remodeling.

Prediction is dependent on identifying specific sets of features that portend the emergence of disease states. Doppler echocardiographic feature sets can be used to make a remarkably accurate prediction based on the relationship of small groupings of interrelated quantifiable features (filling pressure, myocyte relaxation, elastance, etc.). Quantifiable emergent disease is best viewed as a large network of closely connected features. There are an extraordinarily large number of lesser-related features (associated clinical and pathophysiologic features: breathlessness, fatigue, left ventricular mass) and a small number of extensively connected dominant features, which hold the network together (e.g., filling pressure, myocyte relaxation). The consistency, feedback, and memory of the measured dominant features can be used to accurately predict and quantify the severity of emergent cardiovascular disease risk. The severity and emergence of nascent cardiovascular events can be predicted, treated, and modified before the multivariate clinical disease appears.

Prevention of an emergent disease is most successful if treatment is instituted early and focused on dominant features (filling pressure, myocardial relaxation, etc.) and not specifically on associations (variable degrees of breathlessness, wall thickness, etc.). Associations and consequences are commonly mistaken for cause-and-effect relationships (e.g., neither rate nor rhythm control of atrial fibrillation has sufficiently affected associated stroke, quality of life, or death). The objective is to prevent emergent consequences such as heart failure, atrial fibrillation, stroke, and premature death. Although prevention begins with optimization of personal lifestyle and environment, the proportion of adults in the United States engaged in a healthy lifestyle is small. The best prevention is an attacking defense, which tracks down a disease before it causes demonstrable harm and eliminates the likelihood of expression. Holistic risk models based on quantifiable morphologic and physiologic information shift the focus toward tests that are more closely aligned to cause and effect. Treatment should be designed to alter an individual patient's emergent disease toward normality or stabilization. Treatment based on quantifiable features (severity or burden) is capable of individualizing risk and thus reduces overtreatment or undertreatment of the emergent disease. Risk prediction, quantification, and prevention are paramount to the successful lifelong management of adult CHD.

MANAGEMENT OF ADULT CONGENITAL HEART DISEASE

Although noninvasive Doppler echocardiography is recognized as the best means of characterizing and quantifying cardiovascular features, it has received little attention in treatment algorithms. Complexity science teaches one to characterize, manage, and prevent disease by using a portfolio of quantifiable features that can be easily obtained by noninvasive means. Interconnecting features have close similarities to the emergent disease and obey the same fundamental rules. Primary prevention works because treatment of an appropriate feature set (the surrogate model), which is more closely aligned to the cause, is comparable to treating the fully evolved disease.

Multivariate disease states are the consequence of relatively simple rules operating one level below the occurrence of complex disease states. Features simplify general concepts that are determined by natural rules (filling pressure, myocardial relaxation, central aortic pressure, etc.). Just because cardiovascular disease is complicated and multivariate does not mean that it has to arise from a complicated set of rules. Simplicity should be sought within apparently complex states. There is considerable impetus to develop useful multivariate physiologic risk models (disease surrogates) designed to address the enormous public health needs within the constraints of limited medical resources and best serve the individual patient. Noninvasive Doppler echocardiographic pathophysiology is evolving as one of the best means of directing primary prevention of age-associated cardiovascular disease.

Treatment of recognized cardiovascular risk factors is known to be only partially successful in alleviating cardiovascular disease risk.

such as myocardial ischemia and hypertrophic cardiomyopathy. Any condition that interferes with normal regional systolic function (contractility) modifies the distribution of the diastolic intraventricular pressure gradients. Convective deceleration is determined by spatial-temporal filling flow velocity and, particularly, the presence of a normal cone-shaped ventricle (i.e., efficient vortex motor). With distortion of ventricular geometry, as commonly encountered in CHD, the end-diastolic pressure-volume curve is shifted substantially, reflecting the increase in filling pressure. CHD is characterized by abnormal ventricular filling dynamics along with increased left atrial pressure and an inability to increase stroke volume without abnormal elevation of left atrial pressure. Heart failure symptoms are strongly related to the elevation of filling pressure, which accounts for breathlessness, exercise intolerance, and reduced quality of life. Although the increase in filling pressure accounts for the symptoms, it is not directly related to the hemodynamic cause of decreased cardiac output and distorted left ventricular geometry. Decreasing filling pressure decreases symptoms without eliminating the primary problem. Lasting clinical improvement requires reversal of the left ventricular distortion, which is not feasible in many circumstances in chronic operated or unoperated CHD.

PREDICTION AND PREVENTION

CHD is a lifelong multifactorial disease that requires early *prediction* of emergent disease and timely *prevention* with validated management

There is a pressing need to develop safe and cost-effective methods for characterizing and quantifying patients' personal risks to help in the early detection and prevention of age-associated adverse events seen with CHD. Ideally, treatment should be based on the best evidence and, when available, the best evidence should come from statistical research. The use of surrogate models capable of quantifying personal severity promotes primary prevention of emergent cardiovascular risk.

SUGGESTED READING

Bashore TM. Adult congenital heart disease: right ventricular outflow tract lesions. *Circulation.* 2007;115:1933–1947.

Bell SP, Fabian J, Watkins MW, et al. Decrease in forces responsible for diastolic suction during acute coronary occlusion. *Circulation.* 1997;96:2348–2352.

Blacher J, Asmar R, Djane S, et al. Aortic pulse wave velocity as a marker of cardiovascular risk in hypertensive patients. *Hypertension.* 1999;33:1111–1117.

Broberg CS, Ujita M, Prasad S, et al. Pulmonary arterial thrombosis in Eisenmenger syndrome is associated with biventricular dysfunction and decreased pulmonary flow velocity. *J Am Coll Cardiol.* 2007;50:634–642.

Corley SD, Epstein AE, DiMarco JP, et al, AFFIRM Investigators. Relationships between sinus rhythm, treatment, and survival in the Atrial Fibrillation Follow-Up Investigation of Rhythm Management (AFFIRM) Study. *Circulation.* 2004;109:1509–1513.

Courtois M, Kovács SJ, Ludbrook PA. Physiological early diastolic intraventricular pressure gradient is lost during acute myocardial ischemia. *Circulation.* 1990;81:1688–1696.

De Caro E, Trocchio G, Smeraldi A, et al. Aortic arch geometry and exercise-induced hypertension in aortic coarctation. *Am J Cardiol.* 2007;99: 1284–1287.

Diller GP, Gatzoulis MA. Pulmonary vascular disease in adults with congenital heart disease. *Circulation.* 2007;115:1039–1050.

Drenthen W, Pieper PG, Roos-Hesselink JW, et al, ZAHARA Investigators. Outcome of pregnancy in women with congenital heart disease: a literature review. *J Am Coll Cardiol* 2007;49:2303–2311.

Einstein AJ, Henzlova MJ, Rajagopalan S. Estimating risk of cancer associated with radiation exposure from 64-slice computed tomography coronary angiography. *JAMA.* 2007;298:317–323.

Einstein AJ, Moser KW, Thompson RC, et al. Radiation dose to patients from cardiac diagnostic imaging. *Circulation.* 2007;116:1290–1305.

Feinberg WM, Blackshear JL, Laupacis A, et al. Prevalence, age distribution, and gender of patients with atrial fibrillation: analysis and implications. *Arch Intern Med.* 1995;155:469–473.

Fernandes SM, Khairy P, Sanders SP, et al. Bicuspid aortic valve morphology and interventions in the young. *J Am Coll Cardiol.* 2007;49:2211–2214.

Firstenberg MS, Smedira NG, Greenberg NL, et al. Relationship between early diastolic intraventricular pressure gradients, an index of elastic recoil, and improvements in systolic and diastolic function. *Circulation.* 2001;104(suppl 1):I-330–I-335.

Ford ES, Ford MA, Will JC, et al. Achieving a healthy lifestyle among United States adults: a long way to go. *Ethn Dis.* 2001;11:224–231.

Fyfe A, Perloff JK, Niwa K, et al. Cyanotic congenital heart disease and coronary artery atherogenesis. *Am J Cardiol.* 2005;96:283–290.

Gurvitz MZ, Inkelas M, Lee M, et al. Changes in hospitalization patterns among patients with congenital heart disease during the transition from adolescence to adulthood. *J Am Coll Cardiol.* 2007;49:875–882.

Hagens VE, Crijns HJ, Van Veldhuisen DJ, et al, RAte Control versus Electrical cardioversion (RACE) for Persistent Atrial Fibrillation Study Group. Rate control versus rhythm control for patients with persistent atrial fibrillation with mild to moderate heart failure: results from the RAte Control versus Electrical cardioversion (RACE) study. *Am Heart J.* 2005;149:1106–1111.

Hassan W, Malik S, Akhras N, et al. Long-term results (up to 18 years) of balloon angioplasty on systemic hypertension in adolescent and adult patients with coarctation of the aorta. *Clin Cardiol.* 2007;30:75–80.

Hoffman JI, Kaplan S, Liberthson RR. Prevalence of congenital heart disease. *Am Heart J.* 2004;147:425–439.

Holmes KW, Lehmann CU, Dalal D, et al. Progressive dilation of the ascending aorta in children with isolated bicuspid aortic valve. *Am J Cardiol.* 2007;99:978–983.

Johnson NF. *Two's Company, Three Is Complexity: A Simple Guide to the Science of All Sciences.* Oxford: Oneworld Publications; 2007.

Kass DA. Ventricular arterial stiffening: integrating the pathophysiology. *Hypertension.* 2005;46:185–193.

Khairy P, Mackie AS, Ionescu-Ittu R, et al. Changing age distribution of death in congenital heart disease from 1988 to 2005: a population based study [abstract]. *J Am Coll Cardiol.* 2007;49(suppl. 1):268A.

Kostis JB. Treating hypercholesterolemia and hypertension based on lifetime global risk. *Am J Cardiol.* 2007;100:138–142.

Lam YY, Kaya MG, Li W, et al. Effect of chronic afterload increase on left ventricular myocardial function in patients with congenital left-sided obstructive lesions. *Am J Cardiol.* 2007;99:1582–1587.

Little WC. Diastolic dysfunction beyond distensibility: adverse effects of ventricular dilatation. *Circulation.* 2005;112:2888–2890.

Mackie AS, Ionescu-Ittu R, Therrien J, et al. Children and adults with congenital heart disease lost to follow-up: who and when? A population-based study [abstract]. *J Am Coll Cardiol.* 2007;49(suppl. 1):268A.

Marelli AJ, Mackie AS, Ionescu-Ittu R, et al. Congenital heart disease in the general population: changing prevalence and age distribution. *Circulation.* 2007;115:163–172.

Mersich B, Studinger P, Lenard Z, et al. Transposition of great arteries is associated with increased carotid artery stiffness. *Hypertension.* 2006;47: 1197–1202.

Moons P, Van Deyk K, Dedroog D, et al. Prevalence of cardiovascular risk factors in adults with congenital heart disease. *Eur J Cardiovasc Prev Rehabil.* 2006;13:612–616.

Nkomo VT, Gardin JM, Skelton TN, et al. Burden of valvular heart diseases: a population-based study. *Lancet.* 2006;368:1005–1011.

Nieminen HP, Jokinen EV, Sairanen HI. Causes of late deaths after pediatric cardiac surgery: a population-based study. *J Am Coll Cardiol.* 2007;50:1263–1271.

Nieminen HP, Jokinen EV, Sairanen HI. Late results of pediatric cardiac surgery in Finland: a population-based study with 96% follow-up. *Circulation.* 2001;104:570–575.

Niwa K, Perloff JK, Webb GD, et al. Survey of specialized tertiary care facilities for adults with congenital heart disease. *Int J Cardiol.* 2004;96:211–216.

Ohuchi H, Watanabe K, Kishiki K, et al. Heart rate dynamics during and after exercise in postoperative congenital heart disease patients: their relation to cardiac autonomic nervous activity and intrinsic sinus node dysfunction. *Am Heart J.* 2007;154:165–171.

O'Rourke MF, Hashimoto J. Mechanical factors in arterial aging: a clinical perspective. *J Am Coll Cardiol.* 2007;50:1–13.

Ou P, Celermajer DS, Mousseaux E, et al. Vascular remodeling after "successful" repair of coarctation: impact of aortic arch geometry. *J Am Coll Cardiol.* 2007;49:883–890.

Osranek M, Bursi F, Bailey KR, et al. Left atrial volume predicts cardiovascular events in patients originally diagnosed with lone atrial fibrillation: three-decade follow-up. *Eur Heart J.* 2005;26:2556–2561.

Owan TE, Hodge DO, Herges RM, et al. Trends in prevalence and outcome of heart failure with preserved ejection fraction. *N Engl J Med.* 2006;355:251–259.

Packer M. How should we judge the efficacy of drug therapy in patients with chronic congestive heart failure? The insights of six blind men. *J Am Coll Cardiol.* 1987;9:433–438.

Pasipoularides A, Shu M, Shah A, et al. RV instantaneous intraventricular diastolic pressure and velocity distributions in normal and volume overload awake dog disease models. Am J Physiol. 2003;285:H1956–H1965 [erratum in: *Am J Physiol.* 2004;56:H2367].

Rossano JW, Smith EO, Fraser CD Jr, et al. Adults undergoing cardiac surgery at a children's hospital: an analysis of perioperative morbidity. *Ann Thorac Surg.* 2007;83:606–612.

Rovner A, Smith R, Greenberg NL, et al. Improvement in diastolic intraventricular pressure gradients in patients with HOCM after ethanol septal reduction. *Am J Physiol.* 2003;285:H2492–H2499.

Sabet HY, Edwards WD, Tazelaar HD, et al. Congenitally bicuspid aortic valves: a surgical pathology study of 542 cases (1991 through 1996) and a literature review of 2,715 additional cases. *Mayo Clin Proc* 1999;74:14–26.

Seward JB, Chandrasekaran K, Osranek M, et al. Invasive physiology: clinical cardiovascular pathophysiology and diastolic dysfunction. In: Klein AL, Garcia MJ, eds. *Diastolic Heart Failure.* Philadelphia: Elsevier; 2007.

Sundquist K, Li X, Hemminki K. Familial risk of ischemic and hemorrhagic stroke: a large-scale study of the Swedish population. *Stroke* 2006;37: 1668–1673.

Tan JL, Prati D, Gatzoulis MA, et al. The right ventricular response to high afterload: comparison between atrial switch procedure, congenitally corrected transposition of the great arteries, and idiopathic pulmonary arterial hypertension. *Am Heart J* 2007;153:681–688.

The sixth report of the Joint National Committee on Prevention, Detection, Evaluation, and Treatment of High Blood Pressure. *Arch Intern Med* 1997;157:2413-2446 [erratum in: *Arch Intern Med* 1998;158:573].

Topaz O, DeMarchena EJ, Perin E, et al. Anomalous coronary arteries: angiographic findings in 80 patients. *Int J Cardiol.* 1992;34:129–138.

Virmani R, Burke AP, Farb A. Sudden cardiac death. *Cardiovasc Pathol.* 2001;10:211–218.

Walsh EP, Cecchin F. Arrhythmias in adult patients with congenital heart disease. *Circulation.* 2007;115:534–545.

Warnes CA, Liberthson R, Danielson GK, et al. Task Force 1: the changing profile of congenital heart disease in adult life. *J Am Coll Cardiol.* 2001;37:1170–1175.

Whitehead KK, Pekkan K, Kitajima HD, et al. Nonlinear power loss during exercise in single-ventricle patients after the Fontan: insights from computational fluid dynamics. *Circulation.* 2007;116(suppl.):I-165–I-171.

Yotti R, Bermejo J, Antoranz JC, et al. A noninvasive method for assessing impaired diastolic suction in patients with dilated cardiomyopathy. *Circulation.* 2005;112:2921–2929.

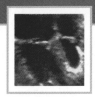

Chapter 36
Evaluation of the Adult With Transposition After Atrial Switch Operation

Frank Cetta • David J. Driscoll • Benjamin W. Eidem

In the current era, the vast majority of infants born with complete transposition of the great arteries (d-TGA) undergo an arterial switch operation soon after birth. The success of this procedure has obviated the need for the right ventricle (RV) to function as a systemic ventricle. However, the majority of patients operated on before 1985 underwent other procedures that resulted in a lifelong commitment of the RV to function as the systemic pump. It is important for the echocardiographer to appreciate the nuances of these techniques when evaluating long-term outcome of these patients. This chapter will be devoted to the evaluation of the adult with d-TGA after an atrial switch (Mustard or Senning) operation. A historical perspective of the evolution of surgery for d-TGA follows.

The evolution of the surgical treatment of complete d-TGA is an important and fascinating story of humans' ingenuity in dealing with a lethal congenital anomaly. Although survival of patients with d-TGA beyond infancy if associated with atrial (ASDs) and/or ventricular septal defects (VSDs) was possible without operation, the majority of patients with d-TGA died in infancy. Those rare infants who survived did so with significant exercise limitation and the morbidity and mortality associated with erythrocythemia and Eisenmenger syndrome. The earliest operation described for d-TGA was the creation of an ASD by Blalock and Hanlon in 1950. This ingenious operation preceded the introduction of the heart-lung machine and was performed on the beating heart. This operation had a relatively high mortality because these infants were very ill and usually quite acidotic. However, it resulted in survival beyond infancy. In 1956, Baffes described a partial repair of d-TGA. The "Baffes" procedure involved connecting the inferior vena cava (IVC) to the left atrium and connecting the right pulmonary veins to the right atrium. Subsequently, Senning (1959) described rerouting of the system and pulmonary venous return that resulted in complete separation of the pulmonary and systemic venous returns. This was accomplished by using right atrial and atrial septal tissue to construct a baffle. In 1964, in a single case report, Mustard described a similar operation using synthetic material that also resulted in complete separation of the pulmonary and system venous returns. However, both atrial switch operations resulted in the RV remaining as the systemic ventricle. Although the "Mustard" operation had the same end result of the "Senning" operation, the former was more popular in the United States. From 1959 to 1975, the Senning and Mustard operations were the mainstay of "physiologic correction" operations for patients with d-TGA and an intact ventricular septum.

In 1975, Jatene and colleagues resurrected the concept of *anatomic* repair of d-TGA and described a number of successful arterial switch procedures. Since the early 1980s, the arterial switch operation has been the operation of choice for patients with d-TGA with or without VSD but without significant pulmonary valve stenosis. In the current era, the Senning and Mustard operations are rarely performed, usually only for patients who are not candidates for an arterial switch or Rastelli procedure. In the late 1970s and early 1980s, the operative mortality for the Senning and Mustard operations actually was lower than that for the Jatene procedure. However, it was anticipated that the operative mortality for the Jatene procedure would decline significantly as surgeons gained experience with the operation and that the long-term results for the Jatene operation would be superior to those of the Senning and Mustard operations. Time has proved that both of these assumptions are true.

The quest for an operation to replace the Senning or Mustard procedure was spurred on because of the long-term complications inherent to these operations. The complications included superior vena cava (SVC) or IVC obstruction (reported in 15% of patients), pulmonary vein obstruction (reported in 5% of patients), arrhythmias,

and right ventricular (systemic ventricle) failure. Systemic ventricular failure and some serious arrhythmias may be amenable only to cardiac transplantation or, very rarely, conversion of the Mustard/Senning to an arterial switch procedure. Cardiac transplantation is costly and is associated with significant mid and long-term morbidity and mortality. Conversion to an arterial switch usually requires banding of the pulmonary artery to prepare the left ventricle (LV). Both the pulmonary banding procedure and the arterial switch operation in these adult patients are associated with significant mortality and the long-term outcome is poorly understood. The late arterial switch has generally been abandoned in adult patients.

Patients who underwent an atrial switch operation (Senning or Mustard) operation for d-TGA encounter unique problems as they enter adulthood. Overall, approximately 80% are alive and generally doing well at 20 years postprocedure. Problems in adulthood include atrial arrhythmia (present in greater than 50%), systemic and pulmonary venous baffle obstruction, and deterioration of the systemic RV. Systemic baffle obstruction is more common after the Mustard operation (SVC is more common than IVC). Pulmonary venous baffle obstruction is more common after the Senning operation. These problems can usually be managed in the cardiac catheterization laboratory with intravascular stent placement or during hybrid minimally invasive surgical/intravascular stent placement procedures. Functional assessment of the systemic RV is challenging and fraught with measurement pitfalls and undependable geometric assumptions. Historically, clinicians have depended on a visual "gestalt" of right ventricular systolic function rather than rigorous quantitation of ejection fraction. Newer techniques to assess function may offer previously unavailable quantitation of systemic RV function.

ASSESSMENT OF THE ADULT AFTER ATRIAL SWITCH OPERATION

After atrial switch operation, not all portions of the systemic venous and pulmonary venous pathways can be visualized in one acoustic window. Standard subcostal, parasternal, apical, and suprasternal windows are used to evaluate these pathways after the Mustard or Senning operation. However, since the vast majority of these patients are currently adults, the subcostal window may have limited utility. Gross visual assessment of right ventricular systolic function should be performed from as many of these windows as available in a given patient. Parasternal long- and short-axis images will typically demonstrate a flattened ventricular septum and a "D"-shaped LV, since the RV is the systemic pump (Fig. 36.1, A and B). The tricuspid regurgitation spectral Doppler signal in these patients represents systemic ventricular pressure and does not indicate pulmonary hypertension. In the apical projection, one can assess the pulmonary venous pathway. This pathway is divided by the SVC systemic venous baffle into a posterior chamber that receives the pulmonary veins and an anterior "right atrium" chamber that contains the inlet of the tricuspid valve. The term "pulmonary venous atrium" is used to describe one or both of these chambers after atrial switch operation. The anatomic connection of the pulmonary veins to the native left atrium is not disturbed during an atrial switch procedure. The flow from the pulmonary veins travels anteriorly and laterally over the SVC baffle to access the tricuspid valve. The complexity of the course of the systemic venous baffles and their relationship to the pulmonary venous flow explains why multiple acoustic windows are needed to fully assess these patients.

The apical four-chamber window provides an excellent assessment of RV dilation and tricuspid regurgitation (Fig. 36.1, C and D). In addition, the pulmonary venous and systemic venous baffles can

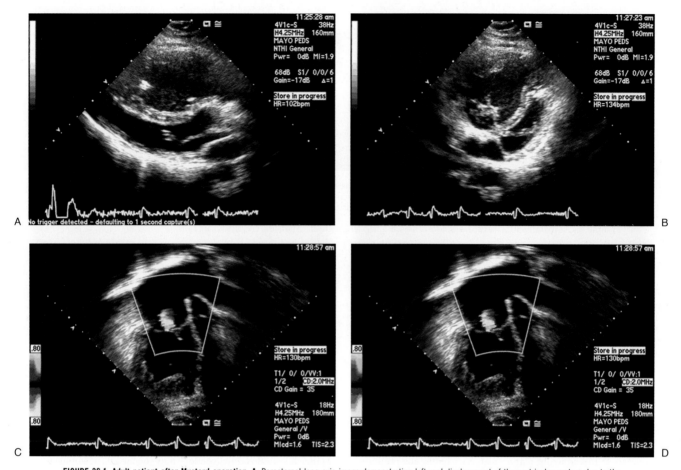

FIGURE 36.1. Adult patient after Mustard operation. A: Parasternal long-axis image demonstrating leftward displacement of the ventricular septum due to the systemic right ventricular (RV) dilation. **B:** Parasternal short-axis image in the same patient demonstrating a "D"-shaped left ventricle (LV) as a result of septal flattening caused by the systemic systolic pressure in the right ventricle. **C:** Apical four-chamber image demonstrating RV dilation in this patient. Varying severity of RV systolic dysfunction is present in these adult patients. **D:** Mild tricuspid regurgitation in the same patient. Progressive tricuspid regurgitation may become a problem as RV systolic dysfunction progresses.

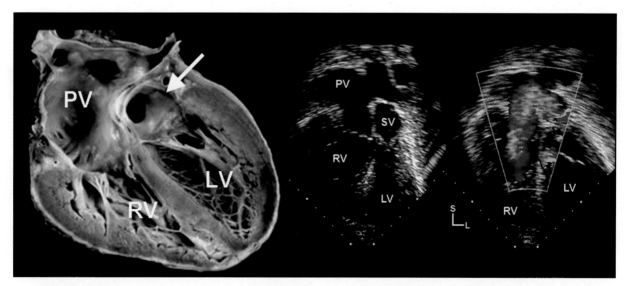

FIGURE 36.2. Pulmonary venous pathway after atrial switch operation in d-TGA. Left: Pathologic specimen cut to demonstrate the pulmonary venous pathway (PV) after atrial switch operation. A small portion of the systemic venous baffle (*arrow*) is demonstrated just above the mitral valve. **Middle:** Apical four-chamber image demonstrating similar anatomy. SV, systemic venous baffle. **Right:** Color Doppler demonstrates laminar flow from the pulmonary veins to the right atrium.

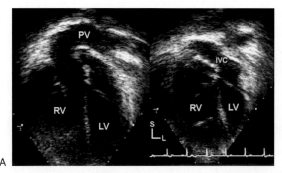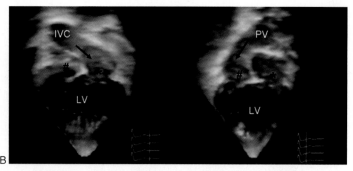

FIGURE 36.3. Systemic venous pathway (IVC) after atrial switch procedure in d-TGA. A: Tilting into a true apical four-chamber view from the more posterior pulmonary venous pathway (PV) (**left**), one can now adequately assess the inferior vena cava (IVC) portion of the systemic venous baffle (**right**). The superior vena cava portion of the systemic venous baffle is not easily visualized in the four-chamber projection. Sometimes the SVC baffle can be partially visualized if one rotates clockwise and tilts anteriorly into the left ventricular outflow tract (LVOT) view. **B:** Three-dimensional images from the apical four-chamber projection demonstrate the PV (**right**) and the IVC baffle (**left**). The relative positions of the right atrium (#) and left atrium (**asterisk**) are noted in each panel.

be assessed from this window. If one begins the scan tilted slightly posterior, the pulmonary venous pathway is readily visualized in most patients (Fig. 36.2). Tilting just anteriorly from the pulmonary venous baffle (returning to a true four-chamber view), so that the mitral valve leaflets are visualized, permits assessment of the IVC portion of the systemic venous baffle (Fig. 36.3). Remembering that the apical four-chamber image is oriented in a posterior plane from superior to apical, the IVC baffle is visualized when the mitral leaflets are seen. Conversely, if one rotates clockwise and tilts slightly anterior into an LV outflow tract view, then sometimes the SVC portion of the systemic venous baffle may come into view. The SVC baffle is best evaluated from the parasternal long-axis projection with medial tilt of the transducer (Fig. 36.4). The portion of the pulmonary venous pathway that is posterior to the SVC baffle can also be evaluated in this imaging plane. If an SVC baffle obstruction is present, the suprasternal notch or high right parasternal views may be helpful to obtain a gradient.

Echocardiography plays an important role in the evaluation of systemic and pulmonary venous baffle obstructions in patients after atrial switch operation. Pulmonary venous pathway obstruction can be detected from the apical four-chamber window (Fig. 36.5). Fig. 36.6 demonstrates an adult who had successful resolution of IVC baffle obstruction with placement of an intravascular stent. The IVC baffle stent is well visualized in the apical four-chamber projec-

tion (Fig. 36.6, A and B). Conversely, relieving pulmonary venous baffle obstruction is technically very challenging in the interventional cardiac catheterization laboratory. Either a transseptal or retrograde aortic approach is needed to access the area of pulmonary venous pathway stenosis. Frequently, stent placement in this region is quite difficult due to the circuitous course of the delivery sheath. Newer hybrid techniques using minimally invasive surgical approaches offer much promise for these patients (Figs. 36.7 and 36.8).

Residual atrial level shunts occur rarely in atrial switch patients and these shunts are usually small. Color Doppler assessment of the pulmonary and systemic venous pathways can demonstrate these shunts. However, since no true atrial septum is present in these patients, the residual shunts, if small, may not be readily apparent with surface echocardiography. Dynamic left ventricular (pulmonary ventricle) outflow obstruction may occur in postoperative atrial switch patients. The obstruction is frequently due to subvalvular fibromuscular obstruction, but valvular pulmonary stenosis also occurs. The morphologic LV is designed inherently to be a high-pressure pump and usually tolerates the left ventricular outflow tract (LVOT) obstruction without significant consequence. Any gradient across the LVOT can usually be evaluated from the apical window when one rotates clockwise into an outflow projection. A small portion of patients who had a late (after 1 year of age) atrial switch or an associated VSD may have pulmonary vascular obstructive disease in adulthood. In these patients, the mitral valve regurgitation signal is useful to evaluate pulmonary ventricle systolic pressure. If left ventricular systolic pressure is elevated, one needs to ensure that LVOT or pulmonary venous pathway obstruction is not present.

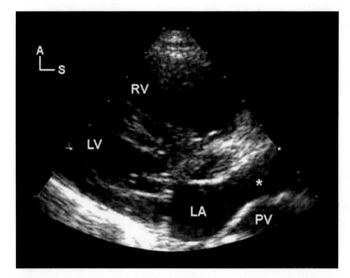

FIGURE 36.4. Parasternal long-axis image demonstrating the superior vena cava (asterisk) portion of the systemic venous baffle as it enters the left atrium (LA). A portion of the pulmonary venous pathway (PV) is also visualized in this image.

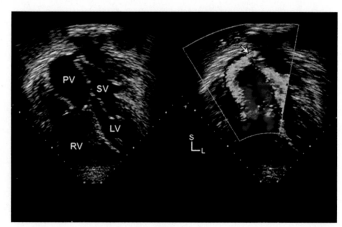

FIGURE 36.5. Apical four-chamber two-dimensional and color Doppler assessment of a patient after Senning operation with significant pulmonary venous pathway (PV) obstruction (*arrow*). The proximal systemic venous baffle (SV) is also visualized.

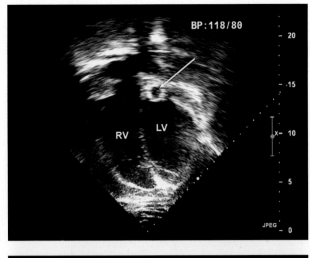
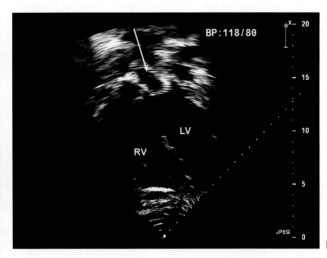

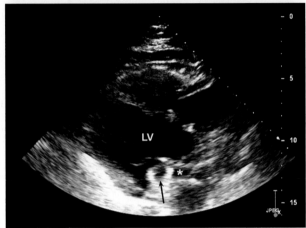

FIGURE 36.6. Stent placement after a Mustard operation with history of IVC baffle obstruction. **A:** Posteriorly tilted apical four-chamber image of a stent (*arrow*) in the inferior vena cava (IVC) baffle. A short-axis view of the proximal stent is visualized in this image. **B:** When one tilts anteriorly to a true apical image, the stent's length (*arrow*) becomes apparent. **C:** Parasternal long-axis image in the same patient demonstrating the IVC stent (arrow) projecting into the systemic venous atrium. A portion of the superior vena cava baffle (*asterisk*) is also visualized in this image.

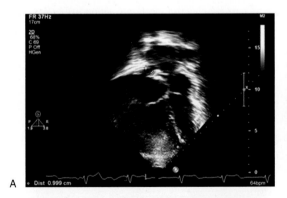
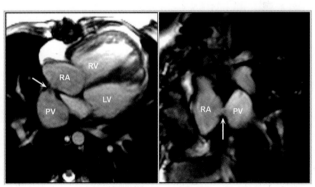

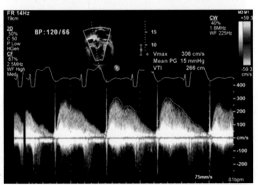

FIGURE 36.7. After a Senning operation, this patient developed pulmonary hypertension due to pulmonary venous pathway obstruction. A: Two-dimensional image from the apical four-chamber projection while tilting the transducer posteriorly. The obstruction is clearly identified measuring less than 1 cm. **B:** Magnetic resonance images in the same patient identifying the obstruction (*arrow*) between the pulmonary venous (PV) portion of the pathway and the native right atrium (RA). **C:** Continuous-wave Doppler assessment of the mean gradient (15 mm Hg) across the pulmonary venous pathway obstruction measured in the same projection as in **A**.

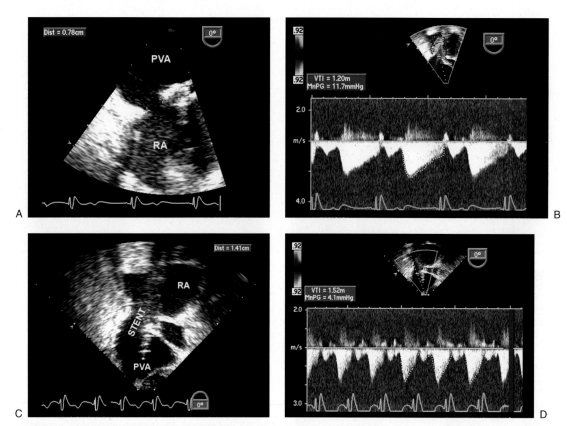

FIGURE 36.8. Intraoperative transesophageal echocardiographic images performed during a hybrid minimally invasive surgery to place a stent in a pulmonary venous pathway obstruction. A: Two-dimensional image demonstrating severe narrowing (8 mm) of the pathway between the pulmonary venous atrium (PVA) and the native right atrium (RA). **B:** *Before stent placement*, continuous-wave Doppler velocity profile demonstrating a mean gradient of 12 mm Hg between the pulmonary venous atrium (PVA) and the native right atrium (RA). **C:** Two-dimensional image status *post placement of a stent* across the stenosis between the pulmonary venous atrium (PVA) and the native right atrium (RA). Pulmonary venous pathway diameter equals 14 mm with the stent deployed. **D:** *After stent placement*, continuous-wave Doppler velocity profile across the pulmonary venous pathway stent. Residual mean gradient equals only 4 mm Hg.

NOVEL TECHNIQUES FOR THE FUNCTIONAL ASSESSMENT OF THE SYSTEMIC RIGHT VENTRICLE

Both the anatomic structure and the physiologic demands of the normal RV and LV are significantly different. Right ventricular chamber geometry is complex with both inlet (sinus) and outlet (conus or infundibulum) components and a contraction pattern that favors longitudinal over radial shortening. Despite the presence of equal right and left ventricular cardiac outputs in the normal circulation, right ventricular physiology is also quite distinct from that of the LV as these ventricles pump to a very different vascular bed. As a result, a different pressure-volume relationship exists and right ventricular external work is approximately 25% of left ventricular work (Fig. 36.9).

Chronic alterations in ventricular loading conditions impart adverse effects on right ventricular performance in the setting of the systemic RV. While many echocardiographic modalities are available to quantitatively evaluate left ventricular systolic and diastolic function, a much more limited armamentarium exists to similarly evaluate right ventricular function (Tables 36.1 and 36.2). In fact, in the clinical setting, the most common approach to the echocardiographic evaluation of right ventricular systolic function is a qualitative visual approach. While three-dimensional echocardiography and cardiac magnetic resonance imaging (MRI) offer a reliable quantitative measure of right ventricular volume and ejection fraction, these modalities are not always readily available. However, they do have distinct advantages over two-dimensional and Doppler echocardiographic approaches, particularly in adults with congenital heart disease and limited transthoracic windows.

Traditional measures of right ventricular function such as fractional area change and ejection fraction are limited because of the complex geometry of the RV. Doppler measures of right ventricular inflow and outflow also may provide valuable information on the systolic and diastolic performance of the RV but are significantly

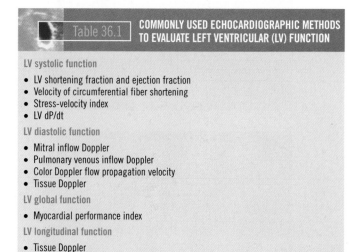

Table 36.1	COMMONLY USED ECHOCARDIOGRAPHIC METHODS TO EVALUATE LEFT VENTRICULAR (LV) FUNCTION

LV systolic function

- LV shortening fraction and ejection fraction
- Velocity of circumferential fiber shortening
- Stress-velocity index
- LV dP/dt

LV diastolic function

- Mitral inflow Doppler
- Pulmonary venous inflow Doppler
- Color Doppler flow propagation velocity
- Tissue Doppler

LV global function

- Myocardial performance index

LV longitudinal function

- Tissue Doppler

LV regional function

- Strain and strain rate imaging
- Myocardial twist and torsion

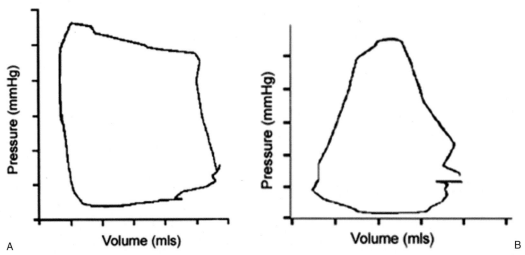

FIGURE 36.9. Pressure-volume relationship of the normal right and left ventricle. Note that the left ventricle **(A)** is a "square wave" pump whose filling and ejection patterns differ significantly from those of the right ventricle. Right ventricular (RV) ejection occurs early during ventricular pressure rise and continues beyond the development of peak RV pressure. **(B)** The relative proportion of left ventricular versus RV work is calculated by measuring the area of each of these pressure volume relationships. (Reprinted with permission from: Redington AN. Right ventricular function. *Cardiol Clin.* 2002;20:341–349.)

influenced by changes in right ventricular filling with respiration. One important Doppler finding, however, that is often helpful in the assessment of right ventricular diastolic function is the presence of antegrade diastolic forward flow into the main pulmonary artery in diastole (Fig. 36.10). Measured with pulsed-wave Doppler distal to the pulmonary valve, this Doppler pattern suggests a "stiff" RV with decreased ventricular compliance. This Doppler pattern may occasionally be present in the normal circulation but is low in velocity (<10 cm/sec) and is not typically present throughout the respiratory cycle. In contrast, patients with a restrictive noncompliant RV have a higher Doppler velocity (>20 cm/sec) that is characteristically present throughout the respiratory cycle.

Additional Doppler measures have been clinically useful to evaluate global and longitudinal right ventricular function in the setting of congenital heart disease with a systemic RV. The myocardial performance index (MPI) incorporates both systolic and diastolic components of right ventricular function and has been shown to be a valuable clinical parameter to serially follow in these patients. Similarly, tricuspid annular plane systolic excursion TAPSE and tissue Doppler imaging (TDI) have provided valuable insights into

longitudinal right ventricular performance in patients with congenital heart disease. In particular, isovolumic acceleration (IVA) has been shown to be a clinically robust measure of right ventricular contractile function that is relatively independent of loading conditions. These more novel Doppler measurements, however, are limited by their angle dependence as well as the impact of cardiac motion and tethering on these velocities.

Recent developments in imaging technology now enable the echocardiographic evaluation of regional myocardial function as well as myocardial twist and torsion with strain and strain rate imaging. Clinical studies in patients with congenitally corrected transposition of the great arteries (CC-TGA) have demonstrated decreased right ventricular global strain and strain rate in a small number of patients with qualitatively normal right ventricular systolic function (Fig. 36.11). A recent study in asymptomatic patients with d-TGA after Senning repair demonstrated distinct changes in right ventricular mechanics and performance in this cohort. Interestingly, the systemic RV had a deformation pattern more similar to the normal LV rather than the normal RV with a shift from longitudinal to circumferential shortening (Fig. 36.12). In addition, there was an almost complete absence of both rotation and global torsion in these systemic RVs (Fig. 36.13). While some changes in the systemic RV appeared to be "adaptive" to the chronic alteration in ventricular load, the lack of myocardial rotation and torsion, coupled with decreases in systolic strain and strain rate, suggests the presence of myocardial

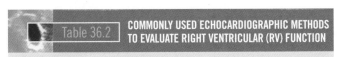

Table 36.2 | **COMMONLY USED ECHOCARDIOGRAPHIC METHODS TO EVALUATE RIGHT VENTRICULAR (RV) FUNCTION**

RV systolic function

- RV fractional area change and ejection fraction
- Three-dimensional echocardiography
- RV dP/dt

RV diastolic function

- Tricuspid inflow Doppler
- Hepatic venous inflow Doppler
- RV outflow tract Doppler
- Tissue Doppler

RV global function

- Myocardial performance index

RV longitudinal function

- Tissue Doppler
- Tricuspid annular plane systolic excursion TAPSE

RV regional function

- Strain and strain rate imaging
- Myocardial twist and torsion

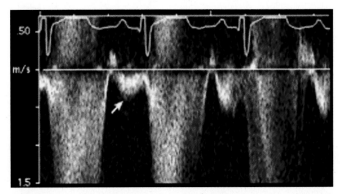

FIGURE 36.10. Restrictive right ventricular (RV) filling in postoperative tetralogy of Fallot. Parasternal short-axis scan with pulsed-wave Doppler interrogation in the main pulmonary artery. Note the antegrade forward flow (*arrow*) into the pulmonary artery with atrial contraction. This Doppler pattern is consistent with decreased RV compliance.

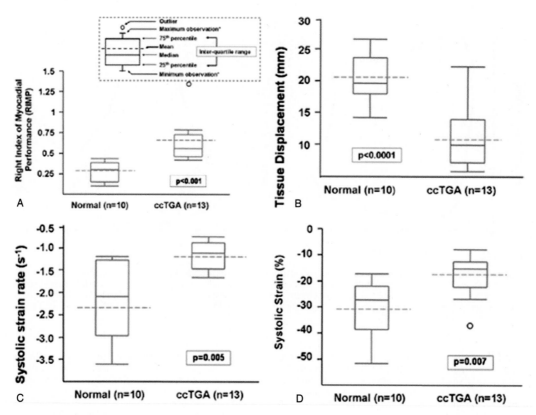

FIGURE 36.11. Evaluation of systemic right ventricular (RV) performance in patients with congenitally corrected transposition of the great arteries (CC-TGA). Note the decreased systolic strain and strain rate in CC-TGA patients compared with control subjects. In addition, an increased RV myocardial performance index and decreased tissue Doppler displacement are consistent with impaired RV function in this cohort. (Reprinted with permission from: Bos JM, Hagler DJ, Silvilairat S, et al. Right ventricular function in asymptomatic individuals with a systemic right ventricle. *J Am Soc Echocardiogr.* 2006;19:1033–1037.)

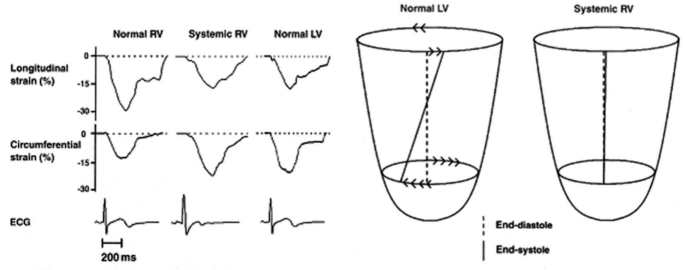

FIGURE 36.12. Right ventricular (RV) strain in the normal right and left ventricles and in patients with transposition of the great arteries (d-TGA). Note the significant change in the strain pattern in the systemic right ventricle to one more similar to a normal left ventricle versus the normal RV pattern of deformation. (Reprinted with permission from Pettersen E, Helle-Valle T, Edvardsen T, et al. Contraction pattern of the systemic right ventricle. *J Am Coll Cardiol.* 2007;49:2450–2456.)

FIGURE 36.13. Ventricular rotation in the normal left ventricle (LV) and the systemic right ventricle (RV). The normal LV has clockwise basal rotation and counterclockwise apical rotation that result in ventricular torsion. Note the absence of basal and apical rotation in the systemic RV, resulting in absence of ventricular torsion in this cohort. (Reprinted with permission from Pettersen E, Helle-Valle T, Edvardsen T, et al. Contraction pattern of the systemic right ventricle. *J Am Coll Cardiol.* 2007;49:2450–2456.)

dysfunction in these apparently "normally" functioning ventricles. Ongoing functional evaluation with these novel echocardiographic modalities as well as cardiac MRI will continue to offer additional important insights into ventricular mechanics in patients with a systemic RV.

SUGGESTED READING

Baffes TJ. A new method for surgical correction of transposition of the aorta and pulmonary artery. *Surg Gynec Obstet.* 1956;102:227.

Blalock A, Hanlon C. The surgical treatment of complete transposition of the aorta and the pulmonary artery. *Surg Gynecol Obstet.* 1950;90:1.

Bos JM, Hagler DJ, Silvilairat S, et al. Right ventricular function in asymptomatic individuals with a systemic right ventricle. *J Am Soc Echocardiogr.* 2006;19:1033–1037.

Ebenroth ES, Hurwitz RA. Long-term functional outcome of patients following the Mustard procedure. *Congenit Heart Dis.* 2007;2:235–241.

Jatene A, Fontes V, Paulista P, et al. Successful anatomic correction of transposition of the great vessels: a preliminary report. *ARQ Bras Cardiol.* 1975;28:461–464.

Mustard WT. Successful two-stage correction of transposition of the great vessels. *Surgery.* 1964;55:469–472.

Pettersen E, Helle-Valle T, Edvardsen T, et al. Contraction pattern of the systemic right ventricle. *J Am Coll Cardiol.* 2007;49:2450–2456.

Redington AN. Right ventricular function. *Cardiol Clin.* 2002;20:341–349.

Senning A. Surgical correction of transposition of the great arteries. *Surgery.* 1959;45:966.

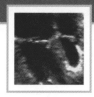

Chapter 37
Tetralogy of Fallot With Pulmonary Regurgitation

Naser M. Ammash

Advances in diagnostic techniques such as echocardiography, cardiac surgery, and anesthesia, as well as improvement in postoperative management, have undoubtedly contributed to the excellent long-term outcome of patients with tetralogy of Fallot (TOF) following surgical repair. However, these patients present unique challenges because of potential residua and sequelae with increasing duration of follow-up. Right ventricular (RV) outflow tract (RVOT) reconstruction often includes infundibular muscle resection, pulmonary valvotomy or valvectomy, and RV outflow augmentation and accounts for the most common long-term postoperative complications. Residual or recurrent RVOT obstruction and pulmonary regurgitation (PR) are important determinants of late morbidity, and the most common reason for reoperation. PR is primarily the result of the surgical ventriculotomy as well as extensive infundibulectomy and transannular patching of the RVOT at the time of surgical repair. This can often result in an RVOT aneurysm. Additional factors also contribute to the development and progression of PR, including (a) residual pulmonary valve (PV) abnormalities, (b) pulmonary annulus size, (c) peripheral pulmonary artery stenosis, (d) increased pulmonary vascular resistance, (e) RV diastolic dysfunction, (f) residual atrial and ventricular septal defects, and (g) acquired cardiovascular and pulmonary diseases including pulmonary hypertension, sleep apnea, systemic hypertension, chronic lung disease, and kyphoscoliosis. Although chronic PR can be tolerated for many years, when left uncorrected, it often leads to progressive RV enlargement and dysfunction, progressive tricuspid valve regurgitation, and eventual right heart failure. PR is also associated with the late development of left ventricular (LV) dysfunction and is recognized as the most important risk factor for atrial and ventricular tachyarrhythmias, as well as sudden death. Assessment of patients with PR following repair of TOF often includes an electrocardiogram, chest radiograph, echocardiogram, exercise testing, cardiac magnetic resonance imaging (MRI), and cardiac catheterization in select patients. This chapter will focus on the echocardiographic assessment of PR following the repair of TOF.

The components of a comprehensive two-dimensional and Doppler transthoracic echocardiographic examination in patients with repaired TOF are summarized in Table 37.1. Each component is essential in the evaluation of patients with TOF to determine outcome and the need for reintervention. In preparation for the echocardiographic examination, it is essential to review the surgical

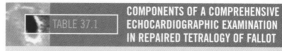

TABLE 37.1 COMPONENTS OF A COMPREHENSIVE ECHOCARDIOGRAPHIC EXAMINATION IN REPAIRED TETRALOGY OF FALLOT

1. Evaluate the etiology and severity of pulmonary regurgitation.
2. Identify residual right ventricular outflow tract obstruction and its level, cause(s), and severity.
3. Evaluate right ventricular size and systolic and diastolic function.
4. Assess the presence and severity of tricuspid regurgitation.
5. Rule out residual atrial or ventricular septal defects.
6. Evaluate left ventricular size and function.
7. Quantitate aortic root and ascending aortic dimensions.
8. Assess the presence and severity of aortic regurgitation.
9. Use Doppler echocardiography to estimate right ventricular systolic and pulmonary artery pressure.

records to obtain an accurate anatomic description of the repair. This ensures adequate understanding of the anatomic variability encountered in these patients and can be very useful as a guide for the echocardiographic examination.

ETIOLOGY AND SEVERITY OF PULMONARY REGURGITATION

PR following repair of TOF is commonly caused by resection of the PV at the time of surgical repair in combination with the concomitant ventriculotomy and transannular patching of the RVOT. These surgical interventions lead to enlargement of the PV annulus and progression to RVOT aneurysm and PR. Alternatively, pulmonary valvotomy, rather than valvectomy, is performed and may result in residual congenital PV abnormalities including stenosis and variable degrees of PR. Bicuspid PV is the most common congenital abnormality of the PV, with a reported incidence of up to 50%, followed by PV dysplasia or hypoplasia. TOF with absent PV occurs in 2% of patients and is associated with severe PR and massive enlargement

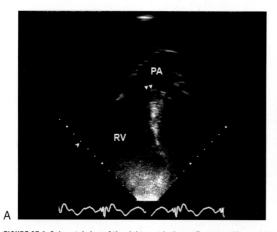
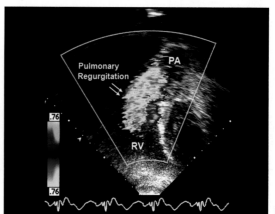

FIGURE 37.1. Subcostal view of the right ventricular outflow tract. Views without (**A**) and with (**B**) color flow Doppler demonstrate the absence of significant outflow tract obstruction (**A**) but severe pulmonary regurgitation.

of the pulmonary arteries. Optimal visualization of the RVOT is needed to assess the etiology and severity of PR. This is accomplished from the parasternal long- and short-axis views of the RVOT. At times, it is possible to image the RVOT from the apical four-chamber or subcostal windows with anterior angulation. These windows are very helpful in the adult patient with emphysema or in patients with poor parasternal windows (Figure 37.1).

Pulmonary valve regurgitation is characterized by abnormalities in the spectral and color flow Doppler analysis of the RVOT. The severity of PR can be semiquantitatively assessed by echocardiographic techniques detailed in Table 37.2.

Color flow Doppler assessment of PR can be qualitative or quantitative. The two most common qualitative signs of severe PR are the presence "free PR" and pulsation of the pulmonary arteries. It is not unusual in patients following TOF repair, and especially in those following PV valvectomy, to have "free" PR, whereby color flow Doppler demonstrates unobstructed bidirectional flow across the PV annulus. This severe regurgitation is often associated with vigorous pulsation of the main pulmonary artery and even the PA branches because of lower pulmonary artery diastolic pressure and a wider pulse pressure. The extent of the diastolic color flow signal caused by PR is often used as an indicator of its severity (Fig. 37.2). Brief flow reversal is normal in the branch pulmonary arteries in systole and early diastole because of the pulmonary artery geometry and differential branching of the right and left pulmonary arteries. This normal diastolic flow reversal is very limited in its duration and extent and is not associated with regurgitation into the right ventricle. On the other hand, the presence of persistent retrograde (>50% of the diastolic phase) PR flow in the branch pulmonary arteries that extends into the right ventricle is consistent with severe PR (Fig. 37.2B).

The RVOT area occupied by the regurgitant color flow Doppler signal can be used to assess PR severity. A PR area index, defined as the maximum area of the PR color jet on the parasternal short-axis imaging plane indexed to body surface area, has been shown to correlate well with the PR regurgitant fraction determined by angiography. Kobayashi demonstrated that the PR area index was 0.36 ± 0.29 in grade 1 angiographic PR, compared with 1.48 ± 0.46 in grade 2 and 2.80 ± 0.94 in grade 3 regurgitation. A significant positive linear correlation was observed between the two methods ($r = 0.84$, $p < 0.001$). However, this technique is limited by two-dimensional image quality, the direction of the PR jet, machine gain settings, and transducer frequency. Given the potential limitations of area measurement, Williams et al. suggested using a linear measurement to assess the severity of PR. The PR jet/annulus ratio is defined as the ratio of the PR color Doppler jet width to the PV annulus dimension in early diastole on the parasternal short-axis view. This ratio has been demonstrated to correlate well with angiographic PR grade. In a study of 26 patients with PR following TOF repair, a PR jet/annulus ratio of 0.4 or less correlated with less than 1+ angiographic PR. On the other hand, a PR jet/annulus ratio of 0.7 separated patients with 2+ from those with 3+ angiographic PR. There was a significant positive correlation between angiographic PR grade and the

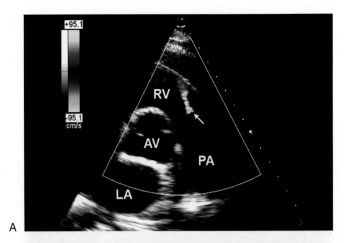

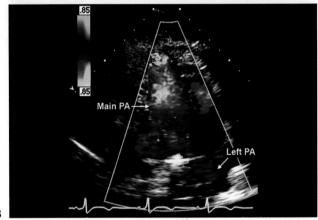

FIGURE 37.2. Parasternal short-axis view demonstrating diastolic color flow Doppler in the right ventricular (RV) outflow tract. The red jet represents (**A**) mild and (**B**) severe pulmonary regurgitation. Notice the difference in the width and extent of the color flow jet that is limited to the RV outflow tract in **A** but extends into the branch pulmonary arteries in **B**.

color jet/annulus ratio ($r = 0.95$, $p < 0.001$). In the same study, the presence or absence of diastolic flow reversal in the branch pulmonary arteries was assessed using pulsed-wave Doppler and/or color Doppler images in the parasternal short-axis view. Retrograde diastolic flow reversal was present in the branch pulmonary arteries in eight of nine patients with more than 2+ angiographic PR but in no patient who had less than 1+ angiographic PR. The positive and the negative predictive values of retrograde diastolic flow reversal in the branch pulmonary arteries for more than 2+ angiographic PR were 100% and 92%, respectively.

Other echocardiographic methods, including pulsed-wave and continuous-wave Doppler, have been used for the assessment of PR severity. Spectral Doppler assessment at the level of the PV in patients with PR demonstrates normal forward flow in systole and reversed flow in diastole (Fig. 37.3). In patients with less than severe PR, the diastolic flow reversal is holodiastolic (Fig. 37.3A) and its peak velocity is characteristically less than 1 m/s in the absence of pulmonary hypertension. The finding of a high-velocity regurgitant signal at end diastole suggests a large difference between pulmonary artery diastolic pressure and RV end-diastolic pressure. On the other hand, in the presence of severe PR, there is early termination of the diastolic flow reversal signal by pulsed- or continuous-wave Doppler assessment (Fig. 37.3B). The regurgitant diastolic velocity peaks early and decreases rapidly as the pressure difference between the pulmonary artery and right ventricle rapidly equilibrates.

This finding is not pathognomonic for severe PR since it is also observed in patients with elevated RV end-diastolic pressure caused by RV diastolic dysfunction, which is not uncommon following TOF repair. However, in the presence of RV diastolic dysfunction, an additional presystolic Doppler forward flow (Fig. 37.4) is often noted. This is the result of end-diastolic RV pressure being higher than the pulmonary artery end-diastolic pressure leading to forward

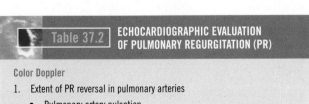

Table 37.2	ECHOCARDIOGRAPHIC EVALUATION OF PULMONARY REGURGITATION (PR)

Color Doppler
1. Extent of PR reversal in pulmonary arteries
   - Pulmonary artery pulsation
2. PR jet width
3. PR jet/annulus ratio

Spectral Doppler
1. PR index
2. PR pressure half-time

Additional techniques
1. PISA
2. Continuity equation
3. Vena contracta

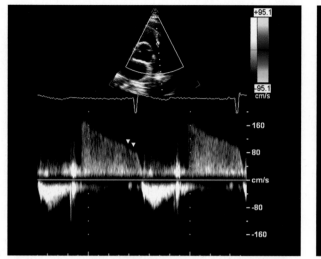

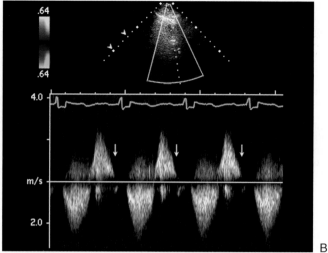

FIGURE 37.3. Continuous-wave Doppler signal at the level of the pulmonary valve in a patient with mild pulmonary valve regurgitation. A: Normal systolic forward flow and reversed flow that continues throughout diastole, indicating mild pulmonary valve regurgitation. The low end-diastolic velocity suggests normal pulmonary artery diastolic pressure. **B:** In patients with severe pulmonary regurgitation, the regurgitant diastolic velocity peaks early and decreases rapidly as pulmonary artery and right ventricular pressures rapidly equilibrate leading to early termination of the continuous-wave Doppler signal, with return of the PR Doppler signal to the baseline.

flow across the PV annulus in late diastole after atrial contraction. This finding helps differentiate RV diastolic dysfunction from isolated severe PR.

Using the continuous-wave PR Doppler signal, further quantification of PR severity can performed by measuring the PV regurgitation index or pressure half-time. Li et al. suggested measuring the ratio of the duration of the continuous-wave PR Doppler signal to total diastolic time (PV regurgitation index) (Fig. 37.5A). This Doppler-derived index correlated closely with cardiac MRI–derived regurgitant fraction ($r = -0.82$, $p < 0.01$) in a study of 53 consecutive patients with PR following TOF repair. Compared to cardiac MRI, a PR index of less than 0.77 had a 100% sensitivity and 85% specificity for identifying a PR fraction greater than 24.5%, with a predictive accuracy of 95%. This study also demonstrated that a PR jet width of greater than 0.98 cm had an accuracy of 90% in identifying the group with a PR fraction greater than 24.5% by MRI. These findings are in agreement with published reports suggesting that severe aortic regurgitation is associated with an LV outflow tract color jet width of greater than 1 cm. Using the same PR velocity profile by continuous-wave Doppler, the pressure half-time can be measured and used for the assessment of PR (Fig. 37.5B). PR pressure half-time was found to be inversely related to PR fraction in the absence of RVOT obstruction and RV diastolic dysfunction. In a prospective study of 34 adult patients with

repaired TOF, Silversides et al. demonstrated that the mean pressure half-time measurements were 181 ± 75 ms in patients with a regurgitant fraction of less than 20% by cardiac MRI and 102 ± 29 ms with a regurgitant fraction greater than 40%.

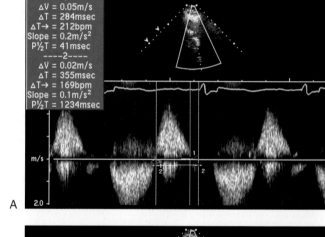

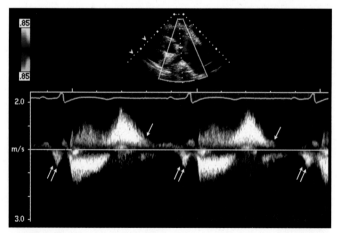

FIGURE 37.4. Assessment of right ventricular diastolic function in patients with pulmonary regurgitation following tetralogy of Fallot repair. Restrictive physiology leads to antegrade forward flow in the pulmonary artery during atrial pedraction (double arrows). This should be noted during all phases of respiration and on five consecutive beats.

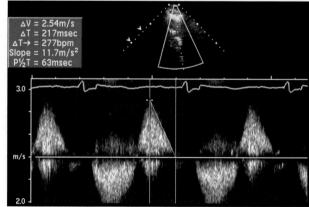

FIGURE 37.5. Continuous-wave Doppler signal across the right ventricular out flow tract demonstrating measurement of the pulmonary valve (PV) regurgitant index. Ratio of duration of the continuous-wave Doppler pulmonary regurgitation (PR) signal to total diastole (**A**) and pressure half-time for the assessment of PR severity (**B**).

A pressure half-time of less than 100 ms demonstrated a high sensitivity and specificity for detecting significant PR.

Additional echocardiographic techniques for the assessment of PR severity include (a) measurement of regurgitant volume, fraction, and effective regurgitant orifice by two-dimensional and color Doppler techniques such as the proximal isovelocity surface area (PISA) and the continuity equation and (b) measurement of the vena contracta. These techniques, however, are not as commonly used in the assessment of PR compared with the assessment of other valvular regurgitation. In addition, each of these techniques has significant limitations. The continuity equation, for example, requires quantitation of the difference between the total forward stroke volume calculated across the PV versus the normal cardiac output calculated across the aortic or tricuspid valve site. Measurement of the PV annular diameter, especially in postoperative patients, has inherent limitations and is subject to significant variability. The presence of tricuspid regurgitation and/or pulmonary stenosis can also affect the accuracy of these measurements. In addition, although PISA appears to be the most reliable method to assess regurgitant volume in patients with mitral and aortic regurgitation, PISA has not gained widespread use in patients with PR because the assumption of a hemispheric shape is not valid in most cases of PR in which flow rates and transorifice pressure gradients are especially low.

 ## RIGHT VENTRICULAR SIZE AND FUNCTION

The right ventricle in patients with TOF is inherently abnormal with significant hypertrophy and fibrosis that persists following surgical repair. Several additional preoperative and postoperative factors are known to contribute to the progressive RV enlargement and dysfunction, including significant tricuspid regurgitation, residual atrial or ventricular level shunts, and residual RVOT obstruction or pulmonary hypertension. RV size and function in repaired TOF are affected by the degree and duration of preoperative cyanosis and pressure overload, as well as factors related to the surgical repair itself including RV injury secondary to a ventriculotomy, possible coronary artery injury, myocardial injury from inadequate myocardial preservation, and transannular patching within the RVOT. All of these factors are important determinants of the adaptive response of the right ventricle to volume overload from chronic PR. As the right ventricle dilates in response to PR, its ejection fraction initially increases because of the increased ventricular volume. With time, the RV ejection fraction decreases and is a reflection of a decrease in myocardial performance of the volume-loaded right ventricle. Progressive deterioration of myocardial function eventually results in decreased stroke volume with further increases in RV end-systolic and end-diastolic volume In the current era, every effort is made to maintain PV competence at the time of surgical TOF repair in an attempt to prevent the potential long-term complications related to chronic PR. Current operative techniques often involve a combined transatrial and transpulmonary approach with a very limited RV incision, if needed, for patch augmentation of the RVOT and/or PV annulus. Under these circumstances, the use of a small stiff patch may provide a more superior hemodynamic result than a large expandable pericardial patch. This strategy may avoid significant PR at the expense of mild to moderate residual RVOT obstruction, which is usually well tolerated.

Assessment of RV size and function is a crucial component of the noninvasive evaluation of patients with repaired TOF. Unfortunately, most quantitative two-dimensional echocardiographic measurements of ventricular size and performance are based on the shape of the elliptical left ventricle; these geometric assumptions do not apply to the right ventricle. The right ventricle has a complex geometric shape with thinner walls and abundant coarse trabeculations that make endocardial border delineation challenging. The right ventricle appears to be crescent shaped in cross section and triangular in the lateral view. In addition, the RVOT is muscular and elongated, ending at the PV, which does not have a true bulbar annulus. These differences in ventricular morphology reflect the hemodynamically different roles of the two ventricles. In our practice, we rely heavily on serial side-by-side comparative assessment of RV size and function. Three-dimensional echocardiography promises an accurate determination of RV volume and function. This technique is currently time consuming and not in widespread clinical use.

Given the limitations as a result of RV geometry, many nongeometric Doppler indices have been proposed that use systolic and diastolic time intervals and tissue Doppler imaging to provide indirect information about RV systolic and diastolic function in repaired TOF.

The Doppler assessment of the instantaneous rate of RV pressure increase (dP/dt) can be measured from the tricuspid regurgitant continuous Doppler velocity profile. dP/dt is measured by calculating the rate of RV pressure gradient increase, for example, from 4 mm Hg (1 m/s) to 16 mm Hg (2 m/s). However, this index is sensitive to changes in afterload and does not accurately reflect RV systolic function in patients with residual RVOT obstruction or pulmonary hypertension.

Tissue Doppler imaging quantitates myocardial velocities. For RV assessment, these velocities are measured at the level of the tricuspid valve annulus near the insertion of the anterior tricuspid valve leaflet. These myocardial velocities are a marker of RV systolic and diastolic longitudinal motion. This relatively volume-independent echocardiographic velocity has been demonstrated to be reduced in patients with repaired TOF compared with controls. Similarly, using tissue Doppler methods, strain and strain rate indices have been used for quantification of regional RV function in patients after repair of TOF.

Another Doppler-derived quantitative index of global ventricular function is the right-sided myocardial performance index (MPI). This index incorporates both systolic and diastolic parameters and is reported to be a measure of global ventricular function. The RV MPI is measured by dividing the sum of RV isovolumic contraction time and isovolumic relaxation time by the ejection time across the PV. Normal values for the RV MPI have been reported in both children (0.32 ± 0.03) and adults (0.28 ± 0.04). This index has been reported to be a valuable noninvasive method to assess RV function in patients with pulmonary hypertension, as well as Ebstein anomaly and, most recently, in repaired TOF. A study by Abd El Rahman et al. suggested that the MPI is affected by the severity of PR as well as the presence of RV diastolic dysfunction in repaired patients with TOF. All patients with PR had a lower than normal isovolumic relaxation time, while those with severe PR also had a prolongation of isovolumic contraction time compared with patients with mild to moderate PR (103 ± 57 versus 27 ± 41 ms, $p < 0.01$). In addition, in the presence of a noncompliant right ventricle, the isovolumic relaxation time was shortened, paradoxically decreasing the RV MPI. Therefore, the sensitivity of the MPI in identifying RV dysfunction may be limited in repaired TOF. However, a recent study by Schwerzmann involving 57 adults with repaired TOF with significant PR demonstrated that an MPI of 0.4 or greater had a 81% sensitivity and a 85% specificity to identify patients with an RV ejection fraction of less than 35%. An MPI less than 0.25 had a 70% sensitivity and a 89% specificity to predict an RV ejection fraction of 50% or greater as determined by cardiac MRI. Yasuoka suggested the use of Doppler tissue imaging in the calculation of the MPI. Fifteen patients (6.3 ± 2.2 years old) with significant PR after TOF repair and 24 age-matched healthy children were analyzed. The MPI obtained by pulsed-wave Doppler was not different in patients with TOF repair compared with normal children (0.30 ± 0.12 versus 0.32 ± 0.07, $p > 0.05$). However, when measured by tissue Doppler imaging, the MPI was significantly greater in patients with TOF than in normal children (0.48 ± 0.07 versus 0.30 ± 0.07, $p < 0.0001$). Therefore, the authors suggest that the MPI measured by TDI is a more sensitive indicator of RV function in these patients and is a promising novel means of assessing global RV function in patients after TOF repair.

Recently, a novel easily reproducible Doppler measurement of systolic RV contractile function that is less dependent on loading conditions has been reported. The isovolumic acceleration index (IVA) is calculated by dividing the myocardial velocity during isovolumic contraction by the time interval from its onset to the time at peak velocity. Frigiola reported that IVA is useful in detecting early preclinical RV dysfunction before the onset of clinical symptoms and may therefore be helpful in determining the optimal timing of PV replacement (PVR). Systolic RV function was evaluated by IVA, peak systolic myocardial velocity, and strain in 124 patients (age, 21 ± 11 years) at a mean of 3.7 years after surgical repair. All of these parameters were noted to be reduced compared with normal controls. Patients with severe PR had a significantly lower isovolumic acceleration than those with mild or moderate PR (whereas systolic myocardial velocity and strain were not different between groups with varying severity of PR). Many of these echo-Doppler methods for assessment of systolic RV function have been used predominantly as research tools; however, their clinical application in the future appears promising.

RV diastolic dysfunction is particularly common in repaired patients with TOF, especially after transannular patch placement. In a study by Munkhammar et al., 47 patients with repaired TOF were evaluated by echocardiography. Restrictive RV physiology was identified by the presence of late diastolic antegrade flow in the pulmonary artery as shown in Fig. 37.4. Ten percent of patients repaired before 6 months of age demonstrated restrictive features at the time of noninvasive follow-up. RV diastolic dysfunction increased to 38% in patients with repair after 9 months of age. Approximately one third of patients with transannular patch repair demonstrated restrictive RV hemodynamics. The patients with restrictive RV hemodynamics had more severe preoperative pulmonary stenosis, were older at the time of TOF repair, and had a less severe degree of PR on serial echocardiographic follow-up. RV diastolic dysfunction is believed to play a protective role from the detrimental effect of severe PR in repaired TOF. RV diastolic dysfunction with elevation in RV diastolic pressure limits the duration of PR and subsequently the degree of RV dilatation. As a result, patients with severe PR and more restrictive RV physiology have smaller RV volume compared with those with severe PR and normal RV diastolic function. Therefore, assessment of RV diastolic function in patients with PR following TOF repair is an integral part of a comprehensive echocardiographic evaluation. However, antegrade late diastolic forward flow into the MPA may be present in normal subjects during inspiration and therefore should be noted in at least five consecutive beats.

The hepatic venous Doppler signal is also very helpful in the identification of RV diastolic dysfunction. Characteristic changes in this setting include higher diastolic forward velocity and a greater reversal of diastolic flow velocity with inspiration.

ADDITIONAL ECHOCARDIOGRAPHIC ASSESSMENT

The presence of residual infundibular, PV, and pulmonary artery branch stenosis, in association with PR, is not uncommon following repair of TOF. Peripheral pulmonary artery stenosis can result from pulmonary artery distortion by previous shunts, extension of the transannular patch to the branch PAs, or secondary to poorly developed distal pulmonary arteries. Downstream obstruction because of branch pulmonary stenosis has been shown to worsen the severity of PR. One important role of echocardiography is to identify and characterize the site and severity of RVOT obstruction. Once the site of obstruction is identified, its severity can be assessed with pulsed-wave and continuous-wave Doppler. Pulsed-wave Doppler should be used to measure flow velocity proximal to the level of obstruction (V_1), while the continuous-wave signal should be used to measure flow accelerating across the site of stenosis (V_2). The peak Doppler gradient across the stenosis is then calculated using the simplified Bernoulli equation with the peak gradient being $4 (V_2 - V_1)^2$. In addition, the Doppler-derived tricuspid regurgitant velocity obtained by CW Doppler can be used to estimate RV systolic pressure using the same Bernoulli principle. The pulmonary artery pressure can then by calculated by subtracting the peak gradient across the PV from the RV systolic pressure. Therefore, echocardiography can be used for the estimation of both RV and pulmonary artery pressures. However, such measurement may be inaccurate because of suboptimal echocardiography windows or the presence of multiple stenosis in series, long tunnel stenosis, or altered pulmonary artery geometry. Under these circumstances, cardiac catheterization with direct pressure measurement as well as angiography is recommended to best assess the location and severity of RVOT obstruction and for determination of pulmonary artery pressures. The presence of pulmonary hypertension in the setting of repaired TOF can be a residua from a previous systemic–to–pulmonary artery shunt (such as the Blalock-Taussig shunt), or may be related to a residual intracardiac shunt. At times, pulmonary hypertension may be related to acquired cardiovascular or chronic lung diseases such as thromboembolism, kyphoscoliosis, emphysema, sleep apnea, systemic hypertension, or left heart failure. The presence of pulmonary hypertension worsens the severity of PR.

Tricuspid valve regurgitation is not uncommon following TOF repair but is rarely severe. Significant TR has been reported in up to 65% of patients following TOF repair. Tricuspid regurgitation can be caused by (a) an intrinsic tricuspid annular abnormality, (b) tricuspid valve dilatation caused by RV volume overload, (c) tricuspid valve damage during retraction during a transatrial surgical approach, and (d) damage to the tricuspid valve and its chordae during placement of the VSD patch. Significant tricuspid regurgitation can contribute to progressive RV enlargement and dysfunction; therefore, echocardiographic assessment of tricuspid regurgitation is an integral part of the noninvasive evaluation of these patients.

The presence of residual atrial or ventricular septal defects should be excluded by color flow with or without contrast echocardiography if needed. Residual ventricular septal defects can occur anywhere along the length of the VSD patch; however, these residual defects are most common in the area of the atrioventricular node where sutures are placed farther apart to avoid damage to the conduction system.

Although the left ventricle is not part of the primary anatomic cardiac defects seen in TOF, patients who have had previous TOF repair have been noted to have varying degrees of LV dysfunction. LV dysfunction plays an important role in the timing of PVR following TOF repair. Factors that are known to contribute to the development of LV dysfunction include (a) the duration of preoperative cyanosis, (b) the preference of LV volume overload from a previously placed systemic–to–pulmonary artery shunt, (c) suboptimal myocardial protection during cardiopulmonary bypass, (d) duration of cardiopulmonary bypass itself, (e) patching of the ventricular septum, (f) myocardial fibrosis, and (g) aortic valve regurgitation secondary to aortic root enlargement. Furthermore, Geva et al. suggested that LV dysfunction could be partly attributed to abnormal septal motion caused by the volume-overloaded right ventricle, as well as its detrimental effects on LV geometry and mechanical performance because of unfavorable ventricular–ventricular interaction. In the absence of abnormal septal motion, LV systolic function can be assessed by the well-standardized conventional M-mode and two-dimensional echocardiographic techniques. An important contributor to LV dysfunction in repaired TOF is the presence of aortic root dilatation with associated aortic regurgitation. Aortic root dilation is believed to be secondary to abnormal intrinsic properties of the aortic root as well as long-standing volume overload prior to TOF repair. Aortic regurgitation may develop secondary to aortic root dilatation or possibly as a result of direct damage during placement of the VSD patch.

Given the concerns about adaptability and the lack of reported symptoms in repaired TOF with severe PR, it is not uncommon for the clinician to rely on exercise stress testing to document significant changes in exercise capacity over time to aid in defining the optimal timing of PVR. Wessel et al. demonstrated that exercise performance was 82% ± 21% of predicted in repaired patients with TOF. Carvalho and coworkers showed significantly reduced duration of exercise in patients after TOF repair as well as a negative correlation between exercise time and the severity of PR. There is also substantial clinical interest in the diagnostic role of brain natriuretic peptide (BNP) in the assessment of patients with PR after TOF repair. Brili et al. reported that patients after repair of TOF had a significantly higher BNP levels than in controls (85.0 ± 87 versus 5.36 ± 1.0 pg/mL, $p < 0.001$) and that this increased BNP level correlated with RV enlargement. Ishii et al. examined the relationship between BNP and RV contractile reserve during exercise in 26 patients after TOF repair compared with 19 age-matched healthy children. Plasma levels of BNP were measured at baseline and at maximum exercise. Echocardiography combined with tissue Doppler imaging was performed at rest and during supine bicycle submaximal exercise. The peak value of the first elevation of RV dP/dT was also measured by continuous wave Doppler. Plasma BNP levels were significantly higher in patients with TOF than in controls (44 ± 34 versus 6 ± 4 pg/mL, P value < 0.01). In addition, a larger increment in BNP was noted after exercise in patients with TOF when compared with normal subjects (15 ± 12 versus 2 ± 2 pg/mL, $p < 0.01$). At peak exercise, systolic myocardial tissue velocity and peak dP/dT values increased significantly in both groups. However, the magnitude of increase in both of these values was significantly less in patients with TOF than in controls (36% ± 19% versus 70% ± 19% and 42% ± 11% versus 81% ± 12%, respectively, with $p < 0.01$). There was significant correlation between the increment in BNP and changes in systolic myocardial tissue velocity and dP/dt values. Furthermore, increments in BNP during exercise were well correlated with severity of PR. Therefore, exercise-induced changes in plasma concentration of BNP may reflect RV contractile reserve in patients with TOF. While it is too early to recommend that stress echocardiography be routinely performed, the future of such innovative techniques to assess anatomic and physiologic changes in repaired patients with TOF with PR appears promising.

COMPLEMENTARY INVESTIGATIVE TECHNIQUES IN PR

Cardiac MRI has emerged as a robust and reliable alternative technique for the quantitative assessment of RV volume, RV function, and PR severity, especially when echocardiographic imaging is suboptimal. MRI offers an advantage over echocardiography in that image quality is not compromised by air, bone, or surgical scar. RV volume calculation by MRI correlates well with angiography. However, significant interobserver and intraobserver variability has been reported primarily because of the complex geometry of the right ventricle. In addition, MRI techniques can underestimate the severity of PR compared with echocardiography. Although cardiac MRI is gaining momentum in the evaluation of patients with repaired TOF, its availability and familiarity compared with echocardiography are lacking. Furthermore, this technique may not provide all the necessary components of the comprehensive echocardiographic examination (Table 37.1).

Impact of Echocardiographic Evaluation on Outcome

PVR remains the only treatment available for postoperative severe PR after TOF repair. PVR has proven long-term benefits, including reduction in RV size and improvement or stabilization of RV function. It has low operative risk when performed at an optimal time and in experienced medical centers. The optimal timing of PVR is determined by many factors including the presence of clinical symptoms such as dyspnea, exercise intolerance, heart failure, and symptomatic or sustained arrhythmias. In addition, the presence of progressive RV enlargement and/or dysfunction, worsening tricuspid regurgitation, a significant residual shunt, or significant RVOT obstruction (right ventricular systolic pressure (RVSP) two-thirds systemic or greater) are indications for PVR with or without intracardiac repair. Furthermore, PVR is also considered when there is a documented decline in functional aerobic capacity on exercise stress testing. Therefore, optimal patient selection for PVR is dependent on the information provided by the comprehensive serial echocardiographic examinations.

Recent advances in interventional cardiology have led to an increased interest in percutaneous PVR using a bovine jugular vein valve mounted on an expandable stent. An important determinant of patient suitability for this technique is the presence of favorable RVOT morphology. Three-dimensional echocardiography has been reported recently to provide additional anatomic details of RVOT anatomy that are incremental to that of two-dimensional echocardiography.

Following PVR, echocardiography is the most commonly used tool for serial assessment of the PV prosthesis, as well as RV size and function. Significant reduction in RV end-diastolic diameter or function is commonly observed. However, considerable residua may persist such as ventricular dysfunction, aortic regurgitation, and pulmonary hypertension. These chronic conditions will need periodic serial echocardiographic assessment. In addition, echocardiography is an optimal technique for ongoing assessment of the PV prosthesis, whether biological or mechanical. These prostheses are almost always located directly retrosternal and are easily visualized by transthoracic echocardiography and at times are palpable on examination. Evaluation of leaflet motion, maximal and mean gradient, and identification of the presence and severity of prosthetic or periprosthetic regurgitation should be routinely performed.

SUMMARY

Assessment of patients following repair of TOF should include a thorough medical history, clinical examination, electrocardiogram, and comprehensive transthoracic echocardiogram to identify all postoperative residua and sequelae. PR is a common postoperative complication associated with progressive RV enlargement and dysfunction. These detrimental changes in RV performance are associated with progressive exercise intolerance, heart failure, tachyarrhythmias, and late sudden death. The echocardiogram plays a key role in identifying the optimal timing of PVR. Ongoing serial echocardiographic evaluation after valve replacement ensures appropriate follow-up in these patients.

SUGGESTED READING

Abd El Rahman MY, Abdul-Khaliq H, Vogel M, et al. Value of the new Doppler-derived myocardial performance index for the evaluation of right and left ventricular function following repair of tetralogy of Fallot. *Pediatr Cardiol.* 2002;23:502–507.

Anwar AM, Soliman O, van den Bosch AE, et al. Assessment of pulmonary valve and right ventricular outflow tract with real-time three-dimensional echocardiography. *Int J Cardiovasc Imaging.* 2007;23:167–175.

Babu-Narayan SV, Kilner PJ, Li W, et al. Ventricular fibrosis suggested by cardiovascular magnetic resonance in adults with repaired tetralogy of Fallot and its relationship to adverse markers of clinical outcome. *Circulation.* 2006;113:405–413.

Borowski A, Ghodsizad A, Litmathe J, et al. Severe pulmonary regurgitation late after total repair of tetralogy of Fallot: surgical considerations. *Pediatr Cardiol.* 2004;25:466–471.

Bouzas B, Kilner PJ, Gatzoulis MA. Pulmonary regurgitation: not a benign lesion. *Eur Heart J.* 2005;26:433–439.

Bove EL, Kavey RE, Byrum CJ, et al. Improved right ventricular function following late pulmonary valve replacement for residual pulmonary insufficiency or stenosis. *J Thorac Cardiovasc Surg.* 1985;90:50–55.

Brili S, Alexopoulos N, Latsios G, et al. Tissue Doppler imaging and brain natriuretic peptide levels in adults with repaired tetralogy of Fallot. *J Am Soc Echocardiogr.* 2005;18:1149–1154.

Carvalho JS, Shinebourne EA, Busst C, et al. Exercise capacity after complete repair of tetralogy of Fallot: deleterious effects of residual pulmonary regurgitation. *Br Heart J.* 1992;67:470–473.

Chaturvedi RR, Kilner PJ, White PA, et al. Increased airway pressure and simulated branch pulmonary artery stenosis increase pulmonary regurgitation after repair of tetralogy of Fallot: real-time analysis with a conductance catheter technique. *Circulation.* 1997;95:643–649.

Cheung MM, Konstantinov IE, Redington AN. Late complications of repair of tetralogy of Fallot and indications for pulmonary valve replacement. *Semin Thorac Cardiovasc Surg.* 2005;17:155–159.

Coats L, Tsang V, Khambadkone S, et al. The potential impact of percutaneous pulmonary valve stent implantation on right ventricular outflow tract reintervention. *Eur J Cardiothorac Surg.* 2005;27:536–543.

Conte S, Jashari R, Eyskens B, et al. Homograft valve insertion for pulmonary regurgitation late after valveless repair of right ventricular outflow tract obstruction. *Eur J Cardiothorac Surg.* 1999;15:143–149.

D'Andrea A, Caso P, Sarubbi B, et al. Right ventricular myocardial dysfunction in adult patients late after repair of tetralogy of Fallot. *Int J Cardiol.* 2004;94:213–220.

Davlouros PA, Karatza AA, Gatzoulis MA, et al. Timing and type of surgery for severe pulmonary regurgitation after repair of tetralogy of Fallot. *Int J Cardiol.* 2004;97(suppl. 1):91–101.

Davlouros PA, Kilner PJ, Hornung TS, et al. Right ventricular function in adults with repaired tetralogy of Fallot assessed with cardiovascular magnetic resonance imaging: detrimental role of right ventricular outflow aneurysms or akinesia and adverse right-to-left ventricular interaction. *J Am Coll Cardiol.* 2002;40:2044–2052.

Davlouros PA, Niwa K, Webb G, et al. The right ventricle in congenital heart disease. Heart. 2006;92(suppl. 1):i27–i38.

Discigil B, Dearani JA, Puga FJ, et al. Late pulmonary valve replacement after repair of tetralogy of Fallot. *J Thorac Cardiovasc Surg.* 2001;121:344–351.

Dolan MS, Castello R, St Vrain JA, et al. Quantitation of aortic regurgitation by Doppler echocardiography: a practical approach. *Am Heart J.* 1995;129:1014–1020.

Eidem BW, Tei C, O'Leary PW, et al. Nongeometric quantitative assessment of right and left ventricular function: myocardial performance index in normal children and patients with Ebstein anomaly. *J Am Soc Echocardiogr.* 1998;11:849–856.

Farzaneh-Far A, Scheidt S. Adult with Repaired Tetralogy of Fallot: Fixed but not cured. *Cardiovasc Rev Rep.* 2003:387–391.

Foster E, Webb G, Human D, et al. The Adult With Tetralogy of Fallot. *ACC Curr J Rev.* 1998;7:62–66.

Frigiola A, Redington AN, Cullen S, et al. Pulmonary regurgitation is an important determinant of right ventricular contractile dysfunction in patients with surgically repaired tetralogy of Fallot. *Circulation.* 2004;110(suppl. 1): II-153–II-157.

Gatzoulis MA, Balaji S, Webber SA, et al. Risk factors for arrhythmia and sudden cardiac death late after repair of tetralogy of Fallot: a multicentre study. *Lancet.* 2000;356(9234):975–981.

Gatzoulis MA, Till JA, Somerville J, et al. Mechanoelectrical Interaction in Tetralogy of Fallot : QRS Prolongation Relates to Right Ventricular Size and Predicts Malignant Ventricular Arrhythmias and Sudden Death. *Circulation.* 1995;92:231–237.

Gatzoulis MA. *Diagnosis and Management of Congenital Heart Disease*: Churchill Livingstone; 2003.

Geva T, Sandweiss BM, Gauvreau K, et al. Factors associated with impaired clinical status in long-term survivors of tetralogy of Fallot repair evaluated by magnetic resonance imaging. *J Am Coll Cardiol.* 2004;43:1068–1074.

Giannopoulos NM, Chatzis AC, Bobos DP, et al. Tetralogy of Fallot: influence of right ventricular outflow tract reconstruction on late outcome. *Int J Cardiol.* 2004;97 Suppl 1:87–90.

Giardini A, Specchia S, Tacy TA, et al. Usefulness of cardiopulmonary exercise to predict long-term prognosis in adults with repaired tetralogy of Fallot. *Am J Cardiol.* 2007;99:1462–1467.

Hazekamp MG, Kurvers MM, Schoof PH, et al. Pulmonary valve insertion late after repair of Fallot's tetralogy. *Eur J Cardiothorac Surg.* 2001;19: 667–670.

Helbing WA, Niezen RA, Le Cessie S, et al. Right ventricular diastolic function in children with pulmonary regurgitation after repair of tetralogy of Fallot: volumetric evaluation by magnetic resonance velocity mapping. *J Am Coll Cardiol.* 1996;28:1827–1835.

Helbing WA, Roest AA, Niezen RA, et al. ECG predictors of ventricular arrhythmias and biventricular size and wall mass in tetralogy of Fallot with pulmonary regurgitation. *Heart.* 2002;88:515–519.

Imanishi T, Nakatani S, Yamada S, et al. Validation of continuous wave Doppler-determined right ventricular peak positive and negative dP/ dt: effect of right atrial pressure on measurement. *J Am Coll Cardiol.* 1994;23:1638–1643.

Ishii H, Harada K, Toyono M, et al. Usefulness of exercise-induced changes in plasma levels of brain natriuretic peptide in predicting right ventricular contractile reserve after repair of tetralogy of Fallot. *Am J Cardiol.* 2005;95:1338–1343.

Jacob R, Stewart WJ. A practical approach to the quantification of valvular regurgitation. *Curr Cardiol Rep.* 2007;9:105–111.

Kang IS, Redington AN, Benson LN, et al. Differential regurgitation in branch pulmonary arteries after repair of tetralogy of Fallot: a phase-contrast cine magnetic resonance study. *Circulation.* 2003;107:2938–2943.

Khambadkone S, Coats L, Taylor A, et al. Percutaneous pulmonary valve implantation in humans: results in 59 consecutive patients. *Circulation.* 2005;112:1189–1197.

Kobayashi J, Nakano S, Matsuda H, et al. Quantitative evaluation of pulmonary regurgitation after repair of tetralogy of Fallot using real-time flow imaging system. *Jpn Circ J.* 1989;53:721–727.

Li W, Davlouros PA, Kilner PJ, et al. Doppler-echocardiographic assessment of pulmonary regurgitation in adults with repaired tetralogy of Fallot: comparison with cardiovascular magnetic resonance imaging. *Am Heart J.* 2004;147:165–172.

Lim C, Lee JY, Kim WH, et al. Early replacement of pulmonary valve after repair of tetralogy: is it really beneficial? *Eur J Cardiothorac Surg.* 2004;25:728–734.

Meluzin J, Spinarova L, Bakala J, et al. Pulsed Doppler tissue imaging of the velocity of tricuspid annular systolic motion; a new, rapid, and non-invasive method of evaluating right ventricular systolic function. *Eur Heart J.* 2001;22:340–348.

Munkhammar P, Cullen S, Jogi P, et al. Early age at repair prevents restrictive right ventricular (RV) physiology after surgery for tetralogy of Fallot (TOF): diastolic RV function after TOF repair in infancy. *J Am Coll Cardiol.* 1998;32:1083–1087.

Murphy JG, Gersh BJ, Mair DD, et al. Long-term outcome in patients undergoing surgical repair of tetralogy of Fallot. *N Engl J Med.* 1993;329:593–599.

Niwa K, Siu SC, Webb GD, et al. Progressive aortic root dilatation in adults late after repair of tetralogy of Fallot. *Circulation.* 2002;106:1374–1378.

Oechslin EN, Harrison DA, Harris L, et al. Reoperation in adults with repair of tetralogy of Fallot: Indications and outcomes. *J Thorac Cardiovasc Surg.* 1999;118:245–251.

Rebergen SA, Chin JG, Ottenkamp J, et al. Pulmonary regurgitation in the late postoperative follow-up of tetralogy of Fallot. Volumetric quantitation by nuclear magnetic resonance velocity mapping. *Circulation.* 1993;88: 2257–2266.

Redington AN, Oldershaw PJ, Shinebourne EA, et al. A new technique for the assessment of pulmonary regurgitation and its application to the assessment of right ventricular function before and after repair of tetralogy of Fallot. *Br Heart J.* 1988;60:57–65.

Schwerzmann M, Samman AM, Salehian O, et al. Comparison of echocardiographic and cardiac magnetic resonance imaging for assessing right ventricular function in adults with repaired tetralogy of Fallot. *Am J Cardiol.* 2007;99:1593–1597.

Silversides CK, Veldtman GR, Crossin J, et al. Pressure half-time predicts hemodynamically significant pulmonary regurgitation in adult patients with repaired tetralogy of Fallot. *J Am Soc Echocardiogr.* 2003;16:1057–1062.

Solarz DE, Witt SA, Glascock BJ, et al. Right ventricular strain rate and strain analysis in patients with repaired tetralogy of Fallot: possible interventricular septal compensation. *J Am Soc Echocardiogr.* 2004;17:338–344.

Stulak JM, Connolly HM, Puga FJ, et al. Should mechanical valves be used in the pulmonary position. *J Am Coll Cardiol.* 2004;43(suppl. 2):A390–A391.

Tei C, Dujardin KS, Hodge DO, et al. Doppler echocardiographic index for assessment of global right ventricular function. *J Am Soc Echocardiogr.* 1996;9: 838–847.

Therrien J, Siu SC, Harris L, et al. Impact of pulmonary valve replacement on arrhythmia propensity late after repair of tetralogy of Fallot. *Circulation.* 2001;103:2489–2494.

Uebing A, Fischer G, Bethge M, et al. Influence of the pulmonary annulus diameter on pulmonary regurgitation and right ventricular pressure load after repair of tetralogy of Fallot. *Heart.* 2002;88:510–514.

van der Wall EE, Mulder BJ. Pulmonary valve replacement in patients with tetralogy of Fallot and pulmonary regurgitation: early surgery similar to optimal timing of surgery? *Eur Heart J.* 2005;26:2614–2615.

van Huysduynen BH, van Straten A, Swenne CA, et al. Reduction of QRS duration after pulmonary valve replacement in adult Fallot patients is related to reduction of right ventricular volume. *Eur Heart J.* 2005;26:928–932.

van Straten A, Vliegen HW, Hazekamp MG, et al. Right ventricular function late after total repair of tetralogy of Fallot. *Eur Radiol.* 2005;15:702–707.

van Straten A, Vliegen HW, Lamb HJ, et al. Time course of diastolic and systolic function improvement after pulmonary valve replacement in adult patients with tetralogy of Fallot. *J Am Coll Cardiol.* 2005;46:1559–1564.

Vliegen HW, van Straten A, de Roos A, et al. Magnetic resonance imaging to assess the hemodynamic effects of pulmonary valve replacement in adults late after repair of tetralogy of Fallot. *Circulation.* 2002;106:1703–1707.

Warner KG, O'Brien PK, Rhodes J, et al. Expanding the indications for pulmonary valve replacement after repair of tetralogy of Fallot. *Ann Thorac Surg.* 2003;76:1066–1072.

Wessel HU, Cunningham WJ, Paul MH, et al. Exercise performance in tetralogy of Fallot after intracardiac repair. *J Thorac Cardiovasc Surg.* 1980;80: 582–593.

Williams RV, Minich LL, Shaddy RE, et al. Comparison of Doppler echocardiography with angiography for determining the severity of pulmonary regurgitation. *Am J Cardiol.* 2002;89:1438–1441.

Yasuoka K, Harada K, Toyono M, et al. Tei index determined by tissue Doppler imaging in patients with pulmonary regurgitation after repair of tetralogy of Fallot. *Pediatr Cardiol.* 2004;25:131–136.

Zahka KG, Horneffer PJ, Rowe SA, et al. Long-term valvular function after total repair of tetralogy of Fallot. Relation to ventricular arrhythmias. *Circulation.* 1988;78(suppl.):III-14–III-9.

Chapter 38
Echocardiographic Evaluation of the Functionally Univentricular Heart After Fontan "Operation"

Sabrina D. Phillips • Patrick W. O'Leary

Patients with functionally single ventricular circulations are challenges to evaluate by any method. The anatomy, physiology, and surgical procedures associated with these malformations are complex and varied. Conventional surgical palliation for the functionally single ventricle is usually focused toward completion of a Fontan "operation." However, the Fontan circulation can be completed using several different surgical techniques. As a result, some of the confusion encountered when evaluating the post-Fontan patient stems from the number of different connections used to create the systemic venous to pulmonary arterial pathway. Therefore, a systematic approach is required if one is to truly understand the circulation of patients after Fontan operations. This chapter will discuss the anatomy of the Fontan circulation, its unique physiology, and an approach to the echocardiographic evaluation of these patients that not only allows a complete delineation of the Fontan circulation but also increases the likelihood of detecting late complications. In conclusion, a number of case studies illustrating the physiology and complications of this type of circulation will be reviewed.

 ## ANATOMY AND PHYSIOLOGY OF THE FONTAN OPERATION

The first step toward understanding the patient with a Fontan circulation is to realize that this procedure is a surgical *palliation*, rather than a "repair." A Fontan operation reduces ventricular workload and eliminates or reduces oxygen desaturation in the patient with a functionally univentricular heart. These goals can be achieved by many different surgical techniques, and the patients who can benefit from the Fontan operation have many different cardiac malformations. Thus, the Fontan is more of a surgical "concept" than it is a specific operative technique. This concept can be summarized as follows: *A Fontan "operation" consists of any combination of surgical procedures that divert the systemic venous return away from the ventricle, eliminate mixing of systemic and pulmonary venous blood, and create a circulation "in series" for patients with functional single-ventricle physiology.* After creation of a Fontan, pulmonary venous flow remains committed to the patient's only functional ventricle. Many types of pathways have been used to create the systemic venous diversion that defines the Fontan circulations. Regardless of how the connections were constructed, superior and inferior vena cava flows bypass the ventricle, and pass through the lungs without the assistance of a ventricular systolic pump.

When the Fontan procedure was first applied, the right atrium was used as the pathway for systemic venous flow and an anastomosis was created between the right atrial appendage and the pulmonary artery provided the outlet from the atrium to the pulmonary arteries. This type of connection is referred to as an "atriopulmonary" Fontan and is illustrated in Figs. 38.1 and 38.2. This approach worked well for patients with tricuspid atresia and others with left atrioventricular valves. However, this approach was difficult to apply to hearts with left atrioventricular valve atresia, hypoplasia, or severe dysfunction. Although atriopulmonary connections have been superseded by newer techniques, there are many patients who still have these connections. Therefore, we need to not only understand how to recognize them but also be aware of the unique complications associated with them. These complications include atrial enlargement and arrhythmias, compression of the pulmonary veins by the enlarged right atrium and atrial thrombus formation within the dilated atrium. Atrial thrombi, sluggish flow in a dilated atrial chamber (with spontaneous echo contrast), blind pouches in communication with the "left" heart (such as a ligated native pulmonary root), and residual right-to-left shunts have all been associated with an increased risk for embolic events.

Over time, less of the right atrium was included in the systemic venous pathway, allowing the right atrioventricular valve to contribute to the systemic circulation. Lateral atrial tunnels or intra-atrial conduits allowed the pulmonary venous return to pass through any atrioventricular valve to reach the ventricle, expanding the spectrum of the Fontan to those with common atrioventricular valves and left atrioventricular valve abnormalities. Recently, the surgical diversions involved in Fontan procedures have bypassed the atrium completely. This has been accomplished by combining direct superior vena cava–to–pulmonary arterial anastomoses (bidirectional Glenn connections) with intracardiac or extracardiac conduits. These nonvalved conduits connect the suprahepatic inferior vena cava to the pulmonary arteries (Fig. 38.3). Fontan circulations that include an extracardiac conduit have been referred to as "extracardiac Fontans" (Figs. 38.4 and 38.5).

Since the early 1990s, many Fontan operations have included a surgical "fenestration." A fenestration is essentially a small, intentional

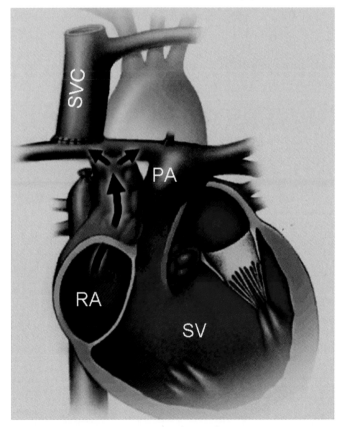

FIGURE 38.1. Diagram of an atriopulmonary Fontan connection. The underlying anatomy is that of a functionally single-ventricle chamber, with right atrioventricular valve atresia and pulmonary stenosis. In this case, the superior vena cava (SVC) has been directly and bidirectionally connected to the right pulmonary artery (a "bidirectional Glenn" anastomosis). The native right atrium (RA) has been converted into a conduit for inferior vena caval flow by closure of the atrial septal defect and a right atrial appendage (black arrow)–to–pulmonary artery (PA) connection. Early atriopulmonary Fontan connections did not involve a separate SVC connection. Both of the venae cavae were left connected to the RA, and the atriopulmonary anastomosis carried all of the systemic venous return. The use of the native RA for at least part of the venous pathway is the hallmark of an atriopulmonary Fontan. The elevated venous and right atrial pressures associated with the Fontan circulation lead to prominent right atrial enlargement after this type of Fontan connection. SV, functional single ventricle.

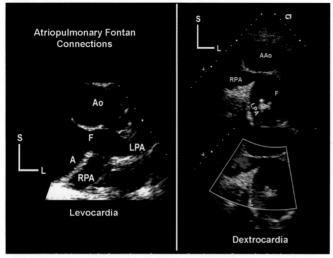

FIGURE 38.2. Parasternal, horizontal plane echocardiographic images demonstrate the tomographic anatomy of atriopulmonary Fontan connection. Left: Taken during an examination of the patient with normally positioned atria and levocardia. The atrial appendage has been surgically opened and connected to the pulmonary arterial confluence, creating the Fontan connection (F). These connections are found posterior to ascending aorta, just superior to the base of the heart. **Right:** Taken during the examination of the patient with atrial situs inversus and dextrocardia. As a result, the anatomy is a mirror image of the left. These images were obtained from the right parasternal border. Scans in the horizontal plane began by demonstrating the dilated native right atrial chamber. The plane of sound was then progressively moved superiorly beyond the semilunar valve to reveal the Fontan connection (F) and the confluence of the right and left pulmonary arteries (RPA and LPA). Regardless of how the surgeon created the connection, a similar progression of scans (beginning with the atrium and moving toward the pulmonary arteries) should allow echocardiographic demonstration of the Fontan anastomosis. A, atrium; AAo or Ao, ascending aorta; L, left; S, superior.

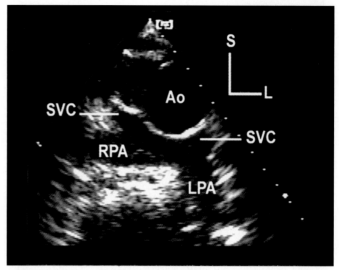

FIGURE 38.4. Horizontal-plane echocardiographic image from a high left parasternal, subclavicular position. It demonstrates bilateral, bidirectional superior vena cava (SVC)–to–pulmonary artery connections. These anastomoses are often referred to as bidirectional Glenn connections or shunts. This type of connection can be used as a part of a Fontan circulation, diverting superior vena caval blood flow away from the heart and into the pulmonary arteries. These connections are often created prior to final Fontan completion, in an attempt to minimize ventricular volume overload in very young patients who would otherwise not tolerate creation of a complete Fontan. In more mature patients, if these connections are not already present, they can be made at the time of Fontan completion. Ao, ascending aorta; L, left; LPA, left pulmonary artery; RPA, right pulmonary artery; S, superior.

residual atrial septal defect (Figs. 38.3 and 38.6). Atrial baffle fenestrations are usually sized between 3 and 5 mm and allow a small, continuous right-to-left atrial shunt, at the expense of mild systemic oxygen desaturation. The physiology of the fenestration's shunt is always right to left. This is because of the absence of a ventricle in the right side of the circulation. As a result, the right atrial/pulmonary arterial pressure must be greater than the functional left atrial

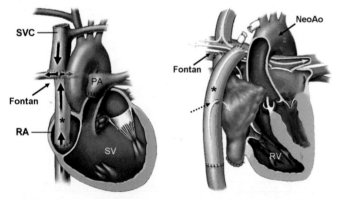

FIGURE 38.3. Diagrams of two types of Fontan circulations that completely bypass the entire heart to create the diversion of superior and inferior vena caval flow to the pulmonary arteries. Left: First use of a nonvalved conduit to complete the Fontan pathway. In this case, the base of an intra-atrial conduit was connected to the inferior vena caval–atrial junction. The superior end of the conduit was then connected to the pulmonary arterial confluence using an incision/anastomosis at the dome of the native right atrium. Although the atrial wall is used to complete the connection, none of the native atrial chamber is actually involved in the venous pathway. The superior vena cava (SVC) has a separate, bidirectional anastomosis to the right pulmonary artery. **Right:** Anatomy of an extracardiac, fenestrated Fontan operation performed in a patient with prior Norwood reconstruction for hypoplastic left heart syndrome. In this case, the inferior vena cava was detached from its native connection to the right atrium and a direct anastomosis was made between the supra diaphragmatic inferior vena cava and a nonvalved conduit (*asterisk*). A superior connection was then made between the conduit and the pulmonary arterial confluence. A 4-mm fenestration (*dashed, black arrow*) was created between the conduit and the lateral wall of the native atrium. This allowed a small residual right-to-left shunt (*white arrow*) to provide a continuous source of extraventricular filling (preload), easing the transition to the Fontan circulation. Two operations had been performed prior to the Fontan completion, as described earlier. The aorta had been reconstructed during the neonatal Norwood operation, enlarging the aortic arch and fusing the hypoplastic native ascending aorta with the native pulmonary root to create a "neoaorta." The SVC had been bidirectionally connected to the right pulmonary artery at an intermediate, second-stage operation. PA, pulmonary artery; RA, native right atrium; RV, right ventricle; SV, functionally single ventricle.

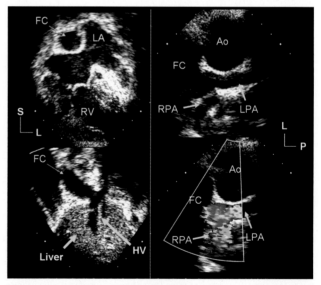

FIGURE 38.5. Echocardiographic images demonstrate the appearance of an extracardiac Fontan operation in a patient with hypoplastic left heart syndrome. Top left: Taken at the cardiac apex; demonstrates how the native left atrial (LA) and right atrial (not labeled) chambers now serve as a combined pulmonary venous chamber, while the extracardiac, Fontan conduit (FC) functions as the patient's new right atrium. **Bottom left:** Inferior connection of the Fontan conduit to the inferior vena cava and hepatic venous confluence (HV). **Top Right:** Superior connection of the Fontan conduit to the pulmonary arterial confluence in a coronal plane. The scans were obtained from the left anterior axillary line with the plane of sound directed toward the patient's right. The Fontan connection and pulmonary arteries are seen just beyond the reconstructed ascending aorta (Ao). There was no evidence of narrowing within the venous pathway or pulmonary arteries. Color flow Doppler interrogation (**bottom right**) revealed laminar flow consistent with widely patent connection from the inferior vena cava, through the Fontan conduit to the pulmonary arteries. L, left; LPA, left pulmonary artery; P, posterior; RPA, right pulmonary artery; S, superior.

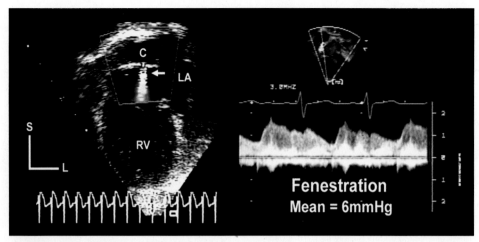

FIGURE 38.6. Echocardiographic images demonstrate an atrial fenestration after completion of a Fontan operation in a patient with asplenia syndrome. Left: An intra-atrial conduit (C) diverted inferior vena caval flow to the pulmonary artery. Color flow Doppler showed a continuous, aliased jet of flow (*white arrow*) from the conduit into the pulmonary venous atrial chamber (LA). **Right:** Continuous-wave Doppler interrogation revealed this flow pattern. Velocities varied during the phase of the cardiac cycle and with respiration. The mean gradient between the conduit and the pulmonary venous atrium was 6 mm Hg, representing a relatively normal transpulmonary gradient after Fontan completion. L, left; RV, right ventricle; S, superior.

pressure, or there would be no driving force for pulmonary blood flow. The purpose of allowing this residual shunt with an atrial fenestration is to provide a relatively continuous source of preload to the systemic ventricle. Prior to creation of a Fontan circulation, functionally single ventricles universally have an increased preload, since they are "filled" by both the systemic and pulmonary venous returns. The extra volume provided to the ventricle by a fenestration eases the transition to the Fontan circulation. It also seems to reduce the duration of pleural drainage in the immediate postoperative period. The disadvantage to a fenestration circulation is that fenestrated patients will remain cyanotic and will face a slightly increased risk for embolic complications compared with the nonfenestrated patient. From an echocardiographer's perspective, a fenestration also provides insight into the patient's pulmonary hemodynamics. The mean pressure gradient across the fenestration can be easily measured by continuous-wave Doppler echocardiography (Fig. 38.6). The fenestration "shunt" originates in the functional right atrium (the Fontan pathway) and (in the absence of stenoses) the pressure in the Fontan pathway is equal to the pulmonary arterial pressure. The fenestration flow is directed into the functionally left atrium. In the absence of pulmonary vein stenosis, the pressure in the functional left atrium will equal the pulmonary venous pressure. Therefore, the mean pressure gradient across the fenestration will reflect the "transpulmonary gradient." This gradient is primarily determined by the patient's pulmonary vascular resistance, a key determinant of outcome in patients with Fontan circulations. Fontan circulations that are functioning well are associated with mean fenestration (transpulmonary) gradients of 5 to 8 mm Hg. Lower values may represent better than average Fontan physiology or may represent dehydration with artificially low right atrial pressures. The higher the gradient, the higher is the total transpulmonary resistance to flow. Gradients greater than 8 mm Hg or that have increased from the patient's historical baseline require explanation, prompting an even more thorough evaluation than usual.

The physiology of the Fontan operation is unique, primarily because the redirected venous flow streams do not benefit from a ventricular pump. Forward flow through the lungs depends upon a combination of residual kinetic energy from the "previous" systemic ventricular contraction, negative intrathoracic pressure (generated by the respiratory muscles), low pulmonary arterial pressure and resistance (involving both large and small vessels), as well as active atrial and ventricular relaxation. Several of these influences are reflected in the pulmonary arterial flow patterns recorded by Doppler echocardiography in Fontan patients (Figs. 38.7 and 38.8). The respiratory influence on flow is reflected by the marked augmentation in the Doppler signal occurring during inspiration. The negative intrathoracic pressure generated during spontaneous inspiration also draws blood forward through the

lungs. Conversely, positive intrathoracic pressures, seen in expiration or with mechanical ventilation, will reduce forward flow. Active ventricular diastolic relaxation also serves to augment forward flow through the lungs. As the atrioventricular valve(s) open, forward flow increases through the pulmonary arteries (Figs. 38.7 and 38.8). Reduced ventricular compliance and elevated ventricular diastolic pressure will blunt this flow, reducing overall cardiac output. Left atrial mechanical activity also affects pulmonary arterial flow in Fontan circulations. Atrial relaxation will augment forward flow by drawing blood out of the pulmonary veins. In contrast, atrial contraction will generally somewhat decrease the forward flow signal. If the ventricle has good diastolic compliance, the increase in pulmonary venous pressure caused by atrial contraction is offset by the increase in ventricular filling and output associated with synchronous atrial rhythms, such as normal sinus rhythm and dual chamber pacing. However, reduced ventricular compliance with elevated diastolic pressure or the atrial contraction is not

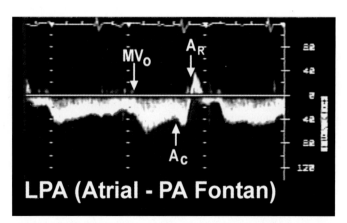

FIGURE 38.7. Pulsed-wave Doppler recording was obtained in the left pulmonary artery of the patient with tricuspid valve atresia and an atriopulmonary Fontan connection. The tracing demonstrates three important phases to "Fontan" flow in this type of connection. Forward flow (below the baseline) is augmented by active ventricular diastolic relaxation when the systemic atrioventricular valve opens (MVO). Since the native right atrial chamber remains in the systemic venous pathway, atrial contraction will also increase forward flow velocity (AC). However, when the atrium relaxes (AR), flow actually reverses out of the pulmonary artery and returns to the atrium (signal now shown above the baseline). This to-and-fro flow contributes to the atrial enlargement seen with this type of Fontan connection. Longer recordings would also demonstrate a respiratory influence on these flows, negative intrathoracic pressure caused by spontaneous inspiration will increase forward flow volume and velocity in the Fontan circulation. Slightly positive expiratory pressures will blunt forward flow. AC, atrial contraction; AR, atrial relaxation; MVO, mitral valve opening; LPA, left pulmonary artery; PA, pulmonary artery.

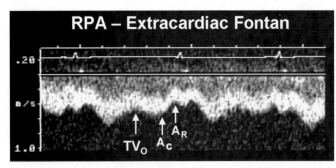

FIGURE 38.8. Pulsed-wave Doppler recording was obtained in the right pulmonary artery of the patient with hypoplastic left heart syndrome and an extracardiac Fontan connection. The tracing also demonstrates phasic flows, but there are important differences to note relative to the flows seen in Figure 38.7. Ventricular diastole and atrioventricular valve opening result in augmented forward flow in both types of Fontan connections. In this recording, this is reflected by the increased forward flow seen in early diastole (TVO). There is no atrial tissue in the extracardiac Fontan pathway. However, left atrial activity can still influence the pulmonary arterial flow pattern. When the left (pulmonary venous) atrium contracts (AC) pulmonary venous pressures rise slightly. This reduces forward flow velocity in the pulmonary artery somewhat. In an extracardiac Fontan, left atrial relaxation (AR) promotes forward flow by drawing blood out of the pulmonary veins and into the atrium. Although pulmonary arterial flow is still phasic in an extracardiac Fontan, the normal flow velocity should rarely decrease to near zero. This is unlike the flow seen in an atriopulmonary Fontan connection, where even flow reversals are common (Fig. 38.7). Intrathoracic pressure changes will produce the same alterations in these flow patterns that were described for the atriopulmonary Fontan connection in Figure 38.7. RPA, right pulmonary artery; TVO, tricuspid valve opening.

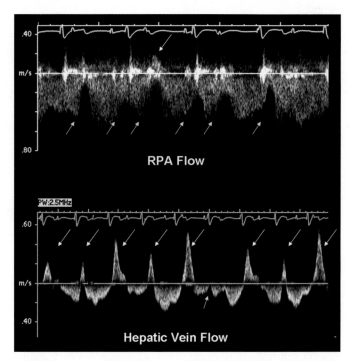

FIGURE 38.9. Pulsed-wave Doppler recordings demonstrate how cardiac rhythm disturbances can also influence flows within the Fontan circulation. These signals were obtained from the right pulmonary artery (**top**) and the hepatic vein (**bottom**) of a patient after extracardiac Fontan operation. These flow patterns are not normal, primarily because of the abnormal cardiac rhythm that is present. Electrocardiography reveals complete heart block with a junctional escape rhythm. The atrium is contracting more often than the ventricle in this case. Since atrial contractions are dyssynchronous in this rhythm, they will produce significant elevations of pulmonary venous pressure (cannon A waves). These pressure increases are reflected not only in the pulmonary arterial flow but are actually transmitted all the way back to the hepatic veins (even though there is no "atrium" within the systemic venous pathway). **Top**, *yellow arrows*: Reductions in forward flow velocity caused by atrial contraction. One of the atrial contractions during this recording occurred so early (*white arrow*) that it actually caused flow reversal in the pulmonary artery. This phenomenon was much more evident when the hepatic venous flows were recorded (*bottom*). Cannon A waves with large flow reversals (*white arrows*) could be seen during nearly every cardiac cycle. *Yellow arrow*, The one cardiac cycle in this recording in which atrial contraction occurred at approximately the "correct" time are relative to ventricular contraction. In this cardiac cycle, there was a slight decrease in forward velocity after atrial contraction, but no reversals were observed.

synchronized with ventricular relaxation (as in junctional rhythms or heart block) and will impair cardiac output. Pulmonary venous pressures and flow reversals associated with atrial contraction in nonsynchronous rhythms are dramatically increased, reducing forward flow (Fig. 38.9). In the setting of an atriopulmonary Fontan connection, the native right atrial contraction and relaxation also alter the pulmonary arterial flow pattern. However, unlike the left atrium, right atrial mechanical activity is inefficient in a Fontan circulation and does not actually alter cardiac output. Any augmentation to forward flow caused by right atrial contraction is counteracted by the accompanying reversal that occurs during atrial relaxation (Fig. 38.7). The only real impact of right atrial contraction in these patients is to create a "to-and-fro" flow through the Fontan connection, which contributes to the progressive atrial dilation common to this type of connection.

The determinants of pulmonary flow as just described provide clues to factors that identify successful Fontan patients and some of the complications that are poorly tolerated by those with Fontan circulations. Ventricular function (both systolic and diastolic) and pulmonary resistance are probably the most critical variables related to the success and/or failure of any Fontan. Table 38.1 outlines these and other factors that combine to create favorable Fontan circulations. If instead there are multiple negative factors, the patient is likely to struggle after the Fontan and is much more likely to develop significant complications.

IMAGING STRATEGIES FOR EVALUATION OF PATIENTS AFTER FONTAN OPERATIONS

Most Fontan patients begin their postoperative follow-up at an older age than other patients with complex congenital heart disease. This is because of the staged nature of this surgical palliation. The fact that Fontan completion was historically performed at even older ages also contributes to this shift in demographics. As a result, the difficulties in this imaging these patients are twofold. The examiner faces not only the complexity of the surgical procedure and underlying congenital heart disease but also the reduction in image quality that is associated with increasing age and multiple prior surgical procedures. Nevertheless, the mainstay of cardiac diagnostic imaging continues to be transthoracic echocardiography. This technique provides convenience, reproducibility, and wide availability. Transesophageal echocardiography, magnetic resonance imaging, computerized tomography, and angiography all play key, but

secondary, roles in obtaining structural and functional information in this patient group. These supplemental imaging strategies should be used when the clinical information required is not adequately outlined by the surface echocardiogram. The most important time to add these alternative imaging techniques to a patient's

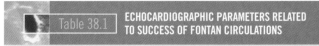

Table 38.1	ECHOCARDIOGRAPHIC PARAMETERS RELATED TO SUCCESS OF FONTAN CIRCULATIONS

- Ventricular systolic performance – normal or nearly normal
- Ventricular diastolic performance – low filling pressures, highly compliant walls
- Pulmonary arterial pressure and resistance – low resistance to flow

  No Fontan connection or pulmonary artery stenosis
  Pulmonary artery size – bigger is better

- Absence of significant atrioventricular and semilunar valve regurgitation, < mild
- Absence of obstructions to systemic inflow and outflow –

  No atrioventricular valve or pulmonary vein stenosis
  No ventricular outlet obstruction (subvalvar or valvar stenosis)
  No coarctation
  No hypertension

- Sinus rhythm or atrioventricular synchrony
  Other rhythms may be tolerated, but are less efficient

evaluation is when he or she is clinically deteriorating, even if the changes are small.

Knowledge of the patient's clinical status is also helpful to choosing an imaging strategy. For example, the patient with increasing fatigue must be evaluated for worsening ventricular systolic or diastolic performance, as well as arrhythmias. The patient with a recent stroke or transient ischemic accident must have a detailed search for source of emboli. While imaging these patients, one must strive to obtain detailed, high-quality images. Unfortunately, we know that after the Fontan, patients often have challenging acoustic windows. When surface echocardiography does not provide adequate detail, transesophageal echocardiography is often useful in visualizing the anatomic areas in question. Transesophageal echocardiography is particularly well suited to evaluating posterior structures such as the atria (to exclude thrombus formation), the Fontan connections (to exclude obstruction), and the atrioventricular valves. Magnetic resonance imaging can be helpful in identifying venous or arterial abnormalities and in quantitating ventricular function, assuming the patient does not have an electronic pacemaker. Cardiac catheterization and angiography still play an important role in the evaluation of a patient's hemodynamic status after the Fontan operation. Catheter-derived hemodynamics remain the gold standard for determination of precise pressure measurements for comparison to the patient's historical baseline and pulmonary vascular resistance.

We will focus the remainder of this chapter on surface echocardiographic evaluations, supplementing the discussion with examples of more invasive imaging strategies, when appropriate.

 ## IMAGE ACQUISITION AND THE ANATOMY OF THE FONTAN RECONSTRUCTION

The most important tool in any assessment of a Fontan patient is the *surgical dictation*. To perform an adequate examination, one must know exactly how the Fontan circulation was created. Early atriopulmonary connections often used the right atrial appendage as the final portion of the pathway for systemic venous flow (Figs. 38.1 and 38.2). The atrial septum was closed in its natural position, and any atrioventricular connection from the right atrium to the ventricle was also closed. Similarly, the pulmonary artery, if present, was ligated and/or divided. Although the atriopulmonary Fontan achieves separation of the systemic and pulmonary venous flow streams, it leaves a large and distensible chamber (the right atrium) in the middle of the systemic venous pathway. Progressive right atrial enlargement, intraatrial thrombi, and persistent atrial arrhythmias have plagued the post-Fontan patient with this type of connection. Intracardiac thrombi can be detected by surface echocardiography (Fig. 38.10). However, transesophageal examinations are more effective in detecting these complications (Fig. 38.11), especially since the transthoracic image quality available in an older Fontan patient is often impaired.

As a result of these problems, more recent surgical connections have been modified and become more streamlined. The most common method used to create a Fontan circulation today combines bidirectional superior vena cava to pulmonary arterial anastomosis(es) with an extracardiac conduit, creating continuity between the inferior vena cava and the pulmonary artery. This type of connection, the extracardiac Fontan, is illustrated in Figures 38.3, 38.4, and 38.5. Not only does an extracardiac Fontan eliminate the dilated right atrial chamber, but it also allows use of both native atria and both atrioventricular valves in the systemic circulation. This approach simplifies creation of a Fontan circulation for patients with anomalous pulmonary venous connections and abnormalities of the atrioventricular valve(s).

These two types of Fontan pathways do not represent the only Fontan connections that are possible. This heterogeneity in surgical approach contributes to making the surgical dictation so valuable. The surgical report also allows the examiner to be confident at the conclusion of the study that all of the components of the Fontan have been assessed.

As with all studies, we tend to begin the examination of the Fontan patient from the subcostal window. Evaluations of the liver, hepatic veins, and inferior vena cava provide an insight into systemic venous pressure (dilated veins suggest elevated pressure). The presence of spontaneous echo contrast is associated with sluggish flow and/or reduced cardiac output. This same acoustic window allows the examiner to then angle the plane of sound superiorly across the diaphragm, producing a subcostal coronal image of the heart. In this position, one can visualize the systemic venous pathway, atria, and usually the dominant ventricle. Although visualization of the

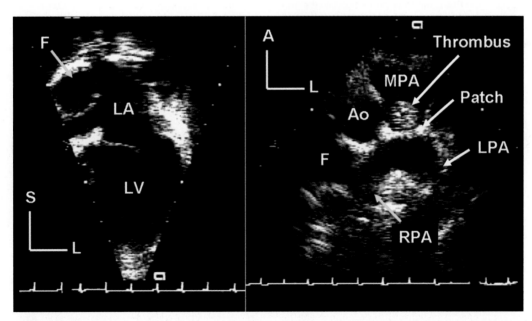

FIGURE 38.10. These images were taken from an examination of a patient with tricuspid valve atresia, normally related great arteries, and restrictive, but patent, ventricular septal defect and a previous lateral tunnel Fontan connection. **Left:** Expected anatomy as observed from the cardiac apex. The Fontan pathway (F) can be seen along the right level border of the native atrium. **Right:** High, left parasternal horizontal plane image. It reveals a relatively large, organized thrombus within the blind ending pouch of the patient's native main pulmonary artery (MPA). The MPA had been "closed" with a patch at the time of Fontan completion. This created an area of limited flow, since the ventricular septal defect allowed some blood flow to reach the pulmonary arterial stump. The Fontan connection to the pulmonary arterial confluence was widely patent. These "blind pouches" create a risk of systemic embolization when thrombi form within them since they retain some potential connections to the aortic circulation. In this case, the patient was anticoagulated, and the thrombus resolved without a complication. A, anterior; F, Fontan pathway/connection; L, left; LA, left atrium; LPA, left pulmonary artery; LV, left ventricle; MPA, main pulmonary artery; RPA, right pulmonary artery; S, superior.

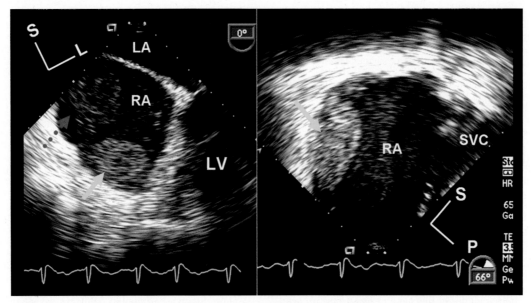

FIGURE 38.11. These images were obtained during an intraoperative transesophageal echocardiogram. The patient had stenosis of his atriopulmonary Fontan connection and had developed massive right atrial enlargement. Surface echocardiography showed spontaneous echo contrast within the atrial cavity but did not reveal the Fontan connection or evidence of organized thrombus. **Left:** Obtained from the distal esophagus, in a "four-chamber" orientation. It shows a large mural thrombus along the lateral right atrial wall (*yellow arrow*). There was also prominent spontaneous contrast noted within the atrium (*dashed red arrow*). **Right:** Sagittal image of the same area, showing the extent of the thrombus (*yellow arrow*) and the position of the superior vena caval–right atrial junction (SVC). L, left; LA, left atrium; LV, left ventricle; P, posterior; RA, right atrium; S, superior.

pulmonary arterial connection is often difficult from this transducer position, the most inferior segments of the pathway—inferior vena cava, the extracardiac conduit, and/or the inferior portion of the atrium—are usually well seen. Sweeps in both the coronal and sagittal planes should be performed. The examination should be geared to detect chamber enlargement, quantitate ventricular wall motion, scan for potential thrombi and intra-atrial shunting, and locate the position of the inferior vena caval pathway to the pulmonary artery. Doppler echocardiography in this transducer position is usually limited to color flow mapping and interrogation of atrial fenestration flow patterns.

The transducer is then transferred to the parasternal area. The majority of the Fontan reconstruction will be visualized from acoustic windows on the anterior chest wall. The atriopulmonary and extracardiac conduit connections can usually be imaged from a parasternal window. The most convenient images of this connection are often found in the horizontal (short-axis) projections (Figs. 38.2, 38.4, 38.5, and 38.10). However, the best visualization of the Fontan reconstruction may not always be obtained from the usual left parasternal location. The examiner should pass the transducer across the entire chest focusing on the left and right parasternal borders, as well as the left anterior axillary line (Fig. 38.12). Repositioning the patient often improves acoustic quality. Images from the left chest are often optimal when the patient is in a left lateral decubitus position. Right parasternal imaging is facilitated by having the patient lie on the right side. Occasionally, simply having the patient in supine position provides the best imaging window.

In addition to routine imaging of the intracardiac structures (focused on the valves, atria, and ventricles), serial images following the inferior vena caval pathway toward the Fontan anastomosis should be obtained. The most convenient way of tracing this pathway is to use a series of horizontally oriented (short-axis) scans obtained by gradually moving the transducer from the inferior costal margin to a more superior position on the chest. When the pulmonary arterial confluence is visualized, the examiner can be confident that the position of the inferior Fontan connection will be slightly below that level. Regardless of how the connection is visualized, it is often found just posterior and slightly to the right of the ascending aorta. If one follows the flow stream beyond the connection, it will lead to the pulmonary arterial bifurcation. Color flow Doppler is often quite helpful not only in tracing the vena caval flow to the Fontan but also in defining the transition between Fontan pathway and the branch pulmonary arteries. Since venous and

pulmonary arterial flows in the Fontan circulation have relatively low velocities, reducing the Nyquist limit to no more than 60 cm/s is recommended.

The scans used to define the inferior pathway to the Fontan can be continued more superiorly to detect any connections from the superior vena cava that may have been performed as a part of the patient's surgical palliation. Once the inferior pathway, pulmonary arteries, and the superior pathway(s) have been identified in horizontal images, the scan planes can be shifted into a more sagittal display to show the long axis of these connections and pathways. Documentation of the venous pathway's diameter at the level

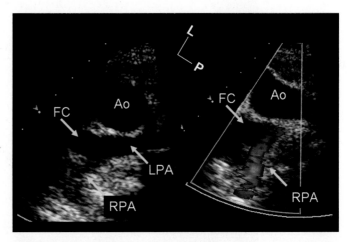

FIGURE 38.12. Echocardiographic images of a nonstandard view of the Fontan connection and pulmonary arterial confluence in a patient after an extracardiac Fontan for "double-inlet left ventricle." As described in the text, the transducer is positioned along the left anterior axillary line just lateral to the pectoralis major muscle group. The image reveals the Fontan connection (FC) and both pulmonary arteries just beyond the aorta (Ao). Since this is a coronal scan originating from the left lateral surface of the chest, the right pulmonary artery (RPA) is seen in the far field. Doppler interrogation of the vessel produces excellent signal quality since RPA flow is parallel to the plane of sound from this transducer position (laminar, blue flow signal, **right**). Resolution of the vessel walls is less optimal. In contrast, the left pulmonary artery (LPA) is clearly seen in the two-dimensional scan on the left, but Doppler flow is difficult to demonstrate since the long axis of the vessel is perpendicular to the imaging plane. L, left; P, posterior.

of the inferior vena cava, the mid-atrium, the pulmonary arteries, and the superior vena cava is helpful in determining whether any significant obstructions are present. Color flow and spectral Doppler interrogation of the suture lines and any fenestrations help define any obstructions and assess the transpulmonary resistance.

Nonstandard acoustic windows can greatly enhance the examination. The "inferior" Fontan connection (atriopulmonary Fontan or extracardiac conduit) can often be visualized using a modified left anterior axillary window. This image is obtained with the transducer positioned just lateral to the pectoralis major muscle, near the axilla. The plane of sound is angled "back" toward the midline, resulting in an imaging plane that is nearly parallel to the long axis of the right pulmonary artery (Fig. 38.12).

Attention is then shifted to the apical window. The long axes of the Fontan connections and venous pathways are often not seen well in this orientation. Some short-axis images of Fontan conduits (extracardiac or intracardiac) and lateral tunnels are usually available at the apex. Residual right-to-left shunts from the Fontan pathway or native right atrium are easily detected by color flow Doppler from this window. Any right-to-left atrial shunt lesions should also be interrogated with continuous-wave Doppler, to determine the mean gradient of that flow. That gradient will reflect the drop in pressure from the Fontan anastomosis to the pulmonary veins or transpulmonary gradient. This value provides crucial insight into the resistance to blood flow within the pulmonary arterial bed.

Finally, the transducer is moved to the high parasternal and suprasternal windows. The upper systemic veins (superior vena cava, jugular, and innominate veins) and aortic arch are evaluated as has been described elsewhere.

ASSESSMENT OF VENTRICULAR PERFORMANCE

The most important variable related to ongoing success of a Fontan operation is ventricular performance. The systemic ventricle must maintain normal (or nearly normal) systolic contractility and low diastolic filling pressure. The complex geometry of functional single ventricles makes use of a single method of assessment impractical. In hearts with primarily left ventricular morphology, standard methods of calculating ejection fraction, circumferential fiber shortening, and wall stress continue to be clinically useful. When ventricular

morphology is more complicated, one must resort to other methods of assessment. An important point to remember is that any method used must be reproducible, both between examiners and over time. In these situations, we have used methods that do not depend on ventricular geometry. Determinations of fractional area change in multiple planes (usually parasternal short-axis and the apical "four-chamber" views) is helpful in documenting ventricular wall motion (Fig. 38.13). Normal values for both right and left ventricular fractional area change are greater than 40%. The myocardial performance index and Doppler-derived systolic rates of ventricular pressure change (dP/dT) can also provide information about ventricular performance. All of these "nonstandard" parameters gain added value when followed over time to outline trends in the same patient.

Detailed discussions of the methodologies used assess ventricular diastolic filling pressure can be found in the previous chapter discussing evaluation of ventricular function. Pulsed-wave Doppler techniques have been validated in patients with single-ventricle physiology. Tissue Doppler and myocardial deformation imaging are likely to provide additional insights but require validation in this group. Pulmonary venous atrial reversal duration and atrioventricular valve diastolic deceleration time have been the most useful diastolic parameters in Fontan patients. Significant prolongation (>28 ms) of the pulmonary venous atrial reversal relative to atrial forward flow duration into the ventricle is a reliable sign of elevated filling pressure even in the Fontan circulation. Reductions in deceleration time have been associated with prolonged chest tube drainage after Fontan creation and increased mortality in patients with protein-losing enteropathy. It is our impression that gradual changes in these parameters provide early warning of impending ventricular dysfunction. Therefore, thorough diastolic filling assessments should be performed regularly and followed serially in these patients.

VENOUS AND ARTERIAL PATHWAY OBSTRUCTIONS

Obstructions at any level are less well tolerated by patients with Fontan physiology than those who have biventricular circulations. Subaortic stenosis, coarctation, and pulmonary arterial distortions represent the most common obstructive problems seen after the Fontan operation. Assessments of ventricular outlet and aortic arch

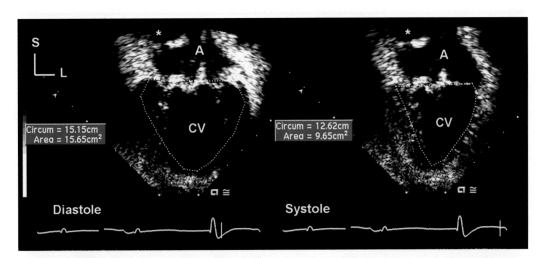

FIGURE 38.13. Diastolic (left) and systolic (right) frames taken from the apex of a common ventricle after Fontan operation. A portion of the extracardiac conduit (*asterisk*) can be seen in the posterior and rightward "corner" of the common atrium (A). Ventricles with mixed or right ventricular morphology do not follow standard geometric conventions. In these cases, an index of ventricular function can be obtained by simply comparing the diastolic and systolic areas of the ventricular cavity. Once these areas are traced, as in the figure, a two-dimensional, systolic fractional area change (FAC) can be calculated by dividing the difference between the two areas by the diastolic area (see formula). This measurement is analogous to the linear systolic shortening fraction determined by M-mode. Similar to shortening fraction and ejection fraction, this will be varied with alterations in preload and afterload, but it offers a simple, reproducible measurement that is related to systolic function even in geometrically complex ventricles. The measurement can be obtained from one or multiple planes and normal values are generally greater than 40%.

FAC = (Diastolic area − Systolic area)/Diastolic area

The ventricle illustrated in this figure had diastolic and systolic areas of 15.7 and 9.7 cm^2, respectively. The difference is 6 cm^2 and the FAC is therefore equal to 6 divided by 15.7 (apical FAC = 38%). L, left; S, superior.

obstructions are performed using the same techniques described in earlier chapters focused on biventricular hearts. However, the examiner needs to recognize that even mild degrees of stenosis can have significant adverse effects in the Fontan patient. Subaortic and arterial obstructions with even the low gradients (15 to 25 mm Hg) can negatively affect cardiac performance and reserve in Fontan patients.

Pulmonary arterial stenosis requires a different method of evaluation in the Fontan patient than in those with biventricular circulations. Since there is no pulmonary ventricular pump, flow in the pulmonary vascular bed is nonpulsatile. Stenoses in the Fontan pathway and pulmonary arteries will display hemodynamics that are more similar to venous obstructions. As a result, Doppler flow gradients are often misleadingly low. Therefore, the focus of the pulmonary arterial examination should be to carefully define the size of the pathways leading to the Fontan connections, the size of the connections themselves, and the size of the pulmonary arteries centrally (Fig. 38.14). Any abrupt decrease in vascular diameter should be considered a potential stenosis. Particular attention should be paid to areas in which the pathway narrows and then enlarges again downstream. These areas should be interrogated with both continuous, and pulsed-wave Doppler. A reduction in flow variability either proximal to (Fig. 38.15) or beyond the narrowing is suggestive of obstruction. If there is an increase in velocity through the narrowed segment, a mean gradient (measured over multiple cardiac cycles) should be calculated (Fig. 38.13). A mean gradient of greater than 3 mm Hg should be considered significant and at a minimum warrants additional evaluation and possibly intervention.

PROBLEMS ASSOCIATED WITH ATRIAL ENLARGEMENT

Older, direct atrial–to–pulmonary arterial Fontan connections can develop complications that are rarely seen with either intra-atrial or extracardiac conduits. The native atrial tissue left in the systemic venous circulation is under a higher than normal distending pressure. In addition, since there are no valves in the Fontan pathways, atrial contraction and relaxation will produce an additional stimulus for atrial enlargement. As a result, these atria will dilate, usually in a progressive fashion. These dilated chambers can compress nearby vascular structures. The pulmonary veins

are most susceptible to this compression, because their distending pressures are lower than those within the Fontan circuit (Fig. 38.16). Pulmonary venous compression/obstruction is poorly tolerated by patients with Fontan physiology. Flow through the segments of lung drained by the compressed pulmonary veins will be reduced. This will certainly reduce the patient's ability to increase cardiac output, and in severe situations may even decrease the resting cardiac output.

The dilated atria seen in patients with atrial pulmonary connections create areas where blood flow is sluggish. These atria are therefore prone to mural thrombosis formation (Figs. 38.10 and 38.11). These thrombi are rarely obstructive but can contribute to embolic disease. Last, it is thought that distended atrial tissue is at increased risk for generating abnormal, reentrant tachyarrhythmias, particularly atrial flutter. These abnormal atrial rhythms can be detected echocardiographically by careful analysis of atrial wall motion or the atrial influences on venous or pulmonary arterial flow patterns (Figs. 38.9 and 38.17).

ECHOCARDIOGRAPHIC CLUES TO A FAILING FONTAN CIRCULATION

A number of echocardiographic findings can provide clues to deteriorating cardiovascular function (Table 38.2). Most of these abnormalities can be detected by standard echocardiographic techniques. The gradual rate at which some of these changes occur make it necessary to track these parameters, particularly chamber sizes, and indices of contractility, consistently over time. When present, these dysfunctional findings should prompt additional investigation, even if the primary problem is not evident to standard interrogations.

A few additional simple scans are required to document the presence or absence of ascites and effusions. The inferior vena cava of Fontan patients will be more prominent than in patients with biventricular circulations. This is because of the expected increase in systemic venous or "right atrial" pressure that accompanies direct connection of the systemic veins to the pulmonary arteries. However, systemic venous pressures will increase even further in the face of decreasing cardiac output or function. Consequently, the inferior vena cava will tend to progressively enlarge in patients with deteriorating cardiac function and progressively elevating right atrial pressures. As a result, serial evaluation of the inferior vena

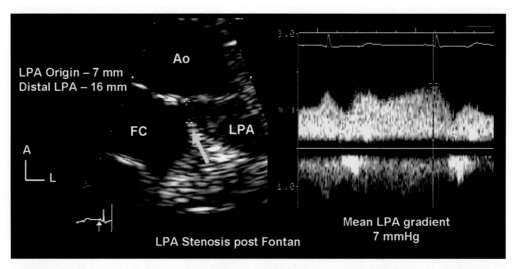

FIGURE 38.14. Branch pulmonary arterial stenosis after an atriopulmonary Fontan operation. The echocardiographic image and Doppler signal demonstrate a discrete, but severe proximal left pulmonary artery (LPA) stenosis (*yellow arrow*). The narrowed segment is short, but the internal pulmonary artery diameter is less than 50% of the diameter downstream. **Right:** Continuous-wave Doppler interrogation of the flow crossing this stenosis resulted in this signal. Flow velocities are elevated, relative to what is usually seen in the Fontan patient. However, maximum flow velocities only reach 1.7 m/s. The mean gradient, averaged over multiple cardiac and respiratory cycles, was 7 mm Hg. Note that although the flow is somewhat phasic, the velocity profile never reverses during atrial relaxation. In fact, it never even approaches the baseline as one would expect in a patient with an atriopulmonary connection. Given the absence of the ventricle in the pulmonary circulation of the Fontan patient, the luminal narrowing, and the pressure gradient it caused, significantly limited the patient's ability to increase his cardiac output and had been associated with a progressively enlarging right atrial chamber. Exercise capacity improved after placement of a left pulmonary artery stent and revision of the Fontan connection using an extracardiac conduit. A, anterior; Ao, aorta; FC, Fontan connection; L, left.

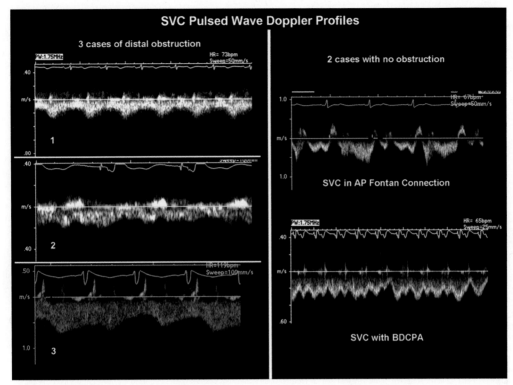

FIGURE 38.15. Alterations in superior vena caval flow patterns in the presence of downstream Fontan obstructions. The best method of determining the presence of or absence of stenosis within a Fontan pathway is to directly visualize the vessels involved. However, image quality after the Fontan operation is often suboptimal. Analysis of venous Doppler flow patterns can provide clues regarding the status of downstream venous connections to the pulmonary circulation. **Left:** Three pulsed-wave Doppler signals were obtained from the mid-portion of the superior vena cava (SVC) in three different patients. All three had significant downstream stenoses in their circulations. The top signal (*1*) was obtained from the patient with near-complete occlusion of the SVC. There is little phasic change in the flow pattern. Flow does increase during ventricular diastole but never returns to baseline. Even respiratory variation is absent; this is extremely abnormal in the venous circulation. The middle (*2*) and bottom (*3*) signals were obtained from patients with less obstruction. There is some respiratory variation and augmentation of forward flow during ventricular diastole. However, similar to the top signal (*1*), flow velocities never return toward the baseline, indicative of a pressure in the SVC, which is constantly greater than the chamber or vessel into which it flows. In a normal situation, illustrated by two signals (**right**), SVC pressure equalizes with downstream pressures, or may occasionally even be less than pressure downstream, resulting in phasic, low-flow velocities or even flow reversal. **Top right:** Signal was obtained in a patient with an atriopulmonary Fontan connection and a widely patent SVC. The patient was in a junctional rhythm during the recording, and as a result the atrial reversals are seen after the QRS complex. Nonetheless, atrial activity is seen to influence the flow pattern in the upper portions of the SVC, confirming a widely patent connection between those two points in the cardiovascular system. **Bottom right:** Signal was obtained from the patient with a bidirectional SVC–to–right pulmonary artery anastomosis. There are no reversals seen, but there is respiratory variation and appropriate reductions and augmentations to forward flow with not only ventricular diastole but also left atrial contraction and relaxation (Fig. 38.8). Evidence of atrial activity in the vena caval flow pattern again confirms the patency of the connection in this case. AP, atriopulmonary; BDCPA, bidirectional cavopulmonary anastomosis.

cava diameter should be included in the postoperative evaluation of all Fontan patients. This evaluation can simply include measurement of expiratory diameter, with adequate two-dimensional visualization to allow exclusion of thrombus and spontaneous contrast. The most convenient approaches for obtaining these images involve acquiring a sagittal plane view of the inferior vena cava from either the central subcostal transducer position or a more lateral transducer position over the body of the liver.

Echocardiographic evaluation of cardiac rhythms is usually confined to the prenatal practice. However, the electrocardiogram of the post-Fontan patient can be difficult to interpret. Therefore, the echocardiographer should report at normal atrial activity when it

is evident. Abnormally rapid or dyssynchronous atrial contractions can often be detected by careful analysis of the venous Doppler flow tracings. Pulmonary venous and arterial flow signals will show an increased number and rate of atrial indentations or reversals in the forward flow pattern when the patient is in atrial flutter (Fig. 38.17). The increased atrial activity can be easily compared with the QRS complex on the simultaneous rhythm strip to determine the cardiac rhythm. Alternatively, if atrial wall motion is evident, M-mode tracings of the atrial appendage can provide the same information.

Pulmonary arterial and hepatic venous flow signals can also provide evidence of atrial contractions. The native right atrium remains in communication with the venae cavae in patients with atriopulmonary connections. In this situation, atrial flow reversals will be seen in the hepatic veins and can be used to assist in determining the rhythm in the same way that was described for the pulmonary veins (Fig. 38.7). However, in atrioventricular dyssynchronous rhythms, like complete heart block and junctional rhythm, hepatic "cannon" atrial reversals caused by left atrial contractions can be present even in patients with extracardiac conduits (Fig. 38.9).

As in all patients, comprehensive examinations of valvar function need to be performed in patients after Fontan procedures. These assessments have been covered elsewhere in this textbook, and detailed discussion of the methods used will not be repeated here.

Table 38.2	ECHOCARDIOGRAPHIC CLUES TO DYSFUNCTION IN A FONTAN CIRCULATION

- Progressive enlargement of the IVC
- Spontaneous echo contrast
- Enlarging ventricular chamber dimension
- Progressive atrial enlargement
- Presence of ascites or pleural effusions
- New onset atrial tachyarrhythmias

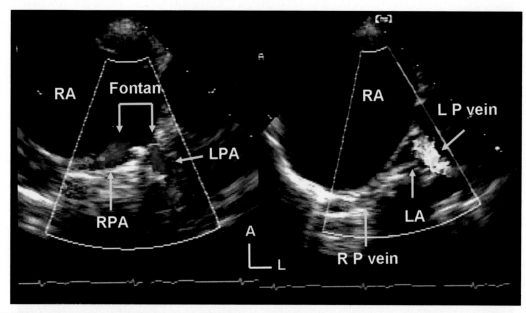

FIGURE 38.16. Pulmonary venous compression secondary to right atrial enlargement. Images display massive right atrial (RA) enlargement in a patient with a very complex past surgical history. The primary lesion was that of the "double-inlet left ventricle." His surgical history included pulmonary arterial reconstructions, subaortic resection, several palliative shunts, and eventually an atriopulmonary Fontan completion. As expected, his ventricular diastolic compliance was poor and led to multiple complications. At the time of this examination, the patient's RA diameter was greater than 7 cm. **Left:** Horizontal-plane image shows the Fontan connection to be widely patent with normal flow seen in both of his pulmonary arteries. **Right:** Relationship of the dilated right atrium to the left atrium (LA). The LA was significantly smaller than the right atrium. Color Doppler detected aliased flow in the left lower pulmonary vein (L P vein), and continuous-wave Doppler revealed a mean gradient of 5 mm Hg between the left pulmonary vein and the LA. The lumen of the right pulmonary vein (R P vein) was difficult to appreciate and Doppler flow could never be detected. This kind of compression severely limits the amount of cardiac output that can pass through the lungs. As might be expected, this patient had symptoms of low cardiac output and tremendous sodium retention with large amounts of ascites and recurrent pleural effusions. Unfortunately, despite an attempted surgical revision of his Fontan pathway, he did not survive. A, anterior; L, left.

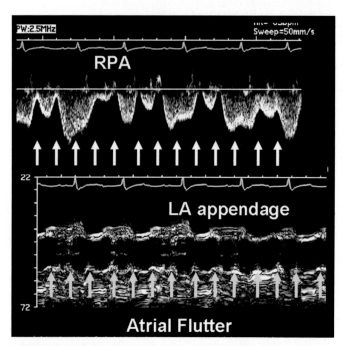

FIGURE 38.17. Detecting atrial arrhythmias using echocardiography. Atrial electrical activity is often difficult to visualize on the standard electrocardiogram of a Fontan patient. The images in this figure were taken from an examination of a patient with hypoplastic left heart syndrome after an atriopulmonary Fontan operation who had developed atrial flutter with 3:1 atrioventricular conduction. Although the rhythm strip does not show discernible P waves, the M-mode tracing (**bottom**) shows multiple contractions of the left atrial appendage during each cardiac cycle (*yellow arrows*). Similarly, the pulsed-wave Doppler flow signal (**top**) shows multiple reductions in forward flow (*white arrows*) that cannot be explained by the cardiac cycle. When a Fontan patient shows rapid narrow complex tachycardia or a relatively constant heart rate with no visible P waves or a prolonged PR interval, one must suspect atrial flutter. Careful analysis of the venous and pulmonary arterial flow patterns or M-mode interrogation of the atrial wall can clarify the origin of the rhythm in these cases. LA, left atrium; RPA, right pulmonary artery.

 ## ILLUSTRATIVE CASES INVOLVING PATIENTS WITH FONTAN CIRCULATIONS

Case 1

These images were taken shortly after creation of an extracardiac, fenestrated Fontan circulation in a 3-year-old with tricuspid valve atresia. The patient has been dismissed from the hospital and was steadily improving. Fig. 38.18 contains apical four-chamber views of the extracardiac conduit (red arrow), pulmonary venous atrium (native right and left atrium), mitral valve, and left ventricle. The aliased color flow signal in the top right panel (yellow arrow) and the continuous-wave Doppler signal in the bottom panel were generated by flow through the fenestration. Both Doppler signals confirm the right-to-left shunt flow. The spectral Doppler tracing shows that the mean "Fontan–to–left atrial" or transpulmonary gradient is 7 mm Hg. The velocity of the right-to-left shunt decreases after left atrial contraction (white arrows), but fenestration flow is continuous as one would expect in a patient after Fontan creation. Fig. 38.19 documents the patency of the anastomosis between the extracardiac conduit and the pulmonary artery. Fig. 38.20 confirms the adequacy of the preexisting bidirectional right superior vena cava–to–right pulmonary artery connection (asterisk) and reveals a normal phasic flow pattern in the superior vena cava (lower pulsed-wave Doppler tracing). The Fontan conduit to inferior vena cava connection is also appreciated in these images (red arrows).

Case 2

These images were taken from an examination of a 7-year-old with hypoplastic left heart syndrome. He had a history of neonatal Norwood operation, followed by bidirectional right superior vena cava–to–right pulmonary artery anastomosis at 7 months of age, and Fontan completion at 3 years of age. Fig. 38.21 shows the apical four-chamber anatomy. Unlike the patient in Case 1, pulmonary venous flow must pass from the native left atrium and cross the

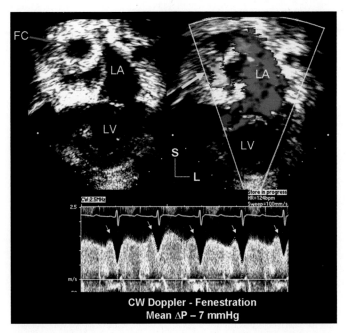

FIGURE 38.18. Case 1. Apical "four-chamber" views and continuous-wave Doppler flow signal generated by the atrial fenestration described in the text and obtained from a patient with tricuspid valve atresia after a fenestrated, extracardiac Fontan completion. CW, continuous wave; FC, Fontan conduit; L, left; LA, left atrium; LV, left ventricle; S, superior; ΔP, pressure gradient.

plane of the resected atrial septum to reach the right atrium and tricuspid valve. The fenestration had spontaneously closed, leaving no evidence of residual intracardiac shunt, but there is a trivial amount of tricuspid valve regurgitation. Pulmonary venous and tricuspid valve pulsed-wave Doppler recordings are consistent with low filling pressure. Ventricular function was normal with an apical fractional area change value of 42%. The arterial reconstruction associated with Norwood operation is seen in Fig. 38.22. The patency of these connections must be confirmed as any residual obstruction will create unnecessary afterload, potentially compromising ventricular function. The connection between the extracardiac conduit and the pulmonary arterial confluence is seen in Fig. 38.23. The connection is not restrictive, although the branch pulmonary arteries are somewhat small (common after the Norwood reconstruction). The pulsed-wave Doppler signal in the bottom panel shows a normal flow pattern within the right pulmonary artery. Appropriate variation is seen with both respiration and "left" atrial and ventricular activity.

Case 3

These images were taken during an examination of the 56-year-old woman with tricuspid valve atresia and normally related great arteries. As a 5-year-old, she had creation of a right Blalock-Taussig shunt. At age 39, an atriopulmonary Fontan was created. Her past history was also remarkable for three episodes of endocarditis prior to the Fontan operation and multiple episodes of atrial tachyarrhythmias, now controlled with chronic amiodarone administration. Her atrial arrhythmias began approximately 12 years after completion of the Fontan. She presented for this examination with increasing fatigue and shortness of breath. Her echocardiogram revealed a distended inferior vena cava with a moderate amount of spontaneous contrast within it. Fig. 38.24 contains the apical four-chamber view. Her right atrium was massively enlarged, the left atrium and ventricle were moderately enlarged, and ventricular ejection fraction was calculated to be 55%. The right panels of Fig. 38.24 show that her atriopulmonary Fontan connection was widely patent and there was no distortion of her proximal pulmonary arteries. Pulsed-wave Doppler interrogation of the right pulmonary artery and hepatic vein showed phasic flow changes because of atrial contraction and relaxation further confirming the patency of the Fontan connection (Fig. 38.25). Doppler interrogation of the mitral inflow tract (Fig. 38.26) revealed limited atrial forward flow duration (yellow arrows) and the presence of a pathologic mid-diastolic L-wave (white arrow, Figure 38.26, top). Pulmonary venous flow pattern (Fig. 38.26, bottom) showed brief early diastolic augmentation (after mitral valve opening) with prominent and prolonged flow reversal after atrial contraction (yellow arrows, Fig. 38.26, bottom). Note that her heart rate was only 45 beats per minute during the examination. Exercise testing showed a blunted heart rate response, reaching a maximum of only 85 beats per minute. This degree of bradycardia is poorly tolerated in the setting of reduced ventricular compliance, since increasing heart rate is one of the few methods available to increase cardiac output in these patients. Since no surgical intervention would have altered her physiology, her regimen was adjusted. Her beta-blocker was discontinued and the amiodarone dose was decreased in an attempt to increase her heart rate. Her diuretic therapy was intensified. These maneuvers resulted in a small improvement in her symptoms, but unfortunately her activities remain limited by her sinus node and severe diastolic dysfunction. Pacemaker implantation is currently being considered as a method to improve her heart rate response to exertion.

Case 4

These transesophageal images were taken during examination of a 31-year-old man with tricuspid and pulmonary valve atresia. He complained of increasing fatigue and exercise intolerance. He had undergone creation of an atriopulmonary Fontan connection

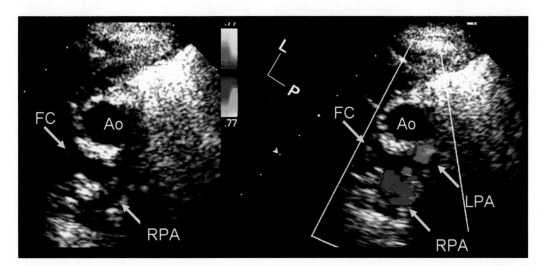

FIGURE 38.19. Case 1. Coronal views of the Fontan connection from the left lateral axillary transducer position. Two-dimensional scans (**left**) and color Doppler (right) showed no narrowing in the Fontan connection (FC) or the pulmonary arteries. Ao, aorta; L, left; LPA, left pulmonary artery; P, posterior; RPA, right pulmonary artery.

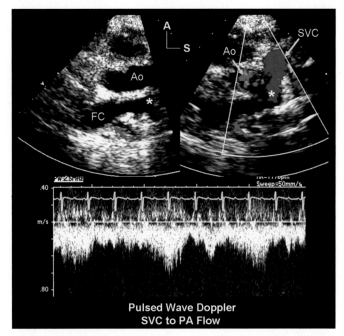

FIGURE 38.20. Case 1. Top: Long-axis (sagittal) images of the superior vena cava (SVC) and Fontan conduit (FC). The preexisting SVC–to–right pulmonary artery anastomosis is marked (*asterisk*). The FC–to–inferior vena cava transition is highlighted (*red arrow*). No narrowings were noted anywhere within the systemic venous diversion. Color flow Doppler profiles and the pulsed-wave Doppler signal from the superior vena cava were normal (**right** and **bottom**). Note the phasic changes in the Doppler signal that relate to both cardiac activity, as well as the respiratory cycle. A, anterior; Ao, ascending aorta; S, superior.

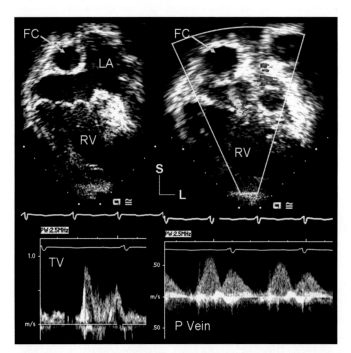

FIGURE 38.21. Case 2. Apical "four-chamber" views and pulsed-wave Doppler flow signals recorded at the tips of the tricuspid valve leaflets and within the right lower pulmonary vein of a patient with mitral valve atresia after a neonatal Norwood operation and eventual fenestrated, extracardiac Fontan completion. The fenestration had spontaneously closed 2 years before this examination. Color flow interrogation of the tricuspid valve showed only mild regurgitation (**top right**). Pulsed-wave Doppler signals at the tricuspid valve and in the pulmonary veins showed normal diastolic filling. Forward flow into the ventricle with atrial contraction was prominent and there was no evidence of reversed flow in the pulmonary vein after the P wave. These findings are consistent with low ventricular filling pressure, a key component of favorable physiology in patients with Fontan circulations. FC, Fontan conduit; L, left; LA, left atrium; P, pulmonary; RV, right ventricle; S, superior; TV, tricuspid valve.

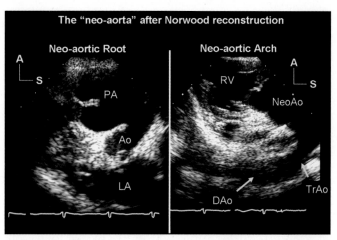

FIGURE 38.22. Case 2. Complex arterial reconstruction involved in the Norwood operation. Examination of these patients both before and after the Fontan operation must confirm the absence of obstruction throughout the thoracic aorta. **Left:** Sagittal-plane image shows the proximal arterial roots near the base of the heart. The native pulmonary artery (PA) and hypoplastic ascending aorta (Ao) have been surgically merged into one functional "neoaortic" root. **Right:** Oblique, high left parasternal transducer position. It shows the native pulmonary valve, ascending "neoaorta" (NeoAo), transverse aorta arch (TrAo), and upper descending aorta (DAo). In this case, the arterial reconstructions were widely patent and the native pulmonary valve showed no evidence of regurgitation. Narrowings of the connection between the native pulmonary artery and the hypoplastic native aorta can compromise coronary blood flow, while residual stenosis in the arch reconstruction (coarctation) causes an unacceptable pressure load on the systemic right ventricle (RV). A, anterior; LA, left atrium; S, superior.

24 years prior to this examination. Before the Fontan completion procedure, he had been palliated with a Waterston shunt. As a result, his pulmonary arterial confluence was significantly distorted. His Fontan connection included a direct right atrial–to–right pulmonary artery anastomosis and placement of a supplemental, 22-mm nonvalved conduit from the right atrium to the left pulmonary artery to bypass the acquired stenosis of his pulmonary arterial confluence. His transthoracic echocardiogram showed

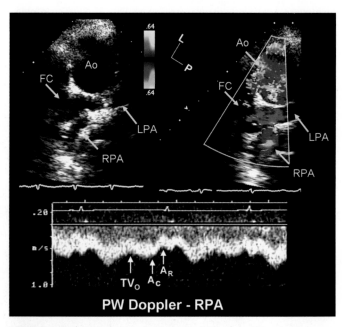

FIGURE 38.23. Case 2. Two-dimensional and color flow images show widely patent Fontan connection (FC) with normal flow in both the proximal right and left pulmonary arteries (RPA and LPA). The pulsed-wave Doppler tracing shows normal phasic activity in the right pulmonary artery as previously described. AC, atrial contraction; Ao, aorta; AR, atrial relaxation; FC, Fontan connection; L, left; LPA, left pulmonary artery; P, posterior; RPA, right pulmonary artery; TVO, tricuspid valve opening.

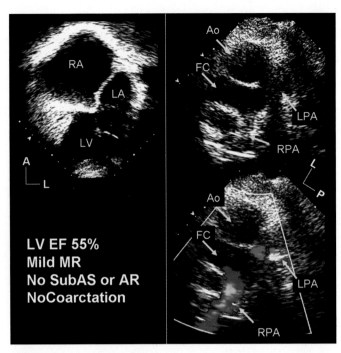

FIGURE 38.24. Case 3. Echocardiographic images show the apical "four-chamber" anatomy, as well as the atriopulmonary Fontan connection and pulmonary arterial confluence in this 56-year-old patient. The right atrium (RA) is tremendously dilated. The Fontan pathway was widely patent. Other pertinent findings are summarized in the text. A, anterior; Ao, aorta; FC, Fontan connection; L, left; LA, left atrium; LPA, left pulmonary artery; LV, left ventricle; P, posterior; RPA, right pulmonary artery.

good ventricular function, mild mitral regurgitation, and a very large right atrium. The Fontan connections could not be visualized by surface echocardiography and a transesophageal echocardiogram was performed. Fig. 38.27 shows two images oriented in the distal esophageal four-chamber view. Scans from this position confirmed satisfactory systolic function and only a mild degree of central mitral valve regurgitation. Fig. 38.28 demonstrates that the right atrial–to–right pulmonary artery connection was quite

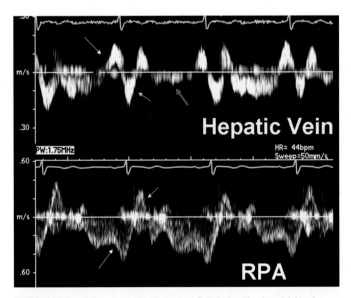

FIGURE 38.25. Case 3. Pulsed-wave Doppler tracings. Both the hepatic vein and right pulmonary artery (RPA) signals show the phasic flows related to atrial contraction and relaxation (arrows) that we expect with patent Fontan connections. However, the degree of forward flow reduction during the expiratory phase of the respiratory cycle was more prominent than usual (red arrow), suggesting elevated systemic venous pressure.

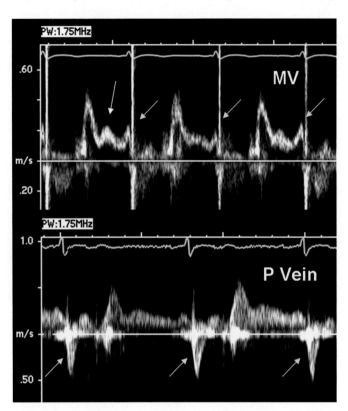

FIGURE 38.26. Case 3. Pulsed-wave Doppler recordings revealed the primary hemodynamic problems afflicting this patient. **Top:** Mitral valve (MV) inflow Doppler signal. Mid-diastolic deceleration time was relatively normal (185 ms), but there was a prominent mid-diastolic L wave (white arrow), indicating significantly abnormal/delayed left ventricular relaxation. The transmitral atrial filling wave (yellow arrows) is abbreviated and ends at approximately the same time as the S wave on the ECG. **Bottom:** Right lower pulmonary vein (P vein). It shows extremely low-velocity diastolic forward flow into a prominent, prolonged atrial reversal (yellow arrows). Venous reversal extends well beyond the S wave. In fact, the reversal duration was 60 ms longer than the atrial forward flow duration. These findings are consistent with reduced diastolic ventricular compliance and significantly elevated ventricular end-diastolic and mean left atrial pressures. One should also note that the patient's heart rate was quite slow (45 bpm). This type of bradycardia may be poorly tolerated in the face of such severe ventricular diastolic dysfunction.

small, measuring only 12 mm in diameter. The color flow signal (Fig. 38.28, top right) showed aliasing at the distal anastomosis. Continuous-wave Doppler revealed reduced variability and an elevated mean gradient (4 mm Hg) across the connection (Fig. 38.28, bottom). The 22-mm conduit could not be identified. However, flow was detected in the area of the left pulmonary artery, just posterior and lateral to the ascending aorta (Fig. 38.29). Cardiac

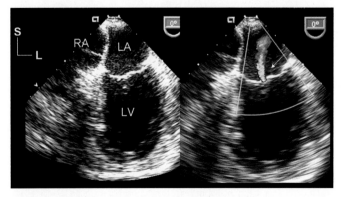

FIGURE 38.27. Case 4. "Four-chamber" views taken from the distal esophageal position during a transesophageal echocardiogram in a patient with tricuspid and pulmonary valve atresia. The atrial septation patch appears to adequately divide the right (RA) and left atrium (LA). All of the cardiac chambers were somewhat enlarged, and color flow Doppler revealed mild mitral regurgitation (**right,** white arrow). L, left; LV, left ventricle; S, superior.

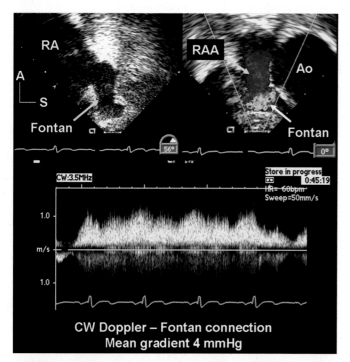

FIGURE 38.28. Case 4. Sagittal plane images (*top*) demonstrate the connection between the dilated right atrium and the pulmonary arterial confluence. The pulmonary arteries are not completely visualized in this plane, but the right atrial appendage "Fontan" connection is well visualized (RAA). The 1.0 × 1.5-cm diameter of this pathway is very small for this 31-year-old man. The color flow signal (**top right**) shows aliasing consistent with elevated flow velocity in this area. As expected, the continuous-wave Doppler signal (**bottom**) shows an abnormal flow pattern. The decreased velocity at either end of the tracing was caused by translational motion and does not reflect the true flow signal. When the Doppler beam was adequately aligned (**center** of the tracing), the flow velocities were elevated and did not reflect the atrial contraction and relaxation patterns expected in this atriopulmonary Fontan connection. The mean right atrial–to–pulmonary artery Doppler gradient was 4 mm Hg. This may seem like a "low" value, but in the unforgiving setting of a Fontan circulation, it represents an important obstruction. A, anterior; Ao, aorta; CW, continuous wave; S, superior.

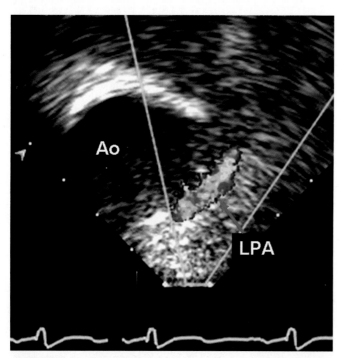

FIGURE 38.29. Case 4. Horizontal-plane image obtained just posterior to the ascending aorta (Ao). The color flow signal outlines the entire diameter and length of the proximal left pulmonary artery (LPA). This vessel was only 5 mm in diameter, clearly too small to provide adequate flow in this adult male. The aliased flow pattern suggests that this stenosis/hypoplasia is causing an additional obstruction to transpulmonary flow (above and beyond that caused by the Fontan obstruction shown in Fig. 38.28). A, anterior; L, left.

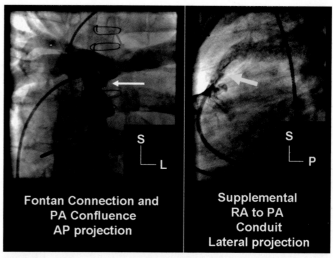

FIGURE 38.30. Case 4. Left: Angiogram shows an anteroposterior (AP) projection of a contrast injection made just proximal to the Fontan anastomosis (*horizontal white arrow*). The Fontan connection is indeed narrow as was seen on the transesophageal echocardiogram (Fig. 38.28). The branch pulmonary arteries bifurcate to the right and left of the Fontan connection. The right pulmonary artery is normal. The left pulmonary artery stenosis, seen in Figure 38.29, can be appreciated here as well (*red arrow*). However, it is now clear that the distal left pulmonary artery is significantly larger and that relief of these narrowings may improve transpulmonary flow. **Right:** Angiogram shows a lateral projection of an injection in the supplemental, 22-mm graft connecting the right atrium to pulmonary artery. This connection could not be detected by any echocardiographic examination and was thought to have been occluded. These injections showed that it was slightly patent (*yellow arrow*) but had narrowed significantly, measuring only 5 to 6 mm in diameter. L, left; P, posterior; PA, pulmonary artery; S, superior.

catheterization subsequently revealed that the stenotic left pulmonary artery retained its connection to the right pulmonary artery, that it was of normal size distally, and that the right atrial–to–left pulmonary artery conduit was actually patent but had an extremely narrow lumen (Fig. 38.30). This case dramatically illustrates the need to use multiple imaging modalities when evaluating a patient with a failing Fontan circulation. Revision of the patient's Fontan connection was recommended. A stent was placed in the pulmonary arterial confluence intraoperatively, enlarging the connection between the right and left pulmonary artery. The Fontan connection was then revised to include an intra-atrial conduit, an enlarged atrial–to–right pulmonary artery connection, and a small atrial fenestration. The images in Fig. 38.31 were taken from the postoperative transesophageal echocardiogram performed during this revision. The left panel shows the

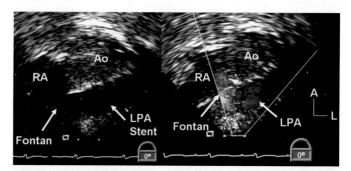

FIGURE 38.31. Case 4. Postoperative transesophageal echocardiogram performed during revision of this patient's Fontan connection. After initiation of cardiopulmonary bypass, an intravascular stent was placed across the left pulmonary artery stenosis and dilated to a 15-mm diameter. An intra-atrial conduit was placed to eliminate the dilated atrial chamber from the Fontan circulation and direct both vena caval flows to the enlarged Fontan connection. **Left:** Much larger communication between the upper portion of the right atrial conduit (RA) and the pulmonary arterial confluence. The left pulmonary artery (LPA) stenosis, posterior to the aorta (Ao), has been completely eliminated. **Right:** Color flow Doppler no longer shows any evidence of aliasing in these areas. A, anterior; L, left.

stent enlarging the left pulmonary artery, and the right panel illustrates the associated improvement in the color flow Doppler pattern within the Fontan connection and proximal left pulmonary artery.

 ## SUMMARY

Understanding and evaluating patients with the Fontan circulation requires a thorough understanding of not only the surgical anatomy but also the unique cardiovascular physiology of these patients. Unfortunately, these patients often have challenging acoustic windows. When surface echocardiography does not provide adequate detail, alternative imaging strategies should be used. The systematic echocardiographic approach described in this chapter allows not only a complete delineation of the cardiovascular anatomy but also the physiology associated with Fontan circulation. Serial, longitudinal follow-up studies using these techniques should increase the likelihood of early detection of late complications of the Fontan operation, leading, it is hoped, to improved therapeutic outcomes.

SUGGESTED READING

Bartz PJ, Driscoll DJ, Dearani JA, et al. Early and late results of the modified Fontan operation for heterotaxy syndrome 30 years of experience in 142 patients. *J Am Coll Cardiol.* 2006;48:2301–2305.

Cetta F, Feldt RH, O'Leary PW, et al. Improved early morbidity and mortality after Fontan operation: the Mayo Clinic experience, 1987 to 1992. *J Am Coll Cardiol.* 1996;28:480–486.

Choussat A, Fontan F, Besse P, et al. Selection criteria for Fontan procedure. In: Anderson FH, Shinebourne EA, eds. *Pediatric Cardiology.* White Plains, NY: Churchill Livingstone; 1978:559–566.

Cook AC, Anderson RH. The functionally univentricular circulation: anatomic substrates as related to function. *Cardiol Young.* 2005;15:7–16.

Earing MG, Cetta F, Driscoll DJ, et al. Long-term results of the Fontan operation for double-inlet left ventricle. *Am J Cardiol.* 2005;96:291–298.

Fontan F, Baudet E. Surgical repair of tricuspid atresia. *Thorax* 1971;26:240–248.

Fyfe DA, Kline CH, Sade RM, et al. Transesophageal echocardiography detects thrombus formation not identified by transthoracic echocardiography after the Fontan operation. *J Am Coll Cardiol.* 1991;18:1733–1737.

Hagler DJ, Seward JB, Tajik AJ, et al. Functional assessment of the Fontan operation: combined M-mode, two-dimensional and Doppler echocardiographic studies. *J Am Coll Cardiol.* 1984;4:756–764.

Harrison DA, Liu P, Walters JE, et al. Cardiopulmonary function in adult patients late after Fontan repair. *J Am Coll Cardiol.* 1995;26:1016–1021.

Huhta JC, Hagler DJ, Seward JB, et al. Two-dimensional echocardiographic assessment of dextrocardia: a segmental approach. *J Am Cardiol.* 1982;50:1351–1360.

Madan N, Robinson BW, Jacobs ML. Thrombosis in the proximal pulmonary artery stump in a Fontan patient. *Heart.* 2002;88:396.

McGoon DC, Danielson GK, Ritter DG, et al. Correction of the univentricular heart having two atrioventricular valves. *J Thorac Cardiovasc Surg.* 1977;74:218–226.

Milanesi O, Stellin G, Colan SD, et al. Systolic and diastolic performance late after the Fontan procedure for a single ventricle and comparison of those undergoing operation at <12 months of age and at >12 months of age. *Am J Cardiol.* 2002;89:276–280.

Olivier M, O'Leary PW, Pankratz VS, et al. Serial Doppler assessment of diastolic function before and after the Fontan operation. *J Am Soc Echocardiogr.* 2003;16:1136–1143.

Rosenthal DN, Friedman AH, Kleinman CS, et al. Thromboembolic complications after Fontan operations. *Circulation.* 1995;92(suppl.):II-287–II-293.

Silvilairat S, Cabalka AK, Cetta F, et al. Protein-losing enteropathy after the Fontan operation: associations and predictors of clinical outcome. *Congenit Heart Dis.* 2008;3:262–268.

Sluysmans T, Sanders SP, van der Velde M, et al. Natural history and patterns of recovery of contractile function in single left ventricle after Fontan operation. *Circulation.* 1992;86:1753–1761.

Van Praagh R, Vlad P. Dextrocardia, mesocardia and levocardia: The segmental approach to diagnosis in congenital heart disease. In: Keith JD, Rowe RD, Vlad P, eds. *Heart Disease in Infancy and Childhood.* 3rd ed. New York: Macmillan; 1978:638.

Chapter 39
Eisenmenger Syndrome

Robert C. Lichtenberg • Frank Cetta

Eisenmenger syndrome as defined by Paul Wood in 1958 refers to any cardiac defect with initial left-to-right shunting that results in the development of pulmonary vascular changes with increased resistance and pulmonary hypertension. The degree of pulmonary hypertension is severe enough to cause the reversal of shunting and subsequent systemic desaturation and central cyanosis. These defects are listed in Table 39.1 and their anatomy and physiology before the development of pulmonary hypertension are covered elsewhere in this text.

The name Eisenmenger refers to Victor Eisenmenger, an Austrian physician who in 1897 described the clinical and pathologic features in a patient with a large ventricular septal defect (VSD). Dr. Eisenmenger described a "powerfully built man of 32 years" in whom cyanosis increased considerably on effort. The patient's clinical course changed to one of cyanosis, clubbing, and a slow progressive decline in functional ability. This was followed by dyspnea and edema with a state of "heart failure." His clinical exam revealed elevated venous pressure, liver distention, and extensive edema. The patient collapsed and died following a large hemoptysis. Autopsy revealed a 2.5-cm membranous VSD with pulmonary but not aortic atherosclerosis. This case demonstrates many salient points for the purpose of this chapter.

- Adult survival
- Pulmonary arteriopathy that includes changes similar to atherosclerosis
- Variable cyanosis, increasing with exercise
- Secondary erythrocytosis (white cells are low normal, platelets are low)
- Hemoptysis
- Thrombosis
- Heart failure
- Sudden death (more than 30% from arrhythmias)

Adults with Eisenmenger syndrome, regardless of the cardiac defect, have similar pulmonary vascular pathology. The pathophysiologic mechanisms contributing to these changes include shear stress, flow, pressure, thrombosis, and inflammation. The grading of the changes was first described by Heath and Edwards. The sequence of these changes subsequently has been shown not to progress from stage I through VI but rather to have an inflammatory component as

described in grade VI that occurs before grades IV and V. The pathologic changes result in elevated pulmonary vascular resistance. It is this abnormality and the presence of a systemic to pulmonary connection that result in the features of Eisenmenger syndrome.

In the current era, congenital cardiac defects are detected and repaired in infancy or childhood. The number of patients at risk for developing Eisenmenger physiology is a decreasing population. However, in older patients, survival without repair is common and Eisenmenger syndrome patients comprise a significant percentage of patients in clinics caring for the adult with congenital heart disease. In an adult congenital heart disease registry from the Netherlands, 58% of adults with an unrepaired septal defect and pulmonary hypertension had Eisenmenger syndrome.

Echocardiography is a critical element in the evaluation of Eisenmenger syndrome patients and aids the clinician in the assessment of these patients, especially those with endocarditis and pump failure. Another important role of echocardiography is the preoperative assessment before the development of pulmonary hypertension. If pulmonary hypertension is present before surgical repair, the pulmonary pressures may regress, remain unchanged, or progress. The assessment is critical in defining the prognosis as well as guiding potential therapy and response to therapy. If the "post-repair" patient still has significant pulmonary hypertension, this can result in critical elevations in RV systolic pressure and right heart failure. In unrepaired patients, the congenital defect functions as a "pop-off" so that the excess flow during increased cardiac output is shunted to the systemic bed where flow is dependent on the difference in resistance between the pulmonary and systemic beds. If a patient with fixed pulmonary vascular obstructive disease undergoes surgery, this "pop-off" is eliminated and may actually shorten survival.

The fate of the adult with congenital heart disease is changing. Longer life expectancy, increasing risk of arrhythmia, and a shift in the cause of death to pump failure are currently observed. The ability of echocardiography to evaluate ventricular performance in these patients is taking on increased importance.

ECHOCARDIOGRAPHIC ASSESSMENT OF THE PATIENT WITH EISENMENGER SYNDROME

The defects associated with Eisenmenger syndrome are described in detail throughout this textbook. This chapter will focus on the assessment of adults with secondary pulmonary hypertension caused by congenital heart disease. Common to all defects is the assessment of pulmonary artery (PA) pressures and ventricular performance.

Pulmonary Artery Pressure

Doppler-derived PA pressure has been shown to be accurate (Fig. 39.1). In the absence of right ventricular (RV) outflow obstruction, the RV systolic pressure (RVSP) and PA systolic pressures (PASP) will be equal and can be calculated using the modified Bernoulli equation. The diastolic pressure within the pulmonary bed can be evaluated by recording the velocity profile of the pulmonary insufficiency jet. The beginning of this signal represents the pressure difference in the PA and the right ventricle at pulmonary valve closure. This corresponds to the dicrotic notch and does *not* represent either the peak systolic or end diastolic pressure. Normally this pressure difference is less than 15 to 20 mm Hg and therefore should have a velocity less than 2 to 2.5 m/s. Fig. 39.2 illustrates the elevated velocity of pulmonary hypertension. The rate of decline of the pulmonary insufficiency jet depends on the

Table 39.1	DEFECTS WITH POTENTIAL FOR THE DEVELOPMENT OF EISENMENGER SYNDROME	

Cardiac Defect	Typical Onset of Pulmonary Hypertension
VSD Large nonrestrictive (>1.0 cm)	Infancy and childhood
PDA Large nonrestrictive (>1.0 cm)	Infancy and childhood
ASD Large nonrestrictive (>2.0 cm)	Adulthood
AVSD	Infancy and childhood
DORV without pulmonary stenosis	Infancy and childhood
Truncus arteriosus	Infancy and childhood
Univentricular heart without pulmonary stenosis	Infancy and childhood
Surgically created shunts: Potts, Blalock-Taussig, Waterston	Variable

ASD, atrial septal defect; AVSD, atrioventricular septal defect; DORV, double-outlet right ventricle; PDA, patent ductus arteriosus; VSD, ventricular septal defect.

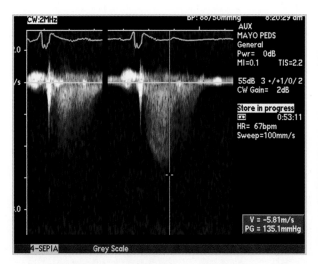 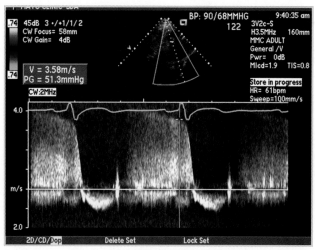

FIGURE 39.1. Spectral continuous-wave Doppler signals demonstrating typical tricuspid and pulmonary regurgitation velocity profiles obtained from an adult with Eisenmenger syndrome.

pressure difference between the PA and right ventricle during the remainder of diastole. The resultant end-diastolic velocity is not always a reflection of the pulmonary diastolic pressure but rather the pressure difference between the PA and RV end diastolic pressures. Equivalent levels of pulmonary pressure can have variable end-diastolic pulmonary insufficiency velocities depending on RV end diastolic pressure. Factors that influence ventricular end-diastolic pressure include:

- Ventricular compliance
- Atrioventricular valve insufficiency
- Pulmonary valve insufficiency

Ventricular Performance in Eisenmenger Patients

Ventricular performance is an important marker of risk stratification for survival as well as potential emerging therapies. Methods of ventricular performance derived by echocardiography include qualitative and quantitative assessment of RV and left ventricular (LV) systolic function. Unfortunately, the traditional assessment of RV systolic function has been a visual estimated ejection fraction based on assessment of multiple two-dimensional imaging planes by experienced echocardiographers. The emergence of high-quality magnetic resonance imaging (MRI) and three-dimensional echocardiography techniques to evaluate RV size and function may bring much-needed precision to the quantification process.

LV dysfunction has been demonstrated to be a marker of mortality in Eisenmenger syndrome patients. Salehian et al. evaluated 122 patients with Eisenmenger syndrome. LVEF was visually estimated and the subgroup with an LVEF less than 50% had increased mortality. Echocardiography measures linear point-to-point dimensions extremely accurately; however, converting these dimensions to a volume measurement (ejection fraction) requires a geometric assumption of ventricular shape. The ventricular geometry in Eisenmenger syndrome introduces error in attempts to calculate the ejection fraction. Septal flattening caused by pressure (systolic) or volume (diastolic) overload on the right ventricle alters the configuration of the left ventricle (Fig. 39.3). This is one limitation of echocardiography that has been a factor in the search for alternative markers of ventricular performance.

Eidem et al. demonstrated the usefulness of the myocardial performance index (MPI) in the assessment of RV function in congenital heart disease. Others have shown a correlation between MPI and brain natriuretic peptide (BNP) levels in adults with congenital heart disease. However, this study did not show a correlation between MPI and visually estimated LVEF or RVEF. MRI evaluation has shown that preserved RV function in Eisenmenger syndrome is associated with improved survival. While MRI has been shown to be the most accurate modality for assessment of RV function, an MPI greater than 0.40 has a 79% sensitivity and 80% specificity to detect an RVEF less than 35%.

Atrial Septal Defect Versus Ventricular Septal Defect in Eisenmenger syndrome

Important hemodynamic differences need to be pointed out between the defects with a shunt above the atrioventricular valve, such as atrial septal defect (ASD) and anomalous pulmonary venous connections, versus those with a shunt at the ventricular or great artery level. As an isolated defect, the ASD, regardless of the type, presents a low-pressure, high-volume overload on the right-sided chambers. The right ventricle is not significantly hypertrophied in childhood and pulmonary pressures are not increased. The degree of shunting is not fixed but variable depending on ventricular compliance. As LV compliance decreases with aging, the degree of left-to-right shunting increases, resulting in further volume overload of the right-sided chambers and pulmonary vascular bed. This results in marked dilation, significantly more so than observed in VSD or patent ductus arteriosus (PDA). As pulmonary hypertensive arteriopathy progresses the degree of left-to-right shunting at the atrial level

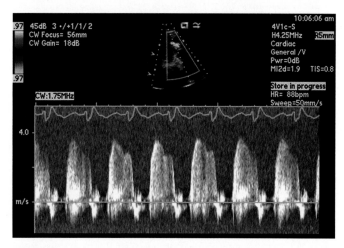

FIGURE 39.2. Continuous-wave Doppler profile of pulmonary regurgitation demonstrating high early and end-diastolic flow velocities consistent with pulmonary hypertension.

decreases until finally RV compliance is less than the left ventricle and the shunt takes on a right-to-left component. The total RV stroke volume is committed to the pulmonary vascular bed. This results in changes in the interventricular septal geometry that affects LV performance (Fig. 39.3).

The age at which shunt volume and direction change is variable. In patients with ASD it is unusual to have fixed pulmonary hypertension and Eisenmenger physiology in the first 3 to 5 decades of life despite the large volume load on the RV. If significant pulmonary hypertension is present in young patients with ASD, other lesions or pathology should also be considered (Table 39.1).

Of all the lesions that could result in Eisenmenger syndrome, the ASD is the one that presents the most difficult diagnostic challenge. An adult with an ASD can have significant pulmonary hypertension but still have reversible pathology within the pulmonary vascular tree. Doppler echocardiography can assist in the hemodynamic assessment of these patients. Fig. 39.4. shows a large secundum ASD with bidirectional shunting and pulmonary hypertension. Balloon occlusion is shown with a trace amount of residual shunting. During ASD occlusion, hemodynamics can be measured by transthoracic echocardiography (TTE), transesophageal echocardiography (TEE), or intracardiac echocardiography (ICE) both at rest and with increased cardiac output during a trial of inotrope (dobutamine) infusion. The failure of pulmonary pressures to drop with signs of right heart failure would indicate prohibitive risk to ASD closure.

When considering older individuals for closure of an ASD, balloon occlusion of the ASD with simultaneous recording of pulmonary capillary wedge pressure (PCWP) is important to insure that the patient will tolerate ASD closure in setting of poor LV compliance. If PCWP approaches or exceeds 20 mm Hg, the patient may be better served by leaving the ASD open. TEE or ICE imaging is an important tool during the interventional cardiac catheterization of these patients.

Ventricular Septal Defect

When the shunt is at the ventricular or great artery level, both vascular beds are available to receive the combined ventricular stroke volume. The availability of the systemic vascular bed to receive a

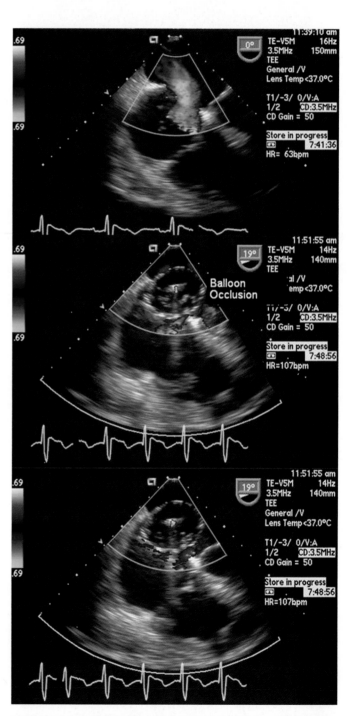

FIGURE 39.4. Transesophageal echocardiography images demonstrating a large secundum atrial septal defect (ASD) with a Q_p/Q_s values of 1.8 and severe pulmonary hypertension. **Top:** Left-to-right shunting during ventricular systole. **Middle, bottom:** Balloon occlusion of the ASD and bidirectional shunting.

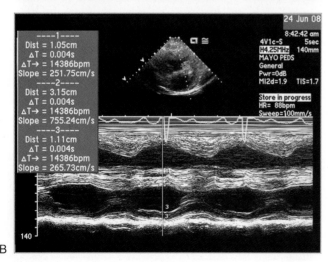

FIGURE 39.3. Parasternal short-axis two-dimensional (A) and M-mode (B) images demonstrating flattening of the interventricular septum consistent with pressure (systole) and volume (diastole) overload in Eisenmenger syndrome.

variable portion of the desaturated systemic venous return unloads the pulmonary vasculature and limits pulmonary pressure to that of systemic level. The findings of the patient with Eisenmenger Syndrome and a VSD are shown in Fig. 39.5. Since the right ventricle is at high pressure since infancy, there has been no thinning of the musculature of the right ventricle. The VSD velocity is not high because of the equal pressures in the ventricles during systole and the net direction of shunting is dependent on ventricular compliance during diastole and vascular bed resistance during systole.

ASSOCIATED ISSUES WITH EISENMENGER PATIENTS

Bleeding and Thrombosis

The cyanotic patient with congenital heart disease is at risk for bleeding. Fatal hemoptysis was a common cause of death for these patients until the past two decades. In current practice, avoidance of phlebotomy has reduced the incidence of hemoptysis dramatically. These patients have thrombocytopenia, abnormal platelet function, activated coagulation cascade with increased fibrin degradation products, and deficiencies of clotting factors and von Willebrand factor.

Despite the predisposition to bleed, many Eisenmenger patients have PA thrombosis. The thrombus is typically found in the proximal PA, which is dilated (Fig.39.6). It has been suggested that pulmonary thrombosis is more common in females as well as in those with lower systemic arterial oxygen saturations. More recently, Broberg et al. studied 55 consecutive patients with Eisenmenger syndrome and found the incidence of detectable pulmonary thrombus to be 20%. Pulmonary thrombosis was associated with older age, lower RV and LV ejection fraction (LVEF), large PA diameter, and lower peak systolic velocity in the PA.

Endocarditis and Brain Abscess

All cyanotic patients with residual shunts should have filters placed on all intravenous lines that are placed. These patients are at increased risk for paradoxical embolization and brain abscess. Endocardium-enhancing contrast agents are generally not used in these patients. Based on the 2007 American Heart Association guidelines, these patients require prophylactic antibiotics when having nonsterile invasive procedures performed. However, they do not usually require antibiotic prophylaxis for TEE. Patients with unrepaired VSD may be at highest risk for development of endocarditis.

Left Coronary Artery Compression

Compression of the proximal left coronary artery is a rare effect of the massive main pulmonary dilation that may occur in Eisenmenger patients. In 2007 Dubois and colleagues described this finding in a patient using angiography and adjunctive MRI (Fig. 39.7). In a patient with LV dysfunction or symptoms of angina, this associated problem should be evaluated.

Echocardiographic Monitoring of Response to Medical Therapy

The pulmonary vascular resistance in Eisenmenger syndrome is markedly elevated. Endothelin-1, a potent vasoconstrictor, has been

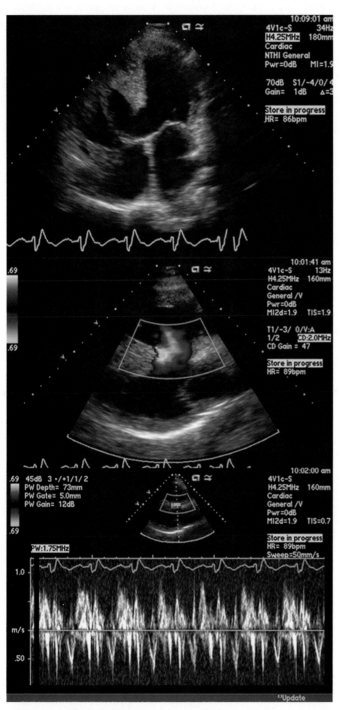

FIGURE 39.5. Transthoracic echocardiography images of a large nonrestrictive ventricular septal defect (VSD) in an adult patient with double-outlet right ventricle. Top: Two dimensional image demonstrating large VSD. Middle: Laminar color Doppler flow representing left-to-right shunt through the VSD during systole. Bottom: Spectral pulsed-wave Doppler sampled in the VSD showing low-velocity bidirectional shunting.

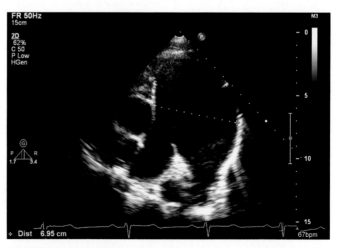

FIGURE 39.6. Massive MPA dilation in an adult with Eisenmenger syndrome. This patient developed a thrombus on the posterior aspect of the proximal right pulmonary artery.

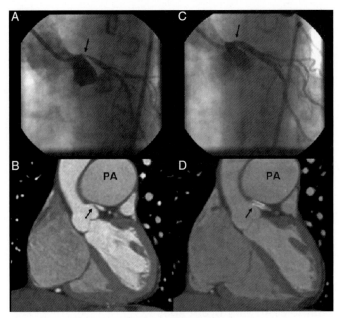

FIGURE 39.7. Left coronary compression (*arrow*) caused by a dilated hypertensive main pulmonary artery in a patient with Eisenmenger physiology. A, C: Coronary angiography before and after coronary stent (*arrow*) placement. **B, D:** Same anatomy with magnetic resonance imaging. (With permission from Dubois CL, Dymarkowski S, Van Cleemput J. Compression of the left main coronary artery by the pulmonary artery in a patient with the Eisenmenger Syndrome. *Eur Heart J* 2007;28:1945.

found to be elevated in these patients. Blockade of endothelin-1 with an endothelin receptor antagonist has been shown to improve the exercise capacity and hemodynamics in patients with Eisenmenger syndrome. Doppler echocardiography can be used to monitor therapy and assess response to therapy. If the defect is unrepaired, therapy with an agent capable of lowering either pulmonary or systemic resistance will result in a change in shunt direction and magnitude. In the BREATHE-5 trial, 54 patients were randomized in a 2:1 ratio to bosentan or placebo for 16 weeks. Bosentan was shown to lower pulmonary vascular resistance index and mean PA pressure while increasing exercise capacity. Sitaxsentan, another endothelin receptor antagonist but selective for endothelin-A, has been studied in patients with Eisenmenger syndrome. Twelve weeks of therapy was associated with an improved pulmonary vascular–to–systemic vascular resistance ratio. This would suggest pulmonary selectivity in these patients. Inhibitors of the cyclic guanosine monophosphate–specific phosphodiesterase enzyme have been tested in postoperative pulmonary hypertension in children with congenital heart disease and adults with primary and secondary pulmonary hypertension, but no data are available on their role and effect in Eisenmenger syndrome. Doppler echocardiography will provide a tool for the follow-up evaluation of these patients and assess not only pressures but also ventricular performance. More recent advances in strain rate imaging and technology also lend insights into early RV dysfunction in patients with pulmonary hypertension. The widespread application of strain rate imaging to Eisenmenger syndrome may be a helpful adjunct to the management of these difficult patients.

SUGGESTED READING

Barst RJ, McGoon M, Torbicki A, et al. Diagnosis and differential assessment of pulmonary arterial hypertension. *J Am Coll Cardiol.* 2004;43:40S–47S.

Broberg CS, Ujita M, Prasad S, et al. Pulmonary arterial thrombosis in Eisenmenger syndrome is associated with biventricular dysfunction and decreased pulmonary flow velocity. *J Am Coll Cardiol.* 2007;50:634–642.

Cacoub P, Dorent R, Maistre et al. Endothelin-1 in primary pulmonary hypertension and the Eisenmenger syndrome. *Am J Cardiol.* 1993;71:448–450.

Cantor WJ, Harrison DA, Moussadji JS, et al. Determinants of survival and length of survival in adults with Eisenmenger syndrome. *Am J Cardiol.* 1999;84:677–681.

Diller GP, Gatzoulis MA. Pulmonary vascular disease in adults with congenital heart disease. *Circulation.* 2007;115:1039–1050.

Duffels MG, Engelfriet PM, Berger RM, et al. Pulmonary arterial hypertension in congenital heart disease: an epidemiologic perspective from a Dutch registry. *Int J Cardiol.* 2006. Epub 2006 Dec 18.

Eidem BW, O'Leary PW, Tei C, et al. Usefulness of the myocardial performance index for assessing right ventricular function in congenital heart disease. *Am J Cardiol.* 2000;86:654–658.

Eisenmenger V. Die angeborenen defekte der kammerscdheidewande des herzens. *Zietschr Klin Med.* 1897;32:1–28.

Fraisse A, Butrous G, Taylor MB, et al. Randomized controlled trial of IV Sildenafil for postoperative pulmonary hypertension in children with congenital heart disease. *Circulation.* 2007;115:1671.

Galie N, Beghetti M, Gatzoulis MA, et al. Bosentan therapy in patients with Eisenmenger syndrome. *Circulation.* 2006;114:48–54.

Gatzoulis MA, Beghetti M, Galie N, et al. Longer-term bosentan therapy improves functional capacity in Eisenmenger syndrome: results of the BREATHE-5 open-label extension study. *Int J Cardiol.* 2008;127:27–32.

Heath D, Edwards J. The pathophysiology of hypertensive pulmonary vascular disease. *Circulation.* 1958;18:533–547.

Kittipovanonth M, Bellavia D, Chandrasekaran K, et al. Doppler myocardial imaging for early detection of right ventricular dysfunction in patients with pulmonary hypertension. *J Am Soc Echocardiogr.* 2008;21:1035–1041.

Mueller J, Cook S. Preserved right ventricular function in Eisenmenger syndrome compared to idiopathic pulmonary hypertension: a possible clue to improved survival. *Circulation.* 2007;114:2109.

Oh JK, Seward JB, Tajik AJ, editors. Pulmonary hypertension. In: *The echo manual.* 2nd ed. Philadelphia, PA: Lippincott Williams & Wilkins; 1999: 215–222.

Perlowski AA, Aboulhosn J, Castellon Y, et al. Relation of brain natriuretic peptide to myocardial performance index in adults with congenital heart disease. *Am J Cardiol.* 2007;100:110–114.

Pietra GG, Capron F, Stewart S, et al. Pathologic assessment of vasculopathies in pulmonary hypertension. *J Am Coll Cardiol.* 2004;43:25S–32S.

Rosenzweig EB. Eisenmenger syndrome in adults: strategies to correct congenital defects before fixed vascular disease develops. *Adv Pulm Hypertens.* 2003;2:13–19.

Salehian O, Schwerzmann M, Rahimbar S, et al. Left ventricular dysfunction and mortality in patients with Eisenmenger syndrome. *Circulation.* 2005;112:564.

Schwerzmann M, Samman AM, Salehian O. Assessment of right ventricular function: adults with repaired tetralogy of Fallot using the myocardial performance index. *Circulation.* 2005;112:539.

Sharma R, Bolger AP, Li W, et al. Elevated circulating levels of inflammatory cytokines and bacterial endotoxin in congenital heart disease. *Am J Cardiol.* 2003;92:188–193.

Silversides CK, Granton JT, Konen E, et al. Pulmonary thrombosis in adults with Eisenmenger syndrome. *J Am Coll Cardiol.* 2003;42:1982–87.

Wood P. The Eisenmenger syndrome: or pulmonary hypertension with reversed central shunt. *Br Med J.* 1958;2:701–79, 755–762.

Chapter 40
Fetal Echocardiography

Anita Szwast • Shobha Natarajan • Jack Rychik

Fetal echocardiography is the ultrasonic imaging of the fetal cardiovascular system, and it is the most important diagnostic tool in the evaluation and management of the heart before birth. The fetus is ideal for ultrasonic imaging as the amniotic fluid lends itself easily to ultrasound energy transmission and reflection. However, the small size of the cardiac structures, the distance of the target organ from the transducer, and the complex position of the fetus can make fetal echocardiography quite a challenge. Interpretation of images can also pose a challenge, as the imaging data must be considered within the context of the age of the fetus because developmental, structural, and functional changes continuously take place as gestation progresses to term. Fetal echocardiography therefore requires a technical operator who has a high level of skill, a sharp eye, flexibility, abundant patience, and a specific and unique fund of knowledge concerning fetal physiology.

In this chapter, we review the technical aspects of performing a fetal echocardiogram, discuss the usefulness of the Doppler evaluation of the fetal cardiovascular system, and highlight key points in the diagnostic imaging of congenital heart disease as well as the impact of anomalies other than congenital heart disease on the fetal cardiovascular system.

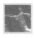

THE FETAL ECHOCARDIOGRAPHIC EXAMINATION

Types of Fetal Ultrasound Examinations

Fetal echocardiography is a high-level ultrasound test targeted specifically at evaluating the fetal cardiovascular system. A variety of fetal ultrasonic tests currently exist and may be performed at different gestational ages. Gestational periods are divided into "trimesters": conception to 13 weeks is the first trimester, 14 weeks to 28 weeks is the second trimester, and 28 weeks to term (40 weeks) is the third trimester. A standard obstetrical ultrasound test to assess for fetal viability, fetal number (single or multiple pregnancy), fetal size, and amniotic fluid volume (standard examination, or level 1 obstetrical ultrasound) is typically performed in the second or third trimester and will usually not include any detailed evaluation of the cardiovascular system beyond the presence of a contracting heart and heart rate. A limited obstetrical ultrasound examination can be performed at any period in gestation to answer a specific question such as fetal gender. A more detailed anatomic "comprehensive" obstetrical ultrasound evaluation (specialized examination, or level II obstetrical ultrasound) is performed in the second or third trimester and is applied when an anomaly is suspected on the basis of history, biochemical abnormalities, or the results of the standard obstetrical examination. Cardiovascular evaluation in this assessment may include a count of the heart chamber number and the outflow tracts, as well as Doppler assessment of vascular structures such as the umbilical cord or ductus venosus.

A commonly used fetal obstetrical ultrasound test is assessment of "nuchal translucency" (NT testing) performed in the first trimester at 11 to 13 weeks' gestation. In this test, the thickness or diameter of the clear space seen behind the fetal neck is measured and is indexed based on gestational age and size (rump-to-crown). Strict guidelines for training have been established to standardize the performance and accuracy of this test. Numerous studies have established a link between increased nuchal translucency in the first trimester and chromosomal abnormality as well as congenital heart disease, independent of aneuploidy. NT testing is increasingly being offered as a screening tool to pregnant women in the United States. Abnormalities on first-trimester NT testing are one of the leading indicators for specialized obstetrical ultrasound examination and referral for fetal echocardiography.

None of the obstetrical ultrasound evaluations just discussed focus extensively on detailed fetal heart anatomy or function, but they can potentially raise concerns that will prompt referral for a more detailed evaluation through a fetal echocardiogram.

Indications for Fetal Echocardiography

The indications for a fetal echocardiogram can be broken down into maternal or fetal indications and are listed in Table 40-1.

Elements of the Fetal Echocardiogram

The fetal echocardiogram is a detailed assessment of fetal heart structure and function. A number of ultrasound systems are commercially available and offer the ability to perform fetal echocardiography through appropriate hardware and software programs. One may choose to adapt obstetrical specific curvilinear probes or more conventional pediatric probes to perform the scan. Ultrasound frequencies used are typically in the 5- to 8-MHz range. The examination includes two-dimensional, color Doppler, and pulsed-wave Doppler echocardiography. Continuous-wave Doppler is used less often than in the pediatric population as increased velocities are less common; however, it should be available for targeted purposes as necessary. Recording of image data for analysis, storage, and review should ideally be as loops of the cardiac cycle in a digital format; however, videotape storage is acceptable.

The American Society of Echocardiography has established key elements of the fetal examination. A series of tomographic planes, views, and sweeps are used to assess the heart with the objective of creating an accurate three-dimensional mental reconstruction of the cardiovascular anatomy. Imaging planes are illustrated in

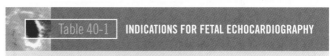

Table 40-1	INDICATIONS FOR FETAL ECHOCARDIOGRAPHY

Maternal Indications

- Family history of congenital heart disease
- Metabolic disorders (eg, diabetes, phenylketonuria)
- Exposure to teratogens
- Exposure to prostaglandin synthetase inhibitors (eg, ibuprofen, salicylic acid, indomethacin)
- Rubella infection
- Autoimmune disease (eg, Sjogren's, systemic lupus erythematosus)
- Familial inherited disorders (Ellis van Creveld, Marfan syndrome, Noonan syndrome)
- In vitro fertilization

Fetal Indications

- Abnormal obstetrical ultrasound screen
- Extracardiac abnormality
- Chromosomal abnormality
- Irregular heart rhythm
- Hydrops
- Multiple gestation and suspicion of twin-twin transfusion syndrome
- Increased first trimester nuchal translucency

Figure 40.1. Although the sequence of imaging views may vary based on fetal position and degree of fetal cooperation, the following are suggested helpful views to obtain.

UMBILICAL CORD, POSITION OF THE FETUS, SITUS – Before starting the assessment of the heart, an evaluation of the number of vessels in the umbilical cord should be performed, with confirmation of the normal presence of two arteries and a single umbilical vein. The position of the fetus as either breech or head down, spine anterior or posterior should be ascertained such that fetal left and right side relative to maternal left and right can be confirmed and the fetal situs established. This is a key aspect of the examination that should be determined at the outset of the scan.

FOUR-CHAMBER VIEW – In this view, the long axis of heart is displayed with either the apex up or down. The atria, ventricles, and atrioventricular valves can be assessed. The conotruncus is not seen in this view; hence, a normal appearing four-chamber view does not rule out a conotruncal anomaly or an abnormality of the outflow tracts (i.e., transposition of the great arteries).

SHORT-AXIS VIEW – This view is obtained at a right angle to the long axis of the heart and allows for visualization of the right ventricular outflow tract as it normally wraps around the aorta and left ventricular outflow. Conal (infundibular) deviation such as in tetralogy of Fallot can be easily seen in this view. Sweeping cephalad will allow visualization of the branch pulmonary arteries, while sweeping caudad provides a short axis of the left and right ventricles.

CARDIAC LONG-AXIS VIEWS – Aligning the transducer with the left ventricular outflow tract will provide an image of the long axis of the heart. Assessment of mitral-to-aortic fibrous continuity can be made, as well as an evaluation for left ventricular outflow tract obstruction and inspection of the ascending aorta. Sweeping rightward and slightly superiorly allows for visualization of the right ventricular outflow tract and proximal main pulmonary artery.

CAVAL LONG-AXIS VIEW – Alignment of the entry sites for the superior and inferior vena cavae into the right atrium allows for assessment of the venous anatomy and the atrial septum. Normal right-to-left atrial shunting can be confirmed via color Doppler imaging.

DUCTAL AND AORTIC ARCH VIEWS – Imaging of the fetal mediastinum allows for visualization of the two arterial arches in the fetus. The aortic arch has a more acute curvature as it originates from the central portion of the heart, while the ductal arch is wider and originates just beyond the bifurcation of the pulmonary artery. The insertion of the ductus arteriosus into the descending aorta should be visualized and the direction of shunting determined. Normal shunting across the ductus arteriosus in the fetus should always be from the pulmonary artery to the descending aorta.

Counseling and the Transmittal of Information to Expectant Families

The information derived from a fetal echocardiographic examination is of tremendous value and has significant implications for fetal

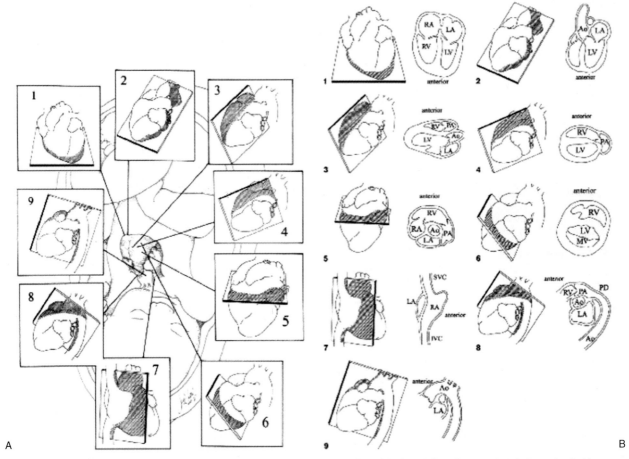

FIGURE 40.1. A and **B.** Tomographic planes used to image the fetal heart and great vessels. Each of the planes in figure A corresponds to the image visualized in figure B, this in a structurally normal heart. Plane 1 is the four-chamber view; plane 2 visualizes the left ventricular outflow tract; plane 3 is the long axis left ventricle outflow view; plane 4 is the long axis right ventricle outflow view; plane 5 is the short axis view at the level of the aortic annulus; plane 6 is the short axis view at the level of the mitral valve; plane 7 is the long-axis view at the level of the superior and inferior vena caval entrance into the right atrium; plane 8 is the ductal arch view; plane 9 is the aortic arch view.

prognosis during what is certainly an extremely stressful period of time. Interpretation of images should not be offered in a vacuum without the ability to provide careful explanation of the findings and their implications to the mother and family. This should be done either by the reader of the fetal echocardiogram or by a knowledgeable colleague. Transmittal of the findings and counseling of the family should be performed immediately after the performance and interpretation of the study. A good understanding of the current management strategies and outcomes for congenital heart disease is mandatory when transmitting these findings to the family. In addition to outlining a strategy for care and management, as objective a portrayal as possible of the findings and prognosis should be made, including notification of legal rights toward termination of pregnancy based on gestational age at the time of study.

DOPPLER EVALUATION OF THE FETAL CARDIOVASCULAR SYSTEM

Doppler echocardiography adds tremendous value to the assessment of the fetal cardiovascular system. Expected normal Doppler flow patterns for the umbilical artery, umbilical vein, middle cerebral artery, ductus venosus, atrioventricular valve inflow, and ductus arteriosus have been well described in the literature at each gestational age. In fetuses with altered hemodynamics secondary to congenital heart disease, intrauterine growth retardation, twin-to-twin transfusion syndrome (TTTS), or significant extracardiac anomalies known to impact the fetal cardiovascular system, Doppler echocardiography can help to quantify the degree of cardiac compromise that is present.

Umbilical Artery and Vein

The umbilical cord is a vital structure linking the fetus to the placenta. It usually consists of two arteries and one vein. The presence of a single umbilical artery may be an isolated finding or may be associated with growth retardation or chromosomal abnormalities, particularly when there are multiple congenital anomalies detected on fetal ultrasonography. Pulsed-wave Doppler interrogation of the umbilical cord is best performed parallel to flow within the midportion of the cord during fetal apnea. Doppler sampling within the umbilical artery reflects downstream resistance within the placenta. Accordingly, the resistance within the umbilical artery is generally quite low to promote blood flow to the placenta so that nutrients and gases may be effectively exchanged. Measures of resistance include (a) the peak systolic/end-diastolic ratio (S/D ratio), (b) the pulsatility index—defined as the peak systolic velocity minus end-diastolic velocity divided by the time-averaged mean velocity, and (c) the resistance index, defined as the peak systolic velocity minus end-diastolic velocity divided by the diastolic velocity. As shown in Figure 40.2A, the Doppler flow pattern within the umbilical artery is characterized by continuous forward flow in both systole and diastole. In cases of intrauterine growth retardation, the diastolic velocity within the umbilical cord decreases and may even be absent (Fig. 40.2B). Indeed, diastolic flow reversal within the umbilical artery has been shown to be a marker for poor outcome and a risk factor for in utero demise.

Doppler assessment of the umbilical vein reflects systemic venous pressure. As systemic venous pressure rises due to heart failure, complete atrioventricular block, or severe tricuspid regurgitation, changes in the Doppler flow patterns are first seen in the inferior vena cava, then in the ductus venosus, and finally in the umbilical vein. Only the most severe derangements in systemic venous pressure are reflected as changes in the umbilical venous Doppler flow pattern. The umbilical venous Doppler flow pattern is usually described as phasic, low-velocity flow. Respiratory variation may be seen if the Doppler sample is not acquired during fetal apnea. With increases in central venous pressure, notching is first seen at end-diastole, corresponding to atrial contraction. In cases of severe compromise, venous pulsations may be seen.

Ductus Venosus

The ductus venosus is a key structure in fetal life, which enables the highly oxygenated blood returning from the umbilical vein to

enter the inferior vena cava, thereby bypassing the liver. Absence of the ductus venosus is associated with an increased incidence of fetal anomalies, including congenital heart disease, chromosomal anomalies, and fetal hydrops—especially in cases where the liver is bypassed entirely and all umbilical venous return is directed into the right atrium. Given its proximity to the heart, abnormalities in the ductus venosus Doppler flow pattern may be seen before any changes within the umbilical vein. The ductus venosus Doppler flow pattern is compromised of s, d, and a waves (Fig. 40.3). After 14 weeks' gestation, flow within the ductus venosus should be entirely antegrade with no reversal occurring with atrial contraction. Over the course of gestation, resistance within the ductus venosus in normal fetuses progressively decreases, so that the pulsatility index in the third trimester is usually less than 1. In fetuses with hemodynamic abnormalities associated with elevated central venous pressure, the a-wave velocity, corresponding to atrial contraction, decreases initially and then can become reversed. Pathologic conditions associated with alterations of ductus venosus Doppler flow pattern include complete atrioventricular block, where the right atrium contracts against a closed tricuspid valve. In this case, there is reversal in the ductus venosus with atrial contraction. Similarly, severe tricuspid regurgitation, as seen in Ebstein's anomaly and in the recipient twins of the TTTS, is associated with reversal of the ductus venosus a-wave velocity.

Middle Cerebral Artery

Doppler assessment of the middle cerebral artery provides important information about overall fetal health as well as about the cerebrovascular resistance. Generally, most of the flow in the middle cerebral artery occurs during systole with only a small amount of flow in diastole. The peak systolic velocity within the middle cerebral artery increases over the course of gestation, ranging from 27 cm/s at 18 weeks' gestation to 59 cm/s at term. An elevated peak systolic velocity within the middle cerebral artery has correctly predicted fetal anemia. In fetuses with normal hemodynamics, the resistance within the cerebral vasculature is greater than the placental resistance. However, in fetuses with chronic hypoxia or inadequate cardiac output, there may be "cephalization" of flow characterized by a ratio of resistance in the middle cerebral artery compared with

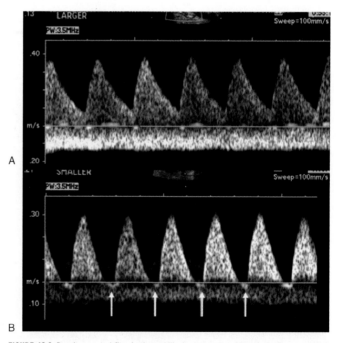

FIGURE 40.2. Doppler spectral flow in the umbilical artery and umbilical vein. Top panel (**A**) is flow in a normal umbilical artery with a good amount of diastolic flow seen relative to systolic flow, reflecting a normal, low vascular resistance. Umbilical venous flow is low velocity and continuous, without any pulsations. Bottom panel (**B**) is umbilical artery flow in a fetus with abnormally elevated placental vascular resistance. Arrows delineate reversal of flow in diastole (below the baseline, layered over the umbilical venous flow tracing)

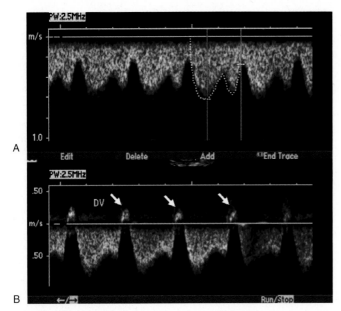

FIGURE 40.3. Doppler spectral flow in the ductus venosus. Top panel (**A**) is a normal, phasic, flow pattern with changes based on temporal aspects of the cardiac cycle. Of note, flow does not reach the baseline, or below it. Bottom panel (**B**) is a tracing from a fetus with abnormal ductus venosus flow. Arrows point out flow below the baseline, which is occurring during atrial contraction. This suggests abnormal right atrial or right ventricular compliance.

the umbilical artery of less than 1, otherwise known as the "brain-sparing effect." Dynamic changes within the middle cerebral artery Doppler flow pattern may occur in response to changes in cardiac output, with an increase in diastolic flow and a decrease in vascular resistance (Fig. 40.4).

Altered flow patterns within the fetal brain have also been described in fetuses with congenital heart disease. Compared with normal fetuses, fetuses with left-sided obstructive lesions have decreased resistance within the middle cerebral artery, likely as a

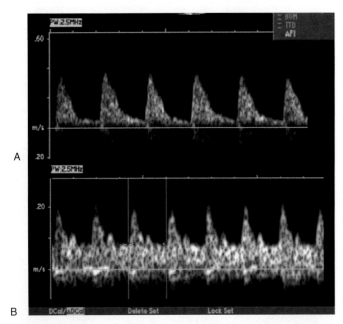

FIGURE 40.4. Doppler spectral flow in the middle cerebral artery. Top panel (**A**) is a normal tracing with a relatively low diastolic velocity in comparison to the systolic velocity reflecting the normal, elevated cerebrovascular resistance. Bottom panel (**B**) demonstrates increased diastolic flow (caliper markers) relative to systolic flow suggesting decreased cerebrovascular resistance in fetus with cardiomyopathy and low cardiac output. This fetus is attempting to increase cerebrovascular flow and preserve perfusion by decreasing resistance. This phenomenon is referred to as "cephalization."

mechanism to improve flow to the brain. In fetuses with hypoplastic left heart syndrome (HLHS) and aortic atresia, all blood flow to the brain is retrograde from the ductus arteriosus into the aortic arch. Whether this abnormal flow pattern affects fetal brain development is an ongoing area of investigation, although abnormalities of the brain have been described in neonates with congenital heart disease even before surgical palliation. Conversely, in fetuses with increased blood flow to the fetal brain secondary to right-sided obstructive lesions, the cerebral vasculature vasoconstricts in an attempt to limit cerebral blood flow. As a consequence, the middle cerebral artery pulsatility index is increased in these fetuses compared with normal fetuses.

Tricuspid and Mitral Inflow

The fetal myocardium is comprised of greater noncontractile elements compared with the mature myocardium. As a consequence of this inherent diastolic dysfunction, there is decreased passive ventricular filling and a greater percentage of ventricular filling during atrial contraction. This, in part, explains why fetuses with complete heart block may develop hydrops fetalis. Without the contribution of atrial contraction to ventricular filling, preload may become compromised, resulting in an overall decreased cardiac output.

In the fetus, typically there is a lower e-wave velocity, representing passive filling, and a dominant a-wave velocity, representing atrial contraction. The ratio of the e wave to the a wave increases over the course of gestation as the relaxation properties of the fetal myocardium improve. With altered ventricular compliance secondary to ventricular hypertrophy, as seen in the recipient twin of the TTTS, or endocardial fibroelastosis, as seen in critical aortic stenosis and evolving HLHS, the normal biphasic inflow pattern may fuse into a single peak inflow.

Ductus Arteriosus

While in utero, the placenta is the site of oxygenation and ventilation. Consequently, the ductus arteriosus enables the oxygen-poor blood pumped by the RV to bypass the fetal lungs and return to the placenta via the descending aorta. The ductus arteriosus should be large and unrestrictive to avoid passage through the fetal lungs, which are under high resistance during fetal life. Constriction of the ductus arteriosus imposes greater afterload on the RV, which can lead to right ventricular hypertrophy, tricuspid regurgitation, and, ultimately, right ventricular failure and intrauterine fetal demise. Numerous medications, most notably, corticosteroids, high-dose aspirin, and prostaglandin synthetase inhibitors, have been implicated as causing ductal constriction. Investigators have defined mild ductal constriction as a pulsatility index between 1.5 and 1.9, moderate ductal constriction as between 1 and 1.5, and severe ductal constriction as less than 1. Long-standing closure of the ductus arteriosus in utero with evidence of right ventricular failure should prompt the clinician to consider delivery to prevent in utero fetal death.

Branch Pulmonary Arteries

Doppler investigation of the branch pulmonary arteries provides important information about the health of the pulmonary vasculature. In many different types of congenital heart disease, cardiopulmonary interactions play a critical role in the pathophysiology of the disorder. In HLHS with a restrictive interatrial communication, tetralogy of Fallot with absent pulmonary valve syndrome, or severe Ebstein's anomaly with massive cardiomegaly and evidence for lung hypoplasia, assessment of the pulmonary vasculature can be of increasing importance in predicting the health of the fetus at birth. Typical Doppler flow patterns have been described for the main pulmonary artery, the distal extraparenchymal pulmonary artery, and the intraparenchymal artery at the first branching point within the fetal lung. In lesions known to cause lung hypoplasia, such as congenital diaphragmatic hernia, kidney abnormalities manifested by agenesis or multicystic degeneration of the kidneys, or chronic premature rupture of membranes, investigators have identified abnormal Doppler spectral patterns within the pulmonary arteries. An increased pulsatility index was shown to be the best parameter to detect flow abnormalities in these fetuses with lethal pulmonary hypoplasia.

Rasenen and colleagues demonstrated that the normal fetal pulmonary vasculature is under acquired vasoconstriction. In response to maternal hyperoxygenation with 60% oxygen, they showed a 20% decline in the pulsatility index within the branch pulmonary arteries, but only after 31 weeks gestation. We recently investigated whether maternal hyperoxygenation testing would be of benefit in predicting critical hypoxemia in fetuses at risk for significant pulmonary vasculopathy at birth, namely in fetuses with HLHS and a restrictive interatrial communication. Maternal hyperoxygenation testing correctly predicted the need for urgent intervention on the interatrial septum at birth secondary to severe neonatal hypoxemia. No fetuses with vasoreactivity within the branch pulmonary artery, defined as a decline of at least 10% in pulsatility index in response to maternal hyperoxygenation after 31 weeks gestation required intervention on the interatrial septum (Fig. 40.5). Assessment of the branch pulmonary artery Doppler flow pattern in response to maternal hyperoxygenation is of value in select diseases and will become an increasingly used assay in the future to best assess fetal lung development.

Assessment of Fetal Cardiac Function via Doppler-Derived Techniques

A number of Doppler-derived techniques assist in the determination of overall fetal ventricular performance and help improve understanding of complex disease processes.

MYOCARDIAL PERFORMANCE INDEX – The myocardial performance index, or Tei index, is a Doppler-derived technique that assesses both systolic and diastolic function. It is defined as the sum of the isovolumic contraction time plus the isovolumic relaxation time divided by the semilunar valve ejection time. In essence, it is the time from atrioventricular cessation of flow to the time of atrioventricular onset of flow minus the ejection time, with this value divided by the ejection time. Atrioventricular valve inflow and semilunar valve outflow may be acquired on the same Doppler tracing or on different Doppler tracings. A higher myocardial performance index value corresponds to a greater degree of total ventricular dysfunction but does not distinguish between systolic or diastolic dysfunction.

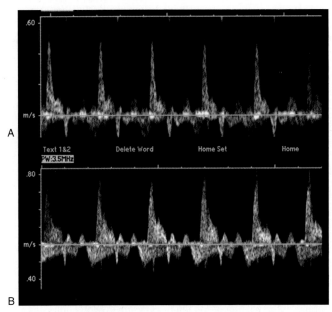

FIGURE 40.5. Doppler spectral tracing from the distal right pulmonary artery of a fetus with hypoplastic left heart syndrome and a wide open atrial septal defect. Top panel (**A**) is flow in room air (21%). Note the very rapid upstroke and sharp downstroke of flow with a very narrow base to the tracing. This reflects a normal healthy, high pulmonary vascular tone, as typically seen in the fetal pulmonary vasculature. Bottom panel (**B**) is flow at the same site of the distal right pulmonary artery but while the mother is breathing 100% oxygen for 20 minutes (maternal hyperoxygenation test). Note the increase in peak velocity as well as a broadening of the waveform base with more flow noted in diastole, all as a consequence of pulmonary vasoreactivity in response to maternal hyperoxygenation. This response reflects a healthy lung vasculature.

Normal values for the right ventricular and left ventricular myocardial performance index have been published. In the fetus, the right ventricular myocardial performance index ranges from 0.35 ± 0.06 to 0.43 ± 0.05, while the left ventricular myocardial performance index ranges from 0.035 ± 0.06 to 0.53 ± 0.13. Abnormalities of the myocardial performance index have been demonstrated in different pathologic conditions. For example, the right ventricular myocardial performance index is elevated in ductal constriction, congenital cystic adenomatoid malformation, fetuses of diabetic mothers, cardiomyopathy, recipient twins of TTTS, and HLHS. In addition, the left ventricular myocardial performance index is elevated in cardiomyopathy, severe tricuspid valve disease, and severely affected twin recipients of the TTTS. Although further studies are needed to correlate the myocardial performance index with clinical outcome, serial assessment of the myocardial performance index may yield important information regarding the impact of treatment in fetuses with ventricular dysfunction.

VENTRICULAR EJECTION FORCE – The ventricular ejection force describes the acceleration of blood across the pulmonic or aortic valve over a specific time interval, and is a reflection of systolic ventricular performance derived from Newton's laws. A higher value corresponds to greater force exerted in ejecting the ventricular volume of blood during systole. Ventricular ejection force is calculated as (1.055 × the cross-sectional area of the valve × the velocity-time integral during the acceleration phase of the cardiac cycle) × (the peak systolic velocity of the Doppler envelope/time to peak velocity), where 1.055 represents the density of blood. The ventricular ejection force increases over the course of gestation. We recently studied ventricular ejection force in twin pairs of the TTTS and consistently found significantly decreased ventricular ejection forces in donor twins, likely as a consequence of decreased ventricular preload. Furthermore, Rizzo et al. demonstrated that fetuses with intrauterine growth retardation and ventricular ejection forces less than the fifth percentile for gestational age were at significantly increased risk for intrauterine death or urgent delivery secondary to fetal distress.

COMBINED CARDIAC OUTPUT – Combined cardiac output, as calculated by Doppler flow techniques, adds to the assessment of the fetal cardiovascular system. It is determined by summing the right and left cardiac outputs, individually calculated according to the formula: semilunar valve cross sectional area × fetal heart rate × velocity-time integral across the valve in systole divided by the estimated fetal weight in kilograms. Determination of the combined cardiac output has been used clinically in a variety of volume-loading conditions, such as fetuses with a sacrococcygeal teratoma and the "pump twin" in the twin-reversed arterial perfusion (or "TRAP sequence"). In our experience, a combined cardiac output greater than 800 mL/kg per minute is a significant risk factor for the development of hydrops fetalis or fetal death. As a result, these fetuses are referred for invasive procedures, such as fetal surgery, or, as in the case of twin-reversed arterial perfusion, selective cord photocoagulation.

EVALUATION OF CONGENITAL HEART DISEASE: KEY POINTS IN DIAGNOSTIC IMAGING FROM THE FETAL PERSPECTIVE

Atrial Septal Defects

A critical component of the normal fetal circulation is the patent foramen ovale, a communication in the central portion of the atrial septum that shunts blood from the right atrium to the left atrium, allowing oxygenated blood from the placenta to bypass the pulmonary circulation and flow to the left side of the heart. The septum secundum forms the superior ridge of this defect on the right atrial side and the septum primum forms the thin flap valve of this defect on the left atrial side. If an atrial communication occupies more than one third of the atrial septum, or if the flap valve of the foramen ovale is absent, then a true secundum atrial septal defect (ASD) may be present. Large sinus venosus defects are best visualized in a sagittal bicaval view of the right atrium and septum. A defect in septum primum is best imaged in the four-chamber view at the level of the inflow. A primum defect is in the spectrum of endocardial cushion defects and the atrioventricular canal must be evaluated during imaging (see later). In most cases, the presence of an atrial communication during normal fetal development makes it difficult to rule out a true ASD in the fetus, and this limitation must be emphasized in counseling sessions.

Ventricular Septal Defects

Ventricular septal defects (VSDs) are much less common in utero compared with postnatal prevalence studies. Complete two-dimensional sweeps of the septum through the long- and short-axis planes must be obtained to image all parts of the ventricular septum. Ideally, the ventricular septum should be imaged perpendicular to the ultrasound beam to minimize dropout and false identification of a defect. True defects often have T-artifact, echo-bright spots that delineate the edges of the defect.

Doppler imaging across an isolated VSD demonstrates bidirectional, low-velocity shunting due to similar pressures in both ventricles in utero. Small defects will also have low-velocity flow. Therefore, it is often difficult to determine whether color flow across the septum represents a true defect versus color-speckling onto the septum. Confirmation with two-dimensional imaging is essential. Smaller defects can be overlooked, and this limitation must be emphasized in counseling sessions.

VSDs can be associated with other cardiac abnormalities and can affect overall prognosis. Malalignment of the conal septum with a VSD is associated with size discrepancy of the semilunar valves and obstruction of one of the outflow tracts. Short-axis views of the base of the heart and the right anterior oblique view can demonstrate anterior deviation of the conal septum, as seen with tetralogy of Fallot. Posterior malalignment is often subtle. Long-axis views may demonstrate "pinching in" of the left ventricular outflow tract. Once a posterior malalignment defect is identified, an assessment for aortic arch obstruction or interruption must be performed. On color Doppler imaging, a unidirectional shunt across the VSD indicates obstruction at the level of the outflow tracts or great arteries.

Both ASDs and VSDs are tolerated well in utero and rarely cause fetal compromise unless associated with other cardiac, extracardiac, or genetic abnormalities. Small VSDs, particularly those in the muscular septum, can close during the course of gestation or within the first year of life.

Atrioventricular Canal Defects

Endocardial cushion defects result in a spectrum of abnormalities ranging from a primum ASD with cleft mitral valve to complete atrioventricular canal defects with large ASDs and VSDs. Absence of septum primum (the inferior third of the atrial septum) and/or the inlet portion of the ventricular septum, as well as lack of offset between the tricuspid and mitral valves on four-chamber imaging, all raise concern for an endocardial cushion defect. Imaging of the mitral valve in the short-axis plane can demonstrate a cleft in the anterior leaflet.

With a single common atrioventricular valve, relative balance over both ventricles can be determined from the four-chamber view and left anterior oblique views of the valve. Color Doppler interrogation of atrioventricular inflow in the four-chamber view can be used to qualitatively assess the relative flows to each ventricle. An unbalanced atrioventricular canal defect can limit inflow to one ventricle, potentially causing ventricular hypoplasia and single ventricle circulation. Atrioventricular canal defects can also be associated with heterotaxy syndromes, tetralogy of Fallot, and aortic coarctation. Therefore, a thorough evaluation of the cardiovascular anatomy is imperative for proper patient counseling and management. Serial fetal echocardiograms through gestation should assess for progression of atrioventricular valve regurgitation, which, in rare cases, can lead to heart failure and nonimmune hydrops. Ventricular hypoplasia can also develop over time depending on the degree of unbalance.

Conotruncal Defects

Abnormal conotruncal development results in defects involving the ventricular outflow tracts and great arteries. The four-chamber view may demonstrate a leftward shift in the axis of the heart but otherwise often appears normal. It is critical to sweep anteriorly and superiorly to assess the outflow tracts and great arteries. Parallel exit of the great vessels from the heart signifies transposition of the great arteries. Transposition of the great arteries can be associated with a VSD. Override of the aorta across an anterior malalignment VSD signifies tetralogy of Fallot. In the setting of a single semilunar valve overriding a VSD, both tetralogy of Fallot with pulmonary atresia and truncus arteriosus need to be considered. A dysplastic semilunar valve with stenosis or insufficiency suggests truncus arteriosus versus tetralogy of Fallot with pulmonary atresia. In transposition of the great arteries, assessment for restriction across the ASD (pathway for oxygenated blood to flow to the aorta postnatally) is important.

Starting from the outflow tracts of the heart, a further superior sweep reveals the "three-vessel view," which normally demonstrates cross-sectional views of the superior vena cava, aorta, and pulmonary artery, arranged sequentially from posterior and rightward to anterior and leftward. In tetralogy of Fallot, the aorta is larger than the pulmonary artery. If the pulmonary valve size is less than 60% of the aortic valve size, the baby will likely have significant right ventricular outflow tract obstruction at birth. In truncus arteriosus, there is only one large great vessel and often the pulmonary arteries can be demonstrated arising from the ascending aorta during the superior sweep. In transposition of the great arteries, the aorta is anterior to the pulmonary artery. From the three-vessel view, arch sidedness can also be assessed by determining toward which side of the spine the aortic arch descends. Anatomy of the patent ductus arteriosus and direction of shunt can also be evaluated. A vertically oriented patent ductus arteriosus and/or a left-to-right shunt indicate significant pulmonary outflow obstruction. In truncus arteriosus, a patent ductus arteriosus is usually not present unless there is an interrupted aortic arch.

The pulmonary arteries in conotruncal defects can be discontinuous, hypoplastic, or absent. It is critical to define their anatomy for prognosis and postnatal management of pulmonary blood flow. The short-axis view of the base of the heart and the three-vessel view can often be helpful. In tetralogy of Fallot, the pulmonary arteries can be discontinuous and arise either from the aorta or directly from a ductus arteriosus. Pulmonary arteries in this defect can also be hypoplastic; therefore, visualizing the pulmonary veins, which travel adjacent to the pulmonary arteries, can help to identify them. In tetralogy of Fallot with pulmonary atresia, the true pulmonary arteries may be absent with pulmonary blood flow provided by aortopulmonary collaterals. In a sagittal view of the aorta, these collaterals usually arise from the anterior surface of the thoracic descending aorta and have continuous flow. They can also arise from the innominate or subclavian arteries. In truncus arteriosus, the pulmonary arteries are usually of normal size. They arise from the common trunk either from a main pulmonary artery segment from the trunk itself or from separate orifices.

Conotruncal defects can be associated with chromosomal abnormalities including deletion in chromosome 22q11. Clues to this diagnosis in the setting of tetralogy of Fallot and truncus arteriosus are a right aortic arch, an aberrant subclavian artery, and an absent thymus. In the "three-vessel view," proximity of the vascular structures to the anterior chest wall suggests the absence of thymic tissue.

Pulmonary Stenosis/Atresia

Right ventricular outflow tract obstruction can progress over the course of gestation. Consequently, fetuses that present with mild forms of pulmonary stenosis early in gestation may progress to more severe forms of pulmonary stenosis or even pulmonary atresia by the end of gestation, supporting the role of serial fetal echocardiography. Diagnosis of pulmonary stenosis depends on careful inspection of pulmonary valve morphology, the size of the pulmonary annulus compared with the aortic annulus, and pulsed-wave Doppler interrogation of the pulmonary valve. In the fetus, the pulmonary annulus should always be larger than the aortic annulus. In addition, a peak Doppler velocity greater than 1 m/s across the pulmonary valve is abnormal and should alert the clinician to the possibility of pulmonary valve stenosis. With moderate to severe pulmonary stenosis, right ventricular hypertrophy, tricuspid regurgitation, and poststenotic dilation of the main pulmonary artery may be seen. Flow within the ductus arteriosus may be reversed to augment pulmonary blood flow, which suggests that the fetus is likely to be ductal dependent at birth. With severe degrees of obstruction, right ventricular filling pressures may be high, leading to increased right-to-left shunting across the patent foramen ovale and dilation of the left side of the heart as a consequence. In fetuses with critical pulmonary stenosis and a severely hypertrophied RV, coronary cameral fistulous communications may form. In fetuses with severe degrees of obstruction, the patent foramen ovale should be assessed, because restriction at the atrial communication places the fetus at risk for the development of hydrops fetalis.

In cases of pulmonary atresia with an intact ventricular septum, there is no antegrade flow across the pulmonary valve. Consequently, all flow across the ductus arteriosus is retrograde, supplying the branch pulmonary arteries. At the atrial communication, there is increased right-to-left shunting, leading to dilation of the left side of the heart. The tricuspid valve annulus should be carefully measured. The size of the tricuspid valve and the degree of tricuspid regurgitation dictates the in utero course. In cases of severe tricuspid regurgitation with a normal tricuspid valve annulus, the right atrium and RV become dilated, placing the fetus at risk for arrhythmia and hydrops fetalis. Marked cardiomegaly with cardiothoracic area ratios greater than 0.60 may compromise pulmonary vascular and lung development. In these cases, the prognosis is particularly poor. Conversely, in cases of severe tricuspid stenosis with little tricuspid regurgitation, the RV becomes severely hypertrophied and noncompliant and fistulous communications between the RV and coronary arteries may form. Various investigators have shown that a tricuspid valve annulus Z-score less than −3 and the presence of coronary cameral fistulous communications predict a postnatal single ventricle palliation.

Ebstein's Anomaly

In Ebstein's anomaly of the tricuspid valve, the septal leaflet of the tricuspid valve is displaced toward the apex of the RV. There is tethering of the leaflet to the ventricular septum and the portion of the RV above the valve annulus is "atrialized" and thin walled. Clinical outcome depends on the degree of apical displacement and regurgitation. When Ebstein's anomaly is diagnosed in fetal life, the degrees of displacement and regurgitation are usually significant.

The four-chamber view demonstrates the displacement of the septal leaflet of the tricuspid valve on two-dimensional imaging. Color Doppler interrogation indicates the degree of regurgitation. Continuous-wave Doppler interrogation of the regurgitation jet will give an estimation of right ventricular pressure. Significant regurgitation can lead to a dilated right atrium, which can be assessed in this view as well. Ebstein's anomaly is also a disease that affects the left heart. Significant regurgitation and an atrialized RV can compress the left heart and decrease overall cardiac output. A compressed LV can appear to be hypoplastic. In fetal presentation of Ebstein's anomaly, it is important to assess whether the LV is apex forming, the mitral valve size and anatomy, and the left ventricular outflow tract.

Multiple views, including the short-axis view at the base of the heart and the right anterior oblique view, will aid in the assessment of the pulmonary valve. Severe tricuspid valve regurgitation can prevent forward flow across the pulmonary valve. This functional pulmonary atresia may not be distinguished from true pulmonary atresia unless pulmonary regurgitation is present. Shunting across the patent ductus arteriosus may be left to right in the setting of decreased pulmonary blood flow. Pulmonary stenosis can also be present and can progress to atresia over gestation.

Severe tricuspid valve regurgitation in the setting of Ebstein's anomaly can progress to heart failure and nonimmune hydrops in the fetus. The degree of right atrial dilation, cardiomegaly (cardiothoracic area ratio > 0.33), ventricular shortening, and left ventricular compression must be followed. Dilation of the heart can lead to compression of the lungs. Flow reversal in the ductus venosus reflects elevated right atrial pressure. If the right atrial pressure is significantly elevated, pulsations can be seen in the umbilical venous Doppler tracing. Pericardial and pleural effusions as well as ascites can develop. Fetal growth may be affected and increased diastolic flow may be detected in the middle cerebral artery Doppler pattern, suggestive of decreased left ventricular cardiac output. Fetal arrhythmias can also develop and can be diagnosed by pulsed-wave Doppler and M-mode assessment. These findings can progress over gestation and lead to fetal death. Early delivery in the third trimester may be

necessary. Therefore, it is essential to monitor the fetus with Ebstein's anomaly closely with serial echocardiographic evaluations.

Left Heart Disease

Left-sided obstructive defects can develop anywhere along the path of blood flow ranging from obstructed total anomalous pulmonary venous connection, mitral valve abnormalities, aortic valve stenosis, and aortic arch obstruction to HLHS. Critical left-sided obstructive defects result in left-to-right flow across the patent foramen ovale and decreased flow through the left heart. Therefore, Doppler assessment may not detect turbulent flow or increased Doppler velocities at the level of left-sided obstruction. Detailed two-dimensional imaging in multiple planes may reveal abnormal valve excursion, abnormal mitral valve chordae, thickened valve leaflets, and annular hypoplasia. There may be multiple levels of obstruction. Therefore, a sequential evaluation of all left heart structures is essential.

In HLHS, the atrial septum may be posteriorly deviated, resulting in a more posterior and leftward position of the ASD. Restriction of flow across the atrial septum in utero may affect the neonatal course and management and is a critical part of the evaluation. The pulsed-wave Doppler pattern in the pulmonary veins near the connection to the left atrium is a reliable way of assessing for restriction. The degree of flow reversal in the pulmonary vein during atrial systole can indicate left atrial pressure and warrants close follow-up in all fetuses with HLHS. Both the four-chamber and sagittal imaging planes can demonstrate atrial septal anatomy and pulmonary vein flow. In HLHS with mitral stenosis/aortic atresia, coronary sinusoids can develop. Using color Doppler with a lower Nyquist limit over the ventricular septum may detect sinusoidal flow.

Ventricular size aids in the diagnosis of left-sided obstruction. The RV is the dominant ventricle in utero and performs 60% of the work of total cardiac output; hence, it is the larger of the two ventricles. Prominent LV-to-RV size discrepancy may be the only clue on fetal echocardiographic imaging for the diagnosis of isolated coarctation of the aorta, because direct inspection of the aortic isthmus can be challenging in the presence of a wide open ductus arteriosus. The aortic arch is best seen in the sagittal plane. In HLHS, hypoplasia of the arch can be demonstrated on two-dimensional imaging. The ductus arteriosus is usually large and provides retrograde flow to the aortic arch, including the head and neck vessels and coronary arteries, as demonstrated by Doppler interrogation of the aortic arch. The diagnosis of interrupted aortic arch can also be made by two-dimensional imaging. Doppler assessment in the arch proximal and distal to the interruption can have different patterns and can offer a clue as to the diagnosis. Continuous antegrade flow in the arch increases the suspicion of coarctation. In counseling sessions, the limitations of fetal echocardiography in diagnosing coarctation of the aorta must be emphasized. Postnatal evaluation of the aortic arch may be warranted, especially in the setting of other left-sided obstructive defects, a large VSD, LV-to-RV size discrepancy, and abnormal flow patterns in the aortic arch.

EVALUATION OF THE IMPACT OF ANOMALIES OTHER THAN CONGENITAL HEART DISEASE ON THE FETAL CARDIOVASCULAR SYSTEM

A number of congenital and developmental abnormalities can have significant secondary impacts on the cardiovascular system, causing serious derangements that may importantly influence management and prognosis.

Congenital Chest Anomalies

CONGENITAL DIAPHRAGMATIC HERNIA – A defect in the diaphragm can result in the extrusion of abdominal contents into the chest cavity, with important impact on the fetal heart. Primary congenital heart malformations can be seen in association with congenital diaphragmatic hernia (CDH). Outcome for these fetuses depends on the degree of pulmonary hypoplasia and the type of congenital heart disease present. CDH can also influence the normal development of the LV, creating an appearance of left-sided heart hypoplasia. A left-sided CDH (more common than right-sided CDH) can extrinsically push on and deviate the LV, thereby altering compliance, and reducing the degree of right-to-left atrial level shunting. Furthermore, CDH reduces lung volume and leads to pulmonary hypoplasia, which results in a reduction in pulmonary venous return, further decreasing the blood volume filling the LV. Distinguishing between true underdevelopment of the LV versus underfilling of the LV is made by careful measurements of the mitral and aortic annuli. These measures may be slightly small but should still be within the range of normal for gestational age for an underfilled LV but will be in the abnormal range for a hypoplastic LV.

Measurement of branch pulmonary artery diameter within the lung parenchyma can be performed in the fetus, as the lungs are collapsed and airless in utero and can therefore be imaged. Branch pulmonary artery size may play a role in predicting the degree of lung hypoplasia in CDH and hence prognosis, but, considering the small size, these measures may have a substantial margin for error.

CONGENITAL CYSTIC ADENOMATOID MALFORMATION – Congenital cystic adenomatoid malformations (CCAM) are primitive fetal lung tumors that may be solid or fluid filled and lack a well-defined bronchial tree. If an arterial connection to the mass is identified, then it is referred to as a "bronchopulmonary sequestration." These tumors can grow in size, creating a mass effect with compression of the fetal heart. Polyhydramnios can occur if the esophagus is obstructed and fetal swallowing is impaired. Hydrops can also be seen as a consequence of cardiac constriction and a "tamponade" effect. Unlike in CDH, where there is free communication between the chest and abdomen, CCAM can lead to increased intrathoracic pressure, bulging of the intact diaphragm caudad, and progressive compression of the heart.

The CCAM mass can be easily identified and is typically of increased echogenicity relative to the normal lung tissue. Fetal echocardiography reveals a small cardiothoracic ratio and small ventricular cavity volumes. Doppler echocardiography can demonstrate changes in diastolic filling properties, reflecting altered compliance. Overall cardiac output measures are decreased. Successful fetal surgical removal of CCAM has been reported, with improvement in cardiac profile.

ARTERIOVENOUS MALFORMATION – Arteriovenous connections, or richly vascular tumors that act as arteriovenous malformations (AVMs), can lead to a substantial increase in venous return to the fetal heart resulting in significant volume load and heart failure. Examples include cerebral AVM and sacrococcygeal teratoma (SCT).

In cerebral AVM, echocardiographic findings include a dilated superior vena cava and dilated right side of the heart, although overall cardiomegaly is commonly seen as the amount of blood volume returning to the heart can be torrential, influencing left-sided heart size as well. Progressive right ventricular dilation will lead to tricuspid annular dilation and development of tricuspid regurgitation, which further results in right-sided enlargement. Doppler evaluation of the aortic arch reveals reversal of flow on color imaging as a cephalad "steal" toward the cerebral circulation is taking place. Scanning of the head with lowering of the color scale will help to visualize the AVM connection itself.

SCT is a highly vascularized tumor found on the lower posterior aspect of the fetus. These tumors can grow to a massive size, exceeding the actual dimensions of the fetal body itself. In SCT, echocardiographic findings include dilation of the inferior vena cava as it carries excess blood volume returning from the tumor, with resultant massive cardiomegaly. Doppler interrogation of the descending aorta may reveal marked antegrade diastolic flow as the SCT contains a very low vascular resistance circulation. If SCT vascular resistance is lower than placental vascular resistance, then a placental "steal" can occur, manifested as alterations in the umbilical arterial Doppler signal with either absent or reversed diastolic flow. Such a finding is quite ominous and may herald impending fetal death.

A valuable echocardiographic technique for assessing and monitoring fetal AVM is serial calculation of combined cardiac output. The normal combined right and left ventricular cardiac output is approximately 400 to 500 mL/min per kilogram and remains relatively stable throughout gestation. In the fetus with AVM, combined cardiac output can rise to levels as high as 1000 mL/min per kilogram or greater. In

our experience, when output exceeds 800 mL/min per kilogram, or umbilical arterial diastolic flow is absent or reversed, the potential for significant fetal hemodynamic instability is at hand.

TWIN-TWIN TRANSFUSION SYNDROME – A rise in the use of assisted reproductive techniques has increased the number of multiple gestation pregnancies. When there is a twin pregnancy with a shared single placenta (monochorionic pregnancy), placental vascular connections develop between the two fetal circulations. Arterial-to-venous connections result in flow from one twin to the other; however, arterial-to-arterial connections compensate and allow for equilibration of volumes. The absence of adequate arterial-to-arterial connections prevents equilibration, with net volume flow from one fetus (donor) into the other (recipient). This phenomenon leads to a complex cascade of events, which are still poorly understood. Donor twin hypovolemia incites the renin-angiotensin system, with the release of a host of mediators targeted at maintaining perfusion and increased vascular tone. These mediators are believed to cross via placental vascular connections to the recipient twin. The recipient therefore receives the combined insults of increased preload volume as well as a whole host of mediators from the donor, all of which result in marked cardiovascular changes leading to a characteristic cardiomyopathy, with a predilection toward right ventricular disease.

The sequelae of this "twin-twin transfusion syndrome" are the development of marked size discrepancy between the twins, oligohydramnios in the donor, polyhydramnios in the recipient, heart failure in the recipient, and neurologic injury or death in one or both twins. Current treatment for TTTS involves laparoscopic laser photocoagulation of placental vascular connections, with substantial improvement in survival. Of great curiosity is the phenomenon in which some recipient fetuses with cardiomyopathy progress to develop pulmonary stenosis or atresia. Morphologic changes progressing from right ventricular hypertrophy and systolic dysfunction to reduced antegrade flow across the pulmonary valve and ultimate pulmonary atresia can be observed with echocardiography over a relatively short period of 4 to 6 weeks of gestation. This phenomenon of "acquired" congenital heart disease in the second trimester of pregnancy reflects the plasticity of the fetal heart late in human development and may yield clues as to the mechanisms of heart malformation in general.

Fetal echocardiography plays a key role in the diagnosis and management of TTTS. A 20-point cardiovascular score for characterization of TTTS has been developed that encompasses the unique aspects of the disorder (Table 40-2). Each of the elements of the score pertain to specific physiologic sequelae seen and provide a means to grade disease severity, gauge response to treatment, and allow for long-term follow-up.

 # FETAL INTERVENTION FOR CONGENITAL HEART DISEASE

Safe invasive techniques have been developed to obtain access directly to the fetus during gestation. Placement of small catheters and shunts to drain pleural effusions is now widely performed. Fetal surgery to repair congenital anomalies such as urinary tract abnormalities, lung lesions, sacrococcygeal teratoma, and meningomyelocele has been reported with improvement in outcome for each of these anomalies. Although controversial, a series of experimental approaches for fetal intervention of congenital heart disease have also been reported. These attempts have focused primarily on the use of balloon valvuloplasty for relief of aortic stenosis to prevent the development of HLHS and opening of the atrial septum in HLHS with intact atrial septum. Deciding on appropriate candidacy for these interventions requires the use of fetal echocardiography and the identification of specific findings that predict poor outcome.

Some fetuses with aortic stenosis and a dilated dysfunctional LV have "arrested" development of the LV and progress to HLHS, reliably predicting which of these will do so is a challenge. Retrospective investigations have identified possible factors such as left-to-right shunting at the atrial level, monophasic inflow across the mitral valve, echo-brightness of the endocardium suggesting endocardial fibroelastosis, and reversal of flow in the transverse aortic arch, which in combination may predict for development of HLHS. Mixed results have been reported in preventing the development of HLHS

| Table 40-2 | CHILDREN'S HOSPITAL OF PHILADELPHIA TWIN-TWIN TRANSFUSION CARDIOVASCULAR SCORE | | |

Recipient

1. Ventricular Elements

Cardiac Enlargement	None (0)	Mild (1)	> Mild (2)
Systolic Dysfunction	None (0)	Mild (1)	> Mild (2)
Ventricular Hypertrophy	None (0)	Present (1)	

2. Valve Function

Tricuspid Regurgitation	None (0)	Mild (1)	> Mild (2)
Mitral Regurgitation	None (0)	Mild (1)	> Mild (2)

3. Venous Doppler

Tricuspid Inflow	2 peaks (0)	1 peak (1)	
Mitral Inflow	2 peaks (0)	1 peak (1)	
Ductus Venosus	All forward (0)	Decreased (1)	Reversal (2)
Umbilical Vein Pulsation	None (0)	Present (1)	

4. Great Vessel Analysis

Outflow Tracts	PA > Ao (0)	PA = Ao (1)	PA < Ao (2)	RVOTO (3)
Pulmonary Insufficiency	None (0)	Present (1)		

Donor

5. Umbilical Arterial Flow	Normal (0)	Decreased Diast (1)	Absent/Reverse Diast (2)

Ao, aorta at level of valve annulus; Diast, diastole; PA, pulmonary artery at level of valve annulus; RVOTO, right ventricle outflow tract obstruction

There are 5 elements to the Score as outlined above. The total maximum value = 20. The Score is a means for characterizing the severity of cardiovascular disease spectrum, and is weighted more heavily towards the recipient – the twin most ostensibly affected by this disorder. Donor placental vascular resistance as reflected by umbilical arterial flow is incorporated. Numbers in parenthesis reflect the numerical value given for the specific grade of each element.

following fetal aortic valvuloplasty, but this exciting work is still in its early stages.

The fetus with HLHS and an intact atrial septum is at risk for severe hypoxemia at birth because pulmonary venous return will not be able to mix with the systemic circulation. In addition, impaired pulmonary venous egress from the left atrium in utero leads to abnormal pulmonary vascular development. Opening of the atrial septum in the fetus with HLHS and intact atrial septum may prevent the development of pulmonary vasculopathy and allow for adequate mixing at birth. Determining which fetuses with a restrictive atrial septum may similarly be at risk is achieved by using Doppler echocardiography to evaluate pulmonary venous return for the degree of flow reversal with atrial contraction. The greater the degree of reversal of flow, the greater is the impediment to left atrial egress. In addition, evaluation of pulmonary vascular reactivity (i.e., vasodilation) in response to maternal hyperoxygenation may play a helpful role in identifying those fetuses at greatest risk. To date, the number of patients who have undergone fetal opening of the atrial septum is quite small; hence, no conclusions can yet be drawn from this experience.

SUMMARY

Fetal echocardiography is a well-established technique for assessment of the fetal cardiovascular system and can be used to evaluate congenital heart disease or the effects of congenital anomalies on the heart. As prenatal diagnostics continues to grow with increasing focus on the fetus as a patient, fetal echocardiography will be the most common way in which congenital heart disease is detected.

SUGGESTED READING

American Institute of Ultrasound in Medicine. Practice guideline for the performance of obstetric ultrasound examinations. *J Ultrasound Med.* 2003;22:1116–1125.

Andrews RE, Tibby SM, Sharland GK, et al. Prediction of outcome of tricuspid valve malformations diagnosed during fetal life. *Am J Cardiol.* 2008;101:1046–1050.

Aoki M, Harada K, Ogawa M, et al. Quantitative assessment of right ventricular function using doppler tissue imaging in fetuses with and without heart failure. *J Am Soc Echocardiogr* 2004;17:28–35.

Bahlmann F, Reinhard I, Krummenauer F, et al. Blood flow velocity waveforms of the fetal middle cerebral artery in a normal population: reference values from 18 weeks to 42 weeks of gestation. *J Perinat Med* 2002;30:490–501.

Berg C, Kamil D, Geipel A, et al. Absence of ductus venosus-importance of umbilical venous drainage site. *Ultrasound Obstet Gynecol* 2006;28:275–281.

Carceller-Blanchard AM, Fouron JC. Determinants of the Doppler flow velocity profile through the mitral valve of the human fetus. *Br Heart J.* 1993;70:457–460.

Chaoui R, Bollmann R, Goldner B, et al. Fetal cardiomegaly: echocardiographic findings and outcome in 19 cases. *Fetal Diagn Ther.* 1994;9:92–104.

Chaoui R, Kalache K, Tennstedt C, et al. Pulmonary arterial Doppler velocimetry in fetuses with lung hypoplasia. *Eur J Obstet Gynecol Reprod Biol* 1999;84:179–185.

Chintala K, Tian Z, Du W, et al. Fetal pulmonary venous Doppler patterns in hypoplastic left heart syndrome: relationship to atrial septal restriction. *Heart.* 2008;94:1446–1449.

Cohen MS, Rychik J, Bush DM, et al. Influence of congenital heart disease on survival in children with congenital diaphragmatic hernia. *J Pediatr* 2002;141:25–30.

Donofrio MT, Bremer YA, Schieken RM, et al. Autoregulation of cerebral blood flow in fetuses with congenital heart disease: the brain sparing effect. *Pediatr Cardiol* 2003;24:436–443.

Dubin J, Wallerson DC, Cody RJ, et al. Comparative accuracy of Doppler echocardiographic methods for clinical stroke volume determination. *Am Heart J.* 1990;120:116–123.

Eidem BW, Edwards JM, Cetta F. Quantitative assessment of fetal ventricular function: establishing normal values of the myocardial performance index in the fetus. *Echocardiography* 2001;18:9–13.

Ertan AK, He JP, Tanriverdi HA, et al. Comparison of perinatal outcome in fetuses with reverse or absent end-diastolic flow in the umbilical artery and/or fetal descending aorta. *J Perinat Med* 2003;40:307–402.

Falkensammer CB, Paul J, Huhta JC. Fetal congestive heart failure: correlation of Tei-index and cardiovascular-score. *J Perinat Med* 2001;29:390–398.

Fernandez PL, Tamariz-Martel MA, Maitre Azcarate MJ, et al. Contribution of Doppler atrioventricular flow waves to ventricular filling in the human fetus. *Pediatr Cardiol* 2000;21:422–428.

Fliedner R, Wiegank U, Fetsch C, et al. Reference values of fetal ductus venosus, inferior vena cava and hepatic vein blood flow velocities and waveform indices during the second and third trimester of pregnancy. *Arch Gynecol Obstet.* 2004;270:46–55.

Friedman D, Buyon J, Kim M, et al. Fetal cardiac function assessed by Doppler myocardial performance index (Tei Index). *Ultrasound Obstet Gynecol.* 2003;21:33–36.

Friedman WF. The intrinsic physiologic properties of the developing heart. *Prog Cardiovasc Dis.* 1972;15:87–111.

Gardiner HM, Belmar C, Tulzer G, et al. Morphologic and functional predictors of eventual circulation in the fetus with pulmonary atresia or critical pulmonary stenosis with intact septum. *J Am Coll Cardiol.* 2008;51:1299–1308.

Hornberger LK, Sahn DJ, Kleinman CS, et al. Antenatal diagnosis of coarctation of the aorta: a multicenter experience. *J Am Coll Cardiol.* 1994;23:417–423.

Hornberger LK, Sahn DJ, Kleinman CS, et al. Tricuspid valve disease with significant tricuspid insufficiency in the fetus: diagnosis and outcome. *J Am Coll Cardiol.* 1991;17:167–173.

Huntsman LL, Stewart DK, Barnes SR, et al. Noninvasive Doppler determination of cardiac output in man. Clinical validation. *Circulation.* 1983;67:593–602.

Inamura N, Taketazu M, Smallhorn JF, et al. Left ventricular myocardial performance in the fetus with severe tricuspid valve disease and tricuspid insufficiency. *Am J Perinatol.* 2005;22:91–97.

Isaaz K, Ethevenot G, Admant P, et al. A new Doppler method of assessing left ventricular ejection force in chronic congestive heart failure. *Am J Cardiol.* 1989;64:81–87.

Jaeggi ET, Fouron JC, Hornberger LK, et al. Agenesis of the ductus venosus that is associated with extrahepatic umbilical vein drainage: prenatal features and clinical outcome. *Am J Obstet. Gynecol* 2002;187:1040–1037.

Jouannic JM, Gavard L, Fermont L, et al. Sensitivity and specificity of prenatal features of physiological shunts to predict neonatal clinical status in transposition of the great arteries. *Circulation.* 2004;110:1743–1746.

Kaltman JR, Di H, Tian Z, et al. Impact of congenital heart disease on cerebrovascular blood flow dynamics in the fetus. *Ultrasound Obstet Gynecol.* 2005;25:32–36.

Khong TY, George K. Chromosomal abnormalities associated with a single umbilical artery. *Prenat Diagn.* 1992;12:965–968.

Leal SD, Cavalle-Garrido T, Ryan G, et al. Isolated ductal closure in utero diagnosed by fetal echocardiography. *Am J Perinatol.* 1997;14:205–210.

Lubusky M, Dhaifalah I, Prochazka M, et al. Single umbilical artery and its siding in the second trimester of pregnancy: relation to chromosomal defects. *Prenat Diagn.* 2007;27:327–331.

Luchese S, Manica JL, Zielinsky P. Intrauterine ductus arteriosus constriction: analysis of a historic cohort of 20 cases. *Arq Bras Cardiol.* 2003;81:405–404.

Mahle WT, Tavani F, Zimmerman RA, et al. An MRI study of neurological injury before and after congenital heart surgery. *Circulation* 2002;106(suppl): I-109–I-114.

Mahle WT, Tian ZY, Cohen MS, et al. Echocardiographic evaluation of the fetus with congenital cystic adenomatoid malformation (CCAM). *Ultrasound Obstet Gynecol.* 2000;16:620–624.

Makikallio K, McElhinney DB, Levine JC, et al. Fetal aortic valve stenosis and the evolution of hypoplastic left heart syndrome: patient selection for fetal intervention. *Circulation.* 2006;113:1401–1405.

Michelfelder E, Gomez C, Border W, et al. Predictive value of fetal pulmonary venous flow patterns in identifying the need for atrial septoplasty in the newborn with hypoplastic left ventricle. *Circulation.* 2005;112:2974–2979.

Miller SP, McQuillen PS, Hamrick S, et al. Abnormal brain development in newborns with congenital heart disease. *N Engl J Med.* 2007;357:1928–1938.

Moise KJ Jr. The usefulness of middle cerebral artery Doppler assessment in the treatment of the fetus at risk for anemia. *Am J Obstet Gynecol.* 2008;198:161–164.

Momma K, Hagiwara H, Konishi T. Constriction of fetal ductus arteriosus by non-steroidal anti-inflammatory drugs: study of additional 34 drugs. *Prostaglandins.* 1984;28:527–536.

Mori Y, Rice MJ, McDonald RW, et al. Evaluation of systolic and diastolic ventricular performance of the right ventricle in fetuses with ductal constriction using the Doppler Tei index. *Am J Cardiol.* 2001;88:1173–1178.

Nicolaides KH, Azar G, Byrne D, et al. Fetal nuchal translucency: ultrasound screening for chromosomal defects in first trimester of pregnancy. *Br Med J.* 1992;304:867–869.

Paladini D, Palmieri S, Lamberti A, et al. Characterization and natural history of ventricular septal defects in the fetus. *Ultrasound Obstet Gynecol.* 2000;16:118–122.

Predanic M, Perni SC, Friedman A, et al. Fetal growth assessment and neonatal birth weight in fetuses with an isolated single umbilical artery. *Obstet Gynecol.* 2005;105:1093–1097.

Rasanen J, Debbs RH, Wood DC, et al. Human fetal right ventricular ejection force under abnormal loading conditions during the second half of pregnancy. *Ultrasound Obstet Gynecol.* 1997;10:325–332.

Rasanen J, Wood DC, Debbs RH, et al. Reactivity of the human fetal pulmonary circulation to maternal hyperoxygenation increases during the second half of pregnancy: a randomized study. *Circulation.* 1998;97:257–262.

Reed KL, Meijboom EJ, Sahn DJ, et al. Cardiac Doppler flow velocities in human fetuses. *Circulation.* 1986;73:41–46.

Rembouskos G, Cicero S, Longo D, et al. Single umbilical artery at 11-14 weeks' gestation: relation to chromosomal defects. *Ultrasound Obstet Gynecol.* 2003;22:567–570.

Rice MJ, McDonald RW, Reller MD. Progressive pulmonary stenosis in the fetus: two case reports. *Am J Perinatol.* 1993;10:424–427.

Rinehart BK, Terrone DA, Taylor CW, et al. Single umbilical artery is associated with an increased incidence of structural and chromosomal anomalies and growth restriction. *Am J Perinatol.* 2000;17:229–232.

Rizzo G, Capponi A, Rinaldo D, et al. Ventricular ejection force in growth-retarded fetuses. *Ultrasound Obstet Gynecol.* 1995;5:247–255.

Roman KS, Fouron JC, Nii M, et al. Determinants of outcome in fetal pulmonary valve stenosis or atresia with intact ventricular septum. *Am J Cardiol.* 2007;99:699–703.

Rychik J, Ayres N, Cuneo B, et al. American Society of Echocardiography guidelines and standards for performance of the fetal echocardiogram. *J Am Soc Echocardiogr.* 2004;17:803–810.

Rychik J, Rome JJ, Collins M, et al. Hypoplastic left heart syndrome with intact atrial septum: atrial anatomy, lung histopathology, and outcome. *J Am Coll Cardiol.* 1999;34:554–560.

Rychik J, Tian Z, Bebbington M, et al. The twin-twin transfusion syndrome: spectrum of cardiovascular abnormality and development of a cardiovascular score to assess severity of disease. *Am J Obstet Gynecol.* 2007;197:392–398.

Rychik J, Tian Z, Cohen MS, et al. Acute cardiovascular effects of fetal surgery in the human. *Circulation.* 2004;110:1549–1556.

Rychik J. Impact of fetal anomalies other than congenital heart disease on the developing cardiovascular system. *Progr Pediatr Cardiol.* 2006;22:109–121.

Salvin JW, McElhinney DB, Colan SD, et al. Fetal tricuspid valve size and growth as predictors of outcome in pulmonary atresia with intact ventricular septum. *Pediatrics.* 2006;118:e415–e420.

Schiessl B, Schneider KT, Zimmermann A, et al. Prenatal constriction of the fetal ductus arteriosus: related to maternal pain medication? *Z Geburtshilfe Neonatol.* 2005;209:65–68.

Shipp TD, Bromley B, Hornberger LK, et al. Levorotation of the fetal cardiac axis: a clue for the presence of congenital heart disease. *Obstet Gynecol.* 1995;85:97–102.

Simpson LL, Malone FD, Bianchi DW, et al. Nuchal translucency and the risk of congenital heart disease. *Obstet Gynecol.* 2007;109:376–383.

Sivan E, Dulitzky M, Lipitz S, et al. The clinical value of umbilical artery Doppler velocimetry in the management of intrauterine growth-retarded fetuses before 32 weeks' gestation. *Gynecol Obstet Invest.* 1995;40:19–23.

Sivan E, Rotstein Z, Lipitz S, et al. Segmentary fetal branch pulmonary artery blood flow velocimetry: in utero Doppler study. *Ultrasound Obstet Gynecol.* 2000;16:453–456.

Sodowski K, Cnota W, Czuba B, et al. Blood flow in ductus venosus in early uncomplicated pregnancy. *Neuro Endocrinol Lett.* 2007;28:713–716.

Szwast A, Tian Z, McCann M, et al. Impact of altered loading conditions on ventricular performance in fetuses with congenital cystic adenomatoid malformation and twin-twin transfusion syndrome. *Ultrasound Obstet Gynecol.* 2007;30:40–46.

Tei C, Ling LH, Hodge DO, et al. New index of combined systolic and diastolic myocardial performance: a simple and reproducible measure of cardiac function—a study in normals and dilated cardiomyopathy. *J Cardiol.* 1995;26:357–366.

Tei C, Nishimura RA, Seward JB, et al. Noninvasive Doppler-derived myocardial performance index: correlation with simultaneous measurements of cardiac catheterization measurements. *J Am Soc Echocardiogr.* 1997;10:169–178.

Todros T, Presbitero P, Gaglioti P, et al. Pulmonary stenosis with intact ventricular septum: documentation of development of the lesion echocardiographically during fetal life. *Int J Cardiol.* 1988;19:355–362.

Toyoshima K, Takeda A, Imamura S, et al. Constriction of the ductus arteriosus by selective inhibition of cyclooxygenase-1 and -2 in near-term and preterm fetal rats. *Prostaglandins Other Lipid Mediat.* 2006;79:34–42.

Tsutsumi T, Ishii M, Eto G, et al. Serial evaluation for myocardial performance in fetuses and neonates using a new Doppler index. *Pediatr Int.* 1999;41:722–727.

Wang KG, Chen CP, Yang JM, et al. Impact of reverse end-diastolic flow velocity in umbilical artery on pregnancy outcome after the 28th gestational week. *Acta Obstet Gynecol Scand.* 1998;77:527–540.

Wladimiroff JW, vd Wijngaard JA, Degani S, et al. Cerebral and umbilical arterial blood flow velocity waveforms in normal and growth-retarded pregnancies. *Obstet Gynecol.* 1987;69:705–709.

Yoo SJ, Lee YH, Kim ES, et al. Three-vessel view of the fetal upper mediastinum: an easy means of detecting abnormalities of the ventricular outflow tracts and great arteries during obstetric screening. *Ultrasound Obstet Gynecol.* 1997;9:173–182.

Index

Note: Page numbers referencing figures are italicized and followed by an "*f*". Page numbers referencing tables are italicized and followed by a "*t*".